Bogert's Nutrition and Physical Fitness

TENTH EDITION

GEORGE M. BRIGGS
University of California at Berkeley

DORIS HOWES CALLOWAY
University of California at Berkeley

1979 W. B. SAUNDERS COMPANY
PHILADELPHIA • LONDON • TORONTO

W. B. Saunders Company: West Washington Square
Philadelphia, Pa. 19105

1 St. Anne's Road
Eastbourne, East Sussex BN21 3UN, England

1 Goldthorne Avenue
Toronto, Ontario M8Z 5T9, Canada

Library of Congress Cataloging in Publication Data

Briggs, George McSpadden, 1919–

Nutrition and physical fitness.

Ninth ed., published in 1973, by L. J. Bogert, G. M. Briggs, and D. H. Calloway.

Includes bibliographies and index.

1. Nutrition. I. Calloway, Doris Howes, joint author. II. Bogert, L. Jean, 1888–1970. Nutrition and physical fitness. III. Title.

TX354.B6 1979 641.1 78–21302

ISBN 0–7216–1987–8

Cover illustration courtesy of Four By Five, Inc., New York, N.Y.

Bogert's Nutrition and Physical Fitness ISBN 0-7216-1987-8

Last digit is the print number: 9 8 7 6 5 4 3 2 1

Preface

The overall aim of this tenth edition is to provide the student, in as simple and interesting a manner as possible, with sufficient knowledge about foods and nutrition for development of good eating habits. This knowledge, along with other good health practices, will greatly help one to have a healthy and vigorous life now and over a lifetime. This has been the overall aim since the first edition was written by the late Dr. L. Jean Bogert in 1931, about *fifty years* ago. Since that time each edition has not only included the years of cumulated experience of, and experimentation by, the authors and the discoveries of nutritionists throughout the world, but also has benefited greatly by suggestions which have come from teachers and students.

The book is written primarily for college students taking their first course in nutrition. It is written so that it may be useful and readily understood not only by the food, dietetics, and nutrition majors, but also by nonmajor students who are interested in what to eat for a healthy life but who are in other fields such as health sciences, mathematics, physical education, history, English, chemistry, agriculture, sociology, humanities, and other nonnutrition areas.

The book does not require the student to have knowledge of biology, chemistry, or biochemistry (though such subjects will be of help to students majoring in foods and nutrition or such fields as health sciences, and the like). Portions of the book which are useful to students with a biology background are given in smaller type, such as in Chapters 7 to 12, and could be omitted when the text is used by nonscience majors or the interested lay person. Formulas are given in the appendix rather than the text for the most part.

Fortunately, because of increased emphasis on science in secondary schools, most present-day college students have already acquired some knowledge of fundamental scientific terms and concepts through courses (general science, biology, chemistry, physics) in high school or even at grade school levels. Hence, college students may be expected to comprehend a presentation of nutrition which relies on an elementary understanding of science.

We firmly believe that only by thoroughly knowing basic facts about foods and nutrition can one build a real understanding of applied nutrition topics and the ability to sort out and accept new developments certain to come along in this field. Only with a strong background can one learn to handle by one's self new claims, fads, and even frauds which continually reach the mass media. This, for instance, is why the first half of the book is primarily a presentation of the "basic facts."

Research in nutrition has concentrated more and more on the study of the basic life processes—the chemistry of the cell, the chemical changes that take place in the various tissues, and the role of enzymes, vitamins, and mineral elements in catalyzing these processes. This deeper inquiry into the need for and functions of the various nutrients is often a team effort, involving the collaboration of biochemists with physiologists and microbiologists. Looking at the vast amount of data and numerous fundamental discoveries which have been accumulated by this type of research, it becomes apparent that even though this material may be somewhat difficult to translate into terms which are understandable to less advanced college students, it cannot be ignored; to be as meaningful as it should be, nutrition must be treated in greater depth than was formerly the case.

The dependence upon the scientific method for providing proven facts about foods and nutrition is often a difficult concept for today's student to accept. Though we could not exist in America without a responsible food industry, the student today has seen evidence of certain segments of the food industry putting the consumer at the low end of the priority list. The student has learned, rightly or wrongly, to mistrust certain intentional food additives, highly processed foods, foods treated with "synthetic chemicals," certain food advertising, high food prices, and even college teachers of a different generation. We recommend that teachers using this book in classes comprised mainly of nonscience-trained students spend the first few days or so of class discussing the meaning of science, the scientific method, a controlled experiment, the placebo, and the difference between a true scientific publication (with its system of peer review) and a scare magazine or newspaper article. (Chapter 1 will assist you somewhat in this.)

Many improvements have been made in this edition, including the addition of Chapter 18, Food Nonnutrients, Enrichment, and Labels, and Chapter 25, Malnutrition: A Global Perspective. Extensive revisions have been made throughout the text with much totally new material on the basic nutrients—amino acids, carbohydrates, fiber, energy concepts, vitamins, and minerals. The subject of alcohol has been expanded. The applied nutrition section is greatly improved and consolidated. In these sections especially we have focused directly on nutrition problems existing today that concern students' own lives and future careers.

One of the greatest strengths of this book, we feel, is that current issues and references to the literature are as accurate and up to date as possible within publication time lags. We have supplied a list of "additional readings" in the current literature that should be readily accessible for use by the student interested in gaining more information about a subject than can be found in the book (which, because it is introductory, must necessarily leave out many important facts). These literature citations will provide important leads for student projects. Each edition, because of space, must eliminate most of the older readings. Teachers interested in older literature citations will find it useful to keep older editions for this purpose.

Nutrition as a field is a constantly evolving and controversial topic because of its essentiality to physical fitness and health, because of its economic, ecological, and environmental aspects, and because of the use of food to provide political influence. No textbook can contain the latest information on all nutrition and food topics. We suggest, therefore, that teachers and students wanting the newest information make widespread use of current literature and of the periodicals and agencies listed at the end of Chapter 1. One will need to keep abreast of information on newer Recommended Dietary/Nutrient Allowances as they appear. We suggest especially current issues of such useful publications as the Journal of the American Dietetic Association, American Journal of Clinical Nutrition, CNI Weekly, Journal of Nutrition Education, Journal of Home Economics, New England Journal of Medicine, and the American Journal of Public Health.

We are pleased that instructors' guides for the teacher and study guides for the student are available for this edition of the textbook. We recommend the use of any such reliable guides, but especially those prepared by Kay Franz and Ruth Walker, available from the W. B. Saunders Company.

We have attempted, as did Dr. Bogert, not to straddle the fence on controversial issues but to give our informed opinion on such issues when valid information exists. We hope you will find the book better able to meet your needs than ever before. Your comments are always most welcome.

GEORGE M. BRIGGS
DORIS HOWES CALLOWAY

Acknowledgments

The authors are indebted to many persons who have helped in one way or another in making it possible for this tenth edition to be published. Suggestions from teachers, teaching assistants, and students who have used earlier editions have been especially helpful. We appreciate, too, the help of a number of persons at the W. B. Saunders Company, including Robert E. Lakemacher, Richard H. Lampert (who made the early arrangements), and the copy editor, designer, indexer, artists, printers, proofreaders, and still others who have worked exceedingly well.

The manuscript has been typed by Mrs. Beatrice Myers and Mrs. Joyce Booth, who have also given much help in proofreading and other especially detailed work with references and readings. We are particularly indebted to those who have had a major role in the preparation of various chapters, including: Dr. Marilyn Crim (Chapter 15), Dr. Christine Wilson, Miss Susan McKeehan (Chapter 18, as well as help with certain other sections), Catherine Briggs, M.D. (Chapters 21 and 22), Mr. Leonard Joy (Chapter 25), and Dr. John Tarr (Chapter 8). Much assistance has been given also by Mrs. Lori Moore with Chapter 9, Dr. Diane Bray with Chapter 11, Dr. Judy Turnland with Chapter 12, Mrs. Joyce Booth with the revision of Chapter 16, and Ms. Karen MacEwan with Chapter 17. Ms. Elena Garcia has provided much assistance with the literature citations.

We acknowledge, also, the additional help in reading and proofreading various portions from Mrs. Eleanor Briggs and Ms. Marilyn Briggs. Our thanks, too, go to those who supplied photographs and other material for the text.

George M. Briggs
Doris Howes Calloway

Contents

PART 4 APPLIED NUTRITION

Appendix

Part 1

Nutrients and Their Functions

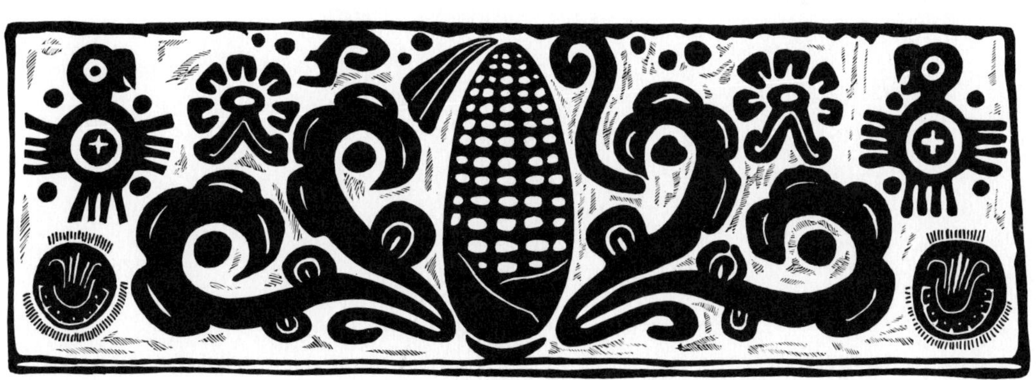

Chapter 1

Food and Its Relation to Physical Fitness

Why do we need to eat? What should we eat? The answers to these questions are what nutrition — and this book — is all about.

The foods we eat contain 42 to 44 highly important substances (the "nutrients") *that each of us must consume in adequate amounts in order to have energy, grow, reproduce, and lead a full healthy life*. The water we drink, another form of food, and the oxygen of the air we breathe are equally essential.

From these rather few essential nutrients that we must get from a source outside the body, our body tissues make literally thousands of substances essential for life and good physical fitness. Most of these substances are far more complicated in structure than the original nutrients. If our bodies could manufacture, in some manner, these essential nutrients that we now get from our food, we would not have to eat at all.

But, of course, this is impossible. In common with green plants and all other forms of life, we must be provided first with water plus 18 or so minerals from some outside source (see Chapters 10 to 12). However, our bodies are more specialized than green plants. We must breathe oxygen, and we must get from our food 24 or more additional nutrients in order to have normal human life and physical fitness as we know it. These additional nutrients (the vitamins, amino acids, fats, and probably several carbohydrates for energy and roughage) are, with few exceptions, rather simple organic chemicals. They are present in foods as part of thousands of organic substances that plants make for themselves, only a few of which are essential for the human body.

These essential nutrients provide fuel, catalysts, and machinery so that we can grow, move about, see, hear, taste, smell, feel, speak, think, learn and remember, sing, walk, run, play, enjoy pleasures, argue, make decisions, love, and be innovative and creative. All of these things, and more, are possible only if we first consume in our food at least minimal amounts of each of the 42 to 44 essential nutrients in some form or another on a regular basis. If an inadequate amount is eaten, or too much of some, these functions will be impaired. Life itself is dependent on what we eat.

Nutrition, then, may be defined as *the science of food as it relates to optimal health and performance.*

Each of us is, or should be, vitally interested in promoting or protecting our own health, since upon it depends our well-being, our work capacity, and even our length of life. How we choose our food, as well as how and where we choose to eat, also affects our budget, our environment, and our social and cultural life. Nutrition is more than just eating the right nutrients — as a field of study it has physiological, biochemical, and behavioral aspects, and reaches into the realms of agriculture, food technology, medicine, economics, ecology, business, politics, and international stability.

Why Study Nutrition?

The rapidly developing science of nutrition has accumulated a mass of facts about how foods are used for building healthy bodies, and what constitutes the best type of diet, within budget limitations.

Some knowledge of the basic facts of nutrition is helpful to anyone who has to make food choices. A more detailed and scientific background of knowledge is essential for those who have the responsibility of feeding others and for those participating in health education — such as homemakers, nurses, doctors, dentists, elementary school teachers, home economists, social workers, health and physical education teachers, extension workers in the field of nutrition, public health workers, food scientists, food industry and advertising personnel, food policy makers, and managers of public eating places and school lunchrooms. Complete training and up-to-date knowledge of nutrition is required by nutritionists at all levels, such as teachers of nutrition, public health nutritionists, dietitians, and nutritional scientists in public and private institutions.

People in the United Nations food and health agencies are concerned with attempting to bring more of the right kinds of food to countries all over the world, many of whose people now exist at a semistarvation level. It should be clear to all, including our national leaders, that no country can achieve the vigor essential for economic, social, and political stability without adequate nutrition for all its people.

People in countries such as our own, with a plentiful supply of a wide variety of foods, do not necessarily choose the right kind and amount of food to eat. Good health resulting from good nutrition cannot be taken for granted. Signs of malnutrition, hunger, and poor eating practices exist all around us. Many of our health problems stem from overeating or from eating too freely of certain types of food (sugar, fats, and alcohol) at the expense of better and lower-calorie foods. This contributes to overweight and the diseases that are often associated with it (diabetes, high blood pressure, heart disease, etc. — see Chapter 24).

Moreover, although proper nutrition provides an essential basis for health, good health also depends on one's lifestyle, heredity, environment, and freedom from disease and accidents. Infection, disease, stress, emotional instability, excessive drugs and alcohol, smoking, and lack of exercise may counterbalance the effects of a good diet. Persons who do not eat luxuriously but whose mode of life involves more exercise may often be more healthy. Less physical work in factory and home, together with the almost universal use of the automobile for getting about, results in the average American getting less exercise than formerly. A survey of pupils in New York City public schools has served to point up the need for regular programs to improve physical fitness. Nearly a third of the pupils failed to qualify at initial testing, but after about 6 weeks of the physical activity program, nearly two-thirds of those who had previously failed were now able to qualify.[1] The young respond quickly to the right conditions; unfortunately, the reconditioning of a sedentary and perhaps overweight adult is of necessity a slower and more gradual process.

Good Nutrition and Good Health

It is true that in many parts of the world peoples who know little or nothing of the science of nutrition have subsisted for generations on diets that maintained strong bodies. Sometimes, with even a limited variety of foods, those available were such that all the requirements for good nutrition were provided. Other primitive peoples were not so fortunate; either the food supply was inadequate or the cultural habits prompted selection of foods that resulted in an improperly balanced diet lacking some factors necessary for growth and health.

McCarrison made some early studies on diets used in different sections of India and their relation to the health of the respective tribes.[2] In the southern sections of the country, the diet consisted chiefly of milled rice, fruits, and vegetables, with little flesh foods or milk; these peoples were of smaller size and inferior strength, and were short-lived, as well. The peoples of tribes farther north, who used unmilled millet or wheat along with goats' milk and butter, had splendid physiques and enough stamina to make good soldiers. In remote sections of the Himalaya Mountains, people were found whose frugal diet was made up mostly of apricots (sun-dried for winter use), vegetables, and goats' milk, with meat eaten only on feast days; these peoples were unusually strong, healthy, and long-lived.

The long-lived Balkan peoples eat little meat, but use whole-grain cereals, cheeses, and the fermented milk known as koumiss. Studies of African tribes have shown that, of two tribes living not far apart, one may have relatively large-sized and healthy bodies, while the other may have bodies that are puny and disease-ridden owing to defective diet[3], though genetic differences may also exist. The diet of many poorer classes in Central and South American countries often comes almost entirely from beans and corn. On such a diet, young children, after weaning, often develop severe nutritional deficiency symptoms, and those who manage to survive may never reach their normal growth potential (Fig. 1–1).

In extensive studies on undernutrition, Keys and coworkers,[4] in classic studies on human volunteers in World War II, showed that changes in behavior and work capacity result from prolonged underfeeding. Today, hundreds of research studies are being conducted in many countries on animals and man that demonstrate clearly that inadequate nutrition can result in lowered intelligence, poor mental health, abnormal behavior, damage to nerve and brain tissue, and poor physical fitness.[4, 5]

Malnutrition Still Widespread Throughout the World

Malnutrition is a term widely used to mean *faulty or poor nutrition in all of its aspects, whether from inadequate intake of nutrients or overconsumption of foods.*

In spite of years of accumulated knowledge of the importance of adequate food and of good nutrition for the health of people, hunger and malnutrition exist throughout the world — even in the so-called "developed" countries.

In the United States, typical of many highly industrialized countries, the nutritional situation is little better today than it was 10 or 20 years ago, if at all.[6] At least 30 percent of the United States population have diets that fail to measure up to standards for one or more nutrients, especially iron, calcium, vitamin A, vitamin C, riboflavin, and calories. Malnutrition can show up as anemia or obesity, or in close association with diseases related to poor nutrition, such as those of the circulatory system (heart disease, hypertension, stroke, etc.), diabetes, severe dental and periodontal disease, digestive diseases, and alcoholism. Especially vulnerable to malnutrition are young children, adolescents, pregnant women, families of the poor, handicapped persons, alcoholics,

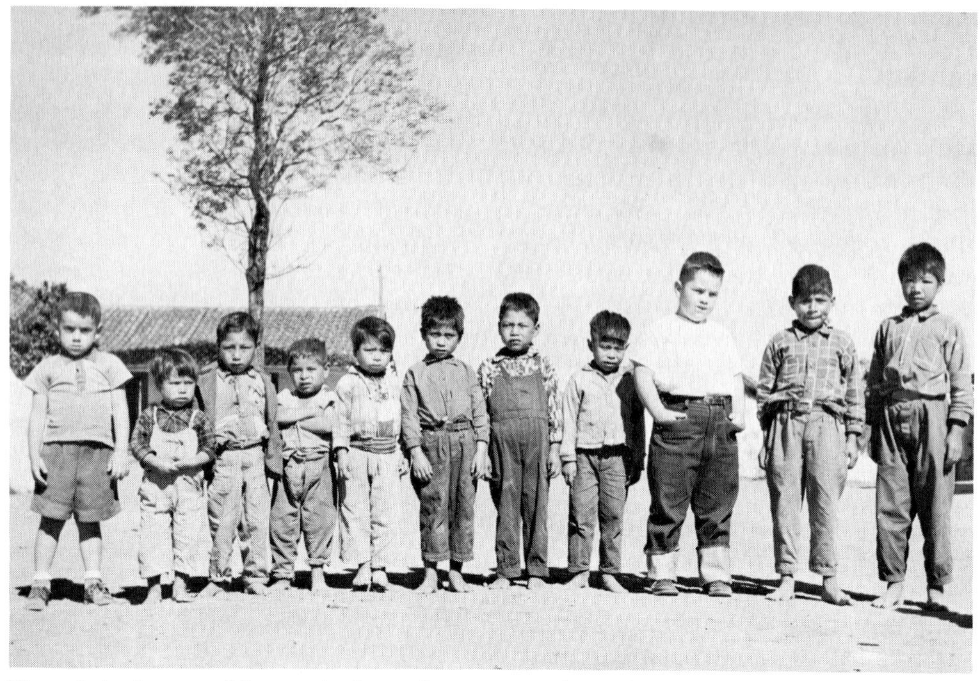

Figure 1–1 A group of Guatemalan boys, showing stunted growth caused by the inadequate native diet, as compared with two boys of the same racial stock who had superior type diet and are of normal weight and height for their age. The boy at left (normal) is 4½ years old, while the four boys next to him range from 5 to 7 years of age. The boy third from right is nearly 7 years old and is of normal height; the three smaller boys beside him are 7–8 and the two boys to his right (approx. same height) are 11 and 12 years old. (Courtesy Dr. Miguel A. Guzmán, Institute of Nutrition for Central America and Panama.)

and people over 65 years of age. Many billions of dollars are wasted each year in the United States from misuse of food.

Our situation in the United States is not much different from most other industrialized countries, such as Canada, the European countries, Australia, and Japan. However, the prevalence of hunger and malnutrition is still much more widespread in most of the nonindustrialized and the developing countries — especially those in the tropical areas of South and Central America and the West Indies, in Africa, in India, and in many other Asian countries, including the numerous islands from the Philippines to New Guinea and the East Indies. In some of these countries hunger unfortunately is widespread. Effects of malnutrition are common, including blindness from vitamin A deficiency, anemia, scurvy, and poor growth of babies and children due to deficiencies of protein, calories, and many other nutrients (Fig. 1–2). Eventually chronic malnutrition in a society can be a direct or indirect cause of high mortality figures at all age levels.

Many national and international groups — such as the World Health Organization (WHO), the United Nations Educational, Scientific, and Cultural Organization (UNESCO), and the Food and Agricultural Organization (FAO) of the United Nations — and many public and private groups are attempting to solve the world malnutrition problem, but the task is immense (see list of supplementary readings at the end of this chapter and Chapter 25).

Factors Affecting What We Eat

Our food habits often stem from prejudices acquired in childhood, either from parental examples or from childish whims that are indulged. *Education* that explains why foods selected should include those needed to supply all the essentials for an adequate diet will provide *motivation* to change old food habits for new ones. This is expecially true when food habits in the home are based on cultural or religious practice. *Deeply rooted food habits*, if bad, can often be overcome by suggesting that larger amounts of certain liked or permitted foods be taken or that new foods be prepared in favorite or familiar styles. *Diet fads and advertising* may also induce a person to subsist on unbalanced diets that furnish too little of certain essential nutrients. The foods we eat are also determined by what we can afford to buy — our *economic* condition.

Complacency, or indifference, is also a strong factor working against change of food habits. Unless a person has a vision of the greater vitality to be attained by improving his food habits, he is apt to believe that he is well enough off as he is. There must be education as to why certain foods are essential for health. Remote goals, including longevity, can strongly influence choice of foods in the diet. With teenagers and young adults, a more immediate objective, such as the physical prowess, athletic ability, and good looks that are associated with buoyant health, may prove more effective in stimulating interest in good food habits. Young college women, as prospective mothers, should be vitally interested in good diets to safeguard their own health and that of their children; instead, they are often careless in eating habits or follow *reducing fads* in order to retain slender figures.

One of the aims of nutrition should be to prolong the vitality of the prime of life into later years. There is still much room for dietary improvement, provided nutritional teaching can convince people that alteration of their dietary habits is worthwhile.

Basic Causes of Hunger and Malnutrition

Why is there so much malnutrition in the supposedly enlightened world of today? Poor food habits and lack of nutrition knowledge are but two reasons. To summarize, a list of basic causes of mal-

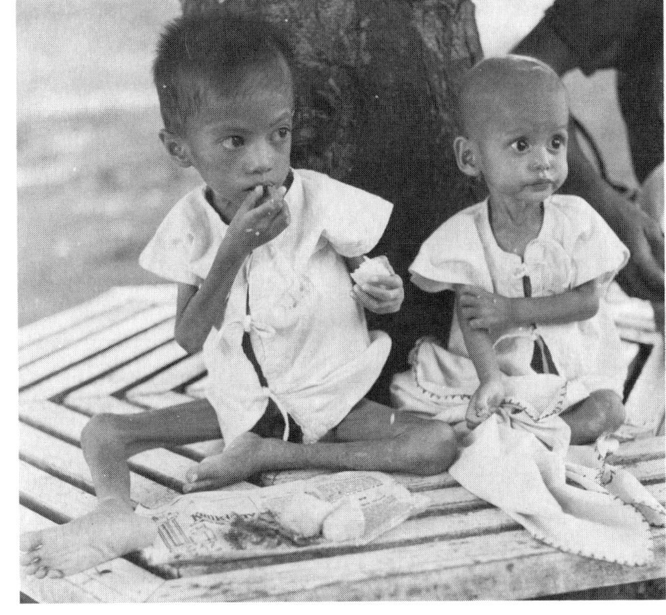

Figure 1–2 Sad and listless, these children show all the signs of advanced malnutrition. Scene is the Southern Islands General Hospital in Cebu, the Philippines. (Courtesy of UNICEF and Mallica Vajrathon. Used with permission.)

nutrition in modern industrial countries includes such factors as:

1. Lack of adequate *nutrition education* in schools and in the home; poor or faulty nutrition knowledge.

2. Complacency, indifference, and poor or misdirected *motivation* to eat properly; lack of goals.

3. *Deeply rooted poor food habits* based on cultural, social, or religious practices; changes in life-styles.

4. *Diet fads* based on unsound nutrition practices.

5. *Unavailability of adequate food* due to poverty, distance from markets, inability to choose or purchase foods for oneself as in the case of those dependent on others (infants, children, severely handicapped persons, and the aged).

6. *Widespread availability of good-tasting, low-value foods,* usually highly processed and containing chiefly energy. Often these are the most heavily advertised.

7. *Inadequate recognition of the importance of good nutrition* by local, state, and national leaders.

8. *Inadequate nutrition training* of physicians, other health professionals, teachers, social workers, food editors of newspapers, and nutrition writers.

You can, no doubt, think of still other reasons for the presence of malnutrition in your own community. Such factors as peer pressures to consume poor foods, improper food labeling, lack of home gardens, ease of obtaining poor foods and candy in vending machines and at store counters and fast-food service establishments, lack of adequately prepared meals in the home, skipped breakfasts and other meals, the low incidence of breast feeding, poor snacking habits, the widespread availability of inferior imitation and fabricated foods, lack of a national food policy (including inadequate enrichment standards and insufficient public service messages on television), and lack of physical activity are all related to poor nutrition.

In developing countries of the world there are many other causes of malnutrition, including *prevailing poverty, overpopulation, illiteracy, social deprivation, poor sanitation and disease, indifference, and the "inability to cope."* Persons working to combat malnutrition in the United States or any place in the world will recognize that working toward the reversal of these causes of malnutrition is necessary if we are ever going to have healthy nations.

Food Is a Basic Human Right

Having sufficient food is a basic need of all individuals — probably more basic than any other human need. Most modern countries, including our own, consider *having sufficient food as a basic human right*. More human effort, on a world basis, goes toward the production, processing, marketing, and consumption of food than toward any other human need, and rightly so.

Functions of Food

We have defined nutrition earlier as the science of food as it relates to optimal health and performance — that is, providing adequately for the body's *growth, maintenance, repair,* and *reproduction*. Except for the *water* we drink and *oxygen* taken in from the air we breathe, the needs of the body must be met by the intake of foods. To nourish the body and to qualify as a food, foods must contain substances that *function* in one or more of *three* ways:

1. Furnish body fuel, substances whose oxidation in the body sets free the *energy* needed for its activities;

2. Provide materials for the *building* or *maintenance* of body *tissues;* and

3. Supply substances that act to *regulate body processes*.

An individual food may fulfill all three of these functions or only one, but all three functions must be served by the diet as a whole in order to maintain the

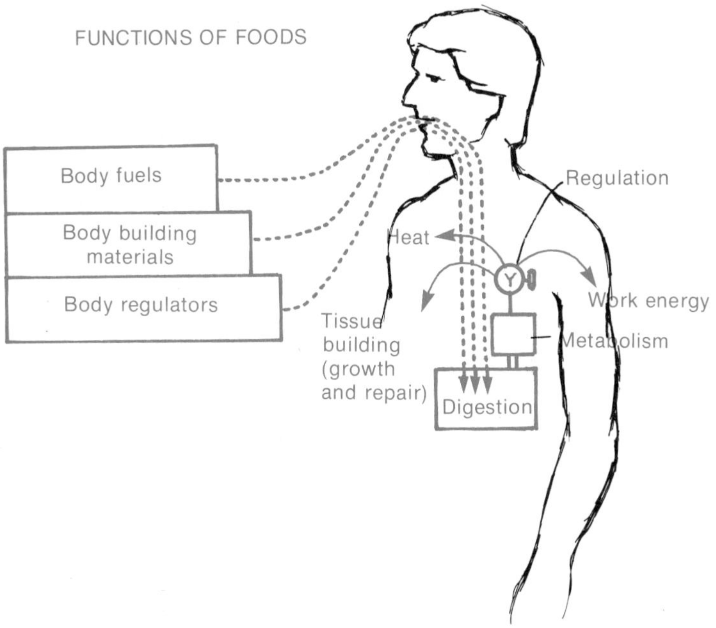

Figure 1–3 Diagram summarizing the functions of foods. To qualify as a food, it must provide substances that act as body fuel to provide energy, serve to build or maintain body tissues, or act as regulators of body processes. Many foods contain substances that serve all three purposes.

body in health. Most foods can fulfill more than one function because they are *mixtures* of a number of chemical substances (see Fig. 1–3).

Other important functions of food, though not essential, are to satisfy our individual requirements of taste, to combat temporary hunger pangs, and to fill certain social needs (discussed in later chapters).

Essential Nutrients

Six general classes, or *kinds of nutrients* found in foods, that are necessary to the body are:

1. Carbohydrates
2. Fats
3. Proteins (amino acids)
4. Vitamins
5. Minerals
6. Water

Carbohydrates, fats, and proteins are often spoken of as the fuel or *energy nutrients,* since they are the only substances that the body can use to supply energy for work and heat. They belong to the great division of chemical substances known as *organic* compounds, which contain *carbon* and are combustible. The *mineral elements* and *water* are sometimes called *inorganic nutrients,* since they do not contain carbon.

Proteins, minerals, and water all enter into the composition of body tissues, and hence are necessary for *building* new *tissues* or repair of those already built. *Vitamins* are chemically diverse organic substances which occur in minute quantities in foods but are essential for normal growth and health. Certain ones may be built into or stored in the tissues, but their chief function is to serve in regulating body processes. Mineral salts and vitamins act as *body regulators* by promoting oxidative processes, normal functioning of nerves and muscles, and vitality of tissues, and are of assistance in many other bodily functions. Water also serves as an important regulating substance in the body. It holds substances in solution in the digestive juices, blood, and tissues, and aids in regulation of body temperature, excretion, circulation, and many other body processes. Vegetable fiber acts along with water to promote intestinal elimination.

The three energy nutrients — carbohydrates, fats, and proteins — can be used by the body more or less interchangeably to supply *energy*, depending on which is more abundant in the diet. Next to water, these three classes of substances are the most abundant nutrients in our food; minerals and vitamins make up a relatively small, or even trace, portion.

For building tissues, different proteins are not completely interchangeable, since the "building blocks," called *amino acids*, that compose them vary in kind and relative amounts. Some nine or ten of these amino acids cannot be made in the body and must be supplied in the diet. Also, the fats eaten must supply an *essential fatty acid*. Some 18 or so different mineral elements must be supplied, in either major or minor amounts. At least 13 or 14 different vitamins are known to be needed. Hence, including water and oxygen, there are actually some 42 to 44 different nutrients known to be essential for normal nutrition, and there are probably others not yet identified.

General Composition of Foods and Units of Measurement

It is important that the nutrition student have a basic understanding of the major differences in the composition of the six classes of nutrients in common foods of distinctly different origins. Table 1–1 shows the composition on a fresh and dried basis of corn (maize), a typical food of plant origin, compared with a typical animal body on the same basis. A column is included for hamburger, a typical animal food. It should become obvious, after study of this table, that a *major characteristic of animals that eat largely vegetable material is the conversion within the body of plant carbohydrates to body fats (after energy needs)*. Along with making this conversion, the animal body accumulates minerals and protein. Only small amounts of carbohydrates are present in animal tissues (see Chapter 3). Knowing the figures in Table 1–1, one can estimate, in a rough, general way, the composition of almost all foods, plant or animal.

The detailed composition of many common foods is given in Table 2 of the Appendix for further comparison. In order to understand food composition tables and to have a clear idea of the *amounts* of foods which we actually need and eat, one must first be at home with the various *units of weight and measurement* commonly used in nutrition. Most countries of the world now use the *metric system*, which is by far the most useful way to describe and measure vitamins and trace minerals, and it makes calculations easier at all levels. A kilogram (metric system) equals 2.2 pounds (visualize, roughly, by thinking of slightly more than 2 pounds of butter or margarine, flour or sugar, or a quart — or liter — of milk). A

Table 1–1 SOME TYPICAL COMPOSITION FIGURES OF PLANT VS. ANIMAL FOODS

Classes of Nutrients	*Corn (Maize) Fresh*	*Corn (Maize) Dried*	*Typical Animal Body (Live Basis)*	*Typical Animal Body (Dried)*	*Hamburger (Fresh)*
	%	%	%	%	%
Water	75.0	12.0	60.0	12.0	50.0
Total carbohydrates	21.0*	73.4*	trace	0.1	trace
Crude fats	1.1	4.0	19.0	41.7	25.0 to 30.0
Crude proteins†	2.5	9.0	17.0	37.0	19.0 to 24.0
Minerals	0.4	1.4	4.0	9.0	1.0
Vitamins	trace	0.2	trace	0.2	trace
Total	100.0	100.0	100.0	100.0	100.0

*Primarily starch and sugars.
†Including small amounts of other compounds containing nitrogen.

Table 1–2 COMMON UNITS USED IN NUTRITION AND IN MEASUREMENT OF FOODS*

Metric units†	1 kilogram (kg) = 1000 grams 1 gram (gm) = 1000 milligrams 1 milligram (mg) = 1000 micrograms (mcg., μg., or γ)	
	Metric	***U.S. Avoirdupois***
Weight	1 kilogram = 1000 gm 0.1 kilogram = 100 gm 0.454 kilogram = 454 gm 0.028 kilogram = 28.4 gm	= 2.2 pounds = 3.52 ounces = 1.0 pound = 1.0 ounce
Volume, liquid	3.785 liters 1.000 liter = 1000 ml 0.946 liter = 946 ml 0.473 liter = 473 ml 0.237 liter = 237 ml 0.015 liter = 14.8 ml 4.9 ml	= 1 gallon = 4 quarts‡ = 1.06 quarts = 1 quart = 2 pints = 1 pint = 2 cups = 1 cup = 16 tablespoons (tbsp) = 1 tablespoon = 3 teaspoons (tsp) = 1 teaspoon
Weight per volume of water§	1 liter = 1 kg 1 milliliter = 1 gm 1 quart = 946 gm 1 cup¶ = 237 gm	 = 1 cubic centimeter (cc) = 8 ounces = ½ pound

*Many of these are approximations only. See Table 5 of the Appendix for more conversion values. (We should use the metric system whenever possible to avoid the confusion demonstrated by the above table, which must be used when we work with two systems.)

†Kilo means × 1000; milli, × $\frac{1}{1000}$; micro, × $\frac{1}{1{,}000{,}000}$. Therefore, kilogram means gram × 1000, milligram means gram × $\frac{1}{1000}$, milliliter means liter × $\frac{1}{1000}$.

‡British Imperial Gallon = 4.545 liters.

§Other liquids may be lighter (e.g., salad oil) or heavier (e.g., honey, corn syrup) than water.

¶A cup is not an official unit of measurement. The values given here are approximations only to help one visualize sizes and weights. The weight of a "cup" depends on what is being measured, of course.

pencil eraser or one lima bean weighs about 1 gram; a penny weighs 3 grams; and a shelled egg about 50 grams. A milligram of sugar would be about the size of a small pinhead — just barely visible.

Useful conversion figures are shown in Table 1–2. We suggest that your understanding of nutrition will be much more complete if you learn these relationships now.

How Composition of Foods Is Studied

What nutrients and how much of each are present in our various everyday foods is usually determined either

1. by chemical analysis, or
2. by biological assay.

Chemical Analysis. This provides useful data as to the approximate distribution of carbohydrates, fats, proteins, minerals, vitamins, and water in any given food. Methods commonly used for determining the relative amounts of the nutrients are briefly discussed in the following outline.

Water is determined by weighing a sample of the food before and after drying to constant weight.

Ash (mineral matter) is determined by completely burning the combustible portion and weighing the noncombustible residue.

Protein is computed by multiplying the nitrogen content of a food (chemically determined) by 6.25, since proteins are known to consist of about 16 percent (one-sixth) nitrogen by weight. This is the classic "Kjehldahl method." Slight errors result both because other nitrogen-containing substances that may be present in the food are included as proteins and because proteins vary somewhat in the amount of nitrogen they contain. This measure, N × 6.25, is often referred to as "crude protein" for this reason.

Fats are determined by extracting a dried sample of the food with ether. With the true fats (weighed after evaporating to dryness the ether extract) will be included small amounts of other ether-soluble substances such as resins, waxes, and coloring matter (pigments). This measure is often called "crude fat," or "ether-extract."

Carbohydrates are usually calculated "by difference"; that is, the remainder of the weight not accounted for under the total of the above headings is assumed to be carbohydrate in nature and is listed as such. Although this residue undoubtedly does consist largely of carbohydrates, it will also include organic acids (in fruits and vegetables), indigestible carbohydrates (cellulose and hemicelluloses, etc.), and various other undetermined substances not carbohydrates.

More accurate figures for individual carbohydrates, such as sucrose or fiber, may be obtained by direct analyses.

Vitamins must be determined individually. Most of the vitamins may be determined by chemical methods: by specific color reactions, by chromatography, or by complicated laboratory equipment using various chemical or physical properties of the vitamins studied. A few vitamins are still measured by biological tests using bacteria or one or more animal species.

Tables of food composition, obtained by the above methods, can never be absolutely accurate for several reasons. First, certain errors are inherent in the methods used or in the manner of calculating results. Then, even in the hands of skilled chemists, small errors occur that are magnified on calculating the composition from the basis of a small sample to a percentage basis for the food as a whole. Lastly, and probably of most importance, foods may vary considerably in composition either in samples from different sections of the country or from soils of different compositions, which may affect trace mineral levels; in different parts of the same sample of food; or especially in cooked foods where moisture and fat content are frequently variable. When a large number of samples of some raw food material, such as flour, milk, or eggs, have been analyzed, *average* values are obtained from which individual specimens probably will not differ much in composition. With cooked foods, fruits, and vegetables, or whenever only a few samples have been analyzed, variations will be larger and figures less accurate.

Biological Assay of Foods. This method involves actual feeding experiments on laboratory animals (usually rats, mice, guinea pigs, or chickens) under controlled conditions. White rats, whose heredity and previous diet history are known, are considered the best "standardized" animals and hence are likely to give the most accurate results. Moreover, the chemistry of their body tissues is, for the most part, reasonably similar to that of man. Also their life cycle is short enough so that one can watch the effects of some special diet on several generations. Such animals are fed a simple diet of known composition that is planned so as to provide plenty of all the essential nutrients *except one.* A certain food is added to this basal diet in known amounts to serve as the sole source of the nutrient in which it is lacking and for which the special food is being tested (see Fig. 1–4).

By such experiments, for example, the existence of *vitamins* in natural articles of food was established. Likewise it was discovered that numerous different vitamins are necessary in the diet for the well-being of both man and animals, and the relative amounts of each vitamin supplied by different foods have been more or less accurately determined. Laboratory feeding experiments also give information, not obtainable by chemical analyses, as to how *efficient* the *protein* content of different foods is for growth or maintaining weight, and how well *absorbed* and utilized the *mineral* content of certain foods may be. Biological assays show us

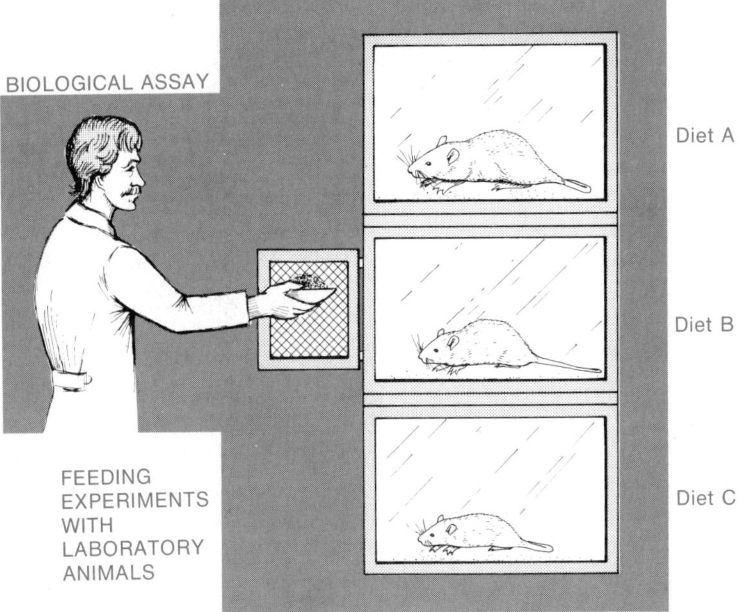

Figure 1–4 Biological assay is used to show how efficient different foods are in supplying body needs for proteins, various mineral elements, or vitamins. The rat is the favorite animal for feeding experiments, and the effectiveness of the diet in supplying body needs is gauged by relative growth and health of animals. In this drawing, the animal fed Diet A obviously got the most complete and adequate diet, while the other two rats either made less growth or show varying degrees of deficiency of one or more essential nutrients. Normally at least 8 to 10 rats would be fed each diet.

how effective different foods really are in supplying the needs of the body for each nutrient.

Each of the vitamins may now be determined by *physical* methods (measurement of absorption spectra, chromatography, fluorescence, turbidity, etc.), by *chemical* methods (chiefly by color reactions), or by *microbiological assay* (influence on growth of bacteria). However, feeding tests with animals retain their usefulness and in some cases are indispensable. Experiments with humans are very costly and require great control and care to protect the health and rights of the subjects. Interpretation of results of human studies is very difficult, partly because of psychic factors, which can affect results. The use of *placebos* as controls (pills that, unknown to the subject, contain a completely inactive substance such as sugar), and *double blind tests* (in which neither the investigator nor the persons directly responsible for the giving of diets or supplements or for diagnosing the subjects know the composition of the dietary variables) should be standard procedures in human nutrition studies. In such studies a code may be used for the various test groups that is disclosed only after the tests are all completed.

Learning About Foods — Food Groups

A simple and convenient way to study the different common foods is to *group them in several classes,* according to the nutrients they supply most abundantly. Thus, there have been in the past the "seven food groups," the "five food groups," and more recently the well-known "four food groups". Foods grouped together in this way are similar in general chemical make-up and hence contribute the same types of nutrients to the diet.

The basis of good nutrition is eating a *variety* of foods from different food groups. No single food group supplies all the essential nutrients in proper proportions to maintain health, but a food plan that includes a suggested number of servings from different groups furnishes at least a major portion of the proteins, minerals, and vitamins needed for an adequate diet. Additional foods may be required to meet the energy needs, and these may be supplied by selecting extra portions of the foods listed in one of the basic groups, or after nutrient requirements have been satisfied, by choosing foods from the "primarily energy", or "fifth" group of "sweets" (sugars, candies, honey, syrups, cakes, jams, etc.) and "fatty foods" (butter, margarine, salad oils, etc.), items not included in usual food guides. These foods are useful chiefly for their fuel value, for pure sugar and fats contribute little except energy value to the diet. (Fats, however, may carry vitamins A and E and essential fatty acids.)

For a very simple daily food guide, the United States Department of Agriculture suggests planning the basic diet around *four* food groups, along with the number of servings from each group that should be included.[7] These four food groups, slightly modified, together with the main contributions in nutrients that each group makes to the diet, are listed in Table 1–3.

The daily "four food groups" guide has, actually, six groups, if we include two subgroups in the vegetable-fruit group. Nevertheless, this guide has the advantages of simplicity and enough freedom of choice to fit individual preferences and different economic levels. However, it is by no means "foolproof." A basic diet, selected in accordance with the rules laid down, may range in essential nutrients from barely adequate (or even inadequate) to one that supplies an extra margin of these nutrients beyond body requirements, depending largely on the *choice of foods* within the four food groups and the *size of the servings* eaten.

Although the foods within a group belong together because they furnish, in general, the same kinds or types of nutrients, these nutrients may be present in quite different quantities or proportion in different foods within the same group. For instance, if only highly milled grain products are eaten (instead of whole-grain or enriched ones), less than adequate amounts of certain minerals and B vitamins may be provided. Within the "meat group," the plant sources of protein (dry beans, peas, and nuts) must be taken in well-balanced proportions or in fairly large amounts to furnish as much good quality protein as an average serving of meat (see Chapter 5).

Finally, the "vegetable and fruit

Table 1–3 DAILY FOOD PLAN BASED ON FOUR FOOD GROUPS

Group and Servings per Day	*Role in Diet*
1. Grain products—bread, flour, cereals, baked goods (whole-grain preferred). (Four or more servings.)	1. Inexpensive sources of energy and proteins Whole-grain or enriched products carry more iron and B vitamins.
2. Meat and vegetable protein group—meats, poultry, fish, shellfish, and eggs; dried beans, peas, and nuts. (Two or more servings.)	2. Valuable sources of proteins and amino acids; also furnish minerals (e.g., iron) and B vitamins.
3. Milk group—milk, cheese, yogurt, ice cream. (Four or more glasses or equivalent for teenagers, two for adults.)	3. Valuable sources of protein, calcium, riboflavin, other minerals, and vitamins.
4. Vegetable-fruit group—all fruits, vegetables, and potatoes. Four or more servings, including:	4. Chiefly important as carriers of minerals, vitamins, and fiber.
a. Leafy, green, and yellow vegetables.	a. High in iron, vitamin A, and folacin.
b. Citrus fruits, tomatoes, raw cabbage, etc.	b. Rich in vitamin C.

group" is widely diversified as to composition. It could well be (and sometimes is) divided into several subgroups — the starchy vegetables (potatoes, peas, beans, etc.); those that are either leafy, green, or yellow; citrus fruits and others that are relatively rich in vitamin C; and succulent fruits and vegetables high in water content—peaches, melons, celery, summer squash, and so forth. To make sure of an adequate intake of certain nutrients, chiefly iron, folacin, and vitamins A and C, the guide specifies serving leafy, green, or yellow vegetables every day, and serving citrus fruits or other fruits or vegetables important for vitamin C daily.

The "four food groups" guide is probably the best teaching device we have, at present, for young students, homemakers, and others just learning about good nutrition practices. However, in addition to the several limitations discussed in the previous paragraphs, nutrition educators know that students become bored hearing year after year about the plan. They begin to want to know *why* certain foods are important to us and to know more about food sources of individual nutrients. Also, the caloric (energy) content of foods and their taste and appeal often seem more important than their nutrient content.

There are two other major disadvantages of the "four food groups" guide. One is that many cultural, religious, and social groups of people here in the United States and in most other parts of the world do not, or cannot, have all the foods in this particular plan readily available to them. For instance, milk products are not universally used or even tolerated. Second, today many manufactured foods are available in the market that do not conveniently fit into one of the four food groups (for instance, pizza, hamburger "with the works," imitation cream products, or complete "meal replacements"). (Also see Chapter 19.)

Alternate Food Plans

It is now clear that there are many ways possible to learn about good food choices. This is a rapidly developing field today. The final selection of food by groups of people depends upon the types of foods readily available and utilized by any group of people, and their level of understanding about nutrition. In the United States we can expect the emergence in the next few years of new and often better guides for teaching about good nutrition. There no doubt will soon be better and more specific guides established for the feeding of infants and children, for different ethnic groups (for instance, Spanish-American and Chinese food guides are now widely available in the United States and elsewhere), for high school and college students, for pregnant women, for partial and complete vegetarians, for elderly persons living alone, and for people living in, or coming from, different countries and cultures.

There is no magic or secret way to good nutrition, nor is it easy. Some degree of nutrition knowledge is essential if an individual is going to ensure good health and physical fitness through good and economical nutrition practices, when so many negative forces are all around us today.

Chapter 17 has a more detailed discussion of various foods and their place in the diet, and Chapter 19 deals with the planning of adequate diets for normal adolescents and adults, while Chapters 20 and 21 discuss the special food needs of pregnancy and of infants and children, respectively.

History of Nutrition

The history of nutrition is fascinating, but the authors believe the subject is enjoyed more when historical matters are tied in with the individual nutrients throughout the book. Nutrition begins with the beginning of mankind on this earth, and many references to food and nutrition exist in man's earliest writings. Early man had to seek the facts for himself, largely by trial and error, as he chose his food from available plants, berries, nuts, roots, grains, fruit, and from the plentiful supply of animal life all around him. All of man's history has been greatly influenced by the distribution, availability, and search for foods and spices.

It was not until the development of modern science in the eighteenth and nineteenth centuries that there began to be an appreciation of the essential nature of certain nutrients. Among the first nutrients to be recognized as essential were protein, oxygen, calcium, iodine, and a scurvy-preventing factor (later identified as vitamin C). Most of these early milestones were in the years 1775 to 1825. Many of the early pioneers in nutrition and the more recent discoverers of the various nutrients will be mentioned later in this book. Students interested particularly in nutrition history will find references on this subject listed at the end of this chapter, and will enjoy reading about the lives and discoveries of such early nutrition pioneers as Lavoisier, Priestley, Liebig, Bernard, Mulder, Spallanzani, Magendie, Davy, E. Fischer, Abderhalden, Beaumont, Voit, Lusk, Rubner, Chittenden, Lind, Lunin, Takeki, Eijkman, Hopkins, Mellanby, Babcock, Hart, Wills, McCollum, Osborne, Mendel, Funk, Elvehjem, Goldberger, Jansen, R. R. Williams, György, Kleiber, Dam, Steenbock, Mitchell, Evans, Forbes, Morgan, Armsby, Burr, Deuel, Best, Kuhn, Murlin, Sherman, Roberts, and many others to whom we owe so much.

Likewise, others living today (though retired) have pioneered in nutrition discoveries which have greatly influenced the course of nutrition history and the health of all of us. Interested students will want to learn more about such nutrition pioneers as King, Castle, R. J. Williams, Folkers, Lepkovsky, C. Williams, Sebrell, Emerson, Zilva, Szent-Györgyi, Rose, Macy-Hoobler, Steibling, Kon, Norris, Waddell, and Almquist, along with many others still active today.

As far as we know, the first professor of human nutrition in the United States was Professor M. Jaffa, in 1908, at the University of California, Berkeley.[8] In 1912 he became chairman of the Department of Nutrition at the Berkeley College of Agriculture. This may also have been the first department of nutrition in America. Since then nutrition departments or divisions have prospered in almost all general colleges and universities of the country and are widely scattered throughout the world, in departments of home economics, animal science, or biochemistry. In the past decade separate nutrition departments or graduate training groups have been formed in at least a dozen universities of the United States, including several medical schools. Unfortunately, though, there are still insufficient nutrition training centers.

Approximately 10,000 research papers are published each year in the world's literature on food and nutrition. The science of nutrition is well established throughout the world, and new important discoveries are being made almost every day. Almost every major country has a nutrition society and publishes its own scientific nutrition journal. Recently the International Union of Nutritional Sciences (IUNS) has become considerably more active and is in the process of setting up international standards for nutrition research, nomenclature, and training.

A list of resource materials on the broader aspects of nutritional sciences may be found at the end of this chapter.

QUESTIONS AND PROBLEMS

1. What is meant by nutrition, a nutrient, an adequate diet?

2. Why do some peoples prosper physcially on diets consisting of only a few types of food, while others show physical degeneration on the limited types of diet that they consume?

3. How is it possible to improve an apparently adequate diet, and what benefits may be expected as a result of doing this? Name the chief motives for making changes in food habits indicated as nutri-

tionally desirable, and some of the factors that stand in the way of changing food habits.

4. What are the three uses of food in the body? What other functions do food serve? Name the six kinds of essential nutrients found in foods. Which of these can serve as body fuel and why? Which are used in the building and repair of tissues? Which are necessary to regulate body processes?

5. Name the four general groups of foods suggested as a basis upon which to plan an adequate diet and the main nutrients contributed by each of these food groups to the diet. How many average servings are recommended from each group daily? Why are green and yellow vegetables and citrus fruits singled out for more frequent use than other fruits and vegetables? Plan a day's diet using foods from *each* of the four main food groups in the following recommended number of servings: grain (four or more), meat (two or more), milk (two or more, for adult), and vegetable-fruit (four or more). What other foods will be needed to round out the diet and satisfy energy needs?

6. Explain what is meant by the biological assay of foods. What information can be obtained by biological assay and how does it supplement facts obtained by chemical analysis? Describe how a food may be assayed for its content of a certain vitamin.

7. Make a record for 3 or 4 days of the kinds of food (including beverages) and the number of servings in each of the four food groups you consume each day. Compare the amounts of each class of food actually consumed against those recommended in Question 5. What foods did you eat in larger or smaller quantities than recommended as the basis for an adequate diet? Did you supplement your diet with additional fuel foods? How could you improve your dietary habits?

8. As a special project, write a report on some aspect of the history of nutrition or on one of the nutrition pioneers.

REFERENCES

1. Jacobziner, H.: Physical fitness in New York City schools. Gen. Prac., *29*:112, 1964.
2. McCarrison, R.: Faulty food in relation to gastro-intestinal disorder. J. Amer. Med. Assoc., *78*:1, 1922.
3. Orr, J. B., and Gilks, J. L.: Studies on nutrition: the physique and health of two African tribes. British Medical Research Council, Special Report No. 155, 1931.
4. Keys, A., et al.: *The Biology of Human Starvation.* Minneapolis, University of Minnesota Press, 1950.
5. Scrimshaw, N. S., and Gordon, E. (eds.): *Malnutrition, Learning and Behavior.* Cambridge, Mass., MIT Press, 1968; (also see references on this topic in the supplementary reading list).
6. See current journals and references in the section on *Nutrition Status, U.S.A. – Policies* in the supplementary reading list.
7. Page, L., and Phippard, E. F.: *Essentials of an Adequate Diet.* Home Economics Research Report No. 3., Washington, D.C., U.S. Department of Agriculture, Government Printing Office, 1957.
8. As cited in the University of California Bulletin of 1908.

SUPPLEMENTARY READING

Nutrition Standards and Food Guides

Ahlström, A., and Räsänen, L.: Review of food grouping systems in nutrition education. J. Nutr. Ed., *5*:13, 1973.

American Institute of Nutrition: Standards for nutritional studies. J. Nutr., *107*:1340, 1977.

Butrum, R. R., and Gebhardt, S. E.: Nutrient data bank: computer-based management of nutrient values in foods. J. Amer. Oil Chem. Soc., *53*:727A, 1976.

Campbell, J. A.: Approaches in revising dietary standards, J. Amer. Dietet. Assoc., *64*:175, 1974.

Canadian Health and Welfare Department: *Dietary Standard for Canada,* 1975. Ottawa.

Davis, D. R., and Williams, R. J.: Potentially useful criteria for judging nutritional adequacy. Amer. J. Clin. Nutr., *29*:710, 1976.

FAO/WHO: Handbook on human nutritional requirements, 1974, Nutr. Rev., *33*:147, 1975.

Food and Nutrition Board: *Recommended Dietary Allowances.* 8th Ed. Washington, D.C., National Research Council, National Academy of Sciences, 1974.

Harper, A. E.: Recommended dietary allowances: Are they what we think they are? J. Amer. Dietet. Assoc., *64*:151, 1974.

Murphy, E. W., Watt, B. K., and Rizek, R. L.: Tables of food composition: availability, uses, and limitations. Food Technol., *27*:40, 1973.

Peterkin, B.: Perspective — the RDA or the U.S. RDA? J. Nutr. Ed., *9*:10, 1977.

Wittwer, A. J., et al.: Nutrient density — evaluation of national attributes of foods. J. Nutr. Ed., *9*:26, 1977.

Yuk, A.W.C.C., Wheeler, E. F., and Leppington, I. M.: Variations in the apparent nutrient content of foods: a study of sampling error. Brit. J. Nutr., *34*:391, 1975.

Nutrition Status, U.S.A. – Policies

Armstrong, H.: Nutritional status of black preschool children in Mississippi. J. Amer. Dietet. Assoc., *66*:488, 1975.

Bass, M. A., and Wakefield, L. M.: Nutrient intake and food patterns of Indians on Standing Rock Reservation. J. Amer. Dietet. Assoc., *64*:36, 1974.

Burgess, H. J. L., and Burgess, A.: A field worker's guide to a nutritional status survey. Amer. J. Clin. Nutr., *28*:1299, 1975.

Cook, R. A., Hurlburt, R. A., and Radke, F. H.: Nutritional status of Head Start and nursery school children. Research, *68*:127, 1976.

Guthrie, H. A., and Guthrie, G. M.: Factor anlysis of nutritional status data from Ten State Nutrition Survey. Amer. J. Clin. Nutr., *29*:1238, 1976.

Hegsted, D. M.: Priorities in nutrition in the United States. J. Amer. Dietet. Assoc., *71*:9, 1977.

Inano, M., and Pringle, D. J.: Dietary survey of low-income, rural families of Iowa and North Carolina. III. Contribution of food groups to nutrients. J. Amer. Dietet. Assoc., *66*:366, 1975.

Larson, L. B., et al.: Nutritional status of children of Mexican-American migrant families. J. Amer. Dietet. Assoc., *65*:29, 1974.

Lowenstein, F. W.: Preliminary clinical and anthropometric findings from the first Health and Nutrition Examination Survey, USA, 1971–1972. Amer. J. Clin. Nutr., *29*:918, 1976.

Marston, R., and Friend, B.: Nutritional review. Natl. Food Situation, USDA, Nov. 1976, p. 25.

O'Neal, R. M., et al.: The incidence of anemia in residents of Missouri. Amer. J. Clin. Nutr., *29*:1158, 1976.

Owen, G., and Lippman, G.: Nutritional status of infants and young children, U.S.A. Ped. Clin. N. Amer., *24*:211, 1977.

Prothro, J., Mickles, M., and Tolbert, B.: Nutritional status of a population sample in Macon County, Alabama. Amer. J. Clin. Nutr., *29*: 94, 1976.

Schlossberg, K.: Symposium: Progress toward a national food policy. Its implications. J. Amer. Dietet. Assoc., *68*:326, 1976.

Select Committee on Nutrition and Human Needs: *Dietary goals for the United States.* 2nd Ed. Washington, D.C., Government Printing Office, 1978.

Walker, M. A., and Page, L.: Nutritive content of college meals: proximate composition and vitamins. J. Amer. Dietet. Assoc., *66*:146, 1975.

Youland, D. M., and Engle, A.: Practices and problems in HANES: dietary data methodology. J. Amer. Dietet. Assoc., *68*:22, 1976.

Malnutrition – World Problems (Also see Chapter 25.)

Berg, A.: Fear of trying. J. Amer. Dietet. Assoc., *68*:311, 1976.

Blaxter, K. L., Chairman: Symposium: Famine. (six papers) Proc. Nutr. Soc., *34*:159, 1975.

Gebre-Medhin, M., and Vahlquist, B.: Famine in Ethiopia — a brief review. Amer. J. Clin. Nutr., *29*:1016, 1976.

Gershoff, S. N.: Science — neglected ingredient of nutrition policy. J. Amer. Dietet. Assoc., *70*:471, 1977.

Goldsmith, G. A.: Food and population. Amer. J. Clin. Nutr., *28*:934, 1975.

Gordon, J. E., and Scrimshaw, N. S.: Field evaluation of nutrition intervention programs. World Rev. Nutr. Dietet., *17*:1, 1973.

McLaren, D. S.: Undernutrition. World Rev. Nutr. Dietet., *16*:141, 1973.

Reutlinger, S., and Selowsky, M.: *Malnutrition and Poverty.* World Bank Staff Occasional Papers No. 23. Baltimore, Johns Hopkins Univ. Press, 1976.

Walter, J. P.: Two poverties equal one hunger. J. Nutr. Ed., *5*:129, 1973.

Nutrition History

Bennion, M.: Food preparation in colonial America. J. Amer. Dietet. Assoc., *69*:16, 1976.

Bing, F. C.: Nutrition research and education in the age of Franklin. A bicentennial study. J. Amer. Dietet. Assoc., *68*:14, 1976.

Day, H. G., Chairman: Symposium: Selected topics in history of nutrition. (four papers) Fed. Proc., *36*:1903, 1977.

Goldblith, S. A., and Joslyn, M.A.: *An Anthology of Food Science,* Vol. 2, *Milestones in Nutrition.* Westport, Conn., Avi Publishing Co., Inc., 1964.

Gurson, C. T.: Historical introduction. In *Textbook of Paediatric Nutrition.* New York, Churchill Livingstone, 1976.

Hertzler, A. A., and Anderson, H. L.: Food guides in the United States. An historical review. J. Amer. Dietet. Assoc., *64*:19, 1974.

Lowenberg, M. E., and Lucas, B. L.: Feeding families and children — 1776 and 1976. J. Amer. Dietet. Assoc., *68*:207, 1976.

McCay, C. M.: *Notes on the History of Nutrition Research.* Berne, Hans Huber Publishers, 1973.

McCollum, E. V.: *A History of Nutrition.* Boston, Houghton Mifflin Co., 1957.

Articles in* Nutrition Reviews (General history references and classics)

Criteria of the monetary value of foods. *31*:211, 1973.

Cicely D. Williams, her life and influence. *31*:331 and 378, 1973.

On the ultimate composition of simple alimentary substances; with some preliminary remarks on the analysis of organized bodies in general. *33*:112, 1975.

Nutrition science: an overview of American genius. *34*:1, 1976.

Paul György—an appreciation. *34*:159, 1976.

Chronology of some events in the development and application of the science of nutrition. *34*:353, 1976.

---

*Nutrition Reviews is published monthly by the Nutrition Foundation, New York.

Recollections of personalities involved in the early history of American biochemistry. *35*:87, 1977.
Kwashiorkor in Africa. *35*:108, 1977.
Todhunter, E. N.: Some aspects of the history of dietetics. World Rev. Nutr. Dietet., *18*:1, 1973.

Nutrition Education and Training

Cho, M., and Fryer, B. A.: Nutritional knowledge of collegiate physical education majors. J. Amer. Dietet. Assoc., *65*:30, 1974.
Frankle, R. T.: Nutrition education for medical students. I. What is it? Where has it been? Why should it be taught? J. Amer. Dietet. Assoc., *68*:513, 1976.
Hart, M. E.: Dietetic education — past, present, and future. J. Amer. Dietet. Assoc., *64*:612, 1974.
Ikeda, J. P.: Expressed nutrition information needs of low-income homemakers. J. Nutr. Ed., *7*:104, 1975.
Johnson, D.: The dietitian — a translator of nutrition information. J. Amer. Dietet. Assoc., *64*:608, 1974.
Manoff, R.K.: Potential uses of mass media in nutrition programs. J. Nutr. Ed., *5*:125, 1973.
Peck, E. B.: The public health nutritionist-dietitian: an historical perspective. J. Amer. Dietet. Assoc., *64*:642, 1974.
Schwartz, N. E.: Nutritional knowledge, attitudes, and practices of high school graduates. J. Amer. Dietet. Assoc., *66*:28, 1975.
Schwartzberg, L., George, C., and Phillips, M. C.: Issues in food advertising — the nutrition educator's viewpoint. J. Nutr. Ed., *9*:60, 1977.
Young, E. A., and Weser, E.: Integration of nutrition in medical education. J. Nutr. Ed., *7*:112, 1975.

Other General References

Berg, A., and Muscat, R.: An approach to nutrition planning. Amer. J. Clin. Nutr., *25*:939, 1972.
Bleibtreu, H. K.: An anthropologist views the nutrition professions. J. Nutr. Ed., *5*:11, 1973.
Correa, H.: Measured influence of nutrition on socio-economic development (a review). World Rev. Nutr. Dietet., *20*:1, 1975.
Dickerson, J. W. T., et al.: Symposium: Interaction of drugs and nutrition. Proc. Nutr. Soc., *33*:191, 1974.
Land, H., et al.: symposium: Social and economic factors in human nutrition. Proc. Nutr. Soc., *33*:39, 1974.
Lloyd-Still, J. D.: *Malnutrition and Intellectual Development.* Littleton, Mass., Publishing Sciences Group, Inc., 1976.
Longhurst, R. W., and Call, D. L.: Scientific consensus, nutrition programs and economic planning. Amer. J. Clin. Nutr., *28*:1177, 1975.
Peters, R. A.: The neglect of nutrition and its perils. Amer. J. Clin. Nutr., *26*:750, 1973.
Popkin, B. M., and Latham, M. C.: The limitations and dangers of commerciogenic nutritious foods. Amer. J. Clin. Nutr., *26*:1015, 1973.
Rechcigl, M., Jr.: Reviews relating to food, nutrition, and health — a selected bibliography. World Rev. Nutr. Dietet., *16*:398, 1973.
Weininger, J., and Briggs, G. M.: Nutrition update, 1974, 1975, 1976, 1977. J. Nutr. Ed., *6*:139, 1974; *7*:141, 1975; *8*:172, 1976; *9*:173, 1977.
Winick, M.: *Malnutrition and Brain Development.* New York, Oxford Univ. Press, 1976.

Articles in Nutrition Reviews

An index of food quality. *31*:1, 1973.
Nutritional quality and food product development. *31*:226, 1973. Present knowledge of the relationship of nutrition to brain development and behavior. *31*:242, 1973.
What is community health? *31*:391, 1973.
Recommended daily dietary allowances (revised 1973). *31*:393, 1973.
The choice of animal species for studies of metabolic regulation. *32*:1, 1974.
Nutrition programs in state health agencies. *32*:65, 1974.
Nutrition Canada — a national nutrition survey. *32*:105, 1974.
Texas tri-county nutrition survey. *32*:222, 1974.
Nutrition in medical education. *32*:360, 1974.
FAO/WHO handbook on human nutritional requirements, 1974. *33*:147, 1975.
Nutrition, food needs and technologic priorities: the World Food Conference. *33*:225, 1975.
Nutrition: toxicology and pharmacology. *34*:65, 1976.
Careers in nutrition from the clinical viewpoint. *34*:97, 1976.
Food science and technology, past, present, future. *34*:193, 1976.
Malnutrition and drug metabolism in man. *34*:237, 1976.
The validity of 24-hour dietary recalls. *34*:310, 1976.
Soil fertility and the nutritive value of crops. *34*:316, 1976.
Dietary goals for the United States. *35*:122, 1977.
Clinical nutrition, an interface between human ecology and internal medicine. (by Olson, R. E.) *36*: 161, 1978.

GENERAL NUTRITION RESOURCES

Journals

Agenda (formerly *War on Hunger*), published monthly by the Agency for International Development, Department of State, Washington, D.C. 20523

American Journal of Clinical Nutrition, published monthly by the American Society for Clinical Nutrition Inc., 9650 Rockville Pike, Bethesda, Maryland 20014.

American Journal of Public Health, published monthly by the American Public Health Association Inc., 1740 Broadway, New York, N.Y. 10019.

British Journal of Nutrition (with the *Proceedings of the Nutrition Society*), published quarterly and semiannually respectively for the Nutrition Society by the Cambridge University Press, Bentley House, 200 Euston Road, London NW 1, or 32 East 57th St., New York, N. Y. 10022.

Cereal Science Today, published monthly by the

American Association of Cereals Chemists, St. Paul, Minnesota 55104.

CERES, FAO Review, published bimonthly by the Food and Agriculture Organization of the United Nations. Available in major cities of the world, including Rome (Via delle Terme de Caracalla, 00100) and New York (UNIPUB, Inc., 650 First Ave., P.O. Box 433).

CNI Weekly Report, published weekly by Community Nutrition Institute, 1146 19th St. N. W., Washington, D.C. 20036

Ecology of Food and Nutrition, published quarterly by Gordon and Breach Science Publishers Ltd., 440 Park Avenue South, New York, N.Y. 10016.

Family Health, published monthly by Family Health Magazine, P.O. Box 2900, Boulder, Colorado 80302.

Federation Proceedings, published bimonthly by the Federation of American Societies for Experimental Biology, 9650 Rockville Pike, Bethesda, Maryland 20014 (containing review articles and abstracts of the American Institute of Nutrition, etc.).

Food Technology, published monthly by the Institute of Food Technologists, Suite 2120, 221 N. LaSalle St., Chicago, Illinois 60601.

Indian Journal of Nutrition and Dietetics, published bimonthly by the SRI Avinashilingan Home Science College, Coimbatore-11, India.

Journal of the American Dietetic Association, published monthly by the American Dietetic Association, 620 North Michigan Ave., Chicago, Illinois 60611.

Journal of the American Medical Association, published weekly by the American Medical Association, 535 North Dearborn, St., Chicago, Illinois 60610.

Journal of Home Economics, published ten times a year by the American Home Economics Association, 1600 20th St. Washington, D.C. 20009.

Journal of Nutrition, published monthly by the American Institute of Nutrition, 9650 Rockville Pike, Bethesda, Maryland 20014.

Journal of Nutrition Education, published quarterly by the Society for Nutrition Education, P.O. Box 931, Berkeley, California 94701.

Nutrition Abstracts and Reviews, published quarterly by the Commonwealth Bureau of Animal Nutrition, Rowett Research Institute, Bucksburn, Aberdeen, AB 2 9SB, Scotland.

Nutrition Reviews, published monthly by the Nutrition Foundation, 99 Park Ave., New York.

Nutrition Today, published bimonthly by Enloe, Stalvey, and Associates, 1140 Connecticut Ave., N. W., Washington, D.C. 20036.

Public and Private Agencies That Provide Nutrition Information

American Dietetic Association, 620 North Michigan Ave., Chicago, Illinois 60611.

American Heart Association, 44 East 23rd St., New York, N.Y. 10010.

American Home Economics Association, 1600 20th Street, N.W., Washington, D.C., 20009.

Cereal Institute Inc., Education Department, 135 So. LaSalle St., Chicago, Illinois 60603.

Food and Agriculture Organization, Rome or New York (UNIPUB, Inc., 650 First Ave., P.O. Box 433). (Publishes various nutrition education materials and booklets. Also has a library for Nutrition workers in developing countries described in J. Nutr. Ed. 8:160, 1976)

Food and Drug Administration, Washington, D.C. (provides miscellaneous consumer information including the "FDA Consumer".)

National Academy of Sciences, Food and Nutrition Board, 2101 Constitution Ave., Washington, D.C.

National Dairy Council, 6300 North River Rd., Rosemont, Illinois 60018. (Publishes a bimonthly "Dairy Council Digest" and quarterly "Nutrition News.")

National Live Stock and Meat Board, 444 North Michigan Ave., Chicago, Illinois 60611. (Publishes a monthly "Food and Nutrition News.")

Nutrition Foundation, Inc., 99 Park Ave., New York, N.Y. 10016.

Public Affairs Committee, Inc., 381 Park Ave., South, New York, N.Y. 10016.

Society for Nutrition Education, 2140 Shattuck Ave., Suite 1110, Berkeley, California 94704. (Has a national clearing house of nutrition education information.)

U.S. Department of Agriculture (Cooperative Extension Service; Food and Nutrition Service; Consumer Marketing Service; Agricultural Research Service; Office of Information; or National Library of Agriculture), Washington, D.C. 20250.

U.S. Department of Health, Education, and Welfare, Washington, D.C. (Children's Bureau; National Institutes of Health; Office of Child Development.)

Chapter 2

The Need for Energy

All living things require energy. In man and other higher animals, the need for energy is second only to the need for air and water, and a critical role of many vitamins and minerals is to facilitate and regulate the utilization of the chief fuel-nutrients — *carbohydrate, fat,* and *protein*. The nutrients that provide energy, together with water, account for almost all the weight of the daily diet.

Energy is defined as the *power to do work*. Energy exists in many different forms, all of which are interconvertible. Heat, light, sound, and electricity are familiar forms of energy, and the fact that they are interconvertible is evident in that electricity is converted to heat and light in a lamp and to mechanical action and sound in an alarm clock. Energy also is stored in chemical forms, as in an automobile battery. Whenever change takes place in a system, energy must be transferred from one part of the system to another to effect the change, but the total amount of energy in the system remains the same. Only its form may be different. It may seem difficult to believe that energy is not simply "used up" in, for instance, riding a bicycle. But if the bicycle wheel is fitted to an electrical generator, it can easily be proved that energy remains and can be used to light a lamp or charge a battery. The fact that energy is neither created nor destroyed during any chemical or physical process is one of the most fundamental tenets of science. It is called the *law of the conservation of energy*.

The energy we use comes to us in the form of the potential chemical energy stored in foods. Ultimately this energy is derived from the sun. Green plants capture light energy through the process of *photosynthesis*, storing this solar energy in the form of organic* compounds that are used by higher animals for their nutrition (see Fig. 2–1). In the basic photosynthetic reaction, carbon dioxide gas (CO_2) from the atmosphere is combined with water (H_2O) to produce a carbohydrate (the typical sugar glucose, $C_6H_{12}O_6$) and gaseous oxygen (O_2), which is given off into the atmosphere. Photosynthesis thus supports animal life in two ways — by adding essential oxygen to the air and by tying up solar energy in the chemical bonds between carbon (C) and hydrogen (H) atoms in a form that we can use to meet our energy needs.

The body needs energy because it has certain indispensable work to perform. Internal work is carried out to maintain life

*Organic compounds are substances that contain the element carbon. Most natural products from plant and animal sources are organic in that they contain carbon. Numerous synthetic chemicals, including drugs, pesticides, and plastics, also are organic in the proper sense of the term, i.e., they contain carbon.

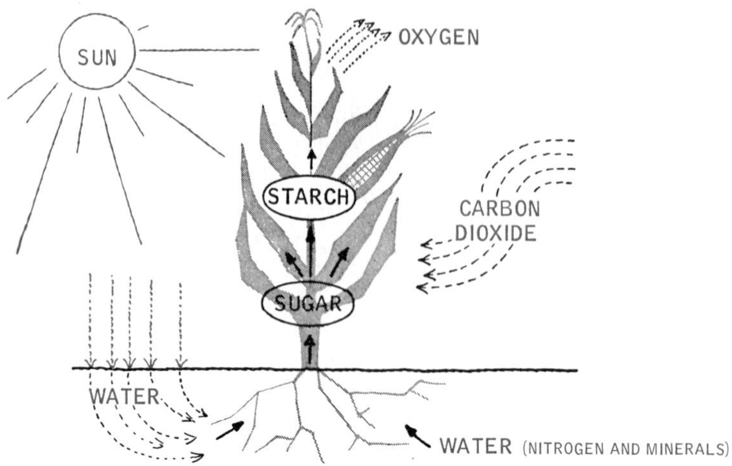

Figure 2–1 Synthesis of sugar from carbon dioxide (CO_2) and water (H_2O) through the agency of sunlight and the green pigment chlorophyll—a process known as photosynthesis. In the typical reaction six molecules of CO_2 are joined with six molecules of H_2O to form one molecule of a sugar ($C_6H_{12}O_6$) and six molecules of oxygen (O_2). To carry out their life processes, plants need light energy from the sun (or a suitable artificial source) and nitrogen (N) and mineral salts present in the soil. Plants cannot use gaseous nitrogen (N_2) found in air. One class of plants, legumes, have associated (symbiotic) bacteria that can fix N_2 into forms available to the plant, but for the most part, plants use the nitrogenous compounds present in animal wastes. Animals also produce the CO_2 needed by plants. Thus, animals and plants exist in a mutually advantageous, balanced system.

processes, even during sleep, in the uncounted numbers of chemical and physical activities of the cells and organs. Muscular work is required for a person to sit and stand erect and to move the body or objects. Energy is also needed to form new tissues during growth and pregnancy or after an injury, to produce milk, and sometimes to heat the body.

ENERGY FOR WORK FROM BURNING BODY FUELS

The body gets energy for its internal and external work in a manner superficially similar to that in which an internal combustion engine uses energy from fuel. In an automobile engine, gasoline vapor is mixed with air, ignited by a spark, and burned (oxidized) with a resultant conversion of chemical energy to work and heat. In the body, the three chief energy nutrients (carbohydrate, fat, and protein) are oxidized in the cells, using oxygen brought to the tissues by the blood, and energy is converted to heat and work. During the process of combustion, carbon and hydrogen bonds in the fuel or energy nutrient are oxidized, that is, changed to the lower energy bonds present in carbon dioxide and water. Since no energy is ever created or lost, the extra energy appears as heat and work.

The body is like a combustion engine in these respects:

1. Energy for work is obtained by *oxidation* of fuel.
2. *Heat* is a *by-product* of the transformations by which energy is released.
3. Both conform to the *law of the conservation of energy.*

Fuel is oxidized in the machine and, to some extent, in the body to provide *mechanical energy* to be utilized in doing work. However, in both cases, more of the energy set free is in the form of *heat* than of mechanical energy. The relative proportion of fuel energy that is converted into mechanical energy is called the mechanical efficiency, which, in the case of a good gasoline engine, is 20 percent; that of a diesel engine is nearly 40 percent. The mechanical efficiency of the body is on the order of 20 percent. This means that to do a given amount of work, about five times as much body fuel must be oxidized as would be represented by the work alone. Since only about one-fifth of the energy of the fuel is transformed into work energy while about four-fifths of it appears as heat, strenuous work has a warming effect on the body. Even the internal work of the body generates enough heat so that temperature regulation of the body is called into play.

The analogy between the body and the combustion engine does have its limitations. In a number of respects the living organism differs radically from the nonvital machine, and in practically all instances these differences represent advantages to the body in adjusting to its environment and varied needs.

In the body, the three primary energy nutrients can be used nearly interchangeably as fuel. The body can also make limited use of alcohol as a fuel source. In contrast, the gasoline engine is dependent on only one kind of fuel. In the body, oxidation is a controlled process during which energy is released slowly in a number of steps rather than in a single instantaneous combustion. (These complex processes are described in Chapter 15.) The internal work of the body never stops. The body needs materials and energy for repairing wear and tear on its tissues and for the continuous upkeep of the other vital internal activities, both of which functions have no counterpart in the machine.

The law of the conservation of energy holds true for the human body. This means that all energy used in the body must come from the burning of energy-yielding foods or of body tissues, and that all energy supplied in food is sooner or later recovered in some form. If a person does not eat enough food to cover the cost of energy expended, he is forced to burn up some of his body tissues and thus loses weight. On the other hand, if his intake of food is in excess of his energy needs, the extra energy is stored in the tissues and he gains weight.

Extra fuel is usually stored in fatty tissue. All of the energy-nutrients can be converted to fat in the body, and an excess of energy eaten as protein or carbohydrate or fat adds to the adipose tissue. Fat deposited in adipose tissue is the body's main long-term energy reserve. The body can store only a very limited amount of carbohydrate as animal starch, or glycogen, in the liver and muscles. This serves as a short-term supply to maintain the sugar level of the blood and to support other cellular processes. Although the body possesses little ability to store extra protein, muscle and internal organs are rich in protein, some of which can be used for fuel if necessary. Protein reserves are not drawn on for energy until the carbohydrate store is exhausted.* In a well-fed adult, the glycogen reserves will last for about 16 to 20 hours of fasting, after which fat and, to a limited extent, protein are available to meet ongoing energy needs. Under ordinary conditions of living, there is a wide margin of safety as to fuel stored in the body, and healthy adults can sustain life without food for several weeks.

ENERGY MEASUREMENT

Naturally, one is interested to know how much energy is needed for the internal and external work of the body. Energy requirements are customarily expressed in terms of calories, a heat unit. One calorie is the amount of energy (heat) required to raise the temperature of one gram of water one degree Celsius†, and is equivalent to 4.184 Joules. (Joule is the energy unit generally accepted by scientists. One

*Some protein components (amino acids) form a normal part of the energy cycle in working muscle (see Chapter 22). Here we refer to general energy needs of the body.

†Centigrade and Celsius, the units of temperature measurement, are the same.

Joule, a work unit, is 10^7 ergs.) The magnitude of human energy requirements makes it awkward to use such a small unit, so the convention of the large Calorie was accepted. The nutritionist's Calorie is 1000 calories and is abbreviated kcal to indicate that it is 1000 times (k for kilo) as large as the calorie. (The abbreviation Cal. is sometimes used and has the same meaning.) Total energy needs vary widely, but for adults 1800 to 3600 kcal (7500 to 15,000 kJoules or kJ) per day would be typical.

Energy expenditure can be measured by the methods of direct and indirect calorimetry. *Direct calorimetry* measures the amount of heat given off as a by-product of energy metabolism. This method was elucidated in 1761 by the Scottish physician Joseph Black, who measured the heat resulting from chemical combustion by melting ice under controlled conditions. During the period 1782 to 1784, the French scientists Lavoisier and Laplace used this principle to demonstrate that animal metabolism is a kind of combustion in which heat is given off, oxygen* is used, and carbon dioxide is produced. With much further refinement, the exact relationships of oxygen usage and heat production were quantified, enabling measurement of energy metabolism indirectly from oxygen utilization, that is, by *indirect calorimetry*.

Proof of these relationships in man was quite a feat. Such experiments had actually been undertaken by Lavoisier (c. 1784), but his research was literally cut short when he was sent to the guillotine by the French Revolutionary tribunal. More than a century passed before Atwater, Benedict, and Rosa constructed the first human respiration calorimeter at Wesleyan University in Connecticut (between 1897 and 1905). Several more of these costly instruments were built later in Bethesda, Md., New York, and Boston. This device, a few of which are still in use, is called a respiration calorimeter because it can measure not only the respiratory exchange (amounts of oxygen used and carbon dioxide produced) but also the amount of heat given off by the human subject. The calorimeter portion of the apparatus consists primarily of a copper box large enough to hold a man comfortably, encased and insulated to prevent any loss of heat through the walls. The heat generated by the subject is carried away by water circulating through a coil of pipe near the roof of the chamber, so that the inner temperature is maintained constant. The heat that is transferred to the water and the heat required to vaporize water in the subject's breath (and perspiration) together represent the total heat production of his body in a given time (*direct calorimetry*).

At the same time, by devices included in the closed circuit of air which the subject breathes, the quantities of oxygen consumed and carbon dioxide given out are measured. From these values, the amount of energy that would have been set free by oxidations within the body can be calculated *(indirect calorimetry)*. Values obtained by the two methods differ by only a fraction of one percent.

Today, human energy expenditure usually is measured by means of a relatively simple apparatus that determines only the respiratory exchange. The use of a portable, easily operated respiration apparatus has made it possible to measure the energy expenditure of patients in bed, of students in the classroom, of people working at a variety of tasks. The early apparatus used (Fig. 2–2) recorded the

*Oxygen was discovered by an English Unitarian minister, Joseph Priestly. He produced the gas from mercuric oxide and showed that mice could live much longer in this gas than in an equal volume of air. Priestly observed that in a closed container a mouse or a burning candle "damaged" the air so that the animal or flame died, and that growing plants would restore the air. He was thus the first to observe (1771) that photosynthesis and animal respiration are counterbalancing processes. He communicated with Lavoisier, and it was the latter who more fully explained the processes and conferred the name "oxygène" on the gas. Priestly emigrated to America in 1793, when life in England was made intolerable for him because he espoused the cause of civil, political, and religious liberty.

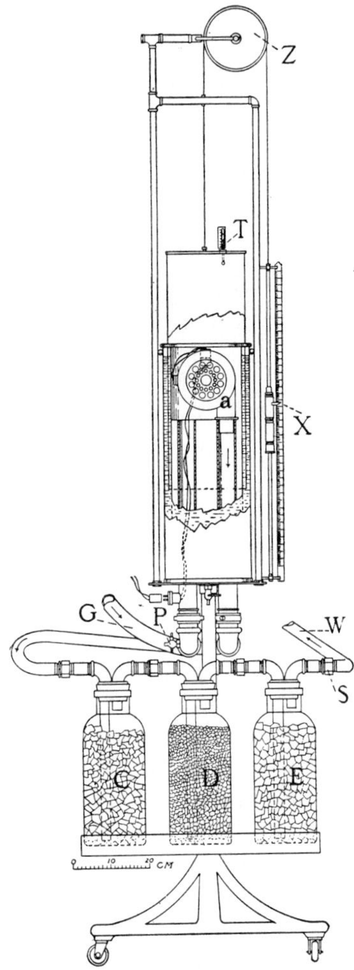

Figure 2–2 Spirometer and absorbing system of portable respiration apparatus developed by F. G. Benedict. G, Large caliber pipe conducting expired air to spirometer; a, air impeller; C, first water absorber; D, carbon dioxide absorber; E, second water absorber; S, point at which rate of ventilation may be tested by disconnecting coupling; W, pipe conducting purified air to subject; P, petcock for introducing oxygen; T, thermometer for obtaining records of temperature of spirometer. The spirometer bell is counterpoised by the weight, X, attached to silk thread passing over aluminum wheel, Z. Scale on which pointer indicates height of spirometer bell is shown at right of X. (Reprinted from the Boston Medical and Surgical Journal, 1918.)

amount of oxygen consumed by the person, at rest, when rebreathing in a closed circuit of oxygen-rich air for 6 to 10 minutes. The heat that would have been produced by this amount of oxidation in the body was then calculated, using the energy value of 4.825 kcal per liter of oxygen. (This figure was derived from extensive studies made in the respiration calorimeter.)

Energy cost of work is now commonly measured by any of several devices (Figs. 2–3 and 2–4) that collect part or all of the air exhaled by a subject during a given time period. By determining the amount of oxygen and carbon dioxide present in the exhaled air and in the atmosphere, the amount of oxygen used and carbon dioxide produced can be computed and, from these values, the amount of energy expended and the nature of the fuels burned. (The significance of the ratio of oxygen used to carbon dioxide produced, the respiratory quotient, will be discussed in Chapter 22.)

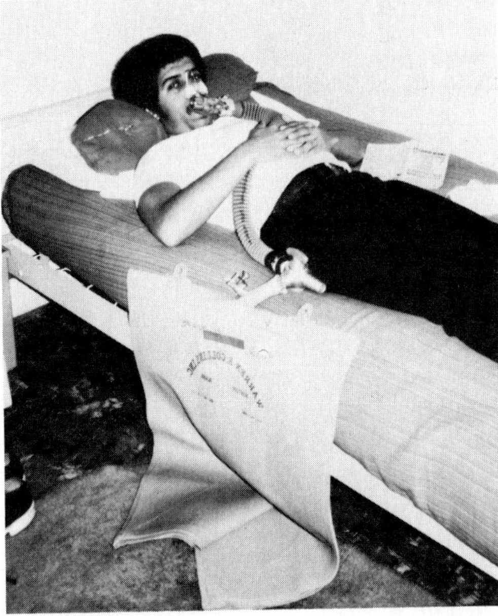

Figure 2–3 Measurement of basal metabolism using a Douglas bag for the collection of expired air. The nasal passages are occluded by a clamp; the subject breathes in room air through a one-way valve while exhaled air passes into the collection bag. Exhaled air is collected within an exact time period, and the volume collected is measured by evacuating the bag through a gas flowmeter. The oxygen and carbon dioxide concentrations in the expired air are measured, and as the composition of the room air is known, the amount of oxygen used and carbon dioxide produced per unit of time can be determined. By using tables previously developed from direct calorimetry, the energy equivalent of the gases exchanged can be calculated. (Courtesy of D. Armstrong, the University of California, Berkeley.)

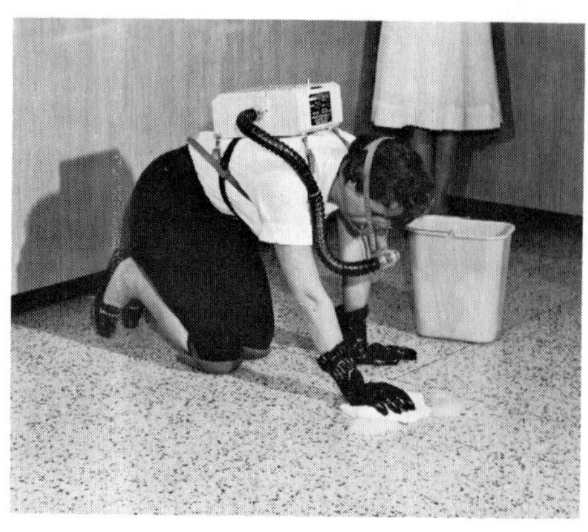

A

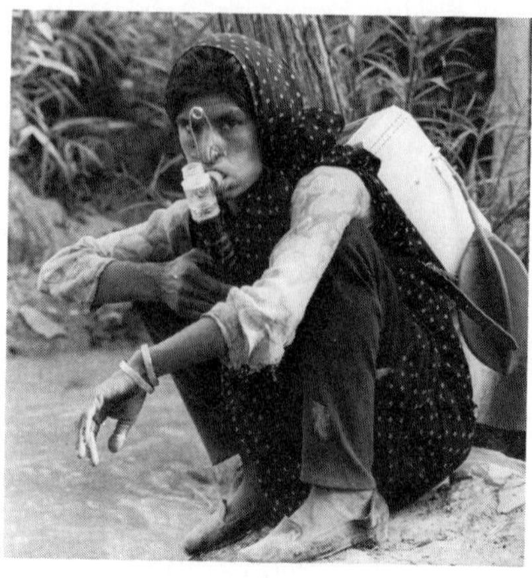

B

Figure 2–4 Energy cost of activities being measured in the laboratory (**A**) and in the field in Iran (**B**) by use of a portable respiration apparatus. The Kofranyi-Michaelis apparatus consists of a lightweight box, which contains a meter that records the volume of expired air. Samples of the expired air are automatically taken at intervals and stored in a small bag attached to the meter. Analysis of the gas in this bag for carbon dioxide and oxygen content gives the necessary data for calculating energy expenditure. (**A**, courtesy of the Ohio State University; **B**, courtesy of C. Geissler-Brun and T. Brun, University of California, Berkeley.)

BASAL METABOLISM

The word *metabolism* is a general term used to cover all the chemical changes that occur in the tissues of the body. Under energy metabolism we include the chemical changes by which fat, carbohydrate, and protein (and alcohol) are broken down and gradually oxidized to release energy or by which they may be synthesized into compounds in which unneeded energy may be stored. Technically we also include the physical changes by which energy is transformed from one kind to another in the body — for example, chemical energy in food and oxygen is set free as work and heat when food is oxidized in the body. Since metabolism includes only chemical changes in tissue cells, it does not include those that occur in digestion of foods.

In a living organism, cells have to be continually active to maintain the life processes, and energy is necessary to maintain these vital processes of the various organs and tissues. The nervous system never stops working, and the activity of the brain alone accounts for about one-fifth of the energy expended by the body at rest. The liver and kidneys constantly work at a high rate; other activities go on at a somewhat lower rate during rest — for example, the beating of the heart, the work of the lungs and of the chest and diaphragm in breathing, the peristaltic movements of the stomach and intestines, and the work of digestive glands in forming their secretions. Even when a person is apparently completely in repose, the tone of the skeletal muscles is maintained.

This internal work of the body is known as *basal metabolism* because upon it are superimposed the other energy needs of the body — the extra amount of energy needed for food intake and muscular work, and at times for adjustment to climate and for the formation of new tissues. Basal metabolism represents the amount of energy required to maintain life at rest — that is, for the internal work of the body. It is defined as the amount of energy expended by the body when lying quietly in a comfortable environmental temperature, relaxed but awake and without food (12 to 15 hours after the last meal). Energy expenditure measured under the same conditions but at different intervals after eating is called resting metabolism. Basal metabolism of adults amounts to about 1200 to 1800 kcal (5000 to 7500 kJ) per day. The basal energy needs are comparatively *constant* for the same individual, but vary slightly at different times and more widely in different persons.

Factors That Influence Basal Metabolism

The *main* factors that determine the basal metabolic energy requirement are:

1. Body size
2. Age
3. Sex
4. Secretions of endocrine glands

The *basal metabolic rate* (BMR) is higher in young people than in older individuals; it increases for some months after birth, then decreases (at first fairly rapidly, but later more gradually) up to and through adolescence. In adults, there is a still slower decline in basal metabolic rate with increasing age. Metabolic rate is also higher in males than in females.

Basal metabolic expenditure varies as a function of body size, but not precisely with weight. When expressed as calories per square meter of body surface area* (or per kilogram of body weight raised to the three-fourths power†), basal metabolic rate of warm-blooded animals ranging in size from mice to elephants is nearly the same. Why these relationships exist is not certain. The close correlation between internal work and surface area, or the three-fourths power of body weight, may be due to a mathematical relationship these measurements have to the active cellular mass of the body. Basal metabolism reflects the activity of all body functions carried on in the resting state (including maintenance of body temperature), and these functions reside in the soft, lean tissues.

Attempts have been made to explain the differences in BMR between people as being due entirely to differences in the amount of lean body mass. (Cell mass can be measured only by indirect methods, of course, so absolute correspondence cannot be proved.) This concept has a certain plausibility when one considers that men have more lean body mass in proportion to fat than do women of the same age, and men have higher BMR than do women. Also, the percentage of body fat rises with age in both sexes, and metabolic rate declines with age. However, while *total* basal energy expenditure does increase with increasing lean body mass, the increase is not linear, because the body tissues do not increase in size proportionately. (See Table 2–1.) In the adult, skeletal muscle is the largest component of the nonbone lean mass, and muscle has a relatively low resting rate of metabolism; the brain, a very active tissue, increases little in weight from infancy to adulthood. Other tissues, such as the liver and kidneys, increase less in size than does the muscle mass during the growth years and constitute about the same percentage of body weight in muscularly well-developed adults as in those who are less fit. Even adipose tissue is not inert metabolically; it has about the same rate of oxidation per unit of protein as does kidney tissue. Of course, adipose tissue, when filled with fat, has only one-third to one-fourth as much protein as does kidney tissue; but fatty tissue may make up about half of the body weight in many adults, so its total contribution to the BMR is not inconsiderable.

For purposes of nutritional planning it is sufficient to remember that the *total* basal energy requirement is greater in persons of larger size than in smaller persons of the same age and sex; and that the *rate* of basal metabolism is higher in men than

---

*Because of the difficulty of actually measuring the body surface area, it is usually computed for man from the body weight and height by means of a mathematical equation. Body surface area (m^2) = Weight $(kg)^{0.425} \times$ Height $(cm)^{0.725} \times 0.007184$[1] or from a nomogram constructed from DuBois' chart by Boothby and Sandiford[2] (Fig. 2–5).

†This weight, often called metabolic body weight, is determined by multiplying the log of body weight by 0.75 and converting to the antilog. Other estimates of the metabolic size may be computed from body weight according to formulas of Brody[3] or Kleiber.[4]

Table 2–1 PERCENTAGE OF BASAL METABOLIC RATE (BMR) DUE TO FIVE MAJOR ORGANS AND THE REST OF THE BODY IN AN INFANT WHOSE BMR IS 540 KCAL PER DAY AND AN ADULT WHOSE BMR IS 1780 KCAL PER DAY*

	10 kg (22 lb) Infant			*70 kg (154 lb) man*		
	Organ Weight	*Organ Metabolism*		*Organ Weight*	*Organ Metabolism*	
Organ	(KG)	KCAL/DAY	% OF BMR	(KG)	KCAL/DAY	% OF BMR
Brain	0.92	240	45	1.4	365	21
Heart	0.05	30	6	0.3	180	10
Kidney	0.07	28	5	0.3	120	7
Liver	0.30	105	19	1.6	560	32
Lung	0.12	24	4	0.8	160	9
Total of above	1.46	427	79	4.4	1385	79
All other	8.64	113	21	65.6	395	21

*In the infant the organs constitute 15 percent of body weight and account for 79 percent of BMR. These organs still account for 79 percent of BMR in an adult of normal weight and leanness but make up only 6 percent of body weight. Thus, BMR does not increase linearly with lean body mass or with total body weight. (Adapted from Holliday et al.[5])

in women and decreases with age. Basal metabolism of healthy men requires about 1600 to 1800 kcal (6500 to 7500 kJ) daily; basal expenditure of women is about 1200 to 1450 kcal (5000 to 6000 kJ) (Fig. 2–5).

The secretions of the *endocrine glands* are the primary regulators of the rate of metabolism of the cells.* The overall rate of cellular oxidation is under the control of the thyroid gland. *Thyroxine,* the iodine-containing hormone secreted by the thyroid, has a very potent influence in speeding up all the oxidative processes of the body. When the thyroid gland is overactive, it forms too much of this substance, and basal metabolism becomes much more rapid than normal. In abnormal conditions, when the thyroid gland is underactive, the amount of thyroxine formed is too small to keep the basal metabolic rate up to what it should be.

Because the hormone thyroxine constitutes the most important single factor influencing the rate of tissue oxidation, or basal metabolism, determination of the level of thyroid hormone in the bloodstream has been used to detect the relative rate of basal metabolism. Thyroxine (tetraiodothyronine) is circulated in the blood in temporary union with blood proteins so that what the chemical test measures is the *protein-bound iodine content of the blood,* which in turn serves as an index of relative activity of the thyroid in releasing its hormone into the blood — hence, the approximate basal metabolic rate. Because this test (PBI, for "protein-bound iodine") is much simpler for both patient and technician, and because many doctors feel it is better suited to clinical purposes, it has largely replaced the measurement of oxygen consumption by respiration apparatus. However, some clinics run both types of tests to compare results of the two methods, and the respiratory method is still used in scientific experiments.

The internal secretion produced by the *adrenals* also exerts an influence on basal metabolism, although not so markedly as does the thyroid hormone. Stimulation of the adrenal glands (such as happens in fright, excitement, and other emotions) causes a temporary rise in the metabolic rate, while it has been shown that cats have a fall of about 25 percent in basal metabolism after an operation to remove these glands. The *pituitary* gland also has an indirect influence on metabolism. (See Chapter 15.)

*The endocrine glands manufacture substances (called hormones) that are absorbed directly into the blood stream and carried to all parts of the body. These glands are more fully discussed in Chapters 13 and 15.

The *sex difference* in metabolism is brought about by the activity of the male and female hormones. The difference in BMR is due partly to the effect these hormones have on body composition, since women have more fatty tissues than do men, and partly to their effects on cell metabolism. During *pregnancy* the BMR increases about 20 percent; this increase is roughly proportional to the increase in body weight of the healthy pregnant woman.

Other Factors Affecting Metabolism at Rest

Several factors may affect the metabolism of a person at rest and, thus, the accuracy of determination of basal metabolic rate, which is why the standardized conditions of measurement include the stipulation that the subject must be awake, but physically and mentally relaxed, in a post-absorptive state (12 to 15 hours after eat-

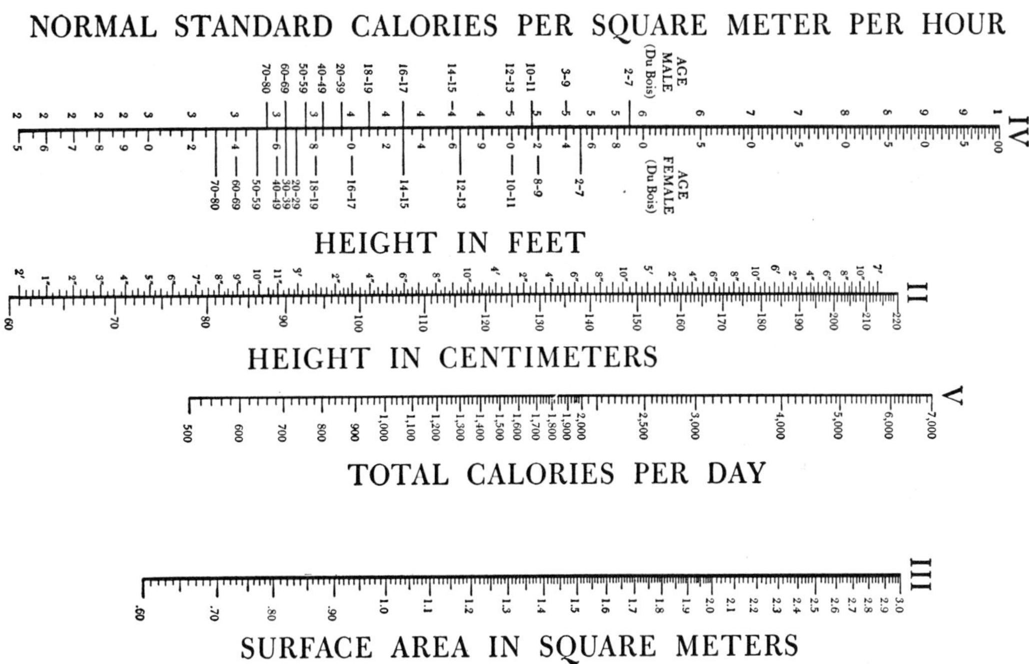

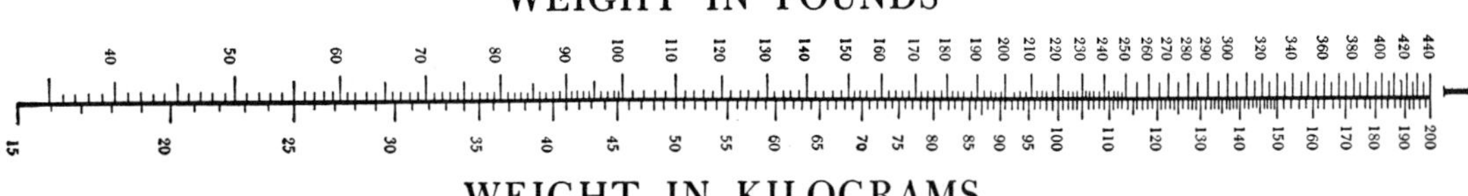

Figure 2–5 This nomogram can be used to derive the basal metabolic expenditure (Scale V, labeled "Total Calories per Day") of normal adults whose height and weight are known. Use only a ruler with a true straight edge. Do not draw lines on the chart but merely indicate their positions by the straight edge of the ruler. Locate the various points by means of needles (pin stuck through the eraser of a lead pencil). Locate the person's normal weight on Scale I and his height on Scale II. The ruler joining these two points intersects Scale III at the person's surface area. Locate the age and sex of the person on Scale IV. A ruler joining this point with the person's surface area on Scale III crosses Scale V at the *basal* energy requirement. To convert Calories (kcal) to kJ, multiply by 4.184. (Nomogram of Boothby and Sandiford,[2] adapted by the Mayo Clinic and reprinted with their permission.)

ing), in a comfortable environment, and free from fever.

Sleep. Individual sleep patterns vary. Some people rest quietly for about an hour and are restless for the remainder of the night, while others rest completely all night. It is not surprising, then, that energy expenditures during a period of sleep may be about the same as in the basal (resting quietly but awake) state, or more or less than that. During the hours of sleep, the internal processes gradually slow down, and may reach a minimum that is 10 percent below basal rate after about 5 to 6 hours (Fig. 2–6). During an 8 hour period of sleep, most adults expend about 400 to 600 kcal (1600 to 2500 kJ).

Muscle Tonus. Most people do not realize that the muscles are never completely relaxed, but that a certain amount of tension (muscular tone or tonus) is maintained even in sleep. The amount of energy required for muscular tension varies considerably with the degree of tenseness or relaxation of the individual, and this amount of energy is of significance because the total amount of muscle tissue is so great. The greatest degree of relaxation will be found on first waking, and muscular tension will increase as the day advances. For this reason, it is best to make tests for determining basal metabolism early in the morning.

Emotions and Mental States. Stimulation of the sympathetic nervous system and the adrenal glands, such as takes place under emotional stress, results in an increased rate of metabolism. In adults such stimulation may increase the BMR by 25 percent or less, but in infants the BMR may be doubled. Another effect of mental strain seems to be an increase in muscular tonus, and the tenseness of the muscles during suspense, anxiety, or excitement, or even during mental work, is a familiar phenomenon.

Transcendental meditation induces a number of physiological changes, including a lowering of the metabolic rate below the resting level. Studies conducted at the University of California (Irvine) and at Harvard showed a 16 percent fall in oxygen utilization during meditation, accompanying a reduced rate of breathing and a fall in blood pressure.[6] This reduction occurred within a few minutes and was twice the magnitude of the decline that followed several hours of sleep in similar individuals (Fig. 2–6). These effects are probably due to a lowered activity of the nervous system, which is, in a sense, the direct opposite of stress reactions.

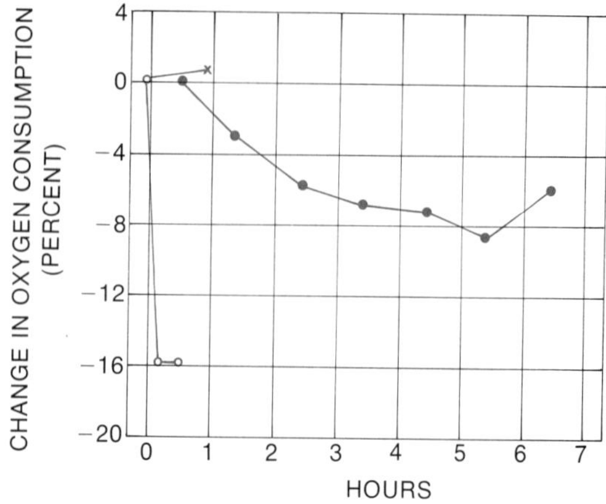

Figure 2–6 Comparison of metabolic rates, measured by consumption of oxygen, that occur during hypnosis, sleep, and meditation. No significant change occurs during hypnosis (which is therefore not represented on the graph). One study shows that oxygen consumption is reduced by about 8 percent after 5 hours of sleep. Meditation causes twice the reduction in a fraction of the time. The "x" represents hypnosis, the colored circles indicate sleep, and the open circles signify meditation. (Redrawn from Wallace, R. K., and Benson, H.: The physiology of meditation. Copyright © 1972 by Scientific American, Inc. All rights reserved.)

In measuring metabolism, relaxation is aided by reassurance that the test will not cause discomfort. Even so, a second test will often give lower figures than the first, and therefore will more truly represent "basal" metabolism.

Exercise. Of course when we are talking of *basal* metabolism, or the energy required for internal processes only, exercise is ruled out, since basal metabolism always means metabolism at rest. However, the aftereffects of severe muscular work persist for a long while after the work has ceased, and the metabolic rate during the night that follows a day of strenuous exercise is higher than after an inactive day. The oxidative recovery processes keep going on in the body for hours after severe muscular effort and for shorter periods after less strenuous work. (See Chapter 22.)

Food. The immediate influence of food is ruled out in measuring basal metabolism, which is always taken 12 to 15 hours after a meal, but the aftereffects of food, like those of exercise, sometimes linger on into the resting period. This is especially true if the food eaten is rich in protein.

Fasting. The internal processes are somewhat slowed down, and the basal energy requirement is lower after a long fast or in an adult whose food supply has been insufficient for his needs for some time. This adjustment of the body to run with greater economy of energy does not occur in a short period of food deprivation.

During World War I, Benedict studied a group of 12 young male students who volunteered for a prolonged period of underfeeding. When they had sustained an average weight loss of 12 percent, there was an average lowering of basal metabolism per unit of body weight by 18 to 20 percent.[7] During World War II at the University of Minnesota, experiments in undernutrition were made, simulating conditions in occupied countries. After 22 weeks, the conscientious objectors who served as subjects showed an average 18 percent reduction in the metabolic rate (together with a lowered expenditure of energy for exercise) on a daily energy intake of 1500 kcal.[8] In undernourished children, however, basal metabolism *per unit of weight* usually is normal and the BMR is increased during recovery.

Fever. In fevers, or when heat loss from the surface of the body is prevented, the temperature of the body itself will rise. Because the rate or intensity of the internal processes is speeded up, there is a rise in temperature, and the basal metabolism will be increased in this event. It has been calculated that the increase in energy expenditure is about 7 percent for every degree Fahrenheit rise in body temperature.[1] A rise in body temperature of 4° F from 98.6° to 102.6° F (or from 37° to 39° C) would increase the basal metabolism by 28 percent, or by 400 to 500 kcal per day for an average-sized person.

MUSCULAR WORK

No person could live for long on the basal level of energy requirement. The ordinary activities of life necessitate moving about, which involves muscular work. Even holding the body in sitting or standing posture requires some muscular work, as do the minor movements that all of us are constantly making even when sitting at rest or during sleep. Some persons take active exercise or must do muscular work in earning their living. What is more, everyone must eat, and the taking of food in itself raises the energy output.

Muscular work is by far the most important of those factors that raise the energy requirement of adults above the BMR. Whenever muscular work is done, energy is used, and the amount required is proportional to the work done. Smaller quantities of energy are needed for maintaining the body in sitting or standing position, while active work, such as walking, climbing stairs, and pushing or lifting objects, requires much more energy. The heavier the person moving about and the greater number or size of muscles involved, the larger the amount of energy that is required. Thus walking, even at a moderate pace, requires more energy than typing rapidly. There is a 100 to 500 percent increase in metabolism with common, everyday activities, or two to six times the basal energy expenditure.

Very hard work with high energy output cannot be kept up for very long at a time, so that the total increase in energy requirement for the day (working 8 hours) may not be more than 100 percent over the maintenance requirement even for active workers. In an inactive (sedentary) man or woman, the distribution of the energy used during the day is usually about two-thirds for the internal work of the body and one-third for visible muscular movements. For example, a small woman might spend a total of 1800 kcal (7500 kJ), with 1200 kcal for basal metabolism and only 600 kcal above that for body movement. As soon as more exercise is taken, however, the energy required for external work mounts rapidly, and the proportion used for physical activity (work) may come to be as much as a half to three-fourths of the whole. Then, the total amount of energy needed will be increased until it may be more than doubled. A young college man during football training might have a basal metabolic rate of 1800 kcal per day but use a total of 4000 kcal (17,000 kJ) or more per day because of his vigorous activity, for instance.

It is difficult to generalize concerning energy needs at various occupations or trades, since not only do the workers vary in body weight and rate of working, but under modern conditions jobs in the same industry often involve widely different amounts of physical exertion. In an automobile factory, a 68 kg (150 lb) man who sits and operates a machine (which does the real work) may require no more than 2500 kcal per day, while an 80 kg (175 lb) man whose job calls for much walking and some lifting obviously uses much more energy — 3700 kcal or even more. Both men belong to the same union and are classed as factory or industrial workers. Furthermore, the way one employs his leisure time affects his total energy need. A sedentary worker, such as an office clerk, by working "out-of-hours" at home (carpentry, painting, gardening) or going in for some active sport, may raise his energy requirement to that of a man whose working day involves more physical exertion but who spends his evenings viewing television or reading.

EFFECTS OF FOOD

DuBois[1] compared the effect of food on metabolism to a tax, deducted at the source, which thus reduces the amount of a man's income; we do not derive the full fuel value of the foods taken in because the metabolic rate rises as a consequence of eating. Part of the increase in metabolism, which begins in a matter of minutes after eating, is due to the energy costs of digestive and absorptive processes, and the remainder is due to effects of the absorbed digestion products on cellular metabolism. The elevation of metabolism is greatest in the first 2 hours after a meal, and values return to the basal level after 3 to 4 hours. The stimulating effect of food on energy production is called *dietary thermogenesis* or, more commonly, *specific dynamic action,* which for convenience is often referred to as SDA.[9, 10]

The rise in metabolism after eating 100 kcal of carbohydrate or fat is about 6 percent, while the rise in metabolism after eating protein is much greater, amounting to about 30 percent. The greater SDA of protein than the other fuel nutrients is thought to be due to the additional processes required to rearrange or remove the nitrogen-containing portion of its components, processes which are carried out primarily in the liver.

If the diet contains a great deal of meat, the day's increase over the basal metabolism may amount to 18 percent, or even more. However, on the ordinary mixed diet, the usual allowance to cover the stimulating effects of the food itself is about 6 to 10 percent, averaged over 24 hours. Thus, in order to have her energy intake equal to output so that weight is maintained, a woman whose energy needs for the day amount to 2200 kcal would probably be spending about 200 kcal to cover the effects of the food.

The energy cost of physical activity usually is measured in individuals who have eaten normal mixed meals within the past several hours. Hence, these values reflect the sum of all processes going on at the same time — work, basal metabolism, and specific dynamic action. As we have pointed out in preceding discussion, "basal metabolism" is arbitrarily defined as energy expended under precise conditions of measurement, conditions that exist only briefly and infrequently. For these reasons, it is customary to determine energy expenditure from oxygen utilization of persons resting quietly at various times of the day, that is, *resting metabolic rate* or RMR (in contrast to BMR), and carrying out representative or actual work tasks at various times of the day. When the RMR is measured 3 to 4 hours after a meal, it is not, of course, significantly different from the BMR.[13] If these practical values are used to estimate energy requirements, there need be no extra allowance for SDA of healthy people eating mixed diets; any error introduced thereby (at the most 6 to 10 percent) is less than the variation in energy expenditure for a given activity measured at different times in different people.

CLIMATE AND HEAT REGULATION

Cold-blooded animals such as fish and frogs have no ability to regulate their body temperature, which accordingly rises and falls as the temperature of their environment changes. Man (and the other warm-blooded animals) possesses a heat-regulating apparatus that keeps the body temperature almost constant at a point usually considerably higher than that of the surroundings. Small variations of body temperature are normal; but variations from the average 98.6° F (37° C) rarely exceed 1° F.

Temperature regulation is ordinarily accomplished in the body without effect on the basal metabolism or total energy needs. Excessive heat loss in a cool environment is prevented by insulation (clothing, shelter), and the heat produced as a by-product of body processes and muscular work is more than sufficient under these circumstances. *Heat regulation is usually a problem of getting rid of the surplus heat produced.* About 80 percent of this excess heat is dissipated by loss at the body surface, or through the skin. Some also is lost through the lungs by evaporation of moisture in the expired air. (For a diagram indicating the various ways of effecting heat balance, see Fig. 2–7.)

Heat is lost from the skin (1) by *radiation or conduction* and (2) by *evaporation* of moisture (invisible or visible perspiration). The relative ease with which heat can be removed by one or the other of these two means depends on the surrounding conditions. Low temperature of the air promotes heat loss by radiation and conduction, whereas high temperature of the air cuts down heat loss by this means and increases loss by evaporation. Low humidity aids evaporation, and high humidity reduces the opportunity for loss of heat through this channel. Wind or circulating currents of air favor heat loss by both conduction and evaporation. A further aid in temperature regulation is the variable amount of blood sent to the surface under different conditions of heat and cold; the skin becomes flushed on a hot day and blanched on exposure to cold.

Under only two conditions do changes in the temperature of the environment have any effect on metabolism. First, if the body surface is insufficiently protected from heat loss and the temperature of the air is sufficiently low, extra fuel must be burned to keep body temperature up to normal. In such a case, there is likely to be shivering (involuntary muscular activity) and increased oxidative processes in the tissues to generate the extra heat needed, so that the rate of metabolism increases. Conversely, under conditions of extreme heat, some energy is required for body cooling because of increased work of the heart and circulatory system and the secretion of sweat.

The main factors that affect the rate at which heat is lost from the body surface are the amount of body surface, the presence or absence of a layer of fat under the skin, and insulation provided from clothing and shelter.

Body Surface. A child has a larger amount of body surface in relation to its

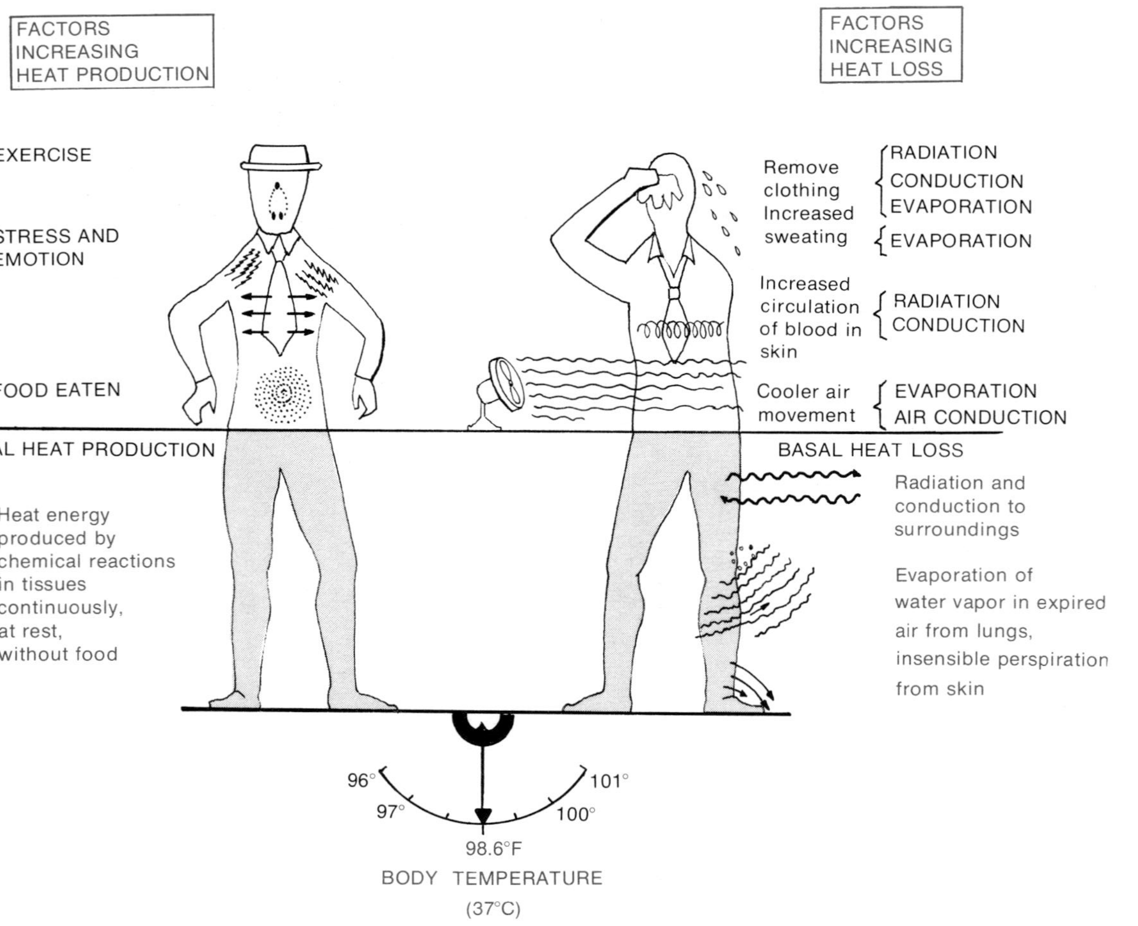

Figure 2–7 Diagram to show balance between factors that cause heat production in and heat loss from the body, thus effecting normal regulation of body temperature.

total size than an adult has, the tiny infant having the largest relative amount of surface for its size. *Shape* of the body also influences the amount of surface. A tall, thin person possesses about one and one-half times as much surface area as a short, fat person of the same body weight. Since heat loss takes place through the surface, the body with a large amount of surface must generate more heat to maintain its normal temperature under conditions of cold than one with a relatively smaller surface exposure. Surface area is a less important factor in adults than in infants and children, in whom there is a larger proportion of surface to volume.

Subcutaneous Fat. A layer of fatty tissue, directly under the skin, is normally present in well-nourished individuals. The extent and thickness of this layer of subcutaneous fat vary considerably in different individuals, according to sex, general build, and dietary habits. Fat is a very poor conductor of heat, or a good insulator, so that persons with a well-developed layer of fat under the skin lose heat to the exterior much less readily than do those who have little subcutaneous fat. Thin people radiate about 50 percent more heat per unit of weight than fat people. This may be an advantage in winter but may not be in hot weather when, because the heat is held within by this layer of insulation, fat people are likely to experience discomfort, especially if they generate any extra heat by exercise.

Clothing and Shelter. In summer, we leave some of the body freely exposed and wear loose clothing of porous weave and light color, which allows heat to escape readily. In cold weather we resort to covering the body with several layers of clothing usually of thicker, less porous material and dark in color, and we use blankets at night. Winter clothing usually helps considerably in conserving body heat. Exposure to cold water involves great heat loss, and even the heat generated by vigorous swimming may be insufficient to maintain body temperature, unless additional fuel is burned for warmth. Scuba divers have learned to wear protective suits, and distance swimmers often apply grease to the body as insulation, but prolonged chilling will increase energy needs.

Even primitive housing conditions protect somewhat from extremes of temperature and from exposure to the elements. With modern conditions of heating houses and suitable indoor clothing, there is seldom a need to burn body fuel for the purpose of maintaining normal temperature. Air conditioning, which permits homes and public buildings to be kept at constant temperatures both winter and summer, is a further factor in ruling out a direct influence of the seasons on body temperature.

Net Effects of Climate

In cold climates, a small extra energy expenditure (2 to 5 percent) may be incurred by reason of the extra weight and hobbling effect of cold weather clothing. If the body is inadequately clothed, body cooling will occur and energy needs will increase because of shivering. In this situation, the heat production with exercise and the SDA due to food are useful in sustaining body temperature. Comfort is maintained longer during sleep in the cold (as for example, outdoors in a sleeping bag) if a small meal is taken at bedtime.

People who live *and perform necessary physical work* at a temperature range of 30 to 40° C (86 to 104° F) may require an extra dietary allowance to compensate for the energy expenditure at such *high temperatures* (increased metabolic rate, lower mechanical efficiency, and efforts to rid the body of excess heat, such as profuse sweating).[11] Under these conditions, energy allowance should be increased at least 0.5 percent for every degree of temperature rise between 30° and 40° C. However, the average individual probably reduces physical activity sufficiently to counterbalance the needs for increased energy just outlined, so that no adjustment in energy allowance is necessary. In fact, total energy expenditure may even be reduced in extremely hot climates.

OTHER FACTORS AFFECTING NEED

Mental Work

Because the brain is always active, *specific mental work does not affect the energy requirement appreciably* except as it may be accompanied by muscular tension. Although the metabolism of nervous tissue is increased slightly by activity, the amount of energy required is so small that the influence of this activity is insignificant. Benedict and Benedict, who found that the effort of complicated mental arithmetic increased metabolism 3 to 4 percent during the short periods it was carried on, compare the relative effects of mental and muscular work as follows: "The professor absorbed in intense mental effort for an hour has an extra demand for food or for calories during the entire hour not greater than the extra need of the maid who dusts off his desk for five minutes."[12]

Growth, Pregnancy, and Lactation

Most adults desire to have the energy intake just about balance the energy requirement so that the body weight will be maintained constant. With children, on the other hand, it is important to provide energy *over and above* that required for the internal work of the body and for muscular activity, in order that additional material may be available for increasing the body weight in *growth*. Rapidly growing infants, 3 to 6 months of age, have been shown to be storing about 15 percent of the energy value of the food taken. This extra energy is stored in the form of newly built tissues. As growth rate diminishes, although the total food requirement is more because of the increased size, the allowance needed per unit of body weight becomes smaller. Adults recovering from a wasting illness also require extra energy for building new tissue. In pregnancy there is also need for energy to build new tissue (growth of fetus and increased size of uterus, mammary glands, etc.), and in lactation to provide for the energy value of the milk secreted. Information concerning the special energy needs of children and pregnant or lactating women is contained in Chapters 20 and 21.

ESTIMATION OF ENERGY REQUIREMENTS

General: Energy Costs According to Habitual Activity Pattern

The total requirement for energy includes amounts needed for resting metabolism and physical activity, and the lesser factors of temperature regulation, growth, and lactation.

Basal metabolism determinations on healthy adults have shown the following normal ranges:

Men
1600–1900 kcal (6500–8000 kJ)
Women
1200–1500 kcal (5000–6000 kJ)

Resting metabolism of healthy adults throughout the day is nearly the same as the BMR in the interval 3 to 4 hours after a meal, but soon after eating it is up to 10 percent greater than the basal level. RMR ranges from 1.1 to 1.4 kcal per minute for men and 0.8 to 1.1 kcal per minute for women (Table 2–2). A rough estimate of the resting metabolic rate of adults of either sex is about *1 kcal per kg of ideal body weight per hour,* with values for women ranging to about 10 percent below this figure and those for men 10 percent above it.* Resting metabolism of a man of

*These values are only approximations. Technically, there should be a small deduction in the day's basal metabolism to allow for the slightly lower metabolic rate during sleep. However, this correction amounts to only 0.1 kcal/kg/hr, or for 8 hours sleep for a 70 kg man, about 56 kcal. Also, the correction for sleep varies with the soundness of sleep and amount of body movement during sleep. Hence, it is ignored in the rough estimation of energy requirement.

Table 2–2 RESTING ENERGY METABOLISM OF ADULTS* ACCORDING TO BODY WEIGHT AND COMPOSITION†

Body Build: Men	Body Build: Women	Body Fat, %	50 (110)	55 (121)	60 (132)	65 (143)	70 (154)	75 (165)	80 (176)	kcal/kg per hr	kcal/kg per day
			kcal per minute								
Thin		5	0.99	1.06	1.12	1.19	1.26	1.32	1.39	1.10	26
Average		10	0.94	1.01	1.08	1.14	1.21	1.28	1.34	1.05	25
Plump	Thin	15	0.89	0.96	1.03	1.09	1.16	1.23	1.30	1.01	24
Fat	Average	20	0.84	0.91	0.98	1.05	1.11	1.18	1.25	0.97	23
	Plump	25	0.80	0.86	0.93	1.00	1.07	1.13	1.20	0.92	22
	Fat	30	–	0.81	0.88	0.95	1.02	1.08	1.15	0.88	21
			kJ per minute							*kJ/kg*	
Average		10	3.93	4.23	4.52	4.77	5.07	5.36	5.61	4.39	105
	Average	20	3.52	3.81	4.10	4.40	4.65	4.94	5.23	4.06	97

Weight, kg (lb) columns: 50 (110) through 80 (176).

*Values for young adults. Metabolic rate declines about 2 to 3 percent per decade over age 30 years, and by age 70 it is about 85 to 90 percent of the BMR of younger adults.

†These values are slightly higher than basal because the subject is not in the strictly postabsorptive conditions (12 hours or more from the last meal). (Adapted from Durnin and Passmore.[13])

average body build and weight (70 kg or 154 lb) is about 1.05 kcal/kg/hr × 70 kg × 24 hr, or 1765 kcal per day. The resting metabolism of an average woman is about 1350 kcal per day (0.97 kcal/kg/hr × 58 kg × 24 hr).

A quick and approximate estimation of an adult's energy requirement may be made, based on resting metabolism (which is based on body weight and age) and the degree of physical activity as the two variables. The *increase above resting* is proportional to the degree of activity in the usual life-style, as follows: For sedentary or maintenance activity, add 50 percent of the resting; for light activity, 60 percent; for moderate activity, 70 percent; for strenuous activity, 100 percent or more. A brief description of what is meant by these varying degrees of activity follows:

Maintenance:*
Sitting most of day; about 2 hours moving about slowly or standing.

Light activity:
Typing, teaching, shop work, laboratory work; some walking but no strenuous exercise.

Moderate activity:
Walking, housework, gardening, carpentry, light industry; little sitting.

Strenuous activity:
Unskilled labor, forestry work, skating, outdoor games, dancing; little sitting.

Very strenuous activity:
Tennis, swimming, basketball, football, running, lumbering; little sitting.

On this basis, a 70 kg male secretary engaged in "light activity" would expend 1.6 times his resting metabolism of 1765 kcal, or a total of about 2820 kcal per day. A 58 kg female gardener, in the "moderate activity" class, would expend 1.7 times her resting rate of 1350 kcal, or about 2300 kcal per day. It should be emphasized that the method of estimating energy needs just discussed gives only a rough approximation and that individuals vary considerably from the average. This is because the amounts of energy required for different occupations included under one level of activity, the vigor with which one works, and the amounts of time devoted to the different activities can vary widely. However, the two factors that have the most influence in determining energy requirement (resting metabolism and level of occupational physical activity) have

*Experimental data indicate that the *maintenance* energy requirement (for constant body weight and composition without any work demanded) of many species (man, rats, cows, sheep, pigs) is about 1.5 × BMR or 105 kcal per kg of body weight to the 0.75 power.[14]

Table 2–3 ENERGY COST OF ACTIVITIES IN RELATION TO RESTING METABOLIC RATE*

Energy Cost Activity Rate ÷ RMR	*Activity*
	RESTING
0.9–1.0	Sleeping, nightly average.
1.0	Lying at ease, 3 to 4 hours after a meal.
	VERY LIGHT WORK
1.2	Sitting at ease, listening to music, reading, hand sewing, knitting.
1.4	Sitting and writing, doing office desk work, repairing watches. Piloting an aircraft, milking by machine.
1.7	Sitting, typing using electric typewriter or using desk calculator; standing and moving around an office. Playing cards; playing woodwind instruments.
1.9	Lower range of domestic and light industrial work, e.g., cleaning shoes, paring vegetables and cooking, painting inside, typing using a mechanical typewriter.
2.1	Sitting and eating. General laboratory work.
	LIGHT WORK
2.3	Lower range of work in transportation, building trades, and mechanized agriculture and forestry, e.g., driving a car or truck with manual shift, or a combine harvester; planting by machine, sharpening a saw. Playing piano or stringed instrument; playing billiards.
2.5	Upper range of light industrial work, e.g., assembly work, machine sewing, bakery tasks. Canoeing 2.5 mph (4.0 km/hr). Horse riding at a walk.
2.7	Walking 2.0 mph (3.2 km/hr) on the level. Dusting, setting a dinner table, washing dishes. Hanging wallpaper.
2.9	Walking 2.0 mph (3.2 km/hr), level, with 22 lb (10 kg) load. Walking 2.5 mph (4.0 km/hr) on the level. Personal care, e.g., dressing, bathing. Lowest range of manual agricultural work, e.g., troweling, transplanting. Repairing shoes, operating a lathe. Playing a pipe organ.
3.1	Milking by hand; weeding and raking. Playing volleyball.
	MODERATE WORK
3.5	Walking 3.1 mph (5.0 km/hr) on the level, usual pace. Light janitorial work, industrial laundry.
3.5 (cont.)	Garage mechanics, washing a car. Bowling.
3.7	Walking 3.1 mph (5.0 km/hr), level, with 22 lb (10 kg) load. Bed-making, vacuuming, scrubbing (kneeling). Cutting wood with power saw.
4.0	Hoeing and weeding, window-cleaning. Cycling at 5.5 mph (8.8 km/hr). Playing with children; table tennis.
4.5	Cutting hedge by hand. Painting outside, plastering. Swimming leisurely, golf, archery.
5.0	Walking 2.0 mph (3.2 km/hr) up a 10% grade. Dancing a waltz.
6.0–6.5	Climbing stairs (70 to 80 kg person) Shoveling, 18 lb (8 kg) load thrown 3.28 ft (1 m) ten times per minute. Canoeing 4.0 mph (6.4 km/hr). Tennis; skiing downhill and using tow-bar uphill. Cycling 10 mph (16 km/hr), usual pace.
6.5–7.0	Walking 2 mph (3.2 km/hr) up a 20% grade. Cutting hard wood with hand saw.
	HEAVY WORK
7.0–7.5	Digging pit in soil; felling, trimming, and barking trees. Weight lifting. Swimming leisurely underwater wearing fins and suit.
7.5–8.0	Upper range of manual work in peasant agriculture and in building, mining, and steel industries. Hockey, basketball, football (game average).
8.0–9.0	Chopping with axe, 1.25 kg head, 35 blows/min. Skiing on the level over hard snow, 3.7 mph (6.0 km/hr). Horse riding at a gallop. Dancing actively, country or folk style.
9.0–10.0	Cross-country running. Climbing, light load and slope. Swimming strenuously. Boxing.
10.0–15.0	Climbing, heavy load and slope. Heaviest occupational work. Football and squash during play.
Over 15.0	Walking in loose snow with a heavy pack. Skiing uphill at maximum speed. Swimming strenuously underwater with full gear. Bicycle racing.

*Derived mainly from energy expenditure data collated by Durnin, J. V. G. A., and Passmore, R.[13, 15]

been taken into account. For application to older age groups, the rate of resting metabolism would have to be adjusted downward by 2 to 3 percent per decade of age, and any decreased vigor of effort due to infirmity would need to be considered.

Any young adult may calculate his or her energy requirement by calculating the resting metabolism, then adding the appropriate percent of the resting metabolism for the level of activity selected by the individual as most typical of his or her daily routine.

Individual: Energy Costs of Activities Estimated

The only way to get a more exact idea of one's individual need for energy is to keep a detailed record of the time spent at different types of activity throughout a representative day and compute the energy used in each activity by means of figures such as those listed in Table 2–3. Values for the energy cost of all kinds of specific tasks (sedentary occupations, walking at different speeds, standing jobs such as ironing or dishwashing, and sports such as tennis or horseback riding) have been determined by numerous research workers.[13, 14] In Table 2–3, these figures are grouped according to levels of activity, ranging from sleeping, through sitting tasks, to those that require moderate or more severe physical exertion, in terms of the elevation above the RMR. As the exertion increases, the energy cost increases gradually from 1.2 times the RMR while sitting at ease, to 10 times the RMR, or more, for tasks or sports that involve strenuous muscular activity (swimming, rowing, track events, etc.). In some activities, body weight is an important factor; for example, a 140 lb man spends 5.2 kcal per minute in walking at 4 mph (7.4 km/hr); but a 180 lb man must move an additional 40 lb and uses 6.4 kcal per minute (Table 2–4). The men's energy requirement for this activity, which is markedly affected by weight, differs by 1.2 kcal/min; but the difference in their RMR's (calculated from Table 2–2) is only about 0.24 kcal/min. Energy cost of a given activity also varies among people according to their body conformation, skill, tension, and the like. Even for sleep there is a 20 percent variation. The values assembled in Table 2–3 are representative of the average young adult, but the range of observed energy costs is substantial. To improve on these estimates would require numerous measurements of the actual energy expenditure of the individual concerned.

The rate of energy expenditure is less for women than for men because of the

Table 2–4 ENERGY COST OF WALKING AS AFFECTED BY BODY WEIGHT AND SPEED OF MOVEMENT*

Speed/hr		*Body Weight*					
		KG: 46	55	64	73	82	91
MI	KM	LB: 100	120	140	160	180	200
		kcal per minute†					
2	3.7	2.2	2.6	2.9	3.2	3.5	3.8
3	5.6	3.1	3.6	4.0	4.4	4.8	5.3
4	7.4	4.1	4.7	5.2	5.8	6.4	7.0

*Adapted from Durnin, J. V. G. A., and Passmore, R.[15] Work is defined as the overcoming of force. In walking, man is using his biological machinery to move his body mass against the force of gravity, and the work done is equal to force × distance. If a mass of 1 gm is accelerated at a speed of 1 cm per second per second, then 1 erg has been expended. One Joule is 10^7 ergs, and 1 kcal is 4.184 kJoules. A woman weighing 55 kg and walking over level ground at a rate of 3.7 km per hour actually expends energy at the rate of 2.6 kcal per minute (equal to 10.9 kJoule or 1×10^{11} ergs). However, only part of this cost is reflected in mechanical work because the body operates with only 20 percent efficiency and internal processes continue during work.

†To convert to kJ, multiply by 4.184.

smaller body weight involved. Not only is basal metabolism less at lower body weight, but in all activities that require moving the body about (walking, climbing stairs, active exercise, etc.), the expenditure required increases as the body mass to be moved increases in size. This means that when the rates of energy expenditure for various activities are given as a combined amount (a single factor that includes basal metabolism, influence of food, and cost of the specific activity), this factor should vary slightly according to sex and body weight. However, the differences are small enough that they are ignored in the table.

In calculating the energy cost of the day's activities, the time accounted for must, of course, add up to 24 hours and the energy factor for activity must then be multiplied by the time spent at each activity. Two examples of computation of individual energy requirements are given in Table 2–5. Both are for students — one, a young man most of whose day is spent in sedentary occupations (meals, classes, study, watching movies or television); the other, a young man whose day is spent fairly similarly except that he takes about 1½ hours of moderately strenuous exercise, which markedly increases his energy requirement. Both spend 3 hours in the classroom; one man drives in a car between home and campus, both walk some about the campus, and the second walks to and from home. In spite of similar class schedules, the energy cost of one's activities is one-fourth less than the other's — 2542 kcal (10,900 kJ) versus 3263 kcal (13,800 kJ).

Keeping accurate diary records of one's activities is difficult; the recording itself becomes a significant "activity," and constant attention may change how time is spent. Also, it is tempting to note that 40 minutes were spent sitting at a desk studying when actually the person may have moved about twice in the interval to consult a dictionary and to use the toilet. In sports, much time spent in getting ready to play, waiting for the ball, and so on, is often recorded as play. The figures in Table 2–3 take some account of this in setting the values for tennis, golf, and the like; but the accuracy is obviously limited. However, for most purposes, no better estimates can be derived for total energy needs, and these values will serve.

The student may find Table 2–3 of interest for comparison of various activities as to their relative energy costs, some of which are rarely listed in the usual tables of activities. The influence of mechanization on energy costs is particularly interesting. For instance, typing 40 words per minute using an electric typewriter is 70 percent above the resting rate (RMR × 1.7), but manual typing at the same rate is 90 percent over the RMR. Milking a cow by machine involves only 1.4 times the farmer's RMR, while hand milking is much more energetic, costing 3.1 times the RMR. Walking on the level at 2 miles per hour takes more than twice as much energy as the average man (70 kg) spends sitting at ease. Modern athletic-type and old-fashioned country dancing are about on a level with other active sports, such as rapid swimming, football, skiing (on level), or cross-country running. For some of the activities, there is a wide range in energy costs, depending on the conditions under which they are performed (speed, whether on level or on incline, etc.).

RECOMMENDED ALLOWANCES VERSUS ACTUAL NEEDS

In the United States, *recommended dietary allowances** have been formulated for some years by the Food and Nutrition Board of the National Research Council (NRC), and these dietary allowances

*The National Research Council's Allowances have for years been called the RDA's. Some confusion has arisen because the Food and Drug Administration now has set nutritional standards for labeling purposes, which it has dubbed the "U.S. RDA's," meaning recommended *daily* allowances.

Table 2–5 CALCULATION OF TOTAL ENERGY REQUIREMENTS OF TWO MALE STUDENTS OF 70 Kg BODY WEIGHT

Activity Diary Record	*Approximate Energy Cost/RMR*	*Student A Time*	*Student B Time*
Sleep (basal)	1.0	450 min	480 min
Dressing, washing, shaving	2.9	15 min	20 min
Eating breakfast	2.1	20 min	30 min
Walking to campus	3.5	20 min	
Driving to campus	2.3		10 min
Sitting in classrooms	1.4	180 min	180 min
Walking to and from classes	3.5	40 min	40 min
Eating lunch	2.1	30 min	45 min
Studying in library	1.2	180 min	180 min
Walking between locations	3.5	30 min	20 min
Playing tennis	6.2	40 min	
Playing cards	1.7		50 min
Walking home	3.5	20 min	
Driving home	2.3		10 min
Eating dinner	2.1	40 min	45 min
Ironing shirt	3.5	15 min	
Driving to and from date	2.3	20 min	
Dancing, active	8.5	40 min	
Eating snack	2.1	30 min	30 min
Sitting and talking to date	1.2	120 min	
Group discussion, watching television	1.2		150 min
Studying	1.2	120 min	120 min
Undressing, showering, etc.	2.9	30 min	30 min

Summation

	Student A Total Time			*Student B Total Time*		
Energy Cost Level	MIN	HR	LEVEL × TIME	MIN	HR	LEVEL × TIME
1.0	450	7.5	7.5	480	8.0	8.0
1.2	420	7.0	8.4	450	7.5	9.0
1.4	180	3.0	4.2	180	3.0	4.2
1.7				50	0.83	1.41
2.1	120	2.0	4.20	150	2.5	5.25
2.3	20	0.33	0.76	20	0.33	0.76
2.9	45	0.75	2.18	50	0.84	2.44
3.5	125	2.08	7.28	60	1.0	3.5
6.2	40	0.67	4.15	—	—	—
8.5	40	0.67	5.70	—	—	—
		24	44.4		24	34.6
			÷24			÷24
Avg. energy level, RMR ×			1.85			1.44

RMR (from Table 2–2) = 1.05 kcal/kg/hr × 70 kg × 24 hr = 1764 kcal/day
Total energy requirement: Student A 1764 × 1.85 = 3263 kcal/day
Student B 1764 × 1.44 = 2542 kcal/day

are revised approximately every 5 years. They include allowances for most of the essential nutrients (for full table, see Appendix, Table 1) for adults, children, and pregnant women. Many other countries have developed similar standards for their own populations, and international standards have been set by the Food and Agricultural Organization (FAO) and the World Health Organization (WHO) of the United Nations.

The NRC's Allowances for energy are lower than those for the "reference" man and woman used by the FAO/WHO for international tables.[14] This is because the degree of physical activity of most adults worldwide is classed as "moderate," while in the United States, where the au-

Table 2–6 VARIATION IN ENERGY ALLOWANCES FOR HEALTHY ADULTS ACCORDING TO AGE, WEIGHT, AND PHYSICAL ACTIVITY

Conditions Specified	*kcal*/day (Weight)* Men	Women	*kcal/kg/day* Men	Women	*Standard ÷ RMR* Men	Women
	International Standards: FAO/WHO[14]					
Ages 20 to 39 yr:	(65 kg)	(55 kg)				
Light activity	2700	2000	42	36	1.58	1.36
Moderately active†	3000	2200	46	40	1.76	1.49
Very active	3500	2600	54	47	2.05	1.76
Exceptionally active	4000	3000	62	55	2.34	2.04
	United States[16]					
Light activity	(70 kg)	(58 kg)				
Ages 23 to 50 yr	2700	2000	38.6	34.5	1.51	1.32
	Canada[17]					
Characteristic activity pattern (by age):	(70 kg)	(56 kg)				
Ages 19 to 35 yr	3000	2100	42.8	37.5	1.68	1.41
Ages 36 to 50 yr	2700	1900	38.6	33.9	1.52	1.32
	Central America and Panama[18]					
Moderate activity	(62.9 kg)	(51.5 kg)				
Ages 19 to 40 yr	2900	2050	46.1	39.8	1.74	1.49

*1 kcal = 4.184 kJ.
†International reference standard.

tomobile is used so freely and adequate exercise is probably the exception rather than the rule, the typical activity pattern is "light" to "sedentary." The Food and Nutrition Board's Recommended Allowances for energy have accordingly been scaled downward.

From Table 2–6 we see that the Food and Nutrition Board has taken as a reference American man and woman individuals 23 to 50 years of age, weighing 70 kg (154 lb) and 58 kg (128 lb) respectively. It is suggested that during the postadolescent period the intake should gradually be adjusted downward from the high allowances for growing boys (15 to 18 years, 3000 kcal) and girls (11 to 14 years, 2400 kcal). The downward adjustment (to cover decreased activity and basal metabolism) beyond age 50 years should reach 90 percent of the typical adult value; greater reductions will be needed if there is a marked decline in activity with advancing age.

The daily energy allowances in Table 2–6 are for men and women whose weight is desirable and suitable for height. (The weight attained at 25 years of age should be maintained throughout later life.) Overweight persons should use the energy allowance appropriate for their ideal weight for height rather than for their actual weight (which has obviously been too high).

The NRC energy allowances (in Table 2–6) are based on the assumption of typical activity patterns and life-styles. Because physical activity is the most important single factor in altering energy requirements, adjustments need to be made for those who take more or less exercise than that assumed as standard. For these allowances the FAO/WHO standards are illustrative (Table 2–6). The international levels are stipulated according to activity and indicate a range from 2000 kcal per day for a woman in the light activity category to 3000 kcal for an exceptionally active person. A moderately active woman (2200 kcal/day) would do general household chores for 8 hours a day or work in light industry; 4 to 6 hours would be spent in only very light activity and not more than 2 hours in walking or active recreation. Very heavy work would involve intensive training, sports, or construction jobs.

Both the Canadian and Central American energy standards (Table 2–6) are consistent with international standards, taking into account the differences in body weights and activity patterns of the populations. This is most readily apparent from comparison of *energy allowances per unit of body weight, which are, for moderately active men and women, 46 and 40 kcal/kg*, and *for light activity, 42 and 36 kcal/kg*, respectively. Only the United States allowances of 38.6 and 34.5 kcal/kg for reference men and women fall below the international standard.

Another interesting observation emerges when the various energy allowances are compared in relation to the resting metabolic rate. For any given activity category, allowances for men are higher than those for women. Partly this is due to the fact that at equal fitness, men have a larger proportion of body weight as muscle than women do, and this has a relatively small effect on resting metabolism but will add to the cost of work involving the movement of body mass. Also, occupational work levels of exceptionally active men may exceed those of women. However, this seems unlikely to be the situation as regards sedentary or light activity levels. Studies of young men and women conducted at the University of California, in fact, indicate that little disparity exists under light activity conditions, and the total energy need *relative to the resting or basal metabolism* is fairly uniform for both sexes. Thus the difference in allowances and standards may reflect a biased view of female work patterns.

The FAO/WHO, in discussing the effects of climate, notes that the impact will vary according to occupation and conditions of clothing and shelter. The agricultural worker in the open has some ability to protect himself against cold, if he is not too poor to purchase clothing, but little opportunity to escape heat. The rich businessman may avoid both. Considering all

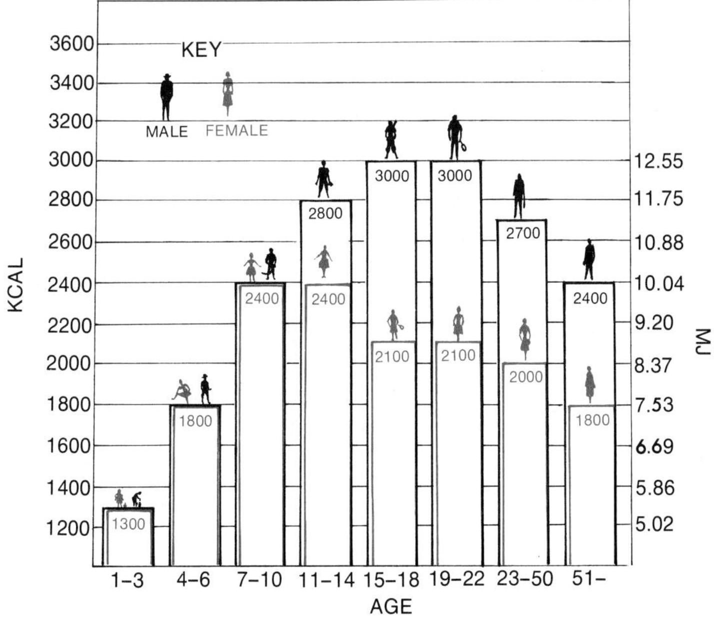

Figure 2–8 Age makes a difference in energy needs. MJ = mega Joule. (Modified from Food and Nutrition Board: *Recommended Dietary Allowances.* 8th Ed. Washington, D.C., National Research Council, National Academy of Sciences, 1974.)

factors, the FAO/WHO concludes that there is no valid basis for adjusting resting and exercise energy requirements according to the climate. If physical activity is restricted by environmental factors, allowances should be selected according to activity level.

It should be evident that the energy allowances set by the various national and international committees are estimates intended for general use and based on the energy needs of so-called average men and women living and working in a comfortable environment (definite weight and arbitrary degree of muscular activity). For persons who vary much from this norm, the energy requirement really needs to be measured individually to achieve any degree of accuracy. The recommended allowances for most other nutrients are purposely set higher than the actual needs (about 30 to 50 percent above), but in respect to energy, the intake should be in balance with the output in order to avoid a loss or gain in body weight. Many persons do not reduce their energy intake sufficiently to compensate for the slightly lower basal metabolism and the far greater influence of decreased activity in later life. Even a relatively small excess of energy foods over the amount needed leads to an accretion of weight over a period of years. Considering the variation in activity from day to day, it is remarkable that body weight can be maintained fairly constant for long periods. The regulatory mechanisms that adjust intake to output are discussed in Chapter 13, and the consequences of failing to adjust adequately in Chapter 24.

ENERGY VALUE OF FOODS

How Fuel Value of Foods Is Determined

The energy value of foods depends primarily upon their chemical composition, i.e., upon the relative amounts of the three primary energy nutrients —carbohydrates, fats, and proteins — and alcohol that they contain. Energy value of a food may be determined by either of the following methods:

1. Complete combustion in a calorimeter.
2. Calculation from its content of the energy nutrients.

The energy value of either a pure nutrient or a natural food may be determined by direct calorimetry, i.e., by complete oxidation in a calorimeter like the one shown in Figure 2–9, in which the energy released is measured by the rise in temperature of a known volume of water.

The average heats of combustion of the *pure energy nutrients,* determined by

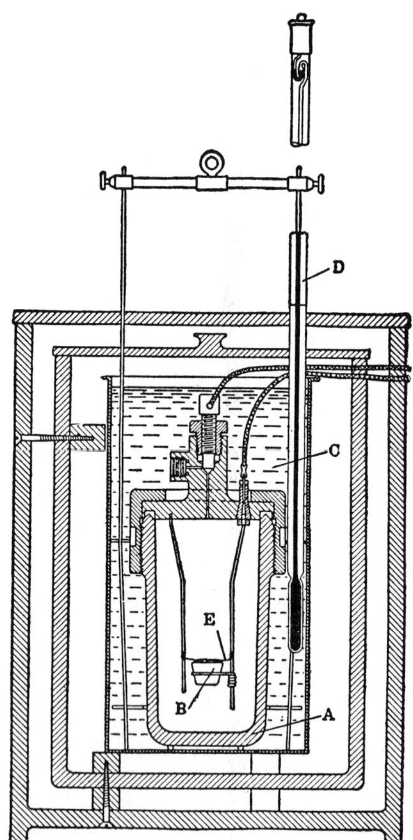

Figure 2–9 Cross-section diagram of the bomb calorimeter used for determination of the fuel value of foods. A weighed sample of the food is placed in the dish B in the inner chamber, which is charged with oxygen and sealed tight. The burning is set off by an electric spark (passed between the wires), and the heat liberated is measured by the rise in temperature of a known volume of the surrounding water; the outer sections are for insulation to prevent loss of heat to exterior. (Courtesy of Emerson Apparatus Co., Boston, Mass.)

numerous experiments, are, in kcal per gram: carbohydrate, 4.1; fat, 9.45; protein, 5.65; and alcohol, 7.1. Fats and alcohol have a higher fuel value because their molecules contain such large amounts of carbon and hydrogen, along with relatively little oxygen; much extra oxygen is required for their burning, and much heat is released. Carbohydrates have enough oxygen in their molecules to combine with all of the hydrogen, so only enough oxygen is required for burning to combine with the carbon and less than half as much heat is liberated. Proteins are intermediate between fats and carbohydrates in energy value, when they are completely oxidized in the calorimeter.

The potential energy value of a food may be computed by multiplying the number of grams of each energy nutrient in a given quantity by the caloric values per gram of carbohydrate, fat, protein, and alcohol. But the energy values that the body can derive from these substances are not identical with those obtained when they are completely oxidized in the calorimeter. There is a small loss entailed due to incomplete digestion and absorption from the intestine. A further deduction must be made in the case of proteins, because these substances are not as completely oxidized in the body as in the bomb calorimeter; the nitrogen-containing products excreted in the urine represent latent heat that amounts, on the average, to 1.3 kcal for each gram of protein burned in the body. When the necessary corrections for these factors are made, the *physiological fuel values* per gram for the three fuel nutrients are as follows:

	Bomb calorimeter value, kcal		*logical energy value*	
			kcal	*kJ*
Carbohydrate	4.1 −2% loss in digestion	= 4.02	4.0	17
Fat	9.45 − 5% loss in digestion	= 8.98	9.0	38
Protein	5.65 − 8% loss in digestion	= 5.20		
	−17% loss in urinary end products	= 4.32	4.0	17
Alcohol	7.1 − small loss in urine and breath	= 7.0	7.0	29

Calculating the Energy Value of Foods

The above general factors — 4, 9, 4 kcal for protein, fat, and carbohydrate, respectively — are sufficiently accurate for practical estimates of the fuel value of any food whose composition is known. For example, the fuel value of milk is calculated as follows:

Milk contains 4.9 gm carbohydrate, 3.5 gm protein, and 3.7 gm fat for every 100 gm.

Each gram of carbohydrate and of protein has a value of 4 kcal, and each gram of fat furnishes 9 kcal.

100 gm of whole milk will have a caloric value of

carbohydrate	$4.9 \times 4 =$	19.6
protein	$3.5 \times 4 =$	14.0
fat	$3.7 \times 9 =$	33.3
total		66.9 kcal

A glassful of milk (8 oz) weighs 244 gm, and hence has a caloric value of 66.9×2.44, or 163 kcal.

During the time of food shortages in World War II, use of the more specific factors derived from tests of individual foods was proposed for calculating the caloric values of food supplies, chiefly grains, available in different countries. For the usual mixture of foods in the American diet, differences between the two methods of calculating are not large. Differences are significant in the case of foods that contain considerable undigestible matter, however. Comparison of the values for white and whole-wheat breads obtained by the two sets of factors are given below as an example.

	kcal per 100 gm computed using:	
	General factors	*Specific factors*
Bread, white, enriched	270	275
Bread, whole wheat	257	240
Beef, pot roast	366	375
Potato, peeled, boiled	69	65

The energy values of foods listed in the most recent tables of food composition issued by the government[19] and in Appendix Table 2 are based on these more specific but more complicated factors.

Foods of High and Low Energy Value

Foods *vary widely in their energy value.* Some are such concentrated sources of fuel that it takes only a small volume of them to yield a considerable amount of energy, or a large number of calories. Others contain so much of non-energy-producing substances, such as water and fiber, and have so low a content of the energy nutrients that they yield only a small number of calories for a comparatively large volume of food.

In general, the foods with *high energy value* are those that are either *rich in fat* or *low in water* content. Thus, all the fatty foods (such as butter, nuts, cream cheese, mayonnaise, bacon) are relatively high in calorie value, as are foods low in moisture content (dried fruits, cookies, candy bars, and the like).

Foods of *low energy value* include most fresh fruits and vegetables, especially green leafy vegetables, since these foods have a high content of both water and fiber. Lean meats, cereal foods, and starchy vegetables are intermediate in energy value.

The *100-kcal portions* of different foods, listed in Table 2–7, show that it takes only a small amount of a high-calorie food to furnish 100 kcal, while a relatively large mass of low-calorie food must be taken to give the same calorie value. The table illustrates the contrasts in concentration of calories between high- and low-energy foods by showing that 1 tablespoonful of any clear fat or 2 chocolate creams furnish the same amount of food energy as ½ cantaloupe or 4 cups of shredded cabbage.

More exact tables of the energy value of foods are required for a fairly accurate check on the number of calories furnished by a day's diet. These have been provided for a wide variety of foods in one government bulletin[19] on a 100 gm basis. The energy values of *average servings* (based on weight in grams) of the more common foods are listed in the table on Nutritive Values of Foods in Table 2 of the Appendix and are also to be found in a recent government bulletin.[20]

QUESTIONS AND PROBLEMS

1. What is the unit used for expressing quantitatively the energy values of foods and energy needs of the body? Define the large calorie and give abbreviations for it. Why is the calorie, a heat unit, used for expressing energy values? What is the factor for converting calories to Joules? Pounds to kilograms?

2. Define basal metabolism. Describe briefly the methods by which it may be determined. How closely do results obtained by the methods compare? Name four main factors that have an influence in determining basal metabolism, explaining how and why each has the effect that it does. If a 70 kg man gains 10 kg of adipose tissue, what will be his original and final resting metabolic rate, in kcal/day? Suppose he goes into training and gains 5 kg of muscle, but his weight does not change; what will be his resting metabolic rate?

3. Name the categories of energy needs that together make up the *total* energy requirement of a normal adult. What factor has by far the greatest effect quantitatively in raising energy expenditure above the level of basal metabolism? Why does mental work have such an insignificant effect on the total energy expended? Under what special circumstances will an adult need an extra allowance of energy for building new tissues?

4. The amount of energy required for muscular work is proportional to the amount and severity of the work done, as illustrated by the following problem: If a man lying quietly requires 77 kcal per hour and his energy need for sitting in a chair is 20 percent higher, how much energy per hour will he need

Table 2–7 100 KCAL (420 kJ) PORTIONS OF SOME FOODS*

Food	*Quantity*
High Energy Value	
Chocolate creams	2 medium-sized
Brazil nuts	4 medium-sized
Almonds	16 medium-sized
Figs	2 large
Dates	4–4½
Cheese, American	1½ in. cube
Peanut butter	1 tbsp
Butter or margarine	1 tbsp
Mayonnaise, or any clear fat	1 tbsp
Cream, thick	1 tbsp, 2 tbsp whipped
Sugar, white or brown	1¾ tbsp
Sweet alcoholic liquors	1 oz
Whiskies, rum	1–1½ oz
Intermediate Energy Value	
Eggs	1¼ med., 1 large
Lean meats, cooked, med. done	2 ounces (lean portion 1 small loin lamb chop)
Bread, white	1½ avg. slices
Breakfast cereals:	
Cooked meals	¾–1 cup
Ready-to-eat, flakes	¾–1 cup
Puffed, rice or wheat	2 cups
Potato, white, baked	1 medium-sized
Banana	1 medium
Apple	1 large
Milk, whole	⅝ cup
Milk, skim	1⅛ cup
Cola, root beer	1 cup
Beer	1 cup
Dry table wine	½ cup
Low Energy Value	
Strawberries, fresh	1 pint
Grapefruit	1 large
Peaches, fresh	2 medium
Tomatoes, raw	4 medium
Cantaloupe	½ melon, 6 in. diam.
Celery	14 large stalks
Asparagus	30 medium stalks
Cabbage, shredded	4 cups
Lettuce (iceberg type)	2 large, firm heads

*See Appendix, Table 2 for energy values of foods.

while sitting at rest? If typewriting rapidly increases the energy need by 90 percent over that required for lying down, how many calories will he use per hour in sitting and typing?

5. Strenuous muscular exertion causes a great rise in energy expenditure over that at the resting level, but when continued for only a short time it does not markedly increase the total day's energy requirements, as illustrated by the following problem: Suppose that a man is sitting in the station quietly; he suddenly realizes his train is about to leave and makes a run for it; after the run that lasted 2 minutes, he relaxes in a seat on the train. If he uses 100 kcal per hour sitting at rest, and 570 kcal per hour while making his dash for the train, how much energy would he use in the 2 minute run?

6. Make a record of your own activities for a sample day, classifying them as nearly as possible under the headings of activities given in Table 2–3. Group the sitting activities, those

that involve standing or walking about the room, those that require light or moderate exercise, and select the nearest comparable figure in Table 2–3 for energy expenditure for each, and multiply by the time involved. Compute energy required for all activities for 24 hours. How does this compare with your resting metabolic rate?

7. What is the energy allowance given in the revised 1973 recommended allowances of the Food and Nutrition Board for your weight (without clothing) and age? (See Table 2–6.) Would you classify your degree of physical activity as sedentary or moderately active? How does your individual energy requirement, as computed in question 6, compare with the general recommendation for your age, weight, and the standard of activity? If your specific requirement differs much from the average, explain what factors cause it to differ (e.g., variations from average in size and degree of muscular activity).

8. How may the energy value of foods be determined? Why is the physiological energy value of the nutrients somewhat less than their value as determined in the bomb calorimeter? What types of food are high in energy value? Low in energy value?

9. Give the general caloric value *per gram* of pure protein, carbohydrate, and fat. Calculate the energy value of 100 gm of each of the foods whose composition is given below (by multiplying the grams of protein, fat, and carbohydrate each by the proper caloric value per gram, and adding these figures).

	Protein, gm	*Fat, gm*	*Carbohydrate, gm*
100 gm of white bread contains	8.7	3.2	50.5
100 gm of butter or margarine contains	0.6	81.0	0.4
100 gm of raw cabbage contains	1.3	0.2	5.4

10. Using the food-energy values in Table 2–7 and Appendix 2, plan a 1 day menu that has as many calories as your own 24 hour resting metabolism. What can you add if you sit for 16 hours and sleep 8 hours in a day? What activity could you add to earn a piece of pie?

REFERENCES

1. Du Bois, E. F.: *Basal Metabolism in Health and Disease*. 3rd Ed. Philadelphia, Lea & Febiger, 1936.
2. Boothby, W. M., et al.: Studies of the energy of metabolism of normal individuals. A standard for basal metabolism with a nomogram for clinical application. Amer. J. Physiol., *116*:468, 1936.
3. Brody, S.: *Bioenergetics and Growth*. New York, Reinhold, 1945.
4. Kleiber, M.: *The Fire of Life*. New York, John Wiley & Sons, Inc., 1961.
5. Holliday, M. A., Potter, D., Jarrah, A., and Bearg, S.: The relation of metabolic rate to body weight and organ size. Pediat. Res., *1*:185, 1967.
6. Wallace, R. K., and Benson, H.: The physiology of meditation. *Sci. Amer., 226*:84, 1972.
7. Benedict, F. G., et al.: Human vitality and efficiency under prolonged restricted diet. Carnegie Institute of Washington, Pub. No. 280, 1919.
8. Keys, A.: Human starvation and its consequences. J. Amer. Dietet. Assoc., *22*:582, 1946.
9. Griffith, W. H., and Dyer, H. M.: Present knowledge of specific dynamic action. Chapter VII in *Present Knowledge in Nutrition*. 3rd Ed. Nutrition Foundation, 1967.
10. Buskirk, E. R., Iampietro, P. F., and Welch, B. E.: Variations in resting metabolism with changes in food, exercise and climate. Metab. Clin. Exptl., *6*:144, 1957.
11. Consolazio, C. F., et al.: Energy requirements in extreme heat. J. Nutr., *73*:126, 1961.
12. Benedict, F. G., and Benedict, C. G.: The energy requirement of intense mental effort. Science, *71*:567, 1930.
13. Durnin, J. V. G. A., and Passmore, R.: *Energy, Work, and Leisure*. London, Heinemann Educational Books, Ltd., 1967.
14. FAO/WHO: Energy and Protein Requirements. WHO Tech. Rpt. No. 522; FAO Nutr. Rpt. No. 52. Geneva and Rome, 1973.
15. Passmore, R., and Durnin, J. V. G. A.: Human energy expenditure. Physiol. Rev., *35*:801, 1955.
16. Food and Nutrition Board: *Recommended Dietary Allowances*. 8th Ed. Washington, D.C., National Research Council, National Academy of Sciences, 1974; 9th Ed. to be published in 1979.
17. Canadian Council on Nutrition: *Recommended Daily Nutrient Intakes*. Revised 1974. Bureau of Nutritional Sciences, Health and Welfare, Canada.
18. Institute of Nutrition of Central America and Panama: *Daily Dietary Recommendations for Central America and Panama*. INCAP Pub. E–709, 1973.
19. Watt, B. K., and Merrill, A. L.: *Composition of Foods — Raw, Processed, Prepared*. U.S. De-

partment of Agriculture Handbook No. 8. Washington, D.C., Government Printing Office, 1963.

20. Adams, C. F.: *Nutritive Value of American Foods in Common Units.* U.S. Department of Agriculture Handbook No. 456. Washington, D.C., Government Printing Office, 1975.

SUPPLEMENTARY READING

Benedict, F. G.: Basal metabolism: The modern measure of vital activity. Sci. Monthly, *27*:5, 1928.

Bradfield, R. B. (ed.): Symposium: Assessment of typical daily energy expenditure. Amer. J. Clin. Nutr., *24*:1111 and 1405, 1971.

Brooke, O. G., and Ashworth, A.: The influence of malnutrition on the postprandial metabolic rate and respiratory quotient. Br. J. Nutr., *27*:407, 1972.

Buskirk, E. R., et al.: Human energy expenditure studies. I. Interaction of cold environment and specific dynamic effect. II. Sleep. Amer. J. Clin. Nutr., *8*:602, 1960.

Buskirk, E. R., Thomson, R. H., and Whedon, G. D.: Metabolic response to cold air in men and women in relation to total body fat content. J. Appl. Physiol., *18*:603, 1963.

Clark, R. G.: Caloric requirements after operation. Proc. Nutr. Soc., *30*:158, 1971.

Flodin, N. W.: The energetic joule. Amer. J. Clin. Nutr., *30*:302, 1977.

Fulton, D. E.: Basal metabolic rate of women. J. Amer. Dietet. Assoc., *61*:516, 1972.

Garrow, J. S., and Hawes, S. F.: The role of amino acid oxidation in causing "specific dynamic action" in man. Brit. J. Nutr., *27*:211, 1972.

Givoni, B., and Goldman, R. F.: Predicting metabolic energy cost. J. Appl. Physiol., *30*:429, 1971.

Glick, Z., et al.: Absence of increased thermogenesis during short-term overfeeding in normal and overweight women. Amer. J. Clin. Nutr., *30*:1026, 1977.

Grisola, S., and Kennedy, J.: On specific dynamic action, turnover and protein synthesis. Perspect. Biol. Med., *9*:578, 1966.

Groen, J. J.: An indirect method for approximating caloric expenditure for physical activity. A recommendation for dietary surveys. J. Amer. Dietet. Assoc., *52*:313, 1968.

Haisman, M. F.: Energy expenditure of soldiers in a warm humid climate. Brit. J. Nutr., *27*:375, 1972.

Harrison, S. L.: Body weight-gain equivalents of selected foods. J. Amer. Dietet. Assoc., *70*:365, 1977.

Hegsted, D. M.: Energy needs and energy utilization. Nutr. Rev., *32*:33, 1974.

Hunscher, H. A.: Pertinent factors in interpreting metabolic data. J. Amer. Dietet. Assoc., *39*:209, 1961.

Jaya Ras, K. S., and Khan, L.: Basal energy metabolism in protein-calorie malnutrition and vitamin A deficiency. Amer. J. Clin. Nutr., *27*:892, 1974.

Kleiber, M.: Joules vs. calories in nutrition. J. Nutr., *102*:309, 1972.

Konishi, F.: Food energy equivalents of various activities. J. Amer. Dietet. Assoc., *46*:186, 1965.

Koong, L. J.: A new method for estimating energetic efficiencies. J. Nutr., *110*:1724, 1977.

Kraut, H. A., and Muller, E. A.: Caloric intake and industrial output. Science, *104*:495, 1946.

McGandy, R. B., Barrows, C. H., et al.: Nutrient intakes and energy expenditure in men of different ages. J. Gerontol., *21*:581, 1966.

Moore, T.: The calorie versus the Joule. J. Amer. Dietet. Assoc., *59*:327, 1971.

NAS/NRC: Biological Energy Interrelationships and Glossary of Energy Terms. Pub. 1411, 1966.

Richardson, M., and McCracken, E. C.: Energy expenditures of women performing selected activities. U.S. Department of Agriculture Home Econ. Res. Rept. No. 11. Washington, D.C., Government Printing Office, 1960.

Schmidt-Nielsen, K.: Energy metabolism, body size and problems of scaling. Fed. Proc., *29*:1524, 1970.

Shipman, W. G., Oken, D., and Heath, H. A.: Muscle tension and effort at self-control during anxiety. Arch. Gen. Psychiatry, *23*:359, 1970.

Southgate, D. A. T.: Assessing the energy value of the human diet. Nutr. Rev., *29*:131, 1971.

Southgate, D. A. T., and Durnin, J. V. G. A.: Calorie conversion factors. An experimental reassessment of the factors used in the calculation of the energy value of human diets. Brit. J. Nutr., *24*:517, 1970.

Spurr, G. B., Maksud, M. G., and Barac-Nieto, M.: Energy expenditure, productivity, and physical work capacity of sugarcane loaders. Amer. J. Clin. Nutr., *30*:1740, 1977.

Swindells, Y. E.: The influence of activity and size of meals on caloric response in women. Brit. J. Nutr., *27*:65, 1972.

Symposium: The application of human and animal calorimetry. Proc. Nutr. Soc., *37*:1, 1978.

Thompson, A. M., and Billewicz, W. Z.: Height, weight and food intake in man. Brit. J. Nutr., *15*:241, 1961.

U.S. Department of Agriculture, Agricultural Research Service: *An Evaluation of Basal Metabolic Data for Children and Youth in the United States.* Home Econ. Res. Rept. No. 14. Washington, D.C., Government Printing Office, 1961.

Warnold, I., et al.: Energy intake and expenditure in selected groups of hospital patients. Amer. J. Clin. Nutr., *31*:742, 1978.

Articles in Nutrition Reviews

The neglected field of heat loss (by DuBois, E. F.). *1*:385, 1943.

Are all food calories equal? *22*:177, 1964.

Variability in basal metabolic rate (BMR). *25*:13, 1967.

Malnutrition and metabolic rates. *28*:279, 1970.

Assessing the energy value of the human diet. *29*:131, 1971.

Not so "specific" dynamic action. *30*:133, 1972.

Activity and energy intake in Ugandan children. *31*:84, 1973.

Heat production by malnourished babies. *32*:173, 1974.

Chapter 3

Carbohydrates and Alcohol

The three major classes of energy nutrients — carbohydrates, fats, and proteins — are by far the most abundant nutrients in foods. Together they constitute about 85 to 99 percent of the dry matter present in foods; in the natural state the only more abundant constituent of many foods is water. Most natural foods contain all three nutrients but in widely varying proportions. In order to have a clear idea of the nature of and the differences between these three classes of nutrients, we will begin with brief definitions of each, devote the rest of this chapter to discussion of carbohydrates, and treat fats and proteins in the two following chapters. The only other significant dietary source of energy is alcohol, and since it is made from carbohydrates, we will include it in this chapter.

All *carbohydrates* are made up of the elements carbon, hydrogen, and oxygen, with the hydrogen and oxygen almost always present in the same two-to-one proportion as in water — hence carbo (for carbon) and hydrate (for water) is the class name, coined by a German chemist, C. Schmidt, in 1844. Food carbohydrates are either sugars (such as ordinary table sugar, honey, and corn syrup) or more complex compounds formed primarily from the union of many sugar groups, such as the starch in cereals and potatoes — or for that matter, such nonnutritive plant substances as cotton and linen.

Fats are also composed of carbon, hydrogen, and oxygen, but with these elements present in different relative amounts from those in carbohydrates. All true fats are alike in chemical nature and physical properties: They have a greasy feel, are insoluble in water, but are soluble in such solvents as ether and gasoline. Every molecule of a true fat yields on digestion one molecule of glycerol (an alcohol) and three molecules of fatty acids. The origin of the usage of the word fat for this class of compounds is lost in antiquity. (See Chapter 4.)

Proteins consist of carbon, hydrogen, and oxygen, again in different proportions, and in addition they always contain the element *nitrogen*. Most proteins also contain some sulfur, and others contain phosphorus, iron, iodine, or other trace elements in addition to the elements common to all proteins. The "building blocks" of proteins are amino acids, and on digestion each molecule of protein breaks down to yield many molecules of various kinds of amino acids. Proteins characteristically have a "gluey" consistency and are precipitated or coagulate on heating. The word protein, meaning "to come first," originated with a Dutch scientist, G. Mulder (1838), and indicates the primacy of protein as an essential nutrient, beyond its role as an energy source. (See Chapter 5.)

Alcohol is the class name of chemical compounds containing a particular configuration of oxygen and hydrogen (– OH, a hydroxyl group) linked to carbon. The alcohol present in beer, wine, and whiskey is called ethyl alcohol or ethanol in chemical terms and grain neutral spirits in industry.

Kinds of Carbohydrates and Their Occurrence

Carbohydrates are subdivided into several groups, according to the relative complexity and size of their molecules. Simple sugars form the basis for all carbohydrates.

Carbon atoms each have four bonds with which they can link up to other atoms or groups of atoms. All simple sugars have a chain of carbons linked with hydrogen and hydroxyl (alcohol) groups (in the configuration H – C– OH or its mirror image HO – C – H) and one carbon doubly bonded with oxygen (C═O).* The names of the simple sugars all end in -ose, and they are classified according to the number of carbons in the chain. A sugar with three carbons is a triose; a pentose has five carbons, and so forth.† The chief carbohydrates in foods and in the body are either hexoses (6-carbon sugars) or multiples of hexose sugar groups.

The carbohydrates of most interest in the diet and the groups to which they belong are as follows:

Monosaccharides

Pentoses — ribose, xylose, arabinose

Hexoses — glucose, fructose, galactose, mannose

Oligosaccharides

Disaccharides — sucrose, lactose, maltose

Trisaccharides — raffinose

Tetrasaccharides — stachyose

Polysaccharides

Dextrin, starch, glycogen

Cellulose

Pectin

Hemicellulose, pentosans, mannosans

Derivatives of Monosaccharides

Sugar alcohols — glycerol, sorbitol, mannitol

Amino sugars — glucosamine, galactosamine

Uronic acids — glucuronic acid, galacturonic acid

The *monosaccharides* (or simple sugars) consist of one sugar unit; the *disaccharides* are composed of two simple sugar units; the *oligosaccharides* have two or more simple sugar units, but the term is usually reserved for those having three to several units of simple sugars; the polysaccharides have many sugar units. The *sugar alcohols* are reduced forms of sugar, having a hydroxyl group in place of the C═O (aldehyde or ketone) group. The *amino sugars* have an amino (NH_2) group substituted, and the *uronic acids* contain an acid group.

The Chemical Structure of Carbohydrates

It may be helpful at this point to learn how carbon, hydrogen, and oxygen atoms are linked up in a molecule of a typical hexose, *glucose*. Glucose is the sugar that circulates in the blood; it is also the building block from which starches are made, and usual diets contain more of this structure than any other except water. The student should understand that every molecule of a given substance is exactly alike, with the same number of atoms of each element linked to each other in precisely the same arrangement; any variation from this pattern makes it a different substance. Seemingly small differences in a structure, such as whether the C═O group occurs in the middle- or end-piece of the carbon chain and whether the alcohol (hydroxyl) group is on one side or another of

*This is called an aldehyde group when it occurs at the end of the molecule and a ketone group when it is in the inner structure.

†The trioses play an important role in metabolism but are not present in significant amounts in foods. The pentoses also have a vital function in the body; the pentose ribose is a constituent of the cellular material RNA or ribonucleic acid (see Chapter 5). Pentoses are not a major component of foods.

the carbon, have a major effect on properties such as crystal structure, solubility, and transmission of polarized light.*

Each molecule of glucose consists of 6 carbon, 6 oxygen, and 12 hydrogen atoms; in other words, its formula is written as $C_6H_{12}O_6$. In glucose, the carbon atoms are linked with each other in a chain (Fig. 3–1A) or in an irregularly shaped ring (Fig. 3–1B). The characteristic features that make this sugar glucose (rather than another hexose) are the presence of a terminal C═O group, and the exact configuration of the hydroxyl (OH) groups at carbons 2 through 6. The other common hexoses—*fructose* and *galactose*—both have the same formula ($C_6H_{12}O_6$), but the hydrogen and oxygen atoms are held in slightly different arrangements about the 6-carbon chain, which makes them different substances and gives them the different properties that are the basis for identifying the sugars and determining the amount present in foods.

The linkage of sugar groups to form di- and polysaccharides is shown in Figure 3–1D. When two simple sugars unite to form a disaccharide, one loses a hydrogen atom and the other a hydroxyl radical and these combine to form water (H—OH or H_2O). In polysaccharide formation (Fig. 3–1E), one molecule of water is lost for each sugar radical added, so the final formula is always $C_n(H_2O)_{n-1}$, rather than the $C_nH_{2n}O_n$ formula of the simple sugars.

Disaccharides and the more complex carbohydrates must all be broken down by digestion into the simple sugar groups of which they are composed before they can be absorbed and used by the body. The digestible saccharides are split into monosaccharides by hydrolysis, a reaction with water (hydro-, water; -lysis, breaking down). In this change, the water lost in formation of the complex carbohydrate is added back to yield the same simple sugars as were present initially. Starch is made up of glucose units and thus always breaks down into glucose; and so it follows, for example, that a syrup made by hydrolysis of corn starch consists only of glucose or oligosaccharides of glucose.* In animals and in honeybees, hydrolysis is brought about by the action of digestive enzymes (see Chapter 14), but in cookery and industrial processing, usually the reaction is achieved by the action of acid and heat.

*A beam of polarized light passing through a solution of glucose is bent to the right—hence the common synonym for glucose, dextrose, from dextro (on the right) and -ose (sugar).

Food Carbohydrates

Sugars. All the major food carbohydrates are formed in the vegetable kingdom. Because the *sugars* are very soluble in water, they are the form in which plants transport carbohydrate from one part to another in the sap or store it in the juices of fruits. Hence, glucose, fructose, and sucrose are found chiefly in plant juices and in fruits† (Table 3–1). The sweet taste of corn and peas is due to the presence of sugar that will be converted to starch as the immature seed ripens; in some fruits (e.g., bananas) starch is present in the unripe fruit and turns to sugar on ripening. Carrots, beets, onions, winter squash, turnips, and sweet potatoes are vegetables that contain appreciable amounts of sugars.

Our main sugar supply for table use and cooking is *sucrose*, a disaccharide made up of glucose and fructose. It comes chiefly from juices of the sugar cane or sugar beet, and over one-third of our supply is derived from the latter source. The sugar obtained from the sap of the sugar maple tree is also sucrose. Fructose and glucose occur in honey in about 50–50

*Commercial "corn" syrup usually has some sugar cane syrup or derived fructose added for flavor.

†Plants form galactose, but only a trace or none is present as the simple sugar; rather, it is linked with glucose and fructose to form the trisaccharide raffinose, the tetrasaccharide stachyose, and other oligosaccharides. The linkage is made differently from that in common disaccharides and starch, and the digestive system of higher animals cannot break the bond formed, so these sugars are not absorbed.

A. STRAIGHT-CHAIN STRUCTURE OF GLUCOSE

B. RING STRUCTURE OF GLUCOSE

C. GLUCOSE RADICAL

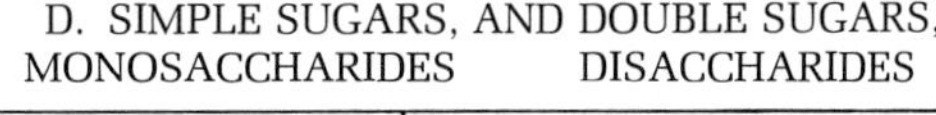
D. SIMPLE SUGARS, MONOSACCHARIDES AND DOUBLE SUGARS, DISACCHARIDES

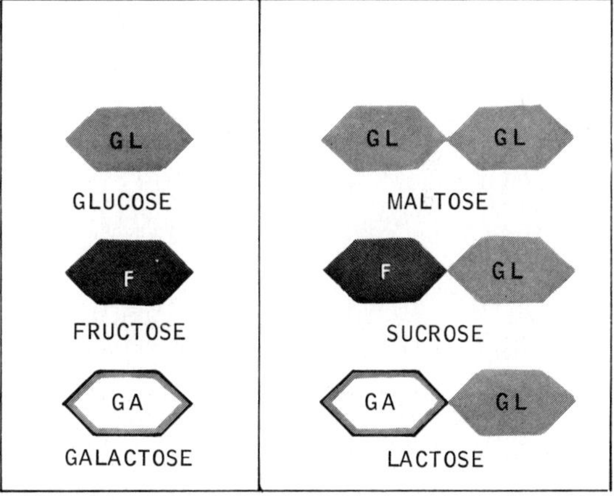

Figure 3–1 Diagram showing arrangement of the atoms in a molecule of the monosaccharide glucose in (A) a straight-chain configuration and (B) a ring configuration, which are freely interchangeable forms of glucose dissolved in water. The carbon atoms have been numbered to show how the ring is arranged. In (C), a glucose radical is shown with two free bonds, each of which could be linked to another monosaccharide. If only one bonding site is used, the resulting compound will be a disaccharide as in (D); or if both bonds are used and many glucose radicals are linked, the resulting compound will be the polysaccharide starch, as in (E). The glucose group, or radical (C), is represented as having lost a hydrogen atom and a hydroxyl radical (OH) in the process of linking up with other sugar groups. When broken apart by hydrolysis (either by digestion or boiling in dilute acid), these component parts of water (H and OH) are taken up again, and glucose molecules are split off.

E. A POLYSACCHARIDE, STARCH (SMALL SECTION OF THE MOLECULE).

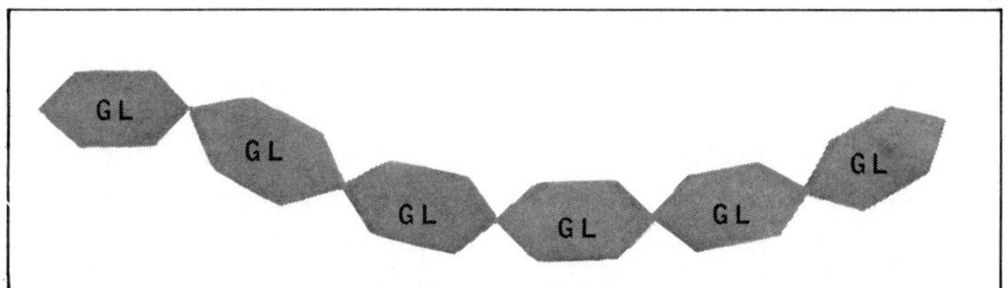

proportion, as it is a digestion product mainly of sucrose from plant nectar.

The sugar *maltose* is formed as an intermediate product during the digestion of starch in the body and is also found in geminated grains such as "malt," and in products prepared from partly digested starch such as corn syrups, malted breakfast foods, and malted milk. It contains two glucose molecules.

Lactose occurs in the milk of most mammals, and serves as a source of energy for the young. On digestion it is broken down into glucose and galactose. All young mammals, except some marine species, can digest lactose, but the enzyme required (lactase) falls to very low levels in most adults. Caucasians of Northern European extraction and some pastoral African groups appear to be an exception to this rule and retain the ability to digest lactose through adulthood. If the digestive enzyme is low or absent, then lactose cannot be absorbed.

The sugars are not all equal in sweetness; in fact, some are barely sweet at all

Table 3–1 FREE SUGARS IN UNPROCESSED FOODS*,†, gm/100 gm

	Total Solids	*Total Carbo-hydrate‡*	*Glucose*	*Fructose*	*Sucrose*	*Other*
Fruits						
Apple	15	15	1.2	6.0	3.8	Maltose, trace
Apricot	15	13	1.9	0.4	5.5	
Banana, ripe	24	22	4.5	3.5	11.9	
Figs, dried	(80)	74	42.0	30.9	0.1	
Grape	18	16	5.4	5.3	1.3	Maltose, 1.6
Orange	14	12	2.5	1.8	4.6	
Peach	13	10	0.9	1.2	6.9	Maltose, 0.1
Prunes, dry	72	67	30.0	15.0	2.0	
Strawberry	9	8	2.1	2.4	1.0	Maltose, 0.1
Vegetables						
Beet (red, root)	11	9	0.2	0.2	6.1	Raffinose/stachyose, traces
Broccoli	12	6	0.7	0.7	0.4	
Lettuce	5	3	0.2	0.5	0.1	
Potato, white	20	17	1.0	1.2	1.7	Raffinose/stachyose, traces
Sweet potato	23	22	0.3	0.3	3.4	
Tomato	5	4	1.1	1.3	trace	
Legumes						
Beans, common, dry seed	89	61			2.4	Raffinose, 0.8 Stachyose, 3.4
Green (snap) beans	8	5	1.1	1.2	0.2	Raffinose, 0.1 Stachyose, 0.2
Peas, green, fresh	26	14		0.1	3.0	Raffinose, 0.1 Stachyose, 0.1
dry, split	91	63	0.2		4.1	Raffinose, 1.8 Stachyose, 8.0
Soybean, dry seed	90	34			4.5	Raffinose, 0.7 Stachyose, 2.7

*Values from Shallenberger, R. S.[1]; Hardinge, M., Swarner, J. B., and Crooks, H. J.[2]; and U.S. Department of Agriculture Handbook No. 8.[3]

†The disaccharide lactose, or milk sugar, makes up 7.5 percent of human breast milk and 4.5 percent of fluid whole cow's milk. Dry skim milk powder is 52 percent lactose, and dry whole milk is 38 percent lactose.

‡By difference; therefore includes fiber.

(Table 3–2). Taking sucrose as the standard (sweetness = 1.0), fructose is nearly twice as sweet and lactose is only one-third as sweet. Other compounds than sugars can evoke the sensation of sweetness; saccharin is a well-known example (sweetness is 500 times that of sucrose) but several of the amino acids also have a very sweet taste. The sugar alcohols, sorbitol and mannitol, are nearly as sweet as glucose; both occur in natural products but not to any major extent. They are used to add sweetness to "sugarless" chewing gum and some dietetic foods. Sorbitol is absorbed more slowly than glucose but has about the same energy value; mannitol is less well absorbed and so it has a lower caloric value.

Polysaccharides. *Starch* is the carbohydrate found in seeds, tubers, and roots, where it functions as an energy store. Starch is formed by union of many molecules of glucose. It has been estimated that the number of sugar groups in the starch molecule may range from 300 up to many thousands. Starch occurs in two types of molecules, one (amylose) consisting of long unbranched chains (wavy or kinked so as to form a three-dimensional spiral), the other type (amylopectin) in highly branched chains. Such large molecules have no sweet taste.

In plants, starch is laid down in "granules" of characteristic size and shape, so that the source of a starch can be determined by microscopic examination.

Starch grains commonly have about 15 to 20 percent amylose and 80 to 85 percent amylopectin. (The waxy varieties of rice and maize corn are very low in amylose, which accounts for the difference in texture.) When subjected to moist heat (as in cooking), starch granules absorb water, swell, and rupture. After such treatment, starch is more easily digested. Before starch can be used as a source of energy, it must first be broken down into the simple sugar groups of which it is composed, each starch molecule yielding many molecules of glucose. *Dextrins* (and the sugar *maltose*) are intermediate products formed in the process of breaking down starch to glucose; dextrins are more soluble than starch, and their molecules may average about one-fifth the size of those of starch.

Cellulose is also a polysaccharide of glucose, but because the glucose units are linked differently, it is much more resistant than starch to degradation. *Hemicelluloses* are not, as one might think, a smaller version of cellulose; they are polysaccharides made up of varying proportions of xylose (a pentose), arabinose, mannose, galactose, other sugars, and uronic acids (derivatives of hexoses). The *pentosans*, made up entirely of pentose units (5-carbon sugars) belong to the class of hemicelluloses. *Pectins*, polysaccharides made up of galacturonic acid, galactose, and arabinose units, are found in small quantities in many fruits and some vegetables; pectin is the agent responsible for the setting of jelly and jam. (See Table 3–3.) Cellulose and hemicellulose (and a noncarbohydrate compound, lignin) make up the structural or fibrous part of plants (leaves, stems, roots, and seed and fruit coverings) and also the cell walls. This group of polysaccharides is not digested by man, so that it is not an energy source.[4] It is used by bacteria and thus serves as an energy source for ruminants.*

Other indigestible or only partially

*Lignin is very resistant to attack, even by microorganisms, which is the reason that wood and sawdust (very high in lignin) are not used for cattle feed.

Table 3–2 SOME SWEET-TASTING SUBSTANCES

Substance	*Relative Sweetness (By Weight)*	*Class*
Neohesperidin dihydrochalcone*	1500	Artificial sweetener
Saccharin (sodium salt)	500	Artificial sweetener
Aspartame (dipeptide)**	160	Artificial sweetener
Cyclamate (calcium salt)†	100	Artificial sweetener
Tryptophan	30	Amino acid
Fructose (levulose)	1.7	Monosaccharide
Invert sugar‡	1.3	Monosaccharide
Sucrose	1.0	Disaccharide
Glycine	0.8	Amino Acid
Glucose (dextrose)	0.7	Monosaccharide
Mannitol		Sugar alcohol
Sorbitol	0.5	Sugar alcohol
Inositol§		Sugar alcohol
Maltose		Disaccharide
Galactose	0.3	Monosaccharide
Lactose		Disaccharide
Raffinose	0.2	Trisaccharide
Starch	~0	Polysaccharide

*New sweetener derived from citrus peel.

**Trade name for a synthetic compound made from two amino acids, phenylalanine and aspartic acid.

†Cyclamate is not allowed in foods because of the possibility that it can lead to cancer. An end-product of cyclamate that can be formed in the body (cyclohexylamine) also is known to raise blood pressure.

‡Invert sugar is a hydrolysis product of sucrose, and is half glucose and half fructose. Honey is also hydrolyzed sucrose and has the same sweetness.

§Inositol is an essential nutrient for some lower animals. See Chapter 8.

Table 3–3 POLYSACCHARIDES AND LIGNIN IN FOODS*,†, gm/100 gm

				Dietary Fiber					
Food	*Total Solids*	*Total Carbo-hydrate*	*Starch*	*Cellulose*	*Hemi-cellulose*	*Pectin*	*Pentosans‡*	*Lignin*	*Crude Fiber*
Fruits									
Apple with skin	15	15		0.7	0.2	2.6		0.2	1.0
Apricot	15	13	0.8		1.2	1.0			0.6
Banana,									
yellow-green	24	22	8.8						
yellow			1.9	0.2	0.1	1.0		0.5	0.5
Orange, peeled	14	12	0	0.3	0.3	1.3	0.3		0.5
Prunes, dry	72	67	0.7	2.8	10.7	0.9	2.0		1.6
Vegetables									
Broccoli	12	6	1.3	0.9	0.9				1.5
Cabbage, raw	8	5		0.8	1.0	0.4		0.1	0.8
Carrot	12	10		1.0	0.5	2.2		0.1	1.0
Lettuce	5	3		0.4	0.6	0.2		0.1	0.5
Potato, white									
(no skin)	20	17	17.0	0.4	0.3	1.4		0.1	0.5
Spinach	9	4		0.3	0.2			0.1	0.6
Sweet potato									
(no skin)	23	22	16.5	0.6	1.4	2.2			0.9
Tomato	5	4		0.2	0.3	0.3		tr.	0.5
Legumes									
Beans, common,									
dry seed	89	61	35.2	3.1	6.4		8.2		4.3
Green or snap beans	8	5	2.0	0.5	1.0	0.5	1.2		1.0
Peas, green, fresh	26	14	4.1	1.1	2.2			0.4	2.0
dry, split	91	63	38.0	5.0	5.1				1.2
Nuts									
Chestnuts, Virginia	48	42	18.6	0.3			2.8		1.1
Peanuts, no skins	95	18	4.0	2.4	3.8			0.2	1.9
Cereals									
Corn (maize),									
fresh sweet	27	22	14.5	0.6	0.9	tr.	1.3		0.7
Corn, dry, whole	88	74	62.0	4.5	4.9		6.2	0.2	1.6
Cornflakes cereal	96	85	60.0	0.4	0.2			0.1	0.7
Rice, polished, dry	88	80	72.9	0.3			1.8		0.3
Wheat, whole grain, dry	87	69	59.0	2.0	5.8		6.6	0.8	2.3
flour, white	88	14	68.8	0.4	0.7		2.1	0.1	0.5
bran†	90	65	17.4	(15)	(32)	3.0	22.1	3.2	8.9

*Values from Hardinge, M., Swarner, J. B., and Crooks, H. J.[2]; and U.S. Department of Agriculture Handbook No. 8[3]. Those in parentheses are estimates from secondary sources.

†Values for wheat bran are from the American Association of Cereal Chemists (Standard bran R07–3691).

‡Pentosans are a constituent of hemicellulose in the usual analytical procedure.

digestible polysaccharides occur less commonly in plant foods. *Inulin,* found in Jerusalem artichokes, is made up entirely of fructose units. *Agar, alginic acid,* and *carrageenan* are polysaccharides present in seaweeds; they are used industrially as thickening agents in ice cream and salad dressing. These carbohydrates plus cellulose, hemicellulose, pectin, and lignin constitute what is generally called "roughage" or "dietary fiber." (A new term, "plantix," has been suggested for this group of compounds, but not yet adopted.) Plants also contain some non-digestible sugars (raffinose, stachyose).

The "crude fiber" value given in most tables of food composition refers to the residue remaining after particular chemical procedures of food analysis; it includes cellulose and lignin but not all the other indigestible carbohydrates. Thus "crude fiber" in ordinary diets is only about one-fifth the value of the physiologically significant dietary fiber. Since most of this material remains undigested, it serves to give bulk to the food residues in the intestine. Further discussion of the function of fiber in the diet is found in Chapter 14.

Glycogen is sometimes called "animal starch" because it is the polysaccharide stored in animal tissues instead of starch. Glycogen molecules are large and seem to vary in size. They are similar to those of the branched form of starch (amylopectin), but they have shorter chains of glucose units and hence a more complicated branched structure. Carbohydrate is an immediate source of fuel for animals. For this purpose animals use glucose, which is the only sugar found in substantial amounts in the blood or tissue fluids. In the postabsorptive state, a man has about 30 gm of glucose in his body, plus about 300 gm of glycogen. Glycogen stored in the liver (about one-third of the total) is used as a reserve supply for keeping up the blood sugar level; muscle glycogen (two-thirds of the total) is used to meet energy needs of the exercising muscle during work.

Only limited amounts of glycogen can be stored in the liver and muscle tissues, and this is used up rapidly during fasting or muscular work. Since animals usually are fasted before slaughter, or may be hunted to exhaustion, there is little glycogen present in our animal foods, such as muscle meats. Liver usually contains about 1.5 to 5 percent glycogen, while shellfish (including oysters) have about 1 to 6 percent.

Animal tissues also contain some heterogenous carbohydrates having substituted acid groupings (uronic acids) or amino groups hexosamines), or linked to proteins or lipids. *Mucopolysaccharides* are present in the fluid around joints and in the eyeball, in blood, and in mucus, skin, nails, cartilage, and the organic structure of bone. Chitin, the organic base of insect skeletons and shells of crustacea, is built up like cellulose but from glucosamine rather than glucose; it is also found in mushrooms and other fungi. The very thick or viscous portion of egg white, ovamucoid, is a *mucoprotein*. Compounds made up of lipids and carbohydrate are chiefly found in the brain and nervous tissue and are called *cerebrosides*.

Carbohydrate Content of Foods

In determining the composition of foods, the amount of water, protein, fat, and mineral (ash) is measured chemically, and the portion of weight not accounted for (the difference between the initial weight and the sum of the four components mentioned) is called "carbohydrate." Thus, the portion listed as carbohydrate in tables of good composition usually includes true carbohydrates plus often substantial amounts of organic acids and lesser weights of flavorants, vitamins, and so on.

The *organic acids*, included in the values for "carbohydrate, by difference," do have some energy value to the body, but less than the sugars. The common organic acids citric and malic provide 2.47 and 2.42 kcal/gm, respectively, in contrast to sugars and starch that yield about 4 kcal/gm. Organic acids contribute about 3 percent of the energy in many vegetables and about 4 to 6 percent in fruits. A notable exception is lemon juice, in which 62 percent of the energy is from this source. Citric acid is a common component of manufactured foods; it is used either for its acid quality (many soft drinks are about 2 to 6 percent solutions of citric acid plus sugar, flavoring, and colorant) or to bind metals that cause off flavors to develop in, for example, processed cheese.

Some typical foods of relatively high carbohydrate content, together with the approximate amount of carbohydrate each contains, are listed in Tables 3–1 and 3–3 and are shown in Figure 3–2. A few highly refined substances — such artificially prepared foods as refined sugar and corn starch — are pure carbohydrate (99.5 and 88 percent respectively, the rest of the weight being mainly due to small amounts of water); but even those foods relatively rich in either sugar or starch contain in their natural state other substances besides carbohydrates. Sugar cane juice, being a plant sap, contains minerals and some vitamins; when sugar is removed by crystallization, the sugar (sucrose) be-

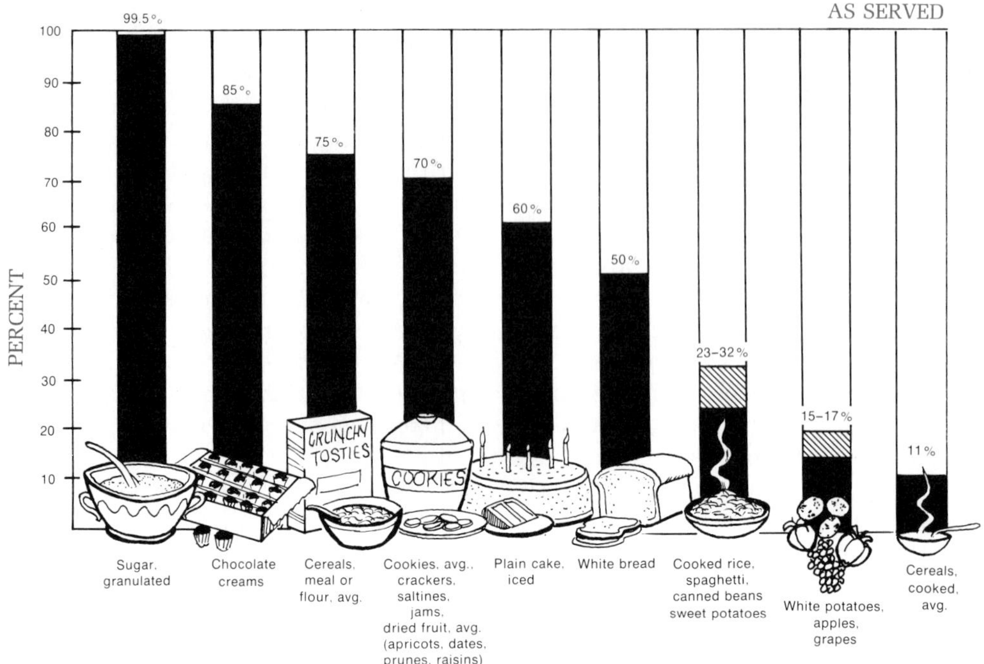

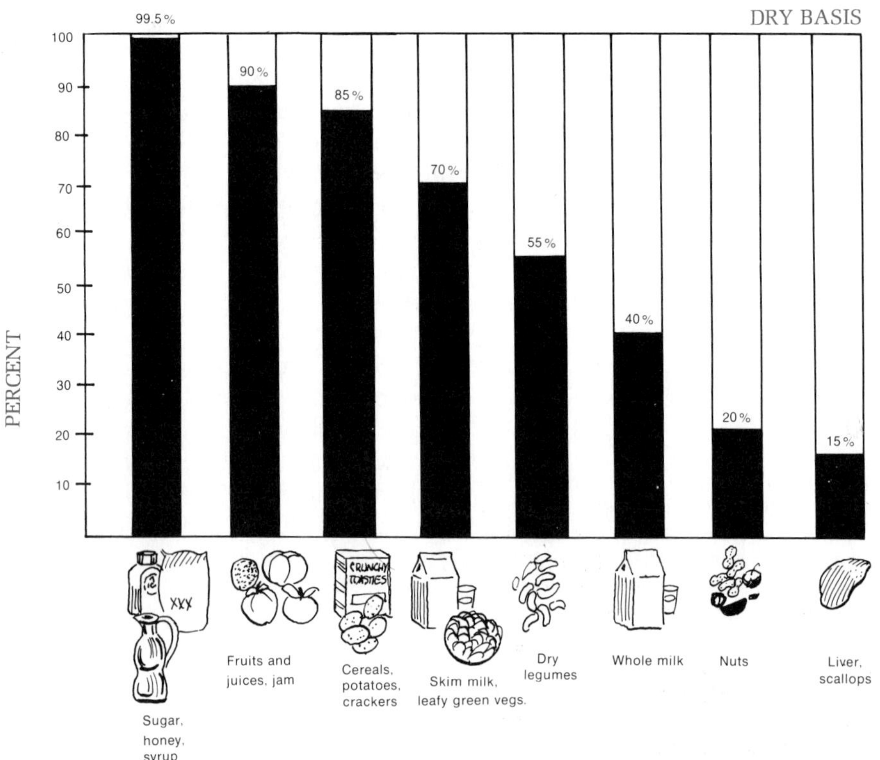

Figure 3–2 Carbohydrate content of common foods.

comes very pure and the nutrient substances left behind are concentrated in the leftover molasses. Honey also contains very small amounts of some nutrients, but these are not nutritionally significant because of the small amount of honey normally eaten. (In the United States, per capita consumption of honey is just over 1 lb/year, or about ¼ tsp/day, while consumption of refined sugar is about 130 gm/day.)

Foods of high sugar content (65 to 99 percent) include table sugars, honey, syrups, candies, cakes, jams, jellies, preserves, and dried fruits (dates, figs, raisins, prunes, apricots); others containing appreciable amounts are fresh fruits (9 to 23 percent) and soft drinks (8 to 10 percent). Taken in considerable quantities, these last two sources may contribute appreciable amounts of energy (calories).

Although highly milled dry rice and white flour are more than four-fifths starch and have a total carbohydrate (starch) content of 81 and 76 percent respectively, they also contain significant amounts of protein (6.5 to 10.5 percent). Whole-grain cereals have somewhat more protein and less starch. Dry peas and beans have over 20 percent of protein along with approximately 60 percent of starch; soybeans differ from other beans in that they contain less starch and more fat. The legumes and whole grains also contain some indigestible fiber, and certain minerals and vitamins.* Starchy roots of the taro and cassava (manioc), which are staple foods in parts of Africa, South America, and the islands of the South Pacific, have very little protein, minerals, or vitamins.

The grains (wheat, corn, rice, rye, barley) and dry products made from them have variable water content, so they range from about 10 to 85 percent carbohydrate as served. Cooked rice, spaghetti, macaroni, and sweet potatoes are 23 to 32 percent carbohydrate, and white potatotes (boiled or baked in skin) are about 17 to 22 percent. Cooked breakfast cereals (e.g., oatmeal and farina) average about 11 percent starch.

*Figures for the carbohydrate content of foods used here and elsewhere in the book are for *total* carbohydrate, by difference, as given by the U.S. Department of Agriculture.[3] These figures are apt to be slightly higher than the actual amount of carbohydrates available to the body.

Place of Carbohydrate-Rich Foods in Diet

We cannot now state that any specific level of carbohydrate intake is most conducive to health. The relative prominence of carbohydrate-rich foods varies widely with individuals and in different parts of the world, depending chiefly on the availability and relative cost of fat- and protein-rich foods (animal products such as meats and dairy products) and the amount of money that can be spent for food. Such foods as grains, starchy roots or tubers, and dried peas or beans are usually the cheapest foods for energy value. In Japan, for example, carbohydrates (rice) contribute four-fifths of the total energy intake, while in the United States, where fats are used more liberally, only one-half or less of the energy intake comes from carbohydrates (Fig. 3–3).

There need be no health hazard in subsisting chiefly on carbohydrate-rich foods, *provided* those foods are not lacking in proteins, minerals, and vitamins or the diet includes some rich source of these nutrients. A major source of concern today is the level of sugars, particularly refined sucrose and syrups, in the diet (Fig. 3–4). In 1972, the total sugar consumption (including that in fruits, milk, etc.) was 200 gm/person/day, of which 130 gm was refined sugar.[1] Intake of sugar has been fairly constant at this level since 1925, but as the total energy consumption has fallen about 200 kcal/day, the percentage contribution of energy from sugar has increased. In the period from 1960 to 1971, use of refined caloric sweeteners has increased by 10 percent, chiefly owing to greater use of manufactured food products, presweetened cereals, and baked goods (Table 3–4). There is no solid

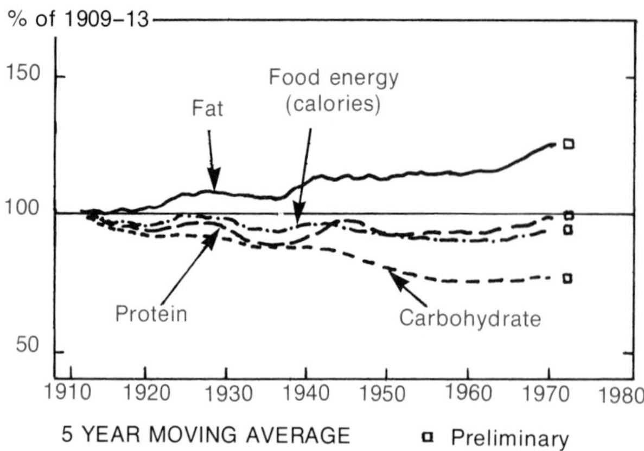

Figure 3–3 Shift in per capita consumption of food energy, protein, fat, and carbohydrate in the United States between 1910 and 1970. Carbohydrate in the national food supply has declined about one-fourth over this period (down from 500 g to 380 g/day) and fat intake has risen steadily. In 1970 per capita consumption of fat was 155 g/day and protein, 100 g/day. (From Page, L., and Friend, B.: Level of use of sugars in the United States. In *Sugars in Nutrition*, ed. H. L. Sipple and K. W. McNutt. New York, Academic Press, 1974. Used with permission.)

evidence that the present intake of sugar is harmful other than as it contributes to obesity and thus to the diseases associated with that condition (diabetes, gallstones, high blood pressure), and to dental caries. In some persons who have a particular genetic make-up, high carbohydrate and often high sucrose intakes cause an undesirable elevation of fatty substances in the blood, but this is ordinarily not severe unless the person is also obese. However, there is great concern that the diet of Americans and Northern Europeans (whose intake of sugar is generally over 100 gm/day) may be low in essential vitamins and minerals because of the displacement of nutritious foods.

There is no clear evidence that more than a very small amount of carbohydrate need be present in the diet if substances from which the body can make sugar are sufficient. Through metabolic processes the body can produce carbohydrate from the sugar alcohol, glycerol, which makes up 10 percent of the weight of fat (see Chapter 4). About half of the amino acids that make up protein can also be converted to carbohydrate. There are limits to these metabolic processes, and if carbohydrate intake is very low, fats are not completely utilized and protein is diverted from its essential roles (see Chapter 5). To prevent these events, the diet should include about 70 to 100 gm of preformed carbohydrate.

In summary, the main contributions to the diet by carbohydrate-rich foods (sugars and starchy foods) are to:

1. Provide an economical energy supply.
2. Furnish some proteins, minerals, and vitamins (whole grains, legumes, and potatoes).
3. Provide fiber (roughage).
4. Add flavor (sugars) to foods and beverages.

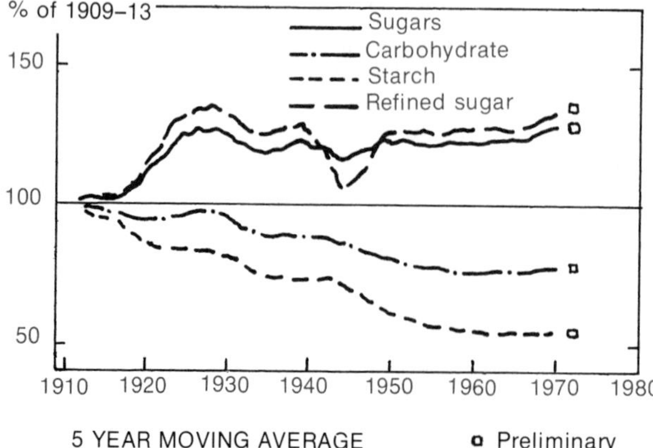

Figure 3–4 Changes in consumption of starch and sugar in the United States between 1910 and 1970. Intake of starch has declined nearly 50 per cent, due to decreased consumption of cereals, legumes, and potatoes, while total sugar intake increased about one-fourth between 1910 and 1925. (From Page, L., and Friend, B.: Level of use of sugars in the United States. In *Sugars in Nutrition*, ed. H. L. Sipple and K. W. McNutt. New York, Academic Press, 1974. Used with permission.)

Table 3–4 EXAMPLES OF SUGAR ADDED TO FOODS*†

Canned or Packaged Food	*Grams of Sugar/ Serving Size*	*Percent of Total Weight*	*Percent of Calories*
Beverages			
Cola type	37/12 oz	10	100
Fruit juice drink	20/6 oz	12	85
Kool-Aid	25/8 oz	11	98
Desserts			
Peaches, light syrup	9/½ c	7	48
heavy syrup	16/½ c	12	61
Pudding, starch type	25/5 oz	18	50
Gelatin dessert	26/5 oz	18	97
Milk chocolate candy	12/1 oz	44	32
Brownies	12/each	50	30
Coconut cream pie	24/¼ pie	68	66
Ready-to-eat cereals			
Corn or wheat flakes	23/1 oz	7–11	11–15
Presweetened, flavored	8–14/1 oz	29–44	26–45
100% Natural	6/1 oz	19	15

*Values from CNI Weekly Report, *4*(18), May 2, 1974.
†Includes cane, beet, and corn sugars, and cornstarch.

ALCOHOL

Probably one of the best-known food processing techniques is fermentation, the production of potable alcohol by the action of yeast on carbohydrate. Almost all cultural groups (some native American tribes were exceptions) have learned to use and control the process. The starting material may be fruit, palm or cactus juices, molasses or sugar, honey, milk, potatoes, or cereal grains; the flavor of the final product will vary accordingly, but the alcohol produced is the same: the simple compound, ethyl alcohol or ethanol, C_2H_5OH.* Because fermentation is a metabolic process, a number of intermediate and alternate compounds may be present; Carbon dioxide (CO_2) is given off as a by-product. If the process is not stopped before the yeast uses all the available carbohydrate, the yeast will begin to convert ethanol to acetic acid (CH_3COOH), making vinegar instead of wine.

Yeast cannot continue to grow if the concentration of alcohol becomes excessive (over about 20 percent), so the hard liquors are produced by distillation, which concentrates the alcohol and separates it from the starting material. Thus, the natural products — beer and wine — contain some nutrients present in the original malted barley and fruit juice, but distilled spirits have no essential nutrients. In terms of dilution of the nutritive quality of the diet, distilled spirits (gin, rum, whiskey, brandy, etc.) have the same effect as refined sugar. It is not surprising, then, that habitual overusers of alcoholic beverages often have poor intakes of vitamins and minerals.

Alcohol is metabolized in the liver, but the capacity is limited. Most individuals can metabolize about 0.1 gm/kg body weight/hr (range, 0.06–0.2 gm). Alcohol yields 7 kcal/gm, so the hourly capacity of a 70 kg man would be $70 \times 0.1 \times 7$, or about 50 kcal/hr from ethanol. In the course of a day of steady drinking, the total energy from this source could reach 1200 kcal, and many regular drinkers consume that much and more. This would amount to some 18 oz (about 520 ml) of 86 proof hard liquor or 1.7 liters (about ½ gal) of wine (Table 3–5).

If alcohol is consumed at a rate faster

*Fermentation of wood pulp results in production of another alcohol, methanol or wood alcohol, which is highly poisonous to man.

Table 3–5 SOCIAL BEVERAGES: CALORIC VALUES AND ALCOHOLIC CONTENT OF PORTIONS COMMONLY USED*

	Approximate Measure	*Weight gm*	*Energy kcal*	*Carbohydrate gm*	*Alcohol† gm*
Distilled liquors					
Liqueurs					
Anisette, Sambuca	1 cordial glass	20	75	7.0	7.0
Apricot brandy	1 cordial glass	20	65	6.0	6.0
Benedictine	1 cordial glass	20	70	6.6	6.6
Creme de menthe	1 cordial glass	20	70	6.0	7.0
Curaçao, Triple sec	1 cordial glass	20	65	6.0	6.0
Brandy or cognac	1 brandy glass	30	75		10.5
Gin, dry, 80 proof	1 jigger, 1½ oz	45	105		15.1
Rum, 80 proof	1 jigger, 1½ oz	45	105		15.1
Whiskey, rye, 90 proof	1 jigger, 1½ oz	45	119		17.2
Whiskey, Scotch, 80 proof	1 jigger, 1½ oz	45	105		15.1
Wines					
California, table wine, red or white	1 wine glass	100	85	4.0	10.5
Champagne, domestic	1 wine glass	120	85	3.0	11.0
Port or muscatel	1 wine glass	100	160	14.0	15.0
Sherry, dry, domestic	1 wine glass	60	85	4.8	9.0
Vermouth, sweet	1 wine glass	100	170	12.0	18.0
Vermouth, dry	1 wine glass	100	105	1.0	15.0
Malt liquors (American)					
Ale, mild	1 bottle, 12 oz	345	150	12.0	13.1
Beer, avg.	Large glass, 8 oz	240	115	10.6	8.9
Beer, avg.	1 bottle, 12 oz	360	175	15.8	13.3
Mixed drinks, cocktails (approx. from recipes)					
Daiquiri	1 cocktail glass	100	125	5.2	15.1
Eggnog, holiday	1 punch cup, 4 oz	123	335	18.0	15.0
High ball	1 glass, 8 oz	240	165		24.0
Manhattan	1 cocktail glass	100	165	7.9	19.2
Martini	1 cocktail glass	100	140	0.3	18.5
Mint julep	1 glass, 10 oz	300	210	2.7	29.2
Old fashioned	1 glass, 4 oz	100	180	3.5	24.0
Planter's punch	1 glass	100	175	7.9	21.5
Rum sour	1 glass	100	165	4.5	21.0
Tom Collins	1 glass, 10 oz	300	180	9.0	21.5
Soft drinks					
Cider, sweet	1 c	250	124	34.4	0
Club soda	12 fl oz	355	0	0	0
Coffee, black	6 fl oz	180	2	0.4	0
Cola type	6 fl oz	180	70	18.5	0
Eggnog	1 c	245	235	17.7	0
Fruit-flavored sodas	12 fl oz	370	170	44.6	0
Ginger ale	6 fl oz	180	55	14.6	0
Hot chocolate, half milk	1 c	220	145	27.1	0
Ice cream soda, chocolate	1 avg.	300	255	46.0	0
Lemonade	10 fl oz	295	105	27.2	0
Postum (cereal-based)	6 fl oz	185	36	8.5	0
Quinine water	6 fl oz	180	55	14.6	0
Root beer	12 fl oz	370	150	39.0	0
Tea, plain	6 fl oz	180	2	0.4	0

*Figure chiefly from Bowes, C. F., and Church, H. N.: *Food Values of Portions Commonly Used.* 12th Ed. Philadelphia, J. B. Lippincott Co., 1975.

†The caloric value of alcohol is approximately 7 kcal per gram, but the body has limited capacity to oxidize it. This gives a physiological reason for sipping rather than gulping down such beverages.

than it can be metabolized (that is, for a 70 kg man, 7 gm/hr, or about half a 12 oz can of beer per hour), then the level of alcohol builds up in body tissues and eventually intoxication and, in the extreme, death results. Alcohol is damaging to the liver, and chronic users have an increased risk of liver disease (cirrhosis). In high concentration, alcohol is damaging to the lining of the intestinal tract; absorption of nutrients is affected adversely, and the risk of cancer of the esophagus increases with alcohol use. Ultimately, overuse leads to degenerative changes in the nervous system. Alcohol abuse is a serious worldwide problem. The World Health Organization reports that in 1970, in the United States, 2.7 percent of persons aged 15 years and older used daily more than 150 ml of alcohol (from all legal beverages consumed); in Canada, the figure is 2.5 percent, and in France it is a staggering 9.0 percent.[6]

On the other hand, alcoholic beverages have a relaxing effect and stimulate the appetite. As long as beer and wine are used in moderation and with awareness of the risks entailed, there seems no reason, other than any religious beliefs, to deny their occasional consumption by nonpregnant women and adult males.

QUESTIONS AND PROBLEMS

1. Define carbohydrates, fats, and proteins. Why are they referred to as the fuel foodstuffs or energy nutrients? Which vital element is supplied in utilizable form only by proteins?

2. Explain the chemical basis for the division of carbohydrates into mono, di-, and polysaccharides. How do the mono- and disaccharides (sugars) differ in properties (taste, solubility, etc.) from polysaccharides (starch, cellulose, etc.)? How are these differences in properties related to the size of the molecules? What are the other classes of carbohydrates?

3. Name three common monosaccharides and some foods in which they are found. Consult the diagram of the molecular structure of glucose in Figure 3–1. How many carbon atoms are there in each molecule; how many hydrogen atoms; how many oxygen atoms? Why are they called *carbohydrates*? Why are the monosaccharides that occur most commonly in nature called hexoses? What is the hexose sugar that occurs in blood and body tissues?

4. When two molecules of monosaccharide link up to form a disaccharide (as two glucose molecules to form one molecule of maltose), what substance is split off at the point of linkage? Does the same thing happen when many molecules of glucose unite to form the polysaccharide starch? What happens when these linkages are broken during digestion or hydrolysis outside the body? Why is this breakdown called hydrolysis?

5. What is the chemical name of common table sugar, and from what sources in nature is it made? Is maple sugar the same or a different substance? Is sugar a relatively expensive or inexpensive source of food energy? Does it carry any other nutrients? What are the disadvantages of using sugar too liberally? Name four common foods of high sugar content.

6. What types or classes of food have a high content of starch? Into what monosaccharide is starch broken down in digestion? Does this process take place gradually or all at once? Why? What polysaccharides found in foods are of no use to the body, and why is this so? Plants store starch in seeds or tubers; what polysaccharide is stored in the body, chiefly in the liver?

7. Make a list of the foods you have consumed in one day, including sugar added at the table and any between-meal snacks. Using the table in the Appendix on Nutritive Values of Foods in Average Servings, calculate your total intake of carbohydrate for the day. At 4 kcal per gram, how much energy did you obtain in the form of carbohydrate? Since the figures for total carbohydrate include indi-

gestible carbohydrate in the form of fiber, how would this affect the total energy actually obtained? Of what use is the fiber in vegetable foods?

8. What are the chief uses of carbohydrate-rich foods in the diet? In what countries and under what economic conditions is the consumption of carbohydrates high? Are there any disadvantages of diets that are made up chiefly of carbohydrate-rich foods? Why is it important that whole-grain or enriched bread and cereal be used when grain products make up a large proportion of the diet? Is there a dietary requirement for carbohydrate? Justify your answer.

9. What is an alcohol? What is ethanol? How is it produced? Do alcoholic beverages have any nutritional value? If so, what? How much alcohol can be utilized? Is it safe to drink alcoholic beverages? Justify your answer.

REFERENCES

1. Sipple, H. L., and McNutt, K. W. (eds.): *Sugars in Nutrition.* New York, Academic Press, 1974.
2. Hardinge, M., Swarner, J. B., and Crooks, H.: Carbohydrates in foods. J. Amer. Dietet. Assoc., *46*:197, 1965.
3. U.S. Department of Agriculture Handbook 8. Revised December, 1963.
4. Mangold, E.: The digestion and utilisation of crude fibre. Nutr. Abstr. Rev. *3*:647, 1934.
5. Spiller, G. A., and Amen, R. J.: *Fiber in Human Nutrition.* New York, Plenum Press, 1976.
6. World Health Organization: Alcohol: a growing danger. WHO Chronicle, *29*:102, 1975.

SUPPLEMENTARY READING

Carbohydrate

Akrabawi, S. S., Saegert, M. M., and Salji, J. P.: Studies on the growth and changes in metabolism of rats fed carbohydrate-deficient, fatty-acid based diets supplemented with graded levels of maize starch. Brit. J. Nutr., *32*:209, 1974.

Anderson, J. W., Herman, R. H., and Zakim, D.: Effect of glucose and high sucrose diets on glucose tolerance of normal men. Amer. J. Clin. Nutr., *26*:600, 1973.

Beyer, P. L., and Flynn, M. A.: Effects of high- and low-fiber diets on human feces. J. Amer. Dietet. Assoc., *72*:271, 1978.

Bierman, E. L., and Nelson, R.: Carbohydrates, diabetes and blood lipids. World Rev. Nutr. Dietet., *22*:280, 1975.

Bing, F. C.: Dietary fiber — in historical perspective. J. Amer. Dietet. Assoc., *69*:498, 1976.

Birch, G. G., and Green, L. F. (eds.): *Molecular Structure and Function of Food Carbohydrate.* New York, Halsted Press, Div. of John Wiley & Sons, Inc. 1973.

Burkitt, D. P.: Epidemiology of large bowel disease: the role of fibre. Proc. Nutr. Soc., *32*:145, 1973.

Calloway, D. H., and Chenoweth, W. L.: Utilization of nutrients in milk- and wheat-based diets by men with adequate and reduced abilities to absorb lactose. 1. Energy and nitrogen. Amer. J. Clin. Nutr., *26*:939, 1973.

Connell, A. M.: Wheat bran as an etiologic factor in certain diseases. Some second thoughts. J. Amer. Dietet. Assoc., *71*:235, 1977.

Danowski, T. S., Nolan, S., and Stephen, T.: Hypoglycemia. World Rev. Nutr. Dietet., *22*:288, 1975.

Duncan, D. L.: The physiological effect of lactose. Nutr. Abstr. Rev., *25*:309, 1955.

Durrington, P. N., et al.: Effect of pectin on serum lipids and lipoproteins, whole-gut transit time, and stool weight. Lancet, *2*:394, 1976.

Fuller, M. F., and Crofts, R. M. J.: The protein-sparing effect of carbohydrate. 1. Nitrogen retention of growing pigs in relation to diet. Brit. J. Nutr., *38*:479, 1977.

Fuller, M. F., Weekes, T. F. C., Cadenhead, A., and Bruce, J. B.: The protein-sparing effect of carbohydrate. 2. The role of insulin. Brit. J. Nutr., *38*:489, 1977.

Grande, F.: Sugar and cardiovascular disease. World Rev. Nutr. Dietet., *22*:248, 1975.

Gray, G. M.: Carbohydrate digestion and absorption. Gastroenterology, *58*:96, 1970.

Grenby, T. H.: The effects of some carbohydrates on experimental dental caries in the rat. Arch. Oral Biol., *8*:27, 1963.

Holloway, W. D., Tasman-Jones, C., and Lee, S. P.: Digestion of certain fractions of dietary fiber in humans. Amer. J. Clin. Nutr., *31*:927, 1978.

Hultman, E., and Nilsson, L. H.: Factors infuencing carbohydrate metabolism in man. Nutr. and Metab., *18* (suppl. 1):45, 1975.

Kelley, J. J., and Tsai, A. C.: Effect of pectin, gum arabic, and agar on cholesterol absorption, synthesis and turnover in rats. J. Nutr., *108*:630, 1978.

Kelsay, J. L.: A review in effects of fiber intake on man. Amer. J. Clin. Nutr., *31*:142, 1978.

Macdonald, I. (ed.): Symposium on dietary carbohydrates in man. Amer. J. Clin. Nutr., *20*:65, 1967.

Mendeloff, A. I.: Dietary fiber. Nutr. Rev., *33*:321, 1975.

Michaelis, O. E., IV, Scholfield, D. J., Nace, C. S., and Reiser, S.: Demonstration of the disaccharide effect in nutritionally stressed rats. J. Nutr., *108*:919, 1978.

Passmore, R., and Swindells, Y. E.: Observations on the respiratory quotient and weight gain of man after eating large quantities of carbohydrates. Brit. Med. J., *17*:331, 1963.

Richardson, J. F.: The sugar intake of businessmen and its inverse relationship with relative weight. Brit. J. Nutr., *27*:449, 1972.

Southgate, D. A. T.: Fibre and the other unavailable carbohydrates and their effects on the energy value of the diet. Proc. Nutr. Soc., *32*:131, 1973.

Spiller, G. A., et al.: Can fecal weight be used to establish a recommended intake of dietary fiber (plantix)? Amer. J. Clin. Nutr., *30*:659, 1977.

Stephenson, L. S., Latham, M. C., and Jones, D. V.: Milk consumption by black and white pupils in two primary schools. J. Amer. Dietet. Assoc., *71*: 258, 1977.

Trowell, H.: Definition of dietary fiber and hypothesis that it is a protective factor in certain diseases. Amer. J. Clin. Nutr., *29*:417, 1976.

Van Soest, P. J., and McQueen, R. W.: The chemistry and estimation of fiber. Proc. Nutr. Soc., *32*:123, 1973.

Wright, E., and Hughes, R. E.: Dietary citric acid. Nutr. (Lond.), *29*:367, 1975.

Yudkin, J.: Sugar and disease. Nature, *239*:197, 1972.

Alcohol

Aylward, F., et al.: Symposium: Alcohol in nutrition. Proc. Nutr. Soc., *31*:77, 1972.

Baker, H., et al.: Inability of chronic alcoholics with liver disease to use food as a source of folates, thiamin and vitamin B-6. Amer. J. Clin. Nutr., *28*:1377, 1975.

Bebb, H. T., et al.: Calorie and nutrient contribution of alcoholic beverages to the usual diets of 155 adults. Amer. J. Clin. Nutr., *24*:1042, 1971.

Bennion, L. J., and Li, T. K.: Alcohol metabolism in American Indians and whites. N. Engl. J. Med., *294*:9, 1976.

Fry, M. M. et al.: Intensification of hypertriglyceridemia by either alcohol or carbohydrate. Amer. J. Clin. Nutr., *26*:798, 1973.

Hanson, J. W., Jones, K. L., and Smith, D. W.: Fetal alcohol syndrome. J.A.M.A., *235*:1458, 1976.

Isselbacher, K. J.: Metabolic and hepatic effects of alcohol. N. Engl. J. med., *296*:612, 1977.

Lieber, C. S.: Alcohol, nutrition and the liver. Amer. J. Clin. Nutr., *26*:1163, 1973.

McDonald, J., and Margen, S.: Wine vs. ethanol in human nutrition. I. Nitrogen and calorie balance. Amer. J. Clin. Nutr., *29*:1093, 1976.

McLaughlan, J. M., et al.: Effect of a low-carbohydrate diet and alcohol on perceptual motor skill. J. Amer. Dietet. Assoc., *68*:138, 1976.

Murdock, H. R., Jr.: Blood glucose and alcohol levels after administration of wine to human subjects. Amer. J. Clin. Nutr., *24*:394, 1971.

Pirola, R. C., and Lieber, C. S.: Hypothesis: energy wastage in alcoholism and drug abuse: possible role of hepatic microsomal enzymes. Amer. J. Clin. Nutr., *29*:90, 1976.

Rubin, E., and Lieber, C. S.: Alcohol-induced hepatic injury in nonalcoholic volunteers. N. Engl. J. Med., *278*:869, 1968.

Smuckler, E. A., et al.: Symposium: The biology of alcohol and alcoholism. Fed. Proc., *34*:2038, 1975.

Soterakis, J., and Iber, F. L.: Increased rate of alcohol removal from blood with oral fructose and sucrose. Amer. J. Clin Nutr., *28*:254, 1975.

Articles in Nutrition Reviews

Carbohydrate

Carbohydrate free diet in rats. *30*:21, 1972.

Effects of different carbohydrates on metabolic levels in saliva. *31*:48, 1973.

Carbohydrate preference in normal and malnourished rats. *31*:161, 1973.

The role of sugars in hyperlipidemia. *32*:340, 1974.

Sucrose, starch and hyperlipidemia. *33*:44, 1975.

Dietary fiber as a binder of bile salts. *35*:183, 1977.

Alcohol

Alcoholic hyperlipidemia. *29*:140, 1971.

Alcoholism and folic acid. *30*:57, 1972.

Alcohol-induced hepatic necrosis. *34*:124, 1976.

Alcohol, gastritis and nutrient absorption. *35*:8, 1977.

Alcohol consumption and blood pressure. *35*:191, 1977.

Fructose treatment of acute alcohol intoxication. *36*: 14, 1978.

Metabolism in alcoholism. *36*:142, 1978.

Chapter 4

Fats and Other Lipids

In Chapter 2 it was noted that fats yield about 900 kcal (3800 kJ) of energy per 100 gm of fat when eaten. This amount is over twice the energy value of the same weight of carbohydrate or protein (400 kcal).

This amount of fat, 100 gm, or about a quarter of a pound, is only slightly less fat than the average per capita intake per day of most persons in industrial societies, including North America. Fat makes up 15 to 20 percent of our food on a weight basis, and over 40 percent of our calories, mostly from isolated oils and meat fat. Also of interest is that the total body tissue of a college-age person, for example, contains from 15 to 25 percent of fat, with women normally having the larger amount. Overweight persons have even more fat in their bodies, up to 40 percent, or more in extreme cases.

Thus, fat as a subject is very important to persons concerned about their weight and body shape. Also, because so much fat is eaten each day (a practice not without nutritional hazards), fat has tremendous economic value. Many billions of dollars' worth of fat is sold and eaten each year in North America. Because of this there are many political and advertising pressures to persuade us to eat one kind of fat or another, or fat-rich foods.

Fats are essential to the life of all cells. As we will learn in more detail, fats are made up of *glycerol combined with fatty acids, at least one of which, linoleic acid, is a dietary "essential fatty acid."* Linoleic acid, an abundant fatty acid easily obtained from food, cannot be made by our bodies — although all the other fatty acids can be made in the body from this one. *A dietary source of linoleic acid, then, is essential for life.* In its absence, a fatty acid deficiency develops, resulting first in minor symptoms such as scaly skin and sore spots. Because linoleic acid has many vital cellular functions, death would result eventually if a person stayed on a linoleic acid-free diet long enough.

Thus, linoleic acid is the first specific nutrient that we will study of about 22 rather small organic chemicals, along with amino acids and vitamins, that are absolutely essential for us to obtain from our foods.

Fats are part of every meal. They are familiar to everyone—butter, margarine, vegetable oils, lard, salad oils, beef fat, and suet being common examples of rich or, in some cases, pure sources. These common fats are also, chemically speaking, *lipids,* a less common word with a broader meaning than the true chemical meaning of "fats." Lipids include many other related substances such as waxes, cholesterol, and phospholipids. The two words (fats and lipids) are often used interchangeably in a classroom or laboratory, with no real problem as long as a "true" fat is not intended, as will be explained. Not all lipids are true fats, but all fats are lipids.

A dietary *oil* — say, corn oil or soybean oil — is a common name for a food fat that is liquid at room temperature (not to be confused with mineral oil, or crude oil used in manufacturing gasoline—they are different chemicals). It is not wrong to speak of "corn fat," for example, or the "fat content of soybeans"; the words *oil* and *fat* are interchangeable for fats that are liquid at room temperature.

All fats and most lipids are distinguished from other food components by feeling greasy to the touch, by leaving a translucent spot on paper, and by being insoluble in water. (This is why we need soap and hot water to clean greasy hands.) All lipids, in addition, are soluble in "fat solvents," such as ether, alcohol, gasoline, trichlorethylene, and the common household cleaning fluids. In fact, *lipids may be defined simply as those organic substances in nature that are extracted by fat solvents.* Even some of the vitamins, as well as many pigments, are lipids.

Discovery and Background

The story of fats goes back to man's earliest history when fats, oils, and tallows were first used for food, for soap manufacture, for lubrication of wheel axles, as a fuel for light and heat, and for cosmetics and medicine. Many Biblical passages refer to fats and oils, as do records surviving from the early Egyptians.

The history of fats includes the classic discoveries of the French chemist M. E. Chevreul, who in 1823 first discovered the chemical nature of fats.[1, 2] The word "margarine" comes from Chevreul's "margaric acid." The word lipid comes from the old Greek word *lipos* for fat. The old Anglo-Saxon word *fāett*, is the source of our word fat; and the word oil is even older, dating back to the Greek word for olive oil, *elaion*. *Glycerol*, a major constituent of all fats, was discovered in 1783 by Karl Scheele, a Swedish chemist. *Phospholipids* have been known since 1844. *Cholesterol*, isolated from gallstones and later named from the Greek words for bile (chole) and solid (stereos), was discovered before 1777 – over 200 years ago.[2] It has become a household word since about 1960 because of its suspected relationship to heart disease.

In the late 1800's physiologists provided proof that excess dietary carbohydrates were readily converted to fats in the body and stored as adipose tissue, a fact experienced and suspected by farmers and laymen centuries earlier. It thus came as a surprise when in 1929 Burr and Burr[3] at the University of Minnesota demonstrated the essential nature of certain fatty acids in the diet.

Composition and Physical Properties of Fats

True fats, or *triglycerides* as they are technically called,* are formed by chemical combination of three *fatty acids* with *glycerol* (commonly known as "glycerin"), as shown in Figure 4–1. The fatty acids contain large amounts of carbon and hydrogen, along with a relatively small amount of oxygen, and hence fats have very high fuel value. Fatty acids exist rarely in the free form in nature. Combined fatty acids (with glycerol) represent the chief form in which animals store extra energy for future use, just as plants store energy as starch. Some plants store fats in fruits, seeds, seed germs, or nuts, which we see as common vegetable oils (from the olive, coconut, peanut, soybean, corn germ, cottonseed, etc.) used for food. Most common nuts contain 50 to 70 percent of fat.

Many food fats are of animal origin: butter, lard, fatty meats and fish, egg yolk, cream, and full-milk cheeses. (See Appen-

---

*Since the word "triglycerides" implies that the molecule has three glyceride units (which, obviously, is not so), a new chemical term for true fats, triacylglycerols, is now more properly used (see Lipids, *12*:455, 1977). Both terms are in use today.

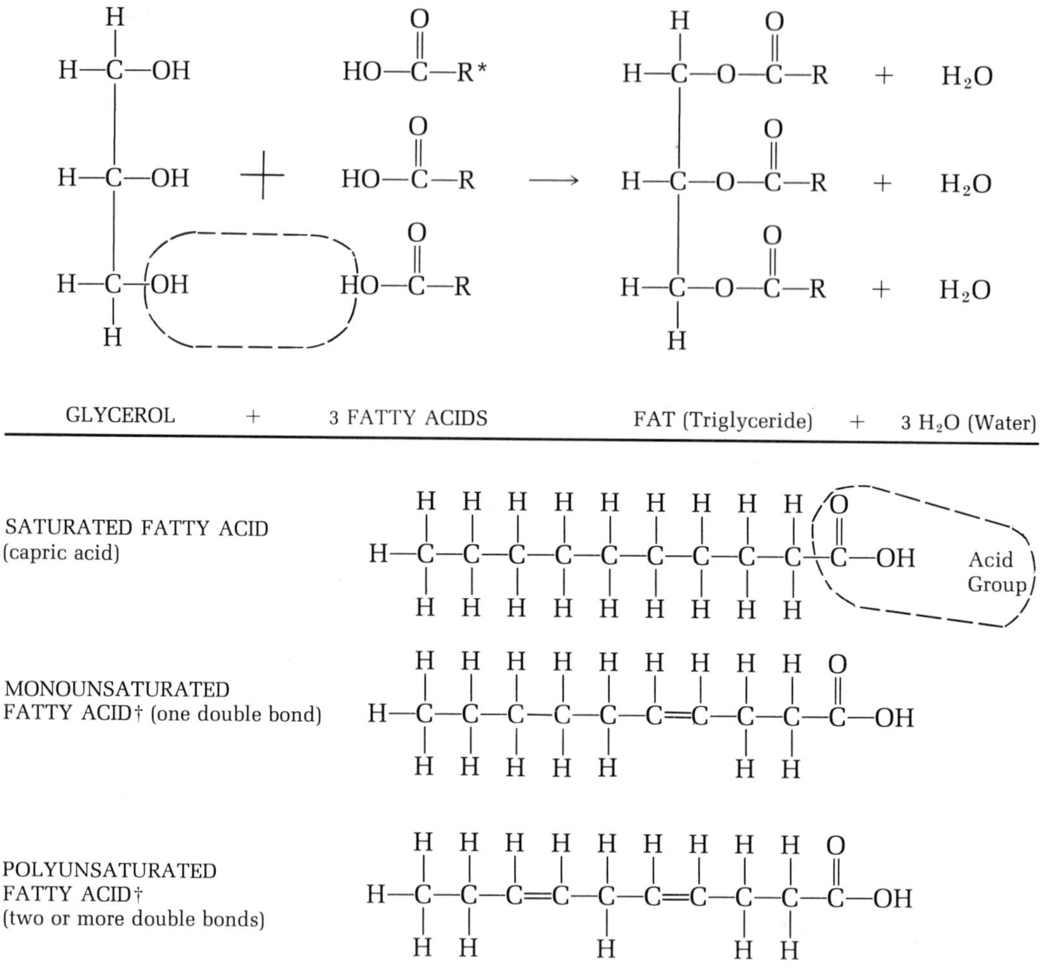

GLYCEROL + 3 FATTY ACIDS → FAT (Triglyceride) + 3 H_2O (Water)

SATURATED FATTY ACID (capric acid) — Acid Group

MONOUNSATURATED FATTY ACID† (one double bond)

POLYUNSATURATED FATTY ACID† (two or more double bonds)

*R = Radical (rest of molecule)
†Type formula (does not exist in nature)

Figure 4–1 Diagrams showing molecular structure of glycerol, fatty acids, fats, and unsaturation of fats. Fatty acid molecules have a chain of carbon atoms with hydrogen attached and at one end of the chain, an organic acid group (COOH). In the fatty acids that occur most commonly in food fats, there are either 15 or 17 carbon atoms in the chain attached to the organic acid group. Saturated fatty acids have only single bonds between carbon atoms in the chain. Unsaturated fatty acids have one or several *double bonds* between carbons and can add on more hydrogen when these double bonds are broken and reduced to single bonds; hence, they are *unsaturated* in respect to hydrogen.

dix, Table 2, for details on the distribution of fat in foods.)

The *physical properties* of fats are important, as they may affect their nutritive value. That fats are insoluble in water and lighter in weight than water is easily apparent from the fact that the fat of cooked meat juices or nonhomogenized milk, for example, rises to the top on standing. The specific gravity of common fats ranges between 0.92 and 0.94. The physical size of fat particles affects its use. *Homogenized fat* goes through a process that breaks up the fat into fine particles that remain evenly distributed (an emulsion), as in homogenized milk for example. Fats that are in small droplets in a fluid, as in milk, beans, and egg yolk, are generally more quickly digested than large amounts of nonemulsified fat, because the tiny droplets can be more readily surrounded and attacked by digestive juices (see Fig. 4–2). Fats that are fluid at body temperature are likewise generally more easily digested than those that have higher melting points. But once they leave the stomach, most common food fats are fully digested, absorbed, and utilized. (See Chapter 14 for more detailed information on fat digestion and absorption.)

Every fat has its characteristic melting point. The oils have low melting points. Butter, lard, coconut fat, and other solid cooking fats melt with only a little heating. Mutton suet, on the other hand, has the highest melting point among the meat fats, most of which are solid at room temperatures.

The physical properties of various fats, such as differences in consistency at room temperature, are due to differences in the *kinds and amounts of fatty acids* that enter into their composition. The melting points of the common fatty acids, their names and formulas, and whether they are *saturated* or *unsaturated* (see next paragraph) are listed in Table 9 of the Appendix. Table 4–1 shows the distribution of major fatty acid groups in various common food fats with different physical properties.

Of the six to eight most common saturated fatty acids, *palmitic acid* and *stearic acid* are most abundant. They have a type formula of $C_nH_{2n}O_2$ and are solid at room temperature. Solid fats contain more of these two fatty acids than do liquid fats or oils. These fatty acids are "saturated" because they cannot accept any more hydrogen. Some fatty acids are "unsaturated" with respect to hydrogen—that is, they have type formulas like $C_nH_{2n-2}O_2$ *(oleic acid) and* $C_nH_{2n-4}O_2$ *(linoleic acid).* They are liquid at room temperature and present in larger amounts in liquid fats or oils of lower melting point.

The more highly unsaturated fatty acids *(linoleic, linolenic,* and *arachidonic acids)* have two, three, and four double bonds, respectively, per molecule; hence, they are said to be "polyunsaturated." These have great nutritional importance. Knowledge of the ratio of polyunsaturated (P) fatty acids to saturated (S) fatty acids, or the P/S ratio, is useful to those persons who have been advised by their physicians to consume a P/S ratio of about one because of an abnormally high level of blood lipids (see page 74).

Oleic acid, with only one double bond, or monounsaturated, is found in relatively large amounts in most vegetable oils (up to 76 percent), along with variable amounts of polyunsaturated fatty acids (see Table 4–1). Animal fats would be more solid at room temperature were it not for an abundant supply of oleic acid in most common animal fats—from 25 to 44 percent. Beef fat and pork fat (lard) have 44 percent of oleic acid, which would surprise those who think of animal fats as saturated fats.

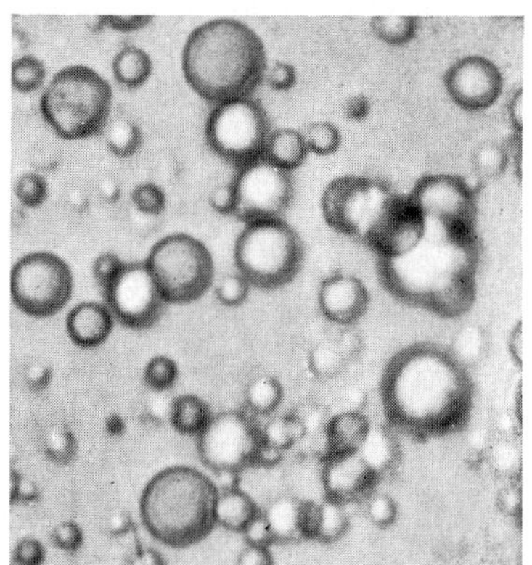

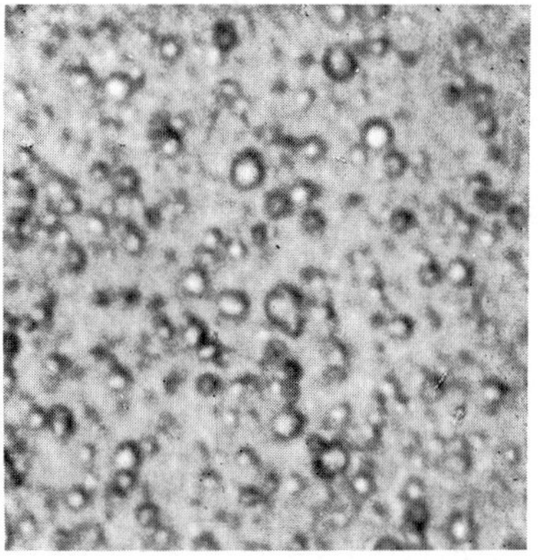

Figure 4–2 *Left*, Fat globules in milk magnified 1000 times. *Right*, The same in evaporated milk, homogenized so fine that the cream does not rise. (Courtesy of Evaporated Milk Association, Chicago.)

Table 4–1 FAT CONTENT AND MAJOR FATTY ACID COMPOSITION OF SELECTED FOODS (IN DECREASING ORDER OF LINOLEIC ACID CONTENT WITHIN EACH GROUP OF SIMILAR FOODS)*

		Fatty Acids†		
			Unsaturated	
Food	*Total Fat*	*Saturated*‡	*Oleic*	*Linoleic*
	PERCENT	PERCENT	PERCENT	PERCENT
Salad and cooking oils				
Safflower	100	10	13	74
Sunflower	100	11	14	70
Corn	100	13	26	55
Cottonseed	100	23	17	54
Soybean§	100	14	25	50
Sesame	100	14	38	42
Soybean, specially processed	100	11	29	31
Peanut	100	18	47	29
Olive	100	11	76	7
Coconut	100	80	5	1
Vegetable fats—shortening	100	23	23	6–23
Margarine, first ingredient on label¶,**				
Safflower oil (liquid)—tub	80	11	18	48
Corn oil (liquid)—tub	80	14	26	38
Soybean oil (liquid)—tub††	80	15	31	33
Corn oil (liquid)—stick	80	15	33	29
Soybean oil (liquid)—stick††	80	15	40	25
Cottonseed or soybean oil, partially hydrogenated—tub††	80	16	52	13
Butter	81	46	27	2
Animal fats				
Poultry	100	30	40	20
Beef, lamb, pork	100	45	44	2–6
Fish, raw††				
Salmon	9	2	2	4
Nuts				
Walnuts, English	64	4	10	40
Peanuts or peanut butter	51	9	25	14
Egg yolk	31	10	13	2
Avocado	16	3	7	2

*From *Fats in Food and Diets*. U.S. Department of Agriculture Information Bulletin No. 361, 1974, p. 5.

†Foods contain other lipids and other fatty acids, so the totals of the last three columns will not generally add up to column one.

‡Includes fatty acids with chains from 8 through 18 carbon atoms.

§Suitable as salad oil.

¶Mean values of selected samples and may vary with brand name and date of manufacture.

**Includes small amounts of monounsaturated and diunsaturated fatty acids that are not oleic or linoleic.

††Linoleic acid includes higher polyunsaturated fatty acids.

Many thousands of different triglycerides are found in foods because of the different possible combinations of fatty acids that may bind with glycerol. It has been calculated that butter contains over 100,000 different triglycerides, for example. Manufactured fats are commonly used by the food industry with specific fatty acids added to the glycerol molecule. MCT, or medium chain (length) triglyceride, is an example of a type used in preparing special foods.

With suitable chemical treatment, the double bonds in the molecules of unsaturated fatty acids may be reduced to single ones, setting free bonds that enable the compound to take up more hydrogen atoms; by this process, oils may be converted to a semisolid or solid state. It is by *hydrogenation* and other chemical modifications that vegetable oils are converted into a semisolid state for use as cooking fats (lard substitutes), margarines, shortening, or thicker peanut butter.*

Value of Fat in Foods

Fats and fat-containing foods are of value in the diet for six main reasons:

1. As a source of essential fatty acid. Linoleic acid and its metabolic derivatives are essential to all cells and tissues of the body (see page 72.) This is the sole *essential* use of fat; the others below are very useful, though not essential.

2. As carriers of fat-soluble vitamins A, D, E, and K, and as an aid to their absorption in the intestine.

3. As a concentrated source of energy and as a builder of fat stores in the body.

4. For satiety value.

5. For making foods appetizing and flavorful.

6. For providing various "functional properties" to cooked and processed foods (see Chapter 17).

The *high energy value* of fats (9 kcal/gm) means that relatively small quantities of fat-rich foods decidedly raise the energy value of the diet. Fats are useful when it is desirable to have a higher intake of food energy without adding unduly to the bulk of the diet. A diet very low in fat often either supplies less energy than the body needs, thereby causing weight loss, or is much more bulky than the customary American or European diet. If one overeats in regard to fats, the diet very likely provides food energy in excess of body needs and causes undesirable weight gains. Excess energy value of the diet, whether taken in the form of fat, carbohydrate, or protein, is converted into body fat and stored in fatty tissues in various parts of the body.

Fat deposits in the human body may be either advantageous or disadvantageous, according to whether they are moderate or excessive. Some deposition of fat, usually under the skin or about the abdominal organs, serves a useful purpose as a *reserve store of fuel* to be drawn on in time of need. Moderate deposits of fatty tissue also serve to *support organs* and protect them from injury and to *prevent undue loss of heat* from the body surface, since fat is a poor conductor of heat, and thus may serve as an "insulation" blanket in times of cold stress. But an overfed person goes on storing fat that he may never need to burn as body fuel; such excessive fat deposits cause undesirable weight gains and place undue strain on the heart and other vital organs. Insurance figures show that overweight persons have a much lower life expectancy than those who maintain normal weight for their height and age (see Chapter 24).

The *satiety value* of fats depends on the fact that fats slow down the digestion and emptying time of the stomach; meals that contain considerable fat remain longer in the stomach and so prevent the early recurrence of the "hunger pangs" that occur when it is empty. When food is scarce or when one is on a reducing diet, small or moderate amounts of fat are a help in preventing hunger. But when too much fat is taken, especially when it is intimately mixed with starch or protein, the meal may stay so long in the stomach as to cause a feeling of discomfort.

Fats incorporated and naturally present in foods give prized *flavor* and make the food more *appetizing* to most people. The flavor varies somewhat with the kind of fat used, individual preference being largely based on habit, culture, and economic conditions. Since certain fats have become scarcer and more costly, the attitude of American consumers has altered to include a greater acceptance of formerly less used but cheaper fats—for example, corn or cottonseed oil instead of olive oil, and margarine instead of butter.

*During hydrogenation, small amounts of "*trans*" *fatty acids* are formed. These isomers make up about 4 percent of our fat intake. In humans, no toxic symptoms are known to result from eating these, but they are being studied to insure safety (see supplementary reading list at the end of the chapter).

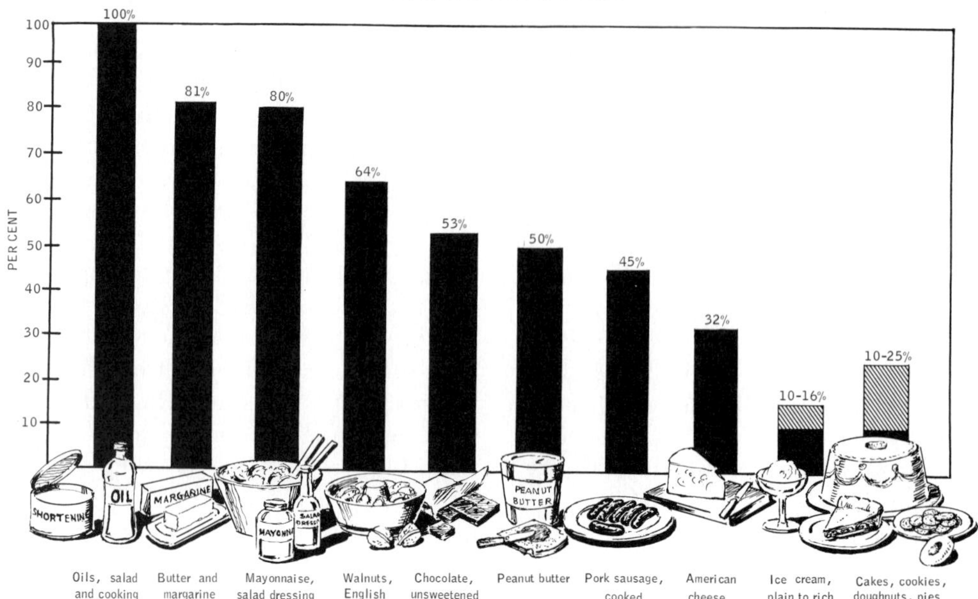

Figure 4–3

Fats in Foods

Some typical fat-rich foods are listed in Figure 4–3, such as butter, lard, margarine, vegetable oils, and cooking fats. These foods are generally used in moderate amounts at a time by being spread on or mixed into other foods low in fat content. Mayonnaise is about 80 percent fat, but other types of salad dressings range between 40 and 60 percent. Foods whose fat content ranges from 20 to 70 percent include cream and full-milk cheeses, fat meats and poultry, chocolate, nuts, and peanut butter. These foods are also generally used in moderation. Olives and avocados contain more fat than other fruits, 16 to 20 percent, but not as much as many common foods (also see Table 4–1).

It must be remembered that foods such as butter, margarine, salad oil, and cooking fats are "visible" fats, and we are conscious of how much of them we use. However, we often fail to recognize that approximately half of our total fat intake comes from the "hidden" fat in such foods as meats, cookies, nuts, cream, ice cream, cheese, and pastries. Even if all visible fat were to be trimmed off meat, the separated lean meat (cooked) still contains 4 to as much as 15 percent "hidden" fat. Often still more is present in choice cuts, in which the flesh is marbled with fat. Whole milk contains about 3.5 to 3.7 percent fat, not a great deal more than "low-fat" or 2 percent (fat) milk. Skim milk has from 0.1 to 0.5 percent fat. A heaping tablespoon full of peanut butter (24 gm) supplies about 12 gm of "hidden" fat. Table 2 in the Appendix gives detailed values for these and other sources of fat in the U.S. diet.

Linoleic Acid, a Dietary Essential

Body tissues possess a marked ability to build (synthesize) complex compounds by combining relatively simple ones. It is well known that excess carbohydrate or protein can be transformed into fat for deposition in fatty tissues. For this purpose, the long carbon chains of saturated fatty acids (and also oleic acid with one double bond) are built by combining simple, 2-carbon groups (acetate radicals). However, the body is not able to synthesize linoleic acid, a dietary *essential fatty*

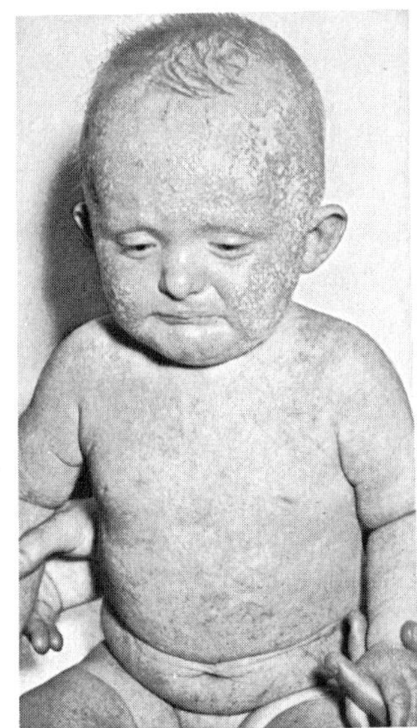
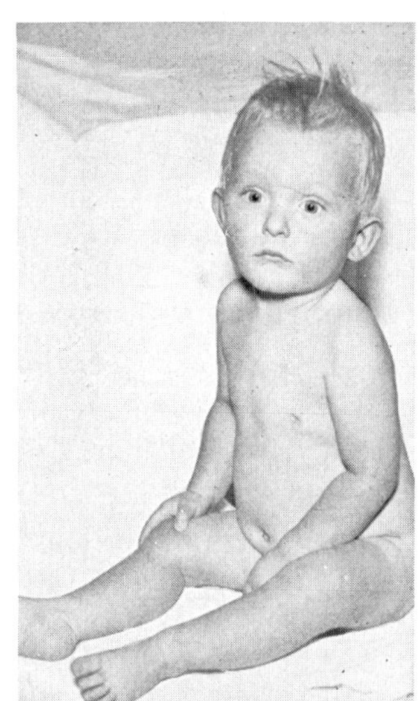

Figure 4–4 Certain fatty acids, found in fats of low melting point, must be furnished in the food. Skin troubles result when these essential fatty acids are lacking. *Left,* Six-month-old infant with very resistant eczema since 2½ months of age. *Right,* The same child 6 months later, after a source of linoleic acid had been included in the diet. (Courtesy of Dr. A. E. Hansen.)

acid. It has to be obtained in the diet for growth and well-being of all species of higher animals, including man. Arachidonic acid, with four double bonds and 20 carbon atoms, used to be included as an essential fatty acid, but since it is found almost only in animal foods (and then only in less than adequate levels), and since it can be readily made in the body from linoleic acid, it is not actually essential in the diet. (However, recent work indicates that members of the cat family may require dietary arachidonic acid).

The discovery of the dietary need for linoleic acid began in 1929, when Burr and Burr demonstrated that rats fed on fat-free diets (adequate as to other nutrients) failed to grow or lost weight, developed a scaly condition of the skin and tail, and developed kidney damage that eventually led to their death.[3] These conditions could be prevented or alleviated by giving linoleic acid. Hansen and coworkers were the first to diagnose symptoms of poor growth and eczematous skin lesions in infants due to a deficiency of essential fatty acids[4] (see Fig. 4–4).

Other workers in this field[5, 6] concur, and place the minimum requirement for infants at 1.4 to 4.5 percent of the calories furnished as linoleic acid, the higher requirement being for premature babies. Human milk and commercially prepared formulas provide a generous allowance of linoleic acid, but formulas based on cow's milk just barely meet the minimum requirement. Hansen and associates established definitely that adults as well as infants require essential fatty acids.[7] The need for dietary linoleic acid by adults has been amply confirmed by recent studies of hospital patients receiving liquid diets by stomach tube or intravenously.

The essentiality for humans of the closely related fatty acid *linolenic acid* with three double bonds is not yet clear. It appears that the body cannot make this from linoleic acid, but the question remains whether a dietary source is necessary for optimal health. At this time there is insufficient evidence to call linolenic acid essential in the diet of humans.

There is no set allowance for essential fatty acids, but the Food and Nutrition Board[6] states that linoleic acid intake equivalent to nearly 2 percent of the total calories in the diet should be sufficient for adults (e.g., about 6 gm per day in a diet of 2700 kcal) and 3 percent of calories for infants. Most Americans at least meet this requirement, and many persons eat much more than needed.[8, 9] Most vegetable oils, such as corn, soybean, cottonseed, safflower, sunflower, and wheat germ oils, are especially rich in linoleic acid; margarines, vegetable shortenings, peanut oil, walnuts, and poultry fat are also good sources.

Metabolic Functions of Fat

The disadvantage of having separate chapters on lipids, proteins, and carbohydrates is that the student may not appreciate how closely related these classes are within the body itself. They are intimately and dynamically related within each body cell and in all body functions. To distinguish certain compounds as being more important than others, metabolically, would be very difficult, and even to study them separately can be misleading unless this close relationship is clearly understood. (See Chapter 14).

The various fats and lipids play extremely important roles, metabolically, in many enzyme reactions, in cell membrane structure, in the synthesis and regulation of certain hormones, in the maintenance of the proper structure of blood vessels, and in energy metabolism, digestion, tissue structure, nerve impulse transmission, memory storage, and other functions. In recent years, for instance, we have learned of the importance of *prostaglandins,* a class of vital hormonelike compounds made in various tissues of the body from arachidonic acid (and other derivatives of linoleic acid) and important in the regulation of such diverse reactions as gastric secretion, pancreatic functions, release of pituitary hormones, and in smooth muscle metabolism.[10] Arachidonic acid appears to be the most important fatty acid, metabolically—more so even than linoleic acid itself.

The amount and kinds of fatty acids in eggs, poultry, and red meats can be influenced to a limited extent by the kinds and amount of dietary fatty acids fed to the animals being raised for food, though this is not a practical means of greatly increasing human linoleic acid consumption.

Fats in Cardiovascular Diseases

From a nutritional point of view it is often important to know the kind of fat one is consuming, and its fatty acid composition. It is expected that improved labeling of manufactured food products will provide more information about this matter in the future. This information becomes especially important to persons "at risk" for atherosclerosis and other forms of heart and cardiovascular diseases (see supplementary reading list).

It is known that the kind and amount of fat eaten can affect blood levels of various fats and lipids. Thus, consumption of fats with a low P/S ratio (see page 69), one with excessive amounts of saturated fat in relation to polyunsaturated fat, can cause an increase in blood cholesterol and other blood lipids. In turn, a desirable ratio of about 1 to 1 is known to be effective in reducing the amount of heart disease in persons at risk. Individuals at risk are those who are overweight, smoke heavily, do not have a regular program of physical fitness, are under work stress, or have a family history of heart disease. Persons with combinations of these risk factors, especially males between 40 and 60 years of age, are particularly susceptible to heart disease.*

In any event, it is prudent for persons at risk for any reason to cut down their fat intake, if high, to no more than 30 percent of the total calories, with a simultaneous reduction of major sources of fats low in linoleic acid. Careful attention to one's diet in these directions is always a desirable goal, whether or not one has obvious risk factors for cardiovascular disease.

---

*Recent interest has focused on how the levels of *high density lipoproteins* (HDL) in the blood can predict risk of subsequent cardiovascular disease. These fatty proteins carry about 20 percent of the cholesterol in the plasma. Persons with *higher* HDL values have *less* risk of cardiovascular disease (see supplementary readings).

Lipids Other Than True Fats

In addition to true fats and fatty acids, *lipids* as a class include some substances chemically related to fats plus some others that are totally unrelated. *Phospholipids,* for example, are composed of glyceryl esters of only two fatty acids and a nonlipid component instead of the usual third fatty acid in a true fat. The phospholipid *lecithin,* which is prominent in egg yolk, is formed by the union of one molecule of glycerol, two molecules of fatty acid, and one molecule each of phosphoric acid and choline, a nitrogenous base. It is readily made by body tissues and is not needed in the diet.

All phospholipids contain phosphoric acid radicals but differ in that other nonfat compounds may take the place of choline or a fatty acid group. Groups may also be attached to a substance other than glycerol in still other types of lipids.

Another class of lipids consists of the *sterols,* which are complex alcohols of high molecular weight. *Cholesterol* is the most prominent member of this group found in the body, while *ergosterol* and *sitosterol* are common sterols found in plants (See Table 4–2 for a list of cholesterol-containing foods.) *Bile acids,* such as cholic acid, which are secreted in the intestine in large amounts, are lipids also.

Phospholipids and sterols are widely distributed in small amounts in foods and are normal constituents of body tissues. They are concentrated especially in the liver and in lesser amounts in the blood and other tissues. Cholesterol, a normal body constituent making up about 0.3 percent of body weight, gives rise to an

Table 4–2 CHOLESTEROL CONTENT OF COMMON MEASURES OF SELECTED FOODS (IN ASCENDING ORDER)*

Food	*Amount*	*Cholesterol*
		MILLIGRAMS
Milk, skim, fluid or reconstituted dry	1 c†	5
Cottage cheese, uncreamed	½ c	7
Lard	1 tbsp	12
Cream, light table	1 fl oz	20
Cottage cheese, creamed	½ c	24
Cream, half and half	¼ c	26
Ice cream, regular, approximately 10% fat	½ c	27
Cheese, cheddar	1 oz	28
Milk, whole	1 c	34
Butter	1 tbsp	35
Oysters, salmon	3 oz, cooked	40
Clams, halibut, tuna	3 oz, cooked	55
Chicken, turkey, light meat	3 oz, cooked	67
Beef, pork, lobster, chicken, turkey, dark meat	3 oz, cooked	75
Lamb, veal, crab	3 oz, cooked	85
Shrimp	3 oz, cooked	130
Heart, beef	3 oz, cooked	230
Egg	1 yolk or 1 egg	250
Liver, beef, calf, hog, lamb	3 oz, cooked	370
Kidney	3 oz, cooked	680
Brains	3 oz, raw	more than 1700

*From Feeley, R. M., Criner, P. E., and Watt, B. K.: Cholesterol content of foods. J. Amer. Dietet. Assoc., *61*:134, 1972; and *Fats in Food and Diets.* U.S. Department of Agriculture Information Bulletin No. 361, 1974, p. 6.

†c = cup.

intermediate substance, 7-dehydrocholesterol, from which vitamin D is formed by ultraviolet light when it penetrates the skin. Certain hormones formed in the adrenal cortex and sex glands (such as *cortisone*) are also sterols, closely related chemically to cholesterol, which serves as a precursor in their synthesis. The *bile acids*, likewise derivatives of cholesterol, are formed in the liver and excreted by way of the bile into the intestine, from which some may be reabsorbed and used over again, others being excreted in the feces. The same pathway (bile, intestine, feces) serves for the excretion of cholesterol and other related sterols.

Cholesterol is thus seen to be a substance normal in, and useful to, the body. Approximately 2 gm is synthesized, and metabolized, each day within the body of normal adults. The level of cholesterol in the blood is normally kept constant by a balance between the sum of it taken in the diet plus that manufactured in the body, and the amount used up in the body plus that excreted through the intestine along with the bile. This explains why it is so difficult, and in many cases impossible, to lower the cholesterol level in the blood by restricting cholesterol in the diet.

Waxes are included among the lipids and are normally present in very small amounts in many foods usually of vegetable origin. Comb honey is an example of a rich source of dietary wax.

Place of Fat-Rich Foods in the Diet

The amount of fat in the diet may be varied widely, as is the case for carbohydrate intake, according to personal tastes, money spent for food, and availability of fat-rich foods. Only about 10 percent of the energy in the average diets of Asiatic peoples is furnished by fats. Overpopulation in any country requires that land be used primarily for the production of carbohydrate-rich foods that furnish energy at least cost, instead of for the production of less efficient meat and dairy products (though often range lands or waste byproducts can be utilized for farm animals).

Among people of moderate means in many European countries, fat intake may account for only 10 to 25 percent of their total energy intake. In countries such as Holland, Denmark, New Zealand, Canada, and the United States, meat fats, dairy products, and vegetable oils (or shortenings and spreads made from them) are available at prices most people can afford. Under such conditions, 40 to 45 percent of the energy content of the diet may come from fat-rich foods. A recent study[9] of students from 50 colleges in the United States showed that fat content of meals averaged 126 gm a day, representing 42 percent of total calories. This was made up of 46 gm saturated fatty acids, 48 gm oleic acid, and 17 gm linoleic acid.

Table 4–3 shows the way in which different foods contribute to our U.S. intake.

Fat Toxicity

Few fats in foods are toxic, but there are important exceptions. Fats such as rapeseed oil, castor oil, and impure cottonseed oil contain unusual fatty acids or other lipids that can cause toxic symptoms to various degrees. Most of these substances can be removed or destroyed by proper processing (see Chapter 18).

Of probably greater importance is the possibility of toxins—such as mycotoxins, pesticides, or other toxins—being inadvertently carried along in the food chain by improperly processed or stored fats.

Fats used over and over in cooking or frying may also develop toxic substances. *Rancidity* is a chemical reaction in fat caused by oxidation hastened by heating, storage, or lack of antioxidants such as vitamin E. Mildly rancid fats are not particularly toxic but are distasteful to most of us. In some cultures, small amounts of rancid fats are considered desirable.

Table 4–3 CONTRIBUTION OF MAJOR FOOD GROUPS TO FAT SUPPLIES AVAILABLE FOR U.S. CONSUMPTION, 1978*

Food	*Percent*
Meat (including pork fat cuts), poultry, and fish	32.9
Eggs	4.0
Dairy products, excluding butter	16.6
Fats and oils, including butter	39.5
Citrus fruits	.1
Other fruits	.3
Potatoes and sweet potatoes	.1
Dark green and deep yellow vegetables	—†
Other vegetables, including tomatoes	.4
Dry beans and peas, nuts, soy flour and grits	3.3
Flour and cereal products	1.6
Sugar and other sweeteners	0
Miscellaneous‡	1.4

*From *National Food Review*, U.S. Department of Agriculture, Economics, Statistics, and Cooperative Services, Jan. 1978.

†Less than 0.05 percent.

‡Chocolate liquor equivalent of cocoa beans.

QUESTIONS AND PROBLEMS

1. What physical properties are characteristic of fats? What substances does any true fat yield on hydrolysis (in digestion or outside the body)? Consult the diagrams in Figure 4–1 as to the chemical elements and structure of glycerol and fatty acids. How many molecules of fatty acid does a molecule of glycerol link up with to form one molecule of fat? Do the fatty acids most commonly found in fats consist of long or short chains of carbon atoms? Is the proportion of carbon to the amount of hydrogen and oxygen greater or less in a molecule of fatty acid than in a molecule of glucose? How does this account for the fact that, when fats are burned or oxidized in body tissues, they yield more than twice as much energy as carbohydrates do?

2. What is the difference between a saturated and an unsaturated fatty acid (consult Fig. 4–1)? What is the difference between a *mono*unsaturated and a *poly*unsaturated fatty acid? Is oleic acid a polyunsaturated fatty acid? What is the name of the polyunsaturated fatty acid found most abundantly in fatty foods? How do the kinds of fatty acids (saturated or unsaturated) that predominate determine the consistency (solid, semisolid, or liquid) of foods that are almost pure fat? Name two fatty foods that are solid and two that are liquid.

3. What is meant by an essential fatty acid? What symptoms sometimes occur in infants because of insufficient essential fatty acids in their foods? Does essential fatty acid deficiency ever occur in adults on normal diets? Why? If one wished to increase the intake of polyunsaturated fatty acids, what foods should be included in moderate amounts in the diet?

4. How can unsaturated fatty acids be made to take on more hydrogen—that is, be converted into saturated ones? Does butter carry any unsaturated fatty acids? When a fluid fat such as corn or cottonseed oil is converted to a semisolid by hydrogenation to make cooking fats or margarine, are all the unsaturated fatty acids converted to saturated ones? Consult Table 4–1 and compare the content of unsaturated fatty acids in butter and the various types of margarine.

5. Define lipids, true fats, phospholipids, and sterols. In what body tissues are phospholipids most abundant? What sterol is found in animal tissues and blood? Can it be formed in the body, and if so, where? Is the level of cholesterol in the blood closely related to the amount of it ingested? Does the intake of total calories, the proportion of the caloric intake furnished by fats, or the ratio of saturated to polyunsaturated fats in the diet influence blood cholesterol level? If so, with what results in each case?

6. What are the chief uses of fats in the body? Of fatty foods in the diet? What percentage of the total caloric (fuel) intake is furnished by fats in the average American diet? What are the disadvantages of too high a level of fat in the diet or of very low fat intake? What special foods would you avoid or take in smaller amounts in order to decrease the relative amount of fat in the diet?

REFERENCES

1. McCollum, E. V.: *A History of Nutrition*. Boston, Houghton Mifflin Co., 1957, Chapter 3.
2. McCay, C. M.: *Notes on the History of Nutrition Research*. Vienna, Hans Huber, 1973, pp. 34–57.
3. Burr, G. O., and Burr, M. M.: A new deficiency disease produced by the rigid exclusion of fat from the diet. J. Biol. Chem., *82*:345, 1929 (reprinted in Nutr. Rev., *32*:19, 1974; Burr, G. O., and Burr, M. M.: On the nature and role of the fatty acids essential in nutrition. J. Biol. Chem., *86*:587, 1930. Burr, G. O., and Burr, M. M.: Fed. Proc., *1*:224, 1942.
4. Hansen, A. E.: Serum lipids in eczema and other pathological conditions. Amer. J. Dis. Child., *53*:933, 1937; Hansen, A. E., et al.: Role of linoleic acid in infant nutrition. Pediatrics, *31*:171, 1963.
5. Holman, R. T., et al.: The essential fatty acid requirement of infants and assessment of their dietary intake of linoleate. Amer. J. Clin. Med., *14*:70, 1964.
6. Food and Nutrition Board: *Recommended Dietary Allowances*. 8th Ed. Washington, D.C., National Research Council, National Academy of Sciences, 1974, pp. 33–36, 49–50. (Also see 9th Ed., to be published in 1979.)
7. Wiese, H. F., Gibbs, R. H., and Hansen, A. E.: Essential fatty acids in human nutrition, I and II. J. Nutr., *52*:355 and 367, 1954; and Wiese, H. F., Hansen, A. E., and Adams, D. J. D.: Essential fatty acids in human nutrition. J. Nutr., *66*:345, 1955.
8. Food and Nutrition Board: *Dietary Fat and Human Health*. Washington, D.C., National Academy of Sciences, Pub. 1147, 1966.
9. Walker, M. A., and Page, L.: Nutritive content of college meals. II. Lipids. J. Amer. Dietet. Assoc., *68*:34, 1976.
10. von Euler, U. S., and Eliasson, R.: *Prostaglandins*. New York, Academic Press, 1967; Pickles, V. R.: Prostaglandins, Nature, *224*:221, 1969. (Also see separate list of readings.)

SUPPLEMENTARY READING

General: Books and Reviews

Coniglio, J. G., et al.: Symposium: Essential fatty acids. Fed. Proc., *31*:1429, 1972.

Galli, C., Jacini, G., and Pecile, A. (eds.): *Dietary Lipids and Postnatal Development*. New York, Raven Press, 1973.

IUPAC-IUB Commission on Biochemical Nomenclature: The nomenclature of lipids. Lipids, *12*:455, 1977.

Kunau, W-H., and Holman, R. T., (eds.): *Polyunsaturated Fatty Acids*. Champaign, Ill., Amer. Oil Chem. Soc. Monograph 4, 1977.

Lech, J. J.: Symposium: Control of endogenous triglyceride metabolism in adipose tissue and muscle. Fed. Proc., *36*:1984, 1977.

National Academy of Sciences: *Fat Content and Composition of Animal Products*. Washington, D.C., 1976.

Perkins, E. G., and Witting, L. A. (eds.): *Modification of Lipid Metabolism*. New York, Academic Press, 1975.

Rice, E. E., Chmn.: Symposium: Status of fat in food and nutrition. J. Amer. Oil Chem. Soc., *51*:244, 1974.

Symposium: Lipid metabolism and its control. Nutr. Soc. U.K. Proc. Nutr. Soc., *34*:203, 1975.

Vergroesen, A. J. (ed.): *The Role of Fats in Human Nutrition*. New York, Academic Press, 1975.

Vranic, M., Chairman: Symposium: Turnover of free fatty acids and triglyceride. Fed. Proc., *34*:2233, 1975.

Fats in Foods: Composition

Anderson, B. A., et al.: Comprehensive evaluation of fatty acids in foods.
- I. Dairy products. J. Amer. Dietet. Assoc., *66*:482, 1975.
- II. Beef products. J. Amer. Dietet. Assoc., *67*:35, 1975.
- III. Eggs and egg products. J. Amer. Dietet. Assoc., *67*:111, 1975.
- IV. Nuts, peanuts, and soups. J. Amer. Dietet. Assoc., *67*:351, 1975.
- V. Unhydrogenated fats and oils. J. Amer. Dietet. Assoc., *68*:224, 1976.
- VI. Cereal products. J. Amer. Dietet. Assoc., *68*:335, 1976.
- VII. Pork products. J. Amer. Dietet. Assoc., *69*:44, 1976.
- VIII. Finfish. J. Amer. Dietet. Assoc., *69*:243, 1976.
- IX. Fowl. J. Amer. Dietet. Assoc., *69*:517, 1976.
- X. Lamb and veal. J. Amer. Dietet. Assoc., *70*:53, 1977.

Brown, H. B., et al.: Polyunsaturated meat and dairy products in fat-modified food patterns for hyperlipidemia. J. Amer. Dietet. Assoc., *69*:235, 1976.

Carpenter, D. L., et al.: Lipid composition of selected vegetable oils. J. Amer. Oil Chem. Soc., *53*:713, 1976.

Consumers Union: Cooking oils and fats. Cons. Rpts., Sept. 1973, p. 553.

Feeley, R. M., Criner, P. E., and Slover, H. T.: Major fatty acids and proximate composition of dairy products. J. Amer. Dietet. Assoc., *66*:140, 1975.

Lacroix, D. E., Mattingly, W. A., Wong, N. P., and Alford, J. A.: Cholesterol, fat, and protein in dairy products. J. Amer. Dietet. Assoc., *62*:275, 1973.

Nazir, D. J., Moorecroft, B. J., and Mishkel, M. A.: Fatty acid composition of margarines. Amer. J. Clin. Nutr., *29*:331, 1976.

Tracey, M. V.: Altering fatty acid composition of ruminant products. Cereal Foods World, *20*:77, 1975.

U.S. Department of Agriculture: *Nutritive Value of American Foods in Common Units*. Agricultural Handbook 456, Agric. Res. Service, Washington, D.C., 1975. (Also see U.S.D.A. Handbook 8, Composition of Foods, 1963. Revisions of portions of this have started to be available in 1977.)

Walker, M. A., and Page, L.: Nutritive content of

college meals. J. Amer. Dietet. Assoc., *68*:34, 1976.

Weihrauch, J. L., Posati, L. P., Anderson, B. A., and Epler, J.: Lipid conversion factors for calculating fatty acid contents of foods. J. Amer. Oil Chem. Soc., *54*:36, 1977.

Fat: Digestion, Absorption

Clement, J.: Nature and importance of endogenous fatty acids during intestinal absorption of fats. World Rev. Nutr. Dietet., *21*:281, 1975.

Hamosh, M., Klaeveman, H. L., Wolf, R. O., and Snow, R. O.: Pharyngeal lipase and digestion of dietary triglyceride in man. J. Clin. Invest., *55*: 908, 1975.

Hofmann, A. F., et al.: Symposium: Gastroenterology: physical events in lipid digestion and absorption. Fed. Proc., *29*:1317, 1970.

Holt, P. R.: The roles of bile acids during the process of normal fat and cholesterol absorption. Arch. Intern. Med., *130*:574, 1972.

Mansbach, C. M.: Conditions affecting the biosynthesis of lipids in the small intestine. Amer. J. Clin. Nutr., *29*:295, 1976.

Prottey, C., Hartop, P. J., and Press, M.: Correction of the cutaneous manifestations of essential fatty acid deficiency in man by application of sunflower-seed oil to the skin. J. Invest. Dermatol., *64*:228, 1975.

Schmitt, M. G., Soergel, K. H., and Wood, C. M.: Absorption of short chain fatty acids from the human jejunum. Gastroenterology, *70*:211, 1976.

Essential Fatty Acids: Deficiency and Metabolism

Cuthbertson, W. F. J.: Essential fatty acid requirements in infancy. Amer. J. Clin. Nutr., *29*:559, 1976.

Fleischman, A. I., et al.: Beneficial effect of increased dietary linoleate upon in vivo platelet function in man. J. Nutr., *105*:1286, 1975.

Fleming, C. R., Smith, L. M., and Hodges, R. E.: Essential fatty acid deficiency in adults receiving parenteral nutrition. Amer. J. Clin. Nutr., *29*:976, 1976.

Friedman, Z., et al.: Rapid onset of essential fatty acid deficiency in the newborn. Pediatrics, *58*:640, 1976.

Lamptey, M. S., and Walker, B. L.: A possible essential role for dietary linolenic acid in the development of the young rat. J. Nutr., *106*:86, 1976.

Privett, O. S., et al.: Studies of effects of trans fatty acids in the diet on lipid metabolism in essential fatty acid deficient rats. Amer. J. Clin. Nutr., *30*:1009, 1977.

Richardson, T. J., and Sgoutas, D.: Essential fatty acid deficiency in four adult patients during total parenteral nutrition. Amer. J. Clin. Nutr., *28*:258, 1975.

Vergroesen, A. J.: Physiological effects of dietary linoleic acid. Nutr. Rev., *35*:1, 1977.

Williams, M. A., et al.: Hydrogenated coconut oil and tissue fatty acids in EFA-depleted and EFA-supplemented rats. J. Nutr., *102*:847, 1972.

Arachidonic Acid: Prostaglandins

Goldberg, V. J., and Ramwell, P. W.: Role of prostaglandins in reproduction. Physiol. Rev., *55*:325, 1975.

Horton, E. W., and Poyser, N. L.: Uterine luteolytic hormone: a physiological role of prostaglandin $F_{2}\alpha$. Physiol. Rev., *56*:595, 1976.

Lee, J. B., Patak, R. V., and Mookerjee, B. K.: Renal prostaglandins and the regulation of blood pressure and sodium and water homeostasis. Amer. J. Med., *60*:798, 1976.

MacDonald, P. C., et al.: Initiation of human parturition. I. Mechanism of action of arachidonic acid. Obstet Gynecol., *44*:629, 1974.

Marx, J.: Blood clotting: the role of the prostaglandins. Science, *196*:1072, 1977.

Needleman, P., and Kaley, G.: Cardiac and coronary prostaglandin synthesis and function. N. Engl. J. Med., *298*:1122, 1978.

Ramwell, P. W., Leovey, E. M. K., and Sintetos, A. L.: Regulation of the arachidonic acid cascade. Biol. Reprod., *16*:70, 1977.

Rivers, J. P. W., et al.: Inability of the cat to desaturate essential fatty acids. Nature, *258*:171, 1975.

Seyberth, H. W., et al.: Prostaglandins as mediators of hypercalcemia associated with certain types of cancer. N. Engl. J. Med., *293*:1278, 1975.

Weeks, J. R., et al.: Symposium: Prostaglandins. Fed. Proc., *33*:37, 1974.

Sterols: Dietary Cholesterol

Feeley, R. M., Criner, P. E., and Watt, B. K.: Cholesterol content of foods. J. Amer. Dietet. Assoc., *61*:134, 1972.

Green, M. H., et al.: Cholesterol turnover and tissue distribution in the guinea pig in response to dietary cholesterol. J. Nutr., *106*:515, 1976.

Itoh, T., Tamura, T., and Matsumoto, T.: Sterol composition of 19 vegetable oils. J. Amer. Oil Chem. Soc., *50*:122, 1973.

Mellies, M., et al.: Plasma and dietary phytosterols in children. Pediatrics, *57*:60, 1976.

Potter, J. M., and Nestel, P. J.: The effects of dietary fatty acids and cholesterol on the milk lipids of lactating women and the plasma cholesterol of breast-fed infants. Amer. J. Clin. Nutr., *29*:54, 1976.

Reiser, R.: Fat has less cholesterol than lean. J. Nutr., *105*:15, 1975.

Slater, G., et al.: Plasma cholesterol and triglycerides in men with added eggs in the diet. Nutr. Rpts. Internatl., *14*:249, 1976.

Subbiah, M. T. R.: Dietary plant sterols: current status in human and animal sterol metabolism. Amer. J. Clin. Nutr., *26*:219, 1973.

Tanaka, N., and Portman, D. W.: Effect of type of dietary fat and cholesterol on cholesterol absorption rate in squirrel monkeys. J. Nutr., *107*:814, 1977.

Weihrauch, J. L., and Gardner, J. M.: Sterol content of foods of plant origin. J. Amer. Dietet. Assoc., *73*: 39, 1978.

Cardiovascular Diseases: Serum Lipids, Saturated Fats

Anderson, J. T.: Independence of the effects of cholesterol and degree of saturation of the fat in the diet on serum cholesterol in man. Amer. J. Clin. Nutr., *29*:1184, 1976.

Bruce, T. C., et al.: Serum cholesterol levels of Seventh-Day Adventists. Arterial Wall *III*:175, 1976.

Diet, energy balance, and genes — and serum cholesterol. Brit. Med. J., *6064*:789, 1977.

Hill, P., and Wynder, E. L.: Dietary regulation of serum lipids in healthy, young adults. Research, *68*:25, 1976.

Kummerow, F. A., et al.: The influence of egg consumption on the serum cholesterol level in human subjects. Amer. J. Clin. Nutr., *30*:664, 1977.

Margolis, S.: Treatment of Hyperlipemia. J.A.M.A., *239*:2696, 1978.

Mattson, F. H.: Effect of hydrogenated fat on the plasma cholesterol and triglyceride levels of man. Amer. J. Clin. Nutr., *28*:726, 1975.

Nestel, P. J., and Poyser, A.: Changes in cholesterol synthesis and excretion when cholesterol intake is increased. Metabolism, *25*:1591, 1976.

Nichols, A. B., Ravenscroft, C., Lamphiear, D. E., and Ostrander, L. D.: Independence of serum lipid levels and dietary habits: the Tecumseh study. J.A.M.A., *236*:1948, 1976.

Porter, M. W., Yamanaka, W., Carlson, S. D., and Fly, M. A.: Effect of dietary egg on serum cholesterol and triglyceride of human males. Amer. J. Clin. Nutr., *30*:490, 1977.

Reiser, R.: Saturated fat in the diet and serum cholesterol concentration: A critical examination of the literature. Amer. J. Clin. Nutr., *26*:524, 1973.

Sacks, F. M., et al.: Plasma lipids and lipoproteins in vegetarians and controls. N. Engl. J. Med., *292*:1148, 1975.

Shaper, A. G., and Marr, J. W.: Dietary recommendations for the community toward the postponement of coronary heart disease. Brit. Med. J., *1*:867, 1977.

Slater, G., et al.: Plasma cholesterol and triglycerides in men with added eggs in the diet. Nutr. Rpts. Internatl., *14*:249, 1976.

Truswell, A. S.: Diet and plasma lipids—a reappraisal. Amer. J. Clin. Nutr., *31*:977, 1978.

Walker, W. J.: Changing United States life-style and declining vascular mortality: cause or coincidence? N. Engl. J. Med., *297*:163, 1977.

Wright, I. S.: Correct levels of serum cholesterol: average vs. normal vs. optimal. J.A.M.A., *236*:261, 1976.

Fat Toxicity: Cancer, Contaminants

Alfin-Slater, R. B., Wells, P., and Aftergood, L.: Dietary fat composition and tocopherol requirement: IV. Safety of polyunsaturated fats. J. Amer. Oil Chem. Soc., *50*:479, 1973.

Andia, A. M. G., and Street, J. C.: Dietary induction of hepatic microsomal enzymes by thermally oxidized fats. J. Agr. Food Chem., *23*:173, 1975.

Chan, P-C., Didato, F., and Cohen, L. A.: High dietary fat, elevation of rat serum prolactin and mammary cancer. Proc. Soc. Exp. Biol. Med., *149*:133, 1975.

Cutler, M. G., and Schneider, R.: Malformations produced in mice and rats by oxidized linoleate. Food Cosmet. Toxicol., *11*:935, 1973.

Hara, I., and Kaunitz, H., Chairmen: Symposium: Biological significance of autoxidized and polymerized oils. Lipids, *8*:329, 1973.

Heyden, S.: Polyunsaturated fatty acids and colon cancer. Nutr. Metab., *17*:321, 1974.

Hsieh, A., and Perkins, E. G.: Nutrition and metabolic studies of methyl esters of dimeric fatty acids in the rat. Lipids, *11*:763, 1976.

Kantorowitz, B., and Yannai, S.: Comparison of the tendencies of liquid and hardened soybean oils to form physiologically undesirable materials under simulated frying conditions. Nutr. Rpts. Internatl., *9*:331, 1974.

Kilgore, L., and Windham, F.: Degradation of linoleic acid in deep-fried potatoes. J. Amer. Dietet. Assoc., *63*:525, 1973.

Miller, J., and Landes, D. R.: Effects of feeding oxidized or heated soybean oil on tissue composition and hematological status of rats. J. Food Sci., *40*:545, 1975.

Nolen, G. A.: A feeding study of a used, partially hydrogenated soybean oil, frying fat in dogs. J. Nutr., *103*:1248, 1973.

Reddy, B. S., et al.: Effect of quality and quantity of dietary fat and dimethylhydrazine in colon carcinogenesis in rats. Proc. Soc. Exp. Biol. Med., *151*:237, 1976.

Wilson, R. B., Hutcheson, D. P., and Wideman, L.: Dimethylhydrazine-induced colon tumors in rats fed diets containing beef fat or corn oil with and without wheat bran. Amer. J. Clin. Nutr., *30*:176, 1977.

Wood, R.: Hepatoma, host liver, and normal rat liver phospholipids as affected by diet. Lipids, *10*:736, 1975.

Other Readings: General

Caster, W. O., et al.: Effect of essential and nonessential fatty acids in complex mixture on fatty acid composition of liver lipids. J. Nutr., *106*:1809, 1976.

Clandinin, M. T.: The role of dietary long chain fatty acids in mitochondrial structure and function. J. Nutr., *108*:273, 1978.

Hirono, H., *et al.*: Essential fatty acid deficiency induced by total parenteral nutrition and by medium-chain triglyceride feeding. Amer. J. Clin. Nutr., *30*:1670, 1977.

Ho, K-J. et al.: Alaskan Arctic Eskimo: responses to a customary high fat diet. Amer. J. Clin. Nutr., *25*:737, 1972.

Kummerow, F. A.: Current studies on relation of fat to health. J. Amer. Oil Chem. Soc., *51*:255, 1974.

Marshall, M. W., et al.: Changes in lactate dehydrogenase, LDH isoenzymes, lactate, and pyruvate as a result of feeding low fat diets to healthy men and women. Metabolism, *25*:169, 1976.

Rai, R. M., et al.: Utilization of different quantities of fat at high altitude. Amer. J. Clin. Nutr., *28*:242, 1975.

Schrock, C. G., and Connor, W. E.: Incorporation of the dietary trans fatty acid (C18:1) into the serum lipids, the serum lipoproteins and adipose tissue. Amer. J. Clin. Nutr., *28*:1020, 1975.

Tollenaar, D.: Dietary fat level as affecting running performance and other performance-related parameters of rats restricted or non-restricted in food intake. J. Nutr., *106*:1539, 1976.

Volpe, J. J., and Vagelos, P. R.: Mechanisms and regulation of biosynthesis of saturated fatty acids. Physiol. Rev., *56*:339, 1976.

Whorton, A. R., and Coniglio, J. G.: Fatty acid synthesis in testes of fat-deficient and fat-supplemented rats. J. Nutr., *107*:79, 1977.

Articles in Nutrition Reviews

The effect of diet on lipid metabolism. *29*:36, 1971.

Dietary cholesterol versus total body cholesterol. *29*:199, 1971.

Rat brain fatty acids in essential fatty acid deficiency. *30*:18, 1972.

Composition of human fat from different sites. *30*:40, 1972.

Exogenous fatty acids and triglyceride production in rat liver. *30*:116, 1972.

Effect of unsaturated fatty acid composition on lecithin-cholesterol interactions. *30*:216, 1972.

Diet and coronary heart disease—a joint statement. *30*:223, 1972.

A cytoplasmic protein which binds fatty acids. *30*:255, 1972.

Tissue biosynthesis of prostaglandins. *31*:24, 1973.

Fat controlled diet and mortality from coronary heart disease. *31*:79, 1973.

Dietary effect on liver fatty acid synthetase. *31*:96, 1973.

Nutrition and the pathology of atherosclerosis in monkeys. *31*:100, 1973.

Utilization of linoleic acid by the rat fetus. *31*:103, 1973.

Polyunsaturated ruminants. *31*:209, 1973.

Glucose ingestion and the control of lipogenesis. *31*:287, 1973.

Fat-free parenteral alimentation of infants. *32*:134, 1974.

Essential fatty acid deficiency and the photoreceptors of rat retina. *32*:342, 1974.

Pharyngeal lipase activity in man. *33*:205, 1975.

Growth and cerebral lipid composition in rats fed linoleate and linolenate. *33*:278, 1975.

EFA deficiency in continuous-drip alimentation. *33*:329, 1975.

Lipid peroxidation and gluthathione peroxidase in the liver of cholesterol-fed rats. *34*:50, 1976.

MCT absorption by preterm infants. *34*:71, 1976.

Cholesterol feeding affects microsomal metabolism of steroids. *34*:88, 1976.

A review of the biological function of taurine. *34*:161, 1976.

Factors influencing the size, composition, and metabolism of very low density lipoproteins in the rat. *34*:214, 1976.

Prevention of coronary heart disease. *34*:220, 1976.

Dietary essential fatty acids, prostaglandin formation and platelet aggregation. *34*:243, 1976.

Physiological effects of dietary linoleic acid. *35*:1, 1977.

Essential fatty acid restriction and turnover of retinal rod discs. *35*:20, 1977.

Essential fatty acids and water permeability. *35*:303, 1977.

Some present concepts concerning diet and prevention of coronary heart disease. *36*:194, 1978.

Chapter 5

Protein and Amino Acids

As the name "protein" — meaning "to come first" — suggests, protein was recognized very early in the history of nutrition as being not only an energy source but an essential nutrient as well. We now know that some fatty acids are essential in the diet and that some carbohydrate is desirable, if not absolutely essential, and we recognize a dietary requirement for about 35 vitamins and minerals. Yet the notion of the primacy of protein persists. Protein-rich foods are generally preferred and command a large share of any food budget; and in part this is logical, because natural protein-rich foods are excellent sources of most of the essential nutrients. What accounts for this association of protein and other nutritional factors is that proteins play a vital part in the structural and functional characteristics of every cell in all living tissues, plant and animal. Protein, in a myriad of forms, makes up more than half of all the organic matter in the human body.

Living tissues contain proteins that are peculiar to themselves and that are present in varying amounts according to the types of tissues. The outer layers of skin, the hair, wool and feathers, and nails and horns consist almost entirely of an insoluble protein called *keratin*. The most active and abundant tissues of the animal body — the organs and muscles — are very high in protein content. Muscle contains about 70 percent water, but even on a moist basis, lean skeletal muscle and heart contain about 20 percent of the proteins *myosin, actin,* and *myoglobin,* by far the most abundant solid constituents of muscles. Blood carries the important iron-containing protein *hemoglobin* in red cells and several proteins in the fluid (plasma) portion, including *albumin* and others that transport fatty substances, minerals, and so forth. The red marrow of bones is rich in protein, and even adipose tissue, which acts chiefly as a storage depot for excess fat, has some protein. Protein is stored in eggs to provide for the growth of all these tissues in the young bird. Plants similarly store protein in the seed, and the most metabolically active part of a plant, its leaf, also has a relatively high level of protein. (On a dry weight basis, spinach is about 40 percent protein, soybeans are 35 percent protein, eggs are about 50 percent protein, and lean meat and fish are about 75 percent protein.) Enzymes and many hormones are proteins, and modern theory suggests that every time we learn a new fact we synthesize a new protein.

Proteins are composed of larger and more complex molecules than those of either fats or carbohydrates, and they are the only class of energy nutrients that contain *nitrogen* (in addition to carbon, hydrogen, and oxygen). Most also contain sulfur, and many contain phosphorus, iron, or other minerals. The large molecules of the proteins are made up of great numbers of relatively simple units, the nitrogen-containing compounds called *amino acids*. These basic units all contain at least one organic acid radical (the carboxyl group, COOH) and one amino radical (NH_2) in a typical structure

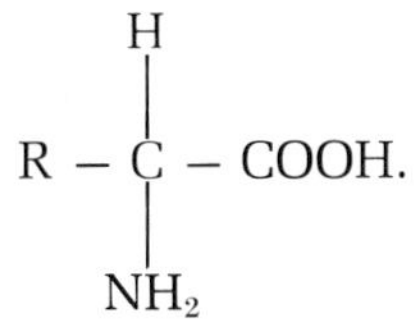

$$R - \overset{\displaystyle H}{\underset{\displaystyle NH_2}{\overset{|}{\underset{|}{C}}}} - COOH.$$

R may be a chain of different lengths or a ring structure, or simply another H, in which case the amino acid (CH_2NH_2COOH) is *glycine*.* A few amino acids contain two acid or two amino groups, and a few amino acids include sulfur in their structures.

Considering all forms of life, it is the element *nitrogen*†, rather than protein, that is indispensable for life, for plants can use the simple nitrogen-containing inorganic compounds in the soil, such as nitrates, to build their own special kinds of protein. Some bacteria can even utilize gaseous nitrogen (N_2) from the air. Animals, however, cannot utilize the simpler sources of nitrogen for the synthesis of proteins, but must get their amino groups preformed, directly from plant foods, from single-celled organisms, or from the proteins in the milk, eggs, or body tissues of other animals. The animal converts the amino acids, which enter the tissues as products of protein digestion, into the special proteins and other nitrogen-containing compounds needed for maintenance of tissues and life processes. The final end-products of protein metabolism in the animal's tissues are simpler compounds that plants can use to build into amino acids and protein. The nitrogen cycle is complete if the excreta of animals and the products of the decay of both plants and animals, which contain nitrates and ammonium compounds, are returned to the soil.

Some 22 different amino acids are known to be present fairly commonly in proteins that occur in nature. The number of different amino acids in the molecules of individual proteins varies from 8 to 18. These amino acids are arranged in an intricate pattern characteristic of each individual protein. Because not only the kinds of amino acids may vary but also the relative quantities of each and their arrangement and sequence, the number of individual proteins that are possible is almost infinite. The molecules of protein are so large that their molecular weight varies from several thousand up to several million.

The manner in which the amino acids link together to form proteins is common to all proteins. This is called *peptide linkage*. Since each amino acid carries a terminal acid group (COOH) and an amino group (NH_2) attached to the carbon atom next to the acid group, the basic amino group of one molecule can react with the acid group of another, linking up by the loss of one hydrogen (H) atom and one OH radical, with the formation of a molecule of water, thus:

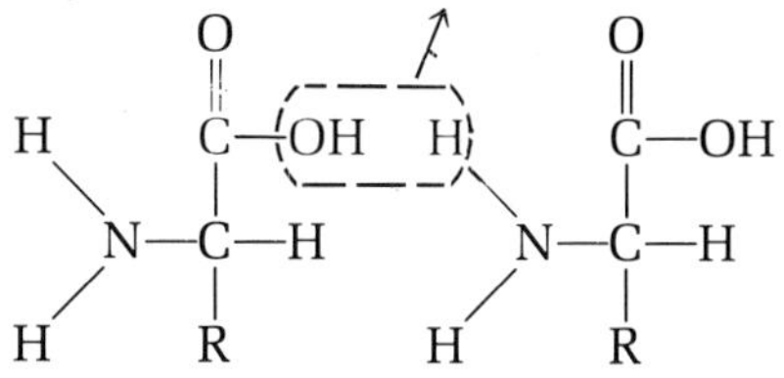

$$\underset{H}{\overset{H}{>}}N-\underset{R}{\overset{O=C-OH}{C}}-H \quad + \quad \underset{H}{\overset{H}{>}}N-\underset{R}{\overset{O=C-OH}{C}}-H$$

When proteins are broken down, as happens in digestion, by reaction with water (hydrolysis) the components of water (H and OH) lost when the peptide link was formed are restored to the individual

*Glycine is known technically as amino acetic acid because its parent compound is CH_3COOH, acetic acid, the sour principle of vinegar. Glycine, on the other hand, is very sweet (see Chapter 3), and its common name comes from the Greek word *glykys*, meaning "*sweet*."

†Discovery of the element nitrogen is usually credited to a British physician. Daniel Rutherford (1772); actually three other men working at about the same time each found it independently. Two were English—Priestly and Cavendish—and the other, Scheele, was Swedish. The French chemist Chapal proposed the name *nitrogène* (1790) (Greek *nitron*) because the gas was generated in reactions involving saltpeter.

amino acids, the peptide linkage is broken, and the protein molecule is broken down into the amino acids from which it was originally formed. Proteins must first be resolved into their constituent amino acids by digestion before they can be absorbed into the blood, and when they are thus carried to the tissues, each tissue utilizes the specific amino acids required to build its own characteristic proteins.

Chemical Classification of Proteins

Proteins are divided into two main categories, simple and conjugated. *Simple proteins* contain only amino acids or their derivatives, while *conjugated proteins* are linked to some nonprotein substance. The simple proteins are subdivided according to their solubility and other properties. The most common ones are:

Albumins: soluble in water, coagulated by heat; e.g., plasma albumin, lactalbumin in milk, egg albumin in egg white.

Globulins: soluble in dilute salt solutions but not in water, coagulated by heat; e.g., myosin in muscle.

Glutelins: soluble in dilute alkali and acid but not in dilute salt solution or water, coagulated by heat; abundant in cereal grains, e.g., wheat glutenin.

Prolamins: soluble in 70 percent alcohol but not in other aqueous solutions; common in cereal grains, e.g., gliadin in wheat, zein in maize corn.

Scleroproteins (albuminoids): insoluble in the common solvents, including alcohol, resistant to digestive enzymes; common in supporting tissues, e.g., collagen, elastin, keratin.

Conjugated proteins are subdivided according to their nonprotein component. Protein molecules may be conjugated with *fat* (lipoproteins in the blood) or *carbohydrate* (glycoproteins, such as are found in the mucus secreted into the digestive tract). Other important conjugated proteins are formed by linkage with *phosphoric acid* (phosphoproteins; milk protein casein is one example); with the lipid *lecithin* (fibrin in clotted blood, vitellin in egg yolk); with an *iron-containing* compound (heme) to form the oxygen-carrying substance *hemoglobin* in the blood; and with *nucleic acid* to form nucleoproteins, which are essential components of cell nuclei and protoplasm.

Amino Acids, Essential and Nonessential

Certain amino acids are known to be *essential* — that is, they must be provided preformed in the food. In reality, all amino acids are essential for the building and upkeep of body tissues, but more than half the number needed can be made in the body. Hence, an amino acid is referred to as *nutritionally essential* or *indispensable* only if it cannot be synthesized in the body out of materials ordinarily available, at a speed that will supply the demands for normal growth. Rose and coworkers at the University of Illinois found that ten different amino acids must be supplied in adequate amounts in the food to support normal growth in young rats, whereas his evidence indicated that only eight of these were essential for maintenance of nitrogen equilibrium in fully grown young men.[1] Subsequently it was shown that a ninth amino acid (histidine) is essential to human infants and, in longer term studies, to adults as well.

An amino acid is nonessential (dispensable from the diet) if its carbon skeleton can be formed in the body, and if an amino group can be transferred to it from some donor compound available, a process called transamination. In the nonessential amino acid *alanine*, the radical represented by R in the typical amino acid formula $RCHNH_2COOH$ is simply CH_3. The body can make this amino acid readily in any amount needed because the carbon chain is a common metabolic product to which the amino group from another common nonessential amino acid, *glutamic acid*, can be added. In *phenylalanine* R represents a ring, or cyclic group called phenyl radical, consisting of six carbon atoms joined in a hexagonal ring with hydrogens attached (C_6H_5) (Fig. 5–1). The carbon skeleton cannot be formed in the human body, so phenylalanine (like several other amino acids) cannot be manufactured but must be supplied preformed in the food. Two other amino acids, *lysine*

$CH_3CH(NH_2)COOH$

Alanine

$C_6H_5{-}CH_2CH(NH_2)COOH$

Phenylalanine

$HO{-}C_6H_4{-}CH_2CH(NH_2)COOH$

Tyrosine

Figure 5–1 Structures of a nonessential amino acid, alanine, and of an essential one, phenylalanine. The carbon chain of alanine can be synthesized in the human body, but that of phenylalanine cannot be. However, the body can make the amino acid tyrosine from phenylalanine, by adding a hydroxyl (OH) group. Tyrosine is needed to make several regulatory substances in the body. Tyrosine is classed as a semi-essential amino acid because it can be made only from the essential amino acid phenylalanine; when tyrosine is present in the diet, the need for phenylalanine is reduced.

and *threonine*, are dietary essentials because their carbon skeletons cannot undergo transamination. In all there are nine amino acids that are essential because the body cannot carry out one or another step necessary for their manufacture. These are listed in Table 5–1.*

*The structural formulas of the amino acids commonly found in foods or tissues are given in Table 13 of the Appendix.

The nonessential amino acids *tyrosine* and *cystine* are an intermediate class, between amino acids that can easily be formed from a number of precursors and those that cannot be made at all. Tyrosine can be made only from the essential amino acid phenylalanine, and the reverse reaction does not take place. Part of the need for phenylalanine in the body is to form tyrosine if the latter is not included in the diet. Thus, the presence of tyrosine will reduce the amount of phenylalanine required in the diet. The nonessential sulfur-containing amino acid cystine can be formed from the essential amino acid methionine, and the reaction is not reversible. The cystine needed in the body (to make hair protein, for example) may be supplied in the diet as cystine, or it will be made from methionine if no cystine is eaten.* Thus, cystine will spare the need for methionine.

Other nonessential amino acids (such as alanine and glycine) can be assembled from carbon chains derived from the metabolism of carbohydrates, fats, or proteins, and amino groups taken from amino acids or other amino-containing com-

*There is some evidence that infants do not have the enzymatic machinery to do this at birth but that the liver develops this capability in the first few weeks of life.

Table 5–1 MINIMUM DAILY REQUIREMENTS OF ESSENTIAL AMINO ACIDS AND ESTIMATED AMOUNTS IN THE AVERAGE AMERICAN DIET

	*Requirements, mg/kg body weight/day**					*In U.S. Food Supply, 1970,‡ gm/day*
Essential Amino Acids†	Infants	School Children‡	Adults	Adult, 70 kg	gm/day 58 kg	
Histidine	28	?	?			
Isoleucine	70	30	10	0.7	0.6	5.3
Leucine	161	45	14	1.0	0.8	8.2
Lysine	103	60	12	0.8	0.7	6.7
Methionine						2.1
and cystine	58	27	13	0.9	0.8	3.5
Phenylalanine						4.7
and tyrosine	125	27	14	1.0	0.8	
Threonine	87	35	7	0.5	0.4	4.1
Tryptophan	17	4	3.5	0.2	0.2	1.2
Valine	93	33	10	0.7	0.6	5.7

*Values from FAO/WHO[2].

†The other amino acid required by rats, arginine, can be made in the human body, but some question remains as to whether the synthesis rate can always keep up with need.

‡NAS–NRC.[3]

pounds. Proteins of the human body include both the essential and nonessential amino acids in their structure, but the nonessential ones can be manufactured, provided the necessary precursors are available.

Functions of Protein in the Body

Protein is required in the diet to provide essential amino acids and enough additional amino groups to make the dispensable ones. The principal uses for amino acids in the body are:

1. For *building new cells and tissues* in growing children, during pregnancy, in athletic training, and after injury.
2. For *upkeep of tissues* already built and for *manufacture of functional and regulatory substances*, such as blood proteins, enzymes, some hormones.
3. For *milk* formation.
4. For *energy*.

Proteins provide the amino acids from which the bases of the genetic information code are made as well as the substance of the cells. By intensive study of the *nucleoproteins* present in the body cells, scientists have made extremely important discoveries concerning the life processes. Nucleoproteins consist of proteins linked to nucleic acids, complex compounds that in turn may be broken down to yield phosphoric acid, a 5-carbon sugar, and cyclic nitrogenous bases. These nitrogenous bases are not proteins,* but they are made in the body from amino acids. The sugar is either ribose or deoxyribose; accordingly, the two types of nucleic acid are known as *ribonucleic acid* (RNA) and *deoxyribonucleic acid* (DNA).

DNA is found in all cell nuclei and is different for each species (even slightly so for individuals within a species). These differences consist of minor rearrangements of sequences among the nitrogenous bases, which constitute a *code* containing all the information on the heritable characteristics of cells, tissues, organs, and individuals. Only four nitrogenous bases are found in DNA; these are adenine, guanine, thymine, and cytosine. The DNA structure is a long, fibrous molecule with two spiral "backbones," consisting of linked sugar and phosphate groups twined about a common axis, forming a double helix (Fig. 5–2). The nitrogenous bases are attached in these spirals so as to extend inward and approach each other in pairs that are joined by a weak hydrogen bond. Of the four bases, adenine can form a pair only with thymine; guanine only with cytosine. The code by which DNA directs the formation and life processes of various cells consists in variations in the kinds and sequences of these pairs.

Ribonucleic acid (RNA) is the messenger that transmits the coded information of DNA. RNA is similar to DNA in structure but differs in two respects — the sugar in the spiral chains is ribose (instead of deoxyribose), and a different nitrogenous base, uracil, is substituted for thymine. The RNA, formed in the cell nuclei under the direction of DNA, migrates to the surface of granules (ribosomes) in the fluid portion of the cell (cytoplasm) (see Chapter 15). Another type of RNA — *transfer* RNA — picks up certain amino acids from the cytoplasm and transfers these amino acids to the messenger RNA, where they are lined up in proper order to form specific enzymes or cell proteins (Fig. 5–3).

We know the composition and structure of DNA and RNA molecules, but the concepts of how they bring about their effects in the cells are chiefly theoretical and are still being revised.

Building New Tissues. The amount of protein needed for these purposes naturally depends on the extent or rapidity of growth and repair processes. For instance, in the rapidly growing infant, as much as one-third of the dietary protein may be retained for building new tissue. Tissues and organs do not all grow at an even rate, so depending on the stage of growth, limitation of dietary protein may have its greatest effect on the brain, on the muscle mass, on the blood supply, and so on. As growth becomes less rapid, the percentage of the protein intake retained in the body for tissue building becomes less, but a plentiful supply of high-quality protein is necessary throughout the growth

*The nitrogenous bases are classed as purines and pyrimidines according to the nature of the ring.

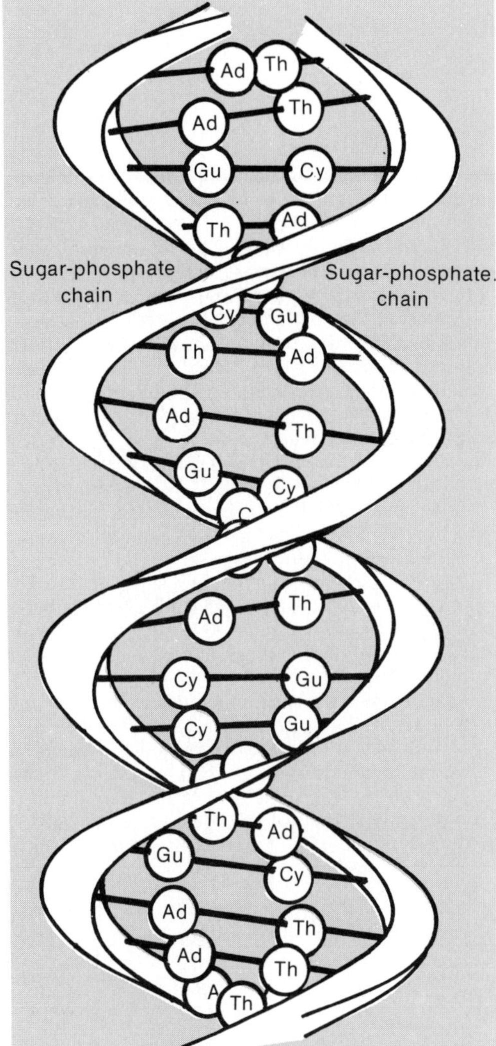

Figure 5–2 The basic building block of life forms on earth is deoxyribonucleic acid, or DNA. It transmits the genetic message of reproduction through the chromosome. The spiral structure of DNA, the Double Helix, was first decoded in 1953 by Francis Crick, James Watson, and Maurice Wilkins. In 1962 these three won the Nobel Prize for physiology and medicine.

Figure 5–2 shows a model of the Double Helix. Only a few of the thousands of turns in the hypothetical DNA molecule are illustrated here. The sugar-phosphate "backbone" is represented by the two ribbons. The third component of the molecule consists of four bases (a base is the nonacid part of a salt) called adenine (Ad), cytosine (Cy), guanine (Gu), and thymine (Th).

period to secure the best possible growth and development. In the later months of pregnancy an extra quota of protein is also needed. Likewise, an athlete in training may require some extra protein for building muscle tissue, because his muscles strengthen and enlarge as a result of exercise.

Excessive destruction of body protein occurs in various periods of stress. Obviously, after severe hemorrhages, extra protein is needed for regeneration of hemoglobin and other blood proteins. Also, after extensive burns, there is excessive loss of protein from the burn surface, as well as need for protein to rebuild damaged skin and muscle tissues. A slow but prolonged loss of nitrogen from extra breakdown of body protein follows bone fractures, and a similar but brief protein loss occurs even after simple surgical operations. Selye's pioneering studies demonstrated that this catabolic reaction of the body to trauma is due to increased output of hormones from the pituitary and adrenal glands.[1] Increased quantities of protein or amino acids are properly given during convalescence, when the metabolic processes become anabolic, to replenish the body protein. A patient who cannot take nourishment by mouth is given intravenous solutions of amino acids (protein hydrolysates), with glucose or emulsified fat added to provide energy and to spare protein.

Maintenance of Structural and Functional Substances. Although the adult does not build new tissues as a child does, there are some tissues that never stop growing, even in the aged. Skin, hair, and nails are obvious examples. The lining of the intestinal tract is renewed about every day and a half; much of this cellular protein is absorbed, but some cells are lost in the fecal matter. Blood cells have a limited life span of 120 days; and if replacement protein is not adequate for formation of new cells and the hemoglobin that they contain, anemia develops. In fact, all the body proteins are constantly being degraded and resynthesized (turning over) at varying rates. So the continuous need for protein to provide for maintenance of tissues already built should not be thought of as due exclusively to death of tissue cells. Functional proteins inside

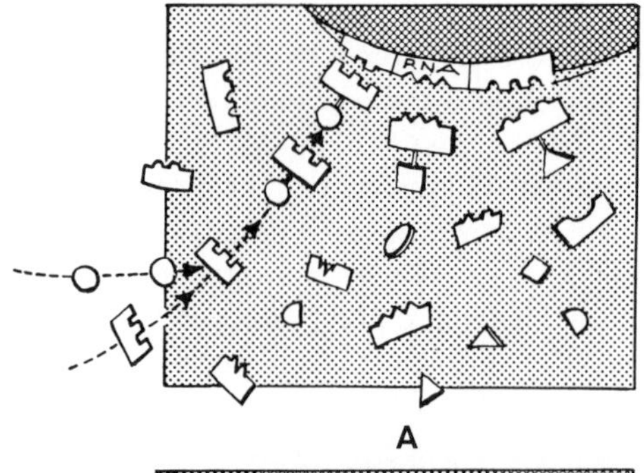

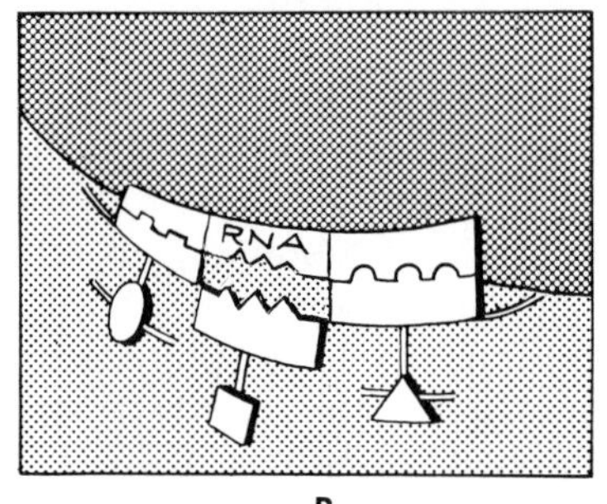

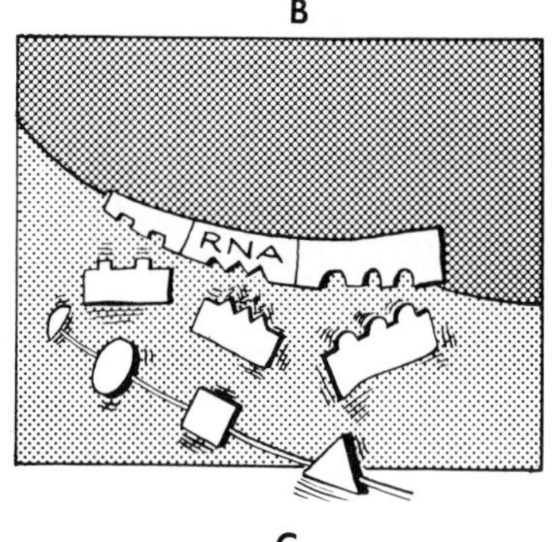

Figure 5–3 Schematic representation of the manner in which RNA functions to bring about synthesis of enzymes and other proteins in the cell. Messenger RNA is made by DNA in the cell nucleus, and then migrates to ribosomes (small, dense particles of cytoplasm outside the nucleus) to whose surface it becomes attached. These three diagrams represent the later stages of protein formation.

A, RNA attached to ribosome (*dark surface*) attracts small sections of another kind of RNA (transfer RNA), each link of which fits into a specific section of the original RNA. Each section of transfer RNA is encoded to attract a specific amino acid from the cytoplasm.

B, The sections of transfer RNA, each carrying a certain amino acid, migrate to the messenger RNA, where they attach themselves in a regular order. The amino acids that the sections of transfer RNA carry are thus brought close together and lined up in a definite order.

C, The amino acids link together and separate from the transfer RNA as a protein chain, thus forming a molecule of some specific protein. The transfer RNA sections are freed from the RNA attached to the ribosome and ready for use in further protein synthesis.

Only a small part of the large molecules of RNA and protein can be shown in the diagrams. The hormone insulin (a relatively simple protein) was the first protein for which the order and arrangement of amino acids is known. In its molecule there are 51 amino acid residues. Myoglobin (a muscle component) consists of an ordered sequence of 153 amino acids and hemoglobin of more than 600 amino acids.

and outside cells continuously turn over in carrying out life processes.

Proteins in the cells are in a state of dynamic equilibrium with the amino acid mixtures (resulting from digestion of protein in foods and catabolism of body proteins) brought to them by the blood and extracellular fluids (Fig. 5–4). The cells transfer some amino acids to the surrounding fluid and take up others from it for utilization in the tissues. This constant flux was discovered by administering

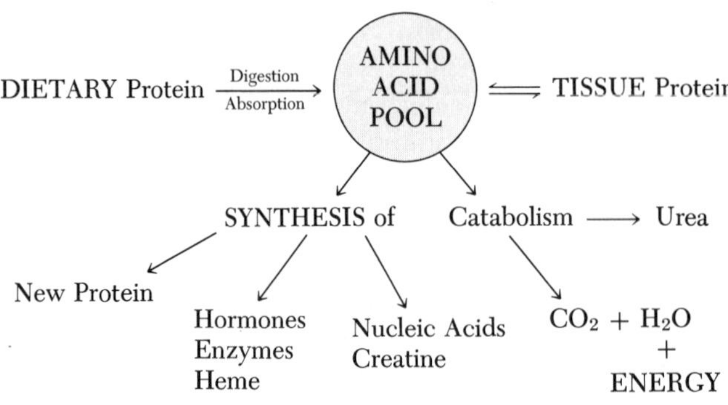

Figure 5–4 Amino acids from food and body tissues enter a common pool, which is drawn upon for synthesis of protein and other compounds or from which amino acids are degraded for energy needs. (From Routh, Eyman and Burton: *Essentials of General, Organic and Biochemistry.* Philadelphia, W. B. Saunders Co., 1977.)

amino acids tagged with nitrogen-15, an isotope of ordinary nitrogen. A good deal of this heavy nitrogen failed to appear in the urine as would have been expected if tissues were static, proving that the labeled amino acids must have been rather freely taken up by tissue cells.[5] Thus, a supply of protein is needed to maintain the body protein pool,* which is indispensable to life.

Proteins in tissue cells and in body fluids, such as the blood, also serve as regulatory substances. Because of their contribution to osmotic pressure, proteins exert an important influence on the exchange of water between tissue cells and the surrounding body fluids, and upon the *water balance* of the body as a whole. For instance, after a prolonged low level of protein intake, the protein content of the blood plasma may be less than normal; under such conditions, extra water is retained in the tissues, which become puffy and swollen, making supply of nutrients to the cells and removal of cellular waste products less efficient. This condition is known as *nutritional edema,* to differentiate it from water accumulation due to disease processes. The ingestion of extra protein sufficient to raise the level of plasma protein to normal is followed by excretion of the excess water by the kidneys and disappearance of the edema. Such retention of extra water in the tissues is often seen in persons who have suffered prolonged undernutrition. A plump-looking malnourished baby is often revealed to be pitifully thin when the refeeding regimen restores normal water distribution and edema disappears.

A second regulatory function of proteins is in maintenance of *acid-base balance* of the blood and tissues. The reaction of blood and tissues is normally maintained very slightly alkaline (pH 7.4) by balance between several different factors, one of which is their protein content. Through the basic amino (NH_2) groups and the organic acid (COOH) radicals present in all amino acids, proteins are able to unite with either acidic or alkaline substances, as these may be taken in or arise in the body from metabolic processes. When these substances are bound by protein, they have little effect on the level of tissue acidity. Considerable amounts of acids formed in metabolism may thus be discharged into the blood stream without any free acid being present to make the reaction of the blood more acid. Hemoglobin and oxyhemoglobin in red cells of the blood also help maintain acid-base equilibrium by forming loose chemical combinations with hydrogen and carbon dioxide from cellular metabolism. (Carbon dioxide in water forms a weak acid, carbonic acid.) Ultimately, carbon dioxide is excreted in expired air.

Smaller but critical amounts of protein are needed for making enzymes* that are essential for digestion and metabolic processes in the tissues. Many potent hormones† are either proteins (e.g., insulin, which is from the pancreas) or smaller peptides (e.g., some of the pituitary and gastrointestinal hormones) or are derived from single amino acids (thyroxine, and epinephrine or adrenaline). The amino acid tyrosine is the precursor from which the pigment of skin and hair is made, which is the reason that in severe protein deficiency dark hair often turns to a pale or reddish color. Tryptophan, tyrosine, glutamic acid, and methionine are direct or indirect precursors of substances in-

*The word "pool" refers to the total amount of a substance present in the body. "Pool" is a concept, rather than a delineated location, mass, or compartment.

*Enzymes are substances formed in living cells that speed up, or catalyze, specific chemical reactions without themselves entering into the reaction. All chemical changes that occur during the digestion of food and in the tissues of the body are brought about through the agency of enzymes, which are themselves proteins.

†Hormones are chemical compounds secreted by the endocrine glands into the blood stream and thus distributed throughout the body. They act to regulate and coordinate body processes or the activity of certain tissues; for example, thyroxine regulates oxidative processes by which body fuel is burned and energy set free (see Chapter 15).

volved in the transmission of messages in the nervous system. The amino acid tryptophan can act as a precursor of niacin, one of the B complex vitamins. The antibodies that help ward off infectious diseases and the substances responsible for clotting of blood are all proteins.

Milk Formation. The proteins of human milk are built by the mammary glands. During lactation a woman needs as much extra protein in the diet as she secretes in her milk plus the amount required for conversion of dietary amino acids to milk protein. This will be discussed in Chapter 20.

Providing Energy. Amino acids are the ultimate precursors from which the nitrogenous base of ATP (adenosine triphosphate, which contains adenine in its structure) is formed, as well as another nitrogenous substance, creatine phosphate, which is present in muscle. These substances are central to the body's energy metabolism (see Chapter 15), but it is not this aspect that is meant in speaking of protein as an energy source. What is referred to in this connection is utilization of the carbon skeleton of the amino acids in much the same way as dietary carbohydrates or fats, with a yield of 4 kcal/gm protein.

If more protein is eaten than is needed for the essential functions listed previously, this extra protein is oxidized, as the body has little capacity to store protein. As is the case with fat and carbohydrate, however, protein is converted to body fat if the total energy intake is excessive. If the energy intake is inadequate, i.e., if the diet does not supply carbohydrates and fats in sufficient quantity to meet the energy needs of the body, proteins are burned for energy, because *energy needs have a higher priority than does maintenance of some of the tissue proteins*. In this event, building or repair processes will suffer.

Nitrogen, which is indispensable as long as protein is used for tissue building, becomes a liability when it is necessary to use protein for energy. Amino (NH_2) groups are split off from the constituent amino acids and formed into simple nitrogen-containing substances (chiefly urea) that are excreted by the kidneys. The nonnitrogenous fragments of amino acids, the carbon chains, are then metabolized along the carbohydrate or fat pathways. Thus about half of the amino acids can provide some glucose when necessary (see Chapter 15).

Since energy is more economically supplied by carbohydrates and fats, the consumption of protein greatly in excess of body need for amino acids is usually disadvantageous. On the other hand, it is certainly unwise to consume a low-energy diet that is likewise low in protein, since the body may then be forced to burn for energy protein needed for tissue building or upkeep. The symptoms of protein deficiency seen in poor people all over the world almost always are due to the fact that these people do not have the means to obtain enough basic food and their diets are too low in energy to make fullest use of whatever protein is eaten. The deficiency state is called protein-calorie malnutrition (PCM, or, more properly, PEM for protein-energy malnutrition) in recognition of its usual origin.

THE PROTEIN REQUIREMENT

Much of the important early work on protein requirements came out of the German school beginning with the French-trained chemist Liebig. His greatest contributions were in the analysis of proteins and their metabolic products. While he appreciated the importance of protein in the diet, he had, however, the erroneous idea that muscle protein was the source of energy for muscular work. (The idea that proteins have some connection with muscular work still persists in the popular mind, in spite of proof that most energy for such work comes from carbohydrate and fat.) With the idea that working men need the most protein, Liebig's student

Voit* studied the diets of German workers and, based on their usual consumption of protein, in 1881 suggested 118 gm of protein daily as a desirable allowance for this nutrient. In 1902, Atwater (a student of Voit, and the American pioneer in nutrition) recommended an allowance of 125 gm of protein, based on studies of protein consumption among men.[6] We know now that these figures are far above the actual *need* for protein but instead reflect the consumption of meats that was customary in the groups surveyed. Today, the consumption of protein is about 100 gm per day in the United States and most other affluent countries.

Chittenden of Yale was among the first to maintain (1904) that such a high intake of protein is not only unnecessary for maintenance of body tissues but might even be disadvantageous to health. For months he studied a volunteer group of athletes and soldiers (men who performed considerable muscular work) given a low-protein diet. He found that 44 to 53 gm of protein daily sufficed to keep them in excellent health, with their physical abilities in no way lessened.[7] Chittenden kept his own protein intake to about 35 gm a day for years and maintained that, as compared with his previous history, he was freer from minor ailments and more vigorous on such a diet. Since he lived to be over 80 years old, he apparently suffered little or no damage thereby. Over 40 years later, Chittenden's findings were confirmed by other investigators, who found that men and women could exist for short periods without apparent harm on 25 to 40 gm of protein a day with generous intakes of energy.[8]

On the other hand, it is no longer widely believed that harm might come from more liberal consumption of protein. It was supposed that the metabolism of such an excess of nitrogen, above the amount needed for tissue maintenance, might overburden the liver (responsible for the conversion of nitrogen into urea) and the kidneys (which must excrete this urea). The Kroghs found that the Eskimos of Greenland, who subsisted almost entirely on a carnivorous diet, had an average protein intake of 280 gm a day, were healthy, had excellent physical endurance, and were free from liver and kidney disease.[9] The explorer Stefansson, who had used a nearly all-meat diet in the Arctic for long periods and found it quite satisfactory, along with his associate Andersen lived for a year under observation by DuBois while they ate a diet exclusively of meats and animal fats (daily intake: 100 to 140 gm of protein, 200 to 300 gm of fat, and only 7 to 12 gm of carbohydrate). They showed no high blood pressure or liver or kidney damage during or after the test.[10] There is laboratory evidence that an exceptionally large intake of protein — 600 gm per day or about 80 to 85 percent of the total energy intake as protein — has undesirable effects on kidney function and results in excessive loss of calcium in the urine.[11] No ordinary diet of natural foods would provide anything like that amount of protein, and there is no indication of harm to healthy adults from consumption of 300 gm of protein daily if enough drinking water is available to take care of the extra urinary wastes and the diet is otherwise well balanced (Chapter 15).

There appears to be a wide range of protein intake to which adults can adapt and be maintained in good health. The consensus now is that a liberal margin over the minimum requirement is good insurance against times of stress, but that superabundant supplies provide no added advantage. Minimal intakes for maintenance of health are of chief interest in parts of the world where protein-rich foods are very scarce or people cannot afford the cost of them. A safe recommendation is that 10 to 15 percent of dietary energy should be derived from protein to avoid risks associated with the very low

---

*Carl van Voit's researches laid the groundwork for many of the important concepts of protein metabolism still held today. He was, for example, the first person to use the nitrogen balance technique effectively. See pp. 92–94.

and very high levels of protein intake just cited.

Nitrogen Balance

Nitrogen balance experiments serve to show whether the amount of protein metabolized in the body is equal to, greater than, or less than the amount taken in from the food. Because nitrogen makes up (on the average) 16 percent of protein, we determine the nitrogen content of foods and multiply these figures by the factor 6.25 (100 ÷ 16) to give the corresponding values in grams of protein. The nitrogen of the urine represents a measure of how much protein has been broken down and oxidized in the body during a day, since nitrogen-containing end-products of protein metabolism leave the body mainly in the urine.* The amount of nitrogen in the feces, consisting of unabsorbed dietary protein, bacteria, and intestinal residues, must also be deducted from intake in estimating balance.† When intake and outgo are practically equal, the body is said to be in *nitrogen* (or protein) *equilibrium* (Fig. 5–5). A *positive* nitrogen balance — intake is greater than output — indicates that new tissue is being built, with consequent retention of nitrogen in the body. If output is greater than intake (*negative* balance), some body protein must have been oxidized in addition to that provided in the food.

An interesting fact about nitrogen balance is that it is usually unrelated to the actual need for protein, because the body can establish nitrogen equilibrium at any level of protein intake that is above *the minimum requirement.* We have noted that protein consumption varies widely in different parts of the world according to foods available. The extremes cited were the low-protein, mainly vegetarian diets common in tropical and less affluent societies (50 gm daily, or less) and the traditional diets of polar regions (about 300 gm daily). Where a variety of protein-rich foods is abundant, protein consumption is usually determined by personal preferences, cultural habits, and the money available for food. Most people seem to prefer a diet in which 12 to 15 percent of energy is from protein. The amount of protein used as an energy source when the energy intake is adequate depends upon the protein intake, and adults will be in nitrogen balance with quite different amounts in the excreta, depending on the amount habitually eaten.

There is little provision for storing protein in the body. Ordinarily a positive nitrogen balance, which indicates protein storage in tissues, is found only in conditions such as growth and pregnancy, when new tissues are being formed. After prolonged undernutrition or serious illness, the protein content of tissues becomes depleted, and on giving plenty of protein, retention of nitrogen continues until the normal protein content of the tissues is restored. Also, on changing from a high level of protein consumption to a diet lower in protein, there is always a few days' lag during which nitrogen balance is negative. Likewise there is a delay in adjusting the balance between the amount metabolized and the intake on changing to a higher protein level, and balance is positive for the first several days. Under these conditions the body nitrogen pool is decreased or increased, reflecting gradual adjustment to a changed protein intake.

It is certain that, when energy intake exceeds body needs (whether from carbohydrate, fat, or protein, or combinations

*A small percentage of nitrogen in urine is present in uric acid and creatinine — products of the metabolism of the nitrogen-containing purines and pyrimidines (from nucleoproteins) and creatine. At customary protein intakes, about 90 percent is urea and ammonium salts — end-products of protein metabolism.

†Small quantities of nitrogen are also lost in perspiration, menstruation and seminal emissions, nail parings, and hair clippings. Except under conditions in which perspiration is excessive or when unusual accuracy is required, these nitrogen losses, amounting to less than 1 gm daily, are usually disregarded.

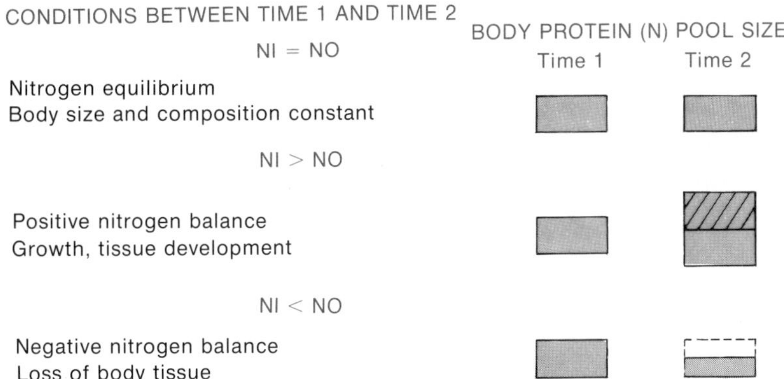

Figure 5–5 The nitrogen balance test is one way to determine an individual's dietary protein requirement. When dietary protein, or nitrogen, intake (NI) equals nitrogen output (NO, amount lost in the urine, feces, sweat, etc.), the adult requirement is met and the individual is neither gaining nor losing body protein. Disequilibrium between NI and NO indicates accumulation or loss of body proteins.

of these energy nutrients), most of the excess is converted to fat and stored in the adipose tissues. Whether or not the body can build true protein reserves is uncertain, but on a liberal protein intake, such tissues as the liver and muscles may have a slightly higher content of protein, amino acids, or other nitrogenous products. This might constitute a reserve that could be drawn on in time of protein lack or extra need. From studies involving tagging of body proteins by feeding amino acids containing isotopic nitrogen or carbon, scientists have shown that part of the protein in cells is more labile — that is, more readily drawn on for metabolic uses in body tissues — while the remainder is more firmly fixed as cellular constituents that cannot be withdrawn without damage to cells. In protein deficiency the liver is the most susceptible to depletion of cellular protein, the muscles are relatively easy to deplete, and the brain is the most difficult. Opinion is divided concerning the functional importance of this labile protein. Some investigators have reported no benefit from a previous high protein intake in rats subsequently deprived of protein, but others reported that pretreatment with protein was beneficial to chicks. The weight of evidence supports the view that liberal protein intakes favor better condition of tissues and perhaps also greater resistance to infections and toxic substances.[12]

Negative nitrogen balance inevitably occurs when the protein intake is reduced below the amount required for maintenance of body tissues — the minimum requirement. However, negative nitrogen balance may occur at levels of protein intake that are above the minimum requirement, if the body is forced to burn protein because the diet furnishes too little carbohydrate and fat to meet the energy requirement. Carbohydrates and fats are both regarded as *protein sparers*, for the presence of a liberal quantity of these foodstuffs in the diet does away with the necessity of using protein for energy. It is especially important that the diet supply sufficient carbohydrate and fatty foods to meet energy needs whenever new tissues are being formed, as in childhood, pregnancy, or recovery from wasting illness. Children can make their best growth only when their food supplies both a liberal quantity of protein, which furnishes all the amino acids needed for tissue building, and, in addition, an amount of fat and carbohydrate entirely adequate to cover their energy needs.

Protein requirement is increased, or tissue proteins are not maintained if only the normal minimum amount is eaten, when the diet is devoid of carbohydrate — even if large amounts of fatty acids are available. Under these conditions, the carbon chains of some of the amino acids are used to supply essential amounts of glucose to the tissues, a function that fatty acids cannot fulfill. (These relationships will be described more fully in Chapter 15.)

Minimum Requirements for Essential Amino Acids

Rose[1] was the first to determine how much of each essential amino acid was needed to meet the minimum requirement by feeding the nitrogen in the form of a well-balanced mixture of all the known *amino acids in pure form* (instead of in proteins) in an otherwise adequate diet (plenty of energy supplied by pure carbohydrate and fat and all needed minerals and vitamins added) (Fig. 5–6). In following periods, the different amino acids were left out of the mixed solution, one at a time, and the effect on nitrogen balance was observed. If the amino acid omitted could be made in the body, no notable results followed; but if the amino acid was one that must be furnished in the food, negative nitrogen balance (denoting inability to build protein for tissue maintenance) developed in the young men. Histidine and arginine, which were essential for rat growth, did not seem to be essential for maintenance of nitrogen balance in young men. Subsequently, histidine was shown to be essential in the diet of infants and there is evidence from studies[13] of longer duration than those of Rose that it is needed by adults as well. The tenth amino acid, arginine, can be synthesized by man, although some doubt remains if it can be manufactured at a sufficiently rapid rate to meet needs under all conditions.

Natural food proteins always contain a spectrum of amino acids, so the total absence of any one amino acid from a

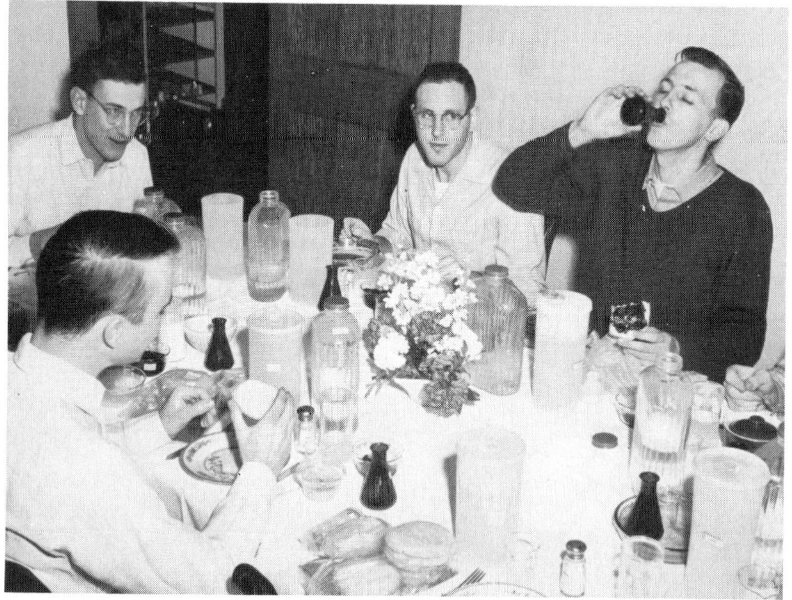

Figure 5–6 Students, volunteers on Dr. Rose's diet squad for determining the amounts of essential amino acids required, shown consuming their experimental diet. The basal diet consisted of pure foodstuffs (sugar, starch, fat). Nitrogen was furnished by a mixed solution of purified amino acids in known amounts (in liquid containers on table). All minerals and vitamins that were known at that time to be needed were given as supplements. Although monotonous, the diet maintained the students in apparent good health. The sophisticated tests now used to identify marginal deficiencies of vitamins and trace elements were largely unknown when this research was done (c. 1935–55). (Courtesy of Dr. W. C. Rose, University of Illinois.)

normal diet would never occur.* For this reason, little direct information exists as to the effects in man of single amino acid deficiencies. There is biochemical evidence for specific roles of some of the amino acids, and absence of any of the essential amino acids from the diet leads, as we have noted, to a loss of body protein. In animals, absence of any of the essentials also causes a prompt reduction in appetite. Some specific attributes of the amino acids will now be listed.

Histidine is present abundantly in muscle as part of a dipeptide, carnosine (the other portion is alanine), whose exact function is unknown but probably relates to muscle contraction. Hemoglobin is high in histidine content, and in the rat, omission of histidine from the diet leads to severe anemia, as well as to dry, scaly skin condition, fatigue, and irritability. The acid or carboxyl group can be removed (a process called decarboxylation) by intestinal bacteria and by tissue enzymes, especially when the tissue is injured, and the compound histamine is left. Histamine causes small blood vessels to expand and is responsible for some of the symptoms noted with injury and with allergies like hay fever; it is a powerful stimulant to acid production in the stomach. Histidine can be used to form glucose. At high concentrations histidine is toxic, and a genetic disease that results in its accumulation in the blood, called histidinemia, results in increased susceptibility to infections and in speech defects.

Isoleucine and *leucine* are oxidized along the same metabolic pathway as fat. Leucine is also one of the precursors of cholesterol. Leucine and isoleucine have branched carbon chains and, together with the other branched-chain essential amino acid, *valine*, share common absorption and excretion mechanisms. The branched-chain amino acids play an important role in energy release during muscular work. A rare genetic disease has been described in which the urine contains partially oxidized acidic end-products of the branched-chain amino acids, which have a peculiar maplelike odor. The disease, called "maple syrup urine disease," causes severe impairment of the nervous system and is fatal early in life. The high degree of specificity of the amino acid sequences in a given protein is illustrated by the fact that in sickle cell anemia, the entire defect in the red blood cells is caused by substitution of just one valine for one glutamic acid in one portion of the hemoglobin molecule. This small change allows the hemoglobin molecule to coil up on itself; its volume is thereby reduced, and the red blood cell changes from the usual disc shape to a sickle shape, which is more fragile than normal and breaks down, resulting in anemia.

Lysine is different from the other essential amino acids in having two amino groups. For this reason it is quite susceptible to being damaged by heat in cooking and processing foods. Most cereal proteins contain relatively little of this amino acid. In addition to its presence in tissue and milk proteins, a hydroxylated form of this amino acid is an important constituent of collagen in the skeleton and connective tissues. In man, its omission from the diet results in negative balances of nitrogen and sulfur and in symptoms that include nausea, dizziness, and increased sensitivity to metallic sounds.

Methionine has two important characteristics, the presence of sulfur in its molecule and of a methyl (CH_3) radical that can easily be transferred to form other needed compounds, such as muscle creatine and the vitamin choline. (See Chapter 8). When choline and methionine are deficient, the liver accumulates an abnormal amount of fat. Methionine is the precursor of numerous important sulfur-containing compounds in the body, including a tripeptide, glutathione, involved in oxidative metabolism, and an amino acid, taurine, needed in bile production. The sulfur-containing amino acid cystine can be made from methionine, so it is not essential in the diet even though it is a major constituent of the hormone insulin (12 percent by weight) and of the protein keratin in hair and nails. Premature babies and the newly born may not have the metabolic machinery fully developed for making cystine from methionine, so it should be included in their diets. Cystine will substitute for about 30 percent of the dietary methionine requirement, and most foods contain both acids. Proteins of legumes and nuts are relatively low in the sulfur-containing amino acids; even in meat and milk these amino acids are the essentials least abundantly supplied relative to human need.

Phenylalanine and its hydroxylated derivative tyrosine are called "aromatic" amino acids in chemical terminology because they contain the phenyl group, a ring structure. About 50 percent of the dietary requirement for phenylalanine is due to the need for tyro-

*The availability of relatively inexpensive pure amino acids (made by chemical synthesis or fermentation) has made it practical to give these orally or intravenously for the treatment of some diseases, so the issue of specific requirements and balances has become a practical matter. It was due to such feeding of amino acids to patients with kidney disease that the need for histidine came to be reevaluated.

sine, and the phenylalanine requirement is accordingly reduced if enough tyrosine is in the diet. Two hormones — thyroxine and epinephrine (adrenaline)—are derivatives of tyrosine, and melanin, the dark pigment of skin and hair, is also made from tyrosine. The addition of a second hydroxyl (OH) group forms the compound *d*ihydr*o*xy*p*henyl*a*lanine, called DOPA; DOPA is then decarboxylated to form the neurotransmitter dopamine. Epinephrine and a similar compound also made from DOPA, norepinephrine, also effect transmission of nerve impulses; the three transmitters can all be grouped in the term catecholamines. Phenylalanine is thus the foundation of three of the six known neurotransmitters, and it is little wonder, then, that the brain is seriously affected by derangement in the metabolism of these compounds. This is the case in the genetic disease PKU (*p*henyl*k*eton*u*ria), in which untreated cases have severe mental retardation. Fortunately, PKU, like most other inborn errors of metabolism, is an uncommon disorder.

Some psychiatric patients are treated with drugs that alter the way the body handles these neurotransmitters. Because their normal control mechanisms are abridged, such patients are very sensitive to the presence of free amines (decarboxylated amino acids) in foods. Blood pressure can be dangerously elevated when these amines are in excess. Tyramine and other free amines occur in aged cheeses owing to action of the bacteria used in cheese manufacture, and in yeast extracts, chianti types of red wine, and less commonly in beer and some legumes.

Threonine was the last one of the essential amino acids to be identified (1935, by Rose and his coworkers), and it was the discovery of threonine that allowed the work on mammalian amino acid requirements finally to proceed. A specific role for threonine, other than as a constituent of proteins where it is commonly a point of attachment for phosphate groups, has not been identified. Its carbon chain can be used to form glucose. After lysine, threonine has the second lowest occurrence in most cereals.

Tryptophan has the lowest quantitative requirement of all the essential amino acids, and as one would suspect, its presence in proteins is commensurately low. One of the B vitamins, niacin, can be manufactured from tryptophan but not in sufficient amounts to meet the total requirement for the vitamin. However, the niacin-deficiency disease, pellagra, is most likely to occur when the diet is low both in the vitamin and in proteins that supply tryptophan. (See Chapter 8.) Tryptophan is the precursor of an important neurotransmitter, serotonin (technically, 5-hydroxytryptamine), which functions in counterbalance to the catecholamines. Cats experimentally deprived of brain serotonin become insomniacs. Administration at bedtime of tryptophan or a protein that supplies it has been reported to improve the duration of sleep in people who have this problem.[14] Consumption of carbohydrate also leads to an elevation of blood tryptophan (under the action of insulin, by mechanisms too complicated to present here), so the custom of having a cup of cocoa or warm milk at bedtime to induce sleep may have some physiological as well as psychological basis. Conversely, rats fed a maize corn diet, which is naturally low in tryptophan, have reduced levels of serotonin in the brain and show behavioral abnormalities.[15]

Serotonin has other effects, notably constriction of the blood vessels, and the release of this amine by blood platelets during clotting contributes to stopping blood flow. Another step along the tryptophan metabolic pathway produces the pineal hormone melatonin, which in part counteracts the influence of the pituitary gland on the adrenal cortex. (See Chapter 13.)

Some of the nonessential amino acids are of special interest. *Arginine,* like lysine, has two amino groups. It is essential for growth in the rat and can be made in the human body, but the rate of synthesis is limited. Even though nitrogen balance was maintained in men fed a diet devoid of this amino acid, one group of investigators has reported a sharp decrease in sperm production. This occurrence has not been confirmed, but it is true that the head of the sperm is extraordinarily high in arginine content. *Glycine* is a precursor for many important compounds, such as the heme portion of hemoglobin, creatine, glutathione, the basis of some nucleic acids (purines), and some compounds present in bile; it is used by the liver to detoxify benzoic acid, a ring-containing organic acid present in some foods (cranberries, plums) and commonly used as a food preservative. *Glutamic acid* is one of the most abundant amino acids, especially high in cereal grains; its salts (monosodium glutamate, or MSG) are used to add a "meaty" flavor in cooking. Physiologically, glutamic acid and glutamine play a key role in the metabolism of amino groups, and glutamic acid is the precursor of a neurotransmitter (gamma-aminobutyric acid). Some individuals are especially sensitive to glutamic acid and experience nausea, tremors, and chest and head pain on eating foods, particularly oriental dishes, high in MSG content. *Hydroxyproline* is the major amino acid component of collagen; gelatin, which is derived from collagen by acid hydrolysis, consequently is very high in hydroxyproline. *Alanine* has an important function in the energetics of exercising muscle.

Sufficient data have been accumulated so that the minimum human requirements for eight of the amino acids essential in the diet can now be stated with fair accuracy. More information is needed as regards histidine in adults, but the infant's requirement is known (Table 5–1). The content in the average American diet of these eight amino acids (based on the average consumption of various foods or food groups) has been calculated and is given in Table 5–1. The intake of each of these essential amino acids is well above the required level stipulated by the FAO/WHO,[2] so there is little danger of their shortage when the diet contains as much of animal proteins as is customary in the United States, Canada, and most European countries.

The intake level of *dispensable* or "nonessential" amino acids cannot be ignored when determining the requirements for specific essential amino acids. To meet the total protein needs, a larger quantity of the dispensable amino acids is needed than of essential ones. For their synthesis, the diet must provide a sufficient amount of amino groups and carbon chains needed to assemble the molecules of these amino acids. These building blocks are drawn from a pool to which all nonspecific amino nitrogen sources (essential and nonessential amino acids, ammonium salts, and urea) contribute. For this reason, one would not be able to determine the absolute *minimum* requirement for essential amino acids under conditions wherein a portion of them must be broken down to provide chemical groups needed for the dispensable or, more correctly, nonspecific amino acids. All of the essential amino acids can be used to supply amino groups for formation of various dispensable amino acids. Hence, the minimal requirements for the various essential amino acids depend upon the adequacy of nonspecific amino nitrogen sources.

A larger requirement for nonspecific amino nitrogen than for essential amino acids has been demonstrated even in infants; the sum of the dietary essential amino acids is only 37 percent of the infant's total protein need.[2] In adults, the essential component is less than 20 percent of the total.[2] Most proteins contain ample amounts of the dispensable amino acids, and ordinarily the concern is to meet the essential amino acid needs of infants and children, from proteins of varying quality.

Nutritional Value of Individual Proteins and Those in Mixed Diets

It should be evident from the preceding discussion that the quality of a protein — that is, its relative usefulness for tissue protein formation — depends on the amount and proportions of amino acids it provides after digestion and absorption into the blood.

Some of the first information on how the amino acid make-up of a protein determines its biological value came from the pioneer experiments of Osborne and Mendel in feeding isolated proteins to rats. They worked at Yale University starting about 1911. Osborne contributed the skill required to obtain proteins in pure form and to analyze them for kinds and amounts of amino acids they contained; Mendel planned and supervised the feeding experiments, so that the rats received a ration adequate in all respects except that only a single protein provided that nutrient (Fig. 5–7). In one series of experiments, young rats were fed diets containing 18 percent protein in the form of either casein (a milk protein), gliadin (a wheat protein), or zein (a protein from maize corn). With casein as the sole protein, the rats remained healthy and made excellent growth; those fed gliadin were able to maintain their weight but did not grow much; those whose sole source of protein was zein not only could not grow,

A

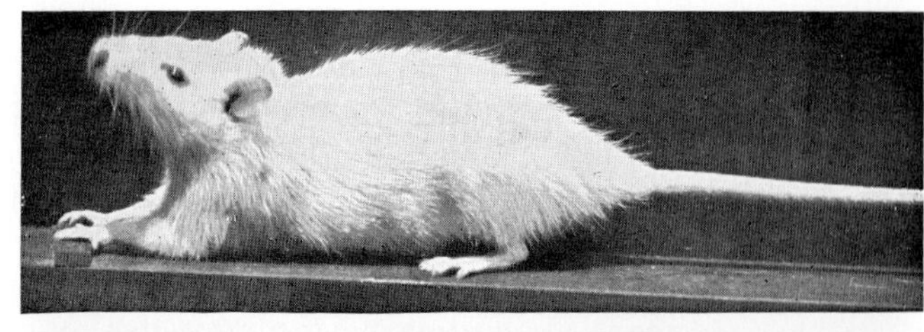

B

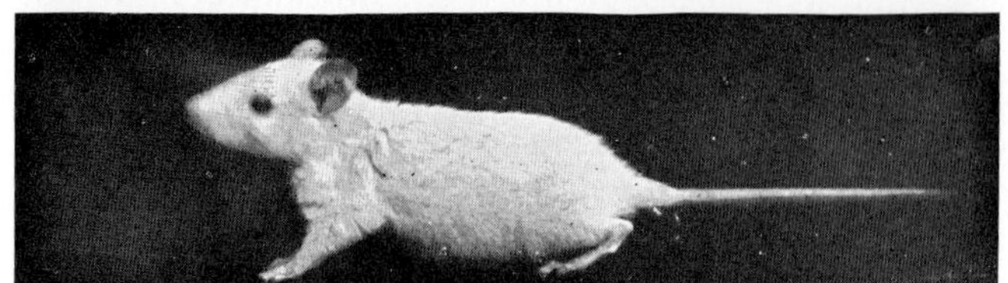

Figure 5–7 Stunting of growth due to feeding an incomplete protein as sole source of protein in the diet. Contrast between two rats of same age kept on diets alike except for the protein, which was a complete protein (casein from milk) in the case of *A*, and an incomplete protein in the case of *B* (gliadin from wheat). (From experiments by Osborne and Mendel, Connecticut Agricultural Experiment Station; pictures reproduced by courtesy of Yale University Press.)

but also lost weight and eventually died if kept on this diet.

Since casein evidently supplied all the amino acids needed for growth, it was said to be a *complete* protein. Gliadin was found to contain too little of the amino acid lysine to support growth; when lysine was added to the ration, the animals grew normally. Since gliadin provided for maintenance but not growth, it was said to be a *partially incomplete* protein. Zein, on the other hand, proved to be an *incomplete*, or *inadequate*, protein that supported neither growth nor maintenance because it was quite low in lysine and tryptophan. When the diet was supplemented with suitable amounts of these two amino acids, the animals grew and thrived. The terms "complete" and "incomplete" still are sometimes used in referring to proteins of good and poor quality, but it should be recognized that a protein almost never is totally lacking in one of the essential amino acids, and in that sense most proteins are not incomplete. Gelatin is an exception because it is produced by treating animal bones with acid, a process that destroys tryptophan completely.

In general, proteins of animal origin (such as those in eggs, dairy products, and meats) yield mixtures of amino acids that are well balanced to suit mammalian requirements, with none of the essential amino acids lacking or in very small amounts. Therefore, they are said to be of higher *biological value* than other proteins. Yet they are not all alike in efficiency for promoting growth. For example, Osborne and Mendel found lactalbumin (one of the proteins in milk) to be quite efficient for promoting growth in rats; only 8 percent of lactalbumin in the diet produced the same weight gain as 12 percent of casein (a second protein in milk) and 15 percent of edestin (found in nuts).

In another experiment, casein at the 18 percent level provided for normal rate of growth, but when it constituted only 9 percent of the diet, the rats grew only half as rapidly. Casein was found to contain relatively small amounts of the sulfur-containing amino acids, and addition of methionine (or cystine) to the diet led to growth at a normal rate. When a protein is low in some needed amino acid, this is said to be the *limiting factor*, for only as much tissue can be built as the smallest amount of necessary tissue ingredient provided. Enough of any protein or mixture of proteins must be taken to furnish the minimum requirement for the amino acid that is in poorest supply or is the limiting factor.

Protein Quality Ratings

The mixtures of proteins found in egg and milk have been judged to be the best quality natural protein for maintenance of tissues and, hence, have received a rating of 100 for comparison with other natural proteins in human assays of protein quality.[2, 3] In standardized feeding tests in the rat, the animal most often used for measuring protein quality, egg protein also rates at the top with an observed value of 94, while the proteins of milk and fish rank about 80, those in meats and soybeans rate about 75, and those of other legumes, vegetables, and cereals are in the range of 60 to 40[16] (Table 5–2). Experience has shown that values obtained in rat assays have good but not unlimited predictive value for human feeding. The rat has a much higher proportional requirement for the sulfur-containing amino acids than man does, so proteins such as milk and meat that are relatively low in methionine plus cystine rank lower in the rat than in man; values for proteins low in lysine and tryptophan match more closely.[23]

Now that requirements for amino acids and their occurrence in foods are better known, it is more common to evaluate protein quality on the basis of amino acid composition. In 1957, the Food and Agricultural Organization published an extensive study of the amino acid content of the different foods used in various countries and proposed an "ideal or reference pattern" of amino acids (limited mostly to essential amino acids) as a measure of the relative nutritive value of the proteins furnished by various foods or combinations of foods in the human diet. This was revised by FAO/WHO in 1973.[2]

Table 5–2 QUALITY OF SOME COMMON FOOD PROTEINS ESTIMATED BY VARIOUS METHODS*

	Food Protein								
Food	% As Purchased	% of Dry Solids	kcal, % of Total kcal	*Digestibility,*† %	*Rat Biological*† *Value,* %	*Net Protein*† *Utilization,* %	*ND_pCal,* %‡	*PER*§	*FAO/WHO Amino Acid Score*¶
Hen's egg, whole	13	48	33	99	94	94	31	3.92	100
Cow's milk, whole	3.5	27	23	97	84	82	19	3.09	98
Fish	19	72	61	98	83	81	49	3.55	100
Beef	18	45	29	99	74	73	21	2.30	100
Soybeans	38	41	39	90	73	66	26	2.32	63
Dry beans, common	22	25	22	73	58	42	9	1.48	46
Peanuts (groundnuts)	26	27	16	87	54	48	8	1.65	55
Green leaves	1.5–4.5	23–31	18–45	85**	64**	54**	6–24	–	c.60
Yeast, brewer's	39	41	54	84	66	55	30	2.24	60
Wheat, whole grain	12	14	13	91	65	59	8	1.53	45
Wheat, white flour	11	12	12	99	52	51	6	0.60	34
Corn, whole grain	10	11	7	90	59	53	4	1.12	42
Rice, brown	8	9	7	96	73	70	5	–	59
Rice, polished, white	7	8	7	98	64	63	4	2.18	58
Potato, white	2	9	7	89	67	60	4	–	48
Cassava (manioc)	2	2	1	No information				–	50

*From FAO Nutrition Studies.[16]

†Determined by rat feeding studies. Digestibility is the amount of fed protein absorbed, and biological value is the portion of absorbed protein that is retained as body tissue. Net utilization is simply digestibility × biological value.

‡Net dietary protein calories as percentage of total calories. The percentage of calories from protein in the food is adjusted according to the net utilization, or quality, of the protein, i.e., (gm protein/100 gm food × NPU × 4 kcal) kcal/100 gm food.

§Protein Efficiency Ratio is the grams of weight gained per gram of protein eaten by the rat.

¶Amino acid score is based on amino acid composition. The amount of the most limiting amino acid present is expressed as a percentage of the amount present in the FAO/WHO reference pattern,[2] corrected for digestibility: 0.85 for coarse, whole-grain cereals, etc.; 0.90 for refined cereals; 1.0 for milk, meat, etc.[17] See Table 5–3.

**Values listed are for kale; net utilization of other leaves may be higher (mustard greens, 60) or lower (cabbage, 35).

Table 5–3 CONTENT OF ESSENTIAL AMINO ACIDS (EAA) IN FOOD PROTEINS,* COMPARED WITH THE FAO/WHO REFERENCE PATTERN†

	Most Common Limiting Amino Acids								*Amino Acids Usually Adequate in the Diet*										
	Lysine		Methionine and Cystine		Threonine		Tryptophan		Histidine	Isoleucine		Leucine		Phenylalanine and Tyrosine		Valine		Total EAA
Estimated Requirement, mg/day‡																		
Adult, 70 kg	840		910		490		245		?	700		980		980		700		
Child, 37 kg (11 yr)	2220		999		1295		148		?	1100		1665		999		1221		
Infant, 7 kg (6 mo)	721		406		609		119		196	490		1127		875		651		
	mg/gm protein	%†	mg/gm protein	%†	mg/gm protein	%†	mg/gm protein	%†	mg/gm§ protein	mg/gm protein	%†	mg/gm protein	%†	mg/gm protein	%†	mg/gm protein	%†	mg/gm protein
FAO/WHO Reference, Pattern†	55	100	35	100	40	100	10	100	—	40	100	70	100	60	100	50	100	360
Individual Food Proteins																		
Hen's egg	70	127	58	166	51	128	15	150	24	62	155	88	126	99	165	68	136	535
Cow's milk	72	131	34	98	44	110	14	140	34	64	160	125	179	131	218	74	148	592
Beef	89	162	40	114	46	115	11	110	34	48	120	81	116	80	133	50	100	479
Gelatin	44	80	10	28	20	50	0	0	?	14	35	30	43	28	47	25	50	
Soybeans	64	116	26	74	39	98	13	130	25	45	112	78	111	81	135	48	96	419
Peanuts (groundnuts)	36	65	24	69	26	65	10	100	24	34	85	64	91	89	148	42	84	349
Cassava leaf	62	113	28	80	47	118	14	140	22	48	120	86	129	94	157	57	114	458
Cassava meal	41	74	27	77	26	65	11	110	21	28	70	39	56	41	68	33	66	201
Potatoes, white	48	87	19	54	38	95	16	160	15	38	95	60	86	67	112	47	94	348
Wheat, whole grain	29	53	40	114	29	72	11	110	23	33	82	67	96	75	125	44	88	351
Wheat, white flour	21	38	40	114	27	68	11	110	21	36	90	70	100	72	120	41	82	339
Corn (maize), whole grain	27	49	35	100	36	90	7	70	27	37	92	125	179	87	145	48	96	429
Rice, brown	38	69	34	97	39	98	12	120	25	38	95	82	117	86	143	55	110	409
Rice, polished	36	65	37	106	33	82	13	130	23	42	105	82	117	80	133	58	116	404
Mixed Proteins																		
1/3 egg, 2/3 potato	55	100	32	91	42	105	16	160	18	46	115	69	99	78	130	54	108	410
1/3 milk, 2/3 white flour	38	69	38	109	33	82	12	120	25	45	112	89	127	92	153	52	104	424
1/3 soybeans, 2/3 white rice	45	82	33	94	35	88	13	130	23	43	108	81	116	80	133	55	110	408
1/3 beef, 2/3 corn	38	69	36	103	39	98	8	80	29	41	102	110	157	85	142	49	98	435
1/3 cassava loaf, 2/3 cassava meal	48	87	27	77	33	82	12	120	21	35	88	55	79	58	97	41	82	330

*FAO/WHO[16], Table I.1. Computed from amino acid content per gram nitrogen × 0.16. Data for gelatin from U.S. Department of Agriculture Res. Rpt. No. 4.[18]

†FAO/WHO[2], Table 21. Percentage given refers to the FAO/WHO reference pattern. The most limiting amino acid is underlined; these scores would, in practice, be lowered to allow for digestibility. See text.

‡FAO/WHO[2], Tables 17, 18, 19.

§Histidine is not included in the FAO/WHO pattern; infant requirement pattern is 14 mg/gm protein.

The present reference pattern of essential amino acids is based on the requirements of preschool children, in relation to their total protein need. Comparing this pattern with the amino acid composition of one or a mixture of food proteins allows computation of an *amino acid score* that depends on the most limiting amino acid (Table 5–3). If the most limiting amino acid (farthest below the level in the reference pattern) is 80 percent of the amount called for in the ideal pattern, then the food or combination of foods in the diet is given a score of 80. Since the reference pattern is based on amino acids that are 100 percent absorbable, the chemical score must be corrected for the factor of digestibility. If digestibility is not known, then for this calculation a figure of 90 percent may be applied to proteins of refined cereals and 85 percent to those of whole-grain cereals, legumes, and coarse vegetables; animal proteins are assumed to be 100 percent digestible.[17]

Complementarity Among Proteins

A protein that may in itself be deficient or low in some amino acid can supplement another protein by furnishing one or more of the amino acids that may be present in insufficient amounts in the other protein. This is illustrated in Table 5–3, by comparing the percentage of amino acids in some typical proteins and mixtures of proteins. The proteins of the cereal grains (wheat, rice, maize corn, sorghum, rye, oats) are low in lysine, but they furnish sulfur-containing amino acids that will supplement the typically low content of these amino acids in soybeans, other legumes, and nuts. These foods contain other amino acids in addition to the ones mentioned, and they may supplement each other in numerous respects. For example, protein of white potato is limiting in the sulfur-containing amino acids with a score of 54 and is below standard in lysine and leucine as well; a mixture of two-thirds potato protein and one-third egg protein is only slightly low in methionine and cystine (score 91), and all other deficits are corrected. Substantial improvements in amino acid pattern always result when a high-quality protein source is added to a diet based on cereals, starchy roots, or tubers (Fig. 5–8).

Imbalance of amino acids in the diet may sometimes have deleterious effects — for example, an excess of a certain amino acid may reduce the utilization of, or increase the need for, another amino acid.[3] For fear of such effects, most nutritionists recommend supplementing a protein low in one or more amino acids with some other food protein known to be rich in those amino acids, rather than simply eating much more of the former protein. The poorer proteins are usually low in more than one amino acid, so it is more expedient to supplement with proteins than with pure amino acids. If the mixed proteins in the diet are of too low a value (probably below a protein score of 60), it is wise to supplement by addition of some protein of higher value, such as egg, milk, meat, legumes, or nuts.

In the American diet, with at least 50 percent of the protein from foods of animal origin, there is little danger of the need to increase quantity of protein intake because of low nutritional value of the combination of proteins in the diet. The vegetable proteins, although they may be low or even lacking in some essential amino acids, contribute other amino acids that supplement those furnished by animal proteins so that the amino acid mixture provided is sufficiently high in quality to more than satisfy the daily requirement for all essential amino acids (Table 5–1).

Other Factors Affecting Dietary Protein Attributes

Another factor that must be considered in practical dietaries is the amount of protein in a food relative to the amount of energy supplied. Foods such as the starchy roots and tubers (potatoes, cassa-

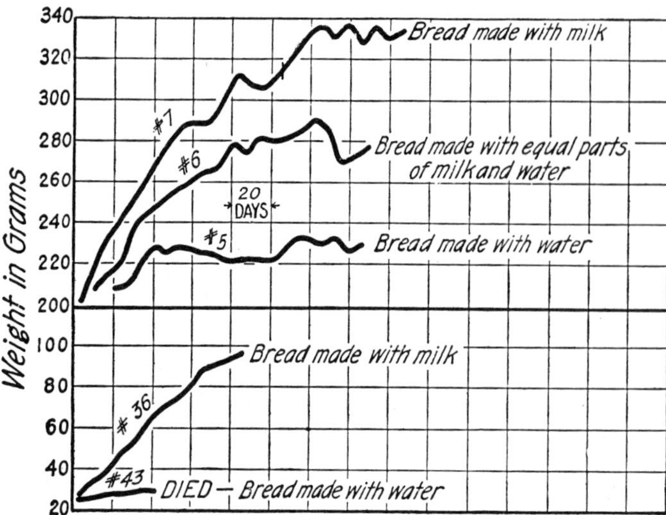

Figure 5–8 Contrasting effects on rat growth of bread made with water and with milk. Milk proteins supplement those of grains in promoting growth. Note that the very young rat (body weight approximately 30 gm) died when fed the bread and water diet, whereas the more mature rat (weight approximately 200 gm) stopped growing but lived. This illustrates that amino acid needs of rapidly growing animals are much higher than those of older animals. (Courtesy of Dr. H. C. Sherman and the *Journal of Biological Chemistry.*)

va, yams) and cereal grains have fairly high energy value, but most of this comes from starch rather than protein (Table 5–2). They may be thought of as "dilute" protein foods, and in order to meet the required amount of *protein*, so much of them would have to be taken that they might provide energy in excess of body needs. Also, the volume of food that would have to be eaten might well exceed the capacity of young children and some adults. This is why protein malnutrition is most commonly seen where foods of relatively low protein content (see Fig. 5–9) form the basis of the diet (such as cassava in Africa and rice in the Orient). It

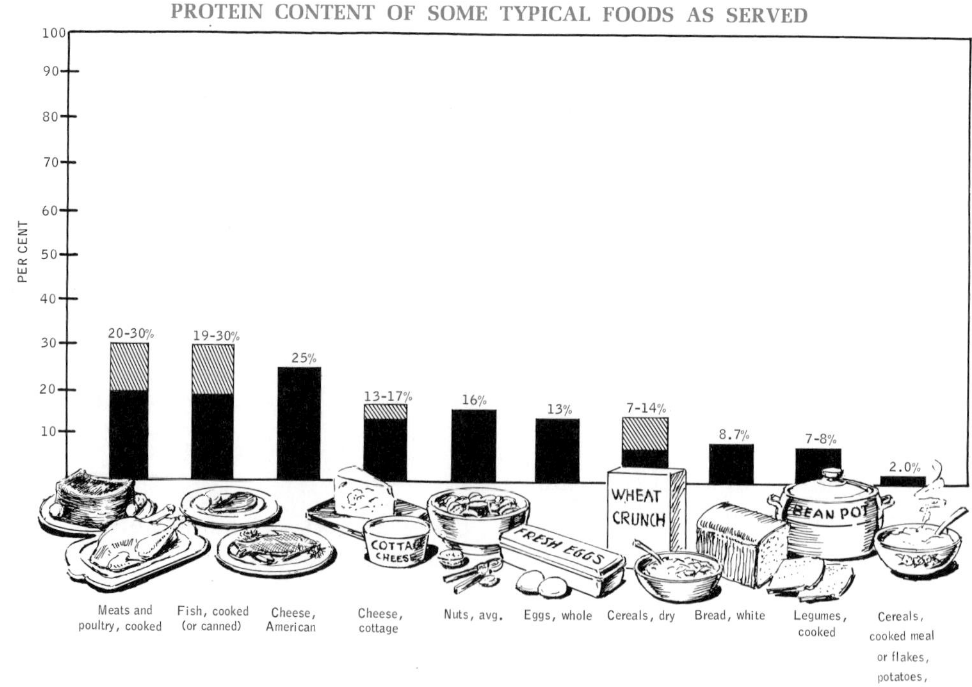

Figure 5–9

is possible to provide an adequate diet from relatively dilute protein sources (such as rice or potatoes) if supplemented with smaller amounts of some foods such as milk or eggs or legumes that are an excellent source of protein of high biological value. Taking one example, to meet the requirement for sulfur-containing amino acids, an 11-year-old child would have to consume 58 gm of potato protein (need 999 mg amino acids/day ÷ 19 mg/gm potato protein, digestibility 90 percent; see Table 5–3). Potatoes have 2.1 percent of protein, so the daily allowance would amount to 2800 gm of boiled potatoes (6.2 lb) and provide 2100 kcal. A mixture of one-third egg protein plus two-thirds potato protein reduces the amount of protein necessary to meet methionine and cystine requirement to 35 gm (999 ÷ 32 × .9), which would be supplied by two very small eggs (89 gm) plus 1100 gm (2.4 lb) of potatoes, in 980 kcal.

Even when the diet contains only high-quality sources, protein may be inadequate. The total amount of protein or *amino nitrogen* may be the limiting factor rather than lack of any essential amino acid—that is, it is possible to run out of total amino acids before reaching a limiting amount of essential amino acids. This has been demonstrated in infants fed milk protein[19] and adults fed egg[20] as the only source of protein.

Digestion and *absorption* are ordinarily not major factors in requirement, unless the diet is very coarse. Proteins that are less completely digested and absorbed than others are less efficient for meeting the body's protein needs on this account. Early experiments of Atwater and Bryant showed that, in an ordinary mixed diet, the proteins from animal foods have a high "coefficient of digestibility"* (i.e., the net percentage digested and absorbed) of about 95 to 99, while those from cereals, fruits, and vegetables have lower values of 85 to 90, and some legumes have values as low as 75 to 80 (Table 5–2). Nitrogen loss in the feces is increased when the diet is composed chiefly of foods that are high in indigestible matter, such as cellulose, pectin, and other fiber, probably because of the increased intestinal bacterial growth these carbohydrates support. Relative to eggs, meat, and milk (the reference protein standard, arbitrarily 100), the digestibility of refined cereals and potatoes and of mixed diets that include animal protein is about 90; diets based on coarse vegetables, whole-grain cereals, and legumes have a relative digestibility of 85.[17]

Another factor that influences the percentage of food protein that is absorbed and retained in the body is the treatment to which the food may have been subjected in cooking or processing. The protein in legumes is rendered more digestible by cooking, but high heating of cereals (as in toasted or puffed breakfast cereals) and milk (as in processing of some canned and dried products) causes adverse structural changes in the protein. Reactions occur between amino acids and carbohydrates with heating that make a portion of the amino acids (especially lysine) unavailable for their essential functions. Processing with acid and heat, as is done in the manufacture of gelatin, completely degrades one amino acid (tryptophan) and damages others. Careful home cooking and commercial processing techniques are required to preserve maximum protein quality.

The distribution of protein foods in the meals throughout the day is also thought to be important. All the essential amino acids must be present at the same time in order to build tissue protein, as well as the nonessential ones that are present in that particular protein. That is, protein formation is an all-or-none reaction, and if one amino acid is missing, no protein is made. To some extent, partially complete mixtures of amino acids may be

---

*Apparent protein digestibility is calculated as the amount of nitrogen in the feces subtracted from the amount eaten, divided by the amount eaten, times 100. For example, with 75 gm protein in diet (12 gm N) and 1.3 gm N in feces, digestibility is (12 − 1.3) ÷ 12 × 100, or 89 percent. To determine true protein digestibility, fecal nitrogen must be corrected for the amount excreted when no protein is fed.

adjusted by contributions from the tissues (such as the intestinal tract), but for assured maximum utilization, balanced protein mixtures should be included in the meal and taken with sufficient calories to prevent the use of protein for energy.

Total Protein Needed to Meet Amino Acid Requirements

How can we determine approximately how much protein must be taken daily to provide for maintenance of body tissues in the average man? Dietary studies to find out how much protein is usually eaten are of no help, for people usually consume more protein than their actual need and adjust to show nitrogen equilibrium at any level of intake above the minimum requirement. If we determine the nitrogen excretion when fasting, this figure is too high because some of the nitrogen excreted will certainly arise from the necessity to burn tissue protein to meet the energy requirement. The way to get a true measure of the protein actually required for tissue upkeep is to determine nitrogen balance on progressively lower levels of protein intake at the same time that *enough carbohydrate and fat are given to meet the energy needs.* A figure slightly above the *protein level at which negative nitrogen balance appears* may be taken as about the intake required for maintenance, or the minimum requirement.

Sherman examined data obtained in this way from 47 different persons and, to make them comparable, calculated each to a common basis of 70 kg body weight.[21] Although there was quite a range of individual values, the average was about 44 gm of protein per day as maintenance requirement for a man of average weight. Sherman estimated that probably 0.5 gm of protein per kg of body weight would suffice to meet the minimum requirement (35 gm daily for a 70 kg man). A summation[8] of all data available 50 years later supports Sherman's estimate, and indicates the normal individual variability to be within ± 15 percent of that value.

Although it would be unwise to limit the protein intake over long periods to the minimum for maintenance, the establishment of such a figure (at about 0.5 gm protein per kg body weight) is useful in permitting us to gauge how much more protein should be included in the diet to provide a suitable margin to cover variations in individual needs, as well as a factor of safety to ensure the best nutritional condition during periods of stress.

We have seen in the preceding pages how many influences come into play to affect the quantity of amino acid intake that is retained in the body for tissue building or upkeep—such as the quantity of carbohydate and fat in the diet; the quantity, quality, and digestibility of the various proteins ingested; the state of the body, and the distribution of the protein over the day's meals—to mention only a few. Since conditions may be more favorable for nitrogen assimilation at one time and much less favorable at another, it is reasonable that the diet should supply some extra protein over the minimum requirement, as a factor of safety to ensure plenty under any condition. How liberal should this extra amount be?

The protein allowance and factor of safety should be especially liberal in conditions of growth or repair of body tissues, such as childhood, pregnancy and lactation, recovery from malnutrition, or conditions in which assimilation of food is poor. A generous factor of safety may also be valuable when proteins of lower biological value make up a large portion of the intake. In setting protein allowances, national and international advisory groups have considered individual and regional variations in needs and have arrived at somewhat different conclusions concerning the magnitude of the necessary margin of safety, as we shall see presently. Other factors that are thought to have a systematic effect on protein need are dealt with separately. These are *body size* and *age*, and the conditions of *pregnancy* and *lactation*.

Size. The total amount of protein needed for tissue upkeep is dependent in part upon the amount of active tissues in the body; for this reason the protein requirement is reckoned as so much *per unit of body weight*. If the minimum requirement is placed at 0.5 gm per kg, a woman who weighs only 44 kg (97 lb) should consume a minimum of 22 gm of protein daily; a tall and muscular man weighing 80 kg (176 lb) would need to take a minimum of 40 gm, which is 5 gm more than the amount (35 gm) for a man of "average" weight (70 kg). Regardless of sex, a person of small body weight requires less, and one of larger than average lean weight needs more than a standard allowance based on average body weight.

Age. The age of the individual is a factor that comes into play chiefly in the younger years when extra protein is needed for building new tissues in growth. Rapidly growing young children may need two to three times as much protein per unit of body weight as adults do, to provide for protein storage in new tissues. The high protein requirement of infants and young children is striking when considered per unit of weight, but the total amount needed by their smaller bodies is, of course, less than the amount needed by an adult. Thus the allowance for a 2-year-old who weighs 13 kg (29 lb), even at 2.5 gm per kg, is only 32 gm of protein daily. The amount of extra protein needed for growth is less per kg body weight as the child is older and enters a period of less rapid growth, reaching adult level after puberty (age 12 to 16 for girls and 14 to 18 for boys). Modern theories give value to liberal (not excessive) protein supplies as one of the factors that favor prolonging vigor into later years. Dietary records of older persons sometimes disclose that they are subsisting on considerably less than optimal protein intakes (e.g., meats may be mostly eliminated because of low income or difficulty in chewing.) It is now advised that, although calories should be somewhat reduced, the level of protein intake for old people should be kept about the same as in younger years of adult life.

Pregnancy and Lactation. Extra protein is needed during pregnancy primarily for the growth of the baby during the second and third trimesters and smaller amounts for the development of maternal supporting tissues and fluids. Additional dietary protein is also required for production of milk. The basis for these recommendations is given in Chaper 20.

Muscular Work Not a Factor in Protein Requirement. Although muscular work is the largest single factor in determining energy needs, it has no appreciable effect on the protein requirement except during initial periods of training when muscular tissue is developing. Careful experiments by Atwater proved that muscular work sufficient nearly to double the energy metabolism showed very little effect on the protein metabolized, as measured by the nitrogen output. Although there is no basis for the popular idea that a man requires extra protein-rich foods such as meats if he is doing muscular work, he does require more carbohydrate and fat in order to provide necessary energy. Since protein is an integral part of many foods, such a working man usually increases his protein intake somewhat when he increases his total food consumption.

Standard Allowances of Protein

The daily allowances of protein recommended by various governmental agencies for adults and teen-agers are as shown in Table 5–4.

The FAO/WHO[2] has expressed protein allowances in terms of egg or milk proteins with the understanding that this will be adjusted according to the quality of local food supplies. The egg-milk allowances for men and women are 0.57 and 0.52 gm per kg respectively. If the local food supply is 70 percent as good as egg when measured by animal growth, nitrogen retention,

Table 5-4 RECOMMENDED DAILY ALLOWANCES OF PROTEIN (IN GRAMS) FOR HEALTHY ADULTS

	Men		*Women*	
Country or Organization	ADOLESCENT*	MATURE ADULT	ADOLESCENT	MATURE ADULT
FAO/WHO[2]				
Per kg body weight				
Egg or milk	0.60	0.57	0.55	0.52
Protein score 70	0.90	0.80	0.80	0.70
United States[22]				
Per kg body weight	0.89	0.80	0.89	0.80
Per day, avg. weight	54 (61 kg)†	56 (70 kg)	48 (54 kg)	46 (58 kg)
Canada[23]				
Per kg body weight	0.84	0.80	0.80	0.73
Per day, avg. weight	54 (64 kg)	56 (70 kg)	48 (54 kg)	41 (56 kg)
United Kingdom[24]				
Percent of energy	10	10	10	10
Per day, for moderately active person	75 (61 kg)	75 (65 kg)	58 (56 kg)	55 (55 kg)

*Range 15 to 18 years.
†Value in parentheses is average or reference body weight.

or chemical score, the allowances would be adjusted as follows:

$$\frac{\text{arbitrary score of egg-milk } 100}{\text{local diet test score } 70} = 1.43\text{, the correction factor.}$$

Then, daily allowances are 1.43 × 0.57 or 0.8 gm per kg for men and 1.43 × 0.52 or 0.7 gm per kg for women.

The United States NRC[22] allowances for normal adults are based on 0.8 gm protein per kg body weight, assuming that the American diet has a score of about 70 to 75. Because variability is substantial, no differentiation was made between allowances for men and women. Authorities agree that such an allowance gives a safety margin of 50 to 100 percent above the normal requirements for maintenance, the margin varying somewhat with individual differences in utilization and body needs. The Canadian Committee on Dietary Standards[23] recommends somewhat less protein for women, 0.73 gm per kg of body weight, allowing a smaller margin of safety.

The protein allowances just given are for adults of average weight. Adults who are markedly under- or overweight should have protein allowances based on the normal weight for their height, rather than on actual body weight.

The allowances for pregnant and lactating women and for children who are growing and maturing provide more protein per kg body weight. A woman in the second and third trimesters of pregnancy should have an additional 30 gm protein daily, and during lactation 20 gm protein above the normal allowance may be required. Allowances for younger children (which usually range from 1.5 to 2.5 gm protein per kg body weight) are found in Chapter 21.

Using a different philosophy, a United Kingdom panel[24] has recommended that the protein intake should furnish 10 *percent of the energy intake.* In making this recommendation, it was observed that the majority of persons in the United Kingdom take between 10 and 15 percent of their energy in the form of protein, that this habitual intake is without apparent harm, and that this level of protein contributes to the palatability of the diet. For persons of normal energy expenditure, an arbitrary allowance of 10 percent of energy intake clearly exceeds minimum requirements by an adequate margin for safety.

On the other hand, we know that muscular exercise is the factor of greatest magnitude in determining need for energy, while it has very little effect on the protein requirement. If a sedentary man had an energy requirement of 2400 kcal, his recommended protein allowance would be calculated as follows: 2400 × 10% = 240 ÷ 4 (caloric value per gm protein) = 60 gm protein. However, if he engaged in hard physical labor, his energy need could be 4400 kcal per day and his allowance would then be 4400 × 10% ÷ 4, or 110 gm protein. If he weighed 70 kg, his allowance on a basis of 0.8 gm per kg would be 56 gm protein. With children, the calculation on percentage of energy can be only approximate, because their high protein needs are accompanied by an increased energy allowance per unit of body weight. Small or very sedentary women and old people may well be allotted too little protein on this basis, because their appetite and energy needs are low but their protein needs will not have decreased correspondingly.

How to Secure Protein Allowance in the Diet

For the average adult sufficient protein of excellent quality will be ensured if the daily diet includes three or four average servings of milk, meat, fish, poultry, eggs, or other protein-rich foods. The "other" protein-rich foods may be legumes such as peas, beans or peanuts, other nuts, cheese, or additional servings of the foods listed.

The protein furnished by the food pattern just given will vary according to the size of the portions of meat, the way it is cooked, and the choice of other protein-rich foods. One should be able to count on an average of at least 30 gm protein from this group of foods.

Grain products and the vegetables needed to make an adequate diet can usually be relied on to provide about 15 to 20 gm protein, which would bring the protein ration to 50 gm, which is about the amount now recommended for the average adult.

To show how this rule might be worked out at three different cost levels and for persons who are either heavy or light meat eaters, foods are listed in Table 5–5 with the number of grams protein they furnish.

It can be seen that the foods in Table 5–5 provide about 50 gm protein (with about 80 percent of it of animal origin), or about the amount needed by a man of average weight. Of course, a vegetarian diet can be made entirely adequate in quality of proteins by the liberal use of legumes and cereal products, and by supplementing vegetable proteins with milk and milk products or with eggs. Meats are one of the most expensive sources of protein, but they furnish it in concentrated form: a 3½ oz (100 gm) serving of meat may be depended on to give 18 to 25 gm protein (depending on its fat and moisture con-

Table 5–5 PROTEIN ALLOWANCE IN THE DIET AT DIFFERENT COST LEVELS*

High Cost		*Moderate Cost*		*Low Cost*	
	Protein (in gm)		Protein (in gm)		Protein (in gm)
Ice cream, ¾ c	4.0	Milk, 1 pt	17.0	Milk, 1 pt (from skim milk powder)	17.0
Roast beef, 5 oz	35.0	Hamburger patty, 3 oz	20.5	Pork and beans, canned, 1 c	16.0
Cheese, Roquefort, ½ oz	3.5	1 egg	6.0	Peanut butter, 2 tbsp	8.0
	42.5		43.5		41.0
Whole wheat bread, 1 slice	2.5	1 hamburger bun	3.3	White bread, 2 slices	4.0
Cereal flakes, 1 c	1.0	1 medium potato	2.5	Oatmeal, ⅔–¾ c	2.0
2 medium cupcakes	3.5	Apple pie, ⅙ pie	3.5	Bread pudding with raisins, ⅔ c	5.0
1 medium potato	2.5				
	52.0		52.8		52.0

*Vegetables should contribute another 3 to 6 gm of protein, or more if several large servings are taken. For example, 5 oz of dark leafy greens provides about 5 to 6 gm protein, but ½ cup tomatoes only 1 to 1.5 gm.

Table 5–6 PROTEIN YIELD OF SOME COMMON FOODS AS SERVED

Food	*Serving Size*	
	Household Measure	Cooked Weight, gm
Protein 20 to 25 gm per serving, or nearly 1/2 the adult daily allowance:		
Meat, fish, poultry	3–3 1/2 oz	90–100
Soybeans	1 c	260
Other dry beans, peas	1 1/2 c	400
Protein 5 to 8 gm per serving, or 1/10 the adult daily allowance:		
Milk	1 glass	200–400
Brick-type cheeses	1 oz	30
Cottage cheese	1/4 c	55
Egg	1	50
Nuts	1–1 1/2 oz	30–40
Peanut butter	2 tbsp	30
Macaroni, noodles	1 c	150
Green peas	3/4 c	120
Bean or pea soup	3/4 c	185
Bacon	3 strips	25
Frankfurter	1 medium	50
Custard and cream pies	1/6–1/8 pie	140–160
Puddings, ice cream	2/3–1 c	120–150
Protein 2 to 4 gm per serving, or 1/20 the adult daily allowance:		
Bread	1 slice	25
Dark green vegetables	1/2–2/3 c	70–120
Ready-to-eat cereals	3/4–1 c	25–30
Potato, white or sweet	1 medium	100
Cakes	2 in slice	50–100
Chocolate candy bar	1 oz	30

tent), or about one-fourth to one-third of the adult's daily ration (Table 5–6). Fish, shellfish, and poultry are usually leaner and slightly higher in protein content than the red meats. Among the least expensive foods for protein are dried legumes, cereal products, dark green leafy vegetables, and potatoes. Eggs and milk, especially dried skim milk, are usually low to moderate in cost.

Normally we include protein-rich food in each meal, partly for its satiety value. Breakfast may be an exception for those who eat a hurried or light meal in the morning. In order to promote maximum retention of nitrogen in the tissues, all the essential amino acids should be in the blood stream during the absorptive period following a meal, and energy intake should be sufficient to prevent the need for protein to be used as an energy source. Inclusion of some high-quality protein in each meal is especially important in periods or conditions when storage of protein in tissues is most desirable, such as growth, pregnancy, or recovery from wasting illnesses. The distribution of protein and energy throughout the day is a much more urgent matter if the diet is borderline than if it is liberal in nutrient content.

PROTEIN-CALORIE MALNUTRITION

There are many areas of the world, particularly in the developing and overpopulated countries, where protein-rich foods, especially those of animal origin, are practically unavailable to the poorer segments of the population. Protein is probably the single essential nutrient most commonly deficient worldwide. This is because protein intake itself is marginal but, *more importantly*, because total food consumption and, hence, energy intake is so inadequate that the protein eaten is not spared to function as an essential nutrient.

Those most apt to show marked symptoms as a result of too little food, too little protein, or both, are young children in the years immediately after weaning. Naturally, with too low a supply of amino acids for building tissue protein and with some of the small protein supply burned for energy, there is failure to grow properly and wasting of tissues. In areas where protein-calorie malnutrition is endemic, adult height is reduced below the genetic potential for growth. If food deprivation occurs in the adult after growth has ceased, as happened in concentration and prisoner-of-war camps in World War II, severe emaciation is the obvious result. Depending on the relative deficit of protein to energy in the diet and on other factors (such as liver function), both infants and adults may show marked edema, especially of the legs and abdomen. This symptom results primarily from a decline in the amount of protein in the blood plasma. Anemia is present because of the failure to form hemoglobin and red blood cells. When people are poor and ill-fed, other public health problems abound, so cases of protein-calorie malnutrition are commonly complicated by the presence of infectious diseases and intestinal parasitism; protein deficiency also impairs the ability to resist infections.[25] Because foods carry more than one nutrient, protein-energy deficiency may have superimposed deficiencies of vitamins and minerals. Naturally, a range of different symptoms may be seen in individuals, depending on these other dietary and environmental factors.

The picture in young children may be one of *marasmus*, appropriately named from the Greek word meaning "to waste away," in which the muscles are atrophied and the face has a wizened "old man" look. Others in whom edema is a prominent symptom are said to have *kwashiorkor*. This name comes from the Ga tribe of the African Gold Coast and was popularized by Williams when she described the condition in Ghanaian children.[26] Some say that the word means "red boy," referring to the odd reddish-orange color of the hair as well as a skin rash characteristic of the disease (Fig. 5–10). Other interpretive meanings suggest displacement or jealousy, from the frequency with which the disease occurs in children who are deprived of breast-feeding by birth of a second infant or urbanization and employment of the mother. This disease, or gradations between the two types of symptom complexes, has been known by many many names over the years ("sugar baby," *dystrophie des farineux, Mehlnahrschaden, distrofia pluricarencial infantile*, etc.) but is one entity caused basically by lack of protein and energy.

With the aid of modern medical care, children can often be saved even in extreme stages of malnutrition. Brain growth is impaired by severe protein lack *in utero* and during the first few months of life.[27] Some neurological deficit may be expected to follow deprivation throughout the early years of life, until the nervous system is formed completely, but the probability is lessened with increasing age. A legacy of poor educability and achievement may be one major cost of failure to feed mothers and babies.

For prevention, satisfactory prenatal diets and nutritionally adequate breast-feeding and weaning diets are essential. When milk is not available or is costly to import, other animal protein foods may be used, or an assortment of vegetable foods may be found that supplement each other as to amino acid content of proteins and other essential nutrients. Several special high-protein, low-cost infant foods have been developed by teams of nutritionists and food scientists. These take advantage of locally available foods that have supple-

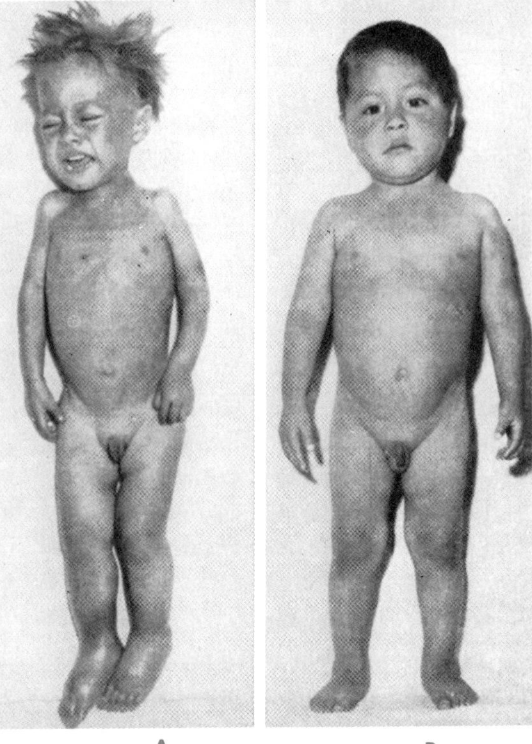

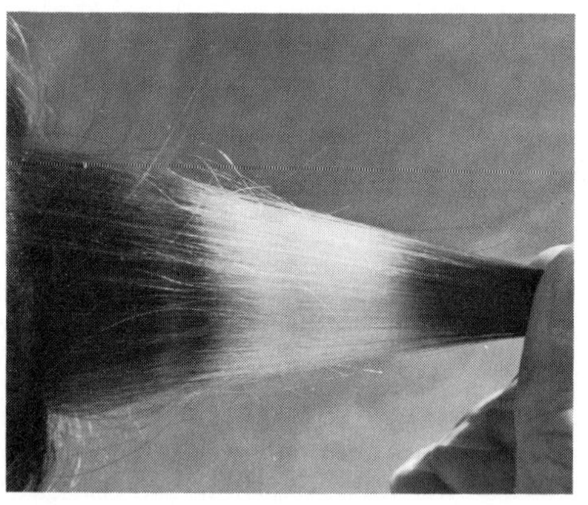

Figure 5–9 Case of protein-calorie malnutrition (PCM). *A*, Child, 2 years 8 months, on admission to hospital. *B*, Same child 19 weeks after treatment with high-protein diet (a special mixture of vegetable proteins). *C*, So-called "flag sign," often seen during recovery from kwashiorkor, when hair is changing from orange color back to black. (Courtesy of Doctors Scrimshaw and Guzmán of the Institute of Nutrition for Central America and Panama, Guatemala City.)

mentary amino acid compositions and conform somewhat to cultural food preferences.

In countries where protein intake is low and most of it is furnished by cereal grains or legumes, some of the essential amino acids are likely to be provided in too small amounts. Lysine, tryptophan, methionine, and threonine are the ones most likely to be lacking in such diets. It has been suggested, and experiments have been made, to fortify cereal foods, such as wheat flour, rice, and corn grits, with the amino acids most apt to be low or lacking in them. Attempts also are being made to improve the amino acid pattern of cereal grains by genetic selection. Actually, supplementation of the diet by more liberal use of some available protein-rich food or by an addition of some vegetable protein mixture is more practical because a mixture of supplementary amino acids is given thereby and, most important, there is usually some degree of energy deficit that the second food will help to correct.

Much effort has been directed by various United Nations and governmental aid agencies and by philanthropic organizations toward securing more adequate diets for people in underdeveloped countries. To make sustained improvement in nutritional state, it is evident that general levels of living must be raised, enabling people to produce or purchase enough food and needed amounts of high-quality protein foods.

QUESTIONS AND PROBLEMS

1. What four chemical elements are combined in proteins? Which one of these is furnished in proteins but not in carbohydrates or fats? What other elements are often or sometimes incorporated in protein molecules?

2. Define amino acids. Can animals synthesize amino acids from simple inor-

ganic compounds of nitrogen? From what simple materials do plants build amino acids, which are later built into plant proteins? What is meant by the "nitrogen cycle" in nature?

3. Where is protein found in the body? Why is an adequate supply of protein so essential for the body welfare? Can protein be burned or oxidized in the body—that is, does protein serve as an energy nutrient as well as a substance used for tissue building and upkeep? Can a liberal supply of carbohydrate or fat in the diet "spare" protein for tissue maintenance?

4. What are nucleoproteins and where are they found in the body? What important biologic functions do they perform? How does DNA differ from RNA in composition and function? How do compound or conjugated proteins differ from simple proteins? What important compound protein is found in red blood corpuscles? Can you name two other proteins found either in the body or in food that are linked up or conjugated with some nonprotein substance?

5. How many different amino acids have been found to occur commonly in proteins? How many are "essential" in the sense that they must be furnished preformed in the food? How many of these are needed for the growth of young rats? To maintain tissue proteins in human adults? Is it likely or unlikely that some arginine may also be needed by humans during periods of growth, and if so, why? Does the body need the other amino acids listed as "dispensable" to build and maintain tissues? If so, why do we not list them as "essential"? What is meant by the statement that a low supply of any essential amino acid may be a "limiting factor"?

6. Define adequate or complete proteins and inadequate or incomplete proteins. Which class of proteins is furnished by foods of animal origin? Are there any exceptions? Explain how incomplete proteins may be supplemented by complete proteins in a mixed diet. Why do cereals with milk furnish a well-balanced mixture of amino acids?

7. What foods or types of food contribute the largest amount of protein in the average diet? Which other types of food contribute less, but valuable, amounts of protein? Which foods are the most expensive and which are the least expensive sources of protein? If you had a choice of maize corn or rice or cassava as the staple crop, which would you choose for protein value? Why? What other factors would you have to consider in deciding which to plant if you are a farmer?

8. How prominent a place in the diet should be given to protein-rich foods? What proportion of the energy is it usually suggested that proteins should contribute? What physical symptoms occur when the diet is deficient in protein? What is marasmus? Kwashiorkor?

9. List the foods in your diet for one day and (from the Table of Nutritive Values of Foods in the Appendix) figure out how may grams of protein you consumed and what relative proportion of the total energy this furnished. Compare this with your standard allowance for protein, and if your protein intake was as much as 20 percent lower than that recommended, make suggestions as to how to bring your protein intake up to a desirable level. Does it matter if you are eating more protein than the standard allowance? If so, why; if not, why not? Under what conditions would your answer be different?

10. Plan a day's diet for a vegetarian that excludes meat and eggs but includes milk or cheese, or both, and that furnishes 50 gm protein. Calculate the amount of lysine and sulfur-containing amino acids provided by the diet as you planned it and with legumes substituted for the milk and cheese. Do these diets meet adult requirements for these amino acids? Children's requirements?

REFERENCES

1. Rose, W. C., et al.: Amino acid requirement of adult men. Nutr. Abstr Rev., *27*:631, 1957.
2. FAO/WHO: *Energy and Protein Requirements.* FAO Nutr. Rpt. No. 52; WHO Tech. Rpt. No. 522. Rome and Geneva, 1973.
3. Committee on Amino Acids, NRC: *Improvement of Protein Nutriture.* Washington, D.C., National Academy of Sciences, 1974.
4. Selye, H.: *The Physiology and Pathology of Exposure to Stress.* Montreal, Acta, Inc., 1950.
5. Schoenheimer, R.: *The Dynamic State of Body Constituents.* Cambridge, Mass., Harvard University Press, 1942.
6. Atwater, W. A., and Bryant, M. S.: Bulletin No. 28. Washington, D.C., U.S. Department of Agriculture, 1902.
7. Chittenden, R. H.: *Physiological Economy in Nutrition.* New York, Stokes, 1904.
8. Irwin, M. J., and Hegsted, D. M.: A conspectus of research on protein requirements of man. J. Nutr., *101*:385, 1971.
9. Krogh, A., and Krogh, M.: Meddelser om Grönland, *51*:1, 1914–15.
10. McClellan, W. S., and DuBois, E. F.: Clinical calorimetry. XLV. Prolonged meat diets with a study of kidney function and ketosis. J. Biol. Chem., *87*:651, 1930.
11. Calloway, D. H., and Margen, S.: Human response to diets very high in protein. (abstract). Fed. Proc., *27*:725, 1968.
12. Munro, H. N., and Allison, J. B.: *Mammalian Protein Metabolism,* Vol. II. New York, Academic Press, 1964, pp. 21–24.
13. Kopple, J. D., and Swenseid, M. E.: Evidence that histidine is an essential amino acid in normal and chronically uremic man. J. Clin. Invest., *55*:881, 1975.
14. Hartman, E.: L-Tryptophan: a possible natural hypnotic substance (editorial). J.A.M.A., *230*:1680, 1974.
15. Fernstrom, J. D., and Wurtman, R. J.: Effect of chronic corn consumption on serotonin content of rat brain. Nature (New Biol.), *234*:62, 1971.
16. FAO Nutritional Studies: *Amino Acid Content of Foods and Biological Data on Proteins.* No. 24, Rome, 1970.
17. FAO/WHO: Recommendations on "protein and energy requirements." Food and Nutr. *1*:(2):11, 1975.
18. Orr, M. I., and Watt, B. K.: *Amino Acid Content of Foods.* Home Econ. Res. Rpt. No. 4. Washington, D.C., U. S. Department of Agriculture, 1957.
19. Snyderman, S. E., et al.: "Unessential" nitrogen: a limiting factor for human growth. J. Nutr., *78*:57, 1962.
20. Scrimshaw, N. S., Young, V. R., Schwartz, R., Piche, M. L., and Das, J. B.: Minimum dietary essential amino acid to total nitrogen ration for whole egg protein fed to young men. J. Nutr., *89*:9, 1966.
21. Sherman, H. C.: Protein requirement of maintenance in man. J. Biol. Chem., *41*:97, 1920.
22. Food and Nutrition Board: *Recommended Dietary Allowances.* 8th Ed. Washington, D.C., National Research Council, National Academy of Sciencies, 1974; 9th Ed. to be published in 1979.
23. Canadian Council on Nutrition: *Recommended Daily Nutrition Intakes.* Revised 1974. Bureau of Nutritional Services, Health and Welfare, Canada.
24. *Recommended Intakes of Nutrients for the United Kingdom.* Dept. Health and Soc. Sec. Rpt. No. 120, 1969.
25. McLaren, D. S.: A fresh look at protein-calorie malnutrition. Lancet, *2*:485, 1966.
26. Williams, C. D.: Kwashiorkor: nutritional disease of children associated with maize diet. Lancet, *2*:1151, 1935.
27. Read, M. S.: Malnutrition, hunger and behavior. I. Malnutrition and learning. II. Hunger, school feeding programs and behavior. J. Amer. Dietet. Assoc., *63*:379, 386, 1973.

SUPPLEMENTARY READING

Abernathy, R. P., Ritchey, S. J., and Gorman, J. C.: Lack of response to amino acid supplements by preadolescent girls. Amer. J. Clin. Nutr., *25*:980, 1972.

Alais, C., and Blanc, B.: Milk proteins: biochemical and biological aspects. World Rev. Nutr. Dietet., *20*:66, 1975.

Alford, B. B., and Onley, K.: The minimum cottonseed protein required for nitrogen balance in women. J. Nutr., *108*:506, 1978.

Anand, C. R., and Linkswiler, H. M.: Effect of protein intake on calcium balance of young men given 500 mg calcium daily. J. Nutr., *104*:695, 1974.

Arroyave, G.: Comparative sensitivity of specific amino acid ratios versus "essential to nonessential" amino acid ratio. Amer. J. Clin. Nutr., *23*:703, 1970.

Beaton, G. H., and Swiss, L. D.: Evaluation of the nutritional quality of food supplies: prediction of "desirable" or "safe" protein: calorie ratios. Amer. J. Clin. Nutr., *27*:485, 1974.

Brasnett, W. R., Powrie, W. D., and March, B. E.: The effect of heat-treatment on the protein quality of granola. J. Inst. Can. Sci. Tech. Aliment., *8*:217, 1975.

Bressani, R., Valiente, A. T., and Tejada, C. E.: All-vegetable protein mixtures for human feeding. VI. The value of combinations of lime-treated corn and cooked black beans. J. Food Sci., *27*:394, 1962.

Briskey, E., Cassens, R. G., and Trautman, J. C. (eds.): *The Physiology and Biochemistry of Muscle as a Food.* Madison, University of Wisconsin Press, 1970.

Butterworth, C. E., Jr.: Interactions of nutrients with oral contraceptives and other drugs, J. Amer. Dietet. Assoc., *62*:510, 1973.

Calloway, D. H.: Nitrogen balance of men with marginal intakes of protein and energy. J. Nutr., *105*:914, 1975.

Calloway, D. H., and Spector, H.: Nitrogen balance as related to caloric and protein intake in active young men. Amer. J. Clin. Nutr., *2*:405, 1954.

Cheng, A. H. R., et al.: Comparative nitrogen balance study between young and aged adults using three levels of protein intake from a combination wheat-soy-milk mixture. Amer. J. Clin. Nutr., *31*: 12, 1978.

Chopra, J. G., Forbes, A. L., and Habicht, J.-P.: Protein in the U.S. diet. J. Amer. Dietet. Assoc., *72*:253, 1978.

Clark, H. E., Stuff, J. T., Moon, W-H., and Bailey, L. B.: Nitrogen retention and plasma amino acids of men who consumed isonitrogenous diets containing egg albumen or mixtures of amino acids. Amer. J. Clin. Nutr., *28*:316, 1975.

Dalgliesh, C. E.: Time factor in protein biosynthesis. Science, *125*:271, 1957.

Garrow, J. S., and Hawes, S. F.: The role of amino acid oxidation in causing "specific dynamic action" in man. Brit. J. Nutr., *27*:211, 1972.

Gates, J. C., and Kennedy, B. M.: Protein quality of bread and bread ingredients: effect of using nonfat dry milk and lysine. J. Amer. Dietet. Assoc., *44*:374, 1964.

Gray, G. M., and Cooper, H. L.: Protein digestion and absorption. Gastroenterology, *61*:535, 1971.

Hegsted, D. M.: Variation in requirements of nutrients—amino acids. Fed. Proc., *22*:1424, 1965.

Hegsted, D. M.: Balance studies. J. Nutr., *106*:307, 1976.

Hegsted, D. M.: Protein needs and possible modifications of the American diet. J. Amer. Dietet. Assoc., *68*:317, 1976.

Hegsted, D. M.: Safe allowance of protein; Scrimshaw, N. S.: Reply to Dr. Hegsted. Amer. J. Clin. Nutr., *30*:465, 1976.

Inoue, G., Fujita, Y., and Niiyama, Y.: Studies on protein requirements of young men fed egg protein and rice protein with excess and maintenance energy intakes. J. Nutr., *103*:1673, 1973.

Irwin, M. I., and Hegsted, D. M.: A conspectus of research on amino acid requirements of man. J. Nutr., *101*:539, 1971.

Johnson, A. A., Latham, M. C., and Roe, D. A.: An evaluation of the use of hair root morphology in the assessment of protein-calorie malnutrition. Amer. J. Clin. Nutr., *29*:502, 1976.

Kies, C., and Fox, H. M.: Comparisons of dry breakfast cereals as protein resources: human biological assay at equal intakes of cereal. Cereal Chem., *40*:233, 1973.

Kies, C. V., and Linkswiler, H. M.: Effect on nitrogen retention of men of altering the intake of essential amino acids with total nitrogen held constant. J. Nutr., *85*:139, 1962.

Kishi, K., Miyotani, S., and Inoue, G.: Requirement and utilization of egg protein by Japanese young men with marginal intakes of energy. J. Nutr., *108*:658, 1978.

Lappe, F. M.: *Diet for a Small Planet.* New York, Ballantine, 1971.

Leverton, R. M., Schlaphoff, D., and Huffstetter, M.: Blood regeneration in women blood donors. II. Effect of protein, vitamin and mineral supplements. J. Amer. Dietet. Assoc., *24*:480, 1948.

MacLean, W. C., and Graham, G. G.: Growth and nitrogen retention of children consuming all of the day's protein intake in one meal. Amer. J. Clin. Nutr., *29*:78, 1976.

Margen, S., et al.: Studies in calcium metabolism. I. The calciuretic effect of dietary protein. Amer. J. Clin. Nutr., *27*:584, 1974.

Miller, D. S., and Payne, P. R.: Problems in prediction of protein value of diets: the use of food tables. J. Nutr., *74*:413, 1961.

Morgan, H. E. (ed.): Regulation of protein turnover. Fed. Proc., *33*:1091, 1974.

Munro, H. N.: Regulation of body protein metabolism. Proc. Nutr. Soc., *35*:297, 1976.

Munro, H. N., and Allison, J. B.: *Mammalian Protein Metabolism,* Vols. I–IV. New York, Academic Press, 1964.

Murti, V. V. S., and Seshadri, T. R.: Naturally occurring less common amino acids of possible nutritional interest and their simpler derivatives. Nutr. Abstr. Rev., *37*:677, 1967.

Nicol, B. M., and Phillips, P. G.: The utilization of proteins and amino acids in diets based on cassava (*Manihot utilissima*), rice or sorghum (*Sorghum sativa*) by young Nigerian men of low income. Brit. J. Nutr., *39*:271, 1978.

Olson, R. E. (ed.): *Protein-Calorie Malnutrition* New York, Academic Press, 1975.

Orten, J. M., and Orten, A. U.: DNA and inborn errors of metabolism. J. Amer. Dietet. Assoc., *59*:331, 1971.

Özalp, I., Young, V. R., Nagchaudhuri, J., Tontisirin, K., and Scrimshaw, N. S.: Plasma amino acid response in young men given diets devoid of single essential amino acids. J. Nutr., *102*:1147, 1972.

Pant, K. C., Rogers, Q. R., and Harper, A. E.: Food selection studies of rats fed tryptophan-imbalanced diets with or without niacin. J. Nutr., *102*:131, 1972.

Pohlandt, F.: Cystine: a semi-essential amino acid in the newborn infant. Acta Paediatr. Scand., *63*:801, 1974.

Porter, J. W. G., and Rolls, B. A.: *Proteins in Human Nutrition.* New York, Academic Press, 1973.

Prothro, J., MacKellar, I., Reyes, N., Linz, M., and Chou, C.: Utilization of nitrogen, energy, and sulfur by adolescent boys fed three levels of protein. J. Nutr., *103*:786, 1973.

Sachan, D. S.: Effects of low and high protein diets on the induction of microsomal drug-metabolizing enzymes in rat liver. J. Nutr., *105*:1631, 1975.

Scrimshaw, N. S.: Through a glass darkly: discerning the practical implications of human dietary protein-energy interrelationships. Nutr. Rev., *35*:321, 1977.

Simmons, W. K.: Urinary urea nitrogen creatinine ratio as indicator of recent protein intake in field studies. Amer. J. Clin. Nutr., *25*:539, 1972.

Taylor, Y. S. M., Scrimshaw, N. S., and Young, V. R.: The relationship between serum urea levels and dietary nitrogen utilization in young men. Brit. J. Nutr., *32*:407, 1974.

Turk, R. E., Cornwell, P. E., Brooks, M. D., and Butterworth, C. E., Jr.: Adequacy of spun-soy protein containing egg albumin for human nutrition. J. Amer. Dietet. Assoc., *63*:519, 1973.

Waslien, C. I.: Unusual sources of proteins for man. Critical Review in Food Sci. Nutr., June 1975, pp. 77–151.
Waslien, C. I., Calloway, D. H., Margen, S., and Costa, F.: Uric acid levels in men fed algae and yeast as protein sources. J. Food Sci., *35*:294, 1970.
Weiner, J. S., Willson, J. O. C., El-Neil, H., and Wheeler, E.: The effect of work level and dietary intake on sweat nitrogen losses in a hot climate. Brit. J. Nutr., *27*:543, 1972.
Ziegler, E. E., et al.: Nitrogen balance studies with normal children. Amer. J. Clin. Nutr., *30*:939, 1977.

Articles in Nutrition Reviews

Size and nature of the protein gap. *28*:223, 1970.
Malnutrition with early treatment of phenylketonuria. *29*:11, 1971.
The effects of malnutrition on specific amino acids in the serum. *29*:76, 1971.
Protein deficiency and tooth and salivary gland development. *32*:24, 1974.
Effects of protein content on the distribution and properties of rice protein. *32*:85, 1974.
Threonine requirements in young and elderly. *32*:234, 1974.
Adaptation to low protein intakes. *33*:180, 1975.
Dietary substitution of essential amino acids by their α-keto and α-hydroxy analogues. *34*:22, 1976.
Protein deficiency over generations in rats. *34*:86, 1976.
Protein sparing produced by proteins and amino acids. *34*:174, 1976.
Nitrogen intake and tumorigenesis in rats. *35*:80, 1977.
Human protein deficiency—biochemical changes and functional implications. *35*:294, 1977.

Chapter 6

Vitamins — General Information

The most dramatic story within the nutrition saga deals with the discovery of the group of body regulators called *vitamins*. Up to the early 1900's it was generally considered that only carbohydrates, protein, mineral elements, water, and possibly fat were needed for normal nutrition of humans and experimental animals.[1,2] Most investigators had paid little attention to, or missed completely, some of the early hints of the existence of vitamins. Among the first such hints were the experiments in Estonia of Lunin,[3] who in 1880 found that mice died if fed an artificial mixture of all the then known constituents of milk, whereas the mice lived if given milk itself. Lunin concluded, "A natural food, such as milk, must therefore contain besides these known principal ingredients small quantities of unknown substances essential to life."

Discovery

In retrospect, the discovery of the nature of vitamins had to wait until the chemical nature of carbohydrates, fats, and proteins was reasonably well established, which did not occur until the early 1900's. Only then, with the maturity of chemistry as a science, could proof be provided that food contained unidentified organic substances, other than the amino acids, that were necessary for the life of animals (the vitamins). It had been known for centuries that certain foods such as liver (which was advocated as a cure for night blindness by Hippocrates), citrus fruits and fresh vegetables, and cod liver oil were able to prevent or cure specific human disorders.

Credit for the discovery of vitamins cannot be given to any one person. Instead the honor goes to a rather small group of foresighted chemists and physiologists, working independently in several countries, who had the curiosity and ability to study *why* diets made of purified food ingredients were not able to support life of experimental animals.

A few pioneers in vitamin discovery deserve mention. They used chemical techniques to make concentrates of the then unknown essential substances in food that could overcome deficiency signs in animals. The Dutch physician Grijns[4] reported in 1901 that the water and alcohol extract of the outer layer of rice and other grains contained an unknown substance that prevented a deficiency disease in man and animals. Pekelharing,[5] also Dutch, fed small amounts of whey from milk to mice and concluded in 1905 that milk had an unknown essential substance. He stated, "My intention is to point out that there is still an unknown substance in milk which even in very small quantities is of paramount importance to nourishment. If this substance is absent, the organism loses its power to assimulate properly the well-known principal parts of food, the appetite is lost and with apparent abundance the animals die of want. Undoubtedly this substance not only occurs in milk but in all sorts of foodstuffs, both of vegetable and animal origin."

In England, from 1906 to 1912, Hopkins[6] established by careful experiments that rats sickened and died on diets of pure protein, fat, and carbohydrates to which all the presumably necessary mineral matter had been added. Less than one-third of a teaspoonful of milk per day, added to the highly purified diet, made all the difference between life and death for the experimental animals. An alcoholic extract of dried milk or of certain vegetables also enabled the animals on purified diets to live and grow, but the *ash* of milk or vegetables was ineffectual. Thus, Hopkins showed that the essential unknowns that existed in foods in the natural state were *organic* (rather than inorganic) substances that could be dissolved in alcohol. For his part in establishing the existence of the substances we now call vitamins, Hopkins later was awarded a Nobel Prize.

In 1907, Holst and Frolich[7] of Oslo developed the first experimental test in guinea pigs for what we now know to be vitamin C. Hart and coworkers[8] at the University of Wisconsin in 1911 made independent pioneering studies, using whole grains in experiments with cattle that demonstrated the essential nature of unknown substances in corn. Hart, chairman of the then Department of Agricultural Chemistry, had a special genius for attracting good persons on his staff to work on identifying the essential substances in food. In 1909, McCollum, then a young chemist, was hired,* and in just four years (1913) McCollum and Davis[9] had proved the existence of an essential food factor in butter and egg yolk. Miss Davis was a young biologist who had just obtained her bachelor's degree from the University of California and who volunteered to do the rat work for Dr. McCollum without a salary. In 1916, McCollum and Kennedy[10] proposed the terms "fat-soluble A" and "water-soluble B" to distinguish between the essential substances in butterfat and in milk whey. So it was proved that at least one of these organic dietary essentials was soluble in water, while another was insoluble in water but soluble in fats and fat solvents. Thus, it became evident that there must be two or more of these mysterious but potent "accessory food substances" carried by natural food.

Research in the field was stimulated greatly by a young biologist, Dr. Casimir Funk, who in 1912 at the age of 28 coined the word "vitamine" and who, in 1914, wrote the first book on "The Vitamines."[11] He proposed that the then known dietary deficiency diseases of beriberi, scurvy, pellagra, and rickets were caused by a lack in the diet of "special substances which are of the nature of organic bases, which we will call vitamines," short for "vital amines" (an amine is an organic form of nitrogen). This name caught the popular fancy and has persisted, despite the fact that not all the vital substances turned out to be amines.† At the suggestion of Drummond[12] in 1920, the final "e" was dropped to avoid any chemical significance. Also, Drummond suggested that the different vitamins "be spoken of as vitamin A, B, C, etc.," thus combining the "fat-soluble A" and "water-soluble B" nomenclature of McCollum with Funk's proposal. These changes were quickly accepted.

The vitamins, we now know, turned

*Other persons now famous for their discoveries in the vitamin field and whom Hart placed on the Wisconsin staff were Steenbock, Elvehjem, Lepkovsky, Snell, Woolley, Strong, and many others.

†Dr. Funk was not, as some have called him, the "father of vitamins," although he can properly be credited for coining the word and for being one of the early vitamin pioneers. He was born in Poland in 1884, and moved to London in 1910. Funk became an American citizen in 1920 and remained active in research in New York City (with interim positions in Europe) until his death in 1967.

out to be a heterogeneous group of substances that differ widely in their chemical nature and in their physiological action.

Definition

Vitamins may be defined as *organic compounds, other than any of the amino acids, fatty acids, or carbohydrates, that are necessary in small amounts in the diet of higher animals for normal growth, maintenance of health, and reproduction.* All animals need vitamins, but not every vitamin that has been discovered is needed in the diet of each animal species. For example, humans and guinea pigs get scurvy when fed diets that provide no vitamin C, but dogs, cats, rats, and many other species make this vitamin in their bodies and do not need it in their food. Some of the vitamin needs of animals can be supplied from microorganisms growing in the digestive tract, especially in animals with a rumen (cows, sheep, and goats, for instance) or a large cecum (horses or rabbits, for example).

There are differences between the vitamin requirements of human beings and of all the other animal species, but interestingly there are more similarities than differences. The invertebrates, from the protozoa through the insect kingdom, largely depend also on dietary or microbial sources of vitamins. However, by convention, because these organisms often require still other organic substances not required by vertebrates, these are lumped together with the vitamins and called "growth factors." All higher plants can manufacture whatever vitamins they require.*

The action of vitamins is not unlike that of trace inorganic elements, such as iodine and copper, in that the presence or absence of very small amounts of them in the food means the difference between normal and abnormal functioning of the body. The potent effects of very small quantities in regulating body processs also remind us somewhat of the action of the hormones (thyroxine, epinephrine, etc.) that are formed by various ductless glands. Vitamins differ from hormones in that they are not formed within the body but must be supplied from a source outside the body (or in the gut).

*A few lower plant forms, such as bacteria and yeast, need an external source of certain vitamins.

Distribution in Foods

In centuries past, before foods were highly processed and refined and when persons generally ate more food each day (because of higher energy needs), vitamin deficiencies were not as likely to occur in persons who ate goodly amounts of the wide variety of natural foods, including fruits and vegetables, then available. Such foods generally supplement each other in vitamin content, though even so-called "natural foods" are richer in some vitamins and poorer in others. Many of the common foods — most cereal grains, for example — were devoid of one or more vitamins, such as vitamin C, vitamin A, and vitamin D, so just eating a variety of foods by chance did not insure good nutritional fitness (as is also true today).

In the later 1800's and early 1900's, when refined foods such as sugar and highly milled grains assumed a more prominent place in the diet and when more energy-saving devices came into vogue, ill health due to at least borderline deficiencies of certain vitamins became frequent. Now that we know about vitamins, we understand the importance of eating a well-chosen selection of foods containing each of the vitamins. Also, we have come full cycle and are adding some vitamins (and some minerals) to many foods from which they have been removed in the course of food processing — for instance, enriched white bread.

What foods are our chief sources of vitamins? The answer depends chiefly on one's culture and food habits. In North America most persons, other than the nursing infant, depend on a variety of foods of plant or animal origin for their vitamins. The green leaves of the plant are its chemical laboratories in which vitamins are made along with many other substances. Hence, green leafy vegetables are good sources of most vitamins. Seeds, such as legumes, nuts, and whole-grain cereals, also have a good content of certain vitamins. Root vegetables and fruits usually have a lower content of most vitamins, although there are notable exceptions. It should be remembered that the different vitamins are often unevenly distributed in food, and the vitamin content of fruits and vegetables may vary, depending on the variety, on the soil in which they are grown, their stage of ripeness when picked, conditions of storage and cooking, and other factors.

When we eat foods of animal origin, we are obtaining vitamins that these animals ate in their feed or that were produced by microorganisms, as in the rumen of a cow or sheep, and then deposited or stored in the milk, eggs, or meat. The lean flesh of animals (meat, poultry, or fish) is a good source of the water-soluble vitamins except vitamin C. Organ meats such as liver and kidneys are much richer in their vitamin content.

Although facts about the general distribution of vitamins in foods are interesting and useful, there are many exceptions in regard to individual vitamins, so that except for a few generalities each vitamin must be studied separately to determine what foods are needed to furnish it in amount adequate for maintaining good health.

Number and Naming of Vitamins

In the 1920's and early 1930's it became clear, after much painstaking research, that water-soluble "vitamin B" was in reality a mixture of at least several unrelated vitamins. Thus, the term "vitamin B complex" was devised (see Chapter 8). It is used today to describe, collectively, the nine water-soluble vitamins other than vitamin C. The B complex vitamins are distinguished by a combination of traits: being soluble in water, containing nitrogen as part of their chemical structure, and being present in large amounts in liver (used in the early studies as the major source in animal studies).

The naming of individual vitamins at first presented a problem, since little was known about their chemistry. As the vitamins became differentiated, they were designated by the letters of the alphabet, usually in order of their discovery. As the fraction originally known as vitamin B became subdivided into many different chemical substances, they were called vitamin B-1, B-2, and so forth* or by their chemical names. As the chemical identity of the different vitamins was established, chemical names gradually supplanted the earlier designation for specific chemical compounds found to have vitamin activity. However, the letter system is used in referring to groups of closely related substances that show a common vitamin activity.[13, 14] For example, one speaks of the "vitamin A activity" of several active chemicals, and of a "deficiency of vitamin A" when the deficiency can be of more than one vitamin A–active substance in food. Most of the individual vitamins exist in several different chemical forms in nature.

Isolation and Synthesis of Vitamins

Once vitamin researchers knew that vitamins were present in a food, or foods, the long and difficult task of isolating them began. Once they were isolated, next came the task of finding out what the vitamin unknowns consisted of chemically.

*Following nomenclature suggestions of the American Institute of Nutrition and the International Union of Nutritional Sciences,[13] the formerly common use of a subscript, as in "B_1" is abandoned in this text (in connection with the different B vitamins only). This has obvious advantages in typing and printing.

This was followed by learning how to make them in the laboratory (by chemical synthesis). At first these steps seemed impossible tasks, since vitamins were present in foods in such minute traces. The dry weight of a man's food intake for a day is a little over one pound, or about 500 gm, whereas the total vitamins in his food, if separated, would weigh about 200 mg or 1/150th of an ounce (about the size of a very small garden pea), or about one part per 2500 parts of dry food.

To add to the difficulty, vitamins are organic substances and hence liable to destruction by heat, oxidation, and chemical processes used in their extraction. The magnitude of the task and the interesting role of vitamins in nutrition, however, constituted a challenge to chemists and early biochemists, who continued their painstaking labors sometimes for many years before the goal was attained. Dr. R. R. Williams, for example, first became interested in the deficiency disease beriberi and the antiberiberi factor in 1910 while with the Philippine Bureau of Science. He continued his research in his free time while head of the American Telephone Laboratories in New York City and more than 20 years later isolated vitamin B-1, and determined its chemical structure. In 1936 he announced its synthesis and gave it the chemical name of thiamin, a sulfur-containing amine. Other scientists in all parts of the world participated in the effort to transform vitamins from unknown mysterious substances found only as traces in foods into known, *pure chemical compounds* that could be made at will.

The first step was to obtain concentrated preparations of vitamins from materials where they occurred in nature in largest amounts. Vitamins A and D were extracted from fish-liver oils, and the early B complex vitamins from rice polishings, liver, and dried yeast. Vitamin C was first obtained in concentrated form from citrus fruits and red peppers. These crude extracts were further concentrated and purified until small quantities of apparently pure substances (usually crystals) were obtained. These were then tested for vitamin activity in animals or microorganisms and analyzed chemically. Finally, the chemical groupings in the molecule of the pure substance were determined and put together to make the substance in the laboratory by chemical synthesis.

Vitamins Today

All of the vitamins (known today) are now obtainable either in concentrated preparations or as pure chemical substances at pharmacies or various retail stores at prices that vary considerably according to the firm that puts out the preparation. All, however, may be obtained at reasonable prices (though, as you will see, there is seldom reason to buy pure vitamins if you practice good nutrition habits).

The 14 vitamins shown in Table 6–1 have been isolated as chemical compounds or groups of compounds, the com-

Table 6–1 THE 14 KNOWN VITAMINS*

Vitamin
Vitamin A
Vitamin B complex
Thiamin (vitamin B-1)
Riboflavin
Pantothenic acid
Niacin
Vitamin B-6
Biotin
Folacin
Vitamin B-12
Choline†
Vitamin C
Vitamin D
Vitamin E
Vitamin K

*The B complex vitamins and vitamin C are water-soluble; vitamins A, D, E, and K are fat-soluble.

†The need of this vitamin for humans has not been proved. Choline, however, is a vitamin for various animals (see Chapter 8). We have not included inositol in this listing, evidently required in the diet of several species of vertebrate animals, since its status as a vitamin is still not clear. Humans apparently synthesize all they need.

position and structure of which are known. Each of them can be synthesized in the laboratory, though synthesis of vitamin B-12 is very difficult and not a commercial practice. Most are white in color, but three of the vitamins are yellow and one is red; two are oily in nature and liquid at room temperature in the pure form. Many are manufactured in large amounts by the chemical industry for fortification of foods and for vitamin preparations.

Overzealous promoters of "health foods" often speak of certain other substances as being "vitamins" for man, such as "vitamin B-15" (pangamic acid) or "vitamin B-17" (Laetrile), but only those listed in Table 6–1 are recognized by nutritional authorities today. Other vitamins may yet be discovered, though the possibilities that any now unidentified vitamins play more than a minor role remain quite slim (see end of Chapter 8).

Current Vitamin Research

Research on vitamins is now centered on determining (1) how they bring about their characteristic effects on body tissues; (2) how much is needed of each of the individual vitamins in the various stages of life; (3) their distribution in, and addition to, individual diets and foods; (4) the effect of deficiencies on pregnancy, growth and development, learning ability, behavior, metabolic diseases, and aging; (5) possible interrelations among different vitamins and among vitamins and other nutrient substances, such as proteins, carbohydrates, and minerals; and (6) relationships of vitamins to nonfood factors (such as hormones, drugs) and to various common diseases, whether of infectious origin or of still unknown origin (such as cancer and heart disease). Such research, although difficult and slow, offers the same challenge to the nutritionists that determination of the chemical nature of the vitamins offered in former years.

Quantities of Vitamins Needed

The actual amount of each vitamin needed in the diet per day by adults is different for each vitamin. They are measured in microgram and milligram amounts. The actual daily requirements of normal adults for the different vitamins range from as little as 2 to 4 micrograms for vitamin B-12 to as much as 20 to 25 mg of vitamin C per day. *This is roughly a 10,000 fold difference,* but this has no physiological significance. Thus, it is a useless exercise to try to compare the requirement of one vitamin with that of another except to test one's ability to use the metric system. However, the specific daily requirement, or allowance, of a vitamin is an important value to learn. As will be seen in Chapter 12, for purposes of comparison, the requirements for vitamins are generally similar, quantitatively, to the requirements for trace inorganic elements — a fact also without physiological significance.

The actual daily requirement of individual vitamins for man varies somewhat from individual to individual, although approximations can be made. Because of differences of inheritance, of microbiological flora in the intestine, of greatly different food and eating patterns, of stresses and disease, and other factors, the *minimum requirement* of individuals within large populations might vary as much as up to twofold, if not more. As seen in the next section, these and still other factors that require reasonable safety margins are considered in setting recommended daily standards of vitamin intake.

Recommended Dietary Allowances

Various national and international groups who establish standards of vitamin intakes generally allow a considerable additional quantity of intake for any *recommended dietary allowances.* This allows for a wide safety margin to cover all but a very few persons of any population, and sometimes to allow for losses in preparation and storage of food. Recommended allowances for vitamins, then, are generally a generous yardstick and are 25 to as much as 100 percent higher than the actual requirement of most of a population; thus intakes below an allowance do not necessarily indicate too low a vitamin intake. On the other hand, recommended allowances are not necessarily sufficient for persons depleted of vitamins because of prior dietary inadequacies, disease, or traumatic stresses.[15]

It is to be hoped that some uniformity of national standards can eventually be attained by international nutrition bodies. In the meantime, the different standards for the United States, Canada, Great Britain, India, and FAO are given in Table 1A to 1C of the Appendix, for comparison. In developing countries, the recommended levels of intake must often be set very close to the minimum because of the impracticality of obtaining larger amounts in most persons' diets.

The *recommended dietary allowances* (RDA) in the United States represent the most authoritative estimates in this country. They are revised every 5 years by the Food and Nutrition Board of the National Academy of Sciences as new research becomes available.[15] The latest available values are given in the Appendix and include daily recommendations not only for vitamins but also for minerals and other nutrients. Where international standards have not been agreed upon, these RDA values are the vitamin allowances most commonly cited in this book, not because they are necessarily "better" than those set by other countries but for uniformity.* The levels are not too unlike those of other countries, with vitamin C being a major exception.

In the United States, for legal purposes of the Food and Drug Administration, including labeling of food products, the detailed RDA's for vitamins mentioned alone have been condensed (giving rise to some artificially inflated values in some cases) in the form of *United States Recommended Daily Allowances*, known as the USRDA (see Appendix, Table IX). Because these are not as specific as the RDA's, they are useful mainly for food labeling purposes and are not generally referred to in the following chapters.

*As revisions of the RDA's become available in the future (the next one is expected in 1979), we recommend that the new allowances be used to supplement this edition of the textbook. Generally the changes, if any, are not expected to be greatly different from the present figures, thus not invalidating current information appreciably.

General Uses of Vitamins in the Body

Although individual vitamins have special functions, which are taken up in the following chapters, as a group of body regulators most of them share in certain functions, such as:

1. The promotion of growth.
2. The promotion of ability to produce healthy offspring.
3. The maintenance of health, vigor, and long life through promoting:
    a. Normal nutrition, especially utilization of mineral elements, amino acids, fatty acids, and metabolism of energy sources.
    b. Normal functioning of appetite and the digestive tract.
    c. Mental alertness.
    d. Health of tissues and resistance to bacterial infections.

It is worthwhile to keep in mind the above general uses of vitamins, since they recur constantly in the study of the functions of individual vitamins (see Fig. 6–1). Also, it should be emphasized that when several vitamins participate in promoting some function of the body, lack of any one of them can inhibit this function. For example, almost all vitamins have a direct influence in stimulating growth. When any one of these vitamins is supplied in inadequate amounts, growth will be stunted, even though the food contains plenty of the other vitamins needed for growth. In similar manner, damage to reproductive ability, to functioning of the digestive tract, and to the health of various tissues

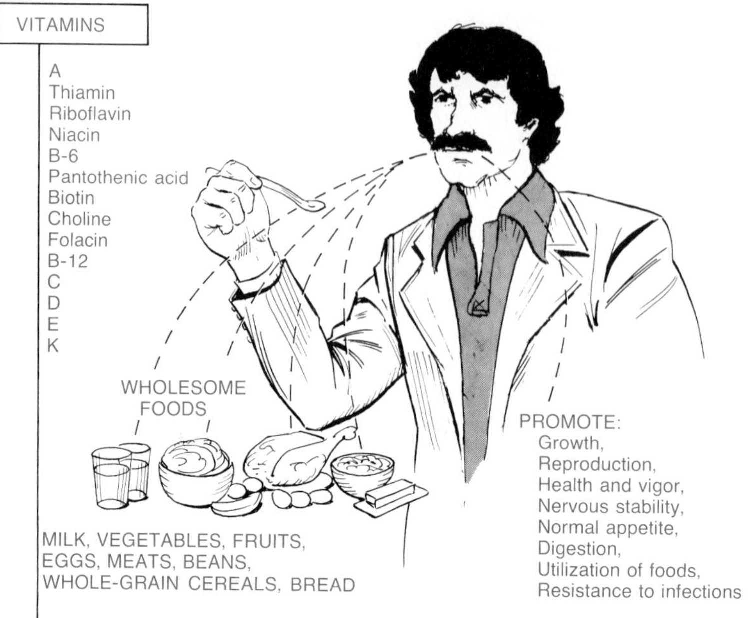

Figure 6–1 Different vitamins found in wholesome foods and their general functions in the body.

may result from lack of any one of several vitamins that are needed for the welfare of these organs or tissues.

It should also be remembered that stunting of growth, lack of appetite, poor utilization of food, and so on may be caused by an insufficiency of nutrients other than vitamins or by medical problems unrelated to the food intake. So some of the more general symptoms of vitamin deficiency are not specific — that is, not due always or solely to vitamin shortages.

Mode of Action of Vitamins

How do vitamins bring about their effects, and why are small amounts of them so indispensable for life? Before the 1930's the life-or-death importance of the presence or lack of these substances in trace amounts seemed mysterious. Research since then has given us much of the answer to this enigma–namely, most vitamins act as an organic catalyst or as a part of a catalyst. A catalyst is a substance that speeds up a chemical reaction without itself taking part in it. Most of the hundreds of chemical reactions taking place in plant and animal tissues, which are essential to the life of the organisms, require catalysts to cause them to occur.

The special types of organic catalysts that promote these reactions in living tissues are known as *enzymes* and *coenzymes*, which aid enzymes in their tasks. Most of the B vitamins occur in the body as part of these enzymes or coenzymes. For instance, cells get much of the energy required for their life processes through oxidation of glucose. This takes place in many intermediate steps, so that energy is set free very gradually instead of all at once (see Chapter 14). The absence of any one of these enzymes means a failure of some indispensable link in the chain of tissue oxidations. Hence the lack of a vitamin that is an essential part of such an enzyme can cripple vital oxidation processes in cells so that tissues all over the body may suffer. Since vitamins, as catalysts, are not generally used up in the reactions they promote, naturally only small amounts of them are needed.

Some of the vitamins occur in enzymes concerned with protein, fat, or mineral metabolism. At least two vitamins are involved in the control of oxidation and reduction (reactions of oxygen and hydrogen) within cells. Although not all vitamins play their role through enzyme action, all act in some manner to promote chemical reactions that are essential for healthy tissues. One vitamin (vitamin D) functions by being converted into a vital hormone, and at least one (vitamin E) serves to prevent abnormal oxidation of fatty acids in the body.

Interrelationship of Vitamins with Other Nutrients

As with the other nutrients, there is a disadvantage to studying the vitamins separately, because one tends to forget that within the body the vitamins are intimately, and very actively, involved in the metabolism and fate of all cellular substances. Most of the B vitamins have some role in energy formation and are essential for proper metabolism of lipids, minerals, or amino acids, or all three.

Several vitamins are closely linked with calcium metabolism, while most could not function at all unless one or more phosphate radicals were attached to the coenzyme form. Additional examples of vitamin interrelationships will be given.

Main Objective of Knowledge of Vitamins

The chief aim of the study of vitamins by the nonspecialist is to be informed about the importance of vitamins in promoting good physical fitness. Much information about vitamins is available to the general public from a variety of sources, some of it good and, unfortunately, some unreliable. There are many facts to learn about vitamins that will assist individuals in making decisions about what to eat.

The need for vitamins begins before birth, since it is important that the diet of a pregnant woman be rich in vitamins if the infant is to start life with a liberal store of these substances in its body. Children must be sufficiently supplied with numerous vitamins in order to build healthy tissues and to achieve maximum growth. In adult life, good health and a longer life cannot be obtained without an adequate supply of all needed vitamins. However, excessive amounts above the "optimal" confer no further benefits.

When vitamins are consumed in our ordinary foods, they are never at a toxic level of intake, but concentrates of vitamins themselves can be toxic when consumed in greater than normal amounts. Fat-soluble vitamins A and D are particularly noted for their toxicity in large doses. Large amounts of vitamins taken as supplements are generally a waste of money and could be toxic. They should be taken only under the direction of a physician.

Although vitamin concentrates and pure, synthetic vitamins are very useful for the cure of conditions in which a person is unable to consume an adequate diet (illness, allergies, or emotional upsets), the objective of nutrition is to have enough of all the needed vitamins in the diet for prevention of disease and promotion of health. Moreover, when we get our vitamins from eating a wide variety of nutritious foods, we obtain in addition all the various other nutrients also essential to health. This is the best way to "get our vitamins" under normal circumstances.

QUESTIONS

1. Why are essential amino acids and fatty acids not classed as vitamins? Why are the "trace" elements, which are needed in very small amounts and must be supplied in food for normal body functioning, not included with the vitamins? Why are hormones, such as epinephrine and thyroxine, not called vitamins?

2. The rat and dog do not have to

have vitamin C (ascorbic acid) supplied in their food, because they can make it in their own body tissues; men, monkeys, and guinea pigs cannot make this substance within their bodies, and hence must get it from foods. Could you say that ascorbic acid is a hormone for rats and a vitamin for man?

3. When was it first known that animals could not be maintained in health, or even survive, on diets of purified nutrients that provided plenty of calories, protein, and all necessary mineral elements? Approximately how long was it before it was recognized that natural foods provided traces of definite *organic substances* that were absent from the purified foodstuffs? When were these substances first called "vitamines"? Who first distinguished between two groups of these substances and called them "fat-soluble A" and "water-soluble B"?

4. What is meant by the following terms that are used in connection with vitamins: biological assay, vitamin concentrates, synthetic vitamins, a milligram, a microgram, minimum requirement, recommended allowance?

5. Why were the vitamins designated by letters of the alphabet? In general, is it better to call a vitamin by its chemical name, when it has been given one, or by a letter, and why?

6. How can the vitamin content of foods be measured? In what types of food are fat-soluble vitamins found? What classes of food are good purveyors of water-soluble vitamins? Name three foods that furnish considerable amounts of some water-soluble and fat-soluble vitamins together. Name five foods that carry few or no vitamins.

7. Give the general uses of vitamins as a whole in the body. Would rats grow on a diet that furnished adequate energy, proteins, minerals, and all of the vitamins except vitamin A? Why? If it is true that vitamins A and C help to prevent infections, would you expect to raise bacterial resistance satisfactorily by taking a diet rich in one of these vitamins and poor in the other? Would taking ten times the recommended allowance of vitamin A be any more effective in raising bacterial resistance than the adequate level?

8. Why is it important that the vitamin intake should be well balanced, i.e., include all of the essential vitamins in the approximate proportions in which they are required by the body? Why is it advantageous to get vitamins in natural foods instead of eating a vitamin-poor diet and taking vitamins in pills or capsules?

REFERENCES

1. McCollum, E. V.: *A History of Nutrition*. Boston, Houghton Mifflin Co., 1957 (Chapters 14–20, 27).
2. Goldblith, S. A., and Joslyn, M. A.: *Milestones in Nutrition*. Westport, Conn., Avi Publishing Co., 1964.
3. Lunin, N.: Dissertation, Univ. Dorpat, 1880 (see page 204 of ref. 1); Zeit. Physiol. Chemie, *5*:31, 1881 (see reprint of this paper on page 99 of ref. 2).
4. Grijns, G.: Geneesk. Tijdschr. v. Ned. Ind. 1, 1901 (see page 216 of ref. 1). Also see Eykman, C.: Arch. Hygiene, *58*:150, 1906.
5. Pekelharing, C. A.: Nederlandsch. Tijdschr. N. Geneesk., *2*:3, 1905 (see page 207 of ref. 1).
6. Hopkins, F. G.: The Analyst, *31*:385, 1906; J. Physiol. (London), *44*:425, 1912 (see reprint of the latter paper on page 109 of ref. 2. Also see excerpts in Nutr. Rev., *31*:19, 1973).
7. Holst, A., and Frolich, J.: J. Hygiene, *7*:634, 1907 (see pages 217 and 255 of ref. 1).
8. Hart, E. B., McCollum, E. V., Steenbock, H., and Humphrey, G. C.: Res. Bull. 17, Wisconsin Agric. Expt. Station, 1911.
9. McCollum, E. V.: *From Kansas Farm Boy to Scientist*. Lawrence, University of Kansas Press, 1964; McCollum, E. V., and Davis, M.: J. Biol. Chem., *15*:167, 1913; *19*:245, 1914.
10. McCollum, E. V., and Kennedy, C.: J. Biol. Chem., *24*:491, 1916.
11. Funk, C.: J. State Med., *20*:341, 1912 (see reprint of this paper on page 145 of ref. 2 and excerpts from the paper in Nutr. Rev., *33*:174, 1975). Funk, C.: *Die Vitamine*. Wiesbaden, 1914 (republished in English in 1922. This is the first complete treatise on the subject of vitamins). Also see Todhunter, E. N.: J. Amer. Dietet. Assoc., *52*:432, 1968.
12. Drummond, J. C.: Biochem. J., *14*:660, 1920 (see reprint on page 177 of ref. 2 and in Nutr. Rev., *32*:209, 1974).
13. IUNS Committee on Nomenclature: J. Nutr., *101*:133, 1971; *107*:7, 1977; Nutr. Abstr. Rev., *40*:395, 1970.
14. Todhunter, E. N.: *A Guide to Nutrition Terminology for Indexing and Retrieval*. Washington, D. C., U.S. Department of Health, Education and Welfare, Public Health Service, 1970.

15. Food and Nutrition Board: *Recommended Dietary Allowances.* 8th Ed., Washington, D.C., National Research Council, National Academy of Sciences, 1974.

SUPPLEMENTARY READING

General, History, and Reviews
(also see refs. 1 to 15)

Adams, C. F.: *Nutritive Value of American Foods in Common Units.* Handbook No. 456. Washington, D.C., U.S. Department of Agriculture, 1975.
Harrow, B.: *Casimir Funk: Pioneer in Vitamins and Hormones.* New York, Dodd, Mead & Co., 1955.
Latham, M. C., McGandy, R. B., McCann, M. B., and Stare, F. J.: *Scope Manual on Nutrition.* Kalamazoo, Mich., The Upjohn Co., 1970.
Lepkovsky, S.: The water-soluble vitamins. Ann. Rev. Biochem., *9*:383, 1940.
Marks, J.: *A Guide to the Vitamins, Their Rolè in Health and Disease.* Baltimore, University Park Press, 1975.
Medical Research Council: *Vitamins, A Survey of Present Knowledge,* Special Reports Series No. 167. London, H. M. Stationery Office, 1932.
Miller, D. F., and Voris, L.: Chronologic changes in the Recommended Dietary Allowances. J. Amer. Dietet. Assoc., *54*:109, 1969.
Robinson, F. A.: *The Vitamin Co-factors of Enzyme Systems.* Oxford, Pergamon Press, 1966.
Rosenberg, H. R.: *Chemistry and Physiology of the Vitamins.* New York, Interscience Publishers, 1942.
Sebrell, W. H., Jr., and Harris, R. S. (eds.): *The Vitamins.* New York, Academic Press, 1967–72 (in 7 volumes; Vols. VI and VII edited by György, P., and Pearson, W. N. Vols. II to V in press. Also see former editions, 1954, for older references).
Seidell, A.: The chemistry of vitamins. Science, *60*:439, 1924.

Other References

Acosta, P. B., et al.: Nutritional status of Mexican American preschool children in a border town. Amer. J. Clin. Nutr., *27*:1359, 1974.
Ahmed, F., et al.: Effect of oral contraceptive agents on vitamin nutrition status. Amer. J. Clin. Nutr., *28*:606, 1975.
Ang, C. Y. W., et al.: Effects of heating methods on vitamin retention in six fresh or frozen prepared food products. J. Food Sci., *40*:997, 1975.
Baker, H., et al.: Vitamin profile of 174 mothers and newborns at parturition. Amer. J. Clin. Nutr., *28*:59, 1975.
Beisel, W. R., et al.: Experimentally induced sandfly fever and vitamin metabolism in man. Amer. J. Clin. Nutr., *25*:1165, 1972.
De Ritter, E.: Stability characteristics of vitamins in processed foods. Food Tech., *30*:48, 1976.
European Nutrition Conference: Recent advances in the assessment of vitamin status in man (symposium proceedings). Proc. Nutr. Soc., *32*:237, 1973.
Food and Drug Administration: FDA Consumer *7*:18 (Sept.), 1973; *8*:4 (Mar.), 5 (May), and 13 (Oct.), 1974 (series of four articles by several authors on vitamins as related to consumer's knowledge and information).
Girdwood, R. H.: Problems in the assessment of vitamin deficiency. Proc. Nutr. Soc., *30*:66, 1971.
Harrill, I., and Cervone, N.: Vitamin status of older women. Amer. J. Clin. Nutr., *30*:431, 1977.
Hegsted, D. M.: Dietary standards. J. Amer. Diet. Assoc., *66*:13, 1975.
Jacob, M., et al.: Biochemical assessment of the nutritional status of low-income pregnant women of Mexican descent. Amer. J. Clin. Nutr., *29*:650, 1976.
Morton, R. A.: Vitamins in Western diets. Proc. Nutr. Soc., *35*:23, 1976.
Schroeder, H. A.: Losses of vitamins and trace minerals resulting from processing and preservation of foods. Amer. J. Clin. Nutr., *24*:562, 1971.
Smith, J. L., and Unglaub, W. G.: Use of specific micronutrients intervention for treatment of malnutrition. J. Agr. Food Chem., *20*:526, 1972.
White, P. L.: Vitamin preparations, proper use in medical practice. Postgrad. Med., *60*:204, 1976.
Young, C. M.: Overnutrition (a review). Food, Nutrition and Health, World Rev. Nutr. Dietet., *16*:179, 1973.

For additional up-to-date vitamin references (since this is a very active research field), see current issues of such publications as:

Amer. J. Clin. Nutr.	J. Nutr.
Brit. J. Nutr.	J. Nutr. Diet. (Japan)
FDA Consumer	J. Nutr. Educ.
Indian J. Nutr. Diet.	New Engl. J. Med.
Int. J. Vit. Nutr. Res.	Nutr. Abstr. Rev.
J. Amer. Dietet. Assoc.	Nutr. Metab.
J. A. M. A.	Nutr. Rev.
J. Biol. Chem.	

Biographies of Early Vitamin Workers in the Journal of Nutrition:

Researcher	*Volume, page, and year*
Cowgill, G. R.	*106*:1227, 1976
Drummond, J. C.	*82*:1, 1964
Eijkman, C.	*42*:3, 1950
Elvehjem, C. A.	*101*:569, 1971
Funk, C.	*102*:1105, 1972
Goldberger, J.	*55*:3, 1955
Grijns, G.	*62*:1, 1957
Hart, E. B.	*51*:3, 1953
Hogan, A. G.	*97*:1, 1969
Holst, A.	*53*:3, 1954
Hopkins, F. G.	*40*:3, 1950
Jansen, B. C. P.	*100*:483, 1970
Lind, J.	*50*:3, 1953
McCollum, E. V.	*100*:1, 1970
Mendel, L. B.	*60*:3, 1956
Osborne, T. B.	*59*:3, 1956
Pekelharing, C. A.	*83*:1, 1964
Spies, T. D.	*102*:1395, 1972
Steenbock, H.	*103*:1233, 1973
Williams, R. R.	*105*:1, 1975
Wolley, D. W.	*104*:507, 1974

Articles in Nutrition Reviews

Oral contraceptive agents and vitamins. *30*:229, 1972.
Control of enzyme levels in vitamin deficiency. *30*:232, 1972.
Importance of accessory factors (a classic, reprinted, by F. Gowland Hopkins). *31*:19, 1973.
The nomenclature of the so-called accessory food factors, (vitamins) (a classic, reprinted, by Jack Cecil Drummond). *32*:209, 1974.
The etiology of the deficiency diseases (a classic, reprinted, by Casimir Funk). *33*:176, 1975.
Reminiscences on the discovery and significance of some of the B vitamins (by Paul György). *34*:141, 1976.

Chapter 7

Fat-Soluble Vitamins

Between 1910 and 1920 it was proved that there were several vitamins in foods. Of the several types found, one was closely associated with certain natural fats and oils — the so-called "fat-soluble A."

"Fat-soluble A" was soon called vitamin A (1920), designated by the first letter of the alphabet. Vitamin A was the first vitamin to have its chemical structure determined — in 1931. Because of these historical facts, and because vitamin A plays a prime role in the vitamin hierarchy, we start discussion of the vitamins with vitamin A. It is logical to include in this chapter the other fat-soluble vitamins, D, E, and K, which are associated with fats in nature. It happens that they are not named in alphabetical sequence. These four vitamins — A, D, E, and K — are unrelated in chemical structure and physiological effects. However, because they are fat-soluble, they do have certain similarities, as described below.

Similarities of the Fat-Soluble Vitamins

The fat-soluble vitamins, as the term implies, are those four vitamins that are found in nature to be generally associated with fatty foods, such as butter, cream, vegetable oils, and the fats of meats and fish — substances usually containing only traces of B vitamins. These four vitamins are all soluble in fat and fat solvents, such as ether. None contain nitrogen in their structure: They are organic compounds of carbon, hydrogen, and oxygen (C, H, O). (See Appendix for structure.)

As knowledge about the fat-soluble vitamins increased, it was found that several forms of the vitamins, especially vitamin K, were present in green, leafy vegetables, which are not considered fatty foods; so the subject became somewhat complicated. As with the other vitamins, we can cover in this chapter only some of the basic highlights about these most interesting and important compounds, and we will attempt to unravel some of the complications.

Though these four vitamins, A, D, E, and K, have quite different properties, they have, in addition to being soluble in fat and containing no nitrogen, certain distinctive similarities:

1. They are *more stable to heat* than the B vitamins and are less likely to be lost in the cooking and processing of foods.

2. Fat-soluble vitamins are *absorbed from the intestine along with fats* and lipids in foods, so that anything interfering with fat absorption results in lowered absorption and body use of this class of vitamins.

3. Because these vitamins are not soluble in water, they are not excreted in the urine. Instead, they are *stored*, to a considerable extent, *in the body*, chiefly in the liver. Hence, deficiency symptoms may be slow in developing, and low-grade shortages may be hard to detect.

There are other similarities shared by

two of these vitamins. The ability of the body to store large amounts of vitamins A and D presents a problem, as toxicity may occur. The body is unable to tolerate excessive amounts of these two vitamins. Certain synthetic forms of vitamin K are also quite toxic, whereas excessive vitamin E appears to be quite well tolerated.

VITAMIN A

Vitamin A is probably the most important of all vitamins, if any single vitamin can be so distinguished from another. Its great importance is demonstrated dramatically in that, more than any other vitamin, *deficiencies of vitamin A are still widespread throughout most developing countries of the world and involve millions of persons, especially children.*

A deficiency of vitamin A causes a weakening of body tissues, resulting in less resistance to infection; a stunting of growth; and, especially, a weakening of eye tissue, resulting in "night blindness." Unfortunately, these conditions are quite common in underdeveloped areas of the world in spite of the fact that the cure can be so easily and cheaply obtained.

Discovery and Identification

Hippocrates, in ancient Greece, knew that the eating of liver was a treatment for night blindness,[1] now known to be caused by a lack of vitamin A. There are many other references to the disease throughout the centuries (as far back as 1500 B.C.) In 1904 Mori, of Japan, found that the night blindness–preventing substance was in fatty foods and suggested the use of cod-liver oil and chicken liver for its treatment in children.[1] He thought the disease was due to a deficiency of fat.

The fact that certain fats contained the substance we now know as vitamin A was detected experimentally by using growth tests with rats. This discovery was made independently by two teams in 1913, by McCollum and Davis and by Osborne and Mendel.[2] Fed on purified foodstuffs with lard as the only fat, rats ceased to grow, developed soreness of the eyes,* and eventually died. With butterfat, ether extract, or egg yolk in the diet, rats were protected from these ill effects. Further experiments showed that cod-liver oil was also very rich in this growth-promoting, health-protecting factor, whereas most commercial fats and oils produced results more like those of lard. Eventually, in 1931, the structure of vitamin A was discovered by Karrer,[3] who received a Nobel Prize for this and for his work with riboflavin, a B vitamin. Several years later, vitamin A was isolated in crystalline form and synthesized in the laboratory. Today, pure inexpensive synthetic forms of vitamin A are readily available and largely replace fish-liver oils as the primary source in food supplements. (See structural formula in the Appendix.)

Vitamin A is rather unique in that, technically speaking, it is only present in animal foods. However, it can be made in the body from yellow provitamins A, i.e., carotene, found largely in foods of plant origin. Hence, pure vegetarians do not eat any "true" vitamin A but eat foods that have, technically, "vitamin A activity" — a term that includes both vitamin A and provitamins A in all food sources.

This use of terms is a result of historical convention. This could be confusing to the student who has been taught in grade schools that carrots, yams, melons, and so on are good sources of "vitamin A." Actually, carrots contain no "true" vitamin A, only vitamin A activity, as will be explained.†

---

*McCollum and Davis did not observe the eye changes at first, but based their conclusions on the growth-promoting properties of the vitamin.

†Generally, when we use the term "vitamin A deficiency" we mean a physiological deficiency of vitamin A, which could refer to a dietary deficiency of either "true" vitamin A or provitamin A. Also, on food labels, in the legal sense in the United States, vitamin A refers to compounds of both sources. The authors have used the recommended nomenclature, but we feel the subject would be easier to understand if carotene and other forms of vitamin A were just considered to be active forms of vitamin A.

Chemical Properties of Vitamin A

Vitamin A is almost *colorless, insoluble in water, soluble in fats* and fat solvents, and fairly *stable to heat*. It may be *destroyed by oxidation,* such as by exposure to ultraviolet light or exposure to air at high temperatures. Fats and oils lose vitamin A content by oxidation as they become rancid. Substances that inhibit this oxidation (antioxidants) are often present in unrefined oils but are usually removed when oils are refined for food use. Hence, we depend mainly on storage in a cool, dark place (refrigerator) and on added antioxidants to protect fats and oils from vitamin A loss.

Several slightly different forms of this vitamin are found in nature. The two most common are *retinol* (formerly called just "vitamin A" or "vitamin A alcohol") and *dehydroretinol* (formerly vitamin A_2).[4] The former is the traditional vitamin A commonly found in all the animal kingdom (but not in plants), whereas the latter occurs only in freshwater fish and in birds that feed on these fish. Since both forms of the vitamin have similar physiological effects, we need make little distinction between them. Both forms of the vitamin exist in nature in alcohol, aldehyde, and acid forms.*

Provitamins A and Total Vitamin A Activity

Animals get their vitamin A either directly or indirectly from plant sources. Plants are the only source in nature of the highly colored *provitamin A carotenoids,* precursors of this vitamin. Fish eat smaller fish or crustaceans, which, in turn, have fed on marine plants that contain the provitamins A. Herbivorous animals eat green plants and convert these substances into the vitamin itself in their bodies. Carnivorous animals get the vitamin from feeding on plant-eating animals. The cow and the hen are efficient in converting the provitamins A in plant foods into the vitamin A in milk fat, eggs, and tissues. Since some provitamin A activity in the diet escapes this conversion, *milk fat, egg yolk,* and other animal products contain a *mixture* of both vitamin A and its plant precursors (which we shall call *total vitamin A activity*). The relative amounts of each depend partly on the food of the animal and partly on its species, or even breed. For instance, milk from Holstein cows contains a higher proportion of vitamin A, and that from Guernsey cows carries less vitamin A and more of the provitamin A, which explains why Guernsey milk is more "golden" in color. Both milks have about the same amount of "total vitamin A activity," however.

Plants As Sources of Provitamin A Carotenoids

As has been stated, vitamin A as such is not found in the plant kingdom. Instead, the provitamin A carotenoids, which are converted to vitamin A in the body, are found in plants. They are bright *yellow* or *orange-yellow* pigments, which give the color to carrots, sweet potatoes, melons, squash, pumpkin, apricots, peaches, and yellow corn. They are also present in all green vegetables, although in these vegetables their color is masked by that of the green pigment chlorophyll. The quantity of these vitamin A precursors roughly parallels that of chlorophyll, being found most richly in thin, green leaves.

---

*Since 1969, new names have been adopted for the various vitamin A compounds.[4] The natural aldehyde form (formerly called vitamin A aldehyde, retinal, or retinene) is now properly termed *retinaldehyde* and the corresponding acid form, *retinoic acid*. Corresponding suffixes are used after the phrase "dehydroretin . . ." in referring to dehydroretinol compounds. Several other active forms of the vitamin exist in nature or as synthetic isomers. In the body, vitamin A exists largely in the form of esters with fatty acids, known as "retinyl esters." When fed to man or animals, the different forms of vitamin A are not necessarily interchangeable in protecting against a deficiency.

Three of these provitamin A carotenoids are known as *carotenes** (alpha-, beta-, and gamma-carotene), and a fourth is *cryptoxanthin,* the yellow pigment of corn. The structures of the carotenes were known several years before it was clear that they were associated with vitamin A.[5] Steenbock and Boutwell first showed that sources of carotene had vitamin A activity in the rat,[6] but this relationship was not fully understood until 1930.[7]

When the carotenes and cryptoxanthin are taken into the body, they are split in half, giving rise to vitamin A. The chief sites of conversion of the provitamins to vitamin A in humans are in the intestinal wall during absorption into the body, and also in the liver. The site of conversion differs from one animal species to another. Although beta-carotene is theoretically capable of being split to give two molecules of vitamin A (twice as much as the other precursors), this is not done very efficiently in the human body. The amount absorbed and utilized depends on many factors — the amount of fat in the diet, the method of food preparation, the rate and completeness of digestion, the presence of vitamin E and the hormone thyroxine, and other factors. Then too, there are wide differences in species and in individuals as to how well they utilize carotenes. It is conservatively estimated that in humans about one-sixth of the carotene intake may be expected to be transformed into vitamin A.[8] This is determined on the basis that only about one-third of the carotene is absorbed and that only about one-half of this (or a total of only one-sixth) has vitamin A activity for humans.

*Carotene is deep red when in pure form and derives its name from carrots, from which it was first isolated and in which it exists at a level of about 0.01 percent.

Effects of Lack of Vitamin A in Man and Animals

A source of vitamin A is essential for growth, for vision, for maintenance of epithelial tissues in a healthy state, and for tooth development. Hence, a diet that contains insufficient amounts of total vitamin A activity to meet the needs of humans will in time cause *stunting of growth, or lack of ability to see well in dim light* (night blindness) or more serious eye troubles. A deficiency also results in diseased conditions of the *skin* and membranes lining the *respiratory passages and the digestive and genitourinary tracts,* and abnormalities in the enamel-forming cells of the *teeth.*

The eye is one of the first organs to show effects of vitamin A deficiency because the vitamin is a *constituent of a pigment in the retina.* When light falls on the normal retina, this pigment — called visual purple (rhodopsin) — is bleached to another pigment known as visual yellow (retinaldehyde; see footnote, p. 129). As a result of this change, images are transmitted to the brain through the optic nerve. In the dark, the vitamin A–containing visual purple is rebuilt, but there is

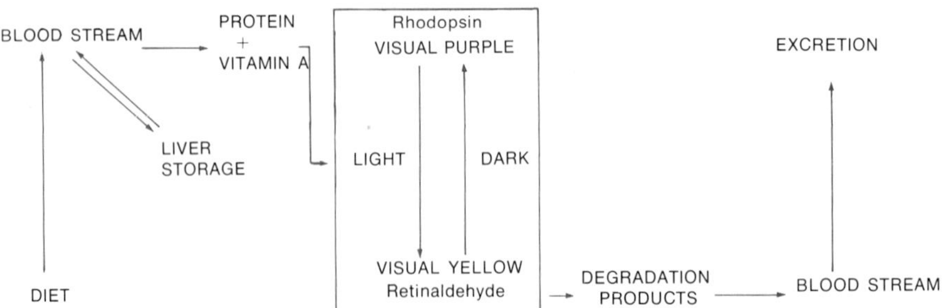

Figure 7–1 Diagram of visual cycle, showing why vitamin A from the blood stream is needed to rebuild the pigment, visual purple, in the eye after exposure to light. (From Gordon, E. S., and Sevringhaus, E. L.: *Vitamin Therapy in General Practice.* Chicago, Year Book Publishers, Inc., 1942.)

always some loss of degradation products, which necessitates new supplies of vitamin A brought by the blood (Fig. 7–1).*

If vitamin A is at a low level in the blood, normal vision will be restored slowly and *dark adaptation* of the eyes will be faulty. Dark adaptation is influenced by too many other factors to be an infallible index of the adequacy of vitamin A in the diet. But lack of vitamin A is one of the common causes of night blindness, and a good many persons with this disorder do respond favorably to extra doses of this vitamin. If a person is suffering from vitamin A deficiency, night driving could prove to be hazardous, because vision would be impaired after exposure to the bright headlights of oncoming cars.

One of the chief functions of vitamin A is to maintain the health of *epithelial tissues* — namely the skin and membranes that line all passages that open to the exterior of the body, as well as glands and their ducts. When deprived of an adequate supply of vitamin A, these tissues undergo changes that lead to a peculiar type of hornlike degeneration called *keratinization.* Damage to the mucous membranes lining the mouth, throat, nose, and respiratory passages is one of the earlier effects of vitamin A deficiency. In addition to general deterioration of the cells, these membranes lack their normal secretions, and there is loss of the little filaments called cilia, which by constant movement aid in keeping the membrane surface clean. As bacteria have easy access to these parts, susceptibility to infections, such as *sinus trouble, sore throat, and abscesses in ears, mouth, or salivary glands,* is a common manifestation of insufficient vitamin A in the diet. Similar damage to membranes lining the alimentary tract may allow bacteria to penetrate into the stomach or intestinal wall, whence they may be carried in the

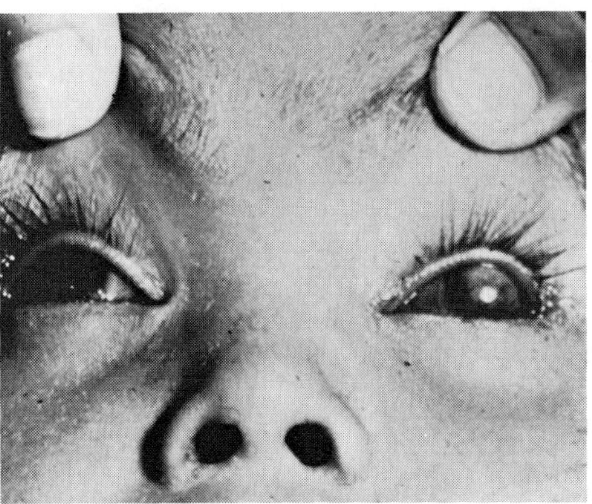

Figure 7–2 Eye changes (xerophthalmia) in a child from a developing country, being examined by a member of a survey team. It costs only a few cents per year to supply this child with adequate amounts of vitamin A. (From *NIH Record.*)

blood stream to other parts of the body. Deficient rats kept under special germ-free conditions live many months longer than similar rats under usual laboratory conditions.

The frequency of such infections (especially of the respiratory tract) in severe vitamin A deficiency has led to the use of concentrated preparations of this vitamin for their prevention and treatment, but obviously vitamin A is useful in such conditions only when they are due to a *deficiency* of vitamin A. Vitamin A shares with other vitamins in promoting health of tissues and is anti-infective only in the sense that it helps to keep healthy the lining membranes that are the first line of defense in preventing entrance of bacteria into the body. If there has been previous deficiency of this vitamin in the diet, extra doses of it are helpful in rebuilding stores of it in the liver and restoring damaged epithelial tissues to health.

A prolonged lack of vitamin A results in dry and scaly skin (follicular hyperkeratosis), with plugs of hornlike material about the hair follicles, and in the eye disease known as *xerophthalmia* (see Figs. 7–2 and 7–3). In this disease, the secretion of tears is stopped, the eyes are sensitive to light, the lids become swollen and sticky with pus, and bacteria may invade the eye itself and cause ulcers of the cornea, which lead to blindness if the dis-

---

*A Nobel Prize in Medicine was awarded in 1967 to Dr. George Wald of Harvard University, who is primarily responsible for these studies on the role of vitamin A in vision.[9]

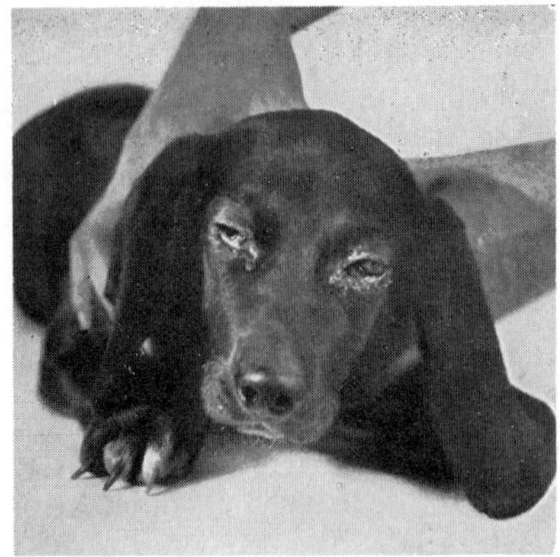

A

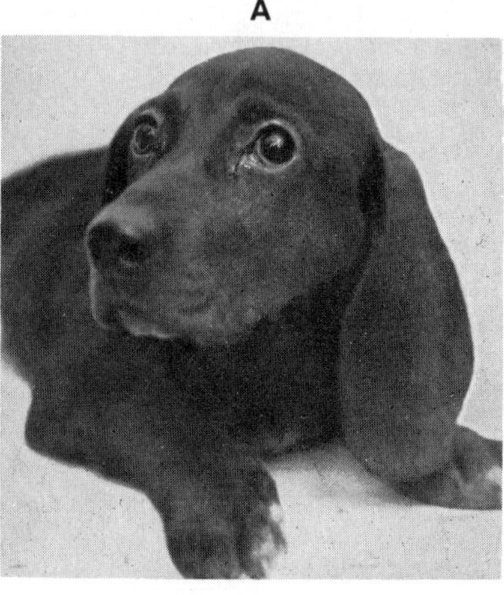

B

Figure 7–3 Xerophthalmia in a pupply due to feeding it a vitamin A deficient diet. **A,** Note the swollen lids and sticky discharge from the eyes. **B,** Full recovery after administration of vitamin A. (Courtesy of Doctors Steenbock, Nelson, and Hart.)

ease is not arrested. Xerophthalmia is a very common disease in *infants* or undernourished *children* in those parts of the world where the deficiency is prevalent, and it may be prevented by including in the diet a good source of vitamin A.

Vitamin A is also essential for proper formation and maintenance of tooth enamel and health of gums, and for health of the sex glands, the uterus, and the membranes that line the bladder and urinary passages. Some investigators have found that nervous lesions develop in animals on vitamin A–deficient diets. It is stated that the bony structure ceases to develop (owing to vitamin A deficiency) before growth of nervous tissue is inhibited, and that the resultant crowding of nerves in the bony cavities of the skull and spinal column is the cause of the nervous lesions. This vitamin is needed to ensure optimum *growth* (Fig. 7–4).

Deficient animals show most, if not all, of the same symptoms that are described in humans. *Reproductive* disorders (Fig. 7–5) are more readily observed in deficient animals with evidence of poor fertilization, abnormal embryonic growth, placental injury, and, in severe deficiency, death of the fetus. Deficiencies have been obtained in all animal species studied — rat, fowl, pig, cow, sheep, dog, guinea pig, and others.

Vitamin A in the Body

Absorption. Chemical and physical methods for detecting and measuring vitamin A in blood and tissues have enabled nutritionists to follow its course within the body. Most of the provitamin A carotenoids are split by a special enzyme in the intestinal wall, and these products, plus any dietary vitamin A itself, are absorbed

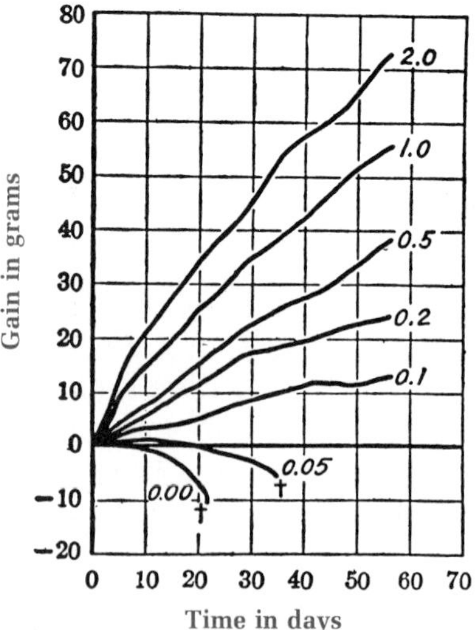

Figure 7–4 Curves of rat growth in pioneer nutrition studies show results due to differences in intake of vitamin A. Figure at end of each curve indicates amount of tomato (in grams) fed to them daily as the sole source of vitamin A. (Courtesy of Dr. H. C. Sherman, Dr. H. E. Munsell, and the *Journal of the American Chemical Society.*)

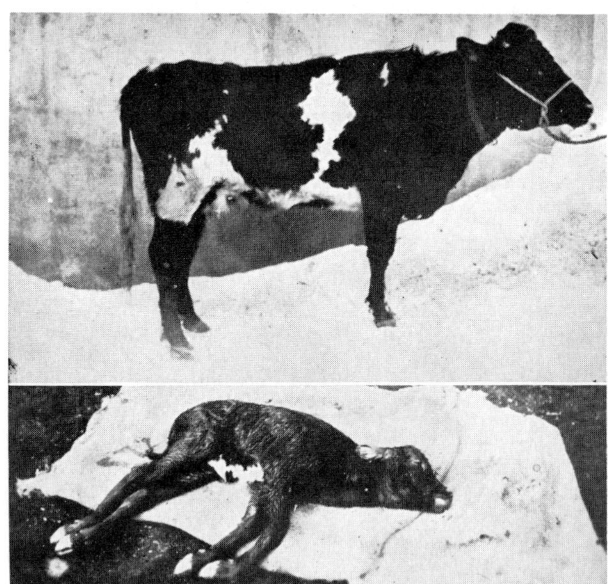

Figure 7–5 A disaster in reproduction caused by feeding this cow a ration, now known to be deficient in vitamin A, made from wheat straw, wheat meal, and wheat gluten, with common salt. In this classic experiment, the cow was shaggy-coated, slow and sleepy in movement, and had a tendency to drag her hind feet. The calf was born prematurely and died later. When the ration was supplemented with bone meal (2 percent), common salt (1 percent), and raw cod-liver oil (2 percent) in another cow, its deficiencies were fully corrected. The cow was in excellent condition and produced twin calves weighing 124 pounds. (From Research Bulletin 17, University of Wisconsin Agricultural Experiment Station, 1911, by Hart, McCollum, Steenbock, and Humphrey.)

along with fats* into the lymph to be emptied later into the blood. The presence of fat and bile favors their absorption. Any factor that lowers fat absorption may affect the absorption of fat-soluble vitamins unfavorably. In disorders such as jaundice and celiac disease, much of the vitamin A value of the diet may fail to be absorbed from the intestine. Bile salts may be given to aid absorption in such cases, or preparations of *water-soluble vitamin A* may be given by mouth as a supplement. Water-soluble vitamin A is an *emulsion* of very finely divided droplets of vitamin A (usually in the form of vitamin A palmitate in a gelatin matrix) in water, and in this state the vitamin is more rapidly absorbed by healthy persons, infants, or patients with faulty fat absorption than when it is given dissolved in oil.

Provitamin A and vitamin A in foods of animal origin are normally completely absorbed. Absorption of the provitamin A carotenoids from fibrous vegetable material is much less efficiently accomplished. Carotenes in green peas are better utilized than those in spinach, but both these vegetables, along with carrots, have much lower vitamin A activity, when taken as food, than equivalent quantities of the vitamin itself taken in cod-liver oil. Other experiments on the relative utilization of carotenes in vegetables showed that the carotenes in kale are about 65 percent available, those in sweet potatoes about 35 percent available, and those in carrots 35 to 40 percent available.[10] The degree to which provitamins in vegetable foods are available later as vitamin A in the body varies not only with the kind of food but also with different individuals.

The very high theoretical total vitamin A activity of some green and yellow vegetables (as listed in tables) may be misleading; owing to incomplete absorption and conversion, they may be expected to yield only one-fourth to one-half as much vitamin A in the body as the listed amount.

The presence of significant amounts of *mineral oil* in the intestine interferes with the absorption of vitamin A, carotenes, and other fat-soluble vitamins, because they dissolve in this oil, which is nonabsorbable; thus they are excreted in the feces.[11] Therefore, mineral oil should not be incorporated in foods (as in salad dressings) or taken too close to mealtimes.

*Vitamin A alcohol (retinol) is esterified in the mucosa of the intestine generally with palmitic acid (a fatty acid) to form retinyl palmitate, an *ester*, in which form it eventually reaches the liver.

Storage and Function in the Body. Both vitamin A (as retinyl palmitate) and any carotenoids not split in the intestinal wall are carried by the lymph system to the blood stream in man.* The *liver* takes up any excess of these substances from the blood and *stores reserves of this vitamin.* These can be released into the blood as retinol, attached to a specific protein† and carried to the tissues later as needed. The level of vitamin A in the blood is thus kept fairly constant and would not be affected by a diet poor in vitamin A until the body reserves were about exhausted. Nearly 95 percent of these reserves are in the liver. How much vitamin A has been stored in the liver depends, of course, on whether the habitual diet has been rich or poor in vitamin A and its precursors. Liver reserves of vitamin A are usually lowest at birth and are built up with advancing years. In diseases of the liver — notably cirrhosis — these stores are markedly reduced.

Because reserve stores of vitamin A exist but are variable in amount in different individuals, it is natural that *symptoms due to a vitamin A deficiency should develop rather slowly* and that the time interval before deficiency symptoms appear differs according to the extent of the body stores available in time of need.

No vitamin A is excreted in the urine because it is not water-soluble, but considerable unabsorbed carotene is normally found *in the feces*. In disorders in which the stools are loose and frequent, or in which bile is lacking, most of the carotene and even some of the vitamin A intake may fail to be absorbed. During lactation, there is a considerable output of vitamin A in the milk secreted, so that the need for extra quantities of this vitamin is greater at this time than at others.

In metabolism, interrelations between vitamin A and other vitamins exist. Vitamin A and provitamin A can lose their potency by oxidation; both vitamin E and vitamin C are thought to spare vitamin A by acting as antioxidants — substances that enhance the preservation of vitamin A in its biologically active form.

Vitamin A appears to be necessary for the formation of *mucopolysaccharides,* which are essential components of mucous membranes and without which epithelial membranes degenerate. Vitamin A appears to be essential for the release of a protein-splitting enzyme necessary for the formation of bone from cartilage, of ribonucleic acid (RNA), and of certain ovarian hormones necessary for reproduction in the rat.

*Some animals, such as the rat, sheep, and pig, absorb no carotene at all.

†The human retinol-binding protein (RBP) in serum is an albumin of low molecular weight rich in tryptophan and specific for this purpose.[12]

Retinol Equivalents and Recommended Allowances

Because the various animal and plant forms of vitamin A and provitamin A have different biological activities and vary among species, to give allowances or food levels of vitamin A in terms of micrograms or milligrams of total vitamin A activity would be quite meaningless. For this reason the *International Unit* has traditionally been used to measure vitamin A activity for convenience, if not for ease of understanding. (International Units are also used for vitamins D and E but not for other vitamins. An International Unit (IU) of vitamin A is defined *on the basis* of rat studies as equal to 0.344 mcg of crystalline retinylacetate (which is equivalent to 0.300 mcg of retinol, or to 0.60 mcg of beta-carotene). These standards were based on experiments that showed that in rats only about 50 percent of the beta-carotene is converted to vitamin A.

In man, however, we know that beta-carotene is not as available as in the rat, owing to poorer absorption in the intestine and other factors. To better quantify vitamin A values for humans within the metric system, therefore, international agencies have now introduced the biological equivalent of 1 microgram (1 mcg) of retinol as the standard.[8, 13] In the long run this will make things much more understandable. However, until better analytical values are available for the provitamin A carotenoids in food, both terms will be used during the years of transition. RDA values are given in both IU's and "retinol equivalents." Since these relationships are based on different standards, they are not equal to each other in terms of "total vitamin A activity"; but the differences are not of great practical importance.

By definition, then, the following relationships hold:

1 retinol equivalent (in humans) =
- 1 mcg retinol (human or rat)
- 6 mcg beta-carotene (human)
- 12 mcg other provitamin A carotenoids (human)
- 3.33 IU of retinol (rat)
- 10 IU of beta-carotene (rat)

These standards are based on beta-carotene being only one-third absorbed and only about one-half converted to vitamin A in humans (unlike the relationship in rats). Thus, for humans, beta-carotene has only about one-sixth the vitamin A activity that retinol has.*

The new retinol equivalent values will be much more useful when good biological assays are available on the total vitamin A activity of different foods using humans as the test subjects, or when tables of food composition are available that have different columns for vitamin A activity: (1) retinol, (2) beta-carotene, (3) other provitamins A, and (4) total mcg retinol equivalents. Until this information is available, we will primarily employ the still widely used IU values.

The average American diet is considered to contain roughly one-half of its total vitamin A activity in the active form and one-half as the provitamin — primarily beta-carotene — according to the Food and Nutrition Board.[8]

Biologically, the active isomers of the pure vitamin A compounds are all in the "trans" form. Various "cis" forms (which are less active than the "trans" forms) of the vitamin and provitamins do exist in foods in smaller amounts. This introduces additional complications, but is not of practical importance except in processed foods.

The most recent recommended allowances of the U.S. Food and Nutrition Board are given in Table 7–1 in both IU and mcg retinol equivalents per day. For additional values for different age groups see Appendix, Table 1. Allowances for infants and children are liberal in terms of minimum requirements in order to provide extra vitamin A for growth and to ensure adequate stores.

Toxicity

Long-continued large doses of vitamin A have a *toxic* effect, and regular moderate intake (5000 to 10,000 IU per

*By use of the above values, then, 5000 IU of vitamin A theoretically should equal about 1500 retinol equivalents. However, because the RDA in IU is based on rat conversion factors and the RDA for retinol equivalents is based on human conversion factors, assuming that about half of the dietary intake is carotene, the two RDA's will not be comparable. The "retinol equivalent" is the better figure to use for humans in the long run.

Table 7–1 RECOMMENDED DIETARY ALLOWANCE FOR TOTAL VITAMIN A ACTIVITY*

Sex	*Age*	*IU Vitamin A*	*mcg Retinol Equivalents*
Females†	11 years and over	4000	800
Males	11 years and over	5000	1000

*From Food and Nutrition Board, 1974.[8]
†The allowance during pregnancy is 5000 IU/day and during lactation 6000 IU/day.

day) is better for building up stores in the liver. Toxic symptoms known as *hypervitaminosis A* may occur in children one to three years of age after they have received 75,000 IU or more of vitamin A daily for at least 6 months (or less, of the water-soluble forms). Such symptoms — which include excessive irritability, swellings over the long bones, and dry and itching skin — are relieved by discontinuing the dosages of supplementary vitamin A. In adults, the early symptoms of toxicity are headache, nausea, and diarrhea; a great excess of vitamin A may also lead to decalcification of bones with consequent bone fragility.

Livers of animals may concentrate so much vitamin A that they may be toxic when eaten in large amounts over long periods.[14] Early explorers in the Arctic, it is said, learned to avoid eating the liver of the polar bear because symptoms of toxicity were observed and were later found to be due to excessive vitamin A. Carotene, in contrast to vitamin A, is not toxic even when consumed at high levels. In humans, the only abnormal sign that might be seen when large amounts of carotene are eaten is a yellow skin (as is seen in some persons who consume large amounts of carrots or red palm oil, for example).

Extent of Vitamin A Deficiency

It is not difficult to get the recommended allowance of total vitamin A activity in daily foods, if good foods are available and are wisely chosen. Although surveys show that it is not uncommon for the diet to fall slightly below the recommended allowance in the United States,[15] marked symptoms of vitamin A deficiency are not seen commonly. The allowances provide a large margin of safety above basic minimum requirements, so diets somewhat below the allowance figure are not necessarily deficient for body needs.

Generally, nutritionists do not become overly concerned unless intakes of vitamin A are less than two-thirds the recommended allowance. In any event, in the United States, it is clear from the references cited[15] that most of us are obtaining sufficient vitamin A in our diets. However, in the diets of teen-age girls, pregnant women, and older persons, the level of vitamin A intake may often be too low to allow for a proper margin of safety. Two studies of diets in several groups of infants indicated the vitamin A intake to be more than ample.[16]

The average amount of vitamin A available to each person per day in the United States has decreased from a level of 8700 IU in 1947–49 to the present level of 8200 IU.[17] These are *available units* and do not include amounts lost in food wastage or in food preparation or processing. When actual United States *intakes* were surveyed in 1971–74, the values were considerably lower, often below recommended amounts.[18]

Vitamin A deficiency, unfortunately, is very widespread throughout the world, especially among children in countries where fat supplies are low and where there are few green vegetables in the diet. Night blindness, xerophthalmia, impaired vision, and blindness as a result of vitamin A deficiency are prevalent throughout Asia, the Middle East, India, Malaysia, and parts of Africa, South America, and Latin America. It has been estimated that throughout the world (excluding Communist China) *about 80,000 children become blind each year from vitamin A deficiency*, and that about one-half of these die.*[19] For instance, in Indonesia, in 82 percent of the blind children below the age of 10, the cause was vitamin A deficiency. Gopalan has stated that in South India, vitamin A deficiency accounts for 25 to 30 percent of all cases of clinical malnutrition and is often seen in association with protein deficiency.[20] In older children and young adults, too low a supply of vitamin A pre-

*To say nothing of the grief and untold misery for parents, and lifetime disability for most of the survivors.

disposes the individual to tuberculosis, which is widespread in a number of countries.

It is difficult to determine when a person is deficient in vitamin A in the absence of the usual symptoms seen in more severe deficiency. Night blindness or dark adaptation tests are not always successful in diagnosing a deficiency. Most useful are measurements of serum vitamin A and carotene values in comparison with known standards. Serum levels of 10 to 19 mcg of vitamin A per 100 ml are considered low, as are 20 to 39 mcg or less of carotene.

Food Sources of Vitamin A Activity

The most important animal sources of vitamin A are *liver, butterfat,* and *egg yolk.* Milk, cream, ice cream, and whole milk or most cheeses all contain vitamin A in smaller amounts. The vitamin A value of these foods varies widely according to the vitamin A value of the food of the animals that produced them. Livers from older animals and from animals fed on green fodder contain much larger stores of vitamin A. Butterfat in the milk of cows is usually yellower and of higher vitamin A value when the animals are grazing in green pastures than when stall-fed in winter. However, improved feeds for dairy cattle, together with their ability to draw on stores of vitamin A in the liver, result in less seasonal variations in vitamin A content of milk and butter than were formerly common. The yellowness of egg yolk and butterfat is not an infallible guide to their vitamin A value, because they contain both yellow carotenoids and colorless vitamin A.

Margarine has been fortified by addition of carotene or vitamin A (also vitamin D) up to the level equal to a year-round average in butter (15,000 IU per lb, or 3300 IU per 100 gm). This makes it fully acceptable nutritionally as a less expensive substitute for butter.

Important plant sources of vitamin A activity are the *green and yellow vegetables.* Some typical food values for total vitamin A activity are given in Table 7–2. As the vitamin A activity of plants is due entirely to yellow carotenoid pigments, either alone or found with chlorophyll, the depth of yellow or green color is a rough index of their potential vitamin A activity. Most thin green leaves, such as spinach, kale, and turnip greens, have a vitamin A value from 5000 to 15,000 IU (average about 8000 IU) per 100 gm. Bleached inner leaves of cabbage and lettuce, as well as bleached asparagus, are of low vitamin A activity. Carrots may vary in vitamin A activity from 2000 to 12,000 IU per 100 gm, and sweet potatoes also vary widely in vitamin A activity (1500 to 7700 IU), according to the depth of their color.

Grains (except for yellow corn), white flour, sugar, and the common colorless vegetable oils carry little or no vitamin A activity, and lean muscle meats, nuts, and many common fruits and vegetables provide only minor quantities. The body fat of animals is usually low in vitamin A, but that of fish may contain considerable amounts.

Combinations of *foods that provide the standard daily allowance of total vitamin A activity for an adult* are given in Table 7–3. Each combination combines animal and plant sources, and furnishes somewhat more than 5000 IU of vitamin A.

There is danger that the diet will provide less than optimum amounts of total vitamin A activity unless green and yellow vegetables are used frequently. In addition, they are inexpensive sources of vitamin A for low-cost diets. This danger of inadequacy of the diet is illustrated by the list of foods in Table 7–4, which might seem to constitute the basis of a normal diet for 1 day, but which falls considerably short of the 5000 IU daily vitamin A allowance.

If one of the vegetables listed in Table 7–4 were of the green or yellow variety, the vitamin A value of this diet would be

Table 7-2 TOTAL VITAMIN A ACTIVITY OF TYPICAL FOODS*

Food	*IU Per 100 Grams, Raw*	*Size of Average Serving*	*IU Per Avg. Serving*
Liver, beef	43,900	2 slices, fried (74 gm)	40,050
Carrots, deep color	11,000	2/3 c, diced, cooked (100 gm)	10,500
Apricots, dried	10,900	1/2 c, cooked, with juice	4200
Sweet potatoes, deep color	8800	1 medium, baked (110 gm)	8910
Green leafy vegetables (4000–15,000), avg.	7870	1/2 c, cooked (100 gm)	7870
Fruits, fresh:			
Apricots	2700	2–3 medium	2700
Nectarines	1650	2 medium	1650
Peaches, avg., yellow	1330	1 medium-large	1330
Cherries	1000	15 large	1000
Watermelon	590	1/16 of 10 × 16 in melon	2530
Others (trace to 400), avg.	135	Avg. serving (100 gm)	135
Squash, winter, boiled	3500	1/2 c, boiled	3500
Cantaloupe, deep color	3400	1/2 melon (200 gm)	6800
Butter (2000–4000), year-round average	3300	1 avg. pat (10 gm)	330
Margarine, fortified	3300	1 avg. pat (10 gm)	330
Broccoli	2500	2/3 c, cooked, or 1 large stalk	2500
Lettuce, green leaf	1900	2 large or 4–5 small leaves	950
Pumpkin	1600	1/2 c, cooked	3840
Prunes, dried	1600	4 medium cooked, 2 tbsp juice	510
Cheese, cream	1540	1 oz avg. serving	460
Cheese, American cheddar	1310	1 oz avg. serving	390
Eggs, whole	1180	1, avg. size (50 gm)	590
Tomatoes	900	1, medium size (150 gm)	1350
Asparagus, green	900	6 stalks, canned (100 gm)	900
Cream, thin, 20%	840	4 tbsp (60 gm)	500
Ice cream, plain, avg.	520	1/6 qt (100 gm)	520
Green vegetables, other than those listed above, avg.	500	Avg. serving (100 gm)	500
Yellow vegetables, other than listed above, avg.	330	Avg. serving (100 gm)	330
Milk, whole, fresh	140	1 pt	740
Other vegetables (10–90), avg.	50	Avg. serving (100 gm)	50

*Figures adapted from U.S. Department Agriculture Handbook No. 8: *Composition of Foods—Raw, Processed, Prepared,* 1963.

raised decidedly, usually up to the 5000 IU level or more, provided the vegetable chosen was strongly colored and an average-sized serving (100 gm) was eaten. Figure 7–6 shows sources of vitamin A in average American diets.

Table 7-3 FOOD COMBINATIONS THAT PROVIDE THE RECOMMENDED DAILY ALLOWANCE OF TOTAL VITAMIN A ACTIVITY FOR AN ADULT*

	Food	*Amount*
1.	Whole milk	1 pt (480 gm)
	Pumpkin pie	4 in wedge (150 gm)
	Vegetable beef soup	1 c
2.	Margarine or butter	2 tbsp
	Broccoli	2/3 c
	Nectarines	2
3.	Eggs	2
	Apricots	2–4
	Tomato juice	6 oz

*Each of these food combinations furnishes somewhat more than 5000 IU of total vitamin A activity.

Effect of Cooking or Processing

Because vitamin A and its precursors (the carotenes) are *insoluble in water* and *stable to heat at ordinary cooking temperatures, most foods lose little of their total vitamin A activity, as measured chemically, in cooking or processing,* unless they are exposed to air. However, the bio-

Table 7–4 A FOOD COMBINATION SUPPLYING AN **INADEQUATE** AMOUNT OF VITAMIN A ACTIVITY FOR DAILY ADULT DIET*

Food	*Amount*
Whole milk	1 pt
Butter or margarine	2 squares
Egg	1
Orange juice	4 oz
Apple	1 medium
Green beans	½ c (3–4 oz)
Coleslaw (cabbage salad)	½ c
Beets	½ c

*This diet contains only about 3000 IU instead of 5000 IU of total vitamin A activity.

logical value of the vitamin A activity of common processed vegetables may be reduced 15 to 20 percent in green vegetables and as high as 30 to 35 percent in common yellow vegetables because of chemical changes in the carotene molecule (some trans forms are changed to other isomers).[21] Drying of eggs, vegetables, or fruits, with exposure to air, sunlight, or high temperatures, may cause serious loss of vitamin A value. Evaporation, pasteurization, or irradiation of milk has little or no effect on its vitamin A content. Vegetables should be stored at low temperatures to conserve their vitamin A value, and, of course, quick freezing is an excellent means to this end. Animal fats should be kept in a cold, dark place, and fish-liver oils should be protected from light by being put in a dark glass bottle.

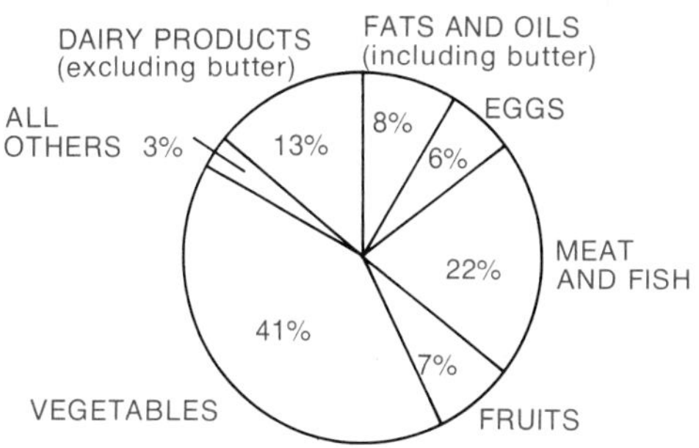

Figure 7–6 Percentages of vitamin A value contributed by various food groups in the average American diet. (From information supplied by U.S. Department of Agriculture, 1978.)

By far the most potent sources of vitamin A today are the synthetic forms; they are also the most inexpensive. Vitamin A costs only a few cents *per gram* of stabilized material (1 million IU), when purchased in large quantities. This is a 200 day supply for one person. The use of synthetic vitamin A and carotene to fortify certain foods accounts today for about 7 percent of all vitamin A intake in the United States. Many tons of synthetic forms of the vitamin are made each year. They are just as effective and safe as the natural forms, though of course they carry no other nutrients with them.

VITAMIN D

History and Identification

Rickets,* a bone disorder also seen in calcium and phosphorus deficiency, has been known since 500 B.C. In industrial England rickets was very common in children in the crowded slums, and it became known as the "English disease." In 1824, cod-liver oil, long used as a "folk medicine," was found to be important in the treatment of rickets, though it was not used universally for this purpose until nearly a century later.

The importance of sunshine for good health of individuals was known by ancient civilizations and is probably one of the bases for sun worship by primitive nations. In the 1890's it was found that sunshine was a specific cure for rickets[22] — though the exact reason for this was not known until the discovery of vitamin D in the 1920's. Ever since, vitamin D has been popularly called "the sunshine vitamin," for good reason.

In 1918 Mellanby of London, in studies with puppies, provided the first experimental proof that rickets was a deficiency

*According to McCollum,[1] the word "rickets" is derived from the old English word *wrikken* (to bend or twist). In 1650 Glisson of Cambridge wrote a treatise about the disease and blamed it on bad home environment and hygiene.[1]

disease. He was able to cure it by feeding them cod-liver oil. McCollum and his coworkers[1, 23] found in 1922 that after destruction (by oxidation) of all the vitamin A in cod-liver oil, it still retained its rickets-preventing potency. This proved the existence of a second fat-soluble vitamin, carried in liver oils and certain other fats, which he called the *calcium-depositing vitamin.*

It is of interest that though McCollum discovered the existence of vitamin D, he did not call it by this name until after the name was in quite common use by others (contrary to many textbook statements).*

The first crystalline vitamin D was obtained in 1931, and it was synthesized shortly thereafter.† Soon it became evident that there appeared to be at least ten natural substances that produce vitamin D–like activity in varying degrees. Only two of these are of practical importance today from the standpoint of their occurrence in foods — *ergocalciferol* (vitamin D_2) and *cholecalciferol* (vitamin D_3). (See formulas in the Appendix.) Because these substances are closely related chemically and produce a like effect on the body, the term vitamin D is used collectively to indicate the *group* of substances that show this vitamin activity.

The vitamin D group belongs to the class of organic substances known as *sterols* — fairly large molecules in plants and animals containing an alcohol group and having the same solubilities as fats. They are very stable compounds, resisting destruction by heat and oxidation, as well as by acids and alkalis. Obviously they are sensitive to light, especially that of shorter wavelengths (ultraviolet). The sterols, except vitamin D, are synthesized in the body and are the precursors of many important hormones, including several hormones made in the body from vitamin D and the sex hormones. Other common sterols are *cholesterol* and the several *bile acids.*

*The term "vitamin D" for the antirachitic vitamin was not suggested until 1924 by Sure (J. Biol. Chem., *58*:693, 1924) and a year later was agreed to by McCollum and coworkers (J. Biol. Chem., *64*:161, 1925). This name was quickly accepted, in spite of the fact that Funk and Dubin (J. Biol. Chem., *48*:437, 1921, and Proc. Soc. Exp. Biol. Med., *19*:15, 1921) had earlier used the term "vitamine D" to describe a new and different water-soluble growth factor for the rat (and for yeast), a suggestion disregarded by others for some reason.

†Crystals of vitamin D were first obtained by the Dutch chemists Reerink and van Wijk (Biochem. J., *25*:1001, 1931).

The Precursors of Vitamin D

Steenbock and Hess, in the 1920's, discovered independently that when certain foods are exposed to ultraviolet light, their ability to protect animals against rickets is increased. This meant that some foods must contain precursors of vitamin D — substances that are altered chemically by light of certain wavelengths (including sunlight) so that they become capable of functioning as vitamins in the body. We now know that there are two major precursors of vitamin D in nature and that each gives rise to a slightly different vitamin D when activated by light. In plants, a substance known as *ergosterol** is converted by light into ergocalciferol (vitamin D_2). In animals, and possibly in some plants, a derivative of *cholesterol* — 7-dehydrocholesterol — is the precursor of cholecalciferol, or vitamin D_3 (as discovered by Waddell in 1934). Birds respond much better to cholecalciferol, but most animals can utilize either type of vitamin D. Cholecalciferol occurs in fish-liver oils and foods of animal origin, such as eggs, butter, milk, and cream. It is also available in a low-cost, synthetic form that is equal in activity to natural forms of the vitamin.

Formation of Vitamin D in the Body by Sunlight

The precursor (7-dehydrocholesterol) of the major form of this vitamin is pres-

*The German chemist Adolph Windhaus received the Nobel Prize in 1928 for his studies on the vitamin activity of irradiated ergosterol. The compound was named from ergot, a black fungus that grows on the rye plant, from which ergosterol was first isolated in 1889.

ent in humans and animals in the oily lubricating material in the skin and on its surface. When *sunlight,* in which there is ultraviolet light of short wavelengths, falls directly on the skin, some of the provitamin is converted into cholecalciferol, the major animal form of vitamin D.[22] The vitamin thus formed in or on the skin is readily taken into the local circulation and carried by the blood to all parts of the body. Amounts formed in excess of immediate body needs can be stored in considerable amounts in the liver and may be found also in the fatty tissues, lungs, spleen, and brain.

Hess found that rickets could be prevented or cured by exposing children (without clothing) to sunlight or the rays of an *ultraviolet lamp,* since they thus were enabled to manufacture vitamin D in their own bodies. Today, however, with the availability of foods enriched with vitamin D and of other low-cost food supplements, ultraviolet lamps or sun lamps are not the most practical way of obtaining this vitamin.

Other animals also generate vitamin D in their bodies on exposure to light. Steenbock kept chicks indoors on a ration low in vitamin D, conditions that led to stunted growth and leg weakness. Exposure to sunlight for a half-hour daily served to protect the chicks against the effects of vitamin D deficiency in the diet (Fig. 7–7). The discovery of cheap dietary sources of vitamin D for farm animals (as substitutes for sunshine) was a major factor in the ability to raise poultry, swine, and cattle indoors and the year around. This resulted in the wide availability of low-cost eggs, milk, and meat in developed countries. Aso, we could not raise cats and dogs as pets in our homes without this discovery of a "sunshine substitute."

Effects of Vitamin D Deficiency

The effects of a lack of vitamin D, as seen most strikingly in children and young animals, are poor growth and lack of normal development of the bones. In the condition *rickets,* the metabolism of calcium and phosphorus is disturbed in such a way that the deposition in the bones of the inorganic salt calcium phos-

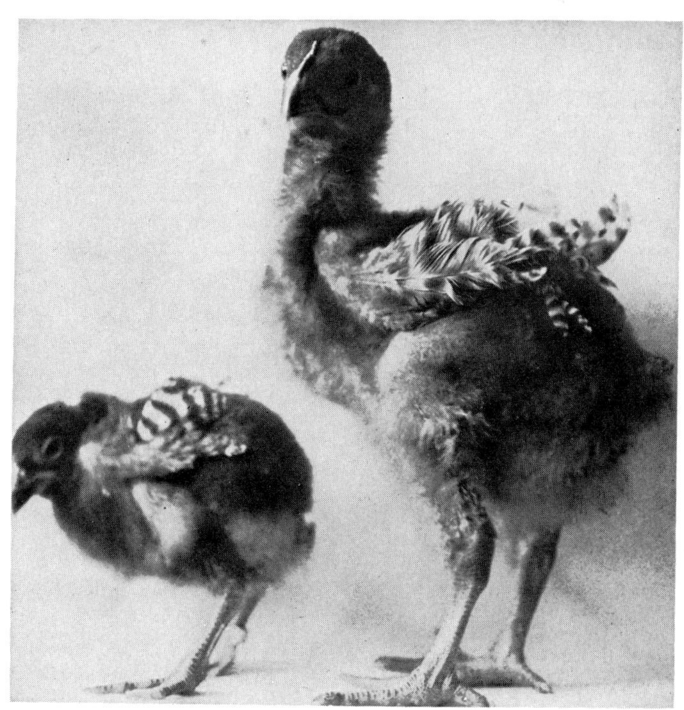

Figure 7–7 Effect of exposure to sunlight in stimulating growth. Both chicks received the same ration, which was poor in vitamin D, but the one on the right was exposed to sunlight one-half hour daily, thus permitting generation of the needed vitamin D in its body. (Courtesy of Dr. H. Steenbock, University of Wisconsin.)

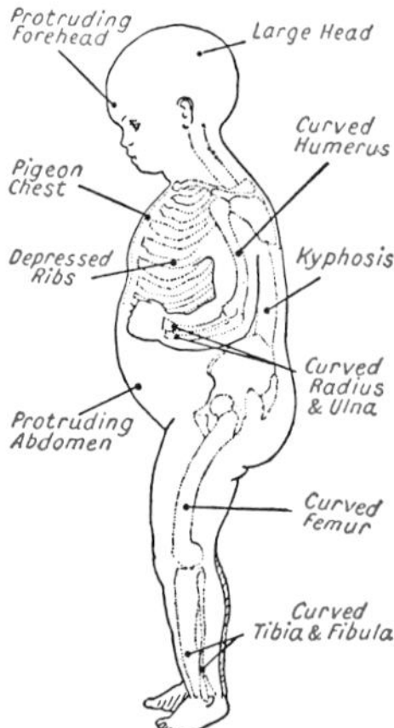

Figure 7–8 Diagram showing deformities that are symptoms of severe cases of rickets. (From Harris, L. J.: *Vitamins in Theory and Practice*. 4th Ed. London, Cambridge University Press, 1955.)

phate, which is responsible for bone rigidity, cannot proceed normally. Hence, this disease is characterized by weak bones, which readily develop curvatures when compelled to carry the weight of the body, and by overgrowth of the softer tissues (cartilage) at the ends of the bones. Rachitic deformities develop, such as *bowlegs*, *knock-knees*, *enlargement of bones* about the *joints*, and a *narrow, distorted chest* with beading of the ribs (Figs. 7–8 and 7–9). These deformities, not themselves causing death, may persist into adult life, at which time the shrunken chest may predispose to lung diseases, and a narrow pelvis may be one of the factors making childbearing difficult for such women. Milder cases of rickets, associated with less severe lack of vitamin D, may be detectable only by blood analyses (showing that either the serum calcium or phosphate, or both, are below normal levels), by failure of bones to grow properly in length, and by x-ray pictures, which show the characteristic failure of normal deposition of calcium phosphate in the ends of the bones. When healing takes place (usually as a result of giving vitamin D), new deposits of calcium phosphate are laid down in the cartilage along the line of demarcation between the head of the bone (*epiphysis*) and the main part or *shaft* of the long bone. This increase of mineral deposit near the ends of the bones is indicated by increased density in x-ray pictures (Fig. 7–10).

Though vitamin D deficiency is not common in adults, it does occur especially during pregnancy, lactation, old age, and in persons eating vitamin D–low diets who do not receive any sunshine. Examples of the latter are certain women in the Middle East and in North Africa who, by

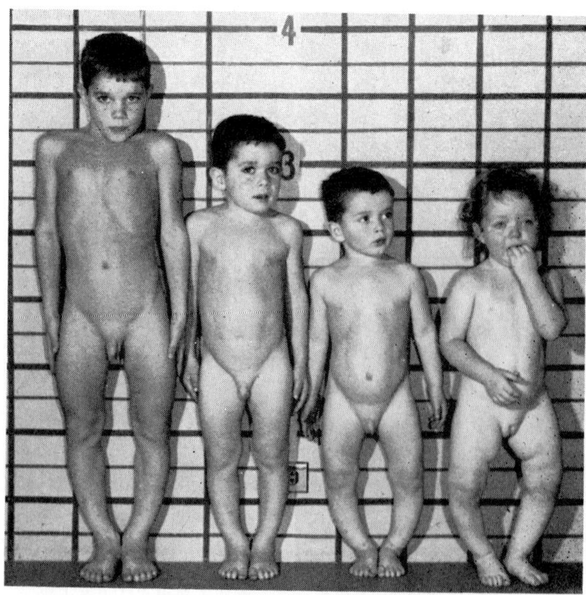

Figure 7–9 Three brothers and a female first cousin with rickets. (These cases were not due to a simple vitamin D deficiency, but the photo illustrates what vitamin D deficiency looks like in children.) (From Fraser, D., and Salter, R. B.:, Pediatr. Clin. North Amer. May 1958.)

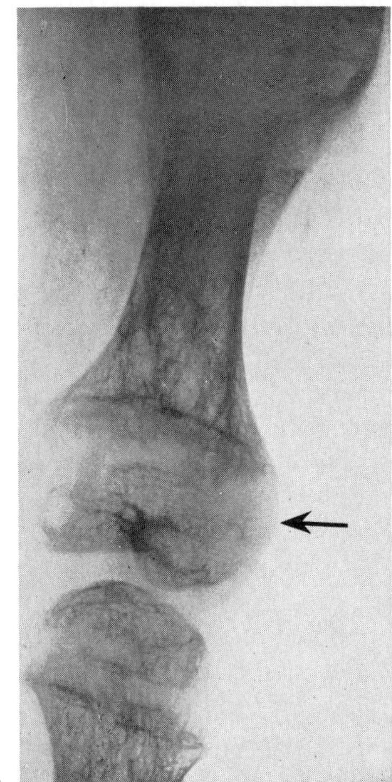

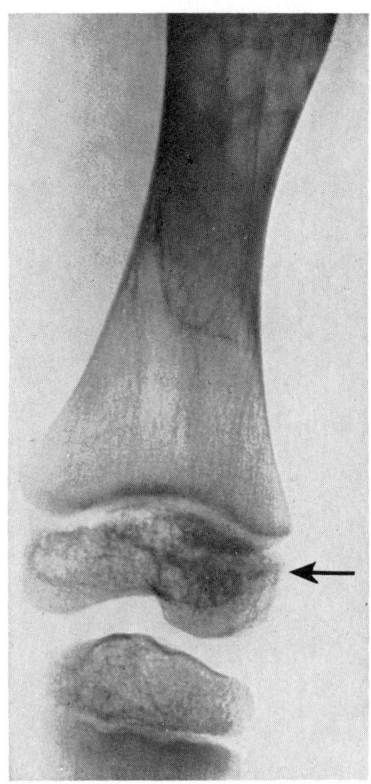

Figure 7–10 X-ray pictures of same joint in a 10-year-old Mexican boy, before and after treatment for rickets. **A,** Rarefication at ends of bones due to failure of normal deposition of calcium phosphate in rickets. **B,** One month later, showing increased density of bones and rapid healing of rachitic changes as the result of very large doses of vitamin D. (From McCune. In Wohl, M. S. (ed.): *Dietotherapy*. Philadelphia, W. B. Saunders Co., 1945.)

the custom of *purdah,* are confined indoors or are heavily clothed when outdoors (see Fig. 7–11). *Adult rickets,* or *osteomalacia* (a form of softening of the bone; see also Chapter 11), is caused by depletion of bone stores of calcium and phosphorus. This may be from poor utilization of these mineral elements associated with vitamin D deficiency — or lack of sunshine — over very long periods, from faulty absorption, from kidney defects, or possibly in old age from changes in activity of certain hormone-producing glands (especially the parathyroid and thyroid glands).

It should be obvious that rickets at any age may be caused also by *lack of either calcium or phosphorus,* since these are the building materials for the calcium phosphate upon which the rigidity and strength of bone depend. No amount of vitamin D will promote normal bone development unless the mineral elements necessary for building strong bones are provided in the diet in adequate quantities. Conversely, if *vitamin D is lacking,* rickets may develop in persons on diets that supply plenty of calcium and phosphorus (e.g., in infants on milk diet). The vitamin D may be supplied in food or an oil concentrate, it may be generated in the body by exposure to sunlight, or some may be obtained from each source. A diet rich in one of the necessary mineral elements and poor in the other predisposes toward development of rickets. The best *protection* against this disease and the most favorable bone growth are secured when calcium and phosphorus are supplied in approximately equal amounts (as in milk) and when liberal quantities of vitamin D are available.

Vitamin D deficiency may also result in poor tooth development, muscular weakness, a protruding abdomen, listlessness, and an enlarged skull.

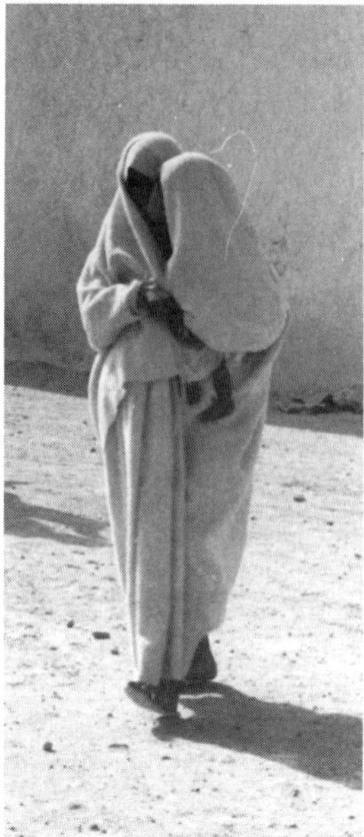

Figure 7–11 An example of *purdah*, a custom of being heavily wrapped in clothes, thus effectively blocking out the sunshine in a land of abundant sunshine. (From World Health, March 1977, p. 20. Courtesy of WHO)

Vitamin D in the Body, and Its Functions

Vitamin D, being fat-soluble, is absorbed from the intestine along with fats. Bile aids in this process, and conditions unfavorable to fat absorption (lack of bile, disorders such as sprue and celiac disease, etc.) may result in poor utilization of vitamin D.

Like other fat-soluble vitamins, vitamin D can be stored in the body to a great extent. It can be passed from the mother's body to build up stores in the child before birth, or into breast milk on which the infant feeds, and in both these ways it may help to protect the infant against rickets. It is noticeable that the age at which rickets is most likely to develop, 1 to 3 years, coincides with a period of rapid growth (high need) and one in which there has been little chance to accumulate large body stores of vitamin D. The gradual accumulation of such stores with age doubtless accounts in large part for the infrequency of any evidence of vitamin D deficiency in adults.

The overall *function* of vitamin D is to produce a vital hormone called 1,25-dihydroxycholecalciferol — known for short as 1,25-dihydroxy D_3 or $1,25(OH)_2D_3$ — or simply "vitamin D hormone." Made by the liver and kidney, this hormone is essential for the overall effects of dietary vitamin D, which include promotion of *growth* and proper *mineralization of the bones and teeth.* There is general agreement that the main result of its action is the *improvement of utilization of calcium and phosphorus* supplied in the food. Vitamin D increases the absorption of calcium, and secondarily also of phosphorus, from the intestinal tract. It is also involved with calcium mobilization from bones and with the preservation of phosphate by control of its excretion from the kidney (see Fig. 7–12). All these reactions help to keep the content of these two elements in the blood up to levels favorable to the deposition of calcium phosphate in the bones. It appears at this time that the only function of dietary forms of vitamin D, such as cholecalciferol, is to serve as a precursor of the hormone form. As far as is known now, vitamin D itself does not function until the two additional OH groups are added in the body.

After vitamin D (cholecalciferol, D_3) is absorbed into the blood, it is carried to the liver by a specific vitamin D carrier protein (a globulin). Here it is changed to an intermediary, more active metabolic form, *25-hydroxycholecalciferol* (25-OH D_3), in which an OH group replaces an H atom on carbon number 25.* This compound is transported in the blood by the same protein to the kidney, where one more OH group is added, forming the compound *1,25-dihydroxycholecalciferol* ($1,25\text{-}(OH)_2D_3$).[24] This appears to be the metabolically active form of vitamin D in the intestine and perhaps the bone. When ingested

---

*Identified by DeLuca and coworkers of Wisconsin (Proc. Nat. Acad. Sci., *61*:1503, 1968; Amer. J. Clin. Nutr., *22*:412, 1969). DeLuca, now in charge of the laboratory of the late Dr. Steenbock, has also shown that ergocalciferol, D_2, is changed to a similar active metabolite in the liver — 25-hydroxyergocalciferol (25-OH D_2).

from food, it acts slightly more efficiently and rapidly than the parent compound.

The active compound (1,25-$(OH)_2$ D_3) is a *hormone,* since it is a vital substance made in the body by one organ (the kidney) and transported in the blood to cells within target tissues. Vitamin D serves as a precursor, whether derived from the food or from the skin as a result of the action of light. (It is comparable, in a sense, to dietary precursors of several hormones, such as thyroxine or those containing essential amino acids).

The new hormone is the metabolically active form of the vitamin used for increasing calcium absorption in the intestine and for serving other vitamin D–dependent functions. For instance, a source of vitamin D is essential through this mechanism for the formation of a specific *ribonucleic acid,* necessary in turn for the formation of several important proteins, including a *calcium-binding protein* in the cells of the intestine. This protein is essential, as is parathyroid hormone, for the absorption and transportation of calcium.

Vitamin D–active compounds appear, also, to be essential for the formation of at least two enzymes — *alkaline phosphatase* in the intestinal lining (involved in calcium transport) and *adenosine triphosphatase,* which appears to be necessary for collagen formation in the bone (necessary for bone matrix). Vitamin D compounds also play a role, somehow, with other hormones, *in the regulation of amino acid levels* in the blood (by protecting against the loss of amino acids through the kidney) and of the *level of citric acid in tissues and bones.* Vitamin D compounds apparently play a part in muscle function and metabolism as well.

In some individuals, vitamin D from the food is not well absorbed, such as in "vitamin D–resistant rickets." The new metabolically active forms of vitamin D have been useful in the treatment of this and similar diseases in which there is a blockage of the conversion of natural vitamin D to the active forms.

International Units

Vitamin D is measured in terms of International Units, as is vitamin A. Crystalline cholecalciferol (vitamin D_3) was adopted in 1949 as the standard reference material. *One International Unit* corresponds to the vitamin activity of *0.025 mcg* of this pure substance, and 400 units equals 10 mcg, a day's allowance, making this one of the most potent vitamins

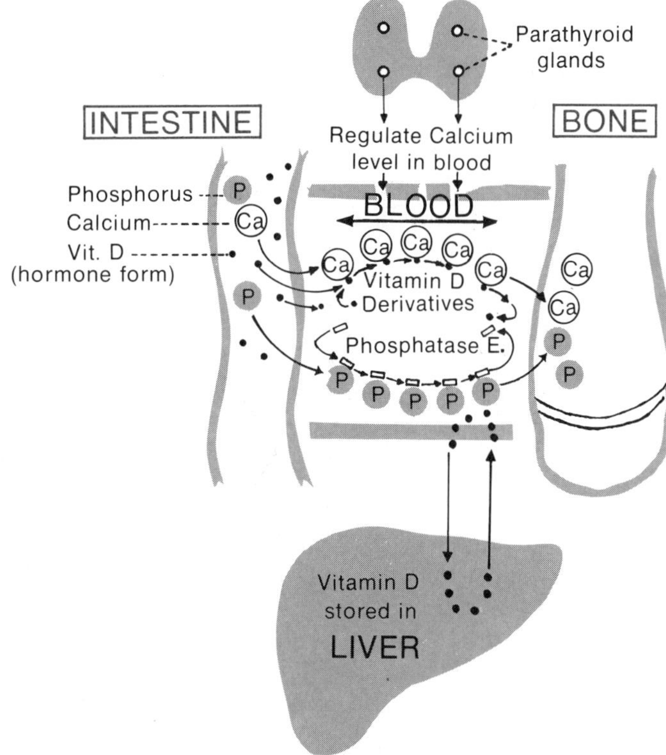

Figure 7–12 Diagram indicating how vitamin D derivatives function in the body by increasing the absorption of calcium and phosphorus from the intestine, thus raising their level in the blood and promoting their deposition in bone. Reserves of vitamin D or their derivatives stored in the liver can be drawn on to keep up the level of this vitamin in blood and tissues during periods of low intake or extra need.

known. The U.S. Pharmacopeia (USP) unit, often used in this country as a standard for potency of medicinal preparations, is the same as the International Unit (as is also true for vitamin A).

Human Requirements

It is impossible to state the vitamin D requirements exactly. The amounts supplied by food can be estimated fairly well, but no one has been able to determine a way of knowing exactly how much extra vitamin D is made in the body under the influence of sunlight.

Jeans and Stearns made extensive studies of the effects of different levels of vitamin D intake on infants[25] They found that 135 IU daily prevents rickets, but that 300 to 400 IU daily results in more rapid growth (especially in length) and earlier eruption of teeth as long as a supply of calcium and phosphorus is available, plentiful, and readily assimilable.

Less is known about the vitamin D requirements of older children than of infants. Jeans and Stearns showed that 300 to 400 IU daily in the form of cod-liver oil favored calcium retention in children from 1 to 12 years of age.[25] They state that in adolescence the need for this vitamin becomes "as universal and as great as in infancy." The Food and Nutrition Board recommends 400 IU of vitamin D daily from birth to 22 years of age, including breast-fed infants.[8]

The Board notes that the vitamin D requirements can readily be satisfied by normal exposure to sunlight or by diets containing vitamin D–fortified foods. However, in environments where sunlight sources are insufficient, dietary sources, up to 400 IU per day, may be necessary.[8]

During pregnancy and lactation, intakes of vitamin D (400 IU daily) should be provided. A liberal supply at these periods is undoubtedly wise, because even though transmission to the fetus and milk is relatively low, the stores of vitamin D in the baby's body and the vitamin D content of milk are appreciably increased by vitamin D in the diet of the mother. In addition, optimum amounts of this vitamin promote the most efficient utilization by the mother of the calcium and phosphorus in her diet.

The amount of vitamin D that is made in the body through exposure to sunlight varies according to the *season*, the *locality* in which one lives, and one's *habits*. In the tropics bright sunlight is available the year round; nevertheless, rickets is still possible. In other parts of the world, sunlight is scarce during the winter months. Sunlight also is richer in ultraviolet rays in summer, and more of these rays get through to the "consumer" when the sun is directly overhead — between 10 A.M. and 2 P.M. On cloudy or foggy days and in cities troubled with "smog," almost all the ultraviolet rays are screened out before light penetrates to the people. Window glass and layers of clothing also effectively prevent ultraviolet rays from reaching the skin. Because only the ultraviolet rays (light of short wavelength and high frequency) have the ability to bring about the chemical change by which vitamin D is formed, persons who live in cities can place little dependence on making this vitamin in their own bodies, especially in winter. Others who live and work outdoors in sunny regions manufacture a considerable amount of vitamin D with the aid of sunlight, and hence are less dependent on food for it. (See Fig. 7–13.)

Estimates of Vitamin D Intake and Nutritional Status

It is very difficult to estimate average vitamin D "intakes" of persons because of the difficulty of measuring that manufactured in the body by the effect of sunlight. Because of the widespread use of fortified milk and other foods, intakes of at least 400 IU daily appear to be commonly eaten by most persons. Filer[26] estimated, from studies with over 2000 6-month-old in-

HOW CHILDREN TODAY
MAY BE DEPRIVED OF
THE SUNSHINE VITAMIN
CLOUDS, SMOG, FOG
SHADE
INDOOR HOME LIFE
WINDOW GLASS
SMOKE AND DUST
DARKENED STREETS
INDOOR WORK OF CITY PEOPLE
CLOTHING

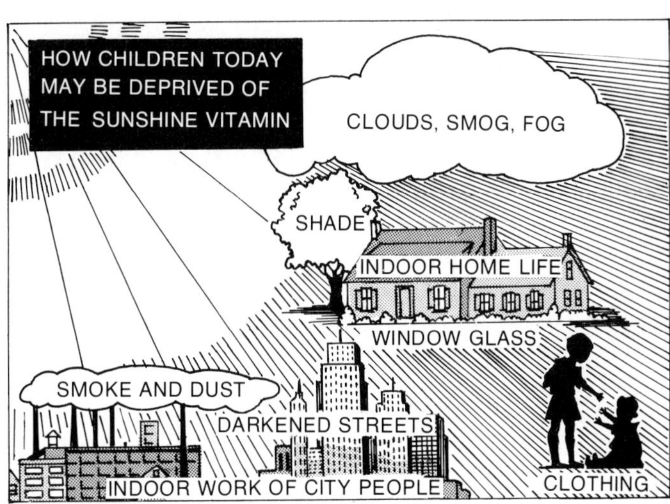

Figure 7–13 People in country districts and in the tropics can make vitamin D in their bodies through the agency of direct sunlight. This drawing shows some of the factors of modern life that screen out ultraviolet light and prevent people from exposure to sunlight, thus at least partially depriving them of the chance of making this vitamin in their bodies. (Courtesy of the Wisconsin Alumni Research Foundation.)

fants, that they were receiving 390 IU from food alone (90 percent from enriched milk and 10 percent from egg). The Committee on Nutrition of the American Academy of Pediatrics pointed out that many older children may be receiving as much as 2000 to 3000 IU per day, owing to the rather wide variety of fortified foods available.[27] This amount is considerably more than necessary.

Since the practice of giving vitamin D concentrates to young children has become widespread, severe cases of rickets are seldom seen in the United States, although mild rickets is still sometimes seen. The value of vitamin D administration is well illustrated by statistics of preschool children in Chicago, obtained from 1926 to 1932. Examination of the children before treatment showed 16 to 21 percent with definite evidence of rickets, but by 1935 the percentage had fallen to 7 percent, with only 0.03 percent having severe rickets. The incidence of severe rickets, on the basis of these 1935 figures, had been reduced to 3 cases per 10,000 children. The American Academy of Pediatrics made a survey in 1962 and found only 4 cases of rickets in every 10,000 pediatric admissions to hospitals.[28] Some of these may have been caused by mineral deficiencies or metabolic disorders, rather than by vitamin D lack. It is clear that rickets as a disease is well on the way to being eradicated in this country, but doubtless very many children do not achieve full growth and proper development of bones and teeth because of lack of optimum amounts of calcium, phosphorus, or vitamin D, or all.

Public health nutritionists, nutrition educators, and all persons in countries who give nutrition advice to normal persons must always be alert to the possibility of indifference and forgetfulness concerning food nutrition habits. Vitamin D supplementation of infant diets is a case in point and has become so routine that the importance of it might readily be forgotten. For instance, in Glasgow, Scotland, in 1963 there was an upswing in the incidence of rickets in infants.[29] Rickets in children has been observed the past decade in Canada (400 cases in only three pediatric hospitals in Montreal and Toronto in 1967 and 1968),[30] Greece (15 percent incidence in 330 infants), France (8 percent in aged persons in one hospital), Japan, South Africa, and Egypt, where it has been observed to a rather large extent in undernourished children in association with caloric deficiency. Fortification of milk and other foods with vitamin D has materially aided in preventing this problem in the United States and elsewhere.

Vitamin D in Foods

Nature's plan seems to have been that man should generate most of his supply of vitamin D by sunlight, for vitamin D is contained in foods more sparsely than any other vitamin. It occurs with other fat-soluble vitamins in such foods of animal origin as egg yolk, butter fat, fatty fishes, and of course in liver, since this is the storage organ for it. The amounts found in these foods are small and vary widely according to the diet of the animal and the extent to which it has been exposed to sunlight. Vegetables, grains, and fruits are generally considered to have little or no vitamin D activity. An important exception is certain shrubs and plants of the *Solanum* family recently found to contain such large amounts of forms of the vitamin D hormone that toxic symptoms (extensive calcification) may be seen in farm animals grazing in overabundance on such plants.* It would be worthwhile if varieties of these plants could be studied for their potential use as a good source of vitamin D for humans. Because vitamin D is stable to heat and insoluble in water, there is little loss of it in the cooking or processing of foods.

Table 7–5 lists some typical food sources of vitamin D with the amount that may be counted on from an average serving, although the content in egg yolk and butter is higher if some rich source of vitamin D has been incorporated in the animals' feed, as is a common practice now. Eggs and dairy products furnish vitamin D in small quantities. Liver and fatty fish (sardines, salmon, mackerel) are good sources, but are infrequently used in United States diets. If the daily diet contains 1 egg, 3 tablespoons of butter, and 1 pint of unenriched milk, one would get only about 65 IU of vitamin D from natural foods. Three ounces of salmon would provide about 300 IU. Most adults , though it is clear they need vitamin D, seem to get along at least fairly well on the small amounts furnished in foods, supplemented with the amounts generated under the influence of sunlight.

Human milk has only about 20 IU of vitamin D per liter, an insufficient amount to prevent rickets, even though calcium intake is adequate. Breast-fed infants require supplementation with vitamin D or exposure to ample sunlight.

*Potatoes and eggplants belong to this family, but these are not known to be a source of vitamin D activity. See the work of Wasserman and others in Science, *194*:853, 1976; Nature, *268*:347, 1977; and J. Biol. Chem., *252*:2580, 1977.

Enriched Foods and Other Rich Sources of Vitamin D

Supplements of vitamin D for infants, usually included with other vitamins and made from synthetic sources of vitamin D, are now readily available, replacing the older, more expensive, and less palatable fish-liver oil concentrates. Synthetic vitamin D can now be purchased in large wholesale lots for only a few cents per million units, sufficient for one person for 7 years. Thus, vitamin D is almost as

Table 7–5 VITAMIN D ACTIVITY OF TYPICAL FOODS

Food	*Size of Serving*	*Avg. Vitamin D, IU*
Fatty fish, canned:		
Herring	1 small fish (100 gm)	330
Salmon	100 gm	314
Tuna	⅝ c solid (100 gm)	200–320
Eggs	1 medium	27
Butter	1 oz or 3 avg. pats (30 gm)	28
Liver, raw	2 large slices (100 gm)	15–45
Cream, light to heavy	1 oz or 2 tbsp	4–8
Milk, whole, fresh (enriched)	1 pt	200

cheap as sunshine itself and much more dependable. The cost of fortifying a quart of milk is therefore negligible (less than 1/100 cent). Vitamin D supplements vary greatly in concentration — often as little as one or two drops supply a full day's requirement. Other foods are quite widely fortified with vitamin D today, so much so that under certain situations there could be danger of getting too much vitamin D (see next section). About 85 percent of all fresh milk is fortified with 400 IU of vitamin D per quart, as is all evaporated milk.[27] Many breakfast foods are fortified (usually from 80 to 400 IU per serving), as are various margarines (125 to 250 IU per ounce) and milk flavorings (from 5 to 150 IU per glass of milk).

Because of the dangers of overconsumption of vitamin D, the Committee of Nutrition of the American Academy of Pediatrics has become concerned about the widespread enrichment programs.[27, 31] Also, because of this, the Food and Drug Administration is attempting to make changes in its regulations by limiting the foods that may be enriched. Obviously when vitamin D–enriched milk is used in the amount of 1 quart daily, no other source of the vitamin is required.

Toxicity

Enough is better than too much as far as vitamin D is concerned, and mothers (especially mothers who believe in the practice of "overinsurance") should be warned of this fact in case they are giving high-potency vitamin D preparations to their children. There is evidence that certain infants are especially sensitive to the toxic action of vitamin D and may be adversely affected by intakes as low as 3000 to 4000 IU per day, as shown by abnormally high calcium levels in the blood, loss of appetite, and retarded growth.[27, 31] With daily doses of 20,000 to 40,000 IU for infants or 75,000 to 100,000 IU for adults, serious toxic symptoms may develop; these include vomiting, diarrhea, weakness, loss of weight, and kidney damage. The serum calcium is elevated to such a degree that deposits of calcium salts may be found in various organs.

Adults should be warned against taking massive doses of this vitamin, or vitamin A, over long periods unless under the direct supervision of a physician. Even moderate overdosage with vitamin D is not wise for the elderly. With water-soluble vitamins overdosage is wasteful but not harmful because the excess is excreted in urine. With fat-soluble vitamins, the excess remains in the body in such quantities that, in the case of vitamin D and to a lesser extent with vitamin A, it may give rise to toxic conditions.

VITAMIN E

Vitamin E is now a common household word. The interest in it is based upon many unjustifiable claims being made for it in the popular press and in the health food literature — especially the unproven popular claim that it will increase one's sexual potency. Unfortunately, much of the current enthusiasm for the vitamin is without experimental basis.

Discovery and Chemical Properties

In 1922, Evans and Bishop, of the University of California, discovered that a third unknown fat-soluble dietary factor (then called *factor X*) in lettuce and wheat germ was essential for *successful reproduction* in rats.[32] Several years later, Sure of the University of Arkansas suggested the term *vitamin E* for the factor, and this was widely accepted.[33] With use of the discovery of Olcott and Mattill that the vitamin was an alcohol and had *antioxidant properties*,[34] Evans* and his coworkers isolated crystalline vitamin E

*Dr. Herbert Evans, who also was codiscoverer of the growth hormone, remained very active until his death in 1971. Dr. Katherine Bishop, a physician, died in 1977 in Berkeley.

Table 7–6 RELATIONSHIPS BETWEEN ALPHA-TOCOPHEROL EQUIVALENTS AND INTERNATIONAL UNITS (IU)*

Compound (1 mg)	*Alpha-Tocopherol Equivalents in 1 mg (Approx.)*	*IU Activity in 1 mg (Approx.)*
d-alpha-tocopherol†	1 mg	1.49 IU
d-alpha-tocopheryl acetate	0.91 mg	1.36 IU
d-alpha-tocopheryl acid succinate	0.81 mg	1.21 IU
dl-alpha-tocopherol	0.74 mg	1.10 IU
dl-alpha-tocopheryl acetate‡	0.67 mg	1.00 IU
d-gamma-tocopherol§	0.10 mg	0.15 IU

*All forms have the same biological activity when expressed in terms of IU or alpha-tocopherol equivalents – or as vitamin E activity.[4,8] Thus it is wrong to say that natural forms are more active than synthetic forms.

†The natural form in foods and the standard for "alpha-tocopherol equivalents," usually just called alpha-tocopherol but in commerce also called RRR-alpha-tocopherol (the RRR refers to the presence of methyl groups at three asymmetrical centers); see Ames, S. R.: IUNS–AIN nomenclature for vitamin E. J. Assoc. Offic. Analyt. Chem., *55*:625, 1972. Vitamin E nomenclature is still tentative.

‡The form of vitamin E most generally used in commerce – a synthetic but more stable form. It is also called "all-rac-alpha-tocopherol" (rac = racemic mixture). This is the standard for International Units.

§The form most abundant in food oils. The activity of other isomers of vitamin E ranges from 1 to 50 percent. See Bieri, J. G.: Nutr. Rev., *33*:161, 1975.

from wheat-germ oil in 1936 and named it *tocopherol*, from Greek words meaning "to bear offspring".[35] The structures of the four natural forms of the tocopherols (alpha, beta, gamma, and delta) were soon determined, and synthesis was accomplished in the laboratory. (See formula of *alpha-tocopherol* in the Appendix. It is, biologically, the most active natural form of vitamin E–active compounds.)

Four other closely related compounds with various degrees of vitamin E activity (from 1 to 50 percent) occur in food: the alpha-, beta-, gamma-, and delta-*tocotrienols*. Foods contain significant amounts of almost all eight natural forms.[36] To avoid confusion about the meaning of an International Unit (IU) of vitamin E, and by agreement of international committees, it is now correct to use milligrams of *alpha-tocopherol equivalents* as a summation term for all vitamin E activity.[8] We continue to use both terms here during this transition period, especially since there is insufficient information on the distribution of active forms in foods (hence current food composition tables generally give values in the old IU terms). See Table 7–6 for the relationships between the new "milligrams of alpha-tocopherol equivalents," used in the new tables of recommended allowances, and the older "IU," still used for labeling food products.

The vitamin E compounds are light yellow, viscous oils, insoluble in water and stable to heat but readily destroyed by oxidation and ultraviolet light. They are not destroyed to any great extent by normal temperatures used in cooking, though some loss occurs in frozen foods and in processing. There are appreciable losses of vitamin E activity in oils heated long periods of times at high temperature, such as in deep fat frying, because rancidity develops.[36]

Because they are capable of taking up oxygen, vitamin E compounds function in the body to protect certain other compounds (such as vitamin A, carotenes, and unsaturated fatty acids) from oxidation by acting as an *antioxidant*. The tocopherols are the chief antioxidants in natural fats and oils and act to prevent fats from becoming rancid. They are often added to food to help stabilize other valuable nutrients.

Vitamin E is available commercially, through chemical synthesis, in over 40 forms with different degrees of activity but most commonly as the active alpha-tocopherol acetate. Where their potency is listed in terms of IU or alpha-tocopherol equivalents, they are all equal in biological value — that is, their activity is the same whether natural or synthetic. None of the forms are especially toxic, even when taken in relatively large amounts.

Effects of Vitamin E Deficiency

Studies by Horwitt and others have shown that man requires vitamin E for normal creatine excretion and for the prevention of blood disorders (including an anemia, and in a laboratory test, the rupturing of isolated red blood cells by oxidizing agents in the so-called "hemolysis" test).[8] There is no convincing evidence that vitamin E deficiency in man causes reduced athletic performance, heart disease, weakened sex drive, muscular dystrophy, sterility, or reduced longevity, as is often claimed.* Deficiencies of this vitamin appear to be very rare, though the requirement is increased considerably by added polyunsaturated fatty acids.

Deficiency Signs in Animals

In rats that have been deprived of vitamin E, the males become permanently sterile, and pregnant females are unable to carry their young to full term, because lack of this vitamin results in death and reabsorption of the embryos in the uterus. Fertility of female rats is not destroyed, however, and when given sufficient vitamin E later, they give birth to normal litters. Young rats, and other animals, after several months on diets deficient in vitamin E, *fail to grow normally* and also develop *weakness and degeneration of the skeletal muscles,* a condition known as *nutritional muscular dystrophy,* which may also be accompanied by paralysis. Lesions have also been found in heart muscle.

Deficiencies of this vitamin have been obtained in many species other than the rat. In the chick, brain lesions and muscular dystrophy occur. Liver damage and a number of other muscular symptoms have been seen in deficient mice, pigs, dogs, and other animals. It is a misnomer to call this the "reproduction vitamin," as is often done, because there are so many more specific symptoms of deficiency and because all vitamins are necessary for reproduction.

Relationship to Selenium

In 1957, a very interesting dietary relationship of vitamin E to a trace mineral was discovered when it became known that extremely low levels of *selenium* could replace the vitamin E need of animals under certain conditions.[37] The full significance of this discovery to the vitamin E needs of humans has not been worked out as yet, but there are large geographic areas in the United States, and in other countries with soils deficient in selenium, where farm animals (usually sheep or cattle) with "white muscle disease" are cured by combinations of selenium and vitamin E (see Chapter 12), which are either injected into the animals or fed to them.

Functions of Vitamin E

Vitamin E deficiency presents such a wide variety of symptoms in so many animals that one might assume that it would be a part of many enzyme systems. However, there is no known specific coenzyme form of the vitamin in tissues (in spite of claims to the contrary), nor does it seem to play a specific role in any enzymatic reaction. Symptoms of a deficiency may be prevented in experimental animals by other antioxidants or by much lower amounts of selenium.

Several generations of animals have been reared without any vitamin E in the diet but with selenium and an antioxidant present. Therefore, the role of vitamin E in the body appears to be related entirely to its antioxidant role at the intracellular

*Nor would the reverse be true. In other words, extra amounts of vitamin E in a diet would not be expected to improve these conditions in man. Also see Amer. J. Clin. Nutr., *28*:1381, 1975, and statement of Food and Nutrition Board — Who needs vitamin E? J. Amer. Dietet. Assoc., *64*:365, 1974.

level. It is highly efficient in preventing cell membrane damage from naturally occurring *peroxides*, forms of toxic *free radicals* formed from fatty acids — substances that have been suggested as playing a role in the aging process.

Most of the vitamin E in the body is associated with the fat content of cells. Vitamin E is carried in the blood stream mainly attached to lipoproteins. The level in the blood is closely associated with the total plasma lipids and hence is influenced greatly by diet and other factors affecting blood lipid values.[8]

Vitamin E protects both vitamin A and carotene from destruction by oxidation, especially in the alimentary tract. In this way, vitamin E spares the supply of vitamin A available to the body, which may be of importance if the intake of vitamin A is barely adequate for body needs.

Requirement for Vitamin E

The Food and Nutrition Board's recommended allowances for young men and women, and older persons, are given in Table 7–7. Figures for other ages are given in Table 1 of the Appendix. These values are considerably lower than the former recommendations, on which the current United States food labeling regulations are legally based.

The requirement of vitamin E for humans is known to vary with other ingredients in the diet, as it does for animals. For instance, the presence of large amounts of *linoleic acid* or other polyunsaturated fatty acids in the diet markedly increases the requirement. This has significance in today's dietary pattern, in which large amounts of vegetable oils are widely used. Also, the presence of rancid fats, oxidizing substances, and selenium would be expected to modify the requirement for vitamin E. The recommended level is generous and should cover all contingencies.

Nutritional Status

Naturally occurring vitamin E deficiencies in adult humans in the United States are extremely unusual. In the classic experiments with men volunteers in Illinois by Horwitt and associates,[38] a deficient diet was consumed for about 3 years before any symptoms became evident. However, low blood or tissue levels of vitamin E, indicative of too low an intake or destruction by excessive polyunsaturated fatty acids, or both, have been observed in infants and adults in this country.[8, 39] This should not be too surprising in light of the losses of vitamin E in food processing and because of high intakes of polyunsaturated fat. Estimates of daily vitamin E intake in the United States appear to average about 8 to 11 mg alpha-tocopherol equivalents (12 to 16 IU),[8] slightly higher than recommended intakes.

Vitamin E in Foods

In a typical American diet, about 66 percent of the intake of vitamin E comes from salad oils, shortening, margarines, and other fats and oils. Normally, then, persons eating extra polyunsaturated fats, who have a higher requirement for vitamin E, will also consume extra vitamin E. The rest of the vitamin E in our diet comes mainly from whole grains, liver, beans, and fruits and vegetables.[40]

Only recently has it been possible to measure with reasonable accuracy the various forms of vitamin E in foods (see Table 7–8 for representative values). However, there is not sufficient knowledge as yet to know the vitamin E activity of many of these various forms, but, generally, non–alpha-tocopherol forms of vitamin E in a mixed diet are considered to supply about 20 percent of the total vitamin E activity. Because of the lack of general availability of figures for vitamin E in food, Table 7–9 gives the alpha-

Table 7–7 RECOMMENDED DIETARY ALLOWANCE FOR VITAMIN E ACTIVITY*

	Age	*Allowance* ALPHA-TOCOPHEROL EQUIVALENTS/DAY (in mg)	IU/DAY
Males	11–14 years old	8	12
	15 years and over	10	15
Females	11 years and over	8	12
	Pregnant	10	15
	Lactating	10	15

*From Food and Nutrition Board, 1974.[8] For additional values see appendix, Table I. These values are lower than the vitamin E values listed on food packages. The U.S. RDA is based on older (1968) estimates.

Table 7–8 SEVERAL COMMON FORMS OF VITAMIN E IN REPRESENTATIVE OILS*

	Alpha-tocopherol	*Beta-tocopherol*	*Gamma-tocopherol*	*Alpha-tocotrienol*	*Delta-tocopherol*
Relative biological potency (estimated)	100	35	10	20–30	1
Food Sources:			mg/100 gm		
Corn oil	20	5	75	5	2
Cottonseed oil	38	–	40	–	1
Palm oil	20	–	20	14	7
Peanut oil	13	1	20	–	2
Safflower oil	30	1	3	–	2
Soybean oil	15	3	100	–	13
Wheat-germ oil	110	40	40	3	27

*Rough averages from incomplete data (recent values given more weight).[36] Also see Slover, H. T., Lipids, *6*:291, 1971; Bieri, J. G., Evarts, R. P., J. Amer. Dietet. Assoc. *66*:134, 1975; Müller-Mulot, W., J. Amer. Oil Chem. Soc. *53*:732, 1976.

Table 7–9 ALPHA-TOCOPHEROL CONTENT OF REPRESENTATIVE FOODS*

Food	*mg/100 gm*	*Food*	*mg/100 gm*
Seeds		*Vegetables and fruits*	
Almond	27.0	Asparagus, fresh	1.8
Barley	0.5	Carrots, fresh	0.5
Corn	0.6	Beans, dry	0.1 to 0.7
Oat	0.5	Mango, ripe	1.0
Rice, white	0.1	Potatoes	0.1
Rice, whole	0.3	Green leafy (most)	1 to 10
Wheat	1.4	Corn, fresh	0.1
Peanuts	10.0	Most fruits, fresh	0.1 to 1.0
Peas	0.5		
		Other foods	
Oils		Potato chips	2.1
Coconut	0.5	Sugar cookie	2.0 to 5.0
Cod-liver	29.0	Eggs	1.0
Corn	11.0	Liver	2.0
Cottonseed	39.0	Codfish	0.2 to 1.2
Olive	5.0	Beef	1.0
Palm	26.0	Lobster	1.7
Peanut	13.0	Butter	2.0
Rapeseed	18.4	Lard	1.2
Safflower	39.0	Margarine	10.0
Soybean	10.0	Shortening (vegetable)	10.0
Sunflower	49.0	Milk (cow's)	0.1
Walnut	56.0	Yeast	0
Wheat germ	133.0	Infant cereals	0.1 to 1.0
		Wheat flour	0.2
		Wheat germ	13.0
		Bread, white	0.2

*Most values adapted from Dicks[40] and Slover (Lipids, *6*:291, 1971). (Values are for alpha-tocopherol only.) Also see Koehler, H. H., Lee, H. C., and Jacobson, M.: J. Amer. Dietet. Assoc., *70*:616, 1977 for values of canned entrees and vended sandwiches.

tocopherol content of representative foods as determined by recent methods. Use of these figures in calculating one's intake will give a conservative value (somewhat lower, in most cases, than the total vitamin E activity), since other, lower potency forms of the vitamin are disregarded. In general, most seeds and oils from these seeds are the best sources of vitamin E. Some vegetables are also good sources, especially green, leafy vegetables. Wheatgerm oil is one of the richest natural sources. Synthetic forms of vitamin E are the least expensive sources, although we recommend that vitamin E be consumed in a regular diet as much as possible, in order to get all the other essential nutrients also.

The vitamin E activity of foods may be considerably reduced in processing, storage, and packaging.[40] For instance, as much as 80 percent or more may be lost in converting whole wheat to white bread. Freezing of vegetables is also known to cause some destruction of vitamin E — a finding rather unique among the vitamins.

VITAMIN K

The fourth, but not the least, of the fat-soluble vitamins was discovered in studies with the chick in 1935 by Dam* of Copenhagen, and a few months later independently by Almquist and Stokstad of the University of California.[41] Because the vitamin is essential for the proper coagulation of blood, Dam proposed that it be called the *Koagulation vitamin* (the Dan-

*Dam, who died in 1976, received the Nobel Prize for this in 1943 with Dr. Doisey of St. Louis (who first determined the structure of vitamin K_2).

ish and German spelling of the word), from which the term *vitamin K* was derived.* Vitamin K was isolated in pure form in 1939, and shortly thereafter it was synthesized and its chemical structure determined. Deficiencies are rare in humans, except in infants or persons receiving antagonists or with clinical problems related to absorption. Considerable use, however, is made of synthetic substances that act as antagonists of vitamin K (such as dicoumarol, an anticoagulant) to prevent clotting of the blood in patients with certain circulatory disorders. The antagonists are also, interestingly enough, used as very potent rat killers (such as warfarin), which destroy the rat by preventing its blood from clotting.

Properties and Distribution

Vitamins K_1 and K_2† are two forms of chemicals known as *quinones* (see formula of vitamin K_1 in Appendix), which exist naturally in plants — especially in green leaves, and in foods that have undergone bacterial fermentation. Several synthetic forms, such as *menadione)* (formerly menaquinone, or vitamin K_3) and its various water-soluble derivatives, are converted to vitamin K_2 in the body, and thus have similar vitamin K activity when fed to animals (but, unlike the natural forms, are toxic when given in large amounts). All forms of the vitamin are yellow and are quite stable to heat, air, and moisture, but not to light. Cooking destroys very little of the vitamin because it is not water-soluble.

Food sources of vitamin K include all the green, leafy vegetables, egg yolk, soybean oil, and liver. Lettuce, spinach, kale, cauliflower, and cabbage are excellent sources; the inner leaves of cabbage have about one-fourth as much as the outer leaves. Very little vitamin K is present in most cereals, fruits, carrots, peas, meats, or highly refined foods.

Effects of Deficiency

The first studies with vitamin K were made with chicks. When vitamin K is absent, they develop delayed blood clotting, causing hemorrhages under the skin, serious internal bleeding, and, if not corrected, death. Deficiencies have also been produced in cattle, pigs, rats, dogs, humans, and all other species studied. Often a drug, such as a sulfa drug or an antibiotic, is added to the diet of the experimental animal in order to reduce biosynthesis of the vitamin by intestinal organisms. Also, experimentally, the animals sometimes are raised in a "germ-free" environment; hence, they have no intestinal flora and no vitamin K synthesis.

Vitamin K deficiency formerly was quite common in commercial poultry flocks in this country becase of the widespread use of sulfa drugs and antibiotics for the prevention of disease and for the promotion of growth. In spite of the many natural foodstuffs that poultry rations contained, they were surprisingly quite low in vitamin K, especially when dried alfalfa was not included. Today, synthetic forms of vitamin K or alfalfa are widely used in such diets for supplementary purposes and successfully prevent signs of deficiency. The lesson of this for human nutrition should be obvious.

Role in the Body

The primary function of vitamin K in the body is the formation in the liver of a protein called *prothrombin,* which is nec-

*Vitamins I and J, now obsolete terms for other vitamins, were proposed also in 1935, so that the use of the latter K was in alphabetical order.

†Most recent nomenclature rules (J. Nutr., *100*:7, 1978) use the chemical name phylloquinone for vitamin K_1 and *menaquinones* for the several vitamins K_2. Vitamin K_1 is the natural form generally found in plant foods, whereas the several vitamins K_2 appear to be the active forms present in bacteria and the animal body.

essary for the clotting, or coagulation, of blood. Several other substances, or "factors,"* needed for blood clotting also depend on vitamin K.

Prothrombin is converted to its active form — *thrombin* — which in turn is necessary for the formation of fibrin, a protein that is the basis for a blood clot, as is illustrated by the simplified diagram at the bottom of the page.

Without vitamin K, or when an antagonist is given, prothrombin and several related substances cannot be formed, and the blood will not clot. Various mechanisms for its clotting action that involve a role in the important cellular enzymes at the ribosome level have been proposed, but a biochemical role is still unknown. One possible function of vitamin K is to promote carboxylation of glutamic acid residues in the prothrombin molecule.[43] Vitamin K appears not to be useful to the body other than its role in clotting. At this time, this is a very active research area.

Requirement and Nutritional Status

No allowance for vitamin K has been set as yet by the Food and Nutrition Board because of synthesis of amounts greater than the requirement by intestinal flora in the gut in normal persons. About 140 mcg would be the amount needed daily if there were no bacterial synthesis.[8] An average mixed diet provided two to three times this amount.

A deficiency is likely to occur in premature or anoxic infants and in those born to mothers receiving anticoagulants. A large, corrective oral dose of 1 to 2 mg usually used for the infant in such cases is probably considerably higher than the minimum requirement.[44] Giving the vitamin to the infant appears to be superior to supplying extra amounts of it to the mother before childbirth.

Deficiencies have been seen in babies receiving drugs for diarrhea or intestinal infections. A normal infant's requirement must be about 15 mcg per day, the amount present in 1 liter of human milk. It is recommended that milk formulas for infants be increased to 100 mcg per liter.[44]

Vitamin K deficiency, as evidenced by internal hemorrhages, has occurred in humans under conditions in which absorption of the vitamin is hindered or prevented, as in any condition in which bile flow is disturbed, such as obstructive jaundice, or after injuries or surgical operations (as with the other fat-soluble vitamins). In such situations, extra doses of vitamin K given with bile salts have proved effective in raising the level of prothrombin in the blood, thus restoring the normal clotting ability of the blood, even though there may be sufficient vitamin K in the diet otherwise. Unless these abnormal conditions exist, vitamin K deficiency would seldom be seen in humans. There appears to be no reason for a normal individual eating a varied diet of traditional foods to feel that his diet does not contain an adequate supply of this vitamin. Vitamin K has proved ineffective in treating hemophilia, an inherited condition causing abnormal hemorrhaging in man.

*Known as Factors VII (proconvertin), IX (Christmas factor), and X (Stuart factor), all proteins apparently. Prothrombin is also known as Factor II.

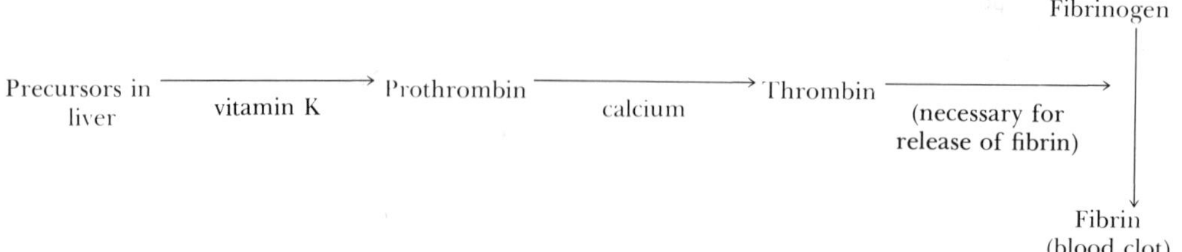

Toxicity

Synthetic menadione and its various derivatives (formerly vitamin K_3) have produced certain toxic symptoms in rats and jaundice in human infants when given in relatively low amounts (over 5 mg).[8, 44] Consequently, the Food and Drug Administration of the United States does not allow any menadione — even 1 mg levels — in any food supplements, including prenatal vitamin capsules. The natural forms of vitamins K_1 and K_2 may still be used for this purpose because they have not produced signs of toxicity even when given in large amounts.

OTHER FAT-SOLUBLE DIETARY FACTORS

No other fat-soluble vitamins are recognized by nutritional science groups in the United States or by international agencies. Certain fat-soluble substances in food are growth factors for lower forms of life, such as *cholesterol* and other *sterols* for insects. *Lecithin,* containing choline (see Chapters 4 and 8), is fat-soluble but is not a vitamin or a necessary dietary ingredient in any sense. Various fatty acids serve as growth factors for lower organisms, and at least one fatty acid is essential (see Chapter 4) for humans, but is not a vitamin.

This is not to say that other health-promoting agents do not occur in natural fats. New facts in this field are difficult to obtain and to confirm. The proposal by the late Dr. Armand Quick, a pioneer in the study of clotting factors, for the existence of a *vitamin Q* is of special interest.[45]

The proposed vitamin Q (in honor of its discoverer) is a phospholipid of unknown composition present in soybeans. It, in addition to vitamin K, appears to be essential for proper functioning of blood clotting mechanisms in humans. Whether it actually is *required in the diet of normal individuals* for this purpose, a basic tenet of vitamin identification, remains to be proved. It is widely distributed in food, and a deficiency in normal persons would no doubt be difficult to obtain, if indeed the so-called vitamin Q is needed (for other proposed vitamins, see the end of Chapters 8 and 9).

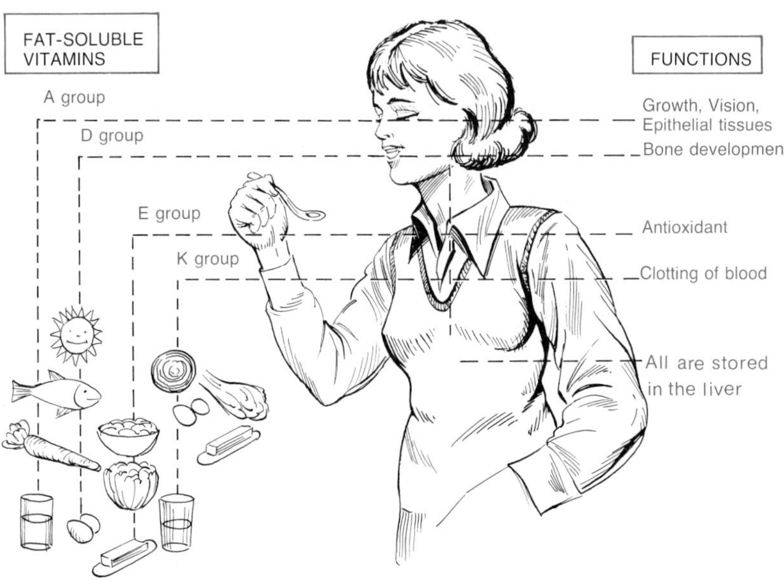

Figure 7–14 Fat-soluble vitamins and their functions.

QUESTIONS AND PROBLEMS

1. Tell in a general way how fat-soluble vitamins differ from water-soluble ones in each of the following respects: solubilities, types of food in which they are carried, losses in cooking and processing of foods, conditions necessary for good absorption from intestine, path or paths of excretion, and ability to be stored in the body.

2. Name four fat-soluble vitamins and give for each one its chief use, or uses, in the body and the effects of moderate and severe lack of it in the diet. How does its function in nutrition account for the type of symptoms that result from an insufficient supply?

3. What is meant by provitamins or vitamin precursors? Name the precursors of vitamin A, and tell in what classes of foods they are found. How and to what extent are they made into vitamin A in the body? What foods contain both the provitamins A and vitamin A? Which contain only provitamins A? What determines whether the vitamin A value of eggs, milk, and butter is high or low? Is the depth of color of egg yolk and milk fat a reliable index of their vitamin A value? Why? Does the depth of color of green and yellow vegetables indicate their relative vitamin A value, and why?

4. List ten vegetables and three fruits of high vitamin A value. List the five foods of animal origin that are the richest sources of vitamin A (consult Table 7–2 and tables in the Appendix for vitamin A values of individual foods).

5. Plan a diet that will furnish 2500 IU of vitamin A (total activity). Modify this diet so that it provides 5000 IU of vitamin A. Substitute foods or add some rich sources of vitamin A, so that the diet as modified supplies 10,000 IU (or more) of vitamin A. Is it difficult to get as much as 5000 IU (recommended daily allowance for adults) in the diet? What will happen if the diet supplies 2500 IU one day and 10,000 IU the next day? Of what advantage is it to have an intake of vitamin A considerably in excess of the minimum requirement?

6. What are the earliest symptoms of vitamin A deficiency? What course would you recommend for getting rid of such symptoms?

7. What are the precursors of vitamin D, and where are they found? By what means are they transformed into vitamin D? Under what circumstances can this vitamin be made in the body? Under what conditions will persons make little of this vitamin in their bodies and so be dependent almost entirely on food sources for their supply of vitamin D? What foods contain small and variable amounts of vitamin D? How may the natural low content of vitamin D in foods be increased? What foods have been reinforced with regard to their vitamin D content?

8. At what periods of life is the need for vitamins A and D relatively high, and why? What rich source (or sources) of these vitamins is usually given at these periods to insure a plentiful supply of vitamins A and D? Why does a baby that is breast-fed derive more benefit if supplementary vitamins A and D are given to it directly than if they are given to its mother?

9. How can rickets be prevented? How can it be cured? Discuss why rickets is no longer a common disease.

10. What are the chief symptoms of deficiency of vitamin E? Of vitamin K? Why are such deficiencies seldom seen in humans? What are the chief functions of vitamins E and K in the body?

11. Which fat-soluble vitamins may be toxic if taken over long periods in large doses?

12. Describe some important research now under way with any of the fat-soluble vitamins.

REFERENCES

Vitamins A and D

1. McCollum, E. V.: *History of Nutrition*. Boston, Houghton Mifflin Co., 1957.
2. McCollum, E. V., and Davis, M.: J. Biol. Chem.,

15:167, 1913; *19*:245, 1914; *23*:181, 1915; Osborne, T. B., and Mendel, L. B.: J. Biol. Chem., *15*:311, 1913, *16*:423, 1913–1914. (Also see reprint in Nutr. Rev., *31*:216, 1973.)

3. Karrer, P., et al.: Helv. Chim. Acta., *14*:1036, 1431, 1931; Chem. Rev., *14*:17, 1934.
4. Nomenclature policy: J. Nutr., *101*:133, 1971; *108*:7, 1978.
5. Karrer, P., et al.: Helv. Chim. Acta., *12*:1142, 1929.
6. Steenbock, H., and Boutwell, P. W.: J. Biol. Chem., *41*:81, 1920; *42*:131, 1920.
7. Moore, T.: Biochem J., *24*:692, 1930.
8. Food and Nutrition Board: *Recommended Dietary Allowances*. 8th Ed. Washington, D.C., National Research Council, National Academy of Science, 1974; 9th Ed. published in 1979. Also see Balsley, M.: J. Amer. Diet. Assoc., *71*:149, 1977.
9. Wald, G., et al.: Vitam. Horm., *1:195, 1943; 18*:417, 1960; Fed. Proc., *12*:607, 1953; Nature, *219*:800, 1968; Science, *162*:230, 1968.
10. Callison, E. C., et al.: J. Nutr., *37*:139, 1949.
11. Rountree, J. L.: J. Nutr., *3*:345, 1931; Dutcher, R. A., et al.: J. Nutr., *8*:269, 1934; Smith, M. C., and Spector, H.: Ariz. Agric. Expt. Stat. Tech. Bull., *84*:375, 1940; Becker, G. L.: Amer. J. Dig. Dis., *19*:344, 1952.
12. Underwood, B. A.: World Rev. Nutr. Dietet., *19*:123, 1974.
13. *Requirement of Vitamin A, Thiamine, Riboflavin, and Niacin.* Report of a joint FAO/WHO Expert Group. FAO Nutr. Meet. Rpt. Ser. No. 41, Rome, 1967; Rao, C. N., and Rao, B. S. M.: Amer. J. Clin. Nutr., *23*:105, 1970.
14. Seawright, A. A., and English, P. B.: Nature, *206*:1171, 1965; Herbst, E. J.: Science *100*:338, 1944.
15. Morgan, A. F.: J. Econ., *52*:631, 1960; Kelsay, J. L.: J. Nutr., *99* (No. 1, Part II, Suppl. 1): 119, 1969; Davis, T. R. A., Gershoff, S. N., and Gamble, D. F.: J. Nutr. Educ., *1* (Fall, Suppl. 1):39, 1969; Schaefer, A. E.: J. Amer. Dietet. Assoc., *54*:371, 1969; Nutr. Today, *4*:2, 1969.
16. Guthrie, H. A.: J. Amer. Dietet. Assoc., *43*:120, 1963; Filer, L. J., Jr., and Martinez, G. A.: Clin. Pediatr., *3*:633, 1964.
17. Marston, R., and Friend, B.: *National Food Review*, U.S. Dept. of Agriculture Issue NFR-1 Washington, D.C. Jan. 1978.
18. Abraham, S., et al.: *Dietary Intake Findings, U.S.* 1971–74. HANES Rpt., Pub. No. (H.R.A.) 77–1647. Hyattsville, Md., U.S. Dept. of Health, Education, and Welfare, National Center for Health Statistics, 1977.
19. Roels, O. A., et al.: Amer. J. Clin. Nutr., *12*:380, 1963.
20. Gopalan, C., et al.: Amer. J. Clin. Nutr., *8*:833, 1960.
21. Sweeney, J. P., and Marsh, A. C.: J. Amer. Dietet. Assoc., *59*:238, 1971; Heierli, C.: Internat. J. Vit. Res., *40*:515, 1970.
22. See reviews by Chick, H.: Lancet, Aug. 13 and 20, p. 325 and 377, 1932; Powers, G. V., et al.: J.A.M.A., *78*:159, 1922; Stein, H. B., and Lewis, R. C.: Amer. J. Dis.. Child., *41*:62, 1931.
23. McCollum, E. V., et al.: J. Biol. Chem., *53*:293, 1922.
24. DeLuca, H. F., et al.: Biochem., *10*:2799, 1971; *10*:2935, 1971; Proc. Nat. Acad. Sci., *68*:803, 1971; Lawson, D., E. M., et al.: Nature, *230*:228, 1971.
25. Jeans, P. C., and Stearns, G.: J. Pediatr., *13*:730, 1938; J.A.M.A., 11:703, 1938; Jeans, P. C.: J.A.M.A., *143*:177, 1950.
26. Filer, L. J., Jr., and Martinez, G. A.: Clin. Pediatr., *3*:633, 1964.
27. American Academy of Pediatrics, Committee on Nutrition: Pediatrics, *31*:512, 1963.
28. American Academy of Pediatrics, Committee on Nutrition: Pediatrics, *29*:646, 1962.
29. Arneil, G. C., and Crosbie, J. C.: Lancet, *2*:423, 1963.
30. Report of Canadian Council on Nutrition: Canadian Nutr. Notes, *24*:85, 1968.
31. American Academy of Pediatrics, Committee on Nutrition: Pediatrics, *40*:1050, 1967.

Vitamins E and K

32. Evans, H. M., and Bishop, K. S.: Science, *56*:650, 1922.
33. Sure, B.: J. Biol. Chem., *58*:693, 1924; *62*:371, 1924; *63*:211, 1925.
34. Olcott, H. S., and Matill, H. A.: J. Biol. Chem., *93*:59, 1931; Olcott, H. S.: J. Biol. Chem., *110*:695, 1935.
35. Evans, H. M., Emerson, O. H., and Emerson, G. A.: J. Biol. Chem., *113*:319, 1936 (reprinted, in part, in Nutr. Rev., *32*:80, 1974).
36. Yuki, E., and Ishikawa, Y.: J. Amer. Oil Chem. Soc., *53*:673, 1976.
37. Schwarz, K., and Folz, C. M.: J. Amer. Chem. Soc., *79*:3292, 1957.
38. Horwitt, M. K.: Amer. J. Clin. Nutr., *8*:451, 1960; J. Amer. Dietet. Assoc., *38*:231, 1961; Fed. Proc., *24*:68, 1964; J. Nutr., *108*:1208, 1978.
39. Horwitt, M. K. (ed.): Symposium: *Vitamin E, biochemistry, nutritional requirements, and clinical studies* (21 papers). Amer. J. Clin. Nutr., *27*:939–1194, 1974.
40. Booth, V. H., and Bradford, M. P.: Brit. J. Nutr., *17*:575, 1963; Bunnel, R. H., et al.: Amer. J. Clin. Nutr., *17*:1, 1965; Dicks, M. W.: *Vitamin E Content of Foods and Feeds for Human and Animal Consumption.* Bulletin 435, Agric. Expt. Stat., Univ. Wyoming, 1965; Dicks-Bushnell, M. W., and Davis, K. C.: Amer. J. Clin. Nutr., *20*: 262, 1967.
41. Dam, H.: Nature, *135*:652, 1935; Biochem. J., *29*:1273, 1935 (reprinted in Nutr. Rev., *31*:121, 1973); Almquist, H. J., and Stokstad, E. L. R.: Nature, *136*:31, 1935; J. Biol. Chem., *111*:105, 1935; Almquist, H. J.: Amer. J. Clin. Nutr., *28*: 656, 1975.
42. H. J. Heinz Co.: *Nutritional Data.* 6th ed. Pittsburgh, 1965, p. 29.
43. Nutr. Rev., *33*:25, 1975; also see Suttie, J. W., and Jackson, C. M.: Physiol. Rev., *57*:1, 1977; Jones, J. P.: J. Biol. Chem., *252*:7738, 1977.
44. American Academy of Pediatrics, Committee on Nutrition: Pediatrics, *48*:483, 1971.
45. Quick, A. J.: Life Sci., *16*:1017, 1975; Wis. Med. J., *74*:85 (Aug.), 1975.

SUPPLEMENTARY READING

Fat-Soluble Vitamins — General

Bauernfeind, J. C., Newmark, H., and Brin, M.: Vitamins A and E nutrition via intramuscular or oral route. Amer. J. Clin. Nutr., *27*:234, 1974.

Bieri, J. G.: Fat-soluble vitamins in the eighth revision of the recommended dietary allowances. J. Amer. Dietet. Assoc., *64*:171, 174.

DeLuca, H. F.: Function of the fat-soluble vitamins. Amer. J. Clin. Nutr., *28*:339, 1975.

Vitamin A

Reviews and History

Beyda, V. (ed.): *Vitamin A Deficiency and Blindness Prevention.* New York, American Foundation for Overseas Blind and Nutrition Foundation, 1974.

DeMaeyer, E. M.: *Assessment of Vitamin A Status.* New York, Nutrition Foundation, Inc., 1976.

International Vitamin A Consultive Group: *Guidelines for the Eradication of Vitamin A Deficiency and Xerophthalmia.* New York, Nutrition Foundation, Inc., 1977.

Pereira, S. M., and Begum, A.: Vitamin A deficiency in Indian children. World Rev. Nutr. Dietet., *24*:192, 1976.

Rietz, P., Wiss, O., and Weber, F.: Metabolism of vitamin A and the determination of vitamin A status. Vitam. Horm., *32*:237, 1974.

Rodriguez, M. S., and Irwin, M. I.: A conspectus of research on vitamin A requirements of man. J. Nutr., *102*:909, 1972.

Roels, O. A.: Vitamin A physiology. J.A.M.A., *214*:1097, 1970.

Shearman, D. J. C.: Vitamin A and Sir Douglas Mawson. Brit. Med. J., *I*; 284, 1978.

Simmons, W. K.: Xerophthalmia and blindness in Northeast Brazil. Amer. J. Clin. Nutr., *29*:116, 1976.

Srikantia, S. G.: Human vitamin A deficiency. World Rev. Nutr. Dietet., *20*:184, 1975.

Underwood, B. A.: The determination of vitamin A and some aspects of its distribution, mobilization and transportation in health and disease. World Rev. Nutr. Dietet., *19*:123, 1974.

Van Veen, A. G., and Van Veen, M. S. Some present-day aspects of vitamin A problems in less developed countries. Ecol. Food Nutr., *3*:35, 1974.

Wolf, G., Chairman: International symposium on the metabolic function of vitamin A. Amer. J. Clin. Nutr., *22*:897, 1969.

Wolf, B.: A historical note on the mode of administration of vitamin A for the cure of night blindness. Amer. J. Clin. Nutr., *31*:290, 1978.

Other References

Araujo, R. L.: Response of retinol serum levels to the intake of vitamin A–fortified sugar by pre-school children. Nutr. Rpts. Internat., *17*:307, 1978.

Bieri, J. G., Thorp, S. L., and Tolliver, T. J.: Effect of dietary polyunsaturated fatty acids on tissue vitamin E status. J. Nutr., *108*:392, 1978.

Fry, P. C., Eitelman, J. D., and Kelly, K.: Vitamin A status of Mexican-American four-year-olds from non-migrant families. Nutr. Rpts. Internat., *11*: 71, 1975.

Furman, K. I.: Acute hypervitaminosis A in an adult. Amer. J. Clin. Nutr., *26*:575, 1973.

Glick, Z., and Reshef, A.: Vitamin A status and related nutritional parameters of children in East Jerusalem. Amer. J. Clin. Nutr., *26*:1229, 1973.

Hypovitaminosis A and its consequences in ophthalmology. Amer. J. Clin. Nutr., *29*:803, 1976.

Mejia, L. A., et al.: Vitamin A deficiency and anemia in central American children. Amer. J. Clin. Nutr., *30*:1175, 1977.

Mitchell, G. V., Young, M., and Seward, C. R.: Vitamin A and carotene levels of a selected population in metropolitan Washington, D. C. Amer. J. Clin. Nutr., *26*:992, 1973.

Mohanram, M., Kulkarni, K. A., and Reddy, V.: Hematological studies in vitamin A deficient children. Internat. J. Vit. Nutr. Res., *47*:389, 1977.

O'Toole, B. A., et al.: Vitamin A deficiency and reproduction in rhesus monkeys. J. Nutr., *104*:1513, 1974.

Raica, N., Scott, J., Lowry, L., and Sauberlich, H. E.: Vitamin A concentration in human tissues collected from five areas in the United States. Amer. J. Clin. Nutr., *25*:291, 1972.

Sinha, D. P., and Bang, F. B.: The effect of massive doses of vitamin A on the signs of vitamin A deficiency in pre-school children. Amer. J. Clin. Nutr., *29*:110, 1976.

Sivakumar, B., and Reddy, V.: Absorption of labelled vitamin A in children during infection. Brit. J. Nutr., *27*:299, 1972.

Smith, F. R., and Lindenbaum, J.: Human serum retinol transport in malabsorption. Amer. J. Clin. Nutr., *27*:700, 1974.

Smith, F. R., et al.: Plasma vitamin A, retinol-binding protein and prealbumin concentrations in protein-calorie malnutrition. III. Response to varying dietary treatment. Amer. J. Clin. Nutr., *28*:732, 1975.

Solon, F. S., Popkin, B. M., Fernandez, T. L., and Latham, M. C.: Vitamin A deficiency in the Philippines: a study of xerophthalmia in Cebu. Amer. J. Clin. Nutr., *31*:360, 1978.

The prevention of blindness, WHO Chronicle, *30*:391, 1976.

Venkataswamy, G., Glover, J., Cobby, M., and Pirie, A.: Retinol-binding protein in serum of xerophthalmic, malnourished children before and after treatment at a nutrition center. Amer. J. Clin. Nutr., *30*:1968, 1977.

Vitamin A deficiency and xerophthalmia. WHO Chronicle, *30*:117, 1976.

Wild, J., Schorah, C. J., and Smithells, R. W.: Vitamin

A, pregnancy, and oral contraceptives. Brit. Med. J., *1*:57, 1974.
Yeung, D. L.: Effects of oral contraceptives on vitamin A metabolism in the human and the rat. Amer. J. Clin. Nutr., *27*:125, 1974.

Articles in Nutrition Reviews

Two physiological forms of human retinol binding protein. *30*:90, 1972.
Vitamin A and spermatogenesis in the rat. *30*:67, 1972.
Synthesis and secretion of retinol-binding protein in vitamin A deficiency. *31*:60, 1973.
Vitamin A deficiency, xerophthalmia and blindness (by Oomen, H.A.P.C.). *32*:161, 1974.
Amelioration of photosensitivity by carotene. *32*:239, 1974.
Retinol-linked sugars in glycoprotein synthesis (by Wolf, G.). *34*:97, 1976.
The transport of vitamin A in hypervitaminosis A. *34*:119, 1976.
Cellular retinol and retinoic acid binding proteins. *35*:146, 1977.
Depression in a rat plasma macroglobulin due to vitamin A deficiency. *35*:179, 1977.
The effect of oral contraceptive agents on plasma vitamin A in the human and the rat. *35*:245, 1977.
Retinol binding protein in man and rat. *35*:253, 1977.
"Turnover" of vitamin A. *35*:310, 1977.
Tissue changes following deprivation of fat-soluble A vitamin (by Wolbach, S. B., and Howe, P. R.). *36*:16, 1978.
Comparative biochemistry and evolution of vitamin A transport in plasma of vertebrates, *36*:187, 1978.

Vitamin D

Reviews and History

Avioli, L. V. (ed.): Vitamin D metabolites: their clinical importance (11 papers). Arch. Intern. Med., *138*:835–886, 1978.
Beale, M. G., Chan, J. C. M., Oldham, S. B., and DeLuca, H. F.: Vitamin D: the discovery of its metabolites and their therapeutic applications. Pediatrics, *57*:729, 1976.
Bergstrom, W. H.: Calcified deficiency here and now. Amer. J. Dis. Child., *129*:1137, 1975.
Bronner, F. (ed.): Symposium: clinical implications of recent advances in vitamin D. Amer. J. Clin. Nutr., *29*:1253, 1976.
DeLuca, H. F.: Recent advances in our understanding of the vitamin D endocrine system. J. Lab. Clin. Med., *86*:7, 1976.
DeLuca, H. F., and Schnoes, H. K.: Metabolism and mechanism of action of vitamin D. Ann. Rev. Biochem., *45*:631, 1976.
Fraser, D. R.: Advances in the knowledge of the metabolism of vitamin D. Proc. Nutr. Soc., *34*:139, 1975.
Haussler, M. R., and McCain, T. A.: Basic and clinical concepts related to vitamin D metabolism and action. N. Engl. J. Med., *297*:974, 1977.
Kodicek, E.: The story of vitamin D from vitamin to hormone. Lancet, *1*:325, 1974.
Neer, R. M.: The evolutionary significance of vitamin D skin pigment and ultraviolet light. Amer. J. Phys. Anthropol., *43*:409, 1975.
Norman, A. W.: Problems relating to the definition of an international unit for vitamin D and its metabolites. J. Nutr., *102*:1243, 1972.
Omdahl, J. L., and Deluca, H. F.: Regulation of vitamin D metabolism and function. Physiol. Rev., *53*:327, 1973.
Symposium: Osteomalacia and rickets (five papers). Proc. Nutr. Soc., *34*:101, 1975.

Other References

Arnaud, S. B., Mathusen, M., Gilkinson, J. B., and Goldsmith, R. S.: Components of 25-hydroxyvitamin D serum of young children in upper mid-western United States. Amer. J. Clin. Nutr., *30*:1082, 1977.
Brickman, A. S., Hartenblower, D. C., Norman, A. W., and Coburn, J. W.: Actions of 1-hydroxyvitamin D_3 and 1,25-dihydroxyvitamin D_3 on mineral metabolism in man. 1. Effects on net absorption of phosphorus. Amer. J. Clin., *30*:1064, 1977.
Chineme, C. N., Krook, L., and Pond, W. G.: Bone pathology in hypervitaminosis D: an experimental study in young pigs. Cornell Vet., *66*:387, 1976.
Dilling, L. A.: Growth and nutrition of preschool Indian children in Manitoba: I. Vitamin D deficiency. Canad. J. Pub. Health, *69*:248, 1978.
Lakdawala, D. R., and Widdowson, E. M.: Vitamin D in human milk. Lancet, *1*:167, 1977.
Lapatsanis, P., Makaronis, G., Vretos, C., and Doxiadis, S.: Two types of nutritional rickets in infants. Amer. J. Clin. Nutr., *29*:1222, 1976.
Norman, A. W.: Evidence for a new kidney-produced hormone, 1,25-dihydroxycholecalciferol, the proposed biologically active form of vitamin D. Amer. J. Clin. Nutr., *24*:1346, 1971.
O'Hara-May, J., and Widdowson, E. M.: Diets and living conditions of Asian boys in Coventry with and without signs of rickets. Brit. J. Nutr., *36*:23, 1976.
Omdahl, J. L., and DeLuca, H. F.: Medication of calcium adaptation by 1,25-dihydroxycholecalciferol. J. Nutr., *107*:1975, 1977.
Tanaka, Y., and DeLuca, H. F.: Role of 1,25-dihydroxyvitamin D_3 in maintaining serum phosphorus and curing rickets. Proc. Nat. Acad. Sci., *71*:1040, 1974.

Articles in Nutrition Reviews

1,25-dihydroxycholecalciferol of biologically active metabolite of vitamin D_3. *30*:14, 1972.

Calcium transport and mobilization mediated by 1,25-dihydroxycholecalciferol. *31*:58, 1973.
Control of vitamin D metabolism. *31*:187, 1973.
A role of 1,25-dihydroxyvitamin D_3 in phosphate metabolism. *32*:247, 1974.
Vitamin D: mode of action and biomedical applications, (by Haussler, M. R.). *32*:257, 1974.
Active vitamin D–like substances in *Solanum Malacoxylon* and other calcinogenic plants (by Wasserman, R. H.) *33*:1, 1975.
Studies on experimental rickets (by McCollum, E. V., Simmonds, N., and Becker, J. E.). *33*:48, 1975.
Hazards of overuse of vitamin D (a statement of the Food and Nutrition Board). *33*:61, 1975.
Recent clinical correlates of vitamin D metabolites and calcium metabolism. *33*:209, 1975.
Genetics and environment in the pathogenesis of nutritional rickets. *34*:266, 1976.
An experimental investigation on rickets (by Mellanby, E.). *34*:338, 1976.
Several classic pre-1930 vitamin D papers are reprinted in part in Nutr. Rev., *31*:280, 1973; *33*:48, 1975; and *34*:338, 1976, a reprint of part of Lancet, *1*:407, 1919.
Vitamin D metabolism in patients with small-bowel resection. *35*:297, 1977.
Vitamin D, calcium-binding protein and the intestinal transport of calcium. *36*:90, 1978.

Vitamin E

Reviews and History

Ames, S. R.: Isomers of alpha-tocopheryl acetate and their biological activity. Lipids, *6*:281, 1971.
Bieri, J. G., and Farrell, P. M.: Vitamin E. Vitam. Horm., *34*:31, 1976.
Horwitt, M. K. (ed.): Symposium: vitamin E, biochemistry, nutritional requirements and clinical studies (22 papers). Part I (939) and Part II (1105). Amer. J. Clin. Nutr., *27*:939, 1974.
Horwitt, M. K.: Vitamin E: a reexamination. Amer. J. Clin. Nutr., *29*:5, 1976.
Mason, K. E.: The first decades of vitamin E. Fed. Proc., *36*:1906, 1977.
Molenaar, I., Vos, J., and Hommes, F. A.: Effect of vitamin E deficiency on cellular membranes. Vitam. Horm., *30*:45, 1972.
Nair, P. P., and Kayden, H. J. (eds.): International conference on vitamin E and its role in cellular metabolism. Ann. N.Y. Acad. Sci., *203*:43, 1972.

Other References

Bieri, J. G., and Poukka-Evarts, R.: Tocopherols and polyunsaturated fatty acids in human tissues. Amer. J. Clin. Nutr., *28*:717, 1975.
Bieri, J. G., Poukka-Evarts, R., and Gart, J. J.: Relative activity of alpha-tocopherol and gamma-tocopherol in preventing oxidative red cell hemolysis. J. Nutr., *106*:124, 1976.
Bunnell, R. H. M., DeRitter, E., and Rubin, S. H.: Effect of feeding polyunsaturated fatty acids with a low vitamin E on blood levels of tocopherol in men performing hard physical labor. Amer. J. Clin. Nutr., *28*:706, 1975.
Chen, C. H., Hsu, S-J., Huang, P-C., and Chen, J-S.: Vitamin E status of Chinese population in Taiwan. Amer. J. Clin. Nutr., *30*:728, 1973.
Christiansen, M. M., and Wilcox, E. B.: Dietary polyunsaturates and serum alpha-tocopherol in adults. J. Amer. Dietet. Assoc., *63*:138, 1973.
Committee on Nutritional Misinformation, Food and Nutrition Board, National Academy of Science, National Research Council: Who needs vitamin E? J. Amer. Dietet. Assoc., *64*:365, 1974.
Davis, K. C.: Vitamin E: adequacy of baby diets. Amer. J. Clin. Nutr., *25*:933, 1972.
Desai, I. D., and Lee, M.: Plasma vitamin E and cholesterol relationship in Western Canadian Indians. Amer. J. Clin. Nutr., *27*:334, 1974.
Farrell, P. M., and Bieri, J. G.: Megavitamin E supplementation in man. Amer. J. Clin. Nutr., *28*:1381, 1975.
Farrell, P. M., et al.: The occurrence and effects of human vitamin E deficiency: a study in patients with cystic fibrosis. J. Clin. Invest., *60*:233, 1977.
Fried, J. J.: The glamour vitamin: E for excess? Family Health, *7*:26, Oct. 1975.
Hodges, R. H.: Vitamin E and coronary heart disease. J. Amer. Dietet. Assoc., *62*:638, 1973.
Lawrence, J. D., Bower, R. C., Riedhl, W. P., and Smith, J. L.: Effects of α-tocopherol acetate on the swimming endurance of trained swimmers. Amer. J. Clin. Nutr., *28*:205, 1975.
Lehmann, J., Marshall, M. W., Slover, H. T., and Iacono, J. M.: Influence of dietary fat level and dietary tocopherols on plasma tocopherols of human subjects. J. Nutr., *107*:1006, 1977.
Leonard, P. J., Doyle, E., and Harrington, W.: Levels of vitamin E in the plasma of newborn infants and of the mothers. Amer. J. Clin. Nutr., *25*:480, 1972.
Leonhardt, E. T. G.: Effects of vitamin E on serum cholesterol and triglycerides in hyperlipidemic patients treated with diet and clofibrate. Amer. J. Clin. Nutr., *31*:100, 1978.
Lewis, J. S., et al.: Effect of long-term ingestion of polyunsaturated fat, age, plasma cholesterol, diabetes mellitus, and supplemental tocopherol upon plasma tocopherol. Amer. J. Clin. Nutr., *26*:136, 1973.
Martin, M. M., and Hurley, L. S.: Effect of large amounts of vitamin E during pregnancy and lactation. Amer. J. Clin. Nutr., *30*:1629, 1977.
Sharman, I. M., Down, M. G., and Sen, R. N.: The effects of vitamin E and training on physiological function and athletic performance in adolescent swimmers. Brit. J. Nutr., *26*:265, 1971.
Steiner, M., and Anastasi, J.: Vitamin E, and inhibitor of the platelet release reaction. J. Clin. Invest., *57*:732, 1976.
Thompson, J. N., Beare-Rogers, J. L., Erdody, P., and Smith, D. C.: Appraisal of human vitamin E requirement based on examination of individual meals and composite Canadian diet. Amer. J. Clin. Nutr., *26*:1349, 1973.
Vobecky, J. S., Vobecky, J., Shapcott, D., and Blan-

chard, R.: Vitamin E and C levels in infants during the first year of life, 1–3. Amer. J. Clin. Nutr., *29*:766, 1976.

Wei-Wo, C. K., and Draper, H. H.: Vitamin E status of Alaskan Eskimos. Amer. J. Clin. Nutr., *28*:808, 1975.

Williams, M. L., Shott, R. J., O'Neal, P. L., and Oski, F. A.: Role of dietary iron and fat on vitamin E deficiency anemia of infancy. N. Engl. J. Med., *292*:887, 1975.

Witting, L. A., and Lee, L.: Dietary levels of vitamin E and polyunsaturated fatty acids and plasma vitamin E; recommended dietary allowance for vitamin E: relation to dietary erthyrocyte and adipose tissue linoleate. Amer. J. Clin. Nutr., *28*:571, 1975.

Articles in Nutrition Reviews

Present knowledge of vitamin E (by Roels, O. A.). *25*:33, 1967.

Compounds with vitamin E activity. *27*:92, 1969.

Pitfalls in calculating the vitamin E content of diets. *30*:55, 1972.

Supplementation of human diets with vitamin E. *31*:327, 1973.

Effects of alpha-tocopherol and analogs on cyclic-AMP systems. *32*:214, 1974.

Elevated xanthine oxidase in vitamin E deficiency. *33*:59, 1975.

Vitamin E (by Bieri, J. G.). *33*:161, 1975.

Vitamin E therapy in premature babies. *33*:206, 1975.

Hypervitaminosis E and coagulation. *33*:269, 1975.

The function of vitamin E as an antioxidant, as revealed by a new method for measuring lipid peroxidation. *36*:84, 1978.

Interactions of lead poisoning and Vitamin E deficiency. *36*:156, 1978.

Vitamin K

Reviews and History

Almquist, H. J.: The early history of vitamin K. Amer. J. Clin. Nutr., *28*:656, 1975.

Anonymous: Oral anticoagulants, vitamin K and prothrombin complex factors. Brit. J. Haematol., *32*:9, 1976.

Dam, H.: Historical survey and introduction. Vitam. Horm. *24*:295, 1966.

Morton, R. A.: Obituary notice of Carl P. H. Dam. Nature, *261*:621, 1976.

Shearer, M. J., Burney, A., and Barkan, P.: Studies on the absorption and metabolism of phylloquinone (vitamin K_1) in man. Vitam. Horm., *32*:513, 1974.

Suttie, J. W., and Jackson, C. M.: Prothrombin structure, activation, and biosynthesis. Amer. Physiol. Soc., *57*:1, 1977.

Symposium on vitamin K (six papers): Mayo Clin. Proc., *49*:911, 1974.

Other References

Aballi, A. J.: Vitamin K deficiency in the newborn. Lancet, *2*:559, 1977.

Bleeding in the newborn (editorial). Brit. Med. J., 915, 1977.

Esmon, C. T., Sadowski, J. A., and Suttie, J. W.: A new carboxylation reaction: the vitamin K–dependent incorporation of $H^{14}CO_3^-$ into prothrombin. J. Biol. Chem., *250*:4744, 1975.

Fernlund, P., Stenflo, J., Roepstorff, P., and Thomsen, J.: Vitamin K and the biosynthesis of prothrombin. J. Biol. Chem., *250*:6125, 1975.

Higard, P.: Experimental vitamin K deficiency and spontaneous metastases. Brit. J. Cancer, *35*:89, 1977.

Hollander, D., Rim, E., and Ruble, P. E., Jr.: Vitamin K_2 colonic and ileal in vivo absorption: bile, fatty acids, and pH effects on transport. Amer. J. Physiol., *233*:E124, 1977.

Hollander, D., Rim, E., and Muralidhara, K. S.: Vitamin K_1 intestinal absorption in vivo: influence of luminal contents on transport. Amer. J. Physiol., *232*:E69, 1977.

Jolly. D. W., Craig, C., and Nelson, T. E., Jr.: Estrogen and prothrombin synthesis: effect of estrogen on absorption of vitamin K_1. Amer. J. Physiol., *232*:H12, 1977.

Jones, J. P., Gardner, E. J., Cooper, T. G., and Olson, R. E.: Vitamin K–dependent carboxylation of peptide-bound glutamate: the active species of "CO_2" utilized by the membrane-bound prothrombin. J. Biol. Chem., *252*:7738, 1977.

Stenflo, J.: A new vitamin K–dependent protein: purification from bovine plasma and preliminary characterization. J. Biol. Chem., *251*:355, 1976.

Articles in Nutrition Reviews

Vitamin K and the newborn. *30*:131, 1972.

A plasma protein which increases with vitamin K deficiency. *30*:211, 1972.

Vitamin K and prothrombin synthesis (by Suttie, J. W.). *31*:105, 1973.

Vitamin K and prothrombin structure. *32:279*, 1974.

Vitamin K and carboxylation of glutamyl residues, *33*:25, 1975.

The functional significance of vitamin K action. *34*:182, 1976.

Interaction between vitamin K_1 and fat absorption. *34*:314, 1976.

Vitamin K reduction precedes epoxidation and prothrombin synthesis. *36*:20, 1978.

Two nutrition "classics" on vitamin K are reprinted in part in Nutr. Rev., *31*:121, 1973 (by Dam, H.), and *32*:244, 1974 (by Campbell, H. A., and Link, K. P.).

Chapter 8

Vitamin B Complex

The identification of the group of water soluble "B vitamins" goes back to the late 1800's and early 1900's (see Chapters 1 and 6). Although no one person can be credited with the total discovery of any specific B vitamin, some names of vitamin pioneers stand out, as will be seen.

Proof for the existence of more than one "vitamin B" came about in the early 1920's. Within a few years, the group of different water-soluble vitamins found in liver and other natural products became known as the "vitamin B complex."* The process of identification of each of the B vitamins was very slow until the pure substance could be isolated, or at least concentrated. Then it could be added routinely to experimental diets — a step necessary for proving the existence of still other unknown vitamins.

Much progress was made in the 1930's with the identification of the vitamin nature of thiamin, then riboflavin, pantothenic acid, niacin, and finally vitamin B-6. During the early 1940's, the vitamin nature of biotin and choline (a compound previously known) was determined. The last two of the B vitamins to be discovered were folacin, in 1945, and vitamin B-12, in 1948.

In contrast to the fat soluble vitamins and vitamin C, each of the nine B vitamins contains the element nitrogen (as well as carbon, hydrogen, and oxygen). Two of the B vitamins, thiamin and biotin, contain the mineral *sulfur* as an essential part of their molecular structure. Vitamin B-12 contains, uniquely, cobalt and phosphorus.

Each of the B vitamins is a vital component of major *coenzymes* in all body cells. Hence, a dietary source of each is necessary for growth, reproduction, nerve and brain function, and nearly every cellular reaction taking place in the body. These mechanisms will be explained briefly later in the chapter.

It should be kept in mind that although all the B vitamins have distinctive properties and, hence, must be studied separately, they are intimately interrelated in the body in cellular reactions.

THIAMIN (VITAMIN B-1)

Discovery

Thiamin was the first of the B complex vitamins to be obtained in pure form, hence the name vitamin B-1, a term proposed by the British in 1927. Various other names were used for short periods, including "antineuritic factor," "antiberiberi factor," "water-soluble B," and simply "vitamin B."

*The first use of the term "vitamin B complex" was by Salmon in 1927.[1]

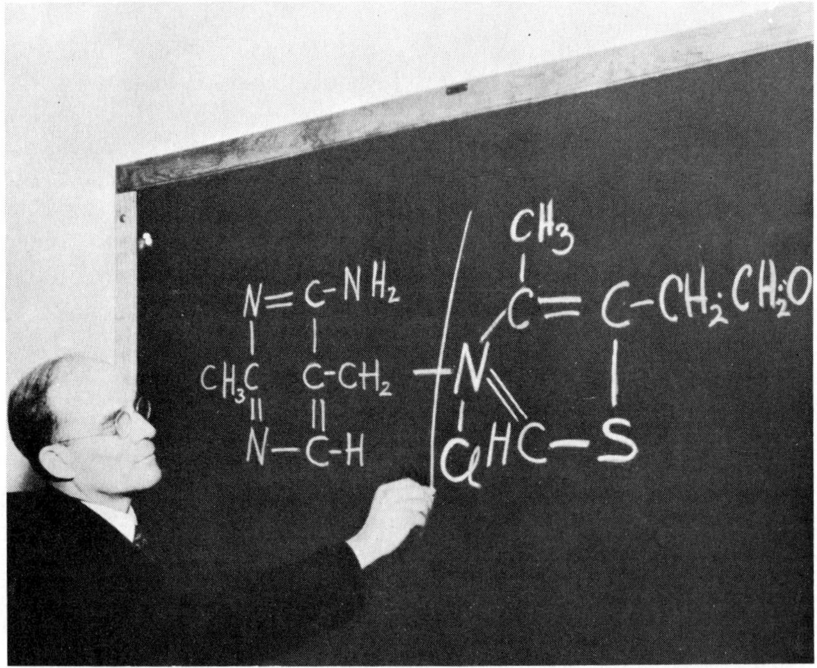

Figure 8–1 Dr. R. R. Williams writing the structural formula of thiamin on blackboard and indicating where the molecule splits on certain chemical treatment. The important sulfur atom is seen in the right-hand part and the amino group (NH_2) in the left-hand part of the molecule. (Courtesy of the late Dr. Williams.)

It took a period of just over 50 years, from 1885 to 1936, to unravel the mystery of the nature of vitamin B-1 and to be able to synthesize it in the chemical laboratory. The first synthesis, along with the establishment of its chemical identity, was made in 1936 by R. R. Williams and coworkers, who gave it the name "thiamine"[2] (from *thio,* meaning sulfur-containing, and *amine;* the final "e" was later dropped). (See Fig. 8–1.)

The search for the cause of the disease *beriberi* in man and the disease *polyneuritis,* its counterpart in poultry, was the start of the discovery of this vitamin. Beriberi had been described in Chinese medical literature before Christ. The word means "I cannot" (since persons with severe beriberi cannot move easily). Its cause was not known to be related to the diet until late in the nineteenth century. In 1880, a Dutch naval doctor, van Leent, reported that death from beriberi was greatly reduced in Indian naval crews when European-type diets were eaten instead of diets consisting primarily of rice. In 1885, Takaki, chief medical officer of the Japanese Navy, reported that beriberi had been eradicated among the sailors as a result of adding extra meat, fish, and vegetables to the regular diet. Before this time, the disease was so common that three out of every ten sailors were likely to have it, and there were many deaths.

In 1890, the young Dutch physician Eijkman, who was assigned to a prision hospital in Java, noticed that a disease similar to beriberi appeared in chickens that had been fed the leftover food from the diet of the hospital patients who had beriberi. This diet consisted of little more than polished rice. He found by careful observation, when his new hospital director forbade him the use of the leftover food, that he could cure the disease in the chickens by feeding whole rice or by returning the hull to the polished rice diet. Eijkman thought that the carbohydrate content of rice produced a toxin, thus missing the true reason for his results.

Later, his work was carried on at the same hospital by another Dutch physician, Grijns, who concluded in 1901[3] that beriberi in man and polyneuritis in chickens were caused by the *absence* in the diet of some unknown substance present in the germ or outer coat of grains, as well as in beans, but not in highly milled grains. These experiments were historically important because they led to the discovery not only of thiamin but also of other B vitamins through studies of deficiencies produced in animals. Shortly thereafter, many other workers in Java, the Philippines, and elsewhere repeated these studies, and found that the disease could be prevented also by feeding subjects concentrates from yeast, wheat germ, and milk.

Between 1911 and 1925, the first serious attempts were made to isolate and identify the "antineuritic factor," as it was then called.[4] These were unsuccessful but helpful to later workers. One extra dividend of these early attempts was the word "vitamine," coined by Funk during his studies on the antineuritic factor (see Chapter 6).

Chemical Identification and Properties

The first pure preparation of what is now known as thiamin was isolated from rice polishings in 1926 by Jansen and Donath[5] of the Dutch East Indian Medical Service in Java in the same laboratory where Eijkman and Grijns did their pioneer work on beriberi in man and polyneuritis in fowl.* This was an important event, since it was the first time any vitamin was obtained from food in crystalline form, thus taking vitamins out of the class of "mysterious substances." However, it was ten years later before Williams was able to announce its structure and synthesis.[2]

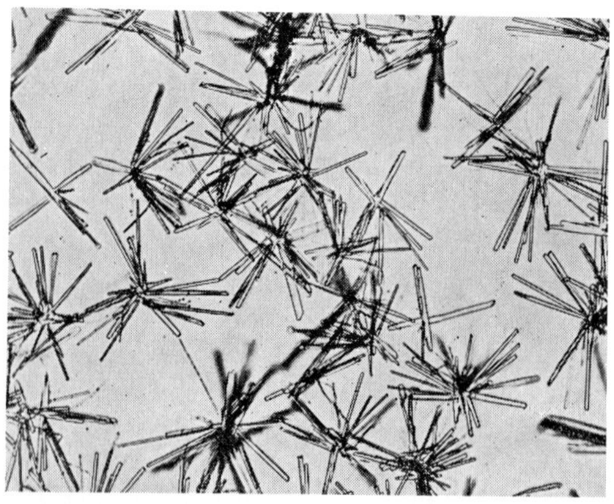

Figure 8–2 Photomicrograph of thiamin hydrochloride, crystalline form. (Courtesy of Merck & Company, Inc.)

Thiamin is a crystalline substance (Fig. 8–2), made up of carbon, hydrogen, oxygen, and sulfur (see formula in Appendix). It is readily soluble in water, slightly soluble in alcohol, and insoluble in fat solvents. Thiamin may be destroyed during storage or by heating in neutral or alkaline solutions, especially by prolonged heating. It is quite stable (not readily destroyed) in the dry state. Synthetic thiamin is usually prepared in the form of one of its salts, such as thiamin hydrochloride or thiamin mononitrate, which are more stable than the free vitamin.

Effects of Lack of Thiamin in Man and Animals

The *symptoms* of beriberi in humans are numbness or tingling in toes and feet, stiffness of ankles and absence of the ankle jerk reflex, cramping pains in legs, difficulty in walking, and finally paralysis of legs with atrophy of leg muscles (see Fig. 8–3). In later stages various nerves may be affected (which gave rise to the terms antineuritic vitamin, and "aneurin" in the early literature), and disturbances of heart function are common. In the form known as *wet beriberi,* dropsical bloating or edema

*They isolated 100 mg of crystals from 100 kg of rice polishings. Of interest is the fact that instead of using pigeons and chickens for their test animals, Jansen and Donath used the native "ricebirds."

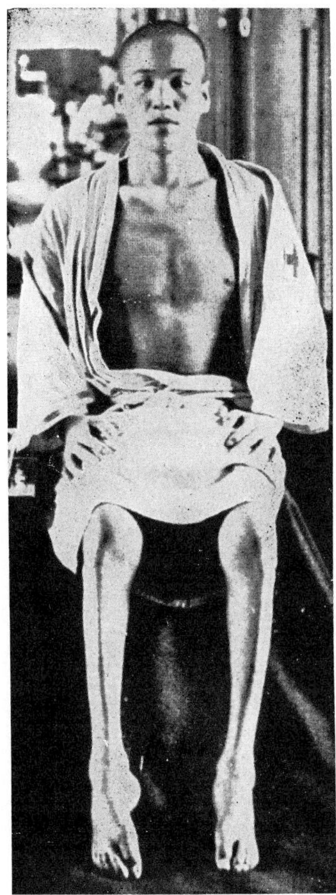

Figure 8–3 Case of "dry" beriberi, showing atrophy of the muscles due to paralysis of the legs. (Courtesy of Herzog and the *Philippine Journal of Sciences.*)

A

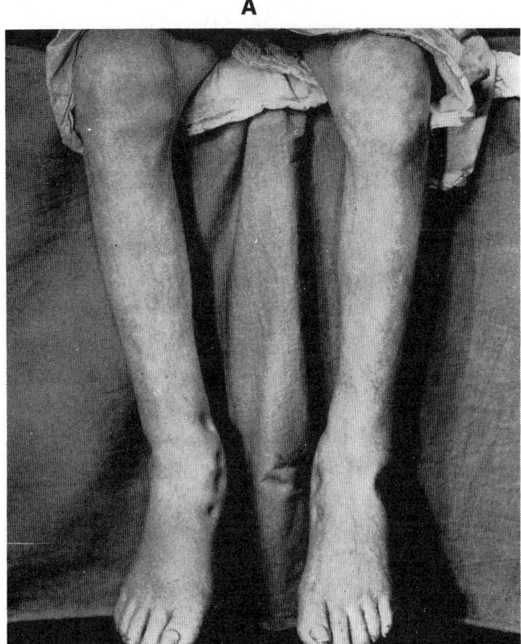

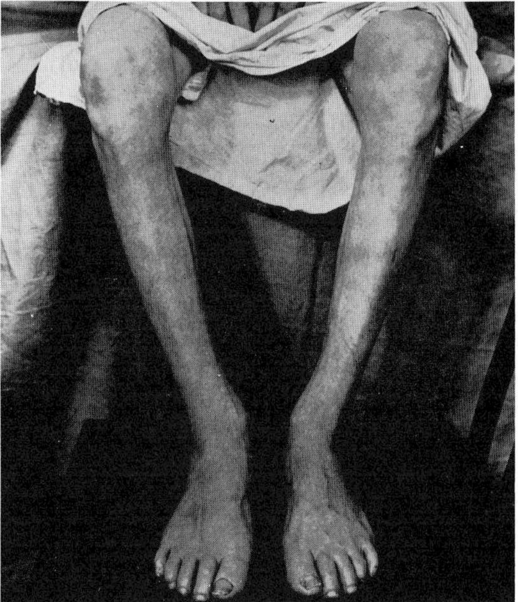

B

Figure 8–4 Patient before and after treatment for vitamin B-1 deficiency (so-called "wet" beriberi). **A,** Swelling of the legs and marked pitting edema in the ankle region. **B,** Ten days after initiation of thiamin therapy; during which the patient lost 40 pounds. Presumably this weight loss was due to the loss of fluid because the general nutritive state was greatly improved. (From Spies: *Rehabilitation Through Better Nutrition.* Philadelphia, W. B. Saunders, 1947.)

(especially of the legs) is a complicating factor due probably to cardiac disturbances (Fig. 8–4). Although the endemic beriberi, so prevalent in the Orient in earlier years, was probably due to a deficiency of several nutrients, there is no doubt that the primary deficiency was that of thiamin. The extensive tissue damage that occurs in beriberi, because of lack of thiamin, makes us realize how important a role this vitamin plays in normal nutrition.

Thiamin plays a part in promoting appetite and better functioning of the digestive tract, effects that have an indirect influence in promoting growth. The emptying time of the stomach and intestines is nearly twice as slow in thiamin-

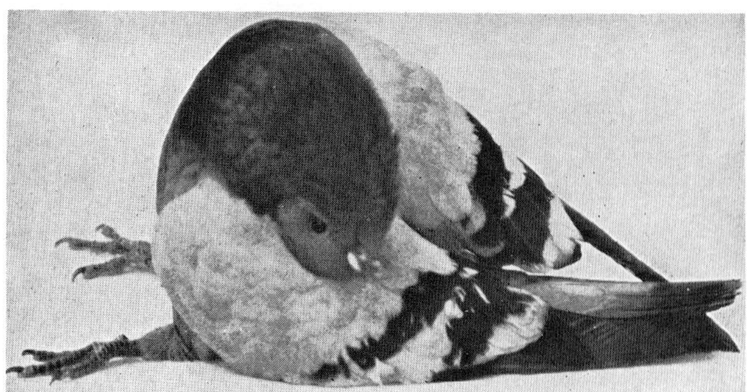

Figure 8–5 Characteristic attitude of pigeon with polyneuritis (avian beriberi) after 3 weeks' feeding with a diet of polished rice. The pigeon was used year after year as a class demonstration, and the extreme effect passed off within a few hours after feeding foods rich in thiamin. (From Morse: *Applied Biochemistry*. Philadelphia, W. B. Saunders, 1927.)

deficient animals as in normal ones. However, most authorities agree that thiamin is not the only vitamin that produces a lack of appetite with a deficiency; other factors may be responsible for the loss of desire for food. Upon reversal of the deficiency, normal appetite is restored. However, large quantities of thiamin do not promote a voracious appetite.

Thiamin has been called "the morale vitamin," because one of the earliest signs of its lack is a lowering of stamina. Studies of people who volunteered to consume a diet moderately low in thiamin demonstrated that after a short time on such a diet (as early as in 10 days) the subjects became depressed and irritable, lacking in ability to concentrate on and to take an interest in their work.[6] In 3 to 7 weeks such symptoms as fatigue, lack of appetite, loss of weight, constipation, muscle cramps, and various pains appeared. The subjects promptly recovered normal health and morale when given larger amounts of thiamin.

Experimental Animals. Without experimental animals to use in studying the counterpart of human deficiencies, it is likely that the discovery of many of the vitamins would have been postponed many years, and the metabolic function of vitamins would be most difficult to study. For this reason and because of the possible use of animals in classroom demonstrations, some attention is given here to vitamin deficiencies in animals, as well as human deficiencies.

In young experimental animals made deficient in thiamin, symptoms may be seen as early as 3 to 6 days after withholding the vitamin. All deficient animals show poor growth, nervous symptoms, and death in severe cases. Pigeons and fowl develop a severe and characteristic head retraction, a form of polyneuritis (Fig. 8–5). Swine develop generalized weakness, vomiting, and dizziness. Rats show reduced growth (Fig. 8–6), convulsions, slowing of the heartbeat, and a loss of appetite. Deficiency signs, generally similar, have been produced also in the dog, monkey, guinea pig, mouse, cat, and, in fact, in every animal tested except those species in which sufficient thiamin is produced by intestinal microorganisms to take care of the animal's requirement. Thiamin is also necessary for normal fertility and lactation in experimental animals.

Most microorganisms are able to synthesize thiamin, which is needed to promote their growth. Microorganisms in the rumen, or large stomach, of cattle, sheep, and goats make sufficient thiamin, and in fact, other B complex vitamins, to take care of the animal's entire need for these vitamins. These are absorbed and utilized in the usual manner. Thus, it is not necessary to give sources of thiamin to these animals except when they are very young before the rumen is functioning. Animals such as rabbits and rats, that routinely eat some of their feces (a practice known as "coprophagy") and thus obtain B vitamins produced by intestinal bacteria, must be kept in cages with screened bottoms in experiments for producing deficiencies, in order to reduce the chance of their eating the feces.

The composition of the diet affects the amount of intestinal synthesis by microorganisms of thiamin in man and animals. In the rat, for instance, a diet high in starch is likely to cause greater synthesis of thiamin by bacteria than a diet high in sucrose. In man some intestinal synthesis of thiamin and other B vitamins by microorganisms also takes place, but the synthesis occurs so low in the tract and in a form so poorly absorbed that it is of little use to the human body.

Functions in the Body

In humans, after thiamin is absorbed, it is distributed widely by the blood throughout the body in all tissues and in somewhat higher concentrations in such organs as the heart, liver, and kidneys. There is limited ability of the body to store thiamin. Tissues are depleted of their normal content of the vitamin in just 1 or 2 weeks if the diet is deficient, so fresh supplies are needed regularly to provide for maintenance of tissue levels. The tissues take up only as much as they need, and because thiamin is freely soluble in water, most of the thiamin intake not required for day-to-day use is excreted in the urine, either as the intact molecule or as split halves.

Of foremost importance is the part thiamin plays in the life processes of individual cells throughout the body. A large part of the energy for the life processes of body tissues comes from the oxidation of carbohydrate, which takes place gradually through the formation of intermediate products and requires enzymes to bring about or catalyze each step of the intricate process. Many enzymes require *coenzymes* to render them active, or make them capable of bringing about a certain chemical change (Fig. 8–7). Thiamin is known to be the active part of the coenzyme *thiamin pyrophosphate,* made in tissue cells by the combining of thiamin with two phosphate groups or radicals.

This very important coenzyme is known to be necessary for at least four different enzyme systems that are needed for the complete oxidation of carbohydrate. Two of these enzymes function by spltting off carbon dioxide in the course of oxidation in the body, or in reverse reactions adding it onto some fragment of metabolism. For example, by such reactions pyruvic acid and other keto acids (intermediates in glucose oxidation) are converted step by step, with the removal of carbon dioxide (decarboxylation), to acetate radicals and eventually to carbon dioxide and water. Hence, thiamin pyrophosphate constitutes an essential link in the chain of the complete oxidation of carbohydrate, thus providing energy to the body. Without a dietary source of thiamin, pyruvic acid and other intermediate compounds may build up in the blood and tissues to a toxic level, and these compounds are presumed to be an important cause of deficiency symptoms.

Thiamin pyrophosphate serves also as a coenzyme in reactions leading to the production of ribose, the important pentose sugar needed by all cells of the body (see sections on DNA and RNA, p. 86). Essential cofactors in these actions of thiamin pyrophosphate are the coenzymes of several other vitamins, such as pantothenic acid and niacin, as well as of magnesium, demonstrating the essential interrelationship in the body of the various vitamins and minerals.

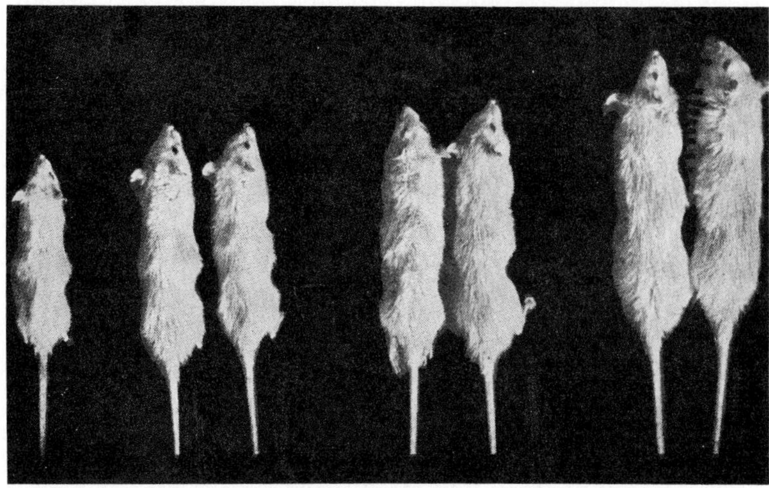

Figure 8–6 Effects on growth of rats of feeding four different levels of thiamin, ranging from none on the left to optimal amounts on the right. (From experiments of Dr. Bertha Bisbey.)

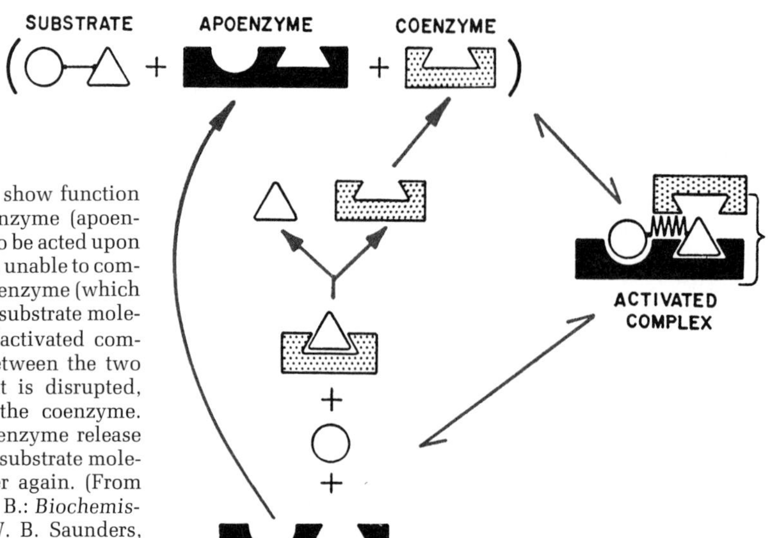

Figure 8–7 Diagram to show function of a coenzyme. The main enzyme (apoenzyme) absorbs the substance to be acted upon on its molecular surface but is unable to complete the reaction until the coenzyme (which is attracted to one part of the substrate molecule) is added to form an "activated complex." Tension is created between the two parts of the substrate and it is disrupted, with one part attached to the coenzyme. Both the apoenzyme and coenzyme release the portions of the disrupted substrate molecule and are free to act over again. (From Cantarow, A., and Shepartz, B.: *Biochemistry*. 3rd Ed. Philadelphia, W. B. Saunders, 1962.)

Requirement and Nutritional Status

American diets provide enough thiamin to prevent the appearance of frank beriberi in this country. However, a good many diets may provide less than optimal amounts, especially in times of body stress caused by growth, pregnancy, lactation, fevers, or surgical operations. Nervous symptoms due to a lack of thiamin are seen often in chronic alcoholic persons in this country, since their diet is often inadequate and their high intake of energy in the form of alcohol increases their requirement for thiamin. Alcohol also reduces thiamin absorption (see page 173).

The presence of a thiamin deficiency, as well as the extent of the deficiency, is determined by measuring urinary levels of thiamin or, more specifically, tissue levels of either thiamin pyrophosphate or *transketolase*, an enzyme requiring thiamin pyrophosphate as a cofactor.

The amount of thiamin required by adults varies according to size, degree of activity, dietary habits, and individual differences in how food is utilized. Since this vitamin takes part in the metabolism of carbohydrate, more of it is needed when the rate of carbohydrate metabolism is high. Persons who do considerable muscular work burn up more energy foods and usually obtain much of this extra energy in the form of starchy foods; hence, they need more thiamin than those who are muscularly inactive. The requirement for thiamin is usually stated in terms of the caloric intake (so much for every 1000 kcal), particularly of the nonfat calories of the diet; with more fat and a lower proportion of calories from carbohydrate, slightly less thiamin is needed. *Growing children* have higher energy needs and therefore have higher thiamin needs per unit of body weight than adults. Women during *pregnancy* have an increased need for thiamin, and *nursing mothers* should have approximately one and one-half times as much thiamin as under normal conditions.

The current recommendations of the U.S. Food and Nutrition Board[7] provide a moderately liberal daily intake of thiamin for normal adults, varying according to the caloric intake recommended for the different age groups, which is greater in younger adults. For college-age women the recommended intake is 1.1 mg per day and for college-age men, 1.5 mg. See Table 8–1 for thiamin allowances of selected age groups (and see

Table 1A in the Appendix for complete details for all age groups).

Daily allowances for adults are calculated on the basis of individual calorie requirements, allowing 0.5 mg per 1000 kcal. The Food and Nutrition Board cautions, however, that older adults who subsist on a calorie intake of less than 2000 should not have less than 1.0 mg of thiamin per day, which is recognized as about the minimum daily requirement. There is no evidence that larger intakes than the recommended allowance will be of any benefit to normal, healthy adults.

Dietary surveys have shown that the average intake of thiamin in the United States is not much higher than the recommended allowance, and we are indebted to the enrichment program for keeping the level as high as it is (see Chapter 18). For example, Williams and coworkers concluded in 1942 that the average American diet, prior to the introduction of enriched bread and cereal foods, provided only about 0.8 mg of thiamin per 2500 kcal, which was dangerously near the minimum requirement.[8] The enrichment of bread and cereals, started during World War II, has increased by about one-third the amount of thiamin available for the average person, most all of this coming from synthetic thiamin at a negligible cost. In 1977 about 2.09 mg of thiamin was available per person per day from the nation's food supply, according to the U.S. Department of Agriculture.[9] This figure is about 30 to 50 per cent higher than the amount actually consumed by the average person, because the U.S.D.A. figure does not take into account either waste of food, use in pet foods, or destruction of thiamin during preparation, cooking, or canning of foods.

It is apparent that many individuals consume levels of thiamin very close to, or even less than, the recommended allowance. However, various food and nutrition surveys[10-13] have shown that in spite of intakes of excessively high amounts of carbohydrate and only borderline amounts of thiamin, few, if any, signs of thiamin deficiency are apparent in large numbers of population groups. Intakes of thiamin in the United States today range from an average of about 1.0 to 1.1 mg per day for females and about 1.4 to 1.5 mg for males.[13] These values are well within the range of amounts needed to protect against a deficiency.

Table 8–1 RECOMMENDED ALLOWANCES FOR THIAMIN*

	Age	*Allowance, mg/day*
Males	11–14 years	1.4
	15–22 years	1.5
	23–50 years	1.4
	51 years and over	1.2
Females	11–14 years	1.2
	15–22 years	1.1
	23 years and older	1.0
	Pregnant	+0.3
	Lactating	+0.3

*From the Food and Nutrition Board.[7]

See Appendix Table 1D for FAO recommendations.

Food Sources of Thiamin

Few foods relatively rich in thiamin are used in quantity in our modern diets unless they are enriched with the synthetic vitamin. Although almost all natural foods contain thiamin, many of them carry only minor amounts, which may be still further reduced by cooking or processing. From available figures (see Appendix, Table 2) it may be seen that the thiamin content of most fruits and vegetables, eggs, milk, and cheese does not generally exceed 0.1 mg per 100 gm.[14] In plants it is concentrated chiefly in *seeds* (whole grains, legumes, and nuts); in animals it is abundant in the *organs* (liver, heart, kidneys). Pork flesh is much higher in thiamin content than other meats, but *meats* and *leafy vegetables* are moderately good sources. In certain processed or refined foods, such as

Table 8–2 EXAMPLES OF GOOD FOOD SOURCES OF THIAMIN*

Food Source	*Thiamin, mg/100 gm*	*Food Source*	*Thiamin, mg/100 gm*
Bacon, Canadian	0.83	Piñon nuts	1.28
Beans, Pinto	0.84	Pork	0.50
Buckwheat flour (dark)	0.58	Rice polish	1.84
Cornflakes with added nutrients	0.43	Rye, whole grain	0.43
Heart, beef	0.53	Sesame seeds	0.98
Kidneys, hog	0.58	Soybeans	1.10
Lentils	0.37	Sunflower seed	1.96
Liver, lamb	0.40	Whole wheat flour	0.55
Oatmeal (dry)	0.60	Wheat flour, enriched	0.44
Peanuts (with skins)†	1.14	Wheat germ	2.01
Milk chocolate with		Yeast	
peanuts	0.25	Baker's, dry	2.33
Peas	0.35	Brewer's	15.61
Pecans	0.86	Torula	14.01

*From U.S. Dept. of Agriculture handbooks.[14] Based on fresh, raw, edible portion, before cooking or roasting.[14]

†Roasted peanuts contain 0.32 mg per 100 gm.

highly milled cereals and sulfured dried fruits, thiamin is present in traces or entirely absent unless these foods have been enriched with added thiamin. There is none in sugar, or in salad oils or other fats.

Our best sources of thiamin —*whole grains, organ meats, pork,* and *legumes* — are not used in quantity in the American diet. However, foods of more moderate thiamin content and thiamin-enriched foods are used in sufficient amounts to provide this vitamin at a fairly safe level. (See Table 8–2.) Of our total thiamin intake about 42 percent comes from bread and cereals; 33 percent from meats, fish, poultry, eggs, legumes, and nuts; 8 percent from milk and other dairy products; and 17 percent from vegetables and fruits.[9] In low-cost diets, in which grain products and potatoes furnish a higher proportion of the diet, it is especially important that bread and cereals be of a whole-grain or enriched variety. Such foods as oatmeal and dried legumes can be an economical source of thiamin. It is significant that beriberi seldom, if ever, develops in countries where meats, dairy products, whole-grain products, fruits, and vegetables are freely used. It should be noted that sucrose and pure fats, most of which is used in making processed foods and which supply over 35 percent of the energy intake of an average American diet, provide no thiamin or other water-soluble vitamins. (See Chapter 17, p. 398.)

Effects of Cooking and Processing

Thiamin in food suffers little destruction on exposure to air at ordinary temperatures. Thiamin, however, is one of the vitamins that may be most easily lost in food preservation and cooking, depending on the methods used.[15] Dry heating at high temperatures, as in preparation of ready cooked cereals or in toasting bread, can cause considerable loss. Moist heat (boiling for not more than an hour) causes little destruction of this vitamin, but its solubility in water means that as much as one-third of the original thiamin content may be lost if cooking water is liberal and is discarded. Thiamin is very unstable in an alkaline medium and is largely destroyed if soda is added in the cooking of vegetables. Meats lose about 20 to 60 percent of thiamin in roasting, depending on the extent of roasting, 30 percent in broiling, and only 15 percent in frying. In baking bread, only 5 to 15 percent of the original thiamin content is lost, while there is no significant loss of this vitamin in cooking cereals in a double boiler. Prolonged cooking, as of dried legumes, results in relatively high losses of their thiamin content. Fresh frozen vegetables maintain as much thiamin as is left in the product after "blanching" to destroy enzyme activity. Canned vegetables suffer a loss owing to solubility of the vitamin in the canning fluid, which is drained away.

Antithiamin Factors in Food

Certain raw fish and seafood, particularly carp, herring, clams, and shrimp, contain the enzyme *thiaminase*, which is capable of splitting the thiamin molecule into its two major chemical groups, thus making it inactive. This effect has been seen in fox farms where the animals were fed raw fish, resulting in severe economic losses. The effect can also be produced in laboratory animals (cats, chickens, etc.) by feeding them raw fish at a level of 10 to 25 percent. This action can be prevented by heating the fish first and destroying the enzyme. In most countries, humans do not normally eat sufficient raw fish or seafood to produce a thiamin deficiency, but it is known that this may be a contributory factor in producing beriberi in certain populations of the world, especially in the Orient.

Other agents are known to affect thiamin levels in the body. For instance, a large amount of live yeast in the diet of man reduces the amount of thiamin absorbed from the intestine. Signs of thiamin deficiency have been seen in Asia in persons who drink large amounts of tea or chew fermented tea leaves or betel nuts, a very common practice. This suggests the presence of antithiamin factors in these substances.[16] Alcohol, in excess, is known to decrease absorption of thiamin in man and animals; thus, it is also an antithiamin substance.[17] Thiamin deficiency is commonly seen in alcoholics.

Thiamin-splitting bacteria have been found in the intestinal tracts of people in Japan who have symptoms of beriberi, but the significance of this is unknown at present.

RIBOFLAVIN

Discovery

In the course of years of experimenting with the growth-promoting factor called "water-soluble B," it became evident between 1917 and 1927 that there must be at least two vitamins in yeast, liver, and the outer coats of grains.[4] It would be difficult to give any one person credit for obtaining the first experimental deficiency of what is now known as riboflavin, but mention should be made of Emmett, of Detroit, who probably provided the first evidence for the existence of a second vitamin B (1917–1920).[18] Severe heating, such as at 120° C in an autoclave for several hours, completely destroyed the anti-beriberi vitamin (thiamin) in yeast, but there remained another vitamin fraction which showed growth-promoting potency. Although this heat-stable fraction is now known to consist of several vitamins, the one first discovered and studied was called *vitamin* B_2 by the British in 1927, or *vitamin G* by Americans. Both of these names are no longer used for riboflavin and the terms have historic significance only.

Chemical Identification and Properties

In 1933, chemists in Germany found that rats grew faster when given a dietary source of a yellow compound called "ovoflavin," which they isolated from egg white (flavus means yellow). It was soon shown that the flavin pigment that had been isolated and that was essential for rats was the same as the pigment associated with the classic "yellow enzyme," isolated by Warburg in Germany in 1931, and similar to the yellow pigment isolated from heart muscle by Szent-Györgyi and coworkers in 1932, which was later shown to be an important coenzyme. This proved to be the *first demonstration of a vitamin-coenzyme relationship* and opened the door to modern nutritional biochemistry. It is of interest that as long ago as 1879 yellowish-green fluorescent pigments were isolated from whey and other biological materials, but the biological significance of such pigments (now known to be riboflavin) had not been established previously.

Other workers in Germany and Switzerland, in most cases before 1933, had isolated similar fluorescent pigments from milk, liver, plant material, and egg yolk, which were given names indicating their source as "lactoflavin" (from milk) or "hepatoflavin" (from liver). It was soon learned that all these substances were similar and the name "riboflavin" was given by Karrer of Switzerland* to the most active compound in 1935 and is in general use today. It was found to have a pentose side chain — *ribitol* (similar to the sugar, ribose) — attached to a flavinlike compound, hence the name riboflavin. Riboflavin was first synthesized in 1935 by two independent groups led by Kuhn of Germany and by Karrer.

Riboflavin is an orange-yellow solid that imparts a greenish-yellow fluorescence to solutions (see formula in Appendix). One of its most important chemical properties is its change to a colorless form on reduction (addition of hydrogen molecules), and its reoxidation (removal of hydrogen) to its orange-yellow color by exposure to oxidizing agents. It is sparingly soluble in water, but it is much more soluble in alkaline solutions. It is stable to heating in neutral or acid solutions, but it may be destroyed by heating in alkaline solution or by exposure to light. In fact, it is so sensitive to light that when someone is using a dilute solution of it in a laboratory — such as when assaying it in foods — it is routine practice to turn off the lights and pull down the shades to darken the room as much as is practical. Riboflavin may also be destroyed by sunlight striking milk kept in glass bottles (see page 180).

Riboflavin (most often in combined forms) is very widely distributed in both plant and animal tissues. It is formed by all higher plants, chiefly in the green leaves, and the younger parts of the plant contain more than older parts. Seeds are rather low in riboflavin, except when sprouting. Also, most microorganisms synthesize this vitamin, and bacteria in the intestinal tract may be a considerable but variable source of it for animals, just as with thiamin. Aside from this undependable source, higher animals must obtain riboflavin from their food.

Effects of Riboflavin Deficiency in Animals and Man

The need of a dietary source of riboflavin was discovered by its effect on *growth* of rats. Experimental animals that receive little or no riboflavin show stunted growth, and when they are fed graded amounts of it, they respond with corresponding increases in growth rate. They also need riboflavin in the diet for maximum health and vigor, maximum ability to bear and suckle offspring, and for delayed senility. Riboflavin is one of the factors essential for successful *reproduction;* rats on diets deficient in this vitamin produced young with abnormal skeletons and other defects.

This vitamin is essential for general health because it is the active constitu-

*Karrer died in 1971. He was also the first to synthesize carotene, discussed in Chapter 7, and made other important discoveries in nutrition. He was awarded the Nobel Prize in 1937 for these studies.

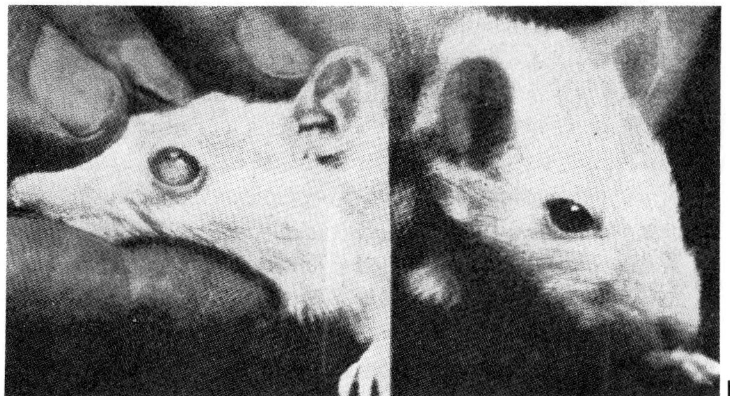

Figure 8–8 Two views of the same rat. **A,** After cataract developed in the left eye as a result of riboflavin deficiency. **B,** Several weeks after administration of riboflavin, the right eye thus being saved. Also note the marked improvement of the rat's general condition as the result of riboflavin administration. (Courtesy of Paul L. Day and the *American Journal of Public Health.*)

ent of several enzymes or coenzymes that are needed for oxidation processes in the various body tissues. It is essential for the health of tissues of ectodermal origin, such as the skin, eyes, and nerves.

In experimental animals (rats), a long-continued lack of riboflavin leads to *sore mouth and nose, falling hair* and *scaly skin, eye symptoms* varying in severity from an inflamed condition of the cornea to its complete opacity in cataract (Fig. 8–8), *digestive disturbances, nervous lesions* (severe cases show paralysis of hind legs), poor utilization of food, increasing weakness, and death.

Deficient chickens show a characteristic *curled toe paralysis,* caused by degenerated nerves, in which the toes curve inward. Eventually, the deficiency causes death unless corrected. This formerly was very common in commercial poultry flocks, but today all poultry rations are routinely fortified with liberal amounts of riboflavin, and the condition is no longer seen. Riboflavin is needed in the diet of all monogastric animals tested, including the mouse, guinea pig, monkey, pig, dog, fox, horse, fish, and even the young calf before the rumen starts to function. Many deficiency signs similar to those seen in the rat are seen in these animals.

In man, symptoms of riboflavin deficiency are similar to those seen in animals, but they are less specific and less severe. In fact, there still is considerable disagreement as to the characteristic signs of deficiency in man; more studies are needed. Sebrell and Butler, who first produced experimental deficiency of this vitamin in human beings, reported as characteristic symptoms reddened, denuded areas on the lips, with cracks at the corners of the mouth — called *cheilosis** (Fig. 8–9).[19] These symptoms were cured when riboflavin was given. Also, other investigators have reported eye disorders in riboflavin-deficient persons, such as dimness of vision and burning of the eyes, and the possibility of cataract. Other skin abnormalities, including a greasy scaly dermatitis around the nose, and particularly on the scrotum in the male, have been seen in riboflavin deficiency. Symptoms of general debility and behavioral changes, similar to those seen in pellagra, may also be associated with a deficient intake of riboflavin.

Ordinarily it takes several months for symptoms of riboflavin deficiency to appear, but Lane and coworkers[20] developed an acute deficiency in man within 10 to 25 days by using a riboflavin *an-*

*The symptoms of cracks in the corner of the mouth seen in riboflavin deficiency, though not specifically so, is called *angular stomatitis.*

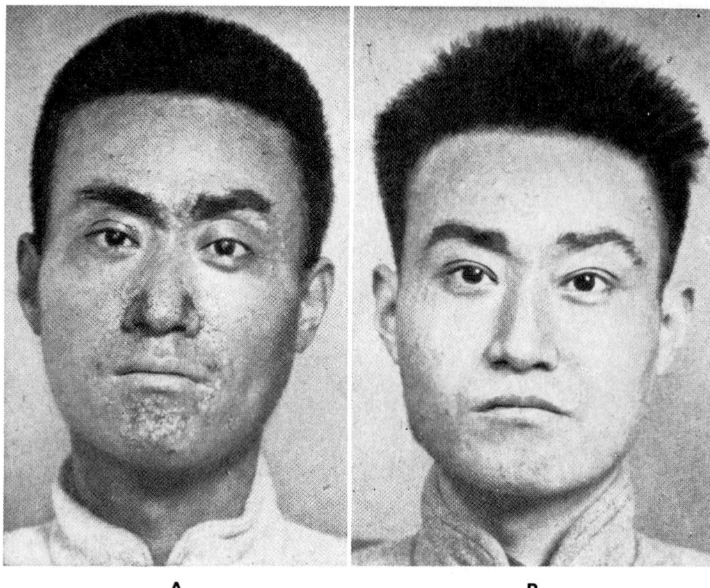

Figure 8–9 Patient before and after treatment for riboflavin deficiency. **A,** Scales and sores on the forehead, nose, cheeks, lips, and chin, and in the folds around nose and mouth. **B,** After treatment with riboflavin, 15 mg the first two days, 10 mg for the next two days, and 5 mg daily for one week. (Courtesy of Bernard Read and H. C. Hou, Shanghai, Wm. Heinemann, Ltd., London, and the *Chinese Medical Journal.*)

*tagonist** in a semisynthetic riboflavin-free diet. The resulting symptoms seen in the six test subjects were: first, sore throat or mouth, followed by reddening and swelling of the mucous membrane of the mouth and throat; cheilosis; *glossitis,* a condition in which the tongue becomes shiny and develops a red-purple color; scaly, greasy dermatitis of the face, ears, and other parts of the body; and anemia. Anemia was a "new" symptom, so it appears that riboflavin deficiency interferes with the production of red blood cells in man, as has been reported in animals. All these symptoms were rapidly and completely reversed after administration of riboflavin.

*A *nutritional antagonist* is a compound whose structure is so similar to a specific nutrient that it can substitute for the nutrient in certain enzyme systems for which the specific nutrient is necessary, thus leading to at least partial inactivity of these systems. Hence, an effect similar to a deficiency is produced in a short time. True nutritional antagonism, or inhibition, can always be overcome by high enough levels of the nutrient in question. The riboflavin antagonist used by Lane et al.[20] was *galactoflavin,* in which galactitol has been substituted for ribotol in the vitamin.

The Role of Riboflavin in the Body

Free riboflavin, such as is found in some foods, must be phosphorylated in the intestinal tract before it can be absorbed. Once it enters the blood, it is distributed to all cells of the body. The chief function of this vitamin is the role it plays in *oxidation-reduction reactions in the tissues.* Riboflavin is contained in a number of different enzymes, called *flavoproteins,* and several coenzymes whose function is to take on hydrogen and pass it on to another substance in the long chain of oxidation-reductions by which hydrogen is finally combined with oxygen to form water (Fig. 8–10). In this way, riboflavin-containing enzymes assist in the metabolism of carbohydrate, of amino acids, and of fats. During this process, energy is released gradually and made available to the cell.

Riboflavin's *biochemical role* revolves chiefly around two important coenzymes in which most of the riboflavin in the body exists — *riboflavin monophosphate* (also called, less correctly, flavin mononucleotide) and the more common but elaborate *flavin adenine dinucleotide*, or "FAD," composed of riboflavin monophosphate with additional phosphate and sugar groups plus adenine, a purine. These coenzymes are attached with various degrees of tenacity to a number of highly important enzymes in the body, the flavoproteins, which catalyze oxidation-reduction reactions. Most of these enzymes act as *hydrogen carriers*, passing this element along from one substance to another until its atoms are finally united with oxygen atoms, by special enzymes, to form molecules of water. It is of interest that several of these enzymes contain a metal — for example, molybdenum or iron — demonstrating again the important interrelationships between vitamins and minerals.

Since one of the enzymes requiring a flavin coenzyme is easily measured (*glutathione reductase* of the red blood cell), a very sensitive test for measuring the degree of riboflavin deficiency in humans is widely used. This is superior to just measuring riboflavin levels in determining the riboflavin status of individuals.

Because riboflavin is essential to numerous chemical changes in tissues, it is natural that deprivation of this vitamin causes damage to many different types of tissues and that sufficient intake of it is necessary to promote the welfare of the body as a whole.

Riboflavin is found in almost all tissues, principally in the form of its coenzymes. There does not appear to be any specialized mechanism for storage of riboflavin, although muscle tissues may retain considerable amounts even in riboflavin deficiency. Unused riboflavin is excreted in the urine.

Requirement and Nutritional Status

We have learned that riboflavin is necessary in the body for energy formation, protein metabolism and many cellular reactions dealing with growth or repair of the body. For practical purposes the daily riboflavin allowances recommended by the Food and Nutrition Board[7] have been based on a value of 0.6 mg of riboflavin for every 1000 kcal consumed for people of all ages. This is about 20 percent over the apparent *minimum requirement* of about 0.5 mg per 1000 kcal, a rather small margin of safety in comparison with the safety margins for many of the other vitamins. This does not allow too great a leeway for "dietary indiscretions" of individuals — at least not over long periods. The RDA for college-age men is 1.8 mg per day, and for college-age women it is 1.4 mg per day (1974). The need for riboflavin increases during pregnancy and lactation, as is true with all B vitamins. See Table 8–3 and Appendix, Table 1A, for more details on allowance values. A minimum of about 1.2 mg per day in adults is necessary to maintain adequate body stores and normal urinary output

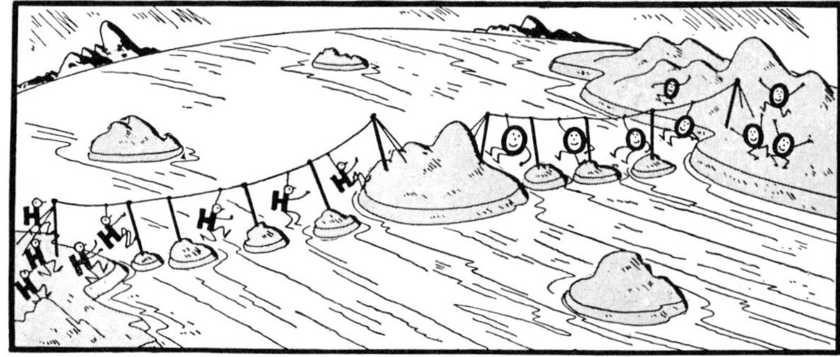

Figure 8–10 Diagram to illustrate how enzymes or coenzymes, which contain vitamins, may act as stepping stones for oxygen or hydrogen atoms in bringing about oxidation-reduction reactions in living tissues. Thiamin, riboflavin, and niacin form part of enzymes and coenzymes that function in this manner. The hydrogen and oxygen atoms, separated by an otherwise formidable barrier, are enabled by the use of stepping stones (enzymes) and the handrails (coenzymes) to move toward each other and ultimately unite to form molecules of water (H_2O). (From W. O. Kermack and P. Eggleton: *The Stuff We're Made of*, Edward Arnold & Co., London.)

Table 8–3 RECOMMENDED ALLOWANCES FOR RIBOFLAVIN*

	Age	*Allowance, mg/day*
Males	11–14 years	1.5
	14–22 years	1.8
	23–50 years	1.6
	51 years and over	1.5
Females	11–14 years	1.3
	15–22 years	1.4
	23–50 years	1.2
	51 years or over	1.1
	Pregnant	+0.3
	Lactating	+0.5

*From the Food and Nutrition Board, 1974.[7]

See Appendix Table 1D for FAO recommendations.

even if the caloric intake is below 2000 kcal.

Riboflavin deficiency once was fairly common in the United States, especially in the South, and wherever milk, the best dietary source, was not consumed. After 1941, the start of the enrichment program (see page 422), cases of severe deficiency of riboflavin in man became very rare. Concentrates of riboflavin, from synthetic or fermentation sources, used in current enrichment programs in the United States contribute an average of 0.33 mg of riboflavin per person per day, which is about one-fourth of the requirement, a very significant amount.* However, not all states have required enrichment programs, and the riboflavin intake of many persons in these and other states is still well below recommended allowances and even below minimum requirements.[10-13] Chronic or "borderline" riboflavin deficiency is most likely to occur to a variable extent in persons with inadequate intake of basic or enriched foods, but is most likely to occur in alcoholics,[21] in the aged when given poor diets,[22] in women of lower socioeconomic levels who are of childbearing age, especially those taking oral contraceptives,[23] and in pregnancy.[24] There is no evidence that the intake of riboflavin need be greater than the RDA for such persons, however. Riboflavin deficiencies also exist in other countries throughout the world. It is important, therefore, that many more efforts be devoted in all countries to increasing intakes of riboflavin and other key nutrients as well, such as vitamin D, folacin, vitamin A, calcium, and iron. To accomplish this, new programs in nutrition education, distribution of free and low cost foods to the poor, and enrichment of foods will be needed.

One of the major reasons for the low consumption of riboflavin in this country, and elsewhere, is that many persons in this country, perhaps 15 to 25 percent, do not use milk in any form, or they use it very sparingly. Since milk supplies about 40 percent of all the riboflavin consumed by persons in the United States, it is clear that people not consuming milk must eat liberal quantities of liver, eggs, leafy vegetables, or legumes, or take vitamin supplements to maintain an adequate intake (see next section).

Because infants generally consume a large amount of breast milk or cow's milk, their average consumption is well above the recommended allowance. Only when milk is not consumed is it necessary to be concerned about an infant's riboflavin intake, and most commercial milk substitutes supply liberal amounts. (See Chapter 21.)

Riboflavin in Foods

Table 8–4 shows that *liver, milk, cheese, eggs, leafy vegetables, enriched bread, lean meat,* and *legumes* are the foods that are among the richest in riboflavin. Dried yeast is a still richer source. Both thiamin and riboflavin are almost universally distributed in foods; only such foods as pure sugars and fats are entirely lacking in them. Riboflavin is

*The cost of riboflavin from such sources is only about 10 cents per 1000 mg (1 gm) — more than a year's requirement for one person.

Table 8–4 EXAMPLES OF GOOD FOOD SOURCES OF RIBOFLAVIN*

Food Source	*Riboflavin, mg/100 gm*	*Food Source*	*Riboflavin, mg/100 mg*
Beans		Meat, lean	0.20
White	0.22	Milk, fluid	
Red	0.20	Whole	0.17
Pinto	0.21	Skim	0.18
Mung	0.21	2% fat, added solids	0.21
Soy	0.31	Pepper, chili, dried	1.33
Beet greens	0.23	Soybean flour	0.31
Cashew nuts	0.25	Spinach	0.20
Cheese, cheddar	0.46	Spleen, beef	0.37
Chicken, dark meat	0.20	Split peas	0.29
Cocoa powder	0.46	Sunflower seeds	0.23
Collards	0.31	Water chestnut	0.20
Egg, white	0.30	Wheat germ, crude	0.68
Heart, calf	1.05	Yeast	
Kale	0.26	Brewer's	4.28
Kidneys, beef	2.55	Torula	5.06
Liver, beef	3.26		

*From U.S. Department of Agriculture tables.[14] Based on fresh, raw, edible portion.

more plentifully supplied in most foods than thiamin, and this is notably true of organ meats, leafy vegetables, eggs, and milk. Milk has about four times as much riboflavin as thiamin (see Fig. 8–11). On the other hand, the whole-grain cereals, which are among the richest sources of thiamin, have only a moderate content of riboflavin. Even when enriched with riboflavin to the level of whole grains, bread and cereals still contribute only about one-seventh the riboflavin in the average American diet.[9] Legumes, nuts, and muscle meats are good sources of both thiamin and riboflavin. Pork, which has five to seven times the thiamin content of other meats, does not differ from other meats in riboflavin content. Eggs are richer in riboflavin than are muscle meats. Vegetables — other than leafy ones and legumes — and fruits contribute less, but still appreciable amounts of, riboflavin.

The riboflavin content of different foodstuffs is not equally available on ingestion. Fortunately, riboflavin is stable enough on heating that little of it is destroyed in ordinary cooking processes, although some may be lost by solution in water in which foods are cooked or canned. Losses also can occur from *exposure to light* if the cooking is done in open vessels. The use of sodium bicarbonate in the cooking of vegetables can also destroy riboflavin. Average losses of riboflavin in cooking are 15 to 20 percent in meats, 10 to 20 percent in vegetables, and 10 percent in baking bread.

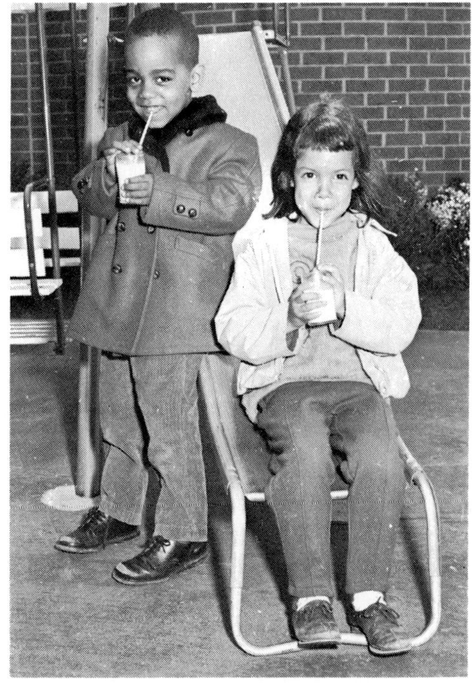

Figure 8–11 Milk supplies about 40 percent of all the riboflavin in the food supply of the United States. (Courtesy of U.S. Department of Agriculture.)

Because of the importance of milk as a dietary source of riboflavin, the possible destruction of this vitamin on exposure of milk to light has been emphasized. Exposure of liquid foods to ordinary daylight may cause considerable losses. Before the 1960's clear glass bottles of milk were delivered on the doorsteps of homes — a practice still very common in many countries. This is now a rare practice in North America, at least, partially because a glass bottle left standing on the doorstep in direct sunlight may lose 50 to 70 percent of its riboflavin potency in two hours.[25] The use of opaque cartons cuts down losses from exposure to sunlight or from display lighting in foodstores. Even so, it is best to keep milk as much as possible in a cool, dark place, such as the refrigerator. Only minor losses of riboflavin occur in pasteurization of milk.

Because of the destructive effect of light on riboflavin, low levels have been observed in newborn infants receiving phototherapy in the treatment of jaundice.[26] This is of interest, but one should not conclude that persons spending long hours in the sun need extra riboflavin.

As with most other B vitamins, large amounts of riboflavin show no toxic symptoms, but we know of no reason for anyone to consume more than the RDA in normal situations.

PANTOTHENIC ACID

Pantothenic acid is a dietary essential for man and animals and plays an unusually important role in the body. However, it is so widely distributed in most foods that a deficiency has not been seen in populations consuming a variety of basic foods.

The name "pantothenic acid," derived from the Greek, meaning "from everywhere," was given in 1933 by R. J. Williams, then of Oregon State, to an unknown factor in various biological materials necessary for the growth of yeast.[27] Dr. Williams, now at the University of Texas, is a brother of the late R. R. Williams, who first synthesized thiamin (page 165). Pantothenic acid was the third member of the vitamin B complex to be clearly differentiated as a vitamin needed by such organisms as yeast, chicks, and rats; hence it is discussed here, after riboflavin.*

Chemical Identification and Properties

After much painstaking research, primarily using the young chick as a test animal, workers at the Universities of California and Wisconsin, in 1939, announced that a highly active preparation of the "chick-antidermatitis factor" and Williams' pantothenic acid had identical growth activity.[28] In 1940, its structure was determined and it was synthesized by Williams (see formula in the Appendix).[29] Stable crystalline salts of pantothenic acid are readily available, such as synthetic sodium or calcium pantothenate.† Pantothenic acid is quite stable to heat but can be destroyed in foods by heating for long periods (2 to 6 days) — far longer than the usual cooking or baking procedures.

Effect of Deficiency in Man and Animals

Deficiency symptoms in man, produced experimentally in volunteers by use of a purified diet and a specific antagonist (see footnote, page 176), include fatigue, headache, sleep disturbances, personality changes, nausea, abdominal distress, numbness and tingling of hands and feet, muscle cramps, impaired coor-

*Pantothenic acid, before its structure was known, was called by several other names, now obsolete, including: filtrate factor, chick antidermatitis factor, factor 2, vitamin B-x, vitamin B-2, and vitamin B-3. Note that the term vitamin B-3, often used in current health food literature for niacin, has no historic significance and is incorrect. (See N. Engl. J. Med., *291*:263, 1974 and niacin section.)

†The D isomer of synthetic salts of pantothenate is the natural active form.

dination, and loss of antibody production.[30] All symptoms are cured by the administration of pantothenic acid. A well-defined deficiency of pantothenic acid has not been observed in man under natural conditions.

Pantothenic acid *deficiency in experimental animals* is readily obtained by using purified diets or natural diets heated over long periods to destroy this vitamin. Deficient chickens have a characteristic dermatitis of the mouth, eyes, and feet. These animals grow poorly, and if not given pantothenic acid, death results in 3 or 4 weeks (see Fig. 8–12). In other animals, a deficiency of pantothenic acid affects many tissues, and, in general, causes poor growth and faulty reproduction. It is of interest that graying of the hair is produced in deficient rats, monkeys, dogs, and foxes; color usually can be restored by added pantothenate in the diet. In humans, this relationship between pantothenic acid intake and graying of hair is not known. (Adding extra amounts of pantothenic acid to human diets does not change the color of gray hair.) In many species, degenerative changes are found in the nervous system and especially in the adrenal glands, which may become enlarged, reddened, and hemorrhagic. The role of pantothenic acid in the activity of the adrenals was found when it was shown to be part of a coenzyme, *coenzyme A*, needed for making certain hormones (cortisone and two related hormones) formed in the outer portion or cortex of these ductless glands. These hormones have important regulatory influences on metabolism and indeed are essential for life.

Biochemical Role of Pantothenic Acid

The *biochemical role* of pantothenic acid is involved primarily with coenzyme A,* one of the most important substances in body metabolism. As part of coenzyme A, pantothenic acid is essential for the intermediary metabolism of

*Coenzyme A, discovered in the 1940's, consists of a complicated molecule, *phosphopantetheine* (composed of pantothenic acid, a phosphate group, and reduced sulfur) plus two additional phosphate groups, a pentose, and adenine (a purine).

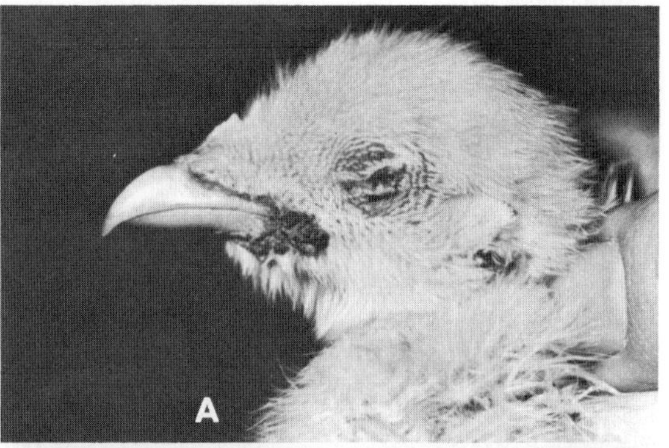

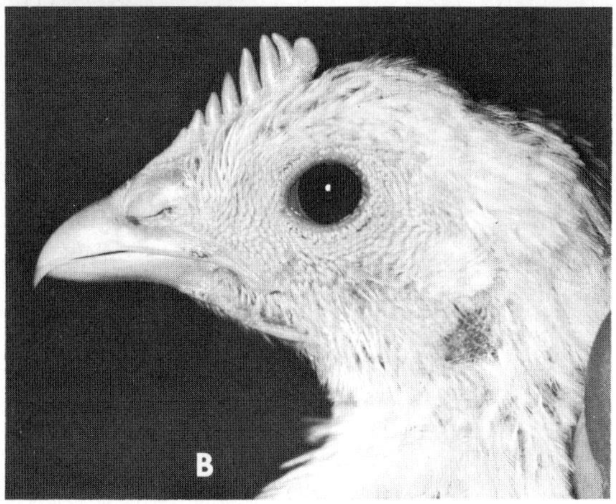

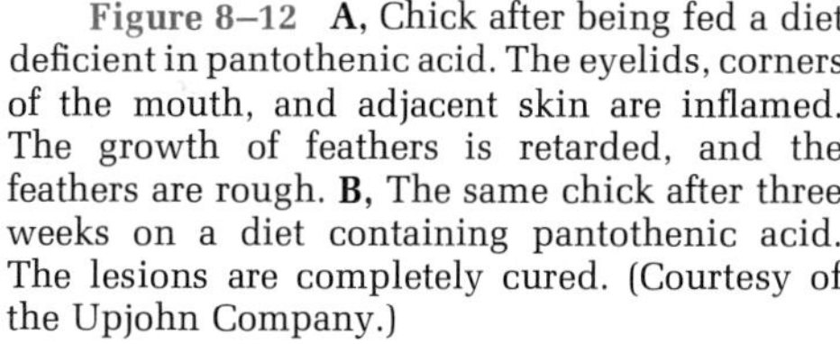
Figure 8–12 **A,** Chick after being fed a diet deficient in pantothenic acid. The eyelids, corners of the mouth, and adjacent skin are inflamed. The growth of feathers is retarded, and the feathers are rough. **B,** The same chick after three weeks on a diet containing pantothenic acid. The lesions are completely cured. (Courtesy of the Upjohn Company.)

carbohydrates, fats, and proteins, for their synthesis, breakdown, and release of energy. It functions primarily by effecting the removal or acceptance of important chemical groups with two, three, four, or more carbon atoms at a time. Coenzyme A is also needed for the formation of such important sterols as cholesterol and the adrenocortical hormones. It is also essential for the synthesis of acetylcholine, an important regulator of nerve tissue, and for making many other important compounds in the body.

Coenzyme A is essential for so many chemical reactions in the body, such as those necessary for energy release and for building many essential complicated compounds out of simpler ones, that pantothenic acid has been said to "sit at the crossroads of metabolism." The diagram found as Figure 15–3 illustrates its strategic position in metabolism.

Pantothenic acid functions also as a component of the enzyme *fatty acid synthetase* involved in fatty acid synthesis in the body. This enzyme contains the important unit *phosphopantetheine* (see footnote on page 181) but not the complete coenzyme A molecule.

In many of these reactions of pantothenic acid, the coenzymes of riboflavin, thiamin, biotin, niacin, and pyridoxal are also involved, as well as the minerals phosphorus, sulfur, magnesium, and manganese, showing again how vitamins and minerals are interrelated.

Requirement and Nutritional Status

A formal "recommended dietary allowance" for pantothenic acid has not been set by the Food and Nutrition Board.[7] However, they state that a "daily intake of 5 to 10 mg is probably adequate for all adults; the upper level is suggested for pregnant and lactating women." A daily intake of 5 to 7 mg by adults appears to be a satisfactory intake from available evidence in balance studies.[31] With such knowledge, and in the absence of enough data to make a recommended allowance, a provisional allowance can be based on normal intakes of a vitamin by a population without signs of deficiency.[7] An average level in "adequate" diets is probably about 7 mg per day and ranges normally between 5 and 20 mg.[7, 31, 32] Instances of intakes as low as 1.1 mg a day have been seen in 2 small samples of teen-age girls (Cohenour and Calloway[31]), a level that would be expected to result in a deficiency eventually, if continued. Human milk has about 2.2 mg of pantothenic acid per liter, so the daily infant requirement would be expected to be less than this. Cow's milk has about 3.4 mg per liter.*

Since processing of food can, in some instances, result in appreciable losses of pantothenic acid (see next section), it is possible that unrecognized borderline deficiencies may exist in human populations, such as in multiple nutritional deficiencies associated with lack of good food for any reason and with alcoholism.[7] Such deficiencies, if they exist, would occur only in connection with other deficiencies in man and would likely escape detection because of emphasis on other nutrients.

Deficiencies of pantothenic acid have been seen, though rarely, in farm animals (swine) fed "natural rations." As a result, synthetic pantothenic acid is often added to commercial swine rations. How a deficiency could develop under such conditions is not clear, but this points out the need for many more studies with this vitamin in human nutrition.

Food Sources and Effects of Processing

Pantothenic acid exists in all cells of living tissues and therefore is present in

*The U.S. RDA for pantothenic acid of 10 mg per day (Chapter 18) based on earlier values appears to be 50 percent or so higher than necessary, and is greater than the amount in average diets.

all natural foods, usually in combined forms. All foods in the four food groups contain pantothenic acid, but foods especially rich in it are yeast, liver, eggs, wheat and rice germ of bran, peanuts, and peas. Moderate to good amounts are contained in such foods as meat, milk, poultry, whole grains, broccoli, mushrooms, and sweet potatoes. Most vegetables and fruits and refined foods contain lesser amounts. White flour, precooked rice, and corn flakes are poor sources of the vitamin, and none is present, of course, in salad oils, shortening, sugar, and similar products. (See detailed values in Table 2 of the Appendix and in the references at the end of the chapter.) Processing and refinement of foods as well as milling of grains can result in considerable losses of pantothenic acid.[33]

Losses of up to 50 percent and even more may occur in processing and storage of frozen vegetables and meats. Similar losses occur in many canned food products.*

Synthetic calcium pantothenate is widely used today in vitamin supplements and to fortify a few breakfast foods, though usually only in trivial amounts. Its cost is about 10 cents per gram. It is not a toxic substance, but there is no reason to consume more than what is found in a good basic diet.

NIACIN

Niacin is a collective term including *nicotinic acid* and *nicotinamide,* both natural forms of the vitamin with niacin activity.

Discovery, and Pellagra

Not until 1937 was this substance established as a member of the group of B vitamins and identified as the long-sought *"pellagra-preventing factor."* The history of its discovery over a search period lasting over 20 years is as interesting as a detective story. Goldberger had demonstrated as early as 1915 that pellagra was directly due to faulty diet, and later that this disease could be prevented or its symptoms relieved by giving liver, yeast, lean meats, or other foods rich in B complex vitamins.[4, 34]

Pellagra had occurred in some parts of Europe for over 200 years, with special prevalence in areas where corn formed a large part of the diet. One of its most typical symptoms is a reddish skin rash, which later makes the skin dark and rough. This gave rise to the name of pellagra in 1771, from the Italian *pelle agra* meaning painful, or rough, skin.

Though a few early physicians were convinced that pellagra was caused by dietary deficiencies, the theory was advanced that it might be due to an infectious agent, or to some toxic substance present in corn, or developed in corn on spoilage. About 1907, pellagra became prevalent in the southern part of the United States, and cases increased in number so rapidly that in 1915 over 10,000 persons died of it. In 1917–1918 there were 200,000 cases of pellagra in this country — not limited to the South, but found throughout the whole country.

This was of great concern to the United States Public Health Service, which instituted special studies of the disease under the direction of Goldberger. At first, opinion was divided as to whether pellagra was due to poor sanitation or diet, but later, when Goldberger had induced the disease solely by feeding a "poor" diet to volunteer convicts and had prevented its incidence in various institutions by improvement of the diet, it was established as a dietary deficiency disease.* Although Goldberger proved

*The results of Schroeder[33] should be considered only preliminary, since the same food item was not used before and after processing.

*Goldberger proved in 1916 that pellagra was not an infectious disease when he and a group of 15 volunteers, in a heroic and crucial experiment, inoculated themselves with blood, swabbed their throats with saliva, and swallowed the excreta of patients severely ill with pellagra. Although some of the volunteers felt a bit squeamish, none became ill with pellagra afterward.[4]

that the preventive factor was a heat-stable substance present in yeast after thiamin had been destroyed by autoclaving, the exact nature of the substance remained a mystery until Elvehjem and coworkers, of the University of Wisconsin, showed in 1937 that blacktongue — an analogous disease in dogs — could be cured by giving nicotinic acid or the closely related nicotinic acid amide (nicotinamide), which they isolated from liver.[35] Administration of these substances was soon shown by several investigators to cure the most striking and characteristic symptoms of pellagra in humans.[36] Even before these discoveries, preventive dietary measures had been instituted in the southern states that resulted in marked decrease in pellagra incidence until, by 1945, acute cases were seldom seen.

Another chapter in the story of pellagra prevention was completed in 1945–1950 when it was discovered that the amino acid tryptophan was converted, in part, to nicotinic acid in the body of man and animals and that sufficient amounts could overcome pellagra in the absence of dietary nicotinic acid (see p. 188).

Chemical Identification and Properties

Nicotinic acid was originally discovered and named in 1867 by Huber (a German chemist). He made it by chemical treatment of nicotine — of the tobacco plant, from which it got its name.* It sat on laboratory shelves untested for many years while thousands of persons were dying from pellagra. No one knew then that there was a relationship, of course. Nicotinic acid and the related compound — nicotinamide — are white compounds, soluble in water and stable to both heating and oxidation, as well as to acids and alkalis. Little is lost in cooking unless the cooking water is discarded. Chemically, these nitrogen-containing compounds are among the simplest of the vitamins (see formulas in the Appendix); one contains an organic acid group (— COOH) and the other has an amino group (— NH_2) substituted in the acid group.

*Nicotine itself has no vitamin activity.

Nicotinic acid had been "rediscovered" many times as a compound present in foods and tissues even before its pellagra-preventive activity was known. For instance, both Funk in England and Suzuki in Japan isolated, and recognized, nicotinic acid from yeast and rice bran in 1912 during their search for the antiberiberi vitamin.[4] In 1935, workers in Germany made the important discovery that nicotinic acid is a part of certain coenzymes needed in energy metabolism.

Goldberger and his coworkers concentrated the active factor from yeast in their studies of dogs with *blacktongue*, or animal pellagra, and used the term "P-factor" (pellagra-preventive) for the substance in their concentrate. Both this term and the term vitamin B-5, once used for this vitamin, are now seldom used.*

The name *niacin* was adopted in 1971 by the American Institute of Nutrition and international agencies for all forms of the vitamin, and the term "niacin activity" for combined activity of nicotinic acid and its derivatives. The word "niacin" was originally coined in 1942 to be used as the popularized form of "nicotinic acid" with the idea of avoiding any possible implication that these normal nutrients are related in activity to nicotine, the alkaloid in tobac-

*Recently this vitamin has been called, wrongly, "vitamin B-3" in certain health food literature. There is no historic basis for this terminology, and its use is to be deplored.

In the early 1930's the name "vitamin B-4" was given to fractions in food found to produce growth activity in rats and chicks. Briggs and coworkers (J. Biol. Chem., 150:11, 1943) showed that vitamin B-4 — at least for chicks — was due to the amino acid content of the fractions. Hence today there is no substance called vitamin B-4, and vitamins B-3 and B-5 are of historic interest only.

co. The word niacin, however, now refers to the two forms of the vitamin. Niacin is present in foods or tissues in either free or combined forms.

Symptoms Due to Lack of Niacin

The tissues that show damage as a result of niacin deficiency are chiefly the skin, the gastrointestinal tract, and the nervous tissues.

The most striking and characteristic *symptoms of pellagra* include a reddish skin rash, especially on the face, hands, and feet when exposed to sunlight, which later makes the skin dark and rough (see Figs. 8–13 and 8–14). There is also a sore mouth and tongue, and inflamed membranes in the digestive tract, with bloody diarrhea in the later stages. There may also be distressing nervous and mental disturbances, such as irritability, anxiety, depression, and in advanced cases, delirium, hallucinations, confusion, disorientation, and stupor. Many mental institutions in this country had large numbers of such persons before the cure was discovered. Physicians sometimes referred to pellagra symptoms as "the three D's — dermatitis, diarrhea, and depression or dementia." Other general effects seen in pellagra are loss of weight, anemia (which may be associated with deficiencies of other B vitamins), and dehydration, from diarrhea. The skin rash always appears on both sides of the body at the same time — that is, it is *bilaterally symmetrical.*

Less acute symptoms of niacin deficiency may be difficult to recognize. Changes in the tongue are among the earliest signs of niacin lack and may be used to detect it. *Latent* or mild pellagra has been reported in infants and children in whom the usual pellagra symptoms were lacking; weakness and failure to grow properly, however, responded favorably to treatment with niacin.[37] Hence, we see that this vitamin is necessary for *growth* and for *health of tissues,* and it also promotes appetite, proper functioning of the digestive tract, and good utilization of foodstuffs in the body.

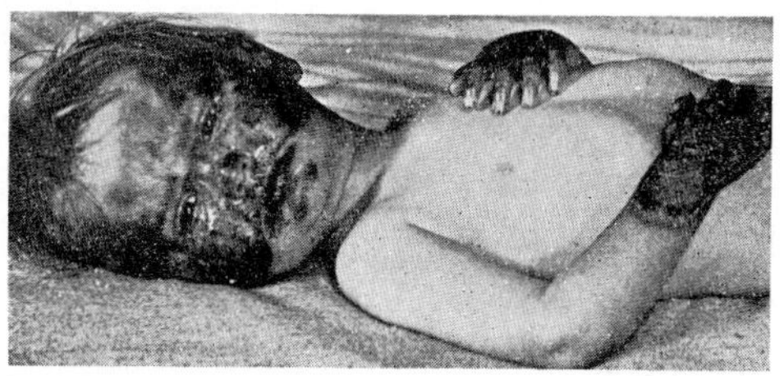

Figure 8–13 Pellagra in a child, showing typical red rash on face and hands. (Courtesy of Dr. John A. McIntosh.)

All experimental animals, except ruminants, need niacin or its equivalent in tryptophan. Deficiency symptoms are often similar to those seen in humans with pellagra, although any mental symptoms are absent or hard to detect. Dogs show a deep reddening or darkening of the tongue and mouth as well as skin rash, bloody diarrhea, wasting, and eventually death. Deficiencies have been produced in the rat, fowl, monkey, rabbit, cat, pig, guinea pig, fish, and many other monogastric animals.

The Pellagra Problem

The wide occurrence, and subsequent conquest, of pellagra in the southern United States affords an interesting example of the relation of nutritional welfare to economic conditions, and also of a dietary deficiency disease that is not due to simple deficiency of one vitamin. The South was a "one crop" region, depending almost entirely on cultivation of cotton and its manufacture into cloth. The cash income of ordinary people was low, especially around the turn of the century, so that they often ate the cheapest foods obtainable and became habituated to a poor diet. Many poor sharecroppers and mill hands lived almost exclusively on corn meal and grits, soda biscuits, corn syrup or molasses, and fatty salt pork — a diet that is deficient

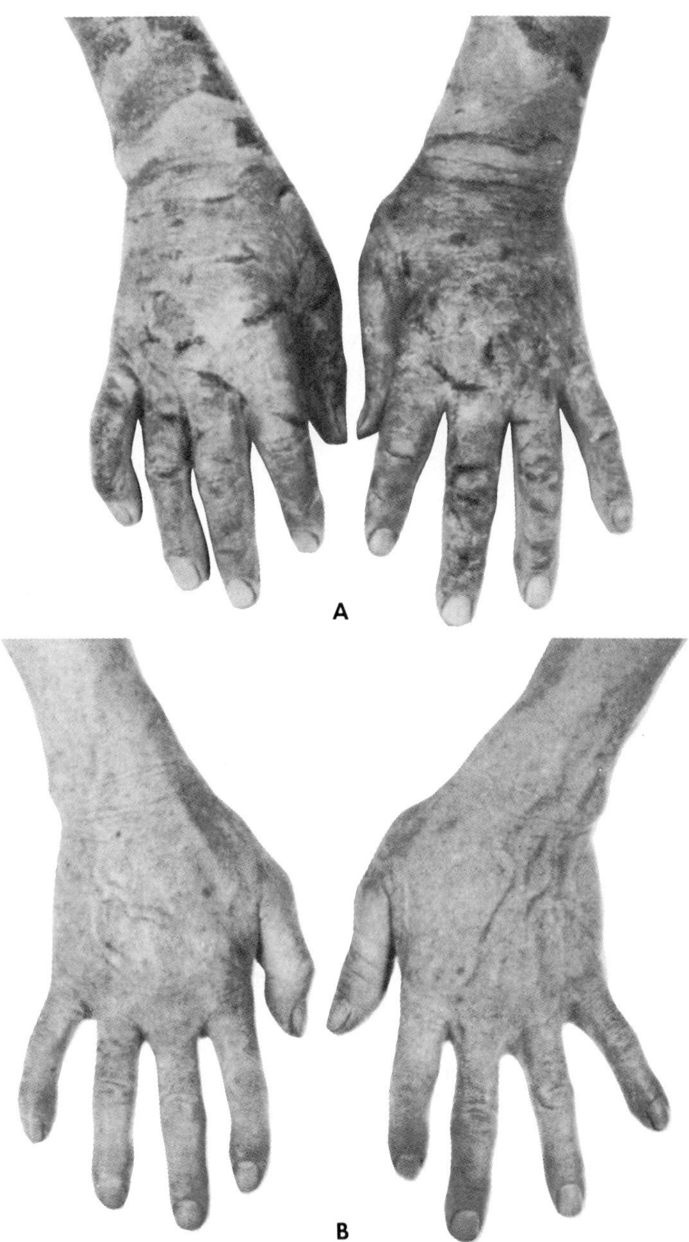

Figure 8–14 Cure of pellagrous lesions on hands of an adult by a diet rich in B vitamins, especially niacin. **A,** Hands of pellagra patient. **B,** Same patient after 2 weeks of corrective diet. (From Spies: *Rehabilitation Through Better Nutrition.* Philadelphia, W. B. Saunders, 1947.)

both as to quality and quantity of protein and in its content of several vitamins and minerals. When pellagra developed because of such diets, although most of the symptoms were due to lack of niacin, the disease was complicated by lack of other B complex vitamins, especially thiamin and riboflavin. Not only the corn products, but any flour and rice used, were degerminated and highly milled; most of the natural content of thiamin, riboflavin, and niacin was removed with the germ and outer coats of the grains. There was almost no lean meat, milk, or eggs to contribute high-quality protein and B vitamins. Riboflavin deficiency is so often associated with niacin deficiency in such diets that it is said to have a bearing on the occurrence and persistence of pellagra. Pellagra is now considered to be a complex dietary deficiency, the major symptoms of which are due to niacin deficiency. Its complete cure requires all-around improvement of the diet, especially of its protein content and intake of all the B complex vitamins (see discussion on tryptophan and its relation to pellagra, page 188).

The campaign to stamp out pellagra thus centered on introducing into the diet certain foods established as effective in preventing the disease. Lean meats, milk, eggs, canned salmon, peanuts, peas, and vegetables were shown to be good foods to add to the diet for preventing pellagra.[38] At the same time, Wheeler and Sebrell commented,[39] "In looking for cases of pellagra, the home surrounded by evidence of good garden, or a cow or two, a few pigs and some poultry may as well be passed up, for the chances are less than one in a thousand that pellagra will be found. On the other hand, the home surrounded only by last year's cotton patch will always bear watching."

Because many families did not have money to buy the needed foods, the campaign was centered on urging them to make home gardens, and to keep a cow and some chickens. In some areas, the Red Cross would lend the family a cow until the health, and with it the earning power, of the people improved sufficiently to enable them to buy the animal. While the educational campaign went on, public health authorities in some states supplied free dried brewer's yeast, which has a higher content of niacin and most other B vitamins than any other food.

The success of this education program was demonstrated by a dietary survey[40] made in two adjacent communities in the Kentucky mountains, one of which had a high incidence of pellagra while the other had almost none. Corn products were eaten in about the same amounts in both districts, but the people in the one which had been freed from pellagra had been influenced by the Frontier Nursing Service to understand the importance of certain foods for health so that they had planted gardens and were keeping cows and chickens.

This campaign to educate the people in change of food habits and increase income levels to make possible the purchase of needed foods was gradually successful. There was a decrease in mortality from pellagra in southern states from 22.4 to 5.1 per 100,000 between 1929 and 1940.[41] Since the discovery of the benefits of treatment with niacin, physicians today seldom see a person with pellagra in this country. However, much remains to be done toward permanent improvement of the nutritive qualities of the diet in socially deprived populations in order to avoid low-grade niacin deficiency and to promote health by making the diet otherwise adequate.

Niacin's Role in the Body

The chief function of niacin in the body is to form the active portion of *coenzymes that play an essential role in tissue oxidations (hydrogen transport)*, and it thus is necessary for the health of all tissue cells. Nicotinamide, in both free and combined form, is carried in the blood and found in all tissues, but most richly in liver, kidney, heart, brain, and muscles.

Niacin's biochemical role revolves around its presence in two important coenzymes essential to all life. These two coenzymes (named from their initials, NAD and NADP*), are known collectively as the *pyridine nucleotides*, and they play several different roles in cellular metabolism. Their most important function is to help bring about the action of enzymes

*NAD, or nicotinamide adenine dinucleotide, was the first coenzyme ever identified (in 1935). It formerly was called "coenzyme I" or "cozymase," and later DPN (for diphosphopyridine nucleotide), terms now obsolete. It contains nicotinamide (a pyridine), two ribose groups, two phosphate groups, and adenine (a purine).

NADP, or nicotinamide adenine dinucleotide phosphate, is similar to NAD but contains an extra phosphate. It formerly was called "coenzyme II" or TPN. These two coenzymes are called NADH and NADPH when they are in the reduced form.

known as *dehydrogenases,* which are essential in the course of oxidation-reduction reactions. For instance, the enzyme *lactic dehydrogenase* in tissues oxidizes lactic acid to pyruvic acid only in the presence of NAD. A second function of the pyridine nucleotides, when in the reduced form, concerns the reduction of riboflavin-containing coenzymes and enzymes. In these reactions, hydrogen is passed along the reduced pyridine nucelotides to a riboflavin-containing coenzyme and then to the cytochromes and eventually to oxygen, with the formation of water. Lack of niacin to form these coenzymes in sufficient quantities handicaps vital chemical processes and may result in injury to tissues throughout the body.

Biosynthesis of Niacin; Role of Tryptophan

Study of the metabolism of niacin and the amounts that should be furnished in the diet is complicated by two facts — it can be synthesized by bacteria in the intestinal flora, and it can be made in the tissues from the amino acid tryptophan. We know that many bacteria can synthesize this and other B vitamins. Because some diets are more favorable for this synthesis than others (a vegetable diet is more favorable for synthesis than some meat diets, for example), the variability of the amounts synthesized may sometimes determine whether or not pellagra occurs when the diet contains borderline quantities of niacin and tryptophan.

Tryptophan has a sparing action on the amount of niacin necessary because it acts as a precursor substance from which niacin can be formed in the body. This was first demonstrated in experiments with rats that were fed diets high in corn and low in niacin by Krehl and his coworkers in 1945.[42] They found that feeding either niacin *or tryptophan* overcame the deficiency. Soon after this discovery, it was shown that man could substitute tryptophan for niacin at a ratio of about 60 parts of tryptophan to one part of niacin.[43] If sufficient tryptophan is eaten (amounts generally higher than in average diets), niacin itself is no longer essential in the diet — all the niacin required would then be made within the body. The pathway of the conversion of tryptophan to niacin in tissues of the body has been worked out, involving a number of biochemical steps.

It had been known for many years that eating diets high in corn (maize) increased the incidence of pellagra in man, but the reason for this was a puzzle to nutritionists. Many persons believed that corn might contain a toxic factor, but following the discovery that tryptophan was an effective substitute for niacin, it was soon discovered by means of animal studies that the simultaneous presence of three conditions was responsible for the detrimental effect of corn: (1) the low amount of available niacin, (2) the low amount of tryptophan, and (3) a dietary imbalance caused by the presence of relatively large amounts of other amino acids in proportion to tryptophan in corn.[44] Other foods low and unbalanced in respect to tryptophan, such as gelatin, give the same effect as corn when fed to experimental animals, as do various mixtures of amino acids devoid of tryptophan. *All three conditions must be present at once to produce pellagra.* The relatively low content of both niacin and tryptophan in corn, as compared to that in wheat, is shown in Table 8–5.

The fact that the body can form niacin from tryptophan also explains why some foods, such as milk and eggs, have far greater pellagra-preventing potency than would be expected from their actual content of niacin.* Such foods are low in niacin but carry proteins that are high in the amino acid tryptophan, thus furnishing the body with protection from pellagra by enabling it to build niacin within the tissues.

---

*Goldberger and other early workers studying pellagra were puzzled many times by this observation. Between 1915 and 1920, Goldberger concluded that certain protein-rich foods low in the "P-P factor" could cure patients with pellagra, and at one time he obtained relief of symptoms by feeding them tryptophan. This work was not followed up, however, when it was found that yeast and liver extracts very low in protein were even more effective.

Table 8–5 RELATIVE AMOUNT OF TRYPTOPHAN AND NIACIN IN CORN AND WHEAT

	Niacin	*Tryptophan*
Whole wheat, per 100 gm	4.3 mg	168 mg
Whole corn, per 100 gm	2.0 gm	55 mg

Niacin Equivalents

It should be evident from the foregoing discussion that the actual *requirement* for niacin varies with the nature of the diet — mainly whether the protein furnishes much or little tryptophan. Allowances are now given in terms of *niacin equivalents* — dietary sources of niacin plus its precursor, tryptophan. Approximately 1 mg of niacin may be expected to be formed for each 60 mg of tryptophan in the diet.*[43] A food that provides a large amount of tryptophan may be an excellent source of niacin equivalents even though its preformed niacin content is not high. A quart of milk daily, for instance, suffices to prevent pellagra, although its content of niacin is relatively low. Its high content of tryptophan may be counted on to furnish additional niacin in the body, which must be added in calculating its "niacin equivalence," as shown in Figure 8–15 [7, 43]

Niacin equivalents of foods, then, can be calculated from food composition tables that give both the niacin and the tryptophan content of foods. In the absence of information on the tryptophan content of foods, one can estimate that most proteins of animal origin, such as milk, eggs, and meat contain about 1.4 percent of tryptophan and most proteins of vegetable origin (cereals and legumes) about 1 percent.[7]

*Thus, one niacin equivalent is defined as 1 mg of niacin or 60 mg of tryptophan (or combinations thereof).

Requirement and Nutritional Status

Recommended allowances for niacin equivalents have been established by the United States Food and Nutrition Board. A college-age woman has an allowance of 14 mg per day of niacin equivalents, and a college-age man 20 mg per day.[7] The allowances decrease somewhat with age because of decreased energy needs. See Table 8–6 for more details on allowances.

The amounts shown in Table 8–6 are approximately 50 percent greater than the minimum requirement — about 10 to 12 mg of niacin equivalents per day. They are based primarily on the energy requirement of an average individual, as is thiamin and riboflavin, because of their essential role in energy formation from carbohydrates and fats. The Food and Nutrition Board has recommended a value of 6.6 mg of niacin equivalent per 1000 kcal (4200 kJ). Even if less than 2000 kcal is consumed per day, the Board states that adults have an allowance of 13 mg per day.[7]

Most diets consumed in the United States supply from 500 to 1000 mg or more of tryptophan daily and 8 to 17 mg of preformed niacin for a total of 16 to 33 mg of niacin equivalents per day, according to the Food and Nutrition Board.[7] The *average* intake, therefore is higher than the recommended allowance, even though it appears that individual diets might be borderline in their content of niacin equivalents. Clinical signs and biochemical and dietary evidence of low niacin intakes are

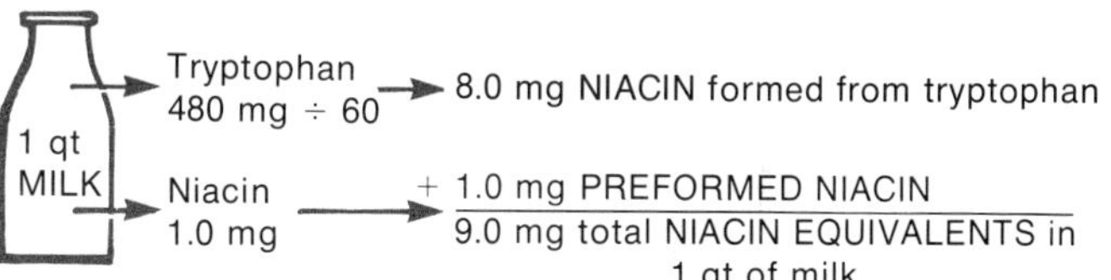

Figure 8–15 Calculating the niacin equivalents in a quart of milk. To the niacin that is carried as such in the milk (1.0 mg per quart) is added the amount that may be expected to be formed in the body from its tryptophan content (480 mg per quart). Assuming that approximately 1 mg of niacin is formed for each 60 mg of tryptophan (480 ÷ 60), 8 mg of niacin might be expected to arise from the tryptophan content of the milk, bringing the total niacin equivalents of a quart of milk up to 9.0 mg.

Table 8–6 RECOMMENDED ALLOWANCES FOR NIACIN EQUIVALENTS*

	Age	Allowance, mg/day
Males	11–14 years	18
	15–22 years	20
	23–50 years	18
	51 years and over	16
Females	11–14 years	16
	15–22 years	14
	23 years and over	13
	Pregnant	+2
	Lactating	+4

*From the Food and Nutrition Board, 1974.[7]

See Appendix Table 1C and 10 for recommendations of other countries and U.N. agencies.

seen in significant numbers of persons in the United States, especially in certain low-income aged groups, where the incidence may be as high as 10 percent or more.[10-13]

Pellagra itself is seldom seen in the United States today. Pellagra may still be seen fairly commonly in certain countries where corn (maize) is a major part of the diet. However, in parts of Latin America and Mexico, where many persons eat large amounts of corn as one of their principal sources of energy, pellagra is seldom seen. This is because it is their common practice to soak the corn in lime, a practice which makes the niacin in corn more available to the body.

Niacin and Niacin Equivalents in Foods

Because niacin can be formed in the body if tryptophan is furnished, the amount of preformed niacin in foods that compose the diet, as has been explained, is not necessarily a measure of the total quantity of this vitamin available to the body. Of greater practical importance are figures showing the niacin equivalents of food (see Table 8–7). It should not be difficult to secure the recommended amounts of niacin equivalents from diets such as are advised for meeting other nutritive requirements.

As for sources of the vitamin forms themselves, in general, animal products contain the vitamin as nicotinamide,

Table 8–7 NIACIN EQUIVALENTS OF SOME REPRESENTATIVE FOODS* (TOTAL NIACIN ACTIVITY PLUS MG TRYPTOPHAN ÷ 60)

Food	Niacin Equivalent mg/100 gm	Food	Niacin Equivalent mg/100 gm
Almond	6.4	Lamb	8.2
Apple	0.2	Milk, cow's, pasteurized	0.9
Asparagus	1.9	Milk, human	0.5
Banana	0.9	Parsley	2.4
Bean, lima	4.7	Pork	5.4
Beef	7.3	Rice, brown	6.3
Beet root	0.7	Rice, milled, parboiled	4.9
Brussels sprouts	1.9	Sesame seed	10.2
Carrot	0.7	Soybean	11.1
Cashew nut	8.1	Spinach	1.2
Cauliflower	1.3	Sunflower seed	8.8
Chicken	10.9	Sweet potato	1.0
Chickpea	4.9	Wheat germ	8.6
Corn, sweet	2.1	Wheat, whole	6.7
Egg, whole	3.2	Yeast, brewer's	45.0
Fish, trout	11.5		

*Calculated from niacin values in Watt, B. K., and Merrill, A. L.,[14] and tryptophan values in FAO: *Amino-Acid Content of Foods and Biological Data on Proteins*, Rome, 1970, and Orr, M. L., and Watt, B. K.: *Amino-Acid Content of Foods*, Washington, D.C., U.S. Department of Agriculture, 1957. Based on fresh, raw, edible portion. Also see ref. 43 (Horwitt) and Paul, A. A.: Nutrition, *23*:131, 1969, and recent food composition tables for additional values.

while in plant products most of it is present as nicotinic acid. Values of niacin activity in foods, as in Table 2 of the Appendix, are of interest in indicating what types of foods are relatively rich in ths vitamin, though such values do not include tryptophan. Foods that are good sources of most other B vitamins, in general, are also high in niacin content — namely liver, lean meats, whole grains, nuts, yeast, and legumes. However, eggs, milk, and cheese are relatively low in niacin (though a good source of tryptophan), while leafy vegetables are not much higher than other vegetables in niacin.

There is very little destruction of niacin in ordinary cooking methods, so figures for cooked foods are omitted.

As with most other vitamins, the most inexpensive source of the vitamin is the synthetic form itself — although, as pointed out elsewhere, persons should depend on traditional foods as their source of nutrients and not on pure compounds, at least for routine purposes. Nicotinic acid is available in wholesale quantities at a price of only about 1 cent per gm, sufficient to supply 25 percent of the daily allowance for one person for 100 days. Obviously, the cost of enrichment of foods with niacin is negligible. The once dreaded pellagra, as a worldwide disease, should be a thing of the past, wherever corn is a basic food.

Toxicity of Niacin

One could eat 30 times the RDA of niacin without the appearance of toxic symptoms. Nicotinic acid, though not the amide form, acts as a drug when taken in large amounts — 2 to 3 gm per day — resulting in vascular dilation or "flushing" of the skin or even a red rash. The compound is often prescribed by physicians for cardiovascular diseases and for treatment of other clinical symptoms, though its value for these purposes is in doubt. High doses should not be used without the advice of a physician.

VITAMIN B-6

More research has been done on vitamin B-6 the past few years than most any other vitamin. Its story is an interesting one.

Identification and Properties

The jigsaw puzzle of the B complex was partially solved by György in 1934, who found that an unidentified substance, to which he gave the name *vitamin B-6*, was necessary in the diet of rats for growth and for prevention of a particular type of skin disorder.[45] This disorder, later called "rat acrodynia," had been described earlier, in 1930, by two British nutritionists, Chick and Copping.[46] Many workers were trying to identify the active compound,* though there was much confusion with the then unknown pellagra-preventive factor (niacin) and other water-soluble growth factors. By 1934 there was evidence for at least five B complex vitamins, none of which had been chemically identified — hence the jigsaw puzzle analogy. As thiamin, riboflavin, pantothenic acid, and niacin were identified, in turn, the solution became possible later.

Biochemists in five different laboratories independently isolated crystals of vitamin B-6 in 1938, using the rat for the biological test, but credit for obtaining the first crystals is widely given to Lepkovsky of the University of California.[47] Vitamin B-6 was synthesized in 1939 by workers in the United States, Germany, and Japan, and it was made freely available to nutritionists, thus making it much easier for the rest of the B complex jigsaw to be assembled within the next few years.

The widely accepted name *pyridoxine*† was suggested in 1939 by György and Eckardt for the first pure substance known

*Also called in the early years Factor Y, rat antidermatitis vitamin; Factor 1, and adermin.

†The name "pyridoxine" was chosen because the compound had a pyridine ring (five carbon and one nitrogen) and three hydroxyl groups.

to have vitamin B-6 activity.[48] Several years later Snell discovered the vitamin B-6 activity of two closely related substances in natural products, which he termed *pyridoxal* and *pyridoxamine*.[49] All three compounds are white solids and have about equal activity when fed to laboratory animals. The pyridoxal and pyridoxamine forms occur mainly in animal products, whereas pyridoxine is found largely in products of vegetable origin (see Appendix for structural formulas of these compounds).

Pyridoxine is much more stable to heat than the other two compounds, but they are all unusually stable to acid and alkali. All three forms may be rapidly destroyed by exposure to light, especially in neutral or alkaline solutions. Pyridoxamine and pyridoxal are considered quite labile compounds when in dilute solutions, being rapidly destroyed by exposure to air and heat. The cooking or processing of foods, especially that from animal sources, may destroy up to 50 percent of their vitamin B-6 activity.[50, 51]

Effect of Vitamin B-6 Deficiency

The question of whether this vitamin is essential for humans was settled in a rather dramatic way. In 1951, babies 6 weeks to 6 months old in various parts of the United States, fed solely on a commercial infant food, suddenly began to develop irritability, muscular twitchings, and convulsions. Those babies who were fed the company's canned liquid product became seriously ill, while others fed a similar formula sold in dry, powdered form were not ill. Kline, then of the United States Food and Drug Administration, recognizing the similarity of these convulsive seizures to those seen in young rats deprived of vitamin B-6, suggested the infants might be ill because of lack of this vitamin. When vitamin B-6 was given to the affected babies, they promptly recovered. The heat used to sterilize the liquid product in cans had been high enough to destroy most of the vitamin B-6, a fact no one had noticed or would have thought important, if known. Because of the proved need for this vitamin in infants' diets,[51] this company and other manufacturers of infant foods take special precautions to make sure that it is present.

Symptoms of vitamin B-6 deficiency in man are similar in some respects to those seen in niacin and riboflavin deficiency.[7, 51-53] In addition to a diet low in this vitamin, an antagonist (see footnote, page 176), deoxypyridoxine, is often used in experiments to develop early deficiency symptoms. A common symptom is a greasy (seborrheic) dermatitis around the eyes, in the eyebrows, and at the angles of the mouth, along with soreness of the mouth and a smooth, red tongue. An early symptom of deficiency is the excretion in the urine of large amounts of *xanthurenic acid*, an abnormal tryptophan derivative, which turns green in the presence of iron salts. Later symptoms include dizziness, nausea, vomiting, weight loss, irritability and confusion, anemia, kidney stones, and severe nervous disturbances including convulsions. All these symptoms, except kidney stones, can be corrected within several days, even within a few minutes for some symptoms, by administering vitamin B-6.

Deficiency signs in animals are similar to those seen in humans, except that the same symptoms do not occur in all species. All species need vitamin B-6 for growth. Deficient *rats* show weight loss, *acrodynia* (a dermatitis affecting the feet, ears, tail, and nose), muscular weakness, edema, peripheral neuritis, and in advanced stages, convulsions. *Dogs* and *pigs* show no skin lesions but develop anemia and later convulsions, with marked changes in nervous tissue seen at autopsy. Deficiency in *fowl* can be obtained in only 4 or 5 days, resulting in poor growth and eventually anemia, decreased clotting time, and convulsions. *Calves* show listlessness, lack of appetite, poor hair coat, and convulsions. Most farm animals are normally protected against vitamin B-6 deficiency by the high content of this vitamin in their natural feed. Cattle and sheep obtain sufficient vitamin B-6 by microbial synthesis in the rumen to avert any such deficiency.

Role of Vitamin B-6 in the Body

The three forms of vitamin B-6 are quite stable in the intestinal tract and are readily absorbed in the upper intestine. Once absorbed, all three forms are converted to *pyridoxal phosphate* — the coenzyme form — which has many important roles in metabolism, particularly in protein and amino acid metabolism. Interestingly, one of the many specific functions of pyridoxal phosphate is as a catalyst in the formation in the body of niacin from tryptophan. Vitamin B-6-deficient animals are unable to do this, which may partially explain why symptoms of vitamin B-6 deficiency in man are similar to those seen in pellagra.

Pyridoxal phosphate is essential for several highly important reactions in the body concerned with amino acid metabolism. The most important of these reactions involving pyridoxal phosphate (and, to some extent, pyridoxamine phosphate) are known as *transamination* and *decarboxylation*. Transamination is the shifting of an amino group (NH_2) from a donor amino acid to an acceptor acid to form another amino acid. By this type of reaction, the building of certain amino acids from nonnitrogen-carrying acids formed in metabolism is made possible.

Decarboxylation is the removal of carbon dioxide (CO_2) from an amino acid. It is necessary for the formation in the body of at least three vital physiological regulators (hormones or similar compounds) from the amino acids, histidine, tryptophan, and tyrosine, as well as for the oxidation of amino acids for energy. Pyridoxal phosphate also catalyzes the removal of SH groups from sulfur-containing amino acids.

As many as 50 specific reactions of amino acids requiring pyridoxal phosphate as a coenzyme have been discovered. It is a part of the enzyme essential in the body for the breakdown of glycogen to glucose (glycogen phosphorylase). In fact, about half the vitamin B-6 in the body is accounted for by its presence in phosphorylases of muscle, which probably explains the low blood glucose seen in deficient experimental animals. Vitamin B-6 may in some way be necessary in metabolism of polyunsaturated fatty acids, for conversion of linoleic acid to arachidonic acid. Judging by the frequency of anemia and severe nervous symptoms in deficiencies, it is clearly involved in red cell regeneration and normal functioning of nervous tissues. The concentration of vitamin B-6 in the brain of mammals is much higher than blood levels — up to 25 to 50 times higher, indicative of many vital functions.

Vitamin B-6–deficient animals show impaired antibody responses. Thus, it must be needed by man for protection against various infections and diseases, although this remains unproved.

Requirement and Nutritional Status

Many studies are now under way to determine the vitamin B-6 requirements with more assurance on the basis of available evidence. The latest available recommended dietary allowance for females aged 15 years and older is 2.0 mg per day with increased amounts during pregnancy and lactation. For male adults the recommended amount is also 2.0 mg per day. See Table 8–8 for a summary of vitamin B-6 recommendations and Table 1 in the Appendix for more details. These allowances for adults are based on an increased need for vitamin B-6 with increased intakes of protein.[7] The allowances for this vitamin suggested by the Canadian Dietary Standard Committee in 1975 are based specifically on a recommendation of a vitamin B-6 intake of 0.02 mg per gram of protein intake for adults.[54] The Canadian allowances are similar to the United States values, though lower for females (1.5 mg per day).

There is no one approved method of measuring the vitamin B-6 deficiency status of an individual or a population.

Table 8–8 RECOMMENDED ALLOWANCES FOR VITAMIN B-6*

	Age	*Allowance, mg/day*
Males	11–14 years	1.6
	15 years and over	2.0
Females	11–14 years	1.6
	15 years and over	2.0
	Pregnant	2.5
	Lactating	2.5

*From the Food and Nutrition Board, 1974.[7]

Dietary intake studies and the occurrence of symptoms, alone, are not reliable. Current biochemical methods being studied include measurements of pyridoxal phosphate levels in blood, red blood cell *transaminase,* or urinary levels of vitamin B-6 and of the levels of metabolites of vitamin B-6 or tryptophan.

There is a concern, as well as ever-increasing evidence, that in more than a few instances our normal diets may be borderline or low in this vitamin.[7, 10, 32] Unfortunately, too few studies have been made on the possible occurrence of vitamin B-6 deficiency in normal persons eating commonly available foods. There is good information showing lower body stores and generally increased needs of this vitamin in pregnancy and lactation, in the elderly, in alcoholics, in various pathologic and genetic disturbances, and in persons receiving high-protein diets or certain common drugs such as isoniazid, penicillamine, and oral contraceptives and other steroids.[7] When there is an increased need, it must be met by a source of vitamin B-6 in some form — often more than the amounts readily available in usual diets — unless foods are enriched with this vitamin or unless they are selected with considerable care.

According to U.S.D.A. figures[9] the overall average per capita availability of vitamin B-6 per day in 1977 was only about 2.3 mg, not including waste or cooking losses. Figure 8–16 shows the percentage contribution of various food groups to this total. Diets of foods commonly available in the United States can be devised with as little as 0.4 to 0.5 mg per day, well below the requirement. In fact, Cheslock and McCully[55] saw signs of vitamin B-6 deficiency in humans fed experimental diets containing cereal products, fruits, milk, vegetables, and other vitamin B-6–low foods (many of which had been highly processed). The actual intake of vitamin B-6 by adults in the United States varies considerably, of course, but ranges somewhere between 0.7 mg to 1.5 mg in poor diets and up to 2 or 3 mg or more in most diets.[7, 32] Many studies show considerable numbers of persons of all ages with low intakes of vitamin B-6 and with biochemical signs of deficiency, not only in the United States but in many other countries as well.[7, 53] (Also see the readings at the end of this chapter.)

Food Sources of Vitamin B-6

The occurrence of vitamin B-6 in foods follows the general distribution of most of the other B vitamins. The best sources are meats — especially liver — some vegetables — including potatoes — wheat germ, wheat bran, and whole grain cereals (Table 8–9; see Table 2 of the Appendix for more details). All these values are given in terms of total vitamin B-6 activity, combining the three naturally occurring forms of the vitamin. For details of the individual distribution in foods of the three forms, pyridoxine, pyridoxal, and pyridoxamine, see Table 2 of Orr.[33] All forms have about equal activity when eaten, so for practical purposes total values provide sufficient information.

In the milling of white flour, more than 75 percent of the vitamin B-6 content of wheat is lost; it is not added in white flour enrichment programs. There are good arguments that this should be done since synthetic pyridoxine is quite inexpensive — about 15 cents a gram.

Sugar and fat, of course, are devoid of this vitamin, as they are of most other vitamins (though they supply over one-third of the energy intake of the average American). Processed or refined foods are generally much lower in vitamin B-6 than the original food, often less than half.[33] Flour, white bread, precooked rice, noodles, macaroni, and spaghetti are quite low in vitamin B-6, and a diet composed solely of these or similar foods would eventually cause a vitamin B-6 deficiency, along with deficiencies of many other nutrients.

It should be obvious that vitamin B-6 is not one of the "lesser vitamins" in terms of its food distribution and its importance to good health. Not only must one choose his food with at least some degree of nutri-

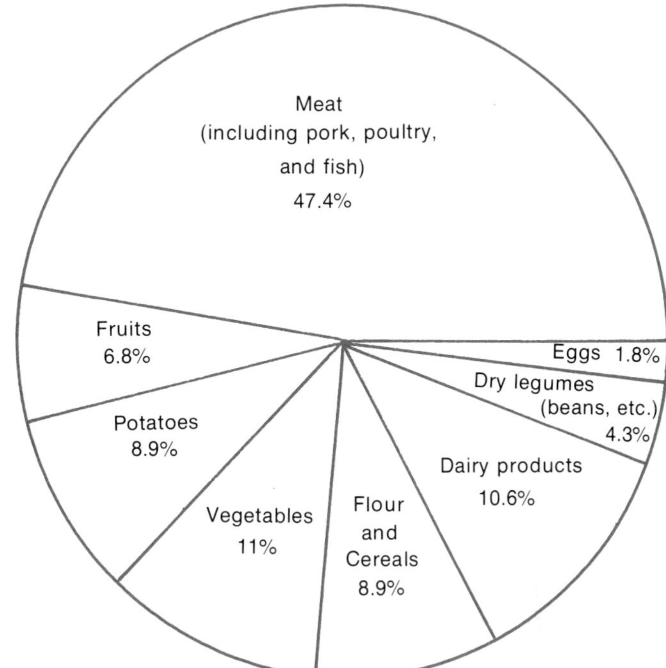

Figure 8–16 Contributions of major food groups to vitamin B-6 supplies. (United States figures for 1977.[9] This includes the amounts supplied by enriched cereals. It does not include 0.3 percent from miscellaneous sources. The total amount available is 2.29 mg per capita per day, before processing and cooking.)

Table 8–9 EXAMPLES OF GOOD FOOD SOURCES OF VITAMIN B-6*

Food Source	*Vitamin B-6 Activity in mg/100 gm (Edible Portion)*	*Food Source*	*Vitamin B-6 Activity in mg/100 gm (Edible Portion)*
Avocados, raw	0.42	Rice, brown, raw	0.55
Bananas, raw	0.51	Salmon steak, raw	0.70
Beans, white, raw	0.56	Soybeans, raw	0.81
Beans, lima, raw	0.58	Spinach, raw	0.28
Beef, raw, lean	0.44	Sunflower seed	1.25
Chicken		Sweet potatoes, raw	0.22
Dark meat	0.32	Trout, raw	0.69
Light meat	0.68	Tuna	
Chickpeas, raw	0.54	Raw	0.90
Cottonseed flour	0.98	Canned	0.42
Crab, cooked or canned	0.30	Turnip greens, raw	0.26
Filberts, shelled	0.54	Veal, raw	0.34
Halibut, raw	0.43	Walnuts	0.73
Kale, raw	0.30	Whole wheat flour	0.34
Liver		Wheat breakfast cereals	
Beef, raw	0.84	Bran, 100 percent	0.82
Chicken, raw	0.75	Germ, toasted	1.15
Peanuts, roasted, shelled	0.40	Shredded	0.24
Pepper, green, raw	0.26	Yeast	
Pork, raw, boned	0.32	Baker's, dry, inactive	2.00
Prunes, dried	0.24	Brewer's, debittered	2.50
Raisins, golden seedless	0.35	Torula	3.00

*Adapted from Orr, M. L., 1969.[33]

tional knowledge in order to have a sufficient amount, but well-planned food enrichment programs with vitamin B-6 will, no doubt, also prove to be useful.

BIOTIN

Symptoms of biotin lack are seldom seen in humans, though deficiencies can, and do, exist. Biotin is just as vital as any other vitamin to body tissues, since they cannot synthesize it. Because, for practical purposes, there is no need to concern one's self about eating greater amounts of biotin than found in normal diets, we will discuss only a few facts about this interesting B vitamin.

Discovery and Properties

Biotin, like pantothenic acid, was known to be a growth factor for yeast before its vitamin nature was discovered. The compound was crystallized in 1936 by Kögl and Tönnis of Germany and given the name "biotin," since it was part of the "bios" factor needed for yeast growth. Its vitamin nature for animals was discovered by György* in 1940.[56] He had previously called it vitamin H — a term no longer used. Another early name was the "anti-egg white injury factor." Biotin was synthesized and its structure determined in 1942 (see Appendix for its formula). It is a white substance and contains sulfur in the molecule as does thiamin. It is quite stable to heat in cooking, processing, and storage.

Producing Biotin Deficiency

A biotin deficiency can be produced in many animal species merely by leaving biotin out of the experimental diet. In rats and monkeys, in which there is a higher degree of intestinal synthesis of biotin, a deficiency can be induced by giving an antibiotic or a sulfa drug or by raising the animal in "germ-free" conditions. These procedures reduce, or eliminate, intestinal microorganisms that produce biotin, similar to the vitamin K story.

In all mammals, including man, the addition of 15 to 30 percent, or more, of raw, dried egg white to a biotin-low diet will induce symptoms of biotin deficiency. This action has been accounted for by discovery in raw egg white of a special protein called *avidin,* which combines with biotin in the intestinal tract, thus rendering the biotin unabsorbable. This so-called "egg white injury" can be overcome by ingesting sufficient biotin, though it takes more than that present in an equivalent number of egg yolks. Cooking egg white, even briefly, destroys the biotin-binding action of avidin.

Effect of Biotin Deficiency and Role in the Body

The fact that biotin is a dietary essential for man was shown in 1942 by use of a diet low in biotin supplemented with dried, uncooked egg white.[57] This resulted in pathologic changes in the skin and tongue, loss of appetite, nausea and a low-grade anemia, lassitude, intense depression, sleeplessness, and muscle pain. Injections of biotin brought marked improvement of symptoms in 3 to 4 days.

Biotin deficiency in animals has been quite widely studied with the use of experimental diets. Deficient rats grow poorly and develop a general dermatitis, muscular incoordination, and hair loss, which occurs, first, around the eye, giving rise to a typical *spectacle-eye* condition (see Fig. 8–17). Deficient fowl develop dermatitis first on the feet, extending to the beak and eyes. Eventually they become weak, show poor growth, and die. In monkeys a deficiency results in poor growth and in a reduction of the amount and color of hair. Deficiencies

*The same Dr. György who was involved in the discoveries of riboflavin and vitamin B-6.

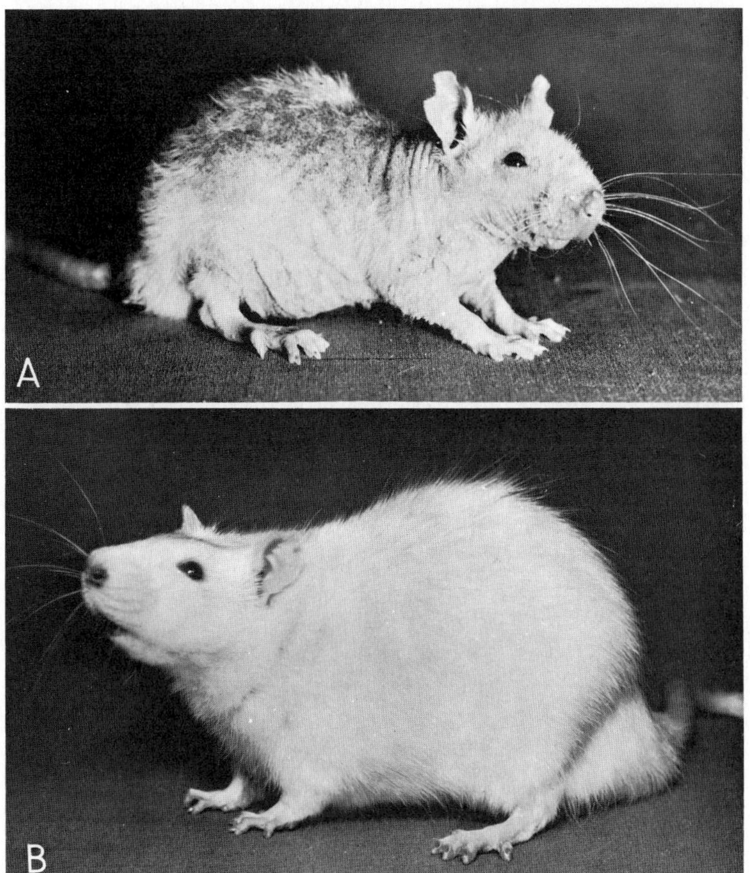

Figure 8–17 **A,** Rat after being fed a diet deficient in biotin, to which raw egg white was added. Growth has been retarded, and there is a generalized inflammation of the skin. **B,** The same rat after three months on a diet containing adequate amounts of biotin. Growth is normal, and the skin lesions are completely healed. (Courtesy of the Upjohn Company.)

also have been produced in dogs, pigs, calves, and many other animal species.

Reactions requiring biotin are very important in the synthesis of fatty acids, in the production of energy from glucose, and in the formation of nucleic acid, glycogen, and several amino acids.

Most biotin in the body is combined in various enzymes by means of chemical union with the amino acid lysine. When thus bound to an enzyme, biotin plays an important role in essential *carboxylation* reactions, in which carbon dioxide is transferred from the enzyme complex to other compounds. These reactions are reversible and are closely involved with those of pantothenic acid (coenzyme A).

Requirement and Nutritional Status

There is insufficient evidence on which to base a recommended allowance for humans. Biotin is not one of the vitamins usually studied in nutrition surveys. Experimental animals require only small amounts of biotin per kilogram of diet, about 100 to 150 mcg. This is equivalent to about 50 to 75 mcg per day for humans, comparatively speaking. The amount supplied by normal diets per day appears to be in the range of 60 to 70 mcg, or possibly slightly more — values below previous estimates.[7, 58] Thus, 70 mcg, or less, is sufficient for normal health, especially since intestinal bacteria produce considerable biotin. It is expected that a "provisional allowance" for biotin will be given by the Food and Nutrition Board in 1979. The level of biotin used as the legal standard for labeling in America is 300 mcg per day for adults (see Chapter 18). This is obviously considerably above actual requirements.

This discussion of requirements is a moot point, since the amount of biotin excreted in the urine and feces of normal adults is greater than the known intake.[59] Synthesis of biotin from microorganisms in the intestinal tract accounts for this difference, though little is known about the availability to the tissues of biotin produced in the lower tract. Biotin deficiency in human populations is not likely to occur except in rare instances, such as when persons might consume large amounts of raw egg whites — 8 to 10 per day — without extra biotin sources. However, the occasional eating of a few raw eggs, as in eggnog, does not provide sufficient avidin to produce a biotin deficiency.

Considerable attention has been given lately to the possibility that a rare clinical condition called seborrheic dermatitis (a skin eruption) in breast-fed infants* may be due to a shortage of biotin in the mother's diet.[60] More research is needed before definite conclusions can be drawn.

Food Sources

Biotin is widely distributed in those foods known to be good sources of other B vitamins. Liver, kidney, yeast, and egg yolks are especially good sources. Whole grains, breads, fish, peanut butter, nuts, beans, meat, and dairy products are also good sources. Vegetables, fruits, and potatoes are rather poor sources.[58, 61] Much needs to be learned yet, about the *availability* of biotin from these food sources. The subject is still relatively young.

*Called Leiner's disease.

FOLACIN

Folacin* (folic acid and related compounds), the next to last of the B vitamins to be discovered, is essential for all vertebrates, including man, for normal growth and reproduction, for the prevention of blood disorders, for important biochemical mechanisms within each cell, and for the prevention of a variety of symptoms in different species. The name "folic acid," the forerunner of the term "folacin" was suggested in 1941 by Mitchell, Snell, and Williams† of Texas, for a highly purified growth factor for bacteria. It is derived from the Latin word for foliage or leaf *(folium)*, because it was first isolated from spinach leaves and was known to be widely distributed in green, leafy plants.

Identification and Properties

The first of the *folacin* group to be obtained in crystalline form was folic acid, known chemically as *pteroylmonoglutamic acid*, isolated from natural materials by two independent groups of workers in pharmaceutical laboratories in the United States in 1943 and 1944.[62] It was first synthesized in 1946 and its structure announced by a team of 16 workers from the American Cyanamid Company.[63] It is a bright yellow powder, quite soluble in slightly alkaline or acid solutions, readily destroyed by heat when in an acid solution, but reasonably stable when in neutral or alkaline solutions — especially in the absence of air.

*According to current international nomenclature rules, the term "folacin," originally proposed by the American Institute of Nutrition in the 1950's, is used here as the generic description for folic acid and related compounds exhibiting the biological activity of folic acid (pteroylmonoglutamic acid). Names of other related compounds have also been changed accordingly. There is no single compound with the name "folacin." The word "folate" is used in biochemical literature for salts of folic acid, and is not properly used in nutrition literature for lack of specificity.

†R. J. Williams, who also coined the word "pantothenic acid."

Its eventual discovery was aided considerably by the previous work (at the Universities of Arkansas, Missouri, California, Wisconsin, Texas, Cornell, and elsewhere) of nutritionists and biochemists who were studying unidentified growth factors for the chicken, monkey, and bacteria, which now appear to have been identical with folacin. The useful term *vitamin B-10* was suggested in the early 1940's for the substance(s) in natural foods with growth activity for young chickens (fed diets which were later found to be deficient in folacin, not available at the time).[64] Vitamin B_c, vitamin M, factors R and U, and *L. casei* factor were other terms used, and although folacin is a recognized member of the B complex, these terms are not used today.

This vitamin exists in several different forms in nature, making up the folacin group of compounds. These different forms have similar activity when fed to higher animals, but they have widely different activities as growth factors for microorganisms. The parent compound, folic acid (pteroylmonoglutamic acid) — which probably does not exist free in nature — is formed by the linkage of three compounds: *pteridine*, a yellow phosphorescent pigment related to the yellow pigment in butterfly wings (the Greek word for wing is *pteron*); *para-aminobenzoic acid* (a growth factor for bacteria),* and *glutamic acid*, an amino acid commonly found in proteins of foods and body tissues. The structural formula of folic acid may be found in the Appendix.

In addition to the parent folic acid with only one glutamic acid group in the molecule, at least two *conjugated* forms of folacin exist in foods with either three or seven glutamic acid groups per molecule *(folic acid glutamates)*. These conjugated forms serve as the major precursors of the vitamin in the diet. The coenzyme form, *tetrahydrofolic acid*, the most common form in the body, is also widely distributed in foods. Another form of folacin which is active metabolically and which occurs in food is *10*-formyltetrahydrofolic acid, a reduced form of folic acid. Methyl derivatives of folic acid are also found in nature. Various synthetic derivatives of folic acid, not present in foods, are antagonists of folic acid and are widely used in the treatment of leukemia and certain other types of cancer.

*Para-aminobenzoic acid has considerable folacin activity when fed to deficient animals in which intestinal synthesis of folacin takes place; in fact, in the rat and mouse dietary para-aminobenzoic acid can completely replace the need for a dietary source of folacin in this manner. This explains why para-aminobenzoic acid was once considered to be a vitamin in its own right. Obviously, since it does exist in the free form in some foods, it can be considered a dietary precursor of folacin, but it is not a vitamin itself, though often listed as one.

Effects of Lack of Folacin

Although all animals require folacin, some species can meet this need by the production of the vitamin through bacterial synthesis in the intestine. Rats, dogs, and rabbits fall into this category, but chicks, monkeys, and men must have folacin supplied in the food in order to avoid deficiency symptoms.

Folacin deficiency in *man* results in a smooth, red tongue, gastrointestinal disturbances, and diarrhea; but the primary symptom is a blood disturbance called *macrocytic anemia*. In this anemia, the mature red blood cells are fewer in number, larger in size, and contain less hemoglobin than normal. The young red blood cells in the bone marrow (megaloblasts) fail to mature during folacin deficiency. Administration of folacin by mouth or injection results in prompt formation and development to maturity of a very large number of new red blood cells. Certain anemias that develop during pregnancy, infancy, and childhood respond well to treatment with folacin, as do those seen in sprue or pellagra due to poor intestinal absorption. Anemias due primarily to dietary lack of iron and certain other causes are not relieved by it. In *pernicious anemia*, there is some initial response with increased level of red cells, but not as marked as after giving much smaller amounts of *vitamin B-12*. The nervous symptoms often seen in this disease cannot be cured by treatment with folacin.

Signs of folacin deficiency in animals include poor growth, faulty reproduction, anemia and other blood disorders, and abnormal biochemical changes within the body. Chicks also show poor pigmentation and faulty structure of the feathers. If rats are prevented from forming folacin through intestinal synthesis by being raised in germ-free conditions or by having sulfa drugs added to the diet, deficiency symptoms will develop including marked decrease in various types of white blood cells. Normal reproduction, lactation, and antibody formation also require folacin. In deficient monkeys, there are loss of weight, anemia, and inflammation and degeneration of the gums. Folacin deficiency has also been developed in the mouse, other fowl, guinea pig, mink, dog, and fox.

Function of Folacin in the Human Body

After absorption, whichever form of folacin is eaten is converted by the body to several active coenzyme forms, the parent form being tetrahydrofolic acid. These coenzyme forms are distributed throughout the body but are most abundant in the liver. Probably their primary function is to serve as carriers for single-carbon groups (specifically, the formyl and hydroxy-methyl groups), which are essential for the building of purines and pyrimidines. These compounds are, in turn, needed for synthesis of nucleic acids, which are vital to all cell nuclei. This explains the important role of folacin in cell division and in animal reproduction. Folacin coenzymes also are responsible for synthesis of certain amino acids, especially glycine and serine, used in the formation of body proteins. These reactions require ascorbic acid for maintaining folic acid in its reduced form, and they also require coenzymes of vitamins B-6 and B-12, again demonstrating the interdependence of various vitamins.

The folacin coenzymes are also necessary for the *breakdown* of many, if not all, amino acids. For instance, in folacin deficiency in man and animals, the amino acid *histidine* is imperfectly utilized, resulting in increased amounts of an abnormal derivative in the urine.*

Coenzymes derived from folacin also serve as a source of carbon and hydrogen atoms in the synthesis of *methyl* groups and thus function with choline, betaine, and methionine in supplying labile methyl groups to the body (see page 207). In most animals, folacin cannot be depended on to supply the entire requirement of methyl groups.

Requirements and Nutritional Status

Folacin deficiency in man is now known to occur under "normal" conditions, especially during the latter stages of pregnancy and lactation when the incidence is often quite marked. A total of 0.4 mg per day of folacin activity is recommended for adult men and women, as seen in Table 8–10 and Table 1 of the Appendix. This takes into account possible losses from cooking, poor absorption, and varying activity of the several forms of folacin in foods. The recommended allowance provides a wide margin of safety, since an intake of about 100 to 200 mcg per day is sufficient to maintain body stores.[7] Many persons in many countries obtain much less than the RDA and ap-

*Formiminoglutamic acid ("FIGLU"). This is the basis for one of the laboratory tests for folacin deficiency.

Table 8–10 RECOMMENDED ALLOWANCES FOR FOLACIN AND VITAMIN B-12*

	Age	*Folacin Activity, mcg/day*	*Vitamin B-12 Activity, mcg/day*
Males	11 years and over	400	3
Females	11 years and over	400	3
	Pregnant	800	4
	Lactating	600	4

*From the Food and Nutrition Board, 1974.[7]

See Appendix Table 1D for FAO recommendations.

pear to be healthy. The Canadian recommended allowance is 200 mcg of free folacin per day,[54] providing a smaller safety margin.

Average American intakes are well over this last amount, although specially low intakes or low tissue levels are often seen in sprue, in infants of low birth weight and infants on unsupplemented milk diets, in various disease states, in certain genetic disturbances, in long-term hospitalized patients, and in alcoholism — as well as in pregnancy.[7, 13, 65] There is no normal need for larger intakes than the RDA or the levels in common foods. Excessive folacin can mask certain symptoms of pernicious anemia.

Food Sources of Folacin

Information about the folacin activity of foods for man is incomplete because of the difficulty of assaying the many different forms of folacin in terms of animal activity.[66] However, the richest sources are liver, yeast, and leafy vegetables, as seen in Table 8–11 and Table 2 of the Appendix. Good sources are dried legumes, green vegetables such as asparagus, lettuce, and broccoli, nuts, fresh oranges, and whole-wheat products.

Poor sources include most meats, eggs, root vegetables, most fruits, white flour and products made with highly milled cereals, most desserts, and processed milks — especially dried milks. Sugar and table fats and oils supply no folacin. Diets made up entirely of natural foods low in folacin have produced folacin deficiencies in animals and in man.[67]

Folacin compounds differ in their ability to cross intestinal barriers, depending on the degree of conjugation with glutamic acid or the nature of other types of binding — generally with protein. Hence, tables of folacin composition in foods, especially in the raw state, should be looked at with a degree of caution.

The folacin content of foods is partially destroyed by heating or processing at high temperatures. Normal cooking temperatures of 110° to 120° C for 10 minutes can cause losses up to 65 percent. Fresh leafy vegetables stored at room temperature for 3 days may lose up to 70 percent of their folacin activity.

A usual western type of diet will generally contain from about 200 to 1500 mcg of folacin per day, making it rather easy to obtain a sufficient amount. As a general guide to ensure ample folacin in a daily diet, the best advice, as with all the nutrients, is to choose one's daily diet from the traditional foods in the four food groups according to energy needs. Obviously the choice of at least one serving of green, leafy vegetables per day contributes significantly to meeting the daily requirement of folacin.

VITAMIN B-12

Vitamin B-12 was the last vitamin to be discovered (1948), thus completing the B complex vitamin jigsaw. Distinguishing characteristics are its red color, the presence in its molecule of cobalt and phosphorus, and, unlike any other vitamin, the inability of higher plants to synthesize it. Its most important deficiency state is called *Addisonian pernicious anemia.*

Pernicious anemia has long been known and was given its name because it arose from some factor inherent in the body, did not respond to any known treatment, and eventually culminated in death. In 1849, Addison, an English physician, gave a detailed description of its symptoms, but no treatment could be found until, in 1926, Minot and Murphy[68] of Boston announced that feeding large amounts of liver (¼ to ½ pound per day) restored a normal level of red blood cells in cases of this disease. This indicated that the disease might well be related to nutritional factors. For this discovery they shared the Nobel Prize with Whipple, who had shown a year previously that liver was of great benefit in blood regeneration in dogs rendered anemic by bleeding. Later concentrates of liver were made available, obviating the necessity of eat-

Table 8–11 EXAMPLES OF FOOD SOURCES OF FOLACIN*

Food Source (in terms of 100 gm)	Per Serving			
	Approximate Measure	Weight	Free Folacin	Total Folacin
		gm	*mcg*	*mcg*
Almonds	1 c	142	47	136
Bananas, raw	1 medium	119	26	33
Bread				
White	1 slice	25	3	10
Whole-wheat	1 slice	28	8	16
Cantaloupe	1 c	145	3	9
Cheddar cheese	1 c, shredded	113	1	20
Collard greens, raw	1 c	55	–	56
Cottage cheese	1 c, packed	245	–	29
Eggs, hard-cooked	1 medium	44	–	22
Garbanzo beans	1 c	200	64	398
Ground beef, cooked	3 oz	85	–	3
Lasagna	10 oz portion	280	–	62
Milk, cow, fluid, whole, pasteurized	1 c	244	12	12
Milk, human	1 fl. oz	31	1	2
Oatmeal, dry	1 c	80	13	42
Orange juice	1 c	248	84	136
Peanuts, roasted	1 c	144	35	153
Pinto beans, cooked	1 c	190	–	112
Pizza, cheese, frozen	1/8 pie	67	–	24
Pork, cooked, lean	3 oz	85	–	4
Potatoes, cooked				
French-fried	10 pieces	50	4	11
Mashed	1 c	210	10	21
Poultry				
Chicken and turkey, dark meat, cooked	3 oz	85	–	6
Rice, brown	1 c	185	22	30
Soybeans, dry	1 c	210	158	359
Spinach, cooked	1 c	180	108	164
Tuna, canned	3 oz	85	7	13
Wheat germ, toasted	1 oz	28	35	118
Yeast				
Baker's dry, active	1 pkg.	7	10	286
Brewer's, debittered	1 tbsp	8	14	313
Yogurt	1 c	245	–	27

*From Perloff, B. P., and Butrum, R. R. Values to be used in the next revision of Handbook 8 of U.S.D.A.[67] Values are also given for "free folacin" in this reference, representing the amount that is available to the assay microorganism (*Lactobacillus casei* generally) before treatment of the food with conjugase enzymes. "Total folacin" shown here represents values more similar to conditions in the intestine of humans and are better values to use in calculating dietary intakes.

ing large amounts of this food. Biochemists began a long series of attempts to isolate the active component present in liver concentrates, which was then called the "antipernicious anemia factor."

Identification and Properties

In 1948 Rickes and coworkers, of Merck and Co., Inc., New Jersey, announced the isolation from a liver concentrate of a crystalline, red pigment, which they called "vitamin B-12."[69] In the same month, E. L. Smith,[69] of England, isolated two similar red, noncrystalline pigments from liver concentrate. In New York, West showed that injections of vitamin B-12 induced a dramatic beneficial response in patients with pernicious anemia.[70] The vitamin was isolated by the Merck group with the use of a convenient test developed at the University of Maryland by Shorb and Briggs.[71] This test, which used

Lactobacillus lactis Dorner (a bacterium), saved much work when compared with the former tests that had to be made with humans with pernicious anemia or with experimental animals.

Vitamin B-12 is the group name for several *corrinoids,* named because of their *porphyrin*like structure.* They are nitrogenous basic substances with very large, complicated molecules. (See formula in Appendix.) The cobalt occupies the center of the molecule and may be attached to various chemical groups including a *cyanide* (CN) group — in which case the compound is called *cyanocobalamin,* or to a *hydroxyl* group (OH), which then is called *hydroxocobalamin,* probably the most common form. A coenzyme form of vitamin B-12 contains an *adenosine*† molecule in place of the cyanide or hydroxyl group and is thought to be the most common form in foods. Methylcobalamin is another form of the vitamin with a coenzyme role. All these forms have about equal vitamin B-12 activity when in the diet.

The structure of cyanocobalamin was first determined in 1955 by Dorothy Hodgkins and coworkers.[72] She later received the Nobel Prize. Vitamin B-12 is the most complicated of all the vitamins and only recently has been synthesized — by Dr. Woodward's group at Harvard using a very complicated and expensive procedure. Fortunately, highly active vitamin B-12 concentrates can be produced inexpensively by the vitamin industry from cultures of certain bacteria and fungi grown in large tanks containing special media. These concentrates are universally used as the source of vitamin B-12 in vitamin supplements and in commercial rations for animals. Neither man nor animals can synthesize vitamin B-12 in their tissues, and unlike any other vitamin, higher plants are unable to synthesize it. Thus, *all the vitamin B-12 available to man and animals comes originally from that produced by bacteria and fungi,* either directly or indirectly. It is present in milk and red meats because of microbial synthesis in the rumen, which provides more than an ample amount. Considerable vitamin B-12 can be made in the intestines of humans as well. Rich soils and cloudy water from farm ponds are often good sources of vitamin B-12 also because of microbial production.

*Porphyrinlike structures are found also in the "heme" part of the hemoglobin in blood and in chlorophyll in plants. They consist basically of four nitrogen-containing rings bound together with a mineral element in the center.

†Adenosine is a nucleoside and consists of a purine (adenine) combined with a pentose sugar, ribose.

Vitamin B-12 Deficiency in Man; Pernicious Anemia

Vitamin B-12 deficiency in man may occur in several ways: as a result of a simple *dietary lack,* possible only in vegetarians or owing to *insufficient absorption* from the intestine no matter how much is eaten. When the latter is due to lack of vitamin B-12–binding proteins in the gut, classic pernicious anemia results. Vitamin B-12 deficiency is occasionally seen also in persons with total or partial removal of the stomach by surgery, those infested with parasites such as the fish tapeworm (not uncommon in some countries), or persons with tropical anemias, sprue, and other conditions in which intestinal absorption is insufficient.

In an uncomplicated dietary deficiency of the vitamin, symptoms such as sore tongue, weakness, loss of weight, back pains, tingling of the extremities, apathy, and mental and other nervous abnormalities may develop. Anemia is rarely seen. On the other hand, in pernicious anemia, anemia and degeneration of the spinal cord are the major signs — though without treatment the other symptoms may appear, and eventually will result in death.

The cause of pernicious anemia was partially explained when Castle, in 1928–1930,[73] described the need for an *intrinsic factor,* formed in the stomach, essential for the absorption of an "extrinsic factor"* from food that prevented the disease in normal persons. The intrinsic factor is formed in the stomach of normal persons, but not in those with pernicious anemia. In many cases the presence of an antibody to intrinsic factor prevents its normal action. The intrinsic factor has been identified as a mucoprotein that binds tightly to vitamin B-12 and facilitates its absorption.

The metabolic defect in pernicious anemia, thought to be inherited, is the inability to secrete the intrinsic factor and usually other gastric juices. This results in inability to absorb vitamin B-12 from the intestinal tract. Hence, there is a low level of vitamin B-12 in the blood and an inability of new red blood cells to develop normally, resulting in *megaloblastic anemia*. Various neurological symptoms may also precede or follow the anemia. As little as 1.5 mcg of vitamin B-12, injected intramuscularly each day† in a pernicious anemia patient, will result in restoration of a normal red cell count and gradual disappearance of all the other symptoms. Because the inherent defect of faulty absorption persists, pernicious anemia patients must continue to receive vitamin B-12 in this manner which by-passes the intestinal tract. Because this treatment is successful, severe symptoms are seldom seen now in pernicious anemia patients. The intrinsic factor, in purified form bound to vitamin B-12, can be used in the treatment of the disease, as can the administration of massive amounts of vitamin B-12 in the diet; but such methods are expensive and are not always successful.

Effects of Lack of Vitamin B-12 in Animals

For years nutritionists had studied the effects on animals of what is now known as vitamin B-12 deficiency in attempting to isolate the active substance in liver. Animals such as chickens, pigs, rats, and mice all require vitamin B-12 for normal growth and reproduction, and develop other symptoms of its lack when fed diets deficient in this factor. As yet no animal has been found to develop the counterpart of human pernicious anemia.

Deficiency symptoms were seen in chickens in the early 1940's when diets made entirely from plant sources were used. These symptoms could be alleviated by adding to this diet animal by-products that provided what was then called the "animal protein factor."[74] After vitamin B-12 was discovered, it was found to replace the need for the previously studied "animal protein factor" and "vitamin B-11" for chicks. "Factor X"* and "zoopherin" for rats, the "anti-thyroid factor" of mice, and the "*Lactobacillus lactis* Dorner factor" for bacteria, as well as the "anti–pernicious anemia factor" for man. With the discovery of vitamin B-12 it became possible, and routine, to raise poultry and swine without the use of scarce and expensive animal by-products.

Deficiencies in rats, fowl, young calves, monkeys, pigs, and many other species are readily obtained merely by leaving the vitamin out of the diet and at the same time preventing the animal from eating litter, soil, or its feces. Deficient animals show poor growth and reproductive disorders, and in severe cases they die. Pigs may show nervous irritability.

Cattle and sheep, grazing on plants grown on cobalt-poor soil (see page 296), develop symptoms of cobalt deficiency, which include loss of weight, weakness, and *anemia*. The injection of vitamin B-12, but not of cobalt, relieves all these symptoms, proving that the cobalt lack resulted in inability of the microorganisms in the rumen to synthesize the vitamin. Because cobalt is one of the constituents of the vitamin B-12 molecule, it is obvious that it is required by all animals that are chiefly dependent on microbial synthesis in the gut for their supply of this vitamin.

*The term "extrinsic factor" is obsolete today, and vitamin B-12 should be used in its place. Castle's so-called extrinsic factor was said to be found in meat, but it was also found in rice polishings, tomatoes, yeast, and wheat germ, none of which, we know now, contain appreciable amounts of vitamin B-12.

†Usually injections are spaced a month or so apart, so that larger amounts are routinely given.

*In fact, it was the specific search for the unknown "Factor X" in milk by U.S.D.A. scientists in the early 1940's that led directly to the bacterial test of Dr. Mary Shorb, later used by the Merck group to isolate vitamin B-12.

Function of Vitamin B-12

Vitamin B-12 is absorbed only to the extent of 30 to 70 percent in normal persons, and none is absorbed in persons with pernicious anemia. Once in the body it is converted to the coenzyme form, if not already in that form. This coenzyme circulates in the blood combined with *trenscobalamin,* a glycoprotein, and it is stored in the liver and kidney. It is essential for the normal functioning of all body cells, particularly those of the bone marrow, the nervous system, and the gastrointestinal tract. However, it is no more active qualitatively than other forms of the vitamin when it is ingested or injected.

The *role of vitamin B-12 in metabolism* is not completely understood, but its most important function is in the formation of nucleic acids by aiding in the synthesis of various purine and pyrimidine intermediates, similar to the function of folacin. Coenzyme B-12 also participates, often with pantothenic acid, in the rather unique but essential *isomerism* reactions, in which several carbon units are rearranged within a molecule, such as in the formation of an amino acid, aspartic acid. It also is involved in the synthesis and transfer of labile methyl groups, along with choline, folacin, and methionine, discussed in the next section — choline.

Food Sources of Vitamin B-12

There is no vitamin B-12 in plant products, such as grains, vegetables, fruits, and so on, except trace amounts that might be absorbed from the soil while the plant is growing, soil being one of the better sources of vitamin B-12 because of its high bacterial content. There is none present in yeast,* the traditional source of other B complex vitamins. Richest sources are liver and organ meats. Muscle meats, fish, eggs, shellfish, milk, and most milk products, except butter, are good sources, while evaporated milk and yogurt are fair sources.[33] (See Table 8–12 for examples of good sources and Table 2 of the Appendix for more values in foods.) The coenzyme form of the vitamin, which accounts for a major portion of vitamin B-12 in food, is not very stable to the heat used in processing procedures or to light. Up to 10 percent is lost in milk during pasteurization, and 40 to 90 percent in evaporated milk.

Meat, including poultry and fish, contributes about 70 percent of the 10 mcg of vitamin B-12 available in the typical United States daily diet; eggs contribute 8 percent, and dairy products 20 percent. A small amount is provided in fortified cereals.[9] Canadian intakes appear to be slightly higher.[54]

The most inexpensive sources of vitamin B-12 are microbial growth concen-

Table 8–12 EXAMPLES OF FOOD SOURCES OF VITAMIN B-12*

Food Source	*Vitamin B-12, mcg/100 gm*
Beef	1.4
Cheese	
Cheddar	1.0
Cottage	1.0
Chicken meat	0.4
Clams, raw, meat only	98
Cod, dehydrated, slightly salted	10
Crab, cooked or canned	10
Eggs, whole	2.0
Herring, Atlantic	
Raw	10
Canned	8
Kidney, raw	
Beef	31
Calf	25
Lamb	63
Liver, raw	
Beef	80
Lamb	104
Mackerel, Atlantic raw	9
Milk,	
Whole fresh	0.4
Yogurt	0.1
Oysters, Eastern, raw	18
Sardines, Atlantic, canned	10
Liverwurst	14

*Adapted from Orr, M. L., 1969.[33] Also see Appendix Table 2.

*However, some special yeasts containing vitamin B-12 are available. They have been grown on media very rich in the vitamin, which is then absorbed in the yeast cell.

trates. One year's supply for one normal person costs about 3 cents. These concentrates have not been used much to enrich man's food, for there has been no demonstrated means of suitably doing this in vegetarian societies.

Requirements and Nutritional Status

The recommended dietary allowance for vitamin B-12 in the United States is 3 mcg per day for adolescents and adults of all ages, assuming that at least 50 percent is absorbed.[7] Allowances in pregnancy and during lactation are slightly higher, as shown in Table 8–10 and Table 1A of the Appendix. Of course, persons with pernicious anemia, who do not absorb the vitamin, will respond to 3 mcg of vitamin B-12 only if it is injected. As little as 0.1 mcg per day can give a small response when injected in anemic persons, making vitamin B-12 one of the most potent compounds known to man.

The vitamin B-12 content of diets in those developing countries where foods of plant origin are more common may be low or borderline, and frank vitamin B-12 deficiencies are not unknown. For instance, vitamin B-12 deficiency in infants can occur frequently in certain areas of the world where intakes of animal products by mothers are low. In studies of pregnant mothers in southern India, Baker and coworkers reported that "babies born and suckled by vitamin B-12–deficient mothers may have lower body vitamin B-12 stores, may receive less vitamin B-12 in breast-milk feeds, and may be in danger of developing frank vitamin B-12 deficiency."[75]

Likewise, children who live exclusively on plant foods ("vegans") may show symptoms of vitamin B-12 deficiency after extended periods. Deficiency signs have also been seen in adults, especially child-bearing women, after eating vegetable and grain diets for several years — even in the absence of pernicious anemia.[76]

All such examples are due to a straightforward deficiency. Normally, the total body stores of vitamin B-12 in well-fed adults are as much as 5 to 10 mg. These reserves are sufficient to last as long as *2 to 3 years*, or much more, even in the absence of a vitamin B-12 supply — but eventually a deficiency will occur.

Vitamin B-12 promises to be one of the most important vitamins for mankind. It is now possible to use plant and cereal foods much more wisely in the human diet in case of future population pressures of famines, and when animal foods are in short supply.

CHOLINE

Choline is an important B vitamin necessary in the diet of many young animals,[7] though its need by man at any stage of life has not been established. Choline, generally combined with other compounds, has several catalytic and metabolic functions in the body. Also it is an essential component of several phospholipids vital in lipid metabolism — notably lecithin and sphingomyelin, which together make up 70 to 80 percent of the phospholipids in the animal body.

Identification and Properties

Choline was isolated from bile in 1862 by a German chemist. *Chole* is the Greek word for bile. Its vitamin nature was not appreciated fully until the early 1940's after studies by Sure and György and Goldblatt,[77] who showed that it is essential for growth of rats and who confirmed in earlier studies that it prevented the accumulation of excessive fat in the liver ("fatty livers") in animals fed choline-low diets.

In 1930 *lecithin*, a phospholipid that contains choline, was shown to prevent fatty livers in dogs. Feeding components of lecithin, Best and his coworkers[78] at Toronto University, between 1932 and 1935, showed that choline was the part of the lecithin molecule that prevented the occurrence of fatty livers in rats fed diets low in protein and high in fat, cholesterol, or sucrose. *Betaine,** a closely related substance in certain foods, acted less efficiently than choline. Best's work was done before any other B complex vitamin was available in pure form, and he considered choline as only an accessory food factor. By 1942, the vitamin nature of choline was fully confirmed by many other workers, who used the rat, chicken, and turkey as experimental animals.[79] This, then, became the seventh B vitamin to be identified. In common with several other B vitamins, it was never given a specific B vitamin number. It is discussed as the ninth B vitamin here because there is no known human requirement for it.†

Choline, a relatively simple molecule, contains three methyl groups (CH_3—) and is strongly alkaline in its free form (see formula in Appendix). It is a water-soluble white syrup that takes up water rapidly on exposure to air (hygroscopic) and readily forms more stable crystalline salts with acids such as choline chloride or choline bitartrate. In foods, it exists primarily in phospholipids or as the water-soluble sulfate or phosphate salts. It is heat-stable and remains at nearly a constant level in dried foods when stored over long periods.

Functions in Body and Deficiency Signs

Choline has many important functions in the body — as a constituent of several phospholipids (primarily lecithin) it aids in the *transport and metabolism of fats;* as a constituent of *acetylcholine* it plays a role in the normal functioning of nerves; and it serves as a source of *labile methyl groups,* which are essential in metabolism.

The methyl group (CH_3—) is found in many organic substances, but in most of them it is fixed and not detachable. When a methyl group is present in such a form that it can be transferred from one compound to another, it is called a labile methyl group and the process is called *transmethylation.* The body has a pool of labile methyl groups contributed from various sources, which it uses for such purposes as the formation of creatine (important in muscle metabolism) and for methylating certain substances for excretion in the urine. These methyl groups are also used in the synthesis of several hormones, such as epinephrine, and have other essential roles. Among the dietary sources of labile methyl are choline (or related substances), the amino acid methionine and, in addition, the vitamins folacin and vitamin B-12.

Mention has been made of dietary factors related to choline that can replace some of its functions or all, in some species. The primary one of these is betaine, which can fully replace choline in preventing fatty liver in some species; in others betaine only supplements choline. Betaine may be considered a *sparing agent* and a member of the "choline group," but is not fully equivalent to choline. To some extent, methionine and vitamin B-12 also spare choline in some animal species. In such cases, an abundance of any of these or other sources of labile methyl groups may be said to "spare" or at least to partially make up for a shortage of one of the others. The action of these substances in preventing fat accumulation in the lever, and in certain other tissues, is said to be a *lipotropic* activity — a term first used by Best.

A *deficiency of choline in rats* resultes in fatty livers in 4 to 6 weeks. In addition, depending on the type of diet and the length of time the deficient diet is fed to them, symp-

*Betaine, which has choline activity, is widely distributed in foods of plant origin. It derives its name from the Latin word *beta,* the beet family, which contain rather large amounts — up to 4 percent in some species. Like choline, it has a nitrogenous base, which contains three methyl groups (CH_3—) in each molecule.

†Lecithin is often added to dietary supplements sold in health food stores and claimed as a nutrient aiding in the utilization of cholesterol, among other claims. There is no evidence that lecithin is a dietary necessity. Of course, it does provide choline and, thus, can overcome a choline deficiency in animals, but is much less efficient in humans.

toms such as poor growth, edema, and an impaired cardiovascular system are seen, the last of which results in hemorrhagic lesions in the kidneys, heart muscles, and adrenal glands. Fatty livers also are seen in deficient dogs, mice, guinea pigs, ducks, rabbits, pigs, calves, cats, and monkeys. Chickens and turkeys are quite immune to fatty livers, but develop *slipped tendon* (a bowing of the legs), which makes walking and getting to the feed supply so difficult that death usually results in 6 to 8 weeks. Borderline deficiencies of choline have occurred in farm animals fed the usual "by-product" feeds low in methionine. Hence choline is added to most animal feeds in this country.

Nutritional Status and "Requirement"

Experimental deficiency of choline in humans has never been obtained, though very few serious studies have been attempted. If choline is needed, one would especially expect infants and young children to show a need, since, generally, it is the young of experimental animals fed deficient diets that are affected primarily. It would not be wise, based on our knowledge of choline, to purposely give infants and children (or adults for that matter) a choline-free diet for any extended time. In fact, a Committee of the American Academy of Pediatrics has recently recommended that choline be added to infant formula diets in amounts similar to breast milk contents as a precaution until more is known about this vitamin.[80]

Fatty infiltration of the liver is seen very commonly, especially in chronic alcoholics or in persons on very low protein diets (e.g., in children with kwashiorkor). Choline and other lipotropic agents have been used by physicians in attempts to cure these disorders, but the results have been inconsistent and disappointing. Other clinical responses to dietary choline or lecithin, or both, are being studied and indicate that these substances have potential use as pharmacological agents for certain nerve disturbances in humans.[81]

The Food and Nutrition Board does not suggest any human allowance for this factor because of this lack of evidence. We estimate that an average mixed diet for adults in the United States contains 500 to 900 mg per day of choline and betaine, or about 0.1 to 0.18 percent of the diet. Human milk contains about 145 mg per liter, nearly 0.1 percent of total solids. These amounts are adequate when compared with known requirements of laboratory animals. Supplementary intake of choline, as in special food supplements, is unnecessary and unwise.

Food Sources of Choline

Choline is present in all foods in which phospholipids occur liberally, as in egg yolk, whole grains, legumes, meats of all types, and wheat germ.[82] Fresh egg yolk contains about 1.5 percent choline — probably the richest natural source — and beef liver contains about 0.6 percent. Legumes, such as soybeans, peas, and beans, contain from 0.2 to 0.35 percent; vegetables and milk have moderate choline activity. Most other foods, including fruits, have little or no choline activity.

ARE THERE OTHER B VITAMINS?

There appear to be no other B vitamins than the nine presented in this chapter and listed in Figure 8–17 (also see Chapter 6). Occasionally, the sugarlike substance *inositol** will be listed among the B complex vitamins on labels, and in textbooks, catalogues, diet-ingredient lists, etc. Inositol is an important constituent of certain phospholipids in the body and is also present in a variety of foods. However, higher animals appear capable of synthesizing all the inositol needed. There is little evidence to confirm earlier conclusions made with diets partially deficient in other vitamins that inositol is a vitamin for either man or higher animals.

*"Inositol" is a group name for several closely related substances. The major one in foods, and the most biologically active, is properly named *myoinositol*.

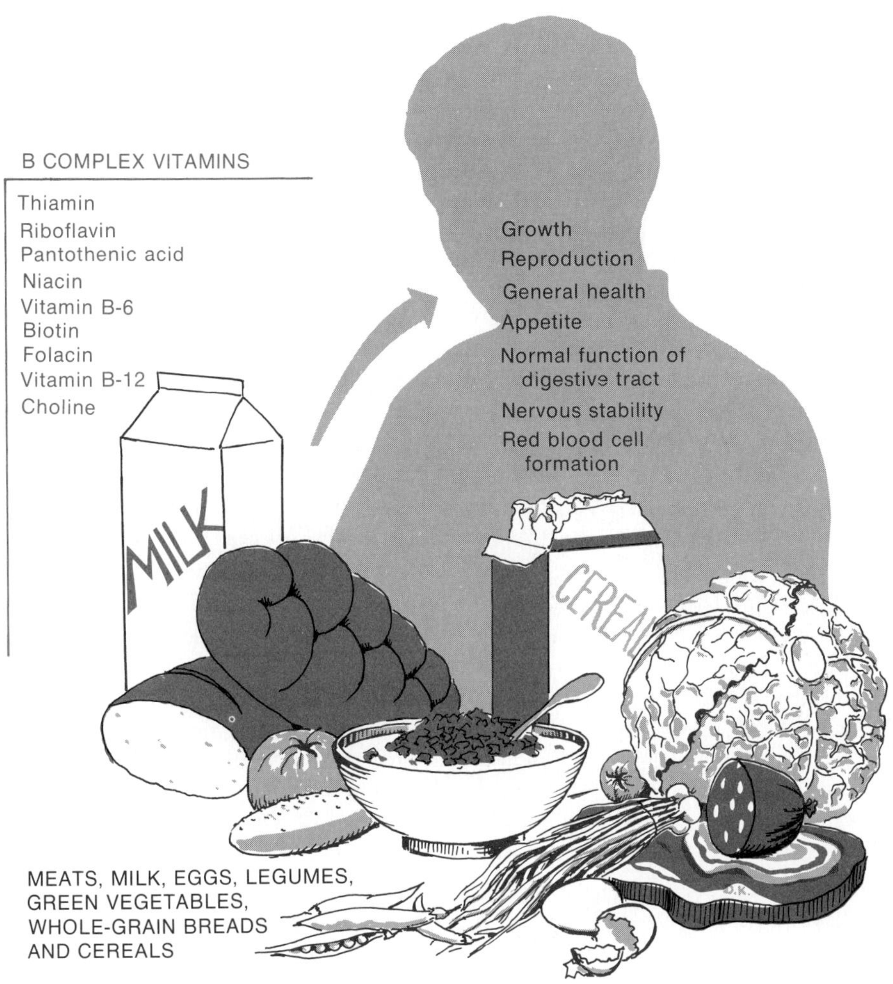
B COMPLEX VITAMINS
Thiamin
Riboflavin
Pantothenic acid
Niacin
Vitamin B-6
Biotin
Folacin
Vitamin B-12
Choline
Growth
Reproduction
General health
Appetite
Normal function of digestive tract
Nervous stability
Red blood cell formation
MILK
CEREAL
MEATS, MILK, EGGS, LEGUMES, GREEN VEGETABLES, WHOLE-GRAIN BREADS AND CEREALS

Figure 8–18

Nevertheless, it still remains an important "growth factor" for certain yeasts (as one of the "bios" group), for many bacteria, and for several lower organisms up to and including several species of fish. The studies at Harvard University[84] that indicate a dietary need of inositol by the female gerbil, a small mammal used as a pet and in laboratory studies, will be watched with interest. Such studies require ample confirmation before inositol can be given full vitamin status.

Another vitaminlike substance receiving much attention recently is *carnitine,* known for many years to be an essential growth factor for certain insects and once called vitamin B_T. Similar in some respects to the story of inositol, carnitine is a vital coenzyme in animal tissues and is involved in fat metabolism. It is widely distributed in foods. It is similar to a vitamin with the exception that in normal conditions higher animals synthesize their total needs within the body. Carnitine is similar to choline and has three active methyl groups in the molecule. It cannot replace choline in preventing a deficiency and is not a vitamin in itself.

Another constituent of foods is *p-aminobenzoic acid,* often listed with B vitamins in the same manner as inositol. This, too, is an important "growth factor" for lower animals, but in higher animals it serves only as a "sparing factor" in the diet for folacin (see page 199). It has no vitamin activity in animals receiving ample folacin and can no longer be considered a vitamin, contrary to its listing in many vitamin preparations on the market.

Over the years during which the B vitamins were developed, it is of historical interest that other numbers were temporarily used to name biologically active fractions of active materials in well-conducted laboratory tests. In this way the names vitamin B-7, B-8, B-10, B-11, B-13, and B-14 have all been used in the literature. Likewise, there has been use of the terms vitamin F, G, H, I, J, L, M, N, P, Q, R, S, T, U, and V in the nutrition literature. None of these are recognized today, for good reasons, by official nomenclature bodies (see references in Chapter 6). Pangamic acid and laetrile, popular fads today, are in no way to be considered as vitamins (see Chapter 6).

This is not to say that there are not biologically active substances in foods essential for health under conditions not recognized now. For instance, there are many other natural, organic "growth factors," other than the vitamins, necessary for lower forms of life — such as lipoic acid, nucleic acids, purines and pyrimidines, "biopterin," peptides, sterols, "hematin," and still others, but none of these fit the definition of a vitamin.

Other compounds that have growth-promoting activity in animals, or some other beneficial effect, probably exist in natural foods or may be synthesized by intestinal bacteria. These compounds are being studied in various laboratories and are conveniently termed "unidentified factors."[85] Whether any of these "unidentified factors" for animals turn out to be B vitamins or whether they will be needed by man remains to be seen. In any event, if such unidentified vitamins actually do exist, they are of no cause for concern as long as one eats a variety of foods from basic foods, which supply ample amounts of all the B vitamins.

QUESTIONS AND PROBLEMS

1. Enumerate nine vitamins that are known as B complex vitamins. For each of the following vitamins, give its chief use, or uses, in the body and the symptoms that are characteristic results of a deficiency of it in the diet: thiamin, riboflavin, and niacin. Are they all needed by humans? Explain.

2. Give three specific examples of a biological relationship between a B vitamin and an amino acid.

3. Is pellagra a clear-cut deficiency disease due to lack of niacin alone? If not, enumerate what other nutritive deficien-

cies are likely to occur as a result of a diet consisting mainly of corn meal and grits, white flour and rice, and fatty salt pork. What foods would you introduce to improve the diets?

4. Either make out a day's menus for what you would consider an attractive diet, or write down your actual food intake for an average day. Specify the amounts of each food consumed. Consult the tables in this chapter and in the Appendix for content of foods in protein, thiamin, riboflavin, and vitamin B-6. Add up the total quantities of each which would be provided in the day's diet that you have planned or consumed.

5. Look up, or calculate as directed in the preceding chapter, the recommended allowance for the above three B vitamins for a person of your sex, size, and degree of activity. How does the intake of each vitamin in the calculated diet compare with the recommended allowance? What foods fairly rich in these three vitamins might be used to increase the thiamin, riboflavin, and vitamin B-6 content of the diet?

6. Give the chief nutritional functions for each of the following vitamins: folacin, vitamin B-12, vitamin B-6, and pantothenic acid. Can you give any examples of interrelations between different B complex vitamins?

7. What types of foods, used freely in the diet, ensure a sufficient intake of the whole group of B vitamins?

REFERENCES

Thiamin

1. Salmon, W. D.: J. Biol. Chem., *73*:483, 1927.
2. Williams, R. R., and Cline, J. K.: J. Amer. Chem. Soc., *58*:1504, 1936.
3. Grijns, G.: Geneesk. Tijdschr. v. Ned. Ind. 1, 1901 (as seen in McCollum, ref. 4).
4. McCollum, E. V.: *A History of Nutrition.* Boston, Houghton Mifflin Co., 1957.
5. Jansen, B. C. P.: Nutr. Abstr. Rev., *26*:1, 1956.
6. Melnick, D., et al.: J. Nutr., *18*:593, 1939; Jolliffe, N., et al.: Amer. J. Med. Sci., *198*:198, 1939; Williams, R. D., et al.: Arch. Intern. Med., *69*:721, 1942; Williams, R. D., et al.: Arch. Intern. Med., *71*:38, 1943; Hulse, M. C., et al.: Ann. Intern. Med., *21*:440, 1944.
7. Food and Nutrition Board: *Recommended Dietary Allowances.* 8th Ed. Washington, D.C., National Research Council, National Academy of Sciences, 1974: 9th Ed. to be published in 1979. Also see Balsley, M. B.: J. Amer. Dietet. Assoc., *71*:149, 1977.
8. Lane, R. L., Johnson, E., and Williams, R. R.: J. Nutr., *23*:613, 1942.
9. U.S. Department of Agriculture: *National Food Review,* Issue NFR–1 (Rm. 0054 S. Bldg.), Washington, D.C., Jan. 1978 (revisions made annually).
10. Kelsay, J. L.: J. Nutr., *99* (No. 1, Part II, Suppl. 1):119, 1969; Davis, T. R. A., Gershoff, S. N., and Gamble, D. F.: J. Nutr. Ed. *1*(Fall, Suppl. 1):39, 1969; Schaefer, A. E.: J. Amer. Dietet. Assoc., *54*:371, 1969; Nutr. Today, *4*:2, 1969.
11. Owen, G. M., et al.: Pediatrics, *53*(No. 4, Part II, Suppl. 1):11, 1974.
12. Lowenstein, F. W.: Amer. J. Clin. Nutr., *29*:918, 1976; Abraham, S., Lowenstein, F. W., and O'Connell, D. E.: U.S. Dept. of Health, Education, and Welfare, Issue No. (HRA) 75–1229, 1975 (National Center for Health Statistics, Rockville, Md.).
13. Abraham, S., et al.: *Dietary Intake Findings, U.S. 1971–1974.* HANES Rpt., Pub. No. (HRA) 17–1647, 1977. Hyattsville, Md., U.S. Dept. of Health, Education, and Welfare (National Center for Health Statistics); Lowenstein, F. W.: Amer. J. Clin. Nutr., *29*:918, 1976.
14. Watt, B. K., and Merrill, A. L.: *Composition of Foods: Raw, Processed, Prepared.* U.S.D.A. Handbook No. 8, Washington, D.C., 1963; Adams, C. F.: *Nutritive Value of American Foods in Common Units.* U.S.D.A. Handbook No. 456, Washington, D.C., 1975.
15. Mulley, E. A., Stumbo, C. R., and Hunting, W. M.: J. Food Sci., *40*:989, 1975; Morrison, M. H.: J. Food Tech., *9*:491, 1974; Oguntona, T. E., and Bender, A. E.: J. Food Tech., *11*:347, 1976; Chaudri, A. B., and Muller, H. G.: J. Food Tech, *9*:123, 1974; Padua, A. B., and Juliano, B. O.: J. Sci. Food Agric., *25*:697, 1974.
16. Vimokesant, S. L., and coworkers: Nutr. Rpts. Internat., *9*:371, 1974; Amer. J. Clin. Nutr., *28*:1458, 1975.
17. Leevy, C. M., and Baker, H.: Amer. J. Clin. Nutr., *21*:1325, 1968; Hoyumpe, A. M.: Amer. J. Clin. Nutr., *31*:938, 1978.

Riboflavin

18. Emmett, A. D., and coworkers: J. Biol. Chem., *32*:409, 1917; *43*:265, 1920; *43*:287, 1920.
19. Sebrell, W. H., and Butler, R. E.: U.S. Pub. Health Rpt., *53*:2282, 1938; *54*:2121, 1939.
20. Lane, M., et al.: J. Clin. Invest., *43*:357, 1964.
21. Rosenthal, W. S., Adham, N. F., Lopez, R., and Cooperman, J. M.: Amer. J. Clin. Nutr., *26*:858, 1973.
22. Vir, S., and Love, A. H. G.: Internat. J. Vit. Res., *47*:336, 1977 (studies made in Ireland).
23. Newman, L. J., et al.: Amer. J. Clin. Nutr., *31*:247, 1978 (studies made in New York).
24. Heller, S., Salkeld, R. M., and Korner, W. F.: Amer. J. Clin. Nutr., *27*:1225, 1974 (studies made in Switzerland); Jacob, M., Hunt, I., Dirige, O., and Swenseid, M. E.: Amer. J. Clin. Nutr., *29*:650, 1976 (studies in low-income

women of Mexican descent in Los Angeles area).
25. Ziegler, J. A.: J. Amer. Chem. Soc., *66*:1039, 1944; Singh, R. P., Heldman, D. R., and Kirk, J. R.: J. Food Sci., *40*:164, 1975.
26. Riboflavin under the lights (editorial, with 11 refs.), Lancet *1*:1191, 1978; Gromisch, D. S., et al.: J. Pediatr., *90*:118, 1977.

Pantothenic Acid

27. Williams, R. J., et al.: J. Amer. Chem. Soc., *55*:2912, 1933; Advanc. Enzymol., *3*:253, 1943; Nutr. Rev., *12*:65, 1954.
28. Jukes, T. H.: J. Amer. Chem. Soc., *61*:975, 1939; Woolley, D. W., Waisman, H. A., and Elvehjem, C. A.: J. Amer. Chem. Soc., *61*:977, 1939.
29. Williams, R. J., and Major, R. T.: Science, *91*:246, 1940; Stiller, E. T., et al.: J. Amer. Chem. Soc., *62*:1785, 1940.
30. Bean, W. B., and Hodges, R. E.: Proc. Soc. Exp. Biol. Med., *86*:693, 1954; Hodges, R. E., et al.: J. Clin. Invest., *37*:1642, 1958; *38*:1421, 1959; Amer. J. Clin. Nutr., *11*:85, 1962; *11*:187, 1962.
31. Cohenour, S. H., and Calloway, D. C.: Amer. J. Clin. Nutr., *25*:512, 1972; Fry, P. C., Fox, H. M., and Tao, H. G.: J. Nutr. Sci. Vitaminol., *22*:339, 1976; Fox, H. M., and Linkswiler, H.: J. Nutr., *75*:451, 1961.
32. Chung, A. S. M., et al.: Amer. J. Clin. Nutr., *9*:573, 1961. (Intakes given for pantothenic acid, vitamin B-6, folacin, and vitamin B-12); Hoppner, K., Lampi, B., and Smith, D. C.: Can. Inst. Food Sci. Tech. J., *11*:71, 1978 (Pantothenic acid, vitamin B-12, and biotin).
33. Orr, M. L.: *Pantothenic acid, Vitamin B_6 and Vitamin B_{12} in Foods.* U.S.D.A., Washington, D.C., Home Econ. Res. Rpt. 36, 1969; Schroeder, H. A.: Amer. J. Clin. Nutr., *24*:562, 1971.

Niacin

34. Goldberger, J., et al.: U.S. Pub. Health Rpt., *30*:3117, 1915; *31*:3159 and 3336, 1916; *33*:2038, 1918; and four reports in *35*:1920. Goldberger was aided considerably by the early work of C. Voegdin (J.A.M.A., *63*:1094, 1914).
35. Elvehjem, C. A., et al.: J. Amer. Chem. Soc., *59*:1767, 1937; J. Biol. Chem., *123*:137, 1938.
36. Fouts, P. J., et al.: Proc. Soc. Exp. Biol. Med., *37*:405, 1937; Smith, D. T., Ruffin, J. M., and Smith, S. G.: J.A.M.A., *109*:2054, 1937; Spies, T. D., et al.: J.A.M.A., *110*:622, and *111*:584, 1938; Ann. Intern. Med., *12*:1830, 1939; Harris, L. J.: Chem. Ind., *56*:1134, 1937.
37. Spies, T. D., et al.: J.A.M.A., *113*:1481, 1939.
38. Sandels, M. R., and Grady, E.: Arch. Intern. Med., *50*:362, 1932; Stiebeling, H. K., and Munsell, H. E.: U.S. Department of Agriculture Technical Bulletin No. 333, 1932; Sebrell, W. H.: U.S. Pub. Health Rpt., *49*:57, 1934.
39. Wheeler, G. A., and Sebrell, W. H.: J.A.M.A., *99*:95, 1932.
40. Kooser, J. H., and Blankenhorn, M. A.: J.A.M.A., *116*:912, 1941.
41. DeKleine, W.: South. Med. J., *35*:992, 1942.
42. Krehl, W. A., Sarma, P. S., Teply, L. S., and Elvehjem, C. A.: Science, *101*:489, 1945; J. Nutr., *31*:85, 1946.
43. Najjar, V. A., et al.: Proc. Soc. Exp. Biol. Med., *61*:371, 1946; Sarett, H. P., and Goldsmith, G. A.: J. Biol. Chem., *177*:461, 1949; Vilter, R. W., Mueller, J. F., and Bean, W. B.: J. Lab. Clin. Med., *34*:409, 1949; Horwitt, M. K., et al.: J. Amer. Dietet. Assoc., *34*:914, 1958; J. Nutr., Suppl., *1*, 1956; Goldsmith, G. A., et al.: Amer. J. Clin. Nutr., *6*:479, 1958; J. Nutr., *73*:172, 1961.
44. Briggs, G. M., et al.: J. Biol. Chem., *161*:749, 1945; *165*:739, 1946; J. Nutr., *32*:659, 1946; *45*:345, 1951; Krehl, W. A., et al.: J. Biol. Chem., *162*:403, 1946; *166*:531, 1946.

Vitamin B-6

45. György, P.: Nature, *133*:498, 1934; Amer. J. Clin. Nutr., *4*:313, 1956.
46. Chick, H., and Copping, A. M.: Biochem. J., *24*;1764, 1930.
47. Lepkovsky, S.: Science, *87*:169, 1938; J. Biol. Chem., *124*:125, 1938.
48. György, P., and Eckardt, R. E.: Nature, *144*:512, 1939.
49. Snell, E. E.: J. Biol. Chem., *154*:313, 1944; *157*:491, 1945; J. Amer. Chem. Soc., *66*:2082, 1944; Harris, S. A., et al.: J. Biol. Chem., *154*:315, 1944; Harris, S. A., Heyl, D., and Folkers, K.: J. Amer. Chem. Soc., *66*:2088, 1944.
50. Lushbough, C. H., Weichman, J. M., and Schweigert, B. S.: J. Nutr., *67*:451, 1959; Tomarelli, R. M., Spence, E. R., and Bernhart, F. W.: J. Agric. Food Chem., *3*:338, 1955.
51. Coursin, D. B.: J.A.M.A., *154*:406, 1954; May, C. D.: Pediatrics, *14*:269, 1954; Nelson, E. M.: Pub. Health Rpt. *71*:445, 1956; Bessey, O. A., Adam, D. J., and Hansen, A. E.: Pediatrics, *20*:33, 1957.
52. Smith, S. G., and Martin, D. W.: Proc. Soc. Exp. Biol. Med., *43*:660, 1960; Mueller, J. F., and Vilter, R. W.: J. Clin. Invest., *29*:193, 1950; Snyderman, S. E., et al.: J. Clin. Nutr., *1*:200, 1953; Vilter, R. W.: Amer. J. Clin. Nutr., *4*:378, 1957; Park, Y. K., and Linkswiler, H.: J. Nutr., *100*:110, 1970.
53. Sauberlich, H. E.: Vit Horm., *22*:807, 1964; Baker, E. M., et al.: Amer. J. Clin. Nutr., *15*:59, 1964.
54. Committee for Revision of the Canadian Dietary Standard: *Dietary Standard for Canada.* Dept. National Health and Welfare, Ottawa, 1975.
55. Cheslock, K. E., and McCully, M. T.: J. Nutr., *70*:507, 1960.

Biotin

56. György, P., et al.: Science, *91*:243, 1940; György, P.: Science, *92*:609, 1940.
57. Sydensricker, V. P., et al.: Science, *95*:176, 1942; J.A.M.A., *118*:1199, 1942; Williams, R. H.: N. Eng. J. Med., *228*:247, 1943.
58. Bonjour, J. P.: Intern. J. Vit. Res., *47*:107, 1977; Hoppner et al. (ref. 32).

59. Oppel, T. W.: Amer. J. Med. Sci., *204*:856, 1942.
60. Messaritakis, J., et al.: Arch. Dis. Child., *50*:871, 1975.
61. Scheiner, J., and De Ritter, E.: J. Agric. Food Chem., *23*:1157, 1978.

Folacin

62. Pfiffner, J. J., et al.: Science, *97*:404, 1943; Campbell, C. J., et al.: J. Biol. Chem., *152*:483, 1944; Stokstad, E. L. R.: J. Biol. Chem., *149*:573, 1943; Hutchings, B. L., et al.: Science, *99*:371, 1944.
63. Angier, R. B., et al.: Science, *103*:667, 1946.
64. Briggs, G. M., et al.: J. Biol. Chem., *148*:163, 1943; *158*:303, 1945; Lillie, R. J., and Briggs, G. M.: Poultry Sci., *26*:289, 1947; Nichol, C. A., et al.: J. Nutr., *39*:287, 1949.
65. Prothro, J., *et al.*: Amer. J. Clin. Nutr., *29*:94, 1976; Herbert, V., *et al.*: Amer. J. Obstet. Gynecol., *123*:175, 1975; Jacob, M., *et al.*: Amer. J. Clin. Nutr., *29*:650, 1976; Daniel, W. A., Jr., *et al.*: Amer. J. Clin. Nutr., *28*:363, 1975.
66. Lillie, R. J., and Briggs, G. M.: Poultry Sci., *26*:289, 1947; Herbert, V.: Ann. Rev. Med., *16*:359, 1965.
67. Perloff, B. P., and Butrum, R. R.: J. Amer. Dietet. Assoc., *70*:161, 1977 (also see other references listed in this paper); Butterfield, S., and Calloway, D. H.: J. Amer. Dietet. Assoc., *60*:310, 1972.

Vitamin B-12

68. Minot, G. R., and Murphy, W. P.: J.A.M.A., *87*:470, 1926.
69. Rickes, E. L., et al.: Science, *107*:396, 1948; *108*:135, 1948; Smith, E. L.: Nature, *161*:638, 1948; *162*:144, 1948.
70. West, R.: Science, *107*:398, 1948.
71. Shorb, M. S.: J. Biol. Chem., *169*:455, 1947; Science, *107*:397, 1948; Shorb, M. S., and Briggs, G. M.: J. Biol. Chem., *176*:1463, Shorb, M. S., and Briggs, G. M.: Univ. Maryland Agric. Exp. Station Bull. A-66, June, 1952.
72. Hodgkin, D. C., et al.: Nature, *176*:325, 1955; *179*:64, 1956.
73. Castle, W. B., et al.: J. Clin. Invest., *6*:2, 1928; Amer. J. Med. Sci., *178*:748, 1929; *180*:305, 1930.
74. Bird, H. R., et al.: J. Biol. Chem., *163*:387, 393, 1946; J. Nutr., *34*:233, 1947; Nestler, R. B., et al.: Poultry Sci., *15*:67, 1936.
75. Baker, S. J., et al.: Brit. Med. J., *5293*:1658, 1962.
76. Saraya, A. K., et al.: Amer. J. Clin. Nutr., *23*:1378, 1970; *24*:622, 1971.

Choline

77. Sure, B.: J. Nutr., *19*:71, 1940; György, P., and Goldblatt, H.: J. Exp. Med., *72*:1, 1940.
78. Best, C. H., and coworkers: Amer. J. Physiol., *101*:7, 1932; J. Physiol., *75*:56 and 405, 1932; *81*:409, 1934; *83*:255, 1935; *84*:38P, 1935; Biochem. J., *29*:2651, 1935; Nutr. Rev., *11*:321, 1953; Fed. Proc., *9*:506, 1950.
79. Jukes, T. H.: Nutr., *20*:445, 1940; *22*:315, 1941; Griffith, W. H., and Mulford, D. J.: Nutr., *21*:633, 1941; Hegsted, D. M., et al.: J. Biol. Chem., *138*:459, 1941.
80. Barness, L. A.: Pediatrics, *57*:278, 1976.
81. Growdon, J. H., et al.: N. Engl. J. Med., *298*:1029, 1978; Boyd, W. D., et al.: Lancet, *II*:711, 1977; Sitaram, N., Weingartner, H., and Gillin, J. C.: Science, *201*:274, 1978; Cohen, E. L., and Wurtman, R. J.: Science, *191*:561, 1976.
82. Hardinge, M. G., and Crooks, H.: J. Amer. Dietet. Assoc., *38*:240, 1961.

Other Factors

83. Yagi, K.: J. Vitamintol., *11*:14, 1965; Anderson, L., et al.: J. Nutr., *64*:167, 1958; Nutr. Rev., *14*:219, 1956.
84. Hegsted, D. M., et al.: J. Nutr., *103*:302, 1973; *104*:588, 1974.
85. Lakhanpal, R. J., et al.: J. Nutr., *89*:341, 1966; Ackerman, C. J.: J. Nutr., *89*:347, 1966; Lofgren, P. A.: Proc. Soc. Exp. Biol. Med., *147*:331, 1974; Blair, R., Scott, M. L., and Young, R. J.: J. Nutr., *102*:1529, 1972.

SUPPLEMENTARY READING

General B Complex Vitamins

(also see refs. 4, 7–14, 32, 33)

Acosta, P. B., Aranda, R. G., Lewis, J. S., and Reed, M.: Nutritional status of Mexican American preschool children in a border town. Amer. J. Clin. Nutr., *27*:1359, 1974.

Baker, H., et al.: Vitamin profile of 174 mothers and newborns at parturition. Amer. J. Clin. Nutr., *28*:59, 1975.

Baker, H., et al.: Inability of chronic alcoholics with liver disease to use food as a source of folates, thiamin and vitamin B-6. Amer. J. Clin. Nutr., *28*:1377. 1975.

Drummond, J. C.: LIX. The nomenclature of the so-called accessory food factors (vitamins). Biochem. J., *14*:1920 (reprinted in Nutr. Rev., *32*:209, 1974, a nutrition classic).

Engler, P. P., and Bowers, J. A.: B-vitamin retention in meat during storage and preparation. J. Amer. Dietet. Assoc., *69*:253, 1976.

Etheridge, E. W.: *The Butterfly Caste: A Social History of Pellagra in the South.* Westport, Conn., Greenwood Publishing Co., 1972.

Johnson, N. E., Nitzke, S., and VandeBerg, D. L.: A reporting system for nutrient adequacy. Home Econ. Res. J., *2*:210, 1974.

Kumar, M., and Axelrod, A. E.: Cellular antibody synthesis in thiamin, riboflavin, biotin, and folic acid–deficient, rats. Proc. Soc. Exp. Biol. Med., *157*:421, 1978.

Marks, J.: *A Guide to the Vitamins: Their Role in Health and Disease.* Baltimore, Md., University Park Press, 1975.

Plaut, G. W. E., Smith, C. M., and Alworth, W. L.: Biosynthesis of water-soluble vitamins. Ann. Rev. Biochem., *43*:899, 1974.

Reddy, K. P., Shahani, K. M., and Kulkarni, S. M.: B-complex vitamins in cultured and acidified yogurt. J. Dairy Sci., *59*:191, 1976.

Roe, D. A.: *A Plague of Corn: The Social History of*

Pellagra. Ithaca, N. Y., Cornell University Press, 1973.

Sims, L. S., and Morris, P. M.: Nutritional status of preschoolers. J. Amer. Dietet. Assoc., *64*:492, 1974.

Vallidevi, A., Ramanuja, M. N., Rao, N. A. N., and Nath, H.: Effect of processing and storage on the thiamins, riboflavin, and nicotinic acid contents of four varieties of Indian pulses. Ind. J. Nutr. Dietet., 9:336, 1972.

Vir, S. C., and Love, A. H. G.: Nutritional evaluation of B groups of vitamins in institutionalised aged. Internat. J. Vit. Nutr. Res., *47*:211, 1977.

Walker, M. A., and Page, L.: Nutritive content of college meals. J. Amer. Dietet. Assoc., *66*:147, 1975.

Thiamin

Reviews, Books, and History

(also see refs. 1–17 and general refs.)

Baldwin, R. S.: Robert R. Williams — a biographical sketch. J. Nutr., *105*:1, 1975.

Evans, W. C.: Thiaminases and their effects on animals. Vit. Horm., *33*:467, 1975.

Fujiwara, M., and Somogyi, J. C. (eds.): Nutritional and clinical problems of thiamine. J. Nutr. Sci. Vit., *22*:1, 1976.

Gulber, C. J., Fujiwara, M., and Dreyfus, P. M.: *Thiamine.* London, John Wiley and Sons, 1976.

Jansen, B. C. P.: Early nutritional researches on beriberi leading to the discovery of vitamin B-1. Nutr. Abstr. Rev., *26*:1, 1956.

Krampitz, L. O.: Catalytic functions of thiamin diphosphate. Ann. Rev. Biochem., *38*:213, 1969.

Peters, R. A.: The neglect of nutrition and its perils. Amer. J. Clin. Nutr., *26*:750, 1973 (some historic notes on thiamin).

Other Readings

Hathcock, J. N.: Thiamin deficiency effects on rat leukocyte pyruvate decarboxylation rates. Amer. J. Clin. Nutr., *31*:250, 1978.

Heller, S., Salkeld, R. M., and Korner, W. F.: Vitamin B-1 status in pregnancy. Amer. J. Clin. Nutr., *27*:1221, 1974.

Kjøsen, B., and Seim, S. H.: The transketolase assay of thiamine in some diseases. Amer. J. Clin. Nutr., *30*:1591, 1977.

Kramer, J., and Goodwin, J. A.: Wernicke's encephalopathy: complication of intravenous hyperalimentation. J.A.M.A., *238*:2176, 1977. Also see Blase, J. P., and Gibson, G. E.: N. Engl. J. Med., *297*:367, 1977. (Wernicke's encephalopathy is a genetic disorder responding to thiamin.)

Mesulam, M-M., Van Hoesen, G. W., and Butters, N.: Clinical manifestations of chronic thiamine deficiency in the rhesus monkey. Neurology, *27*:239, 1977.

Perry, A. K., Peters, C. R., and Van Duyne, F. O.: Effect of variety and cooking method on cooking times, thiamine content and palatability of soybeans. J. Food Sci., *41*:1330, 1976.

Sauberlich, H. E., Herman, Y. F., Stevens, C. O., and Herman, R. H.: Thiamin requirement of the adult human. Amer. J. Clin. Nutr. 1978 (in press).

Trostler, N., Guggenheim, K., Havivi, E., and Sklan, D.: Effect of thiamine deficiency in pregnant and lactating rats on the brain of their offspring. Nutr. Metab., *21*:294, 1977.

Varavithya, W., Dhanamitta, S., and Valyasevi, A.: Bilateral ptosis as a sign of thiamine deficiency in childhood. Clin. Pediatr., *14*:1063, 1975.

Vir, S. C., and Love, A. H. G.: Thiamine status of institutionalised and non-institutionalised aged. Internat. J. Vit. Nutr. Res., *47*:325, 1977.

Warnock, L. G., Nichoalds, G. E., and Burkhalter, V. J.: Erythrocyte transketolase levels in a high school student population by sex and ethnic group. Amer. J. Clin. Nutr., *27*:905, 1974.

Warnock, L. G., Prudhomme, C. R., and Wagner, C.: The determination of thiamin pyrophosphate in blood and other tissues, and its correlation with erythrocyte transketolase activity. J. Nutr., *108*:421, 1978.

Articles in **Nutrition Reviews**

Reversible inactivation of thiaminase 1 by thiamine. *32*:22, 1974.

Thiamine-responsive lactic acidosis. *32*:95, 1974.

Sulfites as food additives. *34*:58, 1976.

Leukocyte transketolase activity an indicator of thiamin nutriture. *35*:185, 1977.

Also see Nutr. Rev., *32*:304, 1974; *33*:211, 1975; *35*:238, 1977 for partial reprints of earlier classic works of Keefer, C. S. (1930); Peters, R. A., and Thompson, R. (1934); and Cline, J. K., Williams, R. R., and Finkelstein, J. (1936).

Riboflavin

(also see refs. 7–14 and 18–26)

Reviews, Books, and History

Bro-Rasmussen, F.: The riboflavin requirement of animals and man and associated metabolic relations. Nutr. Abstr. Rev., Part I, *28*:1, and Part II, *28*:369, 1958.

Rivlin, R. S.: Riboflavin and cancer: a review. Cancer Res., *33*:1977, 1973.

Rivlin, R. S. (ed.): *Riboflavin.* New York, Plenum Press, 1975.

Sebrell, W. H., and Butler, R. E.: Riboflavin deficiency in man. Pub. Health Rpt., *53*:2282, 1938 (reprinted in part in Nutr. Rev., *34*:275, 1976).

Weber, F., Glatzle, D., and Wiss, O.: The assessment of riboflavin status. Proc. Nutr. Soc., *32*:237, 1973.

Other Readings

Buzina, R., et al.: Epidemiology of angular stomatitis and bleeding gums. Internat. J. Vit. Nutr. Res., *43*:401, 1973.

Haralamble, G.: Vitamin B-2 status in athletes and the influence of riboflavin administration on neuromuscular irritability. Nutr. Metab., *20*:1, 1976.

Lakshmi, A. V., and Bamji, M. S.: Regulation of blood pyridoxal phosphate in riboflavin deficiency in man. Nutr. Metab., *20*:228, 1976.

Lopez, R., Cole, H. S., Montoya, M. F., and Cooperman, J. M.: Riboflavin deficiency in pediatric population of low socioeconomic status in New York City. J. Pediatr., *87*:420, 1975.

Sauberlich, H. E., et al.: Application of the erythrocyte glutathione reductase assay in evaluating riboflavin nutritional status in a high school student population. Amer. J. Clin. Nutr., *25*:756, 1972.

Schendel, H., and Gordon, A.: Effect of riboflavin on plasma growth hormone and serum iron in man. Amer. J. Clin. Nutr., *28*:569, 1975.

Stanko, R. T., Mendelow, H., Shinozuka, H., and Adibi, S. A.: Prevention of alcohol-induced fatty liver by natural metabolites and riboflavin. (rat studies) J. Lab. Clin. Med., *91*:228, 1978.

Steier, M., Lopez, R., and Cooperman, J. M.: Riboflavin deficiency in infants and children with heart disease. Amer. Heart J., *92*:139, 1976.

Sterner, R. T., and Price, W. R.: Restricted riboflavin: within-subject behavioral effects in humans. Amer. J. Clin. Nutr., *26*:150, 1973.

Articles in Nutrition Reviews

Riboflavin deficiency in complicated chronic alcoholism. *26*:858, 1973.

The fate of riboflavin in the mammal (by McCormick, D. B.). *30*:75, 1972 (also see *31*:104, 1973).

Erythrocyte glutathione reductase — a measure of riboflavin nutritional status. *30*:162, 1972.

Riboflavin and adrenal cortex. *31*:95, 1973.

Riboflavin metabolism in cancer. *32*:308, 1974.

Riboflavin deficiency, galactose metabolism and cataract. *34*:77, 1976.

The interrelationship between riboflavin and pyridoxine. *35*:237, 1977.

Urinary and serum flavin levels. *36*: 210, 1978.

Pantothenic Acid

(also see refs. 7–14 and 27–33)

History, Books, and Reviews

Krehl, W. A.: Pantothenic acid in nutrition: a review. Nutr. Rev., *11*:225, 1953.

Novelli, G. D.: Metabolic functions of pantothenic acid. Physiol. Rev., *33*:525, 1953.

Sebrell, W. H., Jr., and Harris, R. S. (eds.): Pantothenic acid. In *The Vitamins*, Chapter 11, p. 589. New York, Academic Press, 1954.

Other Readings

Calloway, D. H., and Gibbs, J. C.: Food patterns and food assistance programs in the Cocopah Indian community (a study of pantothenic acid and other vitamins at risk). Ecol. Food Nutr., 5:183, 1976.

Cohenour, S. H., and Calloway, D. H.: Blood, urine, and dietary pantothenic acid levels of pregnant teenagers. Amer. J. Clin. Nutr., *25*:512, 1972.

Hamm, D. J., and Lund, D. B.: Kinetic parameters for thermal inactivation of pantothenic acid. J. Food Sci., *43*:631, 1978.

Hoppner, K., and Lampi, B.: Total pantothenic acid in strained baby foods. Nutr. Rpts. Internat., *15*:627, 1977.

Lederer, W. H., Kumar, M., and Axelrod, A. E.: Effects of pantothenic acid deficiency on cellular synthesis in rats. J. Nutr., *105*:17, 1975.

Mahboob, S., and Estes, L. W.: Effect of pantothenic acid deficiency on rat hepatocytes. Nutr. Metab., *22*:177, 1978.

Srinivasan, V., and Belavady, B.: Nutritional status of pantothenic acid in Indian pregnant and nursing women. Internat. J. Vit. Nutr. Res., *46*:433. 1976.

Tao, H. G., and Fox, H. M.: Measurements of urinary pantothenic acid excretions of alcoholic patients. J. Nutr. Sci. Vitaminol., *22*:333, 1976.

Articles in Nutrition Reviews

Malonyl-CoA and fatty acid synthesis. *31*:129, 1973.

Vitamin level at term in the neonate. *33*:298, 1975.

Reminiscences on the discovery and significance of some of the B vitamins. (By György, P.) A nutrition classic from J. Nutr. (Suppl. II), *91*:5, 1967, and Nutr. Rev., *34*:141, 1976.

Niacin

(also see refs. 7–14 and 33–44)

Reviews, Books, and History

Goldsmith, G. A.: Niacin: antipellagra factor, hypocholesterolemic agent. J.A.M.A., *194*:167, 1965.

Gopalan, C., and Kamala, S. J. R.: Pellagra and amino acid imbalance. Vit. Horm., *33*:505, 1975.

Horwitt, M. K., Harvey, C. C., Rothwell, W. S., Cutler, J. L., and Haffron, D.: Tryptophan-niacin relationships in man. (Studies with diets deficient in riboflavin and niacin, together with observations on the excretion of nitrogen and niacin metabolites.) J. Nutr., *60*:1, 1956.

Sydenstricker, V. P.: The history of pellagra; its recognition as a disorder of nutrition and its conquest. Amer. J. Clin. Nutr., *6*:409, 1958.

Niacin-Tryptophan Relationships

Consolazio, C. F., Johnson, H. L., Krzywicki, H. J., and Witt, N. F.: Tryptophan-niacin interrelationships during acute fasting and caloric restriction in humans. Amer. J. Clin. Nutr., *25*:572, 1972.

Nakagawa, I., et al.: Efficiency of conversion of tryptophan to niacin in humans. J. Nutr., *103*:1195, 1973.

Nakagawa, I., et al.: Effects of excess intake of leucine and valine deficiency on tryptophan and niacin metabolites in humans. J. Nutr., *105*:1241, 1975.

Payne, I. R., Walsh, E. M., and Whittenburg, E. J. R.: Relationship of dietary tryptophan and niacin to tryptophan metabolism in schizophrenics and non schizophrenics. Amer. J. Clin. Nutr., *27*:565, 1974.

Payne, I. R., Lu, G. H. Y., and Meyer, K.: Relationship of dietary tryptophan and niacin to tryptophan metabolism in alcoholics and nonalcoholics. Amer. J. Clin. Nutr., *27*:572, 1974.

Other Readings

Baker, D. H., et al.: Niacin activity in niacinamide and coffee. Nutr. Rpts. Internat., *14*:115, 1976.

Duke, M. L., Kies, C., and Fox, H. M.: Niacin and pantothenic acid excretions of humans fed a low-methionine, plant-based diet. J. Nutr. Sci. Vitaminol., *23*:481, 1977.

Ghafoorunissa, and Rao, B. S. N.: Plasma amino acid pattern in pellagra. Amer. J. Clin. Nutr., *28*:325, 1975.

Mehta, S. K., et al.: Small intestinal deficit in pellagra. Amer. J. Clin. Nutr., *25*:545, 1972.

Miller, D. F.: Pellagra deaths in the United States. Amer. J. Clin. Nutr., *31*:558, 1978.

Mrochek, J. E., Jolley, R. L., Young, D. S., and Turner, W. J.: Metabolic response of humans to ingestion of nicotinic acid and nicotinamide. Clin. Chem., *22*:1821, 1976.

Articles in Nutrition Reviews

Utilization of niacin and niacinamide for NAD formation in rat liver. *30*:139, 1972.

Niacin and myocardial metabolism. *31*:80, 1973.

Conversion of tryptophan to niacin in man. *32*:76, 1974.

Hepatic toxicity of nicotinamide. *32*:94, 1974.

Forms of bound niacin in wheat. *32*:124, 1974.

Niacin (by Darby, W. J., McNutt, K. W., and Todhunter, E. N.). *33*:289, 1975; (also see *33*:310, 1975).

Corn malnutrition, brain serotonin and behavior (by Fernstrom, J. D., and Lytle, L. D.). *34*:257, 1956.

(Also see partial reprints of classic papers on the discovery of niacin in Nutr. Rev., *31*:152, and *31*:184, 1973 (by Goldberger, J.); and *32*:48, 1974 (by Elvehjem, C. A., et al.)

Vitamin B-6

(also see refs. 7, 9, and 45–55)

Reviews, History, and Books

György, P.: *The History of Vitamin B-6*. Vit. Horm., *22*:361, 1964.

György, P.: Developments leading to the metabolic role of vitamin B-6. Amer. J. Clin. Nutr., *24*:1250, 1971.

Holtz, P., and Palm, D.: Pharmacological aspects of vitamin B-6. Pharmacol. Rev., *16*:113, 1974.

Munro, H. N. (Chairman): *Human Vitamin B-6 Requirements*. Committee on Dietary Allowances, Food and Nutrition Board, National Research Council, National Academy of Sciences, Washington, D.C., 1978.

Oral Contraceptives and Vitamin B-6

Driskell, J. A., Geders, J. M., and Urban, M. C.: Vitamin B-6 status of young men, women, and women using oral contraceptives. J. Lab. Clin. Med., *87*:813, 1976.

Leklem, J. E., et al.: Metabolism of methionine in oral contraceptive users and control women receiving controlled intakes of vitamin B-6. Amer. J. Clin. Nutr., *30*:1122, 1977. (Also see earlier papers from this laboratory on this subject in Amer. J. Clin. Nutr., *28*:10, *28*:146, and *28*:872, 1975.)

Lumeng, L., Cleary, R. E., and Li, T-K.: Effect of oral contraceptives on the plasma concentration of pyridoxal phosphate. Amer. J. Clin. Nutr., *27*:326, 1974.

Miller, L. T., Dow, M. J., and Kokkeler, S. C.: Methionine metabolism and vitamin B-6 status in women using oral contraceptives. Amer. J. Clin. Nutr., *31*:619, 1978. (Also see Amer. J. Clin. Nutr., *27*:797, 1974, and *28*:846, 1975.)

Shane, B., and Contractor, S. F.: Assessment of vitamin B-6 status. Studies on pregnant women and oral contraceptive users. Amer. J. Clin. Nutr., *28*:739, 1975.

Brain and Vitamin B-6

Alton-Mackey, M. G., and Valker, B. L.: Physical and neuromotor development of progeny of pyridoxine-restricted rats cross-fostered with control or isonutritional dams. Amer. J. Clin. Nutr., *31*:241, 1978. (Also see Amer. J. Clin. Nutr., *26*:420, 1973, and *31*:76, 1978.)

Driskell, J. A., and Chuang, S-L. L.: Relationship between glutamic decarboxylase activities in brains and the vitamin B-6 requirement of male rats. J. Nutr., *104*:1657, 1974.

Kurtz, D. J., Levy, H., and Kanfer, J. N.: Cerebral lipids and amino acids in the vitamin B-6–deficient suckling rat. J. Nutr., *102*:291, 1972.

Stewart, C. N., Coursin, D. B., and Bhagavan, H. N.: Cortical-evoked responses in pyridoxine-deficient rats. J. Nutr., *103*:462, 1973.

Thomas, M. R., and Kirksey, A.: Postnatal patterns of brain lipids in progeny of vitamin B-6 deficient rats before and after pyridoxine supplementation. J. Nutr., *106*:1404, 1976. (Also see J. Nutr., *104*:111, 1974, and *106*:680, 1976 for similar studies from this laboratory.)

Other Readings

Bapurao, S., and Krishnaswamy, K.: Vitamin B-6 nutritional status of pellagrins and their leucine tolerance. Amer. J. Clin. Nutr., *31*:819, 1978.

Engler, P. P., and Bowers, J. A.: Vitamin B-6 in reheated, held and freshly cooked turkey breast. J. Amer. Dietet., *67*:42, 1975.

Hampton, D. J., Chrisley, B. M., and Driskell, J. A.: Vitamin B-6 status of the elderly in Montgomery County, Virginia. Nutr. Rpts. Internat., *16*:743, 1977.

Heller, S., Salkeld, R. M., and Korner, W. F.: Vitamin B-6 status in pregnancy. Amer. J. Clin. Nutr., *26*:1339, 1978.

Hunter, J. E., and Harper, A. E.: Induction of pyridoxal phosphate–dependent enzymes in vitamin B-6 deficient rats. J. Nutr., *107*:235, 1977.

Kirksey, A., Keaton, K., Abernathy, R. P., and Greger, J. L.: Vitamin B-6 nutritional status of a group of female adolescents. Amer. J. Clin. Nutr., *31*:946, 1978.

Lewis, J. S., and Nunn, K. P.: Vitamin B-6 and 4-pyridoxic acid of children. Amer. J. Clin. Nutr., *30*:2023, 1977.
Nelson, E. W., Jr., Lane, H., and Cerda, J. J.: Comparative human intestinal bioavailability of vitamin B-6 from a synthetic and a natural source. J. Nutr., *106*:1433, 1976.
Potera, C., Rose, D. P., and Brown, R. R.: Vitamin B-6 deficiency in cancer patients. Amer. J. Clin. Nutr., *30*:1677, 1977.
Reinken, L., Zieglauer, H., and Berger, H.: Vitamin B-6 nutriture of children with acute celiac disease, celiac disease in remission, and of children with normal duodenal mucosa. Amer. J. Clin. Nutr., *29*:750, 1976.
Rose, C. S., et al.: Age differences in vitamin B-6 status of 617 men. Amer. J. Clin. Nutr., *29*:847, 1976.
Shin, H. K., and Linkwiler, H. M.: Tryptophan and methionine metabolism of adult females as affected by vitamin B-6 deficiency. J. Nutr., *104*:1348, 1974.
Stone, W. J., Warnock, L. G., and Wagner, C.: Vitamin B-6 deficiency in uremia. Amer. J. Clin. Nutr., *28*:950, 1975.
Vir, S. C., and Love, A. H. G.: Vitamin B-6 status of institutionalised and non-institutionalised aged. Internat. J. Vit. Nutr. Res., *47*:364, 1977.

Articles in Nutrition Reviews

Metabolism of vitamin B-6 in the pregnant rat. *30*:44, 1972.
Conversion of vitamin B-6 in human red blood cells. *30*:119, 1972.
Vitamin B-6 deficiency and brain lipids in the suckling rat. *30*:183, 1972.
Oral contraceptives and vitamin B-6. *31*:49, 1973.
Central nervous system changes in deficiency of vitamin B-6 and other B-complex vitamins. *33*:21, 1975.
Regulation of liver metabolism of pyridoxal phosphate. *33*:214, 1975.
Requirement of vitamin B-6 during pregnancy. *34*:15, 1976.
In what form does vitamin B-6 exist in plasma? *34*:40, 1976.
Pyridoxine and its metabolism in chronic liver disease. *35*:134, 1977.
Phosphorylase response to vitamin B-6 feeding. *36*:55, 1978.

Biotin

(also see refs. 7 and 56–61)

Reviews, History, and Books

Belnave, D.: Clinical symptoms of biotin deficiency in animals: a review. Amer. J. Clin. Nutr., *30*:1408, 1978.
Bonjour, J. P.: Biotin in man's nutrition and therapy: a review. Internat. J. Vit. Nutr. Res., *47*:107, 1977.
Knappe, J.: Mechanism of biotin action. Ann. Rev. Biochem., *39*:757, 1970.
Wood, H. G., and Barden, R. E.: Biotin enzymes. Ann. Rev. Biochem., *46*:385, 1977.

Other Readings

Bhagavan, H. N., and Coursin, D. B.: *In vivo* incorporation of glucose carbon into brain and liver proteins in biotin-deficient rats. J. Nutr. Sci. Vitaminol., *22*:79, 1976.
Klevay, L. M.: The biotin requirement of rats fed 20 per cent egg white. J. Nutr., *106*:1643, 1976.
Marshall, M. W., et al.: Biotin status and lipid metabolism in adult obese hypercholesterolemic inbred rats. Nutr. Metabol., *20*:41, 1976.
Stallings, W. C.: The carboxylation of biotin. Arch. Biochem. Biophys., *183*:189, 1977.
Travis, S., Mathias, M. M., and Dupont, J.: Effect of biotin deficiency on the catabolism of linoleate in the rat. J. Nutr., *102*:767, 1972.

Articles in Nutrition Reviews

Present knowledge of biotin (by Bridges, W. F.). *25*:65, 1967.
Biotin and protein biosynthesis. *29*:93, 1971.
Biotin (by McCormick, D. B.). *33*:97, 1975.
A role of biotin in fatty liver and kidney syndrome in chicks. *34*:217, 1976.

Folacin

(also see refs. 7, 13, and 62–67)

Reviews, History and Books

Babior, B. M.: Folate and aplasia of bone marrow. N. Engl. J. Med., *298*:506, 1978.
Food and Nutrition Board: *Folic Acid: Biochemistry and Physiology in Relation to the Human Nutrition Requirement: A Review.* National Academy of Science, Dept. JH 726, Washington, D.C., 1978.
Herbert, V.: Folic acid deficiency in man: a review. Vit. Horm., *26*:525, 1968.
Herbert, V., and others: Symposium: Folic acid deficiency: a review. Amer. J. Clin. Nutr., *23*:841, 1970.
Malin, J. D.: Folic acid. World Rev. Nutr. Dietet., *21*:198, 1975.
Norris, J. W., and Pratt, R. F.: Folic acid deficiency and epilepsy. Drugs, *8*:366, 1974.
Rosenberg, I. H.: Folate absorption and malabsorption. N. Engl. J. Med., *293*:1303, 1975.
Stokstad, E. L. R., and Koch, J.: Folic acid metabolism: a review. Physiol. Rev., *47*:83, 1967.

Availability from Food

Babu, S., and Srikantia, S. G.: Availability of folates from some foods. Amer. J. Clin. Nutr., *29*:376, 1976.
Grossowicz, N., Rachmilewitz, M., and Izak, G.: Absorption of pteroylglutamate and dietary folates in man. Amer. J. Clin. Nutr., *25*:1135, 1972.
Kaunitz, J. D., and Lindenbaum, J.: The bioavailability of folic acid added to wine. Ann. Intern. Med., *87*:542, 1977.
Racusen, L. C., and Krawitt, E. L.: Effect of folate deficiency and ethanol ingestion on intestinal folate absorption. Amer. J. Dig. Dis., *22*:915, 1977.

Russell, R. M., Ismail-Beigi, F., and Reinhold, J. G.: Folate content of Iranian breads and the effect of their fiber content on intestinal absorption of folic acid. Amer. J. Clin. Nutr., *29*:799, 1976.

Tamura, T., Shin, Y, S., Buehring, K. U., and Stokstad, E. L. R.: The availability of folates in man: effect of orange juice supplement on intestinal conjugase. Brit. J. Haematol., *32*:123, 1976.

Tamura, T., and Stokstad, E. L. R.: The availability of food folate in man. Brit. J. Haematol., *25*:513, 1973.

Other Readings

Akinsete, F. I., and Boyo, A. E.: Studies on folic acid in Nigerian infants and pre-school children. Environ. Child Hlth., *23*:202, 1977.

Asfour, R., et al.: Folacin requirement of children. III. Normal infants. Amer. J. Clin. Nutr., *30*:1098, 1977.

Baker, H., et al.: Inability of chronic alcoholics with liver disease to use food as a source of folates, thiamin and vitamin B-6. Amer. J. Clin. Nutr., *28*:1377, 1975.

Batra, K. K., Wagner, J. R., and Stokstad, E. L. R.: Folic acid compounds in romaine lettuce. Can. J. Biochem., *55*:865, 1977.

Colman, N., et al.: Prevention of folate deficiency by food fortification. IV. Identification of target groups in addition to pregnant women in an adult rural population. Amer. J. Clin. Nutr., *28*:471, 1975.

Hall, C. A., et al.: Variation in plasma folate levels among groups of healthy persons. Amer. J. Clin. Nutr., *28*:854, 1975.

Parker, S. L., and Bowering, J.: Folacin in diets of Puerto Rican and black women in relation to food practices. J. Nutr. Ed., *8*:73, 1976.

Pietarinen, G. J., Leichter, L., and Pratt, R. F.: Dietary folate intake and concentration of folate in serum and erythrocytes in women using oral contraceptives. Amer. J. Clin. Nutr., *30*:375, 1977.

Russell, R. M., et al.: Folate levels among various populations in central Iran. Amer. J. Clin. Nutr., *29*:794, 1976.

Wu, A., Chanarin, I., Slavin, G., and Levi, A. J.: Folate deficiency in the alcoholic — its relationship to clinical and haematological abnormalities, liver disease and folate stores. Brit. J. Haematol., *29*:469, 1975.

Articles in Nutrition Reviews

Present knowledge of folacin (by Vitale, J. J.). *24*:289, 1966.

Intestinal absorption of folates. *30*:179, 1972.

Folate polyglutamates in rat liver. *30*:243, 1972.

Folic acid absorption, anticonvulsant and contraceptive therapy. *32*:39, 1974.

Cerebrospinal folate levels in epileptics and their response to folate therapy. *32*:70, 1974.

The availability of food folate in man. *32*:167, 1974.

Forms of folate in the monkey. *32*:212, 1974.

Folate binder in leukocytes and serum. *33*:9, 1975.

The small intestine in vitamin B-12 and folate deficiency (by Halsted, C. H.). *33*:33, 1975.

Folic acid metabolism in vitamin B-12 deficiency. *33*:118, 1975.

Lengths of poly-gamma-glutamyl chains in natural folate. *33*:115, 1975.

Folic acid, ethanol and jejunal glycolysis. *34*:73, 1976.

Pterin-6-aldehyde production from folic acid by malignant tissues. *35*:169, 1977.

Intestinal enzymes in folate deficiency and tropical sprue. *36*:135, 1978.

Folate-losing gastropathy in giant hypertrophic gastritis. *36*:185, 1978.

Methionine and the "methyl folate trap." *36*:255, 1978.

Vitamin B-12

(also see refs. 7, 9, and 68–76)

Reviews, History, and Books

Babior, B. M. (ed.): *Cobalamin:Biochemistry and Pathophysiology*. New York, John Wiley and Sons, Inc., 1975.

Baker, S. J.: Human vitamin B-12 deficiency. World Rev. Nutr. Dietet., *8*:62, 1967.

Herbert, V., and Das, K. C.: The role of vitamin B-12 and folic acid in hemato- and other cell-poiesis. Vit. Horm., *34*:1, 1976.

Smith, L.: *Vitamin B-12*. New York, John Wiley and Sons, Inc., 1965.

Stadtman, T. C.: Vitamin B-12. Science, *171*:859, 1971.

Weissbach, H., and Taylor, R. T.: Metabolic role of vitamin B-12. Vit. Horm., *26*:395, 1968.

Other Readings

Abe, T., Gibbs, B., and Cooper, B. A.: Forms of vitamin B-12 in blood and bone marrow in patients with pernicious anaemia. Brit. J. Haematol., *31*:493, 1975.

Adams, J. F., McEwan, F., and Wilson, A.: The vitamin B-12 content of meals and items of diet. Brit. J. Nutr., *29*:65, 1973.

Armstrong, B. K., et al.: Hematological, vitamin B-12, and folate studies on Seventh-Day Adventist vegetarians. Amer. J. Clin. Nutr., *27*:712, 1974.

Cullen, P. W., and Oace, S. M.: Methylmalonic acid and vitamin B-12 excretion of rats consuming diets varying in cellulose and pectin. J. Nutr., *108*:640, 1978.

Dastur, D. K., et al.: Interrelationships between the B-vitamins in B-12–deficiency neuromyelopathy. A possible malabsorption-malnutrition syndrome. Amer. J. Clin. Nutr., *28*:1255, 1975.

Doscherholmen, A., McMahon, J., and Ripley, D.: Vitamin B-12 assimilation from chicken meat. Amer. J. Clin. Nutr., *31*:825, 1978.

Ellis, F. R., and Nasser S.: A pilot study of vitamin B-12 in the treatment of tiredness. Brit. J. Nutr., *30*:277, 1973.

Farquharson, J., and Adams, J. F.: The forms of vitamin B-12 in foods. Brit. J. Nutr., *36*:127, 1976.

Herbert, V.: The five possible causes of all nutrient deficiency: illustrated by deficiencies of vita-

min B-12 and folic acid. Amer. J. Clin. Nutr., *26*:77, 1973.
Jacob, E., Herbert, V., and Wong, K.-T. J.: Low serum vitamin B-12 levels in patients receiving ascorbic acid in megadoses: studies concerning the effect of ascorbate on radioisotope vitamin B-12 assay. Amer. J. Clin. Nutr., *31*:253, 1978.
Kark, J. A., Victor, M., Hines, J. D., and Harris, J. W.: Nutritional vitamin B-12 deficiency in rhesus monkeys. Amer. J. Clin. Nutr., *27*:470, 1974.
McCurdy, P. R.: B-12 shots. J.A.M.A., *229*:703, 1974. (Also see J.A.M.A., *231*:289, 1975.)
Newmark, H. L., Scheiner, J., Marcus, M., and Prabhudesai, M.: Stability of vitamin B-12 in the presence of ascorbic acid. Amer. J. Clin. Nutr., *29*:645, 1976.
Santini, R., and Millán, S.: Serum vitamin B-12 levels in Puerto Rico. Amer. J. Clin. Nutr., *29*:689, 1976.
Siddons, R. C., and Jacob, F.: Vitamin B-12 nutrition and metabolism in the baboon. Brit. J. Nutr., *33*:415, 1975.
Tseng, R. Y. L., Cohen, N. L., Reyes, P. S., and Briggs, G. M.: Metabolic changes in golden hamsters fed vitamin B-12 deficient diets. J. Nutr., *106*:77, 1976.

Articles in Nutrition Reviews

The pancreas and vitamin B-12 absorption. *30*:181, 1972.
Rare forms of familial vitamin B-12 malabsorption in children. *31*:149, 1973.
Serum vitamin B-12 binders and human marrow cell uptake of ^{57}Co-vitamin B-12. *31*:277, 1973.
A qualitative platelet defect in severe vitamin B-12 deficiency. *32*:202, 1974.
Abnormal fatty acid synthesis associated with faulty utilization of vitamin B-12. *32*:204, 1974.
Effect of vitamin B-12 deprivation on CoA intermediates related to propionate metabolism. *33*:85, 1975.
Folic acid metabolism in vitamin B-12 deficiency. *33*:118, 1975.
Pernicious anemia and mental dysfunction. *34*:264, 1976.
Origin and function of human plasma R-type vitamin B-12 binding proteins. *34*:148, 1976.
Vegetarian diet and vitamin B-12 deficiency. *36*:24, 1978.
(Also see partial reprints of classic early papers by Minot, Murphy, Castle, Wills, and others reprinted in Nutr. Rev., *36*:50, *36*:80, *36*:113, *36*:149, *36*:245, *36*:246, 1978.

Choline

(also see refs. 7 and 77–82)

Reviews, History, and Books

Barak, A. J., Tuma, D. J., and Sorrell, M. F.: Relationship of ethanol to choline metabolism in the liver. A review. Amer. J. Clin. Nutr., *26*:1234, 1973.
Fernstrom, J. D.: Effects of the diet on brain neurotransmitters. Metabolism, *26*:207, 1977.
Harris, R. S. (ed.): *The Vitamins*. Volume III. New York, Academic Press, 1971.
Lucas, C. C., and Ridout, J. H.: Fatty livers and lipotropic phenomena. In Holman, R. T. (ed.): *Progress in the Chemistry of Fats and Other Lipids*. Volume 10, Part 1. Oxford, Pergamon Press, 1967.

Other Readings

Baker, H.: Assay for free and total choline activity in biological fluids and tissues of rats and man with Torulopsis pintolopessi. Amer. J. Clin. Nutr., *31*:532, 1978.
Carroll, C., and Williams, L.: Influence of dietary fat on fatty livers of choline-deficient rats. J. Nutr., *107*:1263, 1977.
Haubrich, D. R., Wang, P. F. L., Chippendale, T., and Proctor, E.: Choline and acetylcholine in rats: effect of dietary choline. J. Neurochem., *27*:1305, 1976.
Hirsch, M. J., Growdon, J. H., and Wurtman, R. J.: Relations between dietary choline or lecithin intake serum choline levels, and various metabolic indices. Metabolism, *27*:953, 1978.
Keith, M. O., and Tryphonas, L.: Choline deficiency and the reversibility of renal lesions in rats. J. Nutr., *108*:434, 1978.
Monserrat, A. J., Porta, E. A., Ghoshal, A. K., and Hartman, S. B.: Sequential renal lipid changes in weanling rats fed a choline-deficient diet. J. Nutr., *104*:1496, 1974.
Wecker, L., Dettbarn, W.-D., and Schmidt, D. E.: Choline administration: modification of the central actions of atropine. Science, *199*:86, 1978.

Articles in Nutrition Reviews

Lipotropes and fetal growth. *29*:23, 1971.
Choline (by Kuksis, A., and Mookerjea, S.). *36*:201, 1978.
(Also see reprints, in part, of classic papers by Griffith, W. H., duVigneaud, V., and coworkers in Nutr. Rev. *32*:112, and *32*:144, 1974.)

Carnitine and Other Factors

Readings

Andersen, D. B., and Holub, B. J.: The influence of dietary inositol in glyceride composition and synthesis in livers of rats fed different fats. J. Nutr., *106*:529, 1976.
Burton, L. E., and Wells, W. W.: Characterization of the lactation-dependent fatty liver in *myo*-inositol deficient rats. J. Nutr., *107*:187, 1977.
Knopf, K., Sturman, J. A., Armstrong, M., and Hayes, K. C.: Taurine: an essential nutrient for the cat. J. Nutr., *108*:773, 1978.
Mitchell, M. E.: Carnitine metabolism in human subjects. 11. Values of carnitine in biological fluids and tissues of "normal" subjects. Amer. J. Clin. Nutr., *31*:481, 1978. (Also see *31*:293, 1978).
Rigo, J., and Senterre, J.: Is taurine essential for the neonates? Biol. Neonate, *32*:73, 1977.

Shug, A. L., et al.: Changes in tissue levels of carnitine and other metabolites during myocardial ischemia and anoxia. Arch. Biochem. Biophys., *187*:25, 1978.

Tanphaichitr, V., and Broquist, H. P.: Site of carnitine biosynthesis in the rat. J. Nutr., *104*:1669, 1974.

Tsai, A. C., Romsos, D. R., and Leveille, G. A.: Determination of carnitine turnover in choline-deficient and cold-exposed rats. J. Nutr., *105*:301, 1975.

Articles in Nutrition Reviews

Formation of carnitine from lysine in the rat. *30*:117, 1972.

Intestinal lipodystrophy, serum cholesterol levels and inositol deficiency in gerbils. *32*:210, 1974.

Inositol (by Kuksis, A., and Mookerjea, S.). *36*:233, 1978.

Chapter 9

Vitamin C (Ascorbic Acid)

Vitamin C is the very important scurvy-preventing substance found in nature primarily in citrus and other fruits and in fresh vegetables. It has a most interesting history.

The Saga of Scurvy

Serious cases of scurvy, a disease due to prolonged lack of vitamin C, are seldom seen now but the story of its incidence and conquest is of great interest. It led to the discovery that a disease could be caused by lack of some intangible component of the diet and to the eventual isolation of the lacking substance as a vitamin. This is one of the most fascinating stories of achievement in the development of nutrition as a science.*

Scurvy is one of the oldest diseases of mankind; early descriptions are known to exist as far back as about 1500 B.C. Symptoms of gangrene of the gums, loss of teeth, and painful legs in soldiers were described by Hippocrates (about 450 B.C.), and from records of the crusaders, it is evident that they too suffered from scurvy. In the 15th and 16th centuries, it was a scourge throughout Europe, so much so that medical men wondered if all disease might be outgrowths of scurvy. It was particularly prevalent and severe on long voyages of sailing ships, in besieged cities, and in times of crop failures — in short, wherever fresh foods were unavailable. When Vasco de Gama made his long voyage around the Cape of Good Hope, nearly two-thirds of his crew perished from scurvy. The lives of many of the men with the explorer Cartier, when obliged to spend the winter of 1535 in Canada, were saved because they learned from the Indians that a "brew" made from the growing tips of the spruce and other trees was a cure for this malady. (It is obvious now that the "brew" contained vitamin C.)

In 1753, James Lind, a Scottish naval surgeon, published his famous report of experiments made on ships of the British Navy, proving that oranges and lemons prevented or cured the disease.[1] His classic studies generally are considered the first experiments to show that an essential food element can prevent a deficiency disease. The experiences of Lind, Cartier, and others gradually became well known, so that by the time of the historic voyage of Captain Cook (1772–1775), enough was known about the prevention of scurvy to stock the ship with fresh fruits and vegetables at every port visited, thereby keeping captain and crew well throughout the long trip. Cook[2] also recognized that sauerkraut was *antiscorbutic* (prevented

*Persons interested in more detail on this subject will find a list of general references on the history of vitamin C at the end of this chapter.

scurvy) and supplied the ship with large quantities of it, stating that it is "not only a wholesome vegetable food, but, in my judgment, highly antiscorbutic, and spoils not by keeping." It was not until 1795, however, that citrus fruits (lime juice) were made a regulation on ships of the British Navy, providing British sailors with the nickname "limeys."

The explorers of the New World took the potato to Europe and, as potatoes (a good source of vitamin C) became a food staple there, scurvy disappeared. Epidemics of scurvy reappeared on several occasions after disastrous failures of the potato crop in certain regions, as in Norway and in Ireland. While it become generally recognized that citrus fruits and fresh vegetables were preventives against scurvy, nearly 150 years elapsed before the potency of these foods was explained as due to the presence in them of a specific substance known as a vitamin.

Chemical Identification and Properties

By the late 1910's it became clear that there were at least three distinct nutritional deficiencies in man and animals (see Chapter 6). Scurvy had been known for centuries, but as the vitamins were identified, "vitamin C" was arbitrarily given third place in the vitamin alphabet (chiefly because McCollum, who started the use of alphabet letters, was working with rats, which do not get scurvy!).

In 1912, the terms "scurvy vitamine" and "antiscorbutin" were first used in the literature for the scurvy-preventing substance.[3] The first use of the letter "C" for the antiscorbutic factor (or water-soluble C") was in 1918 and 1919 by British workers.[4] This led directly to the use in 1921 of "vitamin C" for the substance by Santos and others,[5] following Drummond's suggestion of combining the word "vitamin" with the letters then in use.[6]

In 1928, Szent-Györgyi, a Hungarian scientist now living in the United States, first isolated what is now known as ascorbic acid (he called it "hexuronic acid") from oranges, cabbages, and adrenal glands,[7] although it was not recognized as vitamin C and was not tried in the treatment of scurvy. In 1932, King and Waugh[8] isolated from lemon juice a crystalline material that possessed antiscorbutic activity in guinea pigs. They found that their compound was identical with the substance isolated by Szent-Györgyi (who, as a result, in 1933 called it *ascorbic acid,* a shortened form of the "*antiscorbutic* factor"[9]). Shortly afterward, the structure of L-ascorbic acid was announced, and it was synthesized in the laboratory, starting with the sugar galactose and later with glucose (Fig. 9–1).

Ascorbic acid is a relatively simple organic acid with six carbon atoms in each molecule, and has a structure fairly similar to the simple six-carbon sugars (see formula in the Appendix). It is the most unstable of all the known vitamins, as it is *easily oxidized* by the loss of two hydrogen atoms per molecule to a substance called *dehydroascorbic acid.* Both forms have vitamin C activity,* although dehydroascorbic acid has only about 80 percent of the biological activity of ascorbic acid. Dehydroascorbic acid can be readily converted in the body to ascorbic acid by reduction (adding hydrogen). Thus both the ascorbic acid and the dehydroascorbic acid in foods contribute to the vitamin C activity in the body. In living plant and animal tissues, this oxidation-reduction between the two substances is *reversible.* When dehydroascorbic acid is further oxidized, however, it loses its vitamin C activity, and the reaction is not reversible — that is, it cannot be reduced to form dehydroascorbic acid again.

---

*International Union of Nutritional Sciences Nomenclature Rules (1976) uses the term *vitamin C* for the combined name of all compounds that exhibit the biological activity of ascorbic acid. Thus, "vitamin C activity" and "vitamin C deficiency" are preferred terms. The term "ascorbic acid" is to be used only for that specific chemical compound, one of several compounds in foods with vitamin C activity.

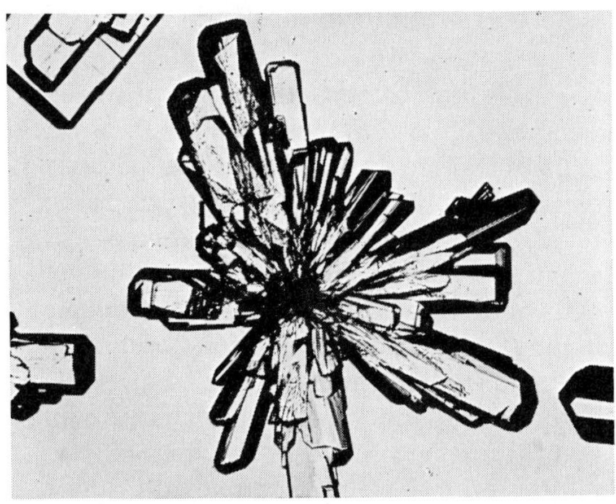

Figure 9–1 Photomicrograph showing crystalline structure of pure ascorbic acid. (Courtesy of Merck & Company.)

The oxidation of ascorbic acid in foods is hastened by an enzyme (ascorbic acid oxidase) that is present in raw fruits and vegetables and that becomes active when leaves or fruits are damaged by drying, bruising, or cutting. In the intact plant, this enzyme is inoperative. Considerable loss of vitamin C activity occurs with the use of heat, alkalis, and catalysts such as copper (e.g., use of copper kettles). Its destruction is slowed down in foods that are acid, by refrigeration, and above all by protection from exposure to air.

Effects of Lack of Vitamin C in Man and Animals

Effects of Acute Lack. The effects of an acute lack of vitamin C have been thoroughly studied by Hodges, Baker, Sauberlich, and others.[10] Five male prisoners volunteered to be placed on a liquid vitamin C–deficient diet for 84 to 97 days. The first symptoms of deficiency seen were *fatigue, rough skin (hyperkeratosis), pink or hemorrhagic skin follicles* (see Fig. 9–2), *hemorrhages in the eye, coiled hairs, and gum changes, followed by pains in the joints, changes in the salivary and tear glands, loss of dental fillings, dental caries, tender mouth, dryness and itching of skin, and excessive loss of hair.* The skin changes were noted as early as 29 days, several weeks before the occurrence of swollen and bleeding gums, contrary to common beliefs. Giving vitamin C overcame all the symptoms eventually (after 3 to 10 weeks).

Acute scurvy presents such a dramatic picture of degeneration in many body tissues (skin, teeth and gums, blood vessel walls, bones, cartilage and muscle tissues) that it is not difficult to recognize. Because these severe symptoms are prevented by taking even moderate amounts of fresh or cooked fruits and vegetables, full-blown scurvy is very seldom encountered.

Effects of Moderate Lack. A condition with less severe symptoms, known as *subacute* or *latent scurvy,* still occurs (though infrequently) among infants fed almost exclusively on heat-treated milk or cereal gruels, when sources of vitamin C are not used or are unobtainable. A deficiency shows up in persons when intake is just below the borderline of sufficiency, when there is greater need of the vitamin (as in growth), or when there are conditions of physiological stress or infection.

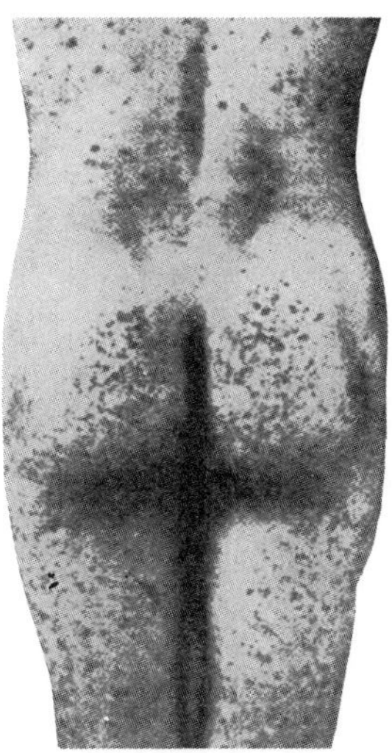

Figure 9–2 A typical case of adult scurvy, showing the numerous petechiae—spots where blood has effused to the skin. (From L. J. Harris: *Vitamins in Theory and Practice.* New York, Macmillan Co., 1955.)

In young children, symptoms of latent scurvy are *failure to grow* properly, weakness, restlessness, irritability, swollen joints, and tenderness of the lower extremities (Fig. 9–3). Signs of vitamin C deficiency in older children and adults are usually listlessness, lack of endurance, fleeting pains in the legs and joints (often mistaken for rheumatism), small hemorrhages under the skin, and gums that bleed easily.

Effects of Deficiency in Animals. Man, monkeys, and guinea pigs are the only common species of higher animals dependent on the vitamin C contained in their food for the prevention of scurvy.* All other common higher animals can synthesize the vitamin C they need in their bodies from glucose and galactose. This *biosynthesis* requires a specific enzyme† not present in the species that develop scurvy.[11]

Deficient guinea pigs, first studied in 1907 by workers in Norway,[13] show loss of weight (within 10 to 16 days), loss of appetite, weakness, lessening of activity, a rough hair coat, hunching with drooping head, stiffening of hind legs, obvious distress when handled, hemorrhage, beading of ribs, and death within 20 to 28 days.

Changes in teeth and gums are readily demonstrated in monkeys with scurvy, because a longer time is required to produce the deficiency, allowing the teeth changes to be produced. Other symptoms are similar to those seen in man and the guinea pig.

Scorbutic symptoms in guinea pigs, for classroom demonstration purposes, can be readily obtained merely by feeding a commercial rabbit feed (containing no added vitamin C) to young guinea pigs. The symptoms are readily cured by giving sources of vitamin C (Fig. 9–4), with no permanent harm to the animal.

*Food sources of vitamin C are also needed by certain species of fish, insects, and bats, and over 15 bird species in India because of the same metabolic block present in primates and guinea pigs. Of the other species that have been investigated, dogs, cats, fowl, cows, horses, snakes, and others do not need a dietary source of vitamin C.

†The missing enzyme is L-gulonolactone oxidase. It is possible that a second enzyme, glucuronate reductase, is also missing in these species.[12]

Role of Vitamin C in the Body

Although the exact manner in which vitamin C functions in metabolism is yet to be explained, it is assumed that because of its instability — its property of being reversibly oxidized and reduced — it plays some part vital to the welfare of cells and tissues throughout the body. As hemoglobin and other iron-containing pigments with a unique function in the body are capable of alternately taking on and giving up oxygen (reversible oxidation-reduction), so ascorbic acid is able alternately to lose and take on hydrogen. It thus can act as a "hydrogen carrier," and as such it may have an essential role in the metabolism of carbohydrates or proteins, or both. Whatever the explanation, the widespread tissue damage seen in scurvy makes it apparent that this vitamin is needed by many kinds of tissues, and hence its role would seem to be a fundamental one.

We get our clues as to many of its functions chiefly from the symptoms seen in scurvy. So many apparently unrelated tissues show damage that only some of its functions can be discussed here.

The main type of tissue showing marked damage in scorbutic animals is connective tissue. This is primarily because *collagen,* a protein important in the formation of skin, tendon, and bone, as well as supportive tissue, is not properly formed when there is vitamin C deficiency. Normally collagen contains the amino acid *hydroxyproline,* which is obtained by conversion from the amino acid *proline.* In vitamin C deficiency, this conversion does not take place. The resulting impairment of connective tissue regeneration is undoubtedly the cause of many characteristic signs of scurvy, including disorganization of bone and tooth calcification and delayed healing of tissue in burns and wounds. Both animal and human studies indicate that a sufficiently low dietary intake of this vitamin results in delayed healing and less strength of the healed wound, whereas administration of

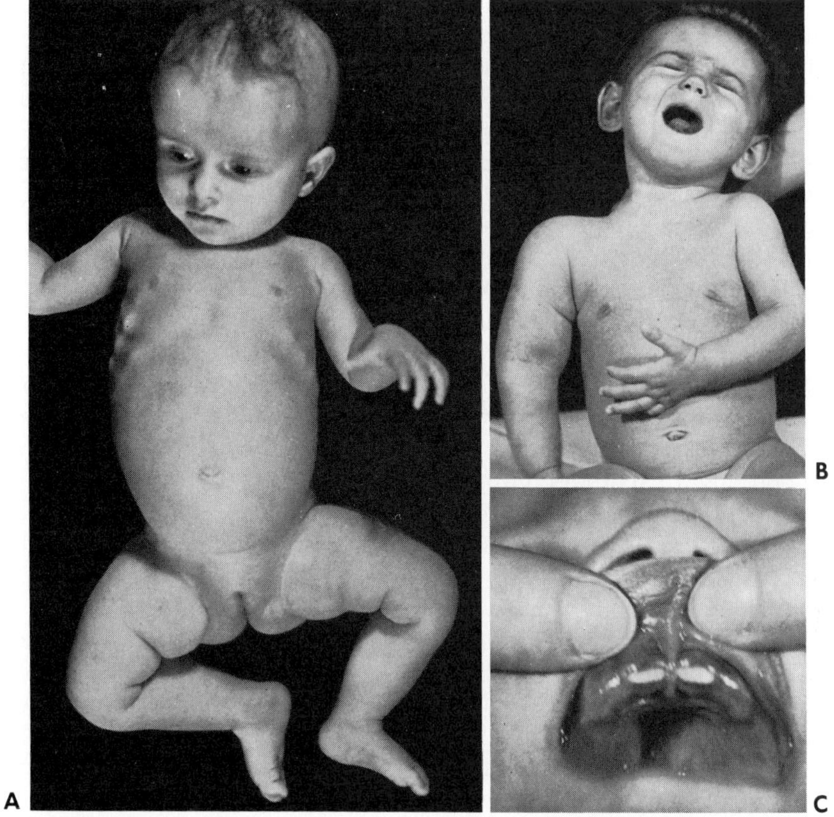

Figure 9–3 Infant scurvy. **A,** The infant becomes irritable when handled. **B,** Characteristic position, with legs flexed at hips and knees, and thighs externally rotated. **C,** Gums are swollen and boggy. (From Cecil-Conn: *The Specialties in General Practice.* 2nd Ed. Philadelphia, W. B. Saunders Co.)

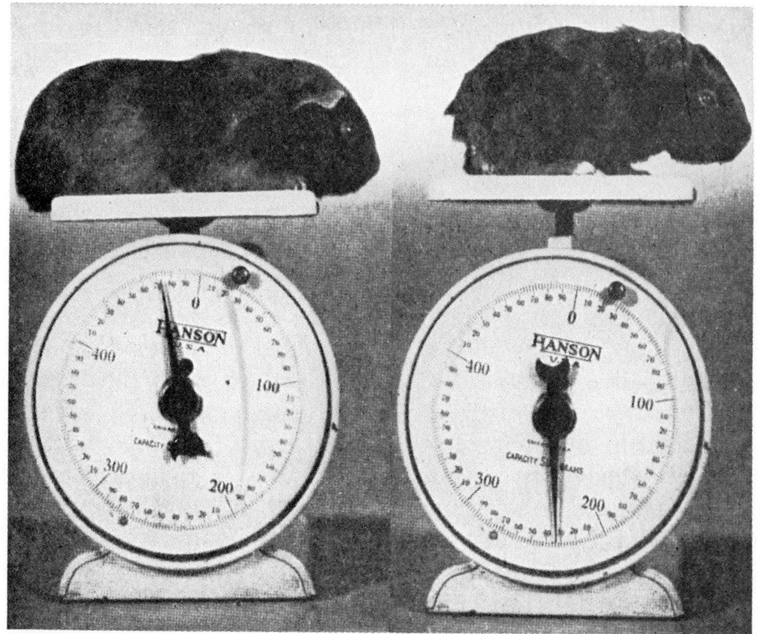

Figure 9–4 Stunting of growth due to lack of vitamin C. The guinea pig at the right, which had a vitamin C–deficient diet, was in poor condition and weighed only 234 gm. The guinea pig at the left, on the same diet plus tomato juice, weighed 473 gm. (Courtesy of Dr. F. F. Tisdall, Toronto.)

vitamin C under such conditions promotes sound healing of wounds. It seems reasonable that vitamin C, which is essential for formation of substances that cement cells together, would function in the reknitting of tissues in wound healing.

Vitamin C appears to function in maintaining strength in blood vessels, a function unrelated to the maintenance of collagen in connective tissue. Small blood vessels under the skin tend to hemorrhage, especially when suction or pressure is applied. This has been used as a test for low-grade lack of vitamin C (the *capillary fragility test*). Examination of the rate of blood flow in scorbutic guinea pigs has revealed a marked sluggishness of the blood flow in vessels that are greatly dilated.

Vitamin C takes part in a number of reactions involving amino acids, such as tyrosine and tryptophan, and the vitamin folacin. It also influences the formation of hemoglobin and deposition of iron in liver tissue. One of the most interesting aspects of vitamin C's influence on iron metabolism is its ability to increase the amount of iron absorbed from the intestine.[14] Thus, vitamin C, when taken with iron supplements or iron-containing foods, will allow more of the iron to be absorbed and available for use by the body.

The adrenal glands contain more vitamin C than most other tissues, and this substance appears to be concerned in some way with the secretion of hormones of the adrenal cortex.

As yet no evidence has been found that this vitamin functions as a specific component of any particular enzyme system, as do many of the other vitamins, but rather its participation appears to be general and is required in the metabolism of many substances in the body. Just how or why vitamin C is concerned in so many and such varied chemical changes that are parts of normal metabolism in the tissues is not yet known, but enough is known to establish it as a very important substance for body welfare.

Vitamin C and Infections

Vitamin C also functions, in some little understood way, in *protecting the body against infections*[15] *and bacterial toxins.*[16] Menten and King fed guinea pigs graded amounts of ascorbic acid, and they found that those which received lower intakes of this vitamin suffered greater injury (loss of weight, tooth damage, etc.) from repeated doses of diphtheria toxin, even though they showed no signs of scurvy.[16] Others have shown that guinea pigs on limited vitamin C intake succumb to inoculations with different strains of bacteria that have little or no effect on animals that received liberal quantities of this vitamin. The lowered resistance to infections in infants with scurvy is notable.

Infections apparently decrease the amount of ascorbic acid in tissues and body fluids; normal recommended intakes of vitamin C are thought to be helpful in enabling the body to combat infections. There is as yet no evidence that amounts greatly in excess of normal recommended intake confer extra benefits, except after deprivation or during periods of unusual physical stress. The possibility suggested by Pauling in 1970,[17] that very large intakes of vitamin C can protect against the common cold, therefore, is without good scientific foundation.[18] Several studies have been done that attempt to define an effect (or lack of effect) of vitamin C on the symptoms and duration of colds. As yet there is no evidence that an intake of vitamin C greater than the recommended dietary allowance will prevent colds. In fact, most of the existing evidence indicates that a high intake of vitamin C is not an effective preventive measure for colds. In any event, the large levels of vitamin C suggested for treatment of colds are far higher than could be normally supplied by natural foods, so any possible beneficial effect (and we know of none) would be a pharmaceutical rather than nutritional effect. (There are toxicological effects known with such high levels of vitamin

C,[19] so any person taking gram levels of the vitamin should do so only with the advice and knowledge of a physician.)

Vitamin C — Smoking and Cancer

Claims have been made over the years that smoking greatly increases vitamin C destruction in the body. Recent research shows there is some truth to this claim, although it is not clear whether this is due to actual destruction or reduced availability of ascorbic acid. Heavy smokers do have lowered blood levels of vitamin C, but the biochemical reason for this has not yet been established.[20] There is no evidence that heavy smokers need more vitamin C than that supplied by the recommended dietary allowances, contrary to many claims in the health food literature.

Recently suggestions have been made that vitamin C may prevent or cure various types of cancer.[21] Since controlled studies investigating any such effects have yet to be done, this claim should not be taken as scientific fact.

Human Metabolism and Nutritional Status

Vitamin C taken in the food is absorbed into the blood stream chiefly from the small intestine within a few hours after it is ingested. The level of vitamin C in the blood plasma is increased only temporarily, because this substance is taken up by the tissues, and any excess is excreted promptly by the kidneys or converted to carbon dioxide and exhaled through the lungs. Intravenously injected ascorbic acid is excreted within 1 to 3 hours. Although there is limited ability to store vitamin C in the body, it is present in higher concentrations in glandular tissues, especially in the adrenal glands. The amount of this substance in the body tissues depends on the quantity in the food and the rate at which it is utilized in and excreted from the body.* About 13 to 30 mg of vitamin C appears to be the amount utilized in the body per day in normal adult men, and 45 mg per day will maintain a normal body pool of about 1500 mg.

There are many surveys of the vitamin C status of samples of the populations of various countries. Unless a survey is recent, it should be regarded with some degree of caution because of changing food habits and new fortification practices. In surveys made in the United States,† including the National Nutrition Survey, borderline (or below) intakes of vitamin C were commonly found (ranging up to 10 to 30 percent of infants, children, and adults, especially in lower income groups). It is one of our most common examples of low vitamin intakes. Frank infantile scurvy is still seen in this country and Canada but in very limited numbers in recent years.

Various estimates have been made recently of the *actual daily intakes* of vitamin C in the United States. Friend states that in 1976, the average vitamin C *available* for consumption was 123 mg per day.[22] This does not take into account loss of vitamin C in food preparation, storage, or wastage, which can be appreciable, so one must conclude that large surpluses of the vitamin do not exist. One encouraging note is the fact that the average daily intakes of vitamin C have been slowly increasing in the United States from the low

*Under normal conditions, higher levels of daily intake of vitamin C result in increased amounts of it both in the body and in the urine. Conversely, low levels of vitamin C in the blood and urine indicate that the daily diet provides little of this vitamin. If a vitamin C–poor diet has been long continued, the tissues become unusually low in, and are said to be "unsaturated" as to, vitamin C. An individual's response to a specific clinical dose of vitamin C therefore reflects the tissue status of that vitamin. A person whose tissues are unsaturated will take up the vitamin into the tissues: there will be "little excess," and a small fraction of the dose will be excreted in the urine. A person whose tissues are saturated will excrete most of the given dose in the urine, since the tissues cannot take up any more. There is no evidence that saturation of the tissues with vitamin C is essential to optimal health.

†See references 10–13, Chapter 8, page 211.

intakes of 1957 to 1959 (about 105 mg). This rise has been attributed to an increase in the consumption of fruit.[22] Obviously from the nutritional status figures, many of our population take in far below these *average* intakes.

Very few normal American diets provide ascorbic acid in such limited amounts as would cause development of scurvy (though the intake may be less than optimal). In fact, since knowledge of the protective action of citrus fruits and other fresh fruits and vegetables has become widespread, actual epidemics of scurvy, as were seen centuries ago, have completely disappeared. Since rice is very low in vitamin C, persons eating extremely simple diets based on rice (such as the "macrobiotic" diet) have been known to develop severe scurvy.

Requirement and Recommended Allowance

The absolute *minimum requirement* of vitamin C per day to prevent scurvy appears to be about 10 mg. To provide a margin of safety, the recommended allowance in Britain is 20 mg per day for adults, and the Canadian and Australian allowance for vitamin C is 30 mg[23] (see Appendix, Table 1C).

Although these levels of vitamin C intake will undoubtedly maintain adults in health and are practical in countries where fresh fruits and vegetables are not abundant, the Food and Nutrition Board of the United States[23] set in 1974 a higher recommended daily allowance at *45 mg per day for adult males* and *45 mg per day for females* in order to provide a generous increment for individual variability and a surplus to compensate for potential losses in food. The Food and Nutrition Board[23] recognizes that the allowances are not necessarily adequate to meet the additional requirement of persons depleted by disease, traumatic stress, or prior dietary inadequacies. For values showing the slightly increased recommendation for pregnancy and lactation and for other details, see Table 9–1 and Table 1A of the Appendix.

Table 9–1 RECOMMENDED ALLOWANCES FOR VITAMIN C*

	Age	*Allowance, mg/day*
Males	infants	35
	1–10 years	40
	11 years and over	45
Females	infants	35
	1–10 years	40
	11 years and over	45
	pregnant	60
	lactating	80

*From Food and Nutrition Board, 1974.[23]

An undetermined amount of vitamin C activity is reaching the American public by way of a common and safe food additive closely related to ascorbic acid, *erythorbic acid (scorbic acid),* an antioxidant. This has about 5 percent of the activity of vitamin C.[24]

Distribution in Foods

For vitamin C we are dependent almost entirely on *fruits* and *vegetables,* and those that may be eaten fresh, uncooked, or previously frozen are the best sources. Milk contains small amounts of vitamin C but is an undependable source, especially if pasteurized. Breast milk provides adequate amounts for infants as long as the mother's intake of vitamin C meets recommended allowances. Most of the vitamin C in meats is destroyed in cooking; eggs, cereal grains, sugar, and fats, nuts, dried legumes, and dried fruits contain either very little or none at all.

Certain kinds of fruits and vegetables are unusually rich in vitamin C (see Table 9–2). Citrus fruits, strawberries, and cantaloupe lead the fruits in vitamin C content, with the exception of two very rich sources rather uncommon in the United States except in "health food" stores. These are a West Indian Cherry, the *acerola,* and a Peruvian jungle fruit called *camu-camu.*[15] (Rose hips are another con-

Table 9–2 FRUITS AND VEGETABLES AS SOURCES OF VITAMIN C*

Food	*Vitamin C (mg/100 gm, Edible Portion)*	*Food*	*Vitamin C (mg/100 gm, Edible Portion)*
Fruits, fresh		Vegetables (cont.)	
Strawberries	59	Cauliflower	78
Oranges (or juice)	50	Spinach	51
Frozen orange juice	45	Cabbage	47
Lemons (or juice)	46	Rutabagas	43
Grapefruit (or juice)	38	Dandelion greens	35
Frozen orange-grapefruit juice	41	Asparagus	33
Cantaloupe	33	Chard	32
Honeydew melon	23	Okra	31
Berries (except strawberries		Beet greens	30
and blueberries)	21	Beans, lima, green	29
Pineapple, fresh	17	string, green	19
Avocados	14	Peas, green	27
Blueberries	14	Radishes	26
Bananas	10	Onions, young, green	25
Cherries	10	mature	10
Apricots	10	Tomatoes	23
Peaches	8	juice, canned	16
Apples }		Squash, summer	22
Grapes }		winter	13
Pears }	7	Sweet potatoes	21
Plums }		Potatoes	20
Watermelon }		Lettuce, green	18
Vegetables		Parsnips	16
Kale, leaves only	186	Corn, sweet	12
Turnip greens	139	Cucumbers	11
Peppers, green	128	Beets	10
Broccoli	113	Celery	9
Brussels sprouts	102	Lettuce, head	6
Mustard greens	97	Eggplant	5
Collards	92	Carrots	8

*Figures are from U.S. Department of Agriculture Handbook No. 8, *Composition of Foods–Raw, Processed, Prepared,* 1963. See Appendix for further details. All values are computed on a raw basis before cooking, unless indicated otherwise.

centrated, though variable, source of vitamin C, but they too are not widely available.) Green leafy vegetables, peppers, broccoli, and cauliflower have a high content of vitamin C and are very good sources of vitamin C, even after cooking. Raw cabbage, turnips, salad greens, and tomatoes (either fresh or canned) are also good sources. Potatoes contribute considerable amounts of ascorbic acid when eaten fresh and in large quantities, and they are still a principal source of dietary vitamin C in areas of the world where other sources are unavailable. Dehydrated potatoes are an undependable source, unless fortified with vitamin C (see Table 9–3). Most cooked and canned vegetables and fruits provide some vitamin C, but in smaller and more variable amounts than the corresponding fresh foods. Freezing, however, preserves most of the vitamin C activity.

Pure ascorbic acid is available in

Table 9–3 RETENTION OF VITAMIN C DURING PROCESSING OF POTATOES*

State of Processing	*Mean Total Vitamin C (Fresh Weight Basis) mg/100 gm*
Raw potatoes	26.5
Fresh mashed	13.6
Reconstituted, dehydrated granules	6.7

*From Bring, S. V., and Raab, F. P.: J. Amer. Dietet. Assoc., 45:149, 1964.

stores wherever vitamins are sold, in very inexpensive form — for as little as 0.5 cent or less per 100 mg (which is more than a day's supply).* This costs less than an equivalent amount in natural foods, but such foods (except for the "acerola" and "camu-camu" berries) also supply a variety of minerals and other vitamins and are to be preferred whenever possible. For this reason, we do not recommend the various high vitamin C, imitation fruit drinks on the market as routine sources of vitamin C for children or adults, except when no other source is available (which would be extremely rare).

It should be understood that there is considerable variability in the vitamin C content of fruits and vegetables, and that the figures given in Table 9–2 represent only approximate mean values. The vitamin C content of plant foods varies greatly with different varieties of the same plant, with soil and climate, and especially with the amount of exposure to sunlight and the degree of ripeness of the fruit. In general, the more mature a plant becomes, the less vitamin C it contains; the more sunlight a plant receives, the more vitamin C it contains. Different varieties of apples and oranges have been found to vary considerably in vitamin C content. Even allowing for variations, it can be seen that certain fruits and vegetables are much richer in this vitamin than others.

Losses in Processing

Further variations in the vitamin C content of table foods must be expected because of losses of this vitamin during *storage*, *processing* (canning or drying), and *cooking*. Vitamin C is very susceptible to destruction during cooking and processing, because it is so water-soluble, is easily oxidized, and is attacked by enzymes. Leafy vegetables (with large surface areas) lose more vitamin C on storage than do root vegetables or tubers. Refrigeration during storage reduces losses, and in markets, more of the vitamin is retained if vegetables are kept in crushed ice than if they are kept in a refrigerator.

In preparation for canning, quick freezing, or drying, a brief blanching with steam favors retention of vitamin C, because this process destroys the enzymes that hasten destruction of the vitamin in raw foods. There is less loss of vitamin C when foods are preserved by quick freezing, as with frozen orange juice, an excellent practical source of vitamin C in countries where refrigerators are available. Most losses occur when foods are preserved by drying, especially if they are exposed to sunlight in the process. Commercially canned foods may compare favorably in vitamin C content with home-cooked products if the fruits or vegetables reach the cannery fresh from nearby fields and are heated quickly in vacuum-sealed cans. The vitamin C content of canned fruit juices will vary considerably, unless fortified with vitamin C or unless it is specially protected in canning.

Because vitamin C is water-soluble, considerable amounts of it may be lost in the liquid in which the food is canned, if this is discarded. In drying fruits, sulfuring before drying and rapid drying (away from sunlight) favor retention of the vitamin content, but dried fruits cannot be counted on as a source of much vitamin C.

In home cooking, there is a great deal of variation in the amount of vitamin C loss that takes place. However, if short boiling times and small amounts of water are used, and if the water is consumed, there is little loss. It has been reported that ascorbic acid in vegetables can be protect-

*If bought in vitamin capsules, which are sold by various pharmaceutical companies, the cost per unit may vary considerably. The natural active form of ascorbic acid is the L-isomer, and this is equal in every way to the synthetic L-isomer, the usual form of commerce. Calcium and sodium salts of ascorbic acid (calcium ascorbate and sodium ascorbate) are also readily available.

for a minute before adding the food. This removes the oxygen dissolved in water, thus preventing oxidative destruction of some of the ascorbic acid.* For example, loss of ascorbic acid from cabbage boiled 15 minutes starting in cold water is 25.5 percent compared with a 1.8 percent loss when cooked in water that has been boiled one minute.[26] The loss in vitamin C content in home cooking also depends on numerous factors, including the nature of the food, its reaction (acid or alkaline), the period and degree of heating, and especially the extent to which the food is exposed to water and to air in the cooking process. Retention of the vitamin is favored by cooking with peel left on or in large pieces and cooking with as much exclusion of air as possible (tightly covered vessel or pressure cooker). Increased losses of the vitamin result from contact with copper or iron in preparing or cooking the food, or from mashing the food and leaving it in a hot place or exposed to the air. The practice of holding cooked foods warm for prolonged periods of time, such as on steam tables in cafeterias, may result in significant (50 to 75 percent) losses of vitamin C.

Practical Suggestions for Conserving Vitamin C in Foods in the Home

It is foolish to allow vitamin C, which is essential for health, to be lost before foods are served. Because this is the most easily destroyed of the vitamins, its conservation presents a special problem. Reasons for the following special *precautions* in handling fresh fruits and vegetables should be self-evident if one keeps in mind that vitamin C is water-soluble and easily destroyed by oxidation, and that heat, alkaline reaction, and, above all, exposure to air hasten its destruction. These practical suggestions are also useful in preserving most water-soluble vitamins in foods in home cooking.

Buy fresh fruits and vegetables in small enough quantities so that they will be used promptly; keep them at low temperature (in refrigerator, if possible).

Prepare them (paring and cutting up) immediately before they are to be cooked or served raw; do not let them stand in water or exposed to air before cooking; serve promptly; *do not keep hot for long* (or reheat) before serving.

Cook in as small a quantity of water and for as short a time as feasible; cook by steaming or broiling (instead of boiling) and with "skins" left on when possible; keep cooking vessels tightly covered.

Never add soda in cooking vegetables and do not use copper cooking vessels if you want to preserve vitamin C (the presence of either alkali or copper hastens vitamin destruction).

Do not allow frozen foods to thaw out before cooking; keep them in refrigerator and start cooking in frozen state in limited amounts of boiling water.

Juices of fresh fruits are best prepared immediately before serving. However, acid juices (orange, grapefruit, tomato) may be left in a covered glass container in the refrigerator several days with little loss in vitamin C value; size of container should be chosen so liquid will about fill it, with minimum of air left above the liquid.

How to Get Allowance of Vitamin C in Diet

The best general rule to safeguard the diet with regard to vitamin C is to include each day one serving of either citrus fruit, tomato, or some other rich source of this vitamin. Other foods included in the normal diet, such as extra fruit and vegetables (both cooked and raw), usually supply sufficient vitamin C to make up the day's allowance. A 6 oz glass of fresh or frozen orange juice supplies 80 to 100 mg of vitamin C, considerably more than the

*Probably practical only where vitamin C is scarce and expensive and the value of one's time in the kitchen is not in question. The monetary value of the vitamin C gained by such a procedure (and which can easily be replaced by some other food or supplementary source) is less than the value of one moment's time in many countries. Of course, the flavor of the food may also be changed by these procedures, which also needs to be considered. (This points out again the necessity of nutrition education for all people who prepare food so that one can weigh these factors oneself.)

recommended daily allowance. Vitamin C is exceedingly well protected in citrus fruit products, because these products contain several constituents that inhibit its oxidation. Ascorbic acid oxidase, the enzyme that causes vitamin C oxidation, is not found in orange juice. Also, citrus fruits do not require cooking, and ordinary refrigerator temperatures prevent loss during short-term storage in the home.

There are many other ways to ensure adequate vitamin C intake (and variety is always to be recommended). This could be fresh strawberries, melon, fresh tomato, or tomato juice, which supply 25 to 60 mg per 100 gm. Vegetables that are good sources of vitamin C may also be used as the main source, or in combination with a second good source (especially if citrus fruit is unavailable or not tolerated). Such vegetables are green peppers, broccoli, cauliflower, Brussels sprouts, and most dark green leafy vegetables. A serving of any of these generally provides the daily allowance for vitamin C.

Table 9–4 EXAMPLES OF FOOD COMBINATIONS THAT FURNISH A GENEROUS DAY'S SUPPLY OF VITAMIN C

Food	*Vitamin C (mg)*
I	
Strawberries, 2/3 cup	60
Cooked summer squash, 1/2 cup	10
	70 mg
II	
Cantaloupe, 1/2 melon, 6 in. diameter	50
Asparagus, 4 stalks	18
	68 mg
III	
Tomato, 1 medium, fresh	35
Sweet potato, 1 medium, baked or boiled with skin	20
	55 mg
IV	
Grapefruit juice, 1/2 cup, canned	41
Lima beans, 1/2 cup cooked	14
Potato, 1 medium, baked or boiled with skin	16
	71 mg

Table 9–2 lists a large variety of foods and their vitamin C content. Table 9–4 illustrates various fruit and vegetable combinations from this list that will furnish 45 mg or more of vitamin C. Combinations I and II represent a more expensive way to obtain vitamin C (i.e., fresh fruits, especially out of season), while combinations III and IV are examples of more economical sources of vitamin C, which are available throughout the year.

Of interest are U.S. Department of Agriculture figures on food sources of vitamin C consumed by the American public in a year* — a reflection of average food habits, whether good or bad! The largest contributors were vegetables, which contributed 51 percent of our vitamin C (potatoes and sweet potatoes — 17, dark green and deep yellow vegetables — 8 and tomatoes and all other vegetables — 26). Citrus fruits supplied 28 percent and all other fruits, including those fortified with synthetic vitamin C, 12 percent for a total of 40 percent. Thus, fruits and vegetables supply 91 percent of our vitamin C intake in foods, which is a demonstration of the importance of this food group.

Similar figures on the percentage of vitamin C intake from synthetic sources are not readily available (but probably range between 20 and 30 percent of the total intake on a per capita basis). This varies considerably with each individual.

Bioflavonoids and Related Substances ("Vitamin P")

Various pigments and related compounds in citrus fruits and other plants are advertised widely in "health food" literature as sources of "vitamin P" — chiefly, certain *bioflavonoids, hesperidin,* and *rutin.* There is *no evidence* today that these compounds in otherwise nutritionally complete diets have activity similar to that of a vitamin, although they may

*1976 figures.

serve as pharmaceuticals (they can protect against capillary fragility, for instance, under special experimental conditions in animals, but this has not been demonstrated to take place in man). Nutritionists in this country and in most countries have not accepted "vitamin P" as either a separate entity or as a significant vitamin C–sparing factor.[27] The term "vitamin P," therefore, must be considered to be obsolete.

QUESTIONS AND PROBLEMS

1. From what materials was ascorbic acid first isolated as a pure substance? What type of chemical compound is it? Why was the name ascorbic acid given to it? Where does it occur in nature? In the human body? How stable is the substance when kept in dry, solid form? In water solution with alkaline reaction? In acid solution? What other conditions affect its stability, and why?

2. Why was scurvy a prevalent disease among crews on long sea voyages and early explorations? Why was it possible for Admiral Byrd to take men into the Antarctic for long periods without fear that any of them would succumb to scurvy? What foods or other substances were known to prevent or cure scurvy long before it was recognized that their efficacy in this respect was due to the presence in all of them of a definite compound that might be classed as a vitamin? Give the symptoms of acute scurvy and explain the widespread tissue damages in the light of one of the chief functions of vitamin C in the body — i.e., the formation and maintenance of intercellular and connective tissue substances.

3. Why do men and guinea pigs develop scurvy when the diet is lacking in vitamin C, while dogs, rats, and other animals do not? Do plants need vitamin C, and if so, how do they get it? Give three characteristic symptoms of subacute or latent scurvy in infants and three symptoms in adults that indicate the diet has furnished too little vitamin C. From consideration of the results of lack of this vitamin, what would you conclude are its main uses in the body?

4. What classes of foods contribute little or no vitamin C in the diet, at least in the condition in which they are eaten? What classes of foods furnish the major part of the vitamin C intake? Consult Table 9–2 and list the five fruits and five vegetables richest in vitamin C in the raw state. List the ten that have the next highest vitamin C content per 100 gm, either fruits or vegetables, in order of their relative vitamin C content when raw. Rearrange these 20 fruits and vegetables in the order of the vitamin C contribution that is made by an *average serving* of each, fruits raw and vegetables with average allowance for loss of vitamin C in cooking, as given in Table 3 of the Appendix.

5. What is the recommended daily allowance of vitamin C for a normal woman? For a teen-age boy? For a pregnant woman? If 10 mg of vitamin C per day protects an adult against scurvy, what is the use of eating the recommended allowance? Is there any point in taking about twice the recommended allowance daily? Is a high level of vitamin C intake practical, or even possible, in some parts of the world? Name three countries in which the available foods and dietary customs make it probable that the average intake of vitamin C is low.

6. List five foods that provide vitamin C at low or moderate cost. Plan a day's diet, at low or moderate cost, that would furnish the RDA of vitamin C for an adult.

7. Plan a day's meals for yourself with some food that is a good source of vitamin C in each meal. Compute how many milligrams of vitamin C this diet would provide and compare with the standard allowance.

8. Give methods of conserving vitamin C in foods during storage and preparation for the table.

REFERENCES

1. Lind, J.: Treatise on Scurvy (first published in 1753). Reprinted, and edited by C. P. Stewart and Douglas Guthrie. Edinburgh University Press, 1953.
2. Editorial: Captain James Cook (1728–1779). J.A.M.A., *209*:1217, 1969.
3. Funk, C.: J. State Med., *20*:341, 1912 (as reprinted in Goldblith, S. A., and Joslyn, M. A.: *Milestones in Nutrition.* Westport, Avi Publishing Co., Inc., 1964, pp. 145–171); Holst, A., and Frölich, J.: Z. Hyg., *72*:1, 1912.
4. Hardin, A., and Zilva, S. S.: Biochem J., *12*:408, 1918; Drummond, J. C.: Biochem. J., *13*:77, 1919.
5. Santos, F. O.: Proc. Soc. Exp. Biol. Med., *19*:2, 1921; McClendon, J. F.: J. Biol. Chem., *47*:411, 1921.
6. Drummond, J. C.: Biochem J., *14*:660, 1920.
7. Szent-Györgyi, A.: Biochem. J., *22*:1387, 1928.
8. King, C. G., and Waugh, W. A.: Science, *75*:357, 1932; Waugh, W. A., and King, C. G.: J. Biol. Chem., *97*:325, 1932; and King, C. G.: Physiol. Rev., *16*:238, 1936.
9. Szent-Györgyi, A., and Haworth, W. N.: Nature, *131*:24, 1933.
10. Hodges, R. E., et al.: Amer. J. Clin. Nutr., *22*:535, 1969; *24*:432, 1971; Baker, E. M., et al.: Amer. J. Clin. Nutr., *19*:371, 1966; *22*:549, 1969; *24*:444, 1971.
11. Sato, P., Nishikimi, M., and Udenfriend, S.: Biochem. Biophys. Res. Comm., *71*:293, 1976.
12. Chaudhuri, C. R., and Chatterjee, I. B.: Science, *164*:435, 1969; Chatterjee, I. B., et al.: Nature, *192*:163, 1961.
13. Holst, A., and Frölich, J.: J. Hyg., *7*:634, 1907.
14. Cook, J. D., and Monsen, E. R.: Amer. J. Clin. Nutr., *30*:235, 1977.
15. Levenson, S. M., et al.: Arch. Int. Med., *110*:693, 1962.
16. Menten, M. L., and King, C. G.: J. Nutr., *10*:141, 1935.
17. Pauling, L.: *Vitamin C and the Common Cold.* San Francisco, W. H. Freeman and Co., 1970; Pauling, L.: Proc. Nat. Acad. Sci., *67*:1643, 1970.
18. Margen, S.: J. Nutr. Educ., *2*:131, 1971: Hodges, R. E.: Amer. J. Clin. Nutr., *24*:383, 1971; Wilson, C. W. M.: Brit. Med. J., *1*:669, 1971; Diehl, H. S.: Amer. J. Public Health, *61*:649, 1971; Consumer Reports, *36*:113, 1971.
19. Mayer, J.: Postgrad. Med., *45*:268, 1969; Goldsmith, G. A.: J.A.M.A., *216*:337, 1971; Lamden, M. P.: New Engl. J. Med., *284*:336, 1971.
20. Brook, M., and Grimshaw, J. J.: Amer. J. Clin. Nutr., *21*:1254, 1968; Pelletier, O.: Amer. J. Clin. Nutr., *23*:520, 1970; *21*:1259, 1968; Pelletier, O.: N.Y. Acad. Sci., *258*:156, 1975.
21. Cameron, E., and Pauling, L.: Supplemental ascorbate in the supportive treatment of cancer. Proc. Natl. Acad. Sci. USA, *73*:3685, 1976.
22. Friend, B.: *National Food Situation.* U.S. Department of Agriculture, Agricultural Research Survey. Washington, D. C., Government Printing Office, Nov. 1976.
23. Food and Nutrition Board: *Recommended Dietary Allowances.* 8th Ed. Washington, D.C., National Research Council, National Academy of Sciences, 1974. (Also see 9th Ed. to be published in 1979.)
24. Wang, M. M., Fisher, K. H., and Dodds, M. L.: J. Nutr., *77*:443, 1962.
25. Derse, P. H., and Elvehjem, C. A.: J.A.M.A., *156*:1501, 1954; Bradfield, R. B., and Roca, A.: J. Amer. Dietet. Assoc., *44*:28, 1964.
26. Roy, J. K., and Biswas, S. K.: Ind. J. Med. Res., *50*:259, 1962.
27. Lee, R. E.: J. Nutr., *72*:203, 1960; Brit. Med. J., *1*:235, 1969.

SUPPLEMENTARY READING

Reviews and History

Beeukwes, A. M.: The prevalence of scurvy among voyagers to America, 1493–1600. J. Amer. Dietet. Assoc., *24*:300, 1948.

Cone, T. E.: History of infantile scurvy in America. In *200 Years of Feeding Infants in America.* Columbus, Ohio, Ross Laboratories, 1976.

Hanck, A., and Ritzel, G. (ed.): Re-evaluation of vitamin C. Internat. J. Vit. Nutr. Res., *47*: 1–309, Supplement 16, 1977.

Harper, A. E.: The recommended dietary allowances for ascorbic acid. Ann. N.Y. Acad. Sci., *258*:491, 1975.

Hess, A. F.: Recent advances in knowledge of scurvy and the antiscorbutic vitamin. J.A.M.A., *98*:1429, 1932.

Irwin, M. I., and Hutchins, B. K.: A conspectus of research on vitamin C requirements of man. J. Nutr. *106*:821, 1976.

King, C. G., and Burns, J. J. (eds.): Second conference on vitamin C. Ann. N.Y. Acad. Sci., *258*:5–546, 1975.

Lorenz, A. J.: The conquest of scurvy. J. Amer. Dietet. Assoc., *30*:665, 1954.

Marks, J.: *A Guide to the Vitamins: Their Role in Health and Disease.* Baltimore, University Park Press, 1975.

Waife, S. O.: Lind, lemons, and limeys. J. Clin. Nutr., *1*:471, 1953.

Yew, M. S.: Biological variation in ascorbic acid needs. Ann. N.Y. Acad. Sci., *258*:451, 1975.

General

Bermond, P.: Clinical symptoms of malnutrition and plasma ascorbic acid levels. Amer. J. Clin. Nutr., *29*:493, 1976.

Bingol, A., et al.: Plasma, erythrocyte, and leukocyte ascorbic acid concentrations in children with iron deficiency anemia. J. Pediatr., *86*:902, 1975.

Boots, L. R., Cornwell, P. E., and Beck, L. R.: Circadian and menstrual cycle variation in serum ascorbic acid levels in baboons. J. Nutr., *106*:329, 1976.

Chatterjee, I. B.: Evolution and the biosynthesis of ascorbic acid. Science, *182*:1271, 1973.

Gatenby-Davies, J. D., and Newson, J.: Low ascorbate status in the Masai of Kenya. Amer. J. Clin. Nutr., *27*:310, 1974.

Keith, M. O., and Pelletier, O.: Ascorbic acid concentrations in leukocytes and selected organs of guinea pigs in response to increasing ascorbic acid intake. Amer. J. Clin. Nutr., *27*:368, 1974.

MacLennan, W. J., and Hamilton, J. C.: The effect of acute illness on leucocyte and plasma ascorbic acid levels. Brit. J. Nutr., *38*:217, 1977.

Murdock, D. S., Donaldson, M. L., and Gubler, C. J.: Studies on the mechanism of the "thiamin-sparing" effect of ascorbic acid in rats. Amer. J. Clin. Nutr., *27*:696, 1974.

Sayers, M. H., et al.: Iron absorption from rice meals cooked with fortified salt containing ferrous sulphate and ascorbic acid. Brit. J. Nutr., *31*:367, 1974.

Schoral, C. J., et al.: Leucocyte ascorbic acid and pregnancy. Brit. J. Nutr., *39*:139, 1978.

Thaete, L. G., and Grim, J. N.: Fine structural effects of L-ascorbic acid on buccal epithelium. Amer. J. Clin. Nutr., *27*:719, 1974.

Distribution, Availability, and Stability

Andrews, F. E., and Driscoll, P. J.: Stability of ascorbic acid in orange juice exposed to light and air during storage. J. Amer. Dietet. Assoc., *71*:140, 1977.

Augustin, J.: Variations in the nutritional composition of fresh potatoes. J. Food Sci., *40*:1295, 1975.

Horowitz, I., Fabry, E. M., and Gerson, C. D.: Bioavailability of ascorbic acid in orange juice. J.A.M.A., *235*:2624, 1976.

Nelson, E. W., Streiff, R. R., and Cerda, J. J.: Comparative bioavailability of folate and vitamin C from a synthetic and a natural source. Amer. J. Clin. Nutr., *28*:1014, 1975.

Pelletier, O., and Keith, M. O.: Bioavailability of synthetic and natural ascorbic acid. J. Amer. Dietet. Assoc., *64*:271, 1974.

Vitamin C and Colds

Clegg, K. M., and Macdonald, J. M.: L-Ascorbic acid and D-isoascorbic acid in a common cold survey. Amer. J. Clin. Nutr., *28*:973, 1975.

Dykes, M. H. M., and Meier, P.: Ascorbic acid and the common cold. J.A.M.A., *231*:1073, 1975.

Miller, J. Z., et al.: Therapeutic effect of vitamin C. J.A.M.A., *237*:248, 1977.

Second Conference on Vitamin C. Part IV. Ascorbic acid and respiratory illness. Ann. N.Y. Acad. Sci., *258*:498, 1975.

Shilotri, P. G., and Bhat, K. S.: Effect of mega doses of vitamin C on bactericidal activity of leukocytes. Amer. J. Clin. Nutr., *30*:1077, 1977.

(*Note*:Various 1977 and 1978 issues of *Nutrition Today* contain interesting but, in some instances, highly controversial papers on vitamin C.)

Other Vitamin C–Related Topics

Dawson, K. P., and Duncan, A.: Ascorbic acid and long-term anticonvulsant therapy in children. Brit. J. Nutr., *33*:315, 1975.

Howald, H., and Segesser, B., and Körner, W. F.: Ascorbic acid and athletic performance. Ann. N.Y. Acad. Sci., *258*:458, 1975.

Hughes, R. E.: Vitamin C and cholesterol metabolism. J. Human Nutr., *30*:315, 1976.

Kerxhalli, J. S., et al.: Effect of ascorbic acid on the human electroencephalogram. J. Nutr., *105*:1356, 1975.

Krumdieck, C., and Butterworth, C. E., Jr.: Ascorbate-cholesterol-lecithin interactions: factors of potential importance in the pathogenesis of atherosclerosis. Amer. J. Clin. Nutr., *27*:866, 1974.

Marquardt, H., Rufino, F., and Weisburger, J. H.: Mutagenic activity of nitrite-treated foods: human stomach cancer may be related to dietary factors. Science, *196*:1000, 1977.

Peterson, V. E., et al.: Quantification of plasma cholesterol and triglyceride levels in hypercholesterolemic subjects receiving ascorbic acid supplements. Amer. J. Clin. Nutr., *28*:584, 1975.

Rivers., J. M.: Oral contraceptives and ascorbic acid. Amer. J. Clin. Nutr., *28*:550, 1975.

Strydom, N. B., et al.: Effect of ascorbic acid on rate of heat acclimatization. J. Appl. Physiol., *41*:202, 1976.

Weininger, J., and King, J. C.: Effect of oral contraceptives on ascorbic acid status of young women consuming a constant diet. Nutr. Rpts. Internat., *15*:255, 1977.

Yeung, D. L.: Relationships between cigarette smoking, oral contraceptives, and plasma vitamins A, E, C, and plasma triglycerides and cholesterol. Amer. J. Clin. Nutr., *29*:1216, 1976.

Articles in **Nutrition Reviews**

Reprints (partial) of various classic papers on vitamin C by Holst, Frolich, Waugh, King, Hess, Wolbach, and others are given in *32*:273, 1974; *34*: 81, 1976; *35*:12, 1977; *35*:299, 1977.

Fish require dietary vitamin C. *29*:207, 1971.

Bioflavonoids as a growth factor for the cricket. *30*:65, 1972.

Ascorbic acid and the catabolism of cholesterol. *31*:154, 1973.

Vitamin C and the common cold. *31*:303, 1973.

New roles for ascorbic acid. *32*:53, 1974.

Vitamin C toxicity. *34*:236, 1976.

New information on synthesis and metabolism of ascorbic acid. *35*:22, 1977.

The function of ascorbic acid in collagen formation. *36*:118, 1978.

Vitamin C and phagocyte function. *36*:183, 1978.

Chapter 10

Water and Minerals: The Electrolytes (Sodium, Potassium, and Chlorine)

The body is composed of *chemical elements* in many different combinations. The chemical elements are thus the basic building blocks of the human body.

Oxygen constitutes over half the body weight, while oxygen and hydrogen together make up three-fourths the body weight (Fig. 10–1). The prominence of these two elements is largely accounted for by the fact that about half the body consists of water. Four nonmetallic elements—oxygen, carbon, hydrogen, and nitrogen — make up 96 percent of the body weight and account for 99 percent of all the atoms in the body. The other elements present in the body are commonly referred to as *minerals* or as inorganic salts. Technically, a salt is the product formed by replacing the hydrogen of an acid with a metal. For example, in ordinary table salt (NaCl), the metal sodium (Na) replaces the hydrogen of hydrochloric acid (HCl). More generally a salt is defined as the combination of any negatively charged element or group, except hydroxyl (OH^-), with any positively charged element or group, except hydrogen (H^+). Sometimes these elements are referred to collectively as ash because they are the portion left after the organic or combustible matter is burned.

Seven minerals that are present in the body in amounts greater than about 0.01 percent of body weight are called the *macrominerals.** These seven — calcium, phosphorus, potassium, sulfur, sodium, chlorine, and magnesium — are essential nutrients and are required in the diet in considerably larger quantities than the essential *trace elements or trace minerals.* Inorganic forms of six of the macrominerals take care of all dietary needs (organic forms are not required); the element sulfur is unique in being required almost exclusively in the form of sulfur-containing amino acids.† The trace ele-

*There is as yet no standard nutritional nomenclature to distinguish macrominerals from trace elements. We use the word "mineral" here in deference to common usage, though whether some of the essential elements are minerals or gases is a moot point. In common usage we generally speak of our "mineral needs" rather than our "element needs," and of "minerals" in foods or diets rather than "elements." The macrominerals are required in the human diet in amounts over 100 mg per day. This serves as a convenient dividing line between macrominerals and trace elements.

†Very limited use can be made of sulfate salts, but most processes require methionine or its derivatives. Nitrogen is, of course, also required in the form of amino compounds; the body cannot use nitrogen as nitrate or nitrite salts. (See Chapter 5.) Carbon as charcoal is not absorbed, and carbonate salts, while entering into the body's acid-base regulation, are not used in most metabolic processes.

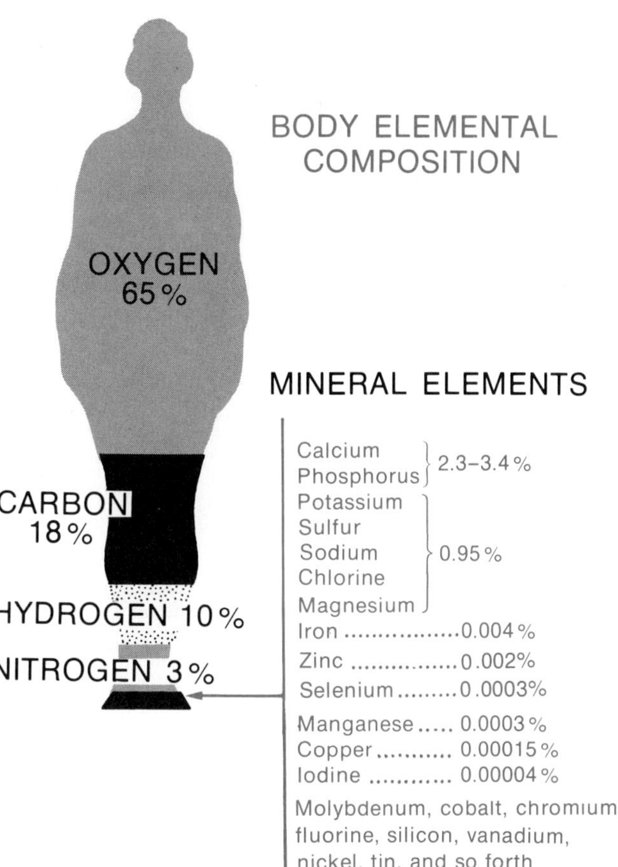

Figure 10–1 The nonmetallic elements oxygen, carbon, hydrogen, and nitrogen together make up 96 percent of the body weight, leaving only 4 percent for all the various mineral elements. Calcium and phosphorus are the mineral elements present in largest amounts, but these amounts vary considerably, depending on the reserves of these two elements stored in the bones. Substantial quantities of potassium, sulfur, chlorine, sodium, and magnesium also are present in the body. These seven elements are referred to as macrominerals, whereas iron, manganese, copper, zinc, cobalt, iodine, and many other elements present in the body in trace amounts are called trace minerals or trace elements.

ments also can be supplied as inorganic salts, with one exception (cobalt is needed as vitamin B-12). Minerals may be more or less effectively utilized in organic form, depending on such factors as solubility, strength of chemical bonds, valence state, and absorbability. By "organic form" we mean bound to or part of the structure of an organic compound, such as iron contained in the protein molecule hemoglobin, and phosphorus linked with protein or lipids. The minerals present in sea salt and crushed oyster shell, while sometimes advertised or sold as "organic" food supplements, are, in fact, inorganic; the various mineral salts in these substances are neither more nor less natural than the same salts in pure form.

While a certain amount of the minerals may exist in foods or tissues as inorganic salts, a considerable quantity of them is found in combination in organic compounds. The bulk of body calcium and phosphorus is concentrated in the mineral salts found in bones and teeth, but the portion — 1 percent of calcium and 20 percent of phosphorus — present in the soft tissues and fluids plays a vital role in the structure and metabolism of all cells. Most metallic elements needed in very small amounts appear to function as a part of enzymes or hormones required to bring about specific chemical reactions in the tissues. The body fluids consist mainly of water in which inorganic salts, protein, and some organic compounds are dissolved.

WATER

Water, a simple compound of two atoms of hydrogen with one of oxygen, has unique features that make it absolutely necessary for life. It has special solvent properties that alter the configuration of

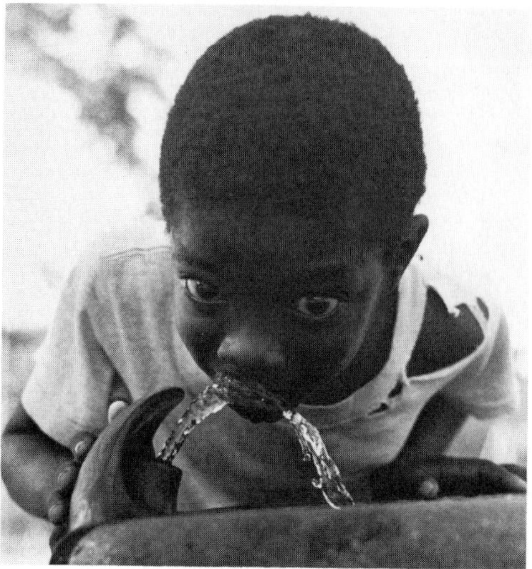

Figure 10–2 The need for water ranks second only to the need for air. Provision of safe public water supplies is an important indirect nutritional measure, by reducing the spread of disease and its concomitant nutritional costs and by freeing women and children from the burden of carrying water. Water can provide some essential minerals, including fluoride, and must be protected from environmental pollutants. (Courtesy of Laurel Stradford, Chicago, 1975.)

substances dissolved in it and thus change their behavior in cellular systems. In spite of its small molecular size, water is liquid at body temperature (by way of comparison, carbon dioxide, a much heavier molecule, is a gas). For these reasons water is an ideal medium for transporting dissolved nutrients and wastes throughout the body. A relatively large amount of heat is needed to vaporize it. It takes about 600 kcal (2500 kJ) to evaporate a kilogram of water, which makes sweating a very effective means of dissipating body heat. Water also participates in some chemical reactions in the body. The splitting of starch into sugar by addition of water is one example.

Water is second only to oxygen in importance to the body (Fig. 10–2). A healthy adult may live for weeks without food but only for a few days without water. A person can lose all reserve carbohydrate (glycogen) and fat, and about half the body protein without real danger, but a loss of 10 percent of total body water is serious, while a loss of 20 to 22 percent is fatal.

When water loss amounts to 1 percent of body weight, the sensation of thirst occurs. If water is not drunk, feelings of discomfort worsen, heart rate and body temperature rise, and the ability to work and to think deteriorates. With a water depletion of up to 10 percent, a person can perform some physical work, but efficiency is low and heat exhaustion takes place. With greater depletion of body water, weakness, disorientation, and circulatory insufficiency preclude physical efforts (Fig. 10–3).

It is common knowledge that the water content of the body must be replenished regularly to make up for continuous loss of this substance. Water is excreted from the body by the kidneys in the urine, by the lungs as water vapor in the expired air, and by the skin as sensible or insensible perspiration (Fig. 10–4). Lesser amounts are regularly lost in the stools. The relative amounts that are excreted through these different channels vary somewhat, as discussed in Chapter 15. Ordinarily more water is excreted in the urine than by other channels, but in hot weather a larger amount is evaporated as perspiration in the effort to regulate the body temperature, and a smaller volume of more concentrated urine is excreted. The amount lost through all channels averages 2 to 2½ liters per day.

Water requirements of infants and children are proportionately higher than those of adults. Both body surface area and metabolic rate per unit of body weight are higher in infants and children than in adults, and water loss under sedentary conditions in a comfortable environment is roughly proportional to the metabolic rate. Children are also more active than many adults and so need additional water to cover the loss of sweat.

In a comfortable environment, the water requirement is on the order of 1 ml per kcal of energy expenditure or 1500 ml

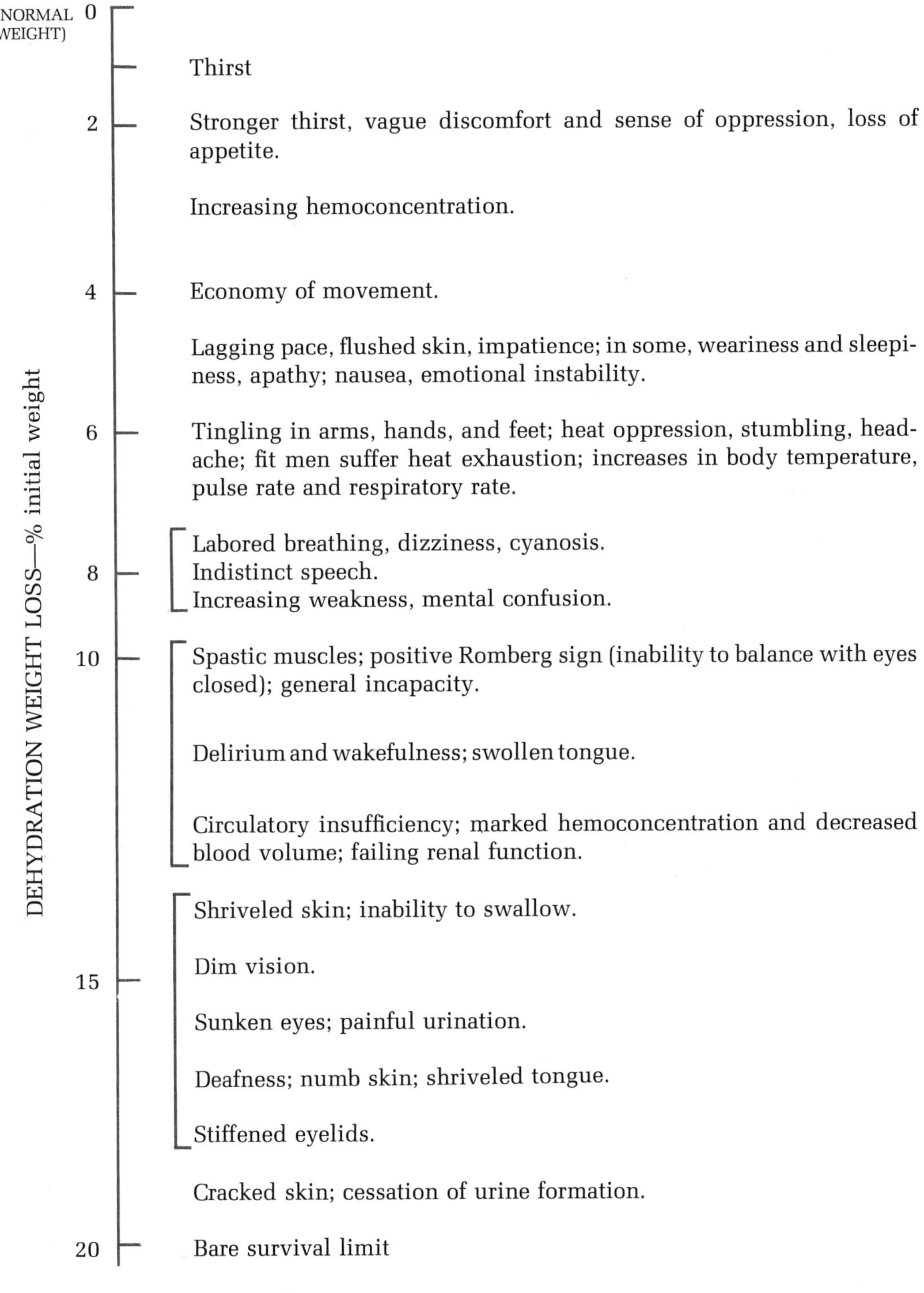

Figure 10–3 Spectrum of dehydration. (After Roth, E. M. (ed.): *Compendium for Development of Human Standards in Space System Design*, Vol. 3. NASA, 1967.)

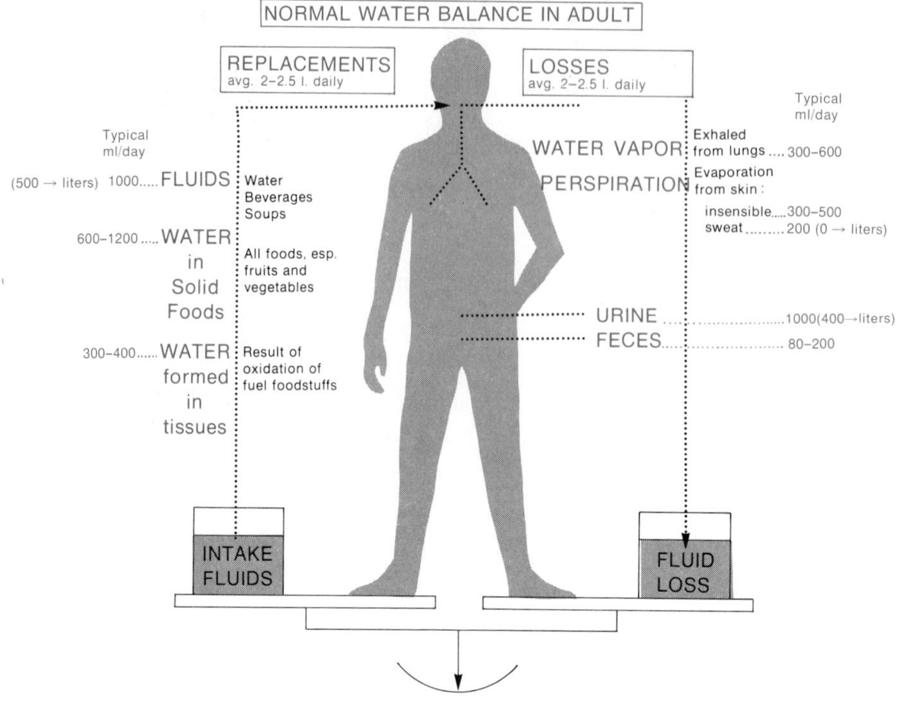

Figure 10–4 Normally the intake and output of water from the body are approximately in balance. If much water is drunk, the volume of urine excreted increases. If water intake is low or the amount lost in perspiration is high (with exercise or in hot weather), the urine will be reduced in volume. With fever, vomiting, or diarrhea, there is excessive loss of water. Any excessive loss should be made up by taking more fluids so that body stores of water are not depleted.

per square meter of body surface area. The requirement is increased in hot environments; if the urine volume is low and the urine appears more concentrated than usual (darker in color, cloudy), it is an indication that fluid intake should be increased.

Water Replacements

Water loss must be made up by the water furnished from three different sources:

1. By the fluids taken (water, beverages, soup, etc.).
2. By the water contained in solid foods.
3. By the water produced in the body as a result of the metabolic processes.

Solid *foods* contain a great deal of water — ranging from about 5 percent in very dry foods such as crackers to over 90 percent in juicy fruits and vegetables such as tomatoes, eggplant, cauliflower, lettuce, strawberries, and watermelon. Even such a solid food as bread contains water to the extent of about 30 to 35 percent of its weight (Table 10–1).

A small amount of water is formed in the body as a product of the oxidative processes necessary to sustain life (see Chapter 15). Water is always one of the products formed when fuel foods are metabolized in the tissues to get energy. Complete oxidation of 1 gm of glucose produces 0.60 gm of water, 1 gm of protein yields 0.41 gm, and 1 gm of fat yields 1.07 gm. With a 2500–3000 kcal energy metabolism, this water of oxidation, or *metabolic water*, amounts to 300 to 400 ml per day.

In addition to the water obtained from these two sources, however, we need to take in *fluids* to replenish the water content of the body. The amount needed is variable, depending on the magnitude of water loss and to some extent on the

Table 10–1 WATER CONTENT OF FOODS*

Food	*Water gm/100 gm*
Fresh vegetables and juices	90–95
Watermelon	93
Soft drinks, beer, soups	88–92
Fresh fruits and juices	85–90
Milk, cow's, whole	87
Potatoes	80
Avocados, bananas, sweet potatoes	75
Eggs	74
Cooked dry beans, cereals	70
Veal, 12% fat (thin)	71
Beef, 24% fat (utility)	62
34% fat (good)	55
46% fat (prime)	45
Tuna fish, canned, drained	60
Bread	30–35
Iced cake	20
Honey	17
Wheat flour	12
Dry beans	10
Crackers, ready-to-eat cereals	2–4
Nuts	2–4

*Data from U.S. Department of Agriculture Handbook No. 8. Washington, D.C., 1963. Values are approximate.

dryness of foods eaten, but usually 5 to 6 glasses daily is sufficient. If a good deal of milk, tea, coffee, or soup is taken, it is not necessary to drink much water. A small excess of water intake over the actual need is a safety factor guarding against constipation and the formation of kidney stones. There is no objection to drinking water with meals. Large quantities of an iced beverage, however, may cause some mild, temporary gastric distress.

Household water supplies are never just pure water; all contain some minerals, and hard water may supply significant amounts of minerals if large quantities are drunk. When hard water is processed by softening, the elements calcium and magnesium are replaced by sodium. Bottled water, sold commercially for use in homes and offices, either is bottled from some natural source or is distilled water to which standard amounts of minerals have been added. Distilled water is produced by converting water (sea water, tap water, etc.) to steam and cooling the steam in a clean collecting system. Dissolved materials remain behind, so that distilled water contains only the substances taken up from the storage containers and pipe systems; its use creates a greater dependency on the diet as the sole source of required elements.

BODY FLUID COMPARTMENTS

At birth, the human body is about 77 percent water. Water content falls to about 63 percent in infants during the first year of life, 59 percent in children, and 45 to 60 percent in healthy young adults. Men have more water and less fat in their bodies than do women, on the average, and both show a steady decline in total body water with advancing age. Men over 60 have about 50 to 54 percent of body weight as water, and women, 42 to 49 percent.

The body water is not a continuous mass but is divided roughly into two main compartments, the *intracellular* fluid and the *extracellular* fluid (Fig. 10–5). About 60 percent of the total body water is found within the cells (the intracellular fluid); the other 40 percent is in various compartments outside the cells (the extracellular fluid). Less than one-fifth of the extracellular fluid is found in the circulatory system; blood plasma constitutes a bit less than 5 percent of body weight in healthy adults, or about 3 to 3.5 liters of fluid. Some of the extracellular fluid is in hollow organs and joints and some is in bone, but by far the largest amount surrounds and bathes the cells. The water inside each cell is also subdivided into yet smaller compartments, which are discontinuous and rather spongelike.[1]

The composition of the fluids within and outside the cells is quite different. The extracellular fluid contains a large amount of sodium and chlorine and is equivalent to a 0.9 percent solution of common salt (sodium chloride). Small amounts of potassium, calcium, magnesium, phosphorus, and sulfur also are present. This composition is about the same as is thought to have been present in the

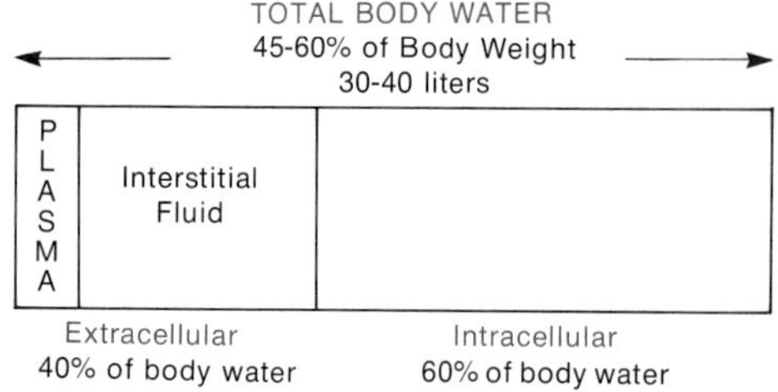

Figure 10–5 The extracellular fluid and intracellular fluid of the body are quite different in composition. Each compartment is maintained in homeostasis by active, energy-requiring body processes. Even though the compositions are different, the compartments are electrically balanced, and both have the same osmotic pressure (except for the plasma, which is slightly higher).

pre-Cambrian sea from which man's remote ancestors emerged to walk on land. When simple life forms emerged, they were surrounded by sea water, with which nutrients and waste products could be exchanged; with increasing complexity, internal cells of the organism were cut off from access to the sea and another means of exchange had to be developed. In higher organisms the internal environment of the extracellular fluid serves this purpose. Over millions of years of evolution, the composition of the extracellular fluid has changed considerably from sea water, but the composition of this fluid compartment does indicate a marine ancestry. Besides the inorganic salts, extracellular fluid contains dissolved carbon dioxide, protein, a small amount of organic acids, and, of course, other organic compounds.

The intracellular fluid is quite dissimilar to extracellular fluid in composition. It is particularly high in potassium and phosphorus content. It contains more magnesium, sulfur, and protein than does the extracellular fluid but less carbon dioxide and much less sodium and chlorine.

It is surprising that the concentration of a substance as freely moving as water is different in these separate compartments. One factor involved is the nature of the membranes that surround the cells. These membranes are semipermeable: That is, they are freely permeable to water, and small molecules like the mineral salts diffuse through them; but other substances with larger molecules (such as proteins) are held back. The membranes within the cells and the nature of the adjacent water layer also play regulatory roles that are only beginning to be understood.[1]

The salt content of the fluids also affects movements of water into or out of the tissues. The salts present in body fluids belong to the class of substances known as *electrolytes.** When in water, the molecules of electrolytes separate into two or more electrically charged particles called *ions,* while nonelectrolytes (such as glucose and urea) do not. The chief electrolytes in body fluids are the positively charged ions (cations), sodium and potassium, plus small amounts of calcium and magnesium, and the negatively charged ion (anion) chloride; there are smaller amounts of the anions sulfate, carbonate, and phosphate. The ionization of sodium chloride may be represented simply as follows:

$$NaCl \rightleftarrows Na^+ + Cl^-$$

Because *osmotic† pressure* is directly proportional to the number of particles in a solution, substances that ionize (separate into two or more particles) have much greater osmotic pressure than do those that do not ionize.

Conditions in a living system are never constant; some products are being

*Electrolytes are substances that will conduct an electric current when they are in solution. When an electric current is passed through an aqueous solution, some elements collect at the positive pole and others at the negative side. This indicates that the elemental particles bear electric charges.

†When a permeable membrane is interposed between two salt solutions of different concentrations, the salt and the water both diffuse from their area of higher concentration to the lower one until equilibrium is attained. If the membrane is semipermeable, the water will move from its area of higher concentration (the dilute solution) more rapidly than will the salt; that is, osmosis will occur. The amount of excess pressure that must be imposed on the solution to prevent the passage of the water through the membrane is called the osmotic pressure of the solution.

formed and others degraded at all times. These products have different electrical charges, and some may ionize and others not. Adjustments are constantly taking place so that within the limits of a dynamic system, fluids in a compartment are balanced with respect to positive and negative ions. The compartments contain different ions and different total amounts of electrolytes and nonelectrolytes, but in spite of these differences in content, the osmotic pressure of the compartments is very nearly the same.

Movement of substances between blood and extracellular fluids, and between these fluids and tissue cells, is due to the influence of osmotic pressure, which in turn is due chiefly to the content of mineral salts.

Both sodium and potassium will diffuse through cell membranes. It is thought that the content of sodium inside the cell is kept low by an active energy-requiring process of pumping out the sodium.[2] The sodium pump, by moving a small number of sodium ions, shifts a large volume of water because of the requirement to achieve equal osmotic pressure. Differences in protein content of the compartments also play a role in osmotic regulation of fluid. Because plasma contains more protein than does the extracellular fluid that is outside the blood vessels, fluid can remain in the circulatory system under the force of pressure needed to circulate the blood, and can re-collect there from the tissues. Thus, fluid moves continuously in and out of cells, carrying in nutrients, oxygen, and other chemical compounds and carrying out wastes and other soluble substances formed by the cells.

There are many other instances in which the exchange of water across body membranes is important and is influenced at least in part by the relative amounts of salts on the two sides of the membrane. These instances include absorption and reabsorption of water across the membrane lining the intestine; passage of water (with dissolved nutrients) from the blood stream into the tissues and from the tissues (laden with waste products or intermediate metabolic products) to the blood stream; and the excretion of water into urinary tubules and its partial reabsorption back into the blood stream. All these processes permit the use of water over and over by the body for various purposes.

Imbalanced Loss of Water and Salt

Loss of body water is always accompanied by some loss of the soluble mineral salts, but under certain circumstances the two may not be commensurate. Suppose a sailor is cut off from his water supply. His water losses continue, and the loss is mainly from the extracellular compartment. The extracellular fluid (ECF) then becomes a more concentrated salt solution, which triggers the sensation of thirst and initiates some hormonal changes that direct the kidney to conserve water and make more concentrated urine. If the water lost is not then replaced, the ECF becomes still more concentrated, and osmosis drives water out of the intracellular compartment until the ECF is diluted to the same concentration as the intracellular fluid (ICF). Both the ECF and ICF compartments are now reduced in size, the cells are dehydrated, and ultimately death will ensue. Present-day sea water is a much more concentrated salt solution than is ECF; it contains 3 to 4 times as much sodium and chloride and 60 times as much magnesium (Table 10–2). Taking in a concentrated salt solution would increase the concentration in the extracellular compartment and lead to further loss of intracellular water, so it is apparent that drinking sea water can only worsen the man's condition.

Excessive sweating at high air temperatures causes loss of water and sodium chloride (salt) from the body. If all the water is replaced and not the salt, the ECF becomes more dilute than normal and water will move from the ECF to the more

Table 10-2 COMPOSITION OF WATER AND SEA SALT

	*Sea Water** *(per kg)*	*North American** *River Waters* *(per liter)*	*Sea Salt†* *(per kg)*
Sodium, gm	10.6	0.009	275
Calcium, gm	0.4	0.020	8.6
Magnesium, gm	1.27	0.005	34
Potassium, gm	0.38	0.001	1.13
Silicon, mg	.02–4.0	9 (SiO_2)	– ‡
Iron, μg	2–20	16	100
Zinc, μg	5	29	0.15
Selenium, μg	4	–	–
Lead, μg	4	–	–
Tin, μg	3	–	–
Cobalt, μg	0.1	4.3	0.1 –1.0
Manganese, μg	1–10	7.1	0.03 –0.3
Molybdenum, μg	0.5	3.9	0.013
Nickel, μg	0.1	–	–
Vanadium, μg	0.3	3.0	–
Copper, μg	3.6	18	20
Chlorine, gm	19.0	0.008	505
Bicarbonate, gm	0.14	0.068	–
Nitrate, mg	.001–0.7	1.0	–
Sulfate, gm	2.65	0.020	18.3(S)
Bromine, mg	65	–	–
Iodine, μg	50	–	1.5
Phosphorus, μg	1–100	–	0.3
Fluorine, mg	1.4	varies	.033

*From Altman, P. L., and Dittmer, D. S.: *Environmental Biology.* Washington, D.C., FASEB, 1966.
†From Kaufman, D. W.: *Sodium Chloride. The Production and Properties of Salt and Brine.* ACS Monograph Series. New York, Reinhold, 1960.
‡Blank indicates no information.

concentrated ICF, and some potassium will be pumped out of the ICF into the ECF. The cells will be overhydrated, and cramps (formerly called *stoker's disease,* after the coal stokers on steamships) may develop because of salt depletion. However, if only enough water is drunk to bring the ECF back to normal osmotic concentration, without taking any salt, the total ECF volume will have shrunk but the state of cellular hydration will be unchanged. When the ECF volume falls, much of the body's protection against water and salt deprivation is gone; and if the loss of ECF is severe, the blood pressure will fall also, to the point of producing faintness.

Sometimes salt is retained excessively, owing to hormonal influences or kidney or liver disease. Then, water is also retained to dilute it, and the ECF volume increases. The tissues may subsequently become edematous because of the large amount of water surrounding the cells.

Edema also results when the protein content of plasma falls, because the force of the blood (hydrostatic) pressure is no longer balanced by the osmotic pressure of extra protein. Fluid is thus lost from the intravascular (within the blood vessels) to the interstitial (surrounding the cells) compartment; the blood volume is diminished, and the tissues have excess fluid. This condition occurs in severe protein deficiency and in some diseases affecting the kidneys or the liver.

OTHER FUNCTIONS OF ELECTROLYTES

Mineral salts have a vital role in maintaining *normal irritability of the nervous tissues and contractility of muscular tissues.* Neither muscles nor nerves function properly unless they are bathed in tissue fluids that contain certain precise amounts of electrolytes. Calcium ions have a stimulating effect, which tends to counterbalance the more or less relaxing or depressing effects of ions of magnesium, sodium, and potassium. Reduced or imbalanced concentrations of these ions can result in paralysis or convulsive movement. Ordinarily, the content of the different salts in the blood and tissue fluids is regulated (chiefly by hormones) to maintain a balance and a constant level so that the muscles and nerves function normally. The rhythmical alternate contractions and relaxations of the heart muscle are an example of this regulation and are dependent on the maintenance of a normal concentration of all the necessary mineral salts in the blood.

The cells function best in a slightly alkaline medium and will be unable to function if the pH* within the cells or in fluids surrounding the cells differs too widely from the optimum. Hence, there are elaborate mechanisms for keeping the blood and tissue fluids within a narrow pH range (7.35 to 7.45). Proteins act as buffer substances capable of uniting with either acids or bases in such a way as to prevent their affecting blood neutrality (see Chapter 5). Mineral elements both affect and regulate body neutrality, in that some of them are acidic and others are basic.

The principal mineral elements may be classified as to their acidic or basic properties (Table 10–3). When sulfur and phosphorus are taken in proteins or other organic compounds, these elements are oxidized to sulfuric and phosphoric acid residues in metabolism. Carbon is oxidized to carbon dioxide whenever organic compounds are burned for energy, and this in turn reacts with water to form carbonic acid (H_2CO_3). These three acidic substances are constantly being formed in tissue metabolism and must be neutralized by basic substances to form salts. Chlorine, another acid-forming element, is taken into the body almost entirely in the form of neutral salts, chiefly common salt or sodium chloride.

Table 10–3 THE CHIEF ACID- AND BASE-FORMING COMPONENTS OF THE DIET

Acid-Forming	*Base-Forming*
ELEMENTS	
Phosphorus	Sodium
Sulfur	Potassium
Chlorine	Calcium
	Magnesium
FOODS	
Meat	Most fruits
Eggs	Vegetables
Cereal products	Milk
Bread	Nuts
Corn	
Cranberries,* plums	

*These are acidic owing to their content of one organic acid, benzoic acid, that yields an acidic end-product in metabolism. Most other organic acids are converted to carbon dioxide and water.

Many basic elements are present in foods in organic combinations, the organic part of which can be oxidized, leaving the basic element free to combine with acids and form salts. For instance, many of the basic elements in fruits are present as salts of organic acids, such as citric and malic acids (e.g., potassium malate in apples). Most of the calcium in milk exists as a salt of the protein casein (calcium caseinate). The carbon chains of protein, organic acids, or other organic matter is oxidized in metabolism to yield carbon dioxide and water, leaving the basic elements free to combine with acids taken in food or formed in metabolism. Thus, it is easier to maintain body neutrality if the acid-forming and base-forming elements in the diet approximately balance each other.

*Acids are compounds containing hydrogen that dissociates to form hydrogen ions (H^+) in aqueous solution. (More precisely, acids are any species capable of accepting a pair of electrons to form a coordinate covalent bond, but these concepts are beyond the scope of this text.) Acidity is, then, a function of the concentration of H ions in solution. In the physiologic range the concentration of H ions is much less than 1 mole per liter, so for convenience in expressing values the pH unit was devised. pH is the negative logarithm of the H ion concentration. pH 7.0 is neutral; values below 7 are in the acid range, and above 7, the alkaline range.

Foods may be classified as acid-forming or base-forming, that is, whether they will furnish a preponderance of acid-forming or base-forming elements after the organic part of the food is oxidized in the tissues. The acid-forming foods usually are high in protein, which contains sulfur and phosphorus; most fruits and vegetables are base-forming because they contain a preponderance of basic elements, either as inorganic salts or as salts of organic acids that can be burned in the body.

The maintenance of pH in the blood and tissues, however, is too important a matter to be left solely to chance selection of diet. In fact, there are several mechanisms for coping with excess acid or base. These are discussed in Chapter 15.

SODIUM

The importance of salt as an item of commerce dates back to ancient times. It was used as a flavoring agent and preservative, and in the making of glass. Sodium (Na), from the word "soda" (or *natrium* in Latin) was first isolated by Davy* in 1807. Elemental sodium is a very active, soft, white, silvery metal that burns on exposure to air. Ordinary table salt (NaCl) and baking soda ($NaHCO_3$) are common and familiar sodium compounds. Although sodium had long been believed to be a dietary essential, final proof was not obtained until after 1905 in experiments with animals.

We have seen that sodium is a key element in regulation of body water and acid-base balance. Because the body has such effective means of conserving sodium when it is scarce and of ridding the body of any excess, it is quite difficult to establish a minimum daily requirement for this nutrient or to set upper limits of tolerance. The average daily American intake is 10 to 15 gm of salt, or about 5 gm of sodium. (Salt is approximately 40 percent sodium and 60 percent chlorine by weight.) There is no evidence as to the desirability of this intake. Where habitual sodium intake is much higher, in Japan, for instance,[3] there is an increased incidence of high blood pressure. In a strain of rats that is prone to develop the condition, a high sodium intake has been proved to induce high blood pressure.[4] This suggests that sodium should be used cautiously, and certainly there is no demonstrated benefit from high intake of sodium in healthy people.

The minimum requirement for sodium can be related to the amount of sodium lost from the body when none is ingested. Under this condition, all available mechanisms are operating maximally to conserve sodium, and excretion falls to less than 200 mg per day. Without question, this amount is not a safe level of intake, by virtue of the fact that it represents output by an individual who is already depleted and it provides no safety margin for changing day-to-day needs. A safe lower intake level is thought to be about 2 to 2.5 gm per day under temperate conditions. Continued sodium depletion leads to shifts in body fluid compartments previously described; there is muscle cramping, loss of appetite, mental apathy, convulsions, and, ultimately, coma and death.

If sweating is profuse, there may be need for additional salt in the diet, but the usual daily intake, 10 to 15 gm of salt, is more than sufficient to cover the loss that occurs with most physical work or moderate heat exposure. Sweat contains up to 1 gm of sodium per liter, so the usual sodium intake (5 gm per day) allows for at least 4 liters of sweat after all other sodium needs are met. For persons who do moderate-to-heavy work in a hot climate *and* under hot conditions, *salt* intake should be increased by about 7 gm per

*Sir Humphry Davy (1778–1829) named and identified not only sodium but also potassium, calcium, chlorine, and boron. He is also recognized as the discoverer of free magnesium and barium. In his home town of Penzance, Cornwall, a statue honors him not for his work with these important elements but rather for his invention of the miner's safety lamp, of greater importance to this mining community.

day.[5] This is best accomplished by salting food heavily or by adding salt to the drinking water that is taken to replace the water lost as sweat. Sweat is *hypotonic;* that is, it contains a lower concentration of salt than the physiologic saline level (0.9 percent), so the fluid drunk for replacement must also be less concentrated than the extracellular fluid. A good solution should have 2 gm of *salt* per liter (2 scant tsp of salt per gal).

Most of the sodium in the diet is added to foods as salt. Not only do we appreciate the taste of salt and have a specific appetite for it (see Chapter 13), but also it is probably the oldest of all chemical preservatives. Even in preindustrial societies, technological processes were developed for providing salt. Natural salt deposits were located, and salt was prepared from saline waters by evaporation. Inland populations traded for salt and also burned green plants to prepare culinary ash. All of these crude salts contain minerals other than sodium chloride, depending on the source from which they were made. Sea salts contain various trace elements (Table 10–2). Plant ash is richer in potassium than in sodium and contains a wide spectrum of essential minerals. Modern commercial salt is nearly pure sodium chloride.

With the increased use of prepared and "convenience" foods, less of an option is open to the individual in setting his own salt intake and there is less salt added to foods in the home.* Other sources of added sodium are monosodium glutamate (MSG), soy sauce, and baking powder. Diets based heavily on processed convenience foods and salted snack foods may contain as much as 25 gm salt; such high salt intake is unwarranted and may be injurious to health. Because of concern over the health aspects of MSG and salt, commercial baby foods are no longer permitted to contain MSG, and their content of salt has been reduced.

Cheese, milk, and shellfish are good natural sources of sodium; and meat, fish, poultry, and eggs make significant contributions (Table 10–4). Cereals, fruits, and vegetables are low in this nutrient unless it is added in processing. Water supplies are quite variable in sodium content but may add significantly to the daily total intake.

*This change in food pattern can reduce the effectiveness of iodization of salt (a public health measure; see Chapter 12) unless both household and commercial salt are fortified with iodine. Proposals have been made to fortify salt with iron and zinc to supplement diets low in these minerals in some regions of the world.

Table 10–4 SODIUM AND POTASSIUM CONTENT OF SOME REPRESENTATIVE FOODS*

Food, 100 gm	*Sodium, mg*	*Potassium, mg*
Apple	1	110
Banana	1	370
Bread, salted	536	273
Bread, unsalted†	38	120
Broccoli, cooked	10	267
Butter, salted	987	23
Butter, unsalted	10	10
Carrot, raw	47	341
Cheese, cheddar	700	82
Chicken, broiled	66	274
Corn, canned, with salt	236	97
Corn, salt-free pack	2	97
Dates, dry	1	648
Egg, cooked in shell	122	129
Hamburger, cooked	47	450
Liver, calf's, fried	118	453
Milk, whole, fluid	50	144
Orange	1	200
Pickle, dill	1428	200
Popcorn, plain	3	660
Popcorn, with oil and salt	1940	512
Potato, French fried	6	853
Potato, French fried, with salt	236	853
Potato chips, salted	up to 1000	1130
Rice, cooked, salted	358	43
Spinach, cooked, no salt	50	324
Tomato, raw	3	244
Tomato juice, canned, with salt	200	227
Wheat, puffed, without salt	4	340
Wheat, puffed, with salt and sugar	161	99

*From Watt, B. K., and Merrill, A. L.: *Composition of Foods: Raw, Processed, Prepared.* Washington, D.C., U.S. Department of Agriculture Handbook No. 8, 1963, except where noted. Where unspecified, values refer to foods cooked without salt.

†Sodium value is for yeast-leavened bread without added salt or sodium propionate (preservative), made with 3 to 4 percent nonfat dry milk solids.

POTASSIUM

Potassium (K) was named in 1807 by Davy, its discoverer, from the word "potash" (Latin *kalium*), the alkaline ash of vegetable substances. Potassium is widely used as a fertilizer for plants and is one of the more abundant elements.

It was not until 1938 that McCollum (using the rat) obtained proof that potassium is an essential nutrient, although this had been suggested earlier.

Potassium is a nearly constant component of lean body tissue, so much so that one method of estimating the amount of lean tissue in a living person is by measuring the amount of potassium present. (This is done by determining the amount of radioactive potassium that is naturally present in a constant ratio to ordinary potassium.) The need for potassium is increased when there is growth or deposition of lean tissue, and potassium is lost whenever muscle is broken down owing to starvation, protein deficiency, or injury. Deficiency of potassium results in muscular weakness or paralysis; the intestinal muscle is also affected, so that normal movement ceases and the abdomen becomes distended with gas. Finally the heart muscle stops. The ordinary diet usually contains enough potassium if energy and protein intake are adequate, because potassium is widely distributed in foods of both plant and animal origin. Deficiency results from a combination of poor diet and excessive loss of potassium due to severe diarrhea, in most cases.* For this reason, potassium deficiency is often present in malnourished children.

Persons given an experimental diet low in potassium excrete about 1.5 gm per day. Most of this is lost in the urine, but there is a substantial amount lost in feces and a little in sweat. A reasonable lower level of intake is thought to be 2.5 gm per day. The usual American diet has about 0.8 to 1.5 gm of potassium per 1000 kcal, little if any above this suggested lower limit.

The same animal model that provides evidence of an adverse effect of sodium on blood pressure (see previous section) shows that blood pressure may be lowered to a more normal level if potassium is increased along with the increased level of sodium in the rat diet. The best response in these rats resulted from a simultaneous increase of potassium and a *reduction* of sodium. It is prudent to maintain a closer ratio of sodium to potassium in the diet than is present in the typical American diet. A more desirable 1:1 ratio can be achieved by either lowering salt intake or increasing potassium intake, or perhaps both.

Meats and other lean muscle tissue are good dietary sources of potassium (Table 10–4). Milk is also a good source, but not cheese, as much of the potassium is lost in whey. Many fruits are outstanding sources of potassium, especially dried dates, bananas, cantaloupe, apricots, and citrus fruits. Tomato juice and the dark green, leafy vegetables are also high in this nutrient. Other vegetables, many fruits, and all cereals make smaller contributions of potassium.

*Dehydration and finally death result from severe diarrhea, owing to the loss of water, sodium, and potassium. Many victims can be saved by oral administration of a simple solution of the following composition:

sodium chloride (table salt)	3.5 gm
sodium bicarbonate (baking soda)	2.5 gm
potassium chloride	1.5 gm
glucose (or honey)	20.0 gm
boiled water to make a total of	1000.0 gm

A child should receive about 1 tsp per minute.

CHLORINE

Chlorine, a common water purifier and bleach, is also an essential element for all higher animals and man. Discovered in 1774 by Scheele and named by Davy in 1810, chlorine (Cl) is a very toxic yellow-green gas in its elemental form. In nature it always exists in a combined form. A common form is salt (NaCl — sodium chloride).

We tend to forget that chlorine is an essential nutrient because it comes into the diet so automatically along with sodium in the salt we add to foods. Chlorine has a special function in forming the hydrochloric acid (HCl) present in gastric juice. This acid is necessary for proper absorption of one of the vitamins (B-12) and iron; it activates the enzyme that breaks down starch, and it suppresses growth of microorganisms that enter the stomach with food and drink. Chloride ion is abundant in the extracellular fluid generally and in the cerebrospinal fluid. In nerve cells, chloride ion tends to stabilize the electrical potential of the membranes. Chloride ion is also involved in the acid-base economy of the body, as noted previously.

Loss of chloride generally parallels that of sodium, and a separate deficiency occurs only when there is loss of chloride due to vomiting. Persons whose sodium intake is severely restricted (owing to diseases of the heart, kidney, or liver) may need an alternative source of chloride; a number of chloride-containing salt substitutes are available for this purpose.

QUESTIONS AND PROBLEMS

1. Which elements are most abundant in the body? What substances are classed as mineral or ash? Why? How much mineral is found in the body?

2. How much water is present in the body? How does water content change with age? Into what compartments is water divided? Is water necessary for building and maintaining tissues? Why? Name and discuss three ways in which water acts as a regulator of body processes.

3. By what routes is water lost from the body? What conditions determine the relative amounts of water lost through the skin and in the urine? What conditions make for excessive loss of water from the body? What is the normal daily (approximate) loss of water from the body? How much heat is required to evaporate 1 kg of water? How much additional water would be needed to compensate for the amount lost as sweat produced from playing tennis for 1 hour indoors? (Use the data on energy cost of activities given in Chapter 2.)

4. Keep a record of your total intake of water for one day — that is, the amount taken as water, soup, tea, coffee, and milk. How does your intake compare with the amount that most persons should take either in beverages or as drinking water? What is meant by "metabolic water"?

5. What is an electrolyte? Which ions are most abundant in the extracellular fluid? The intracellular fluid? How are these differences maintained? What is meant by osmotic pressure? How does it relate to the exchange of substances between fluid compartments?

6. What changes occur in the body when water intake is insufficient? Why must salt and water be replaced when sweating is heavy? What is a good way to take extra salt when it is needed.

7. What foods are high in sodium content? Which are low? How much sodium should be taken daily? What percentage of salt is sodium? What other element is found in common salt? What function does it have in the body?

8. What foods are high in potassium content? Which are low? How does potassium deficiency occur? What are the symptoms? How much potassium should be taken daily?

9. What is meant by acid-base balance? Which elements and foods are acidic? Which basic?

REFERENCES

1. Robinson, J. R.: Water, the indispensable nutrient. Nutrition Today, 5:16, Spring 1970.
2. Schmidt-Nielsen, B.: Symposium: Comparative aspects of transport of hypertonic, isotonic and hypotonic solutions by epithelial membranes. Introduction. Fed. Proc., *30*:3, 1971.
3. Dahl, L. K.: Possible role of chronic excess salt consumption in pathogenesis of essential hypertension. Amer. J. Cardiol., *8*:571, 1961. Salt and hypertension. Amer. J. Clin. Nutr., *25*:232, 1972.
4. Meneely, G. R., and Ball, C. O. T.: Experimental epidemiology of chronic sodium chloride toxicity

and the protective effect of potassium chloride. Amer. J. Med., *25*:713, 1958; Dahl, L. K., Heine, M., and Tassinari, L.: Effects of chronic excess salt ingestion. Evidence that genetic factors play an important role in susceptibility to experimental hypertension. J. Exp. Med., *115*:1173, 1962.

5. Lee, D. H. K.: Terrestrial animals in dry heat: man in the desert. In Code, C. F. (ed.): *Handbook of Physiology,* Section 4, Chapter 35. Baltimore, The Williams & Wilkins Co. for Amer. Physiol. Society, 1964.

SUPPLEMENTARY READING

Adolph, E. F.: Regulation of water intake in relation to body water content. In Code, C. F. (ed.): *Handbook of Physiology,* Section 6, Vol. I, Chapter 12. Baltimore, The Williams & Wilkins Co. for Amer. Physiol. Society, 1967.

Alleyne, G. A. O.: Studies on total body potassium in malnourished infants. Factors affecting potassium repletion. Brit. J. Nutr., *24*:205, 1970.

Baker, E. M., Plough, I. C., and Allen, T. H.: Water requirements of men as related to salt intake. Amer. J. Clin. Nutr., *12*:394, 1963.

Birge, S. J., Jr., Gilbert, H. R., and Avioli, L. V.: Intestinal calcium transport: the role of sodium. Science, *176*:168, 1972.

Bradley, C. C.: Human water needs and water use in America. Science, *138*:489, 1962.

Daly, C., and Dill, D. B.: Salt economy in humid heat. Amer. J. Physiol., *118*:285, 1937.

Denton, D. A.: Salt appetite. In Code, C. F. (ed.): *Handbook of Physiology,* Section 6, Vol. I, Chapter 31. Baltimore, The Williams & Wilkins Co. for Amer. Physiol. Society, 1967.

Ellis, K. J., et al.: Total body sodium and chlorine in normal adults. Metabolism, *25*:645, 1976.

Filer, L. J., Jr.: Salt in infant foods. Nutr. Rev., *29*:27, 1971.

Fitzsimons, J. T.: Thirst. Physiol. Rev., *52*:468, 1972.

Flynn, M. A., Hanna, F. M., and Lutz, R. N.: Estimation of body water compartments of preschool children. Amer. J. Clin. Nutr., *20*:1125, 1967.

Flynn, M. A., et al.: A longitudinal study of total body potassium in normal children. Pediatr. Res., *9*:834, 1975.

Food and Nutrition Board: *Minimal Allowances of Water and Food for Fallout Shelter Survival.* Washington, D.C., National Research Council, National Academy of Sciences, 1962.

Freis, E. D.: Salt, volume and the prevention of hypertension. Circulation, *53*:589, 1976.

Gamble, J. L.: The water requirements of castaways. Proc. Amer. Philosoph. Soc., *88*:151, 1944.

Gozansky, D. M., and Herman, R. H.: Water and sodium retention in the fasted and refed human. Amer. J. Clin. Nutr., *24*:869, 1971.

Holmes, J. H.: Thirst and fluid intake as clinical problems. In Code, C. F. (ed.): *Handbook of Physiology,* Section 6, Vol. I., Chapter 11. Baltimore, The Williams & Wilkins Co. for Amer. Physiol. Society, 1967.

Kirkendall, W. M., et al.: The effect of dietary sodium chloride on blood pressure, body fluids, electrolytes, renal function and serum lipids of normotensive man. J. Lab. Clin. Med., *87*:418, 1976.

Krishnaswami, S. K.: Health aspects of water quality. Amer. J. Public Health, *61*:2259, 1971.

Malhotra, M. S.: Salt and water requirement of acclimatized people working outdoors in severe heat. Indian J. Med. Res., *48*:212, 1960.

Meneely, G. R., and Battarbee, H. D.: Sodium and potassium. Nutr. Rev., *34*:225, 1976.

McKelsen, O., et al.: Sodium and potassium intakes and excretions of normal men consuming sodium chloride or a 1:1 mixture of sodium and potassium chlorides. Amer. J. Clin. Nutr., *30*:2033, 1977.

Miller, R. W.: Carcinogens in drinking water. Pediatr., *57*:462, 1976.

Oexmann-Wannamaker, M. J.: Salt substitutes. Amer. J. Clin. Nutr., *29*:599, 1976.

Perry, H. M., Jr.: Minerals in cardiovascular disease. J. Amer. Dietet. Assoc., *62*:631, 1973.

Pitts, G. C., Johnson, R. E., and Consolazio, C. F.: Work in the heat as affected by intake of water, salt and glucose. Amer. J. Physiol., *142*:253, 1944.

Schmidt-Nielsen, K.: *Desert Animals: Physiological Problems of Heat and Water.* Oxford, Oxford University Press, 1964.

Schuman, S. H., and Williams, G. W.: Biochemical profiles during a Michigan heat wave: suggestion of nutritional disturbance. Ecol. Food Nutr., *3*:117, 1974.

Share, L., and Claybaugh, J. R.: Regulation of body fluids. Ann. Rev. Physiol., *34*:235, 1972.

Spark, R. F., et al.: Renin, aldosterone and glucagon in the natriuresis of fasting. N. Engl. J. Med., *292*:1335, 1975.

Stinebaugh, B. J., Vasquez, M. I., and Schloeder, F. X.: Taste thresholds for salt in fasting patients. Amer. J. Clin. Nutr., *28*:814, 1975.

Tollenaar, D.: Dietary potassium and sodium as affecting work output and other physical performance of rats. Nutr. Rpt. Internat., *15*:483, 1977.

Walker, J. S., et al.: Water intake of normal children. Science, *140*:890, 1963.

Wheeler, E. F., El-Neil, H., Willson, J. O. C., and Weiner, J. S.: The effect of work level and dietary intake on water balance and the excretion of sodium, potassium and iron in a hot climate. Brit. J. Nutr., *30*:127, 1973.

Articles in Nutrition Reviews

Exchangeable potassium and the prediction of fat free body weight. *30*:175, 1972.

Potassium and endocrine pancreatic function. *32*:9, 1974.

Natriuresis of starvation and glucagon. *32*:78, 1974.

Water deprivation and performance of athletes. *32*:314, 1974.

Water and electrolytes in malnutrition. *33*:74, 1975.

Chapter 11

Calcium, Phosphorus, and Magnesium

In the last chapter we discussed the body's need for water and the electrolytes (sodium, potassium, and chlorine). These three elements plus *calcium, phosphorus,* and *magnesium* make up the six important *macrominerals* essential in our diets. They are present in the body in relatively large amounts and are required in the diet in considerably larger quantities than the "trace elements" (Chapter 12).*

CALCIUM

Discovery of Dietary Requirement

Calcium (Ca) was discovered in 1808 by Sir Humphry Davy, the English chemist. The name calcium is derived from the Latin *Calx* or *calcis,* which is also the origin of the word chalk. Calcium exists in nature only in the combined form, often as a phosphate or carbonate in such common substances as chalk, granite, eggshell, seashells, "hard" water, bone, and limestone. All of these substances can serve as a source of calcium in the diet; the knowledge of their antirachitic properties and other health benefits goes back to ancient times, in both the Asian and the Middle Eastern cultures.

*Each of the six macrominerals is required by the human diet in an amount over 100 mg per day. This serves as a convenient dividing line between macrominerals and trace elements.

Calcium was among the first materials known to be essential in the diet. A Frenchman, Chossat, showed experimentally as long ago as 1842 that calcium salts were required by the pigeon. Many other experiments, before 1920, proved the need by all animals for both calcium[1] and phosphorus.[2] Well-controlled experiments with man were not made until more recent years.

Absorption and Retention in Body

The absorption of calcium from the intestinal tract varies with different individuals and under different conditions, but it is not as complete as for some other nutrients. Generally, only 20 to 40 percent of the calcium intake is absorbed. In the first place, any calcium that is in organic combination must be set free in soluble form before it can be absorbed; and second, various substances or conditions in the intestinal tract may contribute to the formation of insoluble (and hence unabsorbable) compounds.

The relative absorption may vary under special conditions or with individual foods.[3] Some of the factors that either

Table 11–1 ABSORPTION OF CALCIUM AND PHOSPHORUS FROM THE INTESTINAL TRACT

Factors Favoring Absorption	*Factors Hindering Absorption*
Acid reaction in upper intestinal tract.	Alkaline reaction in lower intestinal tract.
Normal digestive activity and normal motility of intestinal tract.	Large amounts of fiber in diet.
Calcium and phosphorus in diet in about equal amounts.	Laxatives or any circumstances that induce diarrhea or hypermotility of the intestine.
The fat-soluble vitamin D.	Large excess of either element in comparison with the other (Ca:P ratio unbalanced).
Need for higher amounts of these mineral elements by the body.	With excess calcium present, insoluble Ca salts may be formed with phytin (complex P compound in cereals), oxalic acid (in certain leafy vegetables), and unabsorbed fatty acids.
	Excess of iron, magnesium, or aluminum forms insoluble phosphates.

favor or hinder the absorption of calcium and the closely related mineral phosphorus from the intestinal contents are listed briefly in Table 11–1.

The fact that *oxalic acid* in certain foods (e.g., rhubarb, cocoa, and spinach) forms an insoluble salt with calcium (calcium oxalate) and that *phytic acid* in the outer coats of cereals can tie up much of the calcium and phosphorus in insoluble compounds is not considered of major practical importance, provided the supply of these elements in the diet is liberal enough that sufficient absorbable calcium and phosphorus remain to meet body needs.

Excessive amounts of fatty acids in the intestine can also tie up calcium by forming insoluble "soaps," but this, too, appears to have little practical significance when persons are eating normal diets (see Chapter 19). The amount of *vitamin D* available in the body, however, does play an important role in both the *absorption* and *utilization* of calcium.

Possibly even more critical factors influencing the relative amounts of calcium and phosphorus that are *absorbed* and *retained in the body* are the body's *need* for these elements, especially calcium, and the *level of intake* to which the body has become adapted. If a person regularly takes in large amounts of calcium, his body adjusts by absorbing less calcium. On the other hand, people may adjust to a lower level of calcium intake by more efficient absorption and decreased excretion of this element, thus conserving sufficient calcium for upkeep of body tissues. But in the case of calcium the readjustment process may take many weeks, or months. Again, the amount absorbed is largely dependent on *body need.* In an infant or young child, or during healing of bone fractures, absorption of calcium is relatively more efficient, so that a larger percentage of the intake is available for the building or strengthening of bone tissues. The same is true in pregnancy or in an adult after a fairly long period on a low-calcium intake, in which body stores of this element are likely to be depleted. If higher calcium intake is provided, a relatively larger amount of calcium is absorbed and retained in the body than if the previous diet had furnished calcium in liberal quantities. Thus, the relative amounts of calcium retained in the body vary, depending on the age of the person, his previous dietary habits, and the level of the current supply.

Distribution and Functions in Body

Calcium makes up about 1.5 to 2.2 percent of the human body, more than any other mineral. Ninety-nine percent of this calcium plays a major role in the structure of bones and teeth. A strong, well-developed skeletal system fulfills a number of functions. It gives form to the body, affords protection to the brain and the visceral organs, serves as an anchor for muscles that allow body movement, and is the site of blood formation.

Bone is a connective tissue of which about 30 percent is organic matter (cells and fibers) that is embedded in mineral (70 percent). The mineral part is composed mostly of tiny crystals of calcium phosphate* but includes smaller amounts of magnesium, sodium, and carbonate. The metabolism of bone is so slow that formerly this tissue was thought of chiefly as inert material drawn on only in cases of great need. However, it is now recognized that bone is a living tissue that undergoes remodeling throughout adult life.

The microscopic structure of bone is such that none of the mineral crystals is far from a blood vessel, an arrangement that favors exchange of minerals and nutrients between bone tissues and body fluids. The most readily available supply of calcium and phosphorus in bones is found in the *trabeculae* — columns of crystalline calcium compounds that grow from the inner surface of the cavity at the bone's end and that project toward the center in such a way as to act as braces in strengthening the end of the bone (see Fig. 11–1). The more abundant the supply of calcium in the food, the greater is the development of bone trabeculae; when dietary calcium is inadequate over a considerable period, these structures may be practically absent. Within the cavity, blood vessels and intercellular fluid come into intimate contact with the mineral material in the trabeculae, so that it may be readily taken up by the blood stream to meet minor fluctuations in blood calcium.

Although only 1 percent of the body's calcium is found in the blood, this small amount is of vital physiological importance. Calcium is one of the essential factors for blood clotting, it affects muscle tone and irritability, and it is required for normal nerve transmission. The proper balance between calcium ions on the one hand and sodium, potassium, and magnesium ions on the other is necessary for normal rhythmical contraction and relaxation of the heart muscles. Calcium also activates several enzymes important in metabolism. When the level of blood calcium is subnormal, these functions cannot be fulfilled; the heartbeat becomes erratic, muscles contract spontaneously, and death may result.

Calcium in the blood is maintained at the optimal level through the action of two hormones. When the level rises above normal, *calcitonin* stimulates bone formation, and calcium is removed from blood and deposited in bone. When the level drops below normal, *parathyroid hormone* stimulates bone demineralization, resulting in a movement of calcium from bone to blood. It also stimulates absorption of calcium from the intestines and inhibits loss in the urine. Thus, in addition to its other functions, bone serves as a store of calcium that can be drawn upon for the regulation of the level of this important mineral in blood.

*Similar or identical to hydroxyapatite, $Ca_{10}(PO_4)_6(OH)_2$.

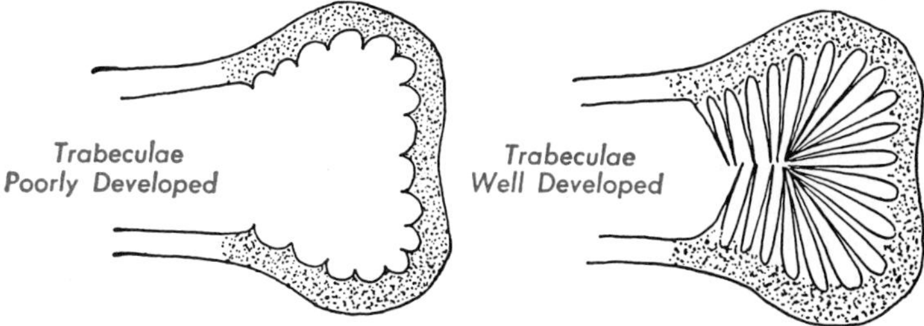

Figure 11–1 Diagrammatic representations of bone trabeculae showing poor or good development according to whether the food calcium intake is low or liberal. (From Sherman, H. C.: *Chemistry of Food and Nutrition.* New York, Macmillan Co., 1952.)

Maintenance Requirement

Calcium is continuously being lost from the body through excretion in the urine and feces, and to a small extent through the skin. The *minimum requirement* in the case of adults is the amount needed to balance these losses.

Attempts to fix a minimum requirement were at first based on balance experiments similar to those described for nitrogen balance (p. 92), but in the case of calcium this method proved to have many drawbacks. While it is possible to obtain some mean value or rather narrow range within which the majority of subjects attain balance, there are many cases in which inexplicable variations occur. Even after 2 or 3 weeks on a basal diet of known calcium content, when the calcium intake is lowered in an attempt to find the minimum requirement, some subjects maintain equilibrium on the lowered intake, while others are in either negative or positive balance. Knowing as we do that absorption of calcium is influenced by body need and that previous patterns of excretion are carried over into the later periods because of slow adaptations to changed levels of intake, this would have to be expected. For instance, when placed on a lower level of calcium intake, a person whose intake was previously liberal has less efficient absorption of calcium and carries over his pattern of high excretion, drawing on his already built-up stores of body calcium (called the *labile calcium pool*) to make up the difference. Hence, he responds to the lowered level by showing a negative balance, although the stores of calcium in his body were excellent.

With such obvious drawbacks in the balance method, investigators have been unable to give an exact figure for the minimum calcium requirement of adults. Estimates of the minimum requirement range from about 400 to 650 mg per day for an adult of average weight with ideal absorption and other ideal conditions.

Several well-known earlier studies[4] have claimed that men can adapt, with time, to lower calcium intakes and maintain calcium balance on intakes as low as 200 to 400 mg daily. Although it is true that a higher proportion of calcium is utilized on a low intake than when it is liberally supplied, most of the national groups cited as in equilibrium on such low calcium intakes live in either tropical or semitropical areas (where abundant sunlight favors calcium utilization by forming vitamin D in the body), or they may have hitherto unrecognized sources of calcium in the diet. These include white clay quite commonly consumed by some cultures (a practice known as *pica*); the lime-steeped corn used for making tortillas in Mexico; and the "stone powder," which is essentially calcium carbonate, added to rice during its milling in Formosa. In a review of the extensive literature on calcium balance experiments, Ohlson states, "Few adults eating diets characteristic of our society are in equilibrium on intakes of less than 500 mg (0.5 gm) per day."[5] It is known that calcium requirements are influenced by levels of protein intake — the greater the protein intake, the greater the calcium loss.

Recommended Allowance for Adults

The Food and Nutrition Board in 1974 kept its *recommended allowance for calcium* at 800 mg per day for adults.[6] This is based on estimates of daily calcium losses in adults of about 175 mg in the urine and 125 mg in the feces, for a total of at least 300 mg. Minor amounts of calcium may be lost in perspiration (at least 20 mg per day), but they need be taken into account only in cases of excessive sweating due to physical activity at high environmental temperatures. Assuming that 40 percent of ingested calcium is absorbed, 800 mg per day are needed in the diet. This allowance provides a factor of safety above the bare maintenance requirement and covers individual differences of need and of the ability to utilize calcium from the diet. Despite the usually

Table 11–2 RECOMMENDED DIETARY ALLOWANCES PER DAY FOR CALCIUM AND PHOSPHORUS*

	Age (yrs)	*Calcium (mg)*	*Phosphorus (mg)*
Males	11–14	1200	1200
	15–18	1200	1200
	19–22	800	800
	23–50	800	800
	51+	800	800
Females	11–14	1200	1200
	15–18	1200	1200
	19–22	800	800
	23–50	800	800
	51+	800	800
	Pregnant	1200	1200
	Lactating	1200	1200

*From Food and Nutrition Board, 1974.[6]

lesser weight and lighter skeletal structure of women, the same amount is recommended for women as for men in order to cover menstrual losses and to provide a reserve store in the body to meet needs of pregnancy and lactation. Table 11–2 gives the recommended dietary allowance for growing children and adults of all ages for both calcium and phosphorus (see more details in Appendix, Table I). The recommended allowances of calcium vary from country to country (see Appendix, Table 1C), ranging from as low as 400 mg a day up to 1000 mg. These differences are to be expected until more research is done on the subject. At this time, we would advise a student to use for himself that figure recommended by the highest nutrition authority in his own country (in the United States it is the Food and Nutrition Board) because of different dietary and environmental conditions in each country.

An FAO/WHO Expert Committee has proposed intakes of calcium between 400 and 500 mg per day as "suggested practical allowances" for adults, especially for countries where calcium-rich foods such as dairy products are either not plentiful or unavailable.[7]

It appears obvious that a large proportion of the population can adjust to levels of calcium intake of 0.5 to 0.6 gm per day without any apparent signs of deficiency, and if their reserves of calcium in skeletal tissue are less than optimum, it is difficult to detect or measure any such depletion. In fact, 10 to 40 percent of the mineral material in bones may be withdrawn for body use before a decrease in bone density can be detected by x-ray pictures. It is evident that the recommended allowance of the United States has a considerable margin of safety for most adults.

Allowances During Childhood, Pregnancy, and Lactation

Adults need calcium and phosphorus only for maintenance of a body already built, but children need also a "growth quota." Extra amounts of these elements are required not only for the *growth* of bones but also for their *strengthening* by further deposits of calcium phosphate. The bones of a newborn infant are more flexible and of lower mineral content than those of an adult, a provision of nature that makes birth easier. As the child grows, the relative proportion of calcium phosphate in the bones must be increased so that they will become stronger and more rigid, in order to bear the weight of the body and to be less easily broken. The teeth are formed and partially calcified in the latter months of fetal life, and their calcification is practically completed by the time the child is 2 to 3 years old. For children from 2 to 6 years of age, the calcium and the phosphorus allowances are the same as for adults (800 mg), and from ages 6 to 10 the allowances are 1000 mg (1 gm). Per unit of weight, growing children may need two to four times as much calcium as does an adult.

Children will continue to grow on diets that supply less than desirable amounts of calcium or phosphorus, but the bones and teeth will not be of as good a quality, or growth may not be so rapid as with a more liberal allowance of these elements. If the quantity of either element is too limited, growth may be stunted. During the rapid growth in the period of preadolescence and puberty (10 to 18 years), a higher intake is recommended (1200 mg; see Table 11–2). At levels of 1 to 1.5 gm daily of each of these elements in the diet, children have shown "maximum retention" — that is, as much calcium and phosphorus is provided as the body can store.[8] Greater amounts would normally be excreted by the body.

Women in the latter half of pregnancy and those who are nursing their babies have considerably higher calcium and phosphorus needs than do normal adults, since the mineral needs of the growing fetus or infant must be met through the mother's body. For mothers, as well as for growing children, there should also be a *plentiful supply of vitamin D,* a vitamin that helps assure good absorption and assimilation of the mineral elements provided in the diet. A liberal intake of calcium is especially important during lactation, in order to provide for the secretion of calcium-rich milk without undue drain on the reserve stores of calcium in the mother's own body (Fig. 11–2). Specific allowances for children of different ages and for pregnant and lactating women are found in Chapters 20 and 21, devoted to diet for these conditions, and also are found in Table 1 of the Appendix.

Effects of Dietary Deficiency of Calcium

A deficiency of calcium is most apparent in the young of any species because of the great demand for this nutrient in bone and teeth formation. The effects of such a deficiency during the growth period are manifested in one or more of the following ways:

1. By stunting of growth.
2. By poor quality of bones and teeth.
3. By malformation of bones (rickets).

When calcium lack has not been too severe, no effect may be noted in the size of the body, but the bones may either be delicate and brittle, or remain soft and pliable because too little mineral salts are deposited in them. The skeleton of the smaller rat in Figure 11–3 shows both stunting in size of bones and their poor quality as exemplified in brittleness and certain deformities. The child suffering from rickets shown in Figure 11–4 evidences the bone deformities peculiar to that disease — narrow chest, enlargement of bones at their ends (seen at knees), and bowlegs resulting from inability of soft bones to bear the body weight. This disease can be caused by lack of either calcium, phosphorus, or vitamin D, or combinations of all three nutrients. The bone deformities of rickets may persist in later life, the narrow pelvic cavity being a complicating factor in pregnancy.

The *teeth* are largely formed during the latter part of fetal life and during infancy. Any lack of calcium during this period is likely to result in malformed teeth and jaws, or in poor-quality teeth that are more subject to decay in later life.

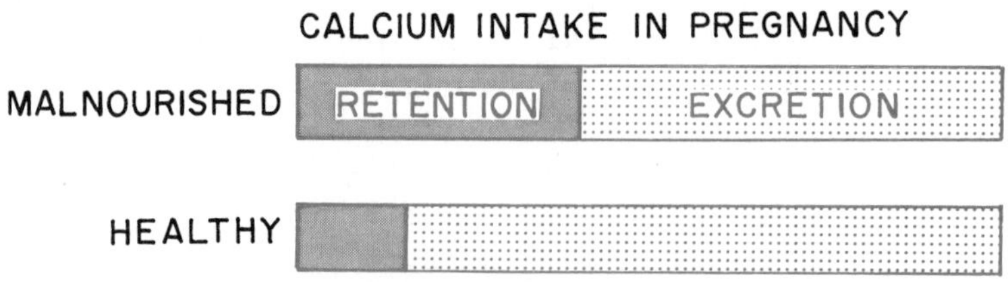

Figure 11–2 Some women enter into pregnancy with too low reserves of those nutrients that can be stored in the body because of previous inadequate diets. Calcium is one of the nutrients most likely to be furnished in less than optimum amounts in American diets. This diagram shows that, when given a relatively rich supply of calcium during pregnancy, the previously malnourished woman retained a good percentage of it, thereby building up her body reserves of this element. The woman whose diet before pregnancy had been adequate and whose stores of calcium were therefore higher had less need to store it and hence retained a smaller percentage of the calcium furnished by the diet than the other woman. (Adapted from Macy and Williams: *Hidden Hunger.* Lancaster, Pa., Jacques Cattell Press, 1945.)

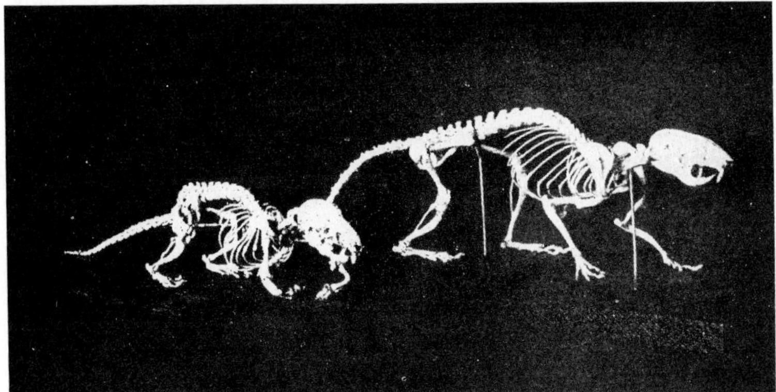

Figure 11–3 Skeletons of twin albino rats, showing influence of calcium content of the diet on the growth and character of the bones. **Right,** This rat, fed a diet adequate in calcium, attained full growth and had strong bones. **Left,** This rat received a diet deficient in calcium. Its growth was stunted, and its bones were soft and fragile, and more or less deformed. (Courtesy of Sherman and MacLeod and the *Journal of Biological Chemistry*.)

Many instances of poor-quality teeth or of teeth crowded too closely in a narrow jaw may be attributable to the mother's insufficient supply of calcium, phosphorus, or other dietary essentials during pregnancy or to the child's receiving an insufficient supply of these dietary essentials during its first years of life. By consuming a good diet in later life, it is difficult to undo the effects of such deficiencies during the formative periods. (See Chapter 23.)

In parts of the world where food supplies and living conditions are poor, conditions that indicate calcium deficiency may be found frequently, both in children and in adults. When milk and meats are scarce or unavailable, a large proportion of the diet must come from vegetable sources, especially cereal grains. Such diets are usually low in calcium, as well as deficient in the quantity and biological value of the proteins supplied. Populations do adapt to low-calcium diets, their children grow, and bone disease is not common among them. However, the children in such countries are often as much as 3 years behind in growth rate, as compared with well-nourished children, and the shorter stature attained by many of the adults suggests strongly that the low level of calcium intake (probably accompanied by other dietary lacks) may have prevented them from growing to the full height of which they were genetically capable. Children of such parents, when given a more nutritionally adequate diet, respond with increased growth rate and by adulthood are considerably taller than their parents.

A lifetime of a low-calcium intake may be a contributing factor to a state of gradual demineralization of bony tissues known as *osteoporosis*. This disorder is characterized by porosity, thinness, and fragility of the bones. Apparently in the continuous remodeling of bone, calcium has been withdrawn for body use or mandatory excretion over a long period and

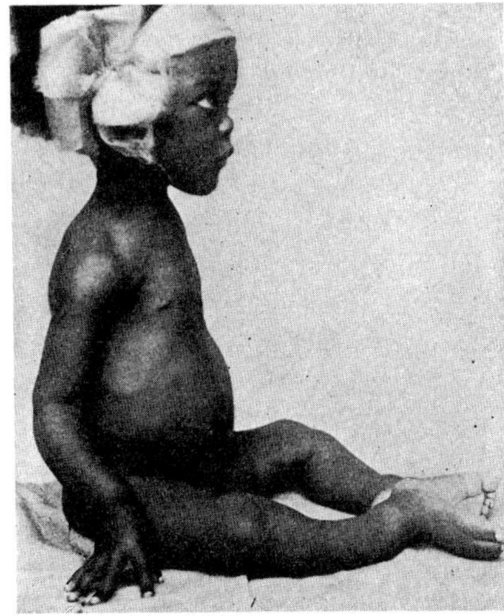

Figure 11–4 Rachitic child—note bowlegs with enlargement of bones about joints, deformity of chest, and enlargement of abdomen. (From Morse: *Clinical Pediatrics*.)

the calcium has not been adequately replaced.

Some persons may respond to an increased calcium intake by showing calcium storage (positive balance), but it seems probable that, in addition to calcium insufficiency, a lack of sex hormones or of protein may be causative factors.

A disease with somewhat similar symptoms, *nutritional osteomalacia*, occurs fairly commonly in parts of the world but is largely due to lack of vitamin D, although calcium or phosphorus, or both, also may be lacking.

Foods as Sources of Calcium

In planning a diet that will furnish enough calcium (or other mineral elements) to meet body needs, one must take into account three main factors:

1. How much of the mineral element is present in different foods?
2. What foods furnish it in an easily utilizable form?
3. Which of the foods are rich enough in it or can be eaten in sufficient quantity to contribute substantially to the daily quota?

Table 11–3 gives examples of foods containing calcium and phosphorus. The first column of figures under each mineral element gives the amount furnished in an *average serving* of each food in the condition in which it is eaten (cooked or raw). The second column shows the number of milligrams present in 100 gm of the food substance. Thus, cheddar cheese ranks high in calcium (750 mg) on a 100 gm basis, but an average serving, or 1 oz portion, would contribute only 225 mg, which is slightly less than the amount furnished by an 8 oz glass of milk. On a weight basis, milk (which is 87 percent water) is not so high in calcium and phosphorus as dried beans or dried figs, but it is at or near the top of the list for both elements in the amount furnished in an average serving. Two other good sources of these minerals do not contribute as much as one might expect in the diet, because dried fruits ordinarily are eaten in small quantities and dried beans increase in water content on cooking. One process used to change regular farina into a quick-cooking product adds nearly 0.5 gm each of calcium and phosphorus per 100 gm of dry product (which is a good demonstration of why nutrient labeling of food products is important).

To generalize, we may group foods according to their contributions of calcium in the ordinary diet as follows:

Excellent sources — hard cheeses, milk, most dark green, leafy vegetables, and soft fish bones.
Good sources — softer cheeses, ice cream, broccoli, baked beans, dried legumes, and dried figs.
Fair sources — cottage cheese, light cream, oranges, dates, salad greens, nuts, lima beans, parsnips, and eggs.
Poor sources — most other fruits and vegetables, grains, and meats.

Eggs and nuts (which are high in phosphorus) are of only moderate calcium content, while meat, poultry, and fish are calcium-poor. Most fruits and vegetables, bread, and breakfast cereals contain relatively minor quantities, but if eaten in considerable quantities, may add appreciably to the calcium intake.

As shown in Table 11–4 and Figure 11–5, about 75 percent of all the calcium in the American food supply comes from dairy products (other than butter). The rest is about equally distributed among meat, eggs, vegetables, beans, and cereals.[9] Enrichment of foods with calcium is not widely done in this country.

How to Get the Recommended Allowance of Calcium in the Diet

Of the various nutrients required, calcium is one of those most likely to be provided by the diet in less than recommended or optimal quantities. However,

Table 11–3 FOODS CONTAINING CALCIUM AND PHOSPHORUS

Calcium (mg)			*Phosphorus (mg)*		
FOOD	PER AVERAGE SERVING	PER 100 GM	FOOD	PER AVERAGE SERVING	PER 100 GM
Sesame seeds, whole, 1/4 c	348	1160	Liver, fried, 2 slices, 75 gm	311	358
Milk, 8 oz glass, 1/2 pt	285	118			
Salmon, red, canned with bones, 2/5 c	259	259	Milk, 8 oz glass, 1/2 pt	227	93
			Cod steak or sole, 100 gm	220	220
Sardines, canned in oil, 2 fish, drained	174	435	Lamb, leg, roast, 2 slices, 100 gm	208	208
			Beef, rib roast, 1 slice, 100 gm	186	186
Cheese, American cheddar, 1 oz	225	750	hamburger, 1/4 lb, 85 gm	165	194
*Leafy vegetables, avg. 1/2 c cooked	140	167	Baked beans, canned, 1/2 c	120	92
			Cheese, American cheddar, 1 oz	140	478
Ice cream, plain, avg. 3/4 c	123	123	Peanut butter, 2 scant tbsp	118	393
†Molasses, medium, 2 tbsp	116	290	Shredded wheat, 1 biscuit	102	360
Artichokes	102	51	Whole-wheat cereal, 1/2 c, cooked	113	83
Broccoli, 2/3 c	88	88	Oatmeal, 2/3–3/4 c, cooked	105	57
Baked beans, canned with			Cottage cheese, 2 round tbsp	108	189
molasses, 1/2 c	82	56	Egg, 1 large	101	210
tomato sauce 1/2 c	70	49	Ice cream, plain, avg., 3/4 c	99	99
Cream, light, 7 tbsp	74	97	Cream, light, 7 tbsp	77	77
Orange, 1 medium	62	40	Broccoli, 2/3 c	76	76
‡Cottage cheese, 2 round tbsp	52	96	Nuts, mixed, 1–12 nuts, 1/2 oz	67	446
String beans, 2/3 c, cooked	50	50	Parsnips, 1/2 c, cooked	62	80
Parsnips, 1/2 c, cooked	44	57			
Lima beans, 1/2 c, cooked	38	47	Lima beans, 1/2 c, cooked	97	121
Salad greens, raw, avg. 2 large or 4–5 small leaves	34	68	Peas, canned, 1/2 c	62	77
			Corn, canned, 1/2 c	43	52
Sesame seeds, hulled, 1/4 c	33	110	Cauliflower, 3/4 c, cooked	42	72
Egg, 1 large	26	54	Leafy vegetables, 1/2 c, cooked, avg.	45	45
Figs, dried, 1 large	25	125			
canned, 3, with juice	13	13	Bread, whole-wheat, 1 slice	60	263
Bread, whole-wheat, 1 slice	23	96	white, 1 slice (4% milk solids)	21	92
white, 1 slice (4% milk solids)	19	79	Apricots, dried, cooked, 3 halves	34	34
Peanut butter, 2 scant tbsp	22	74	Figs, dried, 1 large	33	111
Peas, canned, 1/2 c	20	25	canned, 3, with juice	21	35
Apricots, dried, cooked, 4 halves	20	22	Prunes, 4–5 medium, cooked	27	40
			Dates, 3–4 pitted, 1 oz	18	60
Orange juice, 6 oz	20	25	Orange, 1 small	37	37
Dates, 3–4 pitted, 1 oz	22	72	String beans, 2/3 c, cooked	19	23
Prunes, 4–5 medium, cooked	17	25	Grapefruit, 1/2 medium	16	16
Grapefruit, 1/2 medium	16	16			
Cereal, whole-grain, avg. 2/3–3/4 c, cooked	8–15	9			

*Including dandelion, mustard, turnip greens, collards, and kale, but excluding spinach, beet greens, and chard, in which calcium is in a poorly utilizable form.

†The calcium in molasses is due to addition of lime to neutralize acid in refining sugar; it is in lowest concentration in light molasses and highest in the blackstrap variety.

‡Calcium content of cottage cheese varies according to whether it is made from sour milk or by addition of rennin to sweet milk.

it is not difficult to obtain the recommended allowance of 800 mg daily if one includes 2 cups (1 pint) of milk or its calcium equivalent in milk products other than butter. In Table 11–5, four groups of foods are given, each of which furnishes the recommended calcium allowance for a day, with the amount of milk decreasing in each group from left to right (from 1½ pints, which furnishes more than the day's allowance, to none). It should be noted that, with lesser amounts of milk (or

Table 11-4 SOURCES OF CALCIUM AND PHOSPHORUS BY FOOD GROUPS, SELECTED YEARS*

Food Group	Calcium (Percent)					Phosphorus (Percent)				
	1909–1913	1947–1949	1957–1959	1967	1976†	1909–1913	1947–1949	1957–1959	1967	1976†
Dairy products, excluding butter	67.7	74.2	76.5	76.1	75.0	27.5	37.1	38.3	36.3	34.8
Meat, poultry, fish, including fat pork cuts	4.2	3.5	3.3	3.7	3.8	20.0	21.0	23.0	26.5	28.3
Dry beans, peas, nuts, and soybean products	3.2	2.5	2.6	2.6	3.0	5.4	5.6	5.7	5.7	6.3
Potatoes, sweet potatoes	2.5	1.2	1.0	0.9	0.9	6.9	4.2	3.8	3.7	3.8
Vegetables (excluding potatoes, sweet potatoes)	7.1	7.0	6.2	6.1	6.5	4.5	5.7	5.3	5.4	5.4
Fruit	2.1	2.4	2.1	2.1	2.3	1.7	2.0	1.9	1.8	2.0
Flour and cereal products	7.4	3.3	3.3	3.4	3.4	26.6	15.1	12.9	12.4	12.1
Other foods†	5.7	5.5	5.0	5.0	5.1	6.8	9.2	9.0	8.3	7.2
Total§	100.0	100.0	100.0	100.0	100.0	100.0	100.0	100.0	100.0	100.0
Quantity per capita per day (mg)	817	996	979	946	925	1561	1554	1530	1544	1554

*From Marston, R., and Friend, B.[9]. Values represent availability figures, not including wastage and cooking losses.
†Preliminary.
‡Includes eggs.
§Components may not add to total because of rounding off to closest figure.

with none in group 4), cheese or ice cream, as well as green leafy vegetables and broccoli, are depended on as major sources of calcium.

Other foods in an average diet—some of which are classed as fair, moderate, or even poor sources of calcium—may together contribute significant amounts toward the day's total intake. Two servings each of fruit and vegetables (other than green, leafy ones or broccoli) might contribute somewhere in the neighborhood of 100 to 150 mg calcium, while four to six slices of bread or a serving of cereal might contribute 75 to 150 mg, especially if whole-grain cereals or bread made with added milk solids are used. The typical American dietary pattern of bread and butter, meat and potatoes, other vegetable, salad or fruit, and dessert can be expected to supply about 300 mg of calcium daily. Two cups of milk in the daily diet would bring the total intake up to the recommended allowance, yet less than one-fifth

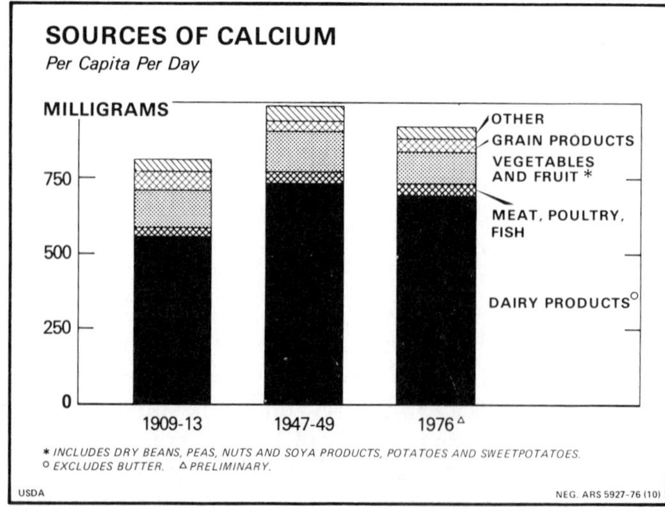

Figure 11-5 Food sources and average *per capita* intake of calcium from 1909 to 1976. (From Marston, R., and Friend, B.: Nutritional review, reprinted from *The National Food Situation*. Hyattsville, Md., U.S. Department of Agriculture Agric. Res. Serv., Consumer and Food Economics Institute Report CFE (Adm.)–299–11, Jan. 1977.)

of the women in a dietary survey had this amount of milk in their diet, even when the milk in cream soups, white sauce, puddings, and ice cream was taken into account.[10]

It is also important to consider which foods carry calcium in forms that are readily absorbed from the intestine and hence available for use in the body. The calcium in milk is highly utilized by man, and its availability is not altered by pasteurization. Broccoli, cauliflower, and kale rank almost with milk in availability of their calcium content, while that in carrots, lettuce, string beans, and almonds has been shown to be only slightly less well assimilated. Leafy vegetables with fairly well-utilized calcium include kale, cabbage, collards, turnip greens, and probably also mustard and dandelion greens. Spinach, chard, and beet greens have much of their calcium in insoluble combination with oxalic acid, and hence in a form unavailable to the body, but this is no menace if there is plenty of absorbable calcium in the diet, and these greens are valuable sources of iron and vitamin A.

The inclusion of at least *a pint of milk daily in the diet of adults is urged as the chief means for obtaining the calcium quota,* as well as for the high-quality proteins and vitamins that milk provides. For those who do not drink milk it should be incorporated in cooked foods wherever possible, and the more common use of cheese would also be advantageous. Hard cheeses have much higher calcium content than soft cheeses with higher water content; cottage cheese has only about one-seventh as much calcium as a hard cheese like cheddar (American), but ½ cup of it can take the place of a scant half cup of milk in calcium value. The wider use of green, leafy vegetables, including salad greens, would help to reinforce the diet in calcium, as well as in other minerals and vitamins.

Nutritional Status

How adequate are freely chosen diets in the United States as to the amount of calcium they supply? The answer to this depends upon which index, or standard, is used and which age and sex group. Then, too, a survey of an *average* population does not mean too much, since adequate calcium intakes are so dependent upon the consumption of milk or milk products by individuals, which varies widely. Whenever milk intake is low, calcium intakes are very likely to be low unless other calcium sources are substituted. Fifteen to 25 percent of the American pop-

Table 11–5 FOODS THAT FURNISH THE ADULT RECOMMENDED CALCIUM ALLOWANCE (800 mg daily)

Group 1	*Calcium, mg*	*Group 2*	*Calcium, mg*	*Group 3*	*Calcium, mg*	*Group 4*	*Calcium, mg*
Milk, 1½ pts	855	Milk, 1 pt	570	Milk, ½ pt	285	Cheese, American cheddar, 1½ oz	337
		Cottage cheese, 2 round tbsp	52	Cheese, American cheddar, 1 oz	225	Ice cream, plain, ⅙ qt	123
		Bread, whole-wheat, 4 slices	92	Bread, whole-wheat, 5 slices	95	Bread, whole-wheat, 4 slices	92
		Orange, 1 medium	62	Orange juice, 8 oz	24	Turnip greens, ¾ c, cooked	138
		Green beans, ¾ c, cooked	45	Broccoli, ⅔ c	88	Beans, baked, with molasses, ½ c	82
			821	Carrots, diced, ⅔ c	33	Egg, 1 medium	27
				Cream, light, 4 tbsp	61	Hamburger, lean, 85 gm	10
					811		809

ulation consume very little, or no, milk, which is directly indicative of the extent of inadequate calcium intakes.

Within a family, fathers and adolescent boys are most likely to eat food that meets the recommended allowances of calcium, while mothers, pregnant and lactating women, and adolescent girls are least likely to do so. Statistics in the United States[11-15] show that girls from age 11 up, on the average, consume less than 75 percent of the recommended allowances of calcium. After age 35 this drops to 66 percent of less.[13] Since this is an *average* figure, it means that there is no question that calcium intakes are too low in many individual females. Males tend to consume more calcium than females at all age periods, no doubt because of their greater total intake of food.

Overall, it appears that at least 10 percent of the American population is consuming less than one-half of the recommended allowance of calcium,[14, 15] an inadequate amount. Anywhere from 15 to 40 percent of men in the population may eat less than two-thirds of the recommended amount of calcium; 50 percent of adolescent girls and 75 percent of women 38 to 80 years of age fall into this category of calcium intake.

Records of growth of children, and osteoporosis (soft bones) in older individuals, are as useful an indicator of calcium (and phosphorus) deficiencies as any available. The extensive Ten-State Survey in the United States[16] showed averages of from 10 to 50 percent of low-income children (6 years or less) in different states with "one or more standard deviations below Iowa growth standards." In a 1970 study in Tennessee on 300 preschool children from poor black families, half of the children were found to be below the twenty-fifth percentile (of "normal" values) for height.[17] These differences are probably largely due to calcium deficiency, though this remains to be proved. The incidence of osteoporosis in older females is known to be very high, but exact figures are not available.

Suggestions have been made for reinforcing the calcium content of some staple foods. The most commonly used of these is the addition of nonfat milk solids to bread in amounts of either 2, 4, or 6 percent. The 6 percent level brings the calcium content nearly up to that of bread made with whole wheat. However, the addition of milk solids is not mandatory, and because of inadequate nutritional labeling of our bread supply (i.e., calcium level per slice or per pound), the consumer has much difficulty in knowing the calcium content of any bread. Even whole-wheat bread does not contribute considerable amounts of calcium.

If calcium is taken in pills (by doctor's advice), it should be in the form of some soluble salt, such as calcium lactate. Unless there is some excellent reason (e.g., an allergy to milk or intolerance to appreciable amounts of lactose), it is far better to revise the diet to include more calcium-rich foods, which furnish, along with calcium, other minerals, vitamins, and amino acids essential for body welfare.

PHOSPHORUS

Discovery of Dietary Requirement

Phosphorus (P), a nonmetallic element, was first identified in urine in 1669 by a German alchemist, Brand. It created much interest, since this element, in the unnatural free form, glows in the dark, is very toxic, breaks into fire spontaneously, and is used in making matches and smoke screens. Fortunately, it exists in nature only in the combined forms (usually with calcium) in such sources as bone and rock phosphates. It is widely used in detergents and in fertilizers. Phosphorus is present in the body at a level of about 1 percent. It is one of the most important nutrients known, taking part in almost every reaction in the body.

Distribution and Function in Body

Phosphorus plays an important role in combining with calcium in the formation and strengthening of bone tissues. In fact, about 80 percent of the phosphorus in the body is in the bones and teeth. The remaining 20 percent, found in the blood and tissues, performs a number of other critical functions.

Inorganic phosphates in the blood act as buffer substances that assist in maintaining blood neutrality and the acid-base balance of the blood (p. 245). Phosphorus (as phosphate radicals) is an essential constituent of nucleic acids and nucleoproteins in cell nuclei and cytoplasm, which play a key role in reproduction, transmission of hereditary traits, cell division, and protein synthesis within the cells. Phosphates are also a component of phospholipids, which promote the emulsification and transport of fats and fatty acids, as well as permeability of cell membranes. Also, phosphorus is indispensable to the oxidation of carbohydrates, by which much of the energy for body processes is obtained; it links with glycogen and glucose to activate them for oxidation, and is a part of several enzymes or coenzymes that are essential to this oxidation. Adenosine mono-, di-, and triphosphates are among the most vital of all body substances for regulating hormone activity and for providing quick release of energy in muscular contraction.

Phosphorus is highly reactive and imparts this property to substances with which it is combined. Phosphorus is present in or combines readily with proteins, lipids, or carbohydrates. Chemically inert substances such as glucose and fats become highly reactive in tissue metabolism and more readily transported in body fluids by combination with phosphate (PO_4^{---}) radicals. From one-half to two-thirds the phosphorus in blood is contained within the red cells.

Maintenance Requirement and RDA

Only in recent years has the Food and Nutrition Board[6] given specific *recommended dietary allowances for phosphorus*. Without other evidence available, the allowances for phosphorus were made the same as for calcium (except for infants). See Table 11–2 and Table 1 of the Appendix. The allowance for a normal adult is 800 mg a day. About twice as much calcium as phosphorus is present in bones and teeth, but because of the much higher amounts of phosphorus in soft body tissues and in our food supply, it is estimated that the requirement is similar to that for calcium. These figures should be considered only as preliminary, since much more research needs to be done in this area before more specific recommendations can be made.

Effects of Phosphorus Deficiency

Phosphorus deficiency sometimes occurs in cattle grazing on soil that has been depleted of phosphates (by crops, leaching, etc.), for the grass grown on such soil is of low phosphorus content. Such a deficiency is evidenced by decrease or distortion of the appetite (desire to eat bones, wood, etc.), emaciation, weakness, and eventually death. Phosphorus deficiency seldom, if ever, develops in normal humans because of its wide distribution in food. Deficiencies are seen in man in certain clinical conditions, in persons receiving antacids over long periods, and in certain stress conditions such as bone fractures. Persons with deficiencies may show weakness, bone pain, demineralization of bone, and loss of calcium.

Food Sources of Phosphorus

Phosphorus is associated chiefly with protein-rich foods and cereal products. It is found in many foods that contribute little calcium, as well as along with calcium in milk and its products. Rich sources of phosphorus in the diet are meats (especially organs), fish, and poultry; eggs; cheese and milk; nuts; legumes; and all

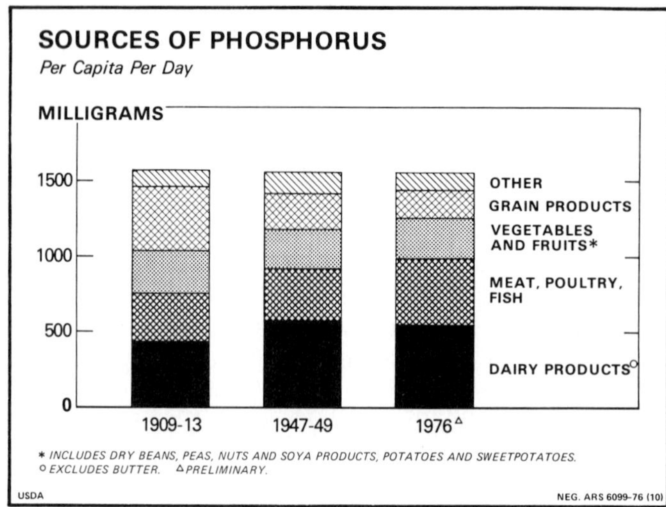

Figure 11–6 Food sources and average *per capita* intake of phosphorus from 1909 to 1976. (From Marston, R., and Friend, B.: Nutritional review, reprinted from *The National Food Situation.* Hyattsville, Md., U.S. Department of Agriculture Agric. Res. Serv., Consumer and Food Economics Institute Report CFE (Adm.)–299–11, Jan. 1977.)

foods made from grains, especially whole grains. Fruits (especially dried ones) and vegetables contribute lesser amounts of phosphorus to the diet. In general, edible roots, stems, and flowerets of plants contain similar amounts of both calcium and phosphorus, but plants concentrate calcium in the green leaves and phosphorus in the seeds (grains). The darker green leaves have higher calcium content than light green ones (e.g., the inner leaves of head lettuce). Phosphorus is carried in foods more liberally than is calcium, and many foods that provide little calcium, such as meats, are excellent sources of phosphorus. Since its distribution follows that of protein, a diet that supplies adequate amounts of protein is usually adequate for phosphorus.

Table 11–4 and Figure 11–6 show that in the American food supply, over 60 percent of the phosphorus comes from dairy products and meat, poultry, and fish. Flour and cereal products contribute 12 percent of the supply. The rest comes largely from eggs, potatoes, vegetables, and beans. Sugar and fats provide only trace amounts of calcium and phosphorus.

Phosphorus deficiency is very uncommon in the United States (except in some clinical conditions and through long-term use of antacids[18]) because of its widespread distribution in food supplies. However, persons consuming typical vegetarian types of diets, especially those low in milk products, might easily be deficient in this element as well as in other nutrients. It is well known that farm animals fed diets composed only of grains, legumes, and green, leafy feeds must have supplementary phosphorus (as well as calcium) in order to have adequate growth and bone structure.

MAGNESIUM

Magnesium (Mg) is a silvery-white metal related closely to calcium and zinc. Much has been learned in nutrition the past few years about this very vital mineral.

Magnesium is the eighth most plentiful element in the earth's crust (2.1 percent) and the third most abundant and lightest structural metal. We see it all about us in a modern world as magnesium alloys (usually containing over 75 percent of this mineral) in airplanes, parts of cars (up to 90 pounds in a Volkswagen), ladders, portable tools, luggage, vacuum cleaners, and as the silverlike material that provides the light in flares, flash bulbs, and fireworks. It is said that more magnesium is in orbit than any other mineral, since it is the major component of spaceships. It is also the major mineral in asbestos, talcum powder, and dolomite limestone — a fertilizer.

More important to nutritionists, magnesium has dozens of essential biological functions in plants and animals. As the central component of *chlorophyll*, the well-known green pigment of all higher plants, it is absolutely essential in plants for making glucose and oxygen from sunlight (energy source), water, and carbon dioxide by the process of photosynthesis. Magnesium is a major mineral component of sea water (0.13 percent), from which life and chlorophyll originally evolved. It is estimated that each cubic mile of sea water, a good industrial source, contains 6 million tons of magnesium, so it appears that we will have enough in the future to take care of our needs!

Discovery and Identification as a Nutrient

We are all familiar with "milk of magnesia" (magnesium hydroxide) and Epsom salts* (magnesium sulfate). Salts of magnesium have been known through the ages for their healing properties. A Roman, whose name is unknown to us, claimed many centuries ago that "magnesia alba" (white magnesium salts from the district of Magnesia in Greece, from which the element was eventually named) cured many ailments. The Scottish chemist Joseph Black, working with this substance (now known to be magnesium carbonate), discovered in 1755 that magnesium was an element. It was first located in 1808 by Sir Humphry Davy, the same person who first isolated many other elements (see p. 246).

Though magnesium was found to be present in the human body in the 1850's, it was not until 1926 that Leroy, in France, could first prove that magnesium is an essential nutrient for the animal body (he used the mouse).[19] Later, McCollum and coworkers[20] described the wide range of deficiency signs in rats and dogs, including *magnesium tetany*, a form of convulsions in which the nerves and muscles are affected. Indications that magnesium was required by man were published shortly thereafter (1933–1944).[21] More complete proof of man's need for the element has since been shown by a number of workers.[6,22] At this time, it is a very active field of research.

*Named after Epsom, a village south of London, found in 1618 to have a water supply with wound-healing properties and a laxative effect. "Epsom salts" were the substance formed after evaporation of the water.

Absorption and Distribution in the Body

Magnesium salts, like those of calcium, are usually rather insoluble, so that their absorption, which occurs in the small intestine, is relatively inefficient. About a third of ingested magnesium is normally absorbed. The use of high levels of salts such as magnesium sulfate as laxatives depends on the fact that they draw much water into the gut by osmosis because they are so poorly absorbed. In active transport across the intestinal membrane, magnesium salts seem to use the same route as calcium salts, so that a high intake of either interferes with the absorption of the other. Unlike calcium, there is little excretion of magnesium through the intestine, except that which is unabsorbed from the food. When extra amounts of magnesium are given after long-continued magnesium-poor diets, a considerable amount is retained and stored in the bones, so the body seems to have reserve stores of magnesium as well as of calcium.*

*Strontium is a nonessential mineral, of the same chemical family as calcium and magnesium, which is also deposited in bone tissue if it is introduced into the body. Normal foods carry only minute amounts of it (not enough to do harm), but much discussion has been raised as to its presence in the atmosphere (strontium-90, radioactive) as an aftermath of an atomic explosion, and toxic effects it might produce if absorbed into foods and then deposited in the bones.

The human body contains about 20 to 28 gm of magnesium, over half of which is found in the complex salts that make up bone. The remainder is chiefly found in the cells of soft tissues (especially the liver and skeletal muscles), where it is second only to potassium in abundance. Small amounts of magnesium are present in the body fluids and take part in the transfer by osmosis of water into and out of the cells; they also take part in the regulation of the acid-base balance of the body. Mostly, magnesium circulates in body fluids in ionic form, but about 35 percent of serum magnesium is bound to protein.

Role in the Body and Deficiency Signs

In animal metabolism, magnesium functions mainly as an activator of various enzymes, especially those which bring about the linking of phosphate groups to glucose in the formation and breakdown of glycogen and release of energy. It is essential for the transfer of "high-energy phosphate groups," as in adenosine triphosphate, ATP. It is essential for maintenance of DNA and RNA structure. Magnesium is necessary also for regulation of temperature of the body, contractions of nerves and muscles, and synthesis of protein. The rate of its excretion in the urine seems to be influenced by aldosterone, one of the hormones of the adrenal cortex.

Symptoms of deficiency in animals are first, failure to grow, followed by pallor, weakness, low level of serum magnesium, excessive irritability of nerves and muscles, irregular heartbeats, heart and kidney damage, and convulsions or seizures (tetany), especially when the animal is suddenly disturbed. Death can result in a few weeks' time in small animals fed magnesium-deficient diets.

In man, similar nervous and muscular excitability is seen in magnesium deficiency. Behavioral disturbances, delirium, and depression are seen, as well as weakness, tremors, vertigo, and tetany (spasms, convulsions, or other forms — similar to that seen clinically in calcium deficiency).

Allowances and Nutritional Status

The magnesium requirement depends upon body size and composition of the diet. A great amount of calcium in the diet, for instance, is known to compete with the absorption of magnesium. Protein, phosphorus, and vitamin D levels also influence the requirement. Requirements are higher during pregnancy and lactation.

The latest RDAs for magnesium are summarized in Table 11–6 and are given in detail in Table 1 of the Appendix. The allowances are from 25 to 50 percent higher than minimal requirements (which range between 200 and 300 mg per day for adults) to allow for individual differences, normal stresses, and variations in diet composition.

Deficiency symptoms are slow to develop in humans because of reserve stores in the body; they have been observed chiefly in alcoholics because of excessive urinary excretion induced by alcohol consumption. Magnesium deficiency also occurs in infants with kwashiorkor. Low

Table 11–6 RECOMMENDED DIETARY ALLOWANCES FOR MAGNESIUM*

	Age (yrs)	*Magnesium (mg/day)*
Males	11–14	350
	15–18	400
	19–22	350
	23–50	350
	51+	350
Females	11–14	300
	15–18	300
	19–22	300
	23–50	300
	51+	300
	Pregnant	450
	Lactating	450

*From Food and Nutrition Board, 1974.[6]

Table 11–7 EXAMPLES OF MAGNESIUM DISTRIBUTION IN COMMON FOOD*

Food	*Magnesium in Edible Portion, mg/100 gm*	*Food*	*Magnesium in Edible Portion, mg/100 gm*
Apples, raw, unpared	8	Lettuce	11
Bananas, raw	33	Liver, beef	13
Beans, white, canned, baked	37	Macaroni, cooked	20
Beans, snap, frozen	21	Milk, whole	13
Beef cuts	18	Oatmeal, cooked	21
Beef, hamburger, broiled	25	Orange juice, frozen	10
Beet greens, raw	106	Peaches, raw	10
Bread, white	22	Peanuts, roasted	173
Bread, whole-wheat	78	Peas	35
Cabbage, raw	13	Potatoes, unpeeled	34
Carrots, raw	23	Rice, brown, cooked	29
Chard, Swiss, raw	65	Rice, white, cooked	8
Cheese, cheddar	45	Soybeans	265
Chicken, white meat, stewed	19	Spinach, raw	88
Chocolate, sweet	107	Sweet potatoes	31
Cocoa, dry powder	420	Tomatoes, raw	14
Coffee, instant, dry powder	456	Turnip greens, raw	58
Corn flakes	16	Walnuts, black	190
Eggs, whole	11	Wheat bran (breakfast cereal)	420
Flour, whole-wheat	133	Wheat germ	336
Flour, all-purpose	25	Yeast, brewer's	231

*Watt, B. K., and Merrill, A. L.: *Composition of Foods: Raw, Processed, Prepared.* Washington, D.C., U.S. Department of Agriculture Handbook No. 8, 1963. See this source for more detailed figures.

serum magnesium levels have been seen in diabetes, in malabsorption conditions, in certain surgical patients with restricted diets, and in patients receiving high levels of diuretics over long periods. The normal kidney is able to conserve magnesium in borderline intakes, thus preventing more deficiencies from occurring. Acute kidney failure is accompanied by the reserve picture — namely, high levels of serum magnesium and depression of the central nervous system, as seen in uremic coma.

Magnesium deficiencies do not occur in normal persons eating a variety of the traditional wholesome foods. Only when one is eating a very limited diet of white rice or a mixed diet consisting only of limited amounts of highly processed foods (such as a "tea and white toast" diet) would magnesium deficiency be possible, and then only in conjunction with deficiencies of many other nutrients. Magnesium deficiency is known to occur in persons who have malfunctioning kidneys or who are alcoholics. Persons eating little or no foods over long periods (as in extreme fasting) are known to become depleted in magnesium.[23]

Food Sources

Distribution of magnesium in foods tends to follow that of protein and phosphorus. Whole grains, nuts, beans, and green, leafy vegetables are good sources. Animal products, including meat and milk, are only poor to fair sources. Processing of foods can result in great losses. Thus, there is little left in rice and white flour (about 20 percent of that in the whole grain) and practically none in sugar, alcohol, or fats and oils. Boiling of vegetables can cause losses if the water is discarded. Table 11–7 gives figures for magnesium distribution in some common foods.

An average American diet provides about 350 mg per day — about the recommended allowance. In such a diet, most of the magnesium comes from milk (22 percent), vegetables — including potatoes (20 percent), cereal products and flour (18 percent), meat and eggs (15 percent), coffee and cocoa (8 percent), fruit (6 percent), and dry beans, nuts, and legumes (12 percent).*

QUESTIONS AND PROBLEMS

1. In what special tissue or tissues is most of the calcium and phosphorus in the body found? What function do they serve in this tissue? In what other tissues do these mineral elements occur, and what are their special roles in these tissues?

2. Can the body build up reserve stores of calcium and phosphorus, provided the diet supplies more than enough to meet current body needs? Where are these elements stored? What are the bone trabeculae, and what is the advantage of having them well developed?

3. Why do growing children store more calcium and phosphorus than adults? In addition to the rate of growth, what other factors influence the relative amount of the calcium intake that is retained in the body? What special advantages are there in a liberal intake of both calcium and phosphorus for young children? Why are the needs for these two elements greater in pregnant women and nursing mothers than in other adults?

4. Describe the relationship of the hormone calcitonin to calcium nutritional needs.

5. Give the minimum requirement and recommended allowance for calcium and phosphorus in normal adults. Explain why the minimum requirement for calcium varies rather widely in different individuals. Why is the recommended allowance for calcium set as high as it is? If it varies with body size and amount of bony tissue, why is the allowance for women the same as for men? Explain how the body may adapt to varying levels of calcium intake.

6. Compare the average extent to which calcium in the food is utilized with the degree of utilization of proteins, fats, and carbohydrates in foods. Why does the absorption of mineral elements tend to be less complete? Name three factors that have a favorable influence and three that have an unfavorable influence on absorption of calcium from the intestinal contents. What vitamin exerts an important influence on the utilization of calcium and phosphorus?

7. Name the two classes of foods that are the richest sources of calcium; of phosphorus. Name five specific foods that are comparatively rich in calcium and five rich in phosphorus. Which foods are used in large enough quantities in the average diet to contribute largely to making up the calcium quota for the day? Which classes of food contribute phosphorus liberally but carry little calcium? Why is the average diet less likely to be high in calcium than in phosphorus?

8. Keep an individual record of all foods eaten in a certain day, with the quantities of each consumed. Using either Table 11–3 or the table in the Appendix that gives nutritive values of average servings or common measures of foods, calculate the quantity of calcium furnished by this day's diet (either in milligrams or grams). How does the total compare with the standard allowance for calcium? If it is lower than the standard, how could the diet best be reinforced as to its calcium content?

9. What symptoms may develop in growing children as the result of a deficient supply of calcium or phosphorus in the diet? Why do adults seldom show recognizable signs of such deficiency? What signs of deficiency may appear in adults after long-continued diets that furnish too little calcium for body needs? At what periods in life is the character of the teeth most affected by any deficiency in these mineral elements?

10. What is the function of magnesi-

*National Food Review, U.S. Department of Agriculture, Jan. 1978. Revisions are made anually. These figures represent the magnesium available in raw foods, before processing and wastage. The coffee and cocoa figure includes miscellaneous and enrichment sources.

um in the body? Is a deficiency likely to occur in your own diet? Why? What common foods contain little or no magnesium, based on your own knowledge of foods?

REFERENCES

1. Osborne, T. B., and Mendel, L. B.: J. Biol. Chem., *34*:131, 1918.
2. McCollum, E. V.: Amer. J. Physiol., *25*:120, 1909; Hart, E. B., McCollum, E. V., and Fuller, J. G.: Univ. Wis. Agric. Exp. Stat. Res. Bull. No. 1, 1909; Plimmer, R. H. A.: Biochem. J., *7*:34, 1913; Forbes, E. B., and Keith, M. H.: Ohio Agric. Exp. Stat. Tech. Ser. Bull. No. 5, 1914.
3. McBean, L. D., and Speckmann, E. W.: Amer. J. Clin. Nutr., *27*:603, 1974.
4. Hegsted, D. M., Moscoso, J., and Collazos, C.: J. Nutr., *46*:181, 1952; Nicolaysen, R., et al.: Physiol. Rev., *33*:424, 1953.
5. Ohlsen, M. A.: J. Amer. Dietet. Assoc., *31*:333, 1955.
6. Food and Nutrition Board: *Recommended Dietary Allowances.* 8th Ed. Washington, D.C., National Research Council, National Academy of Sciences, 1974; Balsley, M.: J. Amer. Dietet. Assoc., *71*:149, 1977.
7. FAO Nutrition Meetings Report: *Calcium Requirements.* Series No. 30. Rome, 1962.
8. Sherman, H. C., and Hawley, E.: J. Biol. Chem., *55*:375, 1922, Daniels, A. L. et al.: J. Nutr., *10*:373, 1935; Stearns, G., and Jeans, P. C.: Proc. Soc. Exp. Biol. Med., *32*:428, 1934; and Stearns, G.: J.A.M.A., *142*:478, 1950.
9. Marston, R., and Friend, B.: Nutritional Review, reprinted from The National Food Situation. Hyattsville, Md., U.S. Department of Agriculture Agric. Res. Serv., Consumer and Food Economics Institute Report CFE(Adm.)–299–11, Jan. 1977.
10. Swanson, P. P., et al.: Fed. Proc., *21*:308, 1962.
11. Morgan, A. F. (ed.): *Nutritional Status, U.S.A.* Calif. Agric. Exp. Stat. Bull. 769, 1959.
12. Ohlson, M. A., and Stearns, G.: Fed. Proc., *18*:1075, 1959.
13. U.S. Department of Agriculture Consumer and Food Economics Res. Div.: *Food Intake and Nutritive Value of Diets of Men, Women, and Children in the United States, Spring 1965* (preliminary report). Washington, D.C., Agric. Res. Serv., Pub. No. ARS 62–18, 1969.
14. Davis, R. A., Gershoff, S. N., and Gamble, D. F.: J. Nutr. Educ., *1* (No. 2, Suppl. 1): 41, 1969; Kelsay, J. L.: J. Nutr., *99* (No. 1, Suppl. 1, Pt. II):123, 1969.
15. Abraham, S., et al.: *Dietary Intake Findings, U.S. 1971–1974,* HANES Rpt., Pub. No. (HRA) 17–1647, 1977, Hyattsville, Md., U.S. Dept. of Health, Education, and Welfare (National Center for Health Statistics); Lowenstein, F. W.: Amer. J. Clin. Nutr. *29*:918, 1976.
16. Center for Disease Control: *Ten-State Nutrition Survey in the United States, 1968–1970* (preliminary report). Washington, D.C., U.S. Department of Health, Education, and Welfare, 1971.
17. Zee, P., Walters, T., and Mitchell, C.: J.A.M.A., *213*:739, 1970.
18. Lotz, M. E., Zisman, E., and Bartter, F. C.: N. Engl. J. Med., *278*:409, 1968.
19. Leroy, J.: C. R. Soc. Biol., *94*:431, 1926.
20. Kruse, H. D., Orent, E. R., and McCollum, E. V.: J. Biol. Chem., *96*:519, 1932; *100*:603, 1933; Orent, E. R., Kruse, H. D., and McCollum, E. V.: Amer. J. Physiol., *101*:454, 1932; J. Biol. Chem., *106*:573, 1934.
21. Hirschfelder, A. D.: J. Clin. Invest., *12*:982, 1933; J.A.M.A., *102*:1138, 1934; Daniels, A. L., and Everson, G. J.: J. Nutr., *11*:327, 1936; Miller, J. F.: Amer. J. Dis. Child., *67*:117, 1944.
22. Flink, E. B.: J.A.M.A., *160*:1406, 1956; Suter, C., and Klingman, W. O.: Neurology, *5*:691, 1955; Vallee, B. L., Wacker, W. E. C., and Ulmer, D. D.: N. Engl. J. Med., *262*:155, 1960; Durlach, J.: Lancet, *1*:282, 1961; Montgomery, R. D.: Lancet, *2*:264, 1960; Leverton, R. M., et al.: J. Nutr., *74*:33, 1961.
23. Drenick, E. J., Hunt, I. F., and Swendseid, M. E.: J. Clin. Endocrinol. Metab., *29*:1341, 1969.

SUPPLEMENTARY READING

General Reviews and History

Bourne, G. H. (ed.): *The Biochemistry and Physiology of Bone,* Vol. II. 2nd Ed. New York, Academic Press, 1972.

Calcium in bone health. Dairy Council Digest, *47*:31, 1976.

Feeley, R. M., et al.: Major mineral elements in dairy products. J. Amer. Dietet. Assoc., *61*:505, 1972.

Greger, J. L., et al.: Calcium, magnesium, phosphorus, copper, and manganese balance in adolescent females. Amer. J. Clin. Nutr., *31*:117, 1978.

Ismail-Beigi, F., et al.: Effects of cellulose added to diets of low and high fiber content upon the metabolism of calcium, magnesium, zinc and phosphorus by man. J. Nutr., *107*:510, 1977.

Kenny, A. D., and Dacke, C. G.: Parathyroid hormone and calcium metabolism. World Rev. Nutr. Dietet., *20*:231, 1975.

Kobayashi, A., et al.: Effects of dietary lactose and a lactase preparation on the intestinal absorption of calcium and magnesium in normal infants. Amer. J. Clin. Nutr., *28*:681, 1975.

Lutwak, L., Singer, F. R., and Urist, M. R.: Current concepts of bone metabolism. Ann. Intern. Med., *80*:630, 1974.

Mazess, R. B., and Mather, W.: Bone mineral content of North Alaskan Eskimos. Amer. J. Clin. Nutr., *27*:916, 1974.

Nordin, B. E. C. (ed.): *Calcium, Phosphate and Magnesium Metabolism.* Edinburgh, Churchill Livingstone, 1976.

Odland, L. M., Mason, R. L., and Alexeff, A. I.: Bone density and dietary findings of 409 Tennessee subjects. I. Bone density considerations. Amer. J. Clin. Nutr., *25*:905, 1972; II. Dietary considerations, Amer. J. Clin. Nutr., *25*:908, 1972.

Schneider, A. B., and Sherwood, L. M.: Calcium homeostasis and the pathogenesis and management of hypercalcemic disorders. Metabolism, *23*:975, 1974.

Seelig, M. S., and Heggtveit, H. A.: Magnesium interrelationships in ischemic heart disease: a review. Amer. J. Clin. Nutr., *27*:59, 1974.

Stewart, R. J. C.: Bone pathology in experimental malnutrition. World Rev. Nutr. Dietet., *21*:1, 1975.

Calcium

Allen, L. H., and Hall, T. E.: Calcium metabolism, intestinal calcium-binding protein, and bone growth of rats fed high protein diets. J. Nutr., *108*:967, 1978.

Anand, C. R., and Linkswiler, H. M.: Effect of protein intake on calcium balance of young men given 500 mg calcium daily. J. Nutr., *104*:695, 1974.

Anderson, M. P., et al.: Long-term effect of low dietary calcium: phosphate ratio on the skeleton of *Cebus albifrons* monkeys. J. Nutr., *107*:834, 1977.

Armbrecht, H. J., and Wassermann, R. H.: Enhancement of Ca^{++} uptake by lactose in the rat small intestine. J. Nutr., *106*:1265, 1976.

Berlyne, G. M., et al.: Bedouin osteomalacia due to calcium deprivation caused by high phytic acid content of unleavened bread. Amer. J. Clin. Nutr., *26*:910, 1973.

Chu, J-Y., Margen, S., and Costa, F. M.: Studies in calcium metabolism. II. Effects of low calcium and variable protein intake on human calcium metabolism. Amer. J. Clin. Nutr., *28*:1028, 1975; also see Nutr. Rpts. Internat., *17*:503, 1978).

Cohn, S. H., et al.: Effects of fluoride on calcium metabolism in osteoporosis. Amer. J. Clin. Nutr., *24*:20, 1971.

Heaney, R. P., Recker, R. R., and Saville, P. D.: Calcium balance and calcium requirements in middle-aged women. Amer. J. Clin. Nutr., *30*:1603, 1977.

Irwin, M. I., and Kienholz, E. W.: A conspectus of research on calcium requirements of man. J. Nutr., *103*:1019, 1973.

Margen, S., Chu, J.-Y., Kaufmann, N. A., and Calloway, D. H.: Studies in calcium metabolism. I. The calciuretic effect of dietary protein. Amer. J. Clin. Nutr., *27*:584, 1974.

Morgan, D. B., Rivlin, R. S., and Davis, R. H.: Seasonal changes in the urinary excretion of calcium. Amer. J. Clin. Nutr., *25*:652, 1972.

Newell, G. K., and Beauchene, R. E.: Effects of dietary calcium level, acid stress, and age on renal, serum, and bone responses of rats. J. Nutr., *105*:1039, 1975.

Pingle, V., and Ramasastri, P. V.: Absorption of calcium from a leafy vegetable rich in oxalates. Brit. J. Nutr., *39*:119, 1978.

Polanska, N., and Wills, M. R.: Factors contributing to osteomalacia in the elderly and in Asian communities. J. Human Nutr., *30*:371, 1976.

Reinhold, J. G., et al.: Decreased absorption of calcium, magnesium, zinc, and phosphorus by humans due to increased fiber and phosphorus consumption as wheat bread. J. Nutr., *106*:493, 1976.

Root, A. W., and Harrison, H. E.: Recent advances in calcium metabolism. II. Disorders of calcium homeostasis. J. Pediatr., *88*:177, 1976.

Walker, A. R. P.: The human requirement of calcium: should low intakes be supplemented? Amer. J. Clin. Nutr., *25*:518, 1972.

Phosphorus

Bell, R. R., et al.: Physiological responses of human adults to foods containing phosphate additives. J. Nutr., *107*:42, 1976.

Draper, H. H., Sie, T-L., and Bergan, J. G.: Osteoporosis in aging rats induced by high phosphorus diets. J. Nutr., *102*:1133, 1972.

Ferraro, C., et al.: Intestinal absorption of phosphate: action of protein synthesis inhibitors and glucocorticoids in the rat. J. Nutr., *106*:1752, 1976.

Kohaut, E. C., et al.: Reduced renal acid excretion in malnutrition: a result of phosphate depletion. Amer. J. Clin. Nutr., *30*:861, 1977.

Krishnarao, G. V. G., and Draper, H. H.: Influence of dietary phosphate on bone resorption in senescent mice. J. Nutr., *102*:1143, 1972.

Moon, W. H., Malzer, J. L., and Clark, H. E.: Phosphorus balances of adults consuming several food combinations. J. Amer. Dietet. Assoc., *64*:386, 1974.

Schoolwerth, A. C., and Engle, J. E.: Calcium and phosphorus in diet therapy of uremia. J. Amer. Dietet. Assoc., *66*:460, 1975.

Sie, T-L., Draper, H. H., and Bell, R. R.: Hypocalcemia. hyperparathyroidism and bone resorption in rats induced by dietary phosphate. J. Nutr., *104*:1195, 1974.

Spencer, H., et al.: Effect of phosphorus on the absorption of calcium and on the calcium balance in man. J. Nutr., *108*:447, 1978.

Tewell, J. E., Clark, H. E., and Howe, J. M.: Phosphorus balances of adults fed rice, milk, and wheat flour mixtures. J. Amer. Dietet. Assoc., *63*:530, 1973.

Magnesium

Anderson, T. W., et al.: Ischemic heart disease, water hardness and myocardial magnesium. Can. Med. Assoc. J., *113*:199, 1975.

Caddell, J. L., Saier, F. L., and Thomason, C. A.: Parenteral magnesium load tests in postpartum American women. Amer. J. Clin. Nutr., *28*:1099, 1975.

Cook, D. A.: Availability of magnesium: balance studies in rats with various inorganic magnesium salts. J. Nutr., *103*:1365, 1973.

George, G. A., and Heaton, F. W.: Changes in cellular composition during magnesium deficiency. Biochem. J., *152*:609, 1975.

McCoy, J. H., and Kenney, M. A.: Depressed immune response in the magnesium-deficient rat. J. Nutr., *105*:791, 1975.

Medalle, R., Waterhouse, C., and Hahn, T. J.: Vitamin

resistance in magnesium deficiency. Amer. J. Clin. Nutr., *29*:854, 1976.

Neafsey, P. J., and Schwartz, R.: Serum and duodenal alkaline phosphatase levels in fed and fasted magnesium deficient rats. J. Nutr., *107*:1061, 1977.

Schwartz, R., et al.: Metabolic responses of adolescent boys to two levels of dietary magnesium and protein. I. Magnesium and nitrogen retention. Amer. J. Clin. Nutr., *26*:510, 1973.

Schwartz, R., et al.: Metabolic responses of adolescent boys to two levels of dietary magnesium and protein. II. Effect of magnesium and protein level on calcium balance. Amer. J. Clin. Nutr., *26*:519, 1973.

Scrivastava, U. S., Nadeau, M. H., and Gueneau, L.: Mineral intakes of university students: magnesium content. Nutr. Rpt. Internat., *18*:235, 1978.

Zieve, F. J., Freude, K. A., and Zieve, L.: Effects of magnesium deficiency on protein and nucleic acid synthesis *in vivo*. J. Nutr., *107*:2178, 1977.

Articles in *Nutrition Reviews*

Hypomagnesemia in protein-calorie malnutrition. *29*:89, 1971.

Effect of bed rest on bone mineral loss. *30*:11, 1972.

Carbonic anhydrase and bone resorption. *31*:101, 1973.

The role of calcium in insulin secretion. *31*:122, 1973.

Dietary phosphorus, PTH, and bone resorption. *31*:124, 1973.

Regulation of 25-hydroxycholecalciferol metabolism by inorganic phosphate. *31*:188, 1973.

Protein and magnesium deficiency. *32*:90, 1974.

Calcium transport in the ileum. *33*:84, 1975.

Clinical correlates of vitamin D metabolites and calcium metabolism. *33*:209, 1975.

Anticonvulsant drugs and calcium metabolism. *33*:221, 1975.

Neonatal calcium homeostasis, vitamin D and parathyroid function. *34*:112, 1976.

On the relation of the parathyroid to calcium metabolism and the nature of tetany (by W. G. MacCallum and C. Voegtlin). *34*:212, 1976.

Relation of zinc to calcium in bone. *34*:294, 1976.

Vitamin D, calcium-binding protein and the intestinal transport of calcium. *36*:90, 1978.

Chapter 12

Trace Elements (Iron, Iodine, Copper, Manganese, Zinc, Fluorine, and Others)

TRACE ELEMENTS GENERAL

The *essential trace elements* can be defined simply as those elements necessary in the diet of humans or animals in trace* amounts — less than 100 mg per. day for humans. This is an arbitrary dividing line, of more use to students and teachers than to the animal body.

The requirements for the trace elements range from milligram quantities for iron, zinc, and manganese down to microgram quantities for some of the newly discovered *micronutrient elements* such as selenium, chromium, and vanadium. They are measured in foods and tissues in concentrations of parts per million (ppm) or sometimes in amounts as low as parts per billion (ppb). One ppm equals 1 mg per kg, and one ppb equals 1 mcg per kg. A combined total of only about 25 to 30 gm of all trace elements, about 1 ounce, exists in the human body as compared with over 1000 gm of calcium alone.

*The word "trace" was given to these elements by early nutritionists before modern methods of analyzing food and tissues were available. The levels present were just barely discernible in a qualitative way only and, therefore, were said to be present in "trace amounts."

The trace element field is one of the most active and interesting areas of nutrition today, with important discoveries constantly being made.

There is no convenient single way to classify trace elements in nutrition because they vary so much in function, distribution, level of need, and chemical properties. To call them the "minor elements" is very misleading. Table 12–1 lists the 13 essential trace elements in about the order of discovery of their nutritional importance, the order we will use in this chapter to study them. Understandably, this happens also to be roughly the order they follow in terms of decreasing quantitative needs, with some exceptions. Iodine, which is needed in less than milligram amounts, was one of the first trace minerals determined to be essential. Silicon, found recently to be essential, may be needed in greater amounts than the other trace elements. Table 12–1 also lists other trace elements that are known to be present in plants and in the animal body but for which no biological function is known.

Because the field is so relatively new, in this chapter we will discuss each trace element known to be essential by any

Table 12–1 TRACE ELEMENTS, ESSENTIAL AND NONESSENTIAL

Trace Elements Essential for Higher Animal Species	*Examples of Trace Elements Present in Food for Which No Essential Role is Known in Higher Animals*	
1. Iron	A. *Element known to have a biological role in plants or lower organisms:*	
2. Iodine	Boron	
3. Copper		
4. Manganese	B. *Possibly essential in animals:*	
5. Zinc	Arsenic	
6. Fluorine*	Tin	
7. Cobalt†	C. *No essential role yet known in plants or animals:*	
8. Molybdenum‡	Aluminum	Lead
9. Selenium‡	Antimony	Lithium
10. Chromium	Barium	Mercury
11. Nickel‡	Bismuth	Rubidium
12. Vanadium‡	Bromine	Silver
13. Silicon‡	Cadmium	Strontium
	Gallium	Titanium
Total: 13 essential trace elements	Germanium	Zirconium
	Gold	Others

*No enzymatic role known. See text.
†Needed by man only in the organic form, as vitamin B-12.
‡The need by man has not yet been proved but can be assumed from the role in animals. See text.

higher animal species, even though its role in human nutrition is not yet proved. Understandably, experiments with humans, when feasible, are much more expensive and difficult than experiments with animals. From past experience, it would be most unlikely for humans not to require a trace element that has a vital function in another higher mammal.[1]

Role in Plant Nutrition — "Organic" vs. Inorganic Foods

Because we hear so much today about "organic" foods (meaning "organically grown" foods),* it is important to look briefly at the role of trace elements in the nutrition of plants used as food sources. Of the essential trace elements listed in Table 12–1, only iron, copper, manganese, zinc, molybdenum, and boron (and rarely, silicon and selenium) are essential for the growth of plants. From these elements in inorganic form, plus inorganic nitrogen, sulfur, calcium, phosphorus, potassium, magnesium, water, carbon dioxide, and sunlight (energy), the plant is able to grow normally and make within its own tissues all the carbohydrates, fiber, protein, fat, vitamins, pigments, and flavors that make up plant foods as we know them.

None of the substances known to be required in the soil for plant growth are needed in the organic form — in fact, organic sources of the elements must first be broken down to inorganic forms before they can be absorbed by the plant root tips. (Certain organic plant hormones in soil can be exceptions.) This explains why the term "organically grown foods" is a misnomer. The term "organic food," especially, is very misleading, because all foods of plant or animal origin are basically organic in the chemical sense.

The confusion that many people seem to have about these terms comes

*Sellers of "organic" foods state that food labeled "organic" is produced with the use of humus and organic fertilizers, and without the use of chemical pesticides, herbicides, hormones, antibiotics, or food additives. There is no easy way to corroborate most of these claims, and except for the possibility that certain trace elements might be present in higher levels, there is no basis for claiming significant nutritional superiority of such foods (see text). "Organic" foods are not likely to be any less free of contamination with filth, mold or bacterial growth, natural toxins, or heavy metals (such as mercury or lead) than the same natural foods sold at regular food stores often at much lower prices.

from the fact that plants, fortunately, have the ability to absorb from the soil into their tissues trace elements that they do not need but that can later serve as sources of these trace elements for animals that eat such plants. Examples of elements carried along from the soil are iodine, fluorine, cobalt, selenium (needed by some plants), chromium, and the macrominerals sodium and chlorine. The level of these trace elements in plant tissues, and to a small extent the level of certain other minerals, protein and vitamins, can be influenced to some extent by the level of these trace elements in the soil. In some cases, such as the levels in food of iodine, copper, zinc, chromium, and selenium, the extent of influence of soil elements can be considerable. Climate, temperature, and other environmental conditions can also affect plant composition.

Thus, theoretically, plant foods raised on soils with "natural" or organic fertilizers containing many trace elements, such as compost and farm manures, could be nutritionally superior in terms of their content of certain trace elements to plant foods raised on trace element–deficient soil. But this possibility is true only if such foods make up a major part of a person's diet over a long period of time and if other sources of these trace elements are not available. This is very unlikely to be the case, practically speaking. In terms of your own nutritional needs, keep in mind that those few trace minerals (such as iodine, chromium, and selenium) affected by the soil:

1. Are generally present in adequate amounts in a mixed diet consisting of a variety of foodstuffs and iodized salt,

2. Are not usually in short supply in farm soils and if they are they can be added as inorganic fertilizers, and

3. Can be added to foods by other means such as enrichment programs (though this is not done now except for iron and iodine).

This is not meant to depreciate the value of compost, farm manures, and other organic fertilizers, since they are very useful, though not necessary, for plant growth and soil texture. However, it needs to be made clear that, nutritionally speaking, "organically grown" foods have no special magic. Furthermore, the amount of organic fertilizer available is greatly insufficient to take care of fertilizer needs (phosphorus, nitrogen, and potassium) in the United States or anywhere in the world.

Distribution in Foods and Effect of Processing

As explained in the last section, the composition of many trace elements in plants, especially the micronutrients, depends to some extent on the soil on which the plant is raised. For that reason we will not attempt to provide tables of distribution in plant foods of most of the trace elements discussed in the following sections. Such information would be quite meaningless. However, as a general rule, since plant cells require certain trace elements for their growth and activity and will not grow without them, the natural plant foods, such as grains, beans, fruits, and vegetables (when eaten as a mixture) are reasonably good sources of all these elements and most always are good sources of the other trace elements not required by plants. Also, animal foods, such as eggs, milk, meat, and fish, are more likely to contain fairly uniform amounts of all essential trace elements because the animal will not grow if they are absent from the diet. This is one of the major reasons nutritionists recommend some animal foods as part of a normal diet.

The processing of foods, if severe and if anything is discarded, can be just as detrimental to trace minerals as to vitamins. Boiling or blanching of foods (and discarding the water) or removal of the endosperm of grains are examples of processes that can remove trace elements. Few trace elements are present in sugar, starch, gelatin, fats and oils, or in foods made from these products, such as soft drinks, desserts, or hard candies.

Absorption and Utilization

As a general rule, except for cobalt, all the trace elements are absorbed (or can be) in the inorganic form before being utilized by the animal body. Some minerals present in organic forms in the food must be split off to the free inorganic form before absorption. Others, such as iron in meat and chromium, are better absorbed in organic forms, though inorganic forms are quite well utilized. It is also a general rule that trace elements in food may not be readily available from the gut and, in such cases, are only partially absorbed. Because such small amounts of trace elements are present in the gut, their availability to the body can be greatly affected by the level of other minerals as well as by the presence of various organic compounds such as *oxalates, phytates,** or other organic *chelating*† compounds (natural or synthetic compounds that can chelate, or "tie up" an element, thus preventing its absorption). Specific exceptions and examples will be discussed individually.

Function in the Body

The trace elements have no common biological role other than that they function in the body at the cellular level, often as constituents of enzymes or as enzyme activators. Their function is not unlike that of vitamins in some ways, except that they can be absorbed by the body in the inorganic form. Most function in the body as constituents of important organic compounds, such as iron in *hemoglobin* and iodine in the hormone *thyroxine.*

*The phytates are especially abundant in whole wheat but also occur in other grains. They are salts or esters of phytic acid containing inositol and phosphates as the base.

†From the Greek, meaning claw of a crab.

The specific role of each element, if known, will be discussed individually. The function of some of the newly discovered essential elements is unknown.

Nutritional Status and Deficiencies of Trace Elements

Iron deficiency (anemia, etc.) is probably the most common deficiency of all nutrients in the United States, and as such illustrates the importance of the trace minerals. Other trace elements known to be of any nutritional importance in the United States are iodine (deficiency results in goiter) and fluorine (needed to prevent tooth decay), since many areas of the country have soils and water supplies low in these elements.

From what we know about the widespread distribution of trace elements in foods and the effect of processing, we can assume that any person eating a varied diet of traditional foods, including animal products, will receive sufficient, if not abundant, amounts of most trace elements. The effects of inadequate intake of iron, iodine, and fluorine have been known for some time. Recent evidence suggests that deficiencies of zinc and chromium in the United States are more prevalent than has been realized.

IRON

Iron* and its alloys such as steel are very familiar substances to everyone. Iron is the major element of the total earth (35 percent, greater than oxygen at 30 percent and silicon at 15 percent), making up the major part of the earth's interior.

Since iron (Fe, its chemical symbol from the Latin *ferrum*) is easy to obtain, its

*The origin of the word "iron" for this mineral is unclear, but similar-sounding root words such as *iran* or *iren* have been used for this metal back to prehistoric European times. A number of common English words in use today are derived from the name of this metal, such as "to iron clothes," golf "irons," and the "iron curtain."

discovery is lost in the history of man, many thousands of years ago. The early Greeks were aware of the health-giving properties of iron. It has been one of the favorite health tonics ever since and a major ingredient in old-time patent medicines (whether based on good reason or not). Iron was found to be a specific treatment for anemia in man as early as the seventeenth century in England.[2] Reasons for its beneficial properties began to become clear in the 1700's, when it was discovered to be a component of the body and, later, the blood.[3] It was soon found that about 3 to 5 gm of iron is present in the human body, most of which is in the blood as an essential component of the red protein *hemoglobin* of the red blood cells (of this color because of the iron content).

Experimental evidence of the *essential nature of iron* in nutrition was provided by the French chemist, Boussingault, in 1867.[3,4] Later, further proof was obtained by many others in Europe and the United States. It became clear, gradually, that as a dietary source, inorganic iron could be as effective as organic forms, thus opening the door to the field of inorganic trace elements in nutrition. Tables on the iron composition of common foods were published late in the nineteenth century.

It is paradoxical that although the need for iron was discovered long ago and although it is the most common and cheapest of all metals, more deficiencies of iron (mainly in the form of anemia) exist in the United States and most other developed countries than of any other nutrient. The extent of the deficiency lies somewhere between 10 and 25 percent of the total population. Refining and processing of our food supply and the great decrease in use of cast-iron cooking equipment in food manufacturing and in our homes have been major reasons for this. Deficiencies of iron in developing countries are also very common. As a result, iron is now one of the most pressing (and popular) topics among nutritionists. Many basic and applied studies are now in progress around the world on how to improve the iron nutriture of humans. Increased food enrichment with iron is one partial solution to the problem. (See Chapter 18.)

Absorption and Availability of Iron

The body guards its iron stores very carefully and reuses any that is broken down in the body over and over again. Only the small amounts of iron lost in the urine, sweat, hair, sloughed-off skin, and nails, and by menstruation need to be replaced — normally only about 1 or 1.5 mg a day.

Because considerable iron is needed when large amounts of blood are lost (as in bleeding from wounds), the body has a unique built-in control mechanism that allows the intestine to absorb more iron when the need is greatest and to inhibit absorption, in part, when there is an excess.[5,6] Normally, only about one-tenth of the iron in the diet is absorbed. This means, for practical purposes, that the amount of iron that must generally be eaten is about ten times the 1 or 1.5 mg a day actually used by the body in its tissues. The rest is excreted in the feces unabsorbed.

The situation is further complicated by the fact that not all dietary forms of iron are equally *available* to the body; that is, their chemical state also affects the amount absorbed over and above the body's normal control mechanism. Many factors are known to affect the availability and absorption of iron, such as the form of iron in food, conditions in the gut, composition of the food, iron status and needs of the body (as in pregnancy), age, sex, and hormonal factors. The presence of infections and parasites — hookworm infection, for example — is known to increase iron requirements greatly.

Both inorganic and some organic forms of iron can be utilized by the body. Hemoglobin iron from red meats (veal, beef, lamb) may be absorbed directly into the mucosal cells before the iron is released. Even elemental iron, when added to the diet in fine enough particles and when ionized in the gut, is available to the body. This explains why cast-iron cooking ware can supply iron to food (as could rust or common nails, if ground fine enough). Iron is more readily absorbed in the less oxidized form — as ferrous rather than ferric iron. Ferrous sulfate, a fully available chemical form, is generally used as a standard in absorption studies, and is usually absorbed at nearly the maximum rate of 20 to 40 percent (not more because of the control mechanisms). Ferric citrate is also a highly available iron source, being converted to the ferrous form before absorption. Factors favorable for absorption are:

1. Normal acidity of the gastric juice secreted in the stomach.
2. The presence of reducing substances (such as ascorbic acid) that can change ferric iron to the more readily absorbable ferrous form.
3. A well-balanced diet in which a fair proportion of the iron is provided in meat or eggs and not too high amounts in fibrous vegetable foods in which the iron is not very available.

Surprisingly, green leafy vegetables, such as spinach, formerly famous for its iron content, are relatively poor sources of iron (only 2 to 5 per cent of its iron is absorbed). Phytic acid, found especially in grains, militates against absorption by forming insoluble compounds with iron, as with calcium. This accounts for the poor absorption of iron from whole wheat (also about 2 to 5 percent), which explains the high incidence of anemia in countries whose population depends on whole wheat as its major carbohydrate source. The iron in rice, corn, and beans (except for soybeans) is likewise poorly absorbed. When these plant foods are eaten with meat, their iron availability is approximately doubled. Because there are wide individual differences in the efficiency of iron absorption and the number of variables affecting absorption of food iron are so numerous, it is difficult to equate the true body requirement with the amount needed in the diet to meet this requirement.

In the small intestine, the epithelial cell lining the intestinal wall (the *mucosal* cell) is the key to the *mechanism of iron absorption* (see Fig. 12–1). This cell takes in iron by regulatory procedures not fully understood — possibly hormonal regulation.

Once iron is inside the mucosal cell,

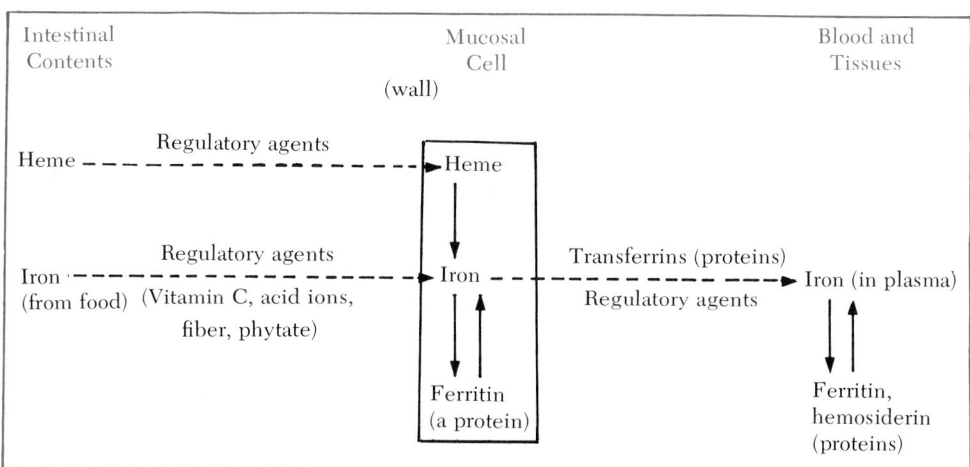

Figure 12–1 Absorption of iron from the intestine (simplified).

it can be either transferred (and later released) to the tissues with the aid of a protein known as *transferrin*,[2, 7] or stored in the mucosal cell or other body cells in the form of unique proteins called *ferritin* and *hemosiderin*.

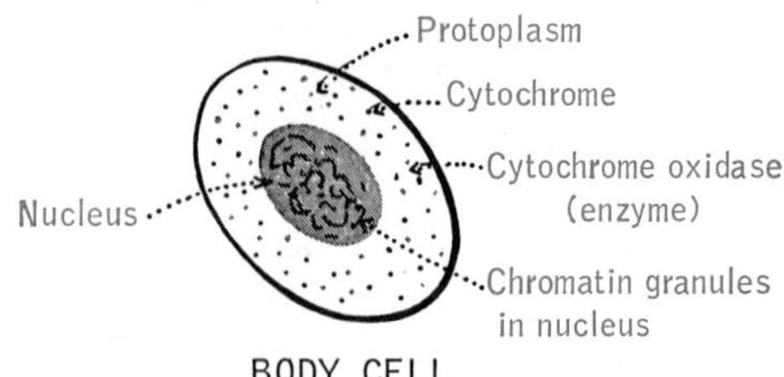

Figure 12–2 Small amounts of iron are found in every tissue cell—in chromatin granules in the cell nucleus and in the protoplasm as the pigment cytochrome and the enzyme cytochrome oxidase. These iron-containing substances are largely responsible for the uptake of oxygen by the cells and for the use of oxygen in their life processes.

Distribution and Role in the Body

Iron, being a component of essential metabolic enzymes in every cell, is distributed throughout the body. The adult human body contains a total of about 3 to 5 gm of iron. Most of this, about 65 to 70 percent, is present in the blood as *hemoglobin* in red blood cells. Hemoglobin is a red compound consisting of two parts: *globin*, a protein tightly connected to a nonprotein substance called *heme*, which contains iron in the ferrous state. Each molecule of hemoglobin can carry four molecules of oxygen and is essential for oxygen transfer in the blood. A total of about 800 to 900 gm (2 pounds) of hemoglobin is present in an adult man. Normally it is present in blood at a level of about 11 to 14 percent (except in anemic persons, in whom the amount is lower — down to as low as 5 to 8 percent in rare instances). Hemoglobin contains about 0.33 percent iron.

The next largest concentration of iron is that stored in combination with proteins (such as ferritin and *hemosiderin*) in the liver, spleen, and bone marrow, which normally constitutes about 25 to 30 percent of that in the whole body.

The minor quantities of iron (about 5 percent) found in other tissues are nevertheless vitally important, as is evidenced by their locations:

1. In the chromatin network in cell nuclei.

2. In *cytochrome* (an iron-containing pigment) in protoplasm of cells, and in numerous enzymes that help catalyze oxidation-reduction processes in body tissues.

3. In *myoglobin* in muscles, which is closely related in chemistry and function to blood hemoglobin but is fixed in muscle tissue (and which constitutes about 3 percent of the total body iron).

In all these sites, the iron-containing compounds are involved in the vital life processes of cells and tissues (Fig. 12–2).

Iron owes its usefulness in the body to its special ability to be reversibly oxygenated — that is, to take on oxygen and later give this oxygen up to other substances. By means of this property, the iron-containing hemoglobin in red blood cells can take on extra oxygen when blood circulates through the lungs, can then carry oxygen to the tissues, and there can pass it on to the tissue cells for oxidative processes necessary to their life. Venous blood, which owes its bluish color to the presence of reduced hemoglobin, takes on excess carbon dioxide (a waste product of tissues) and is returned to the lungs, where it loses carbon dioxide and takes on another load of oxygen, becoming bright red again when *oxyhemoglobin* is formed. When insufficient iron is available to the body, less hemoglobin is formed (anemia), and these oxygen-carrying mechanisms are reduced, giving rise to many physiological problems (see later section).

The iron-containing pigments and enzymes in the tissues serve to bring about transfers of oxygen within cells in much the same manner. The cytochromes and *cytochrome oxidases* (enzymes that contain iron) have been estimated to be responsible for about 90 percent of the energy transfers associated with the oxidative phases of tissue respiration. *Catalase*, another example of an iron-containing enzyme (in the form of heme, also present in hemoglobin), is present in relatively high concentrations in red blood cells and in other tissue cells. The level of catalase in cells is reduced in an iron deficiency.

Among the billions of red blood cells (about 4½ to 5 million per cubic millimeter of blood), there are continual casualties and calls for replacements; the lifetime of such cells has been determined by use of isotopes to be about

4 months. They are formed in the bone marrow and destroyed chiefly in the spleen. Not only is iron needed for their formation, but also protein (for the protein part of hemoglobin) and other materials for the *stroma* — the body of the cell in which hemoglobin is embedded. When the cells disintegrate, the main nonprotein portion of hemoglobin is split into an iron-containing substance *(hematin)* and a pigment *(bilirubin)*. Almost all the iron and much of the bilirubin are saved to be used over again in new red corpuscles.

Only traces of iron are excreted in the urine, and the excreted iron lost to the body in the feces amounts ordinarily to less than 1 mg daily. More than half this loss is from cells sloughed off from the intestinal mucosa and the minimal intestinal blood losses. In girls and women between puberty and menopause, there is an extra loss of iron during menstruation, which needs to be taken into account.

The body has a store of readily available iron, a "labile pool of iron,"[8] made up of recently absorbed iron plus that recently released by the breaking down of red blood cells. This iron is used by preference for hemoglobin in building new red cells. Older stores of iron (as in the liver) may be somewhat less readily available, and the fixed iron in tissue cells is not drawn upon even in times of great need for this element.

Iron Deficiency Symptoms: Anemia

The most common sign of iron deficiency in humans is *iron deficiency anemia*, in which the level of hemoglobin in the red cells is reduced and the red cells themselves are smaller.* Some other symptoms of iron deficiency, though, are now known to occur even in the absence of anemia — such as faulty digestion, measurable changes in levels of various enzymes containing iron, cellular damage, and low iron stores.

Because the body uses iron so economically and has opportunity to build up considerable reserve stores of it over long periods, any deficiency due to an iron-poor diet or to poor absorption of the iron in the food is likely to develop only after a long period or in persons (the infant — see Chapter 21 — and growing child) or conditions (pregnancy, severe loss of blood by hemorrhage) that require an unusually great amount of iron. Diarrhea over long periods, hemorrhoids, peptic ulcers, malignancies, subnormal acidity of the gastric juice (fairly common in older persons), and excessive loss of blood during menstrual periods are clinical situations in humans that can appreciably increase iron needs and the severity of symptoms.

Iron deficiency anemia, like anemias from other causes, reduces the oxygen-carrying capacity of the blood, resulting, if severe, in such symptoms as paleness of the skin, weakness, shortness of breath, lack of appetite, and a general slowing of vital functions of the body. Severe iron deficiency over long periods is known to cause death, as would be expected. Recent evidence suggests that iron deficiency in humans is closely related to the occurrence of infections, though the exact relationships are unclear.[9]

Iron deficiency anemia may be precipitated in young girls whose diets are on the borderline of adequacy for iron when the onset of menstruation results in increased losses of iron from the body. More common than outright anemia in very young women are the low stores of body iron with which they come into the period of possible pregnancy. Pregnancy is a period during which iron deficiency anemias may be precipitated because of the increased need for iron both for blood in the unborn child and for building up a store of iron in the placenta and in the infant's liver. The child may be born with a good store of iron in its own liver, but this may be at the cost of depletion of the mother's store. Repeated pregnancies are especially costly to iron stores in the mother's body. (See Chapter 20.)

Iron deficiency is uncommon in breast-fed infants. While the iron content of breast milk is not higher than that in other infant foods, iron is apparently pres-

*Called technically a *microcytic hypochromic* anemia (small cells and reduced color).

ent in breast milk in a highly available form that is about 50 percent absorbed.[10]

Anemias Due to Blood Losses

Anemias may also be brought about by excessive loss of blood. Average menstrual losses amount to 0.6 mg iron per day, but are highly variable with different individuals. It is estimated that in about 20 percent of women these losses exceed 1 mg per day,[11] and in some they may be considerably higher. Excessive menstrual bleeding may constitute a continual drain on body iron stores, which may be hard to replace unless the diet is high in available iron and iron absorption is relatively efficient.

Unusually high iron needs may be precipitated by hemorrhages (either sudden loss of much blood or long-continued pathological bleeding such as with ulcers) or by the donation of blood for transfusions. Such losses may occur in persons of either sex. The body tends to replace a major loss of iron for hemoglobin building at a rate far in excess of that supplied in the diet and for this it mobilizes stored iron, especially the more labile types. The need for extra iron under these circumstances is far in excess of the amounts supplied by normal absorption of dietary iron from the intestine. This in turn promotes more efficient absorption of food iron. A diet that offers a plentiful supply of all substances needed for rebuilding blood (especially protein and including some rich sources of iron, such as liver, meats, and eggs) often is adequate, provided there are normal reserves of iron in the body.[12] If the previous diet has been too low in iron to provide such reserve stores, or if the current diet is low in iron, extra iron supplements would be needed to promote rapid blood regeneration.

Requirement and Recommended Allowances

It is difficult to fix any exact figure regarding the minimal requirements for iron, because of the many variables that we have mentioned previously. Chiefly because of the very limited absorption and availability of iron, the recommended intake has to be much higher (about ten times) than the actual tissue requirements.

Taking all these variables into consideration, the Food and Nutrition Board recommends a 10 mg per day allowance for men and postmenopausal women and an 18 mg per day allowance for other women.[1] The recommendation, based on an assumed average availability of 10 percent of the iron in food, provides for retention of 1 mg per day for men and postmenopausal women and 1.8 mg per day for other women.

The Food and Nutrition Board feels that its recommendations are reasonable and that a larger margin of safety may make for better health. The recommended iron allowances for both sexes and different periods of life are given in Table 12–2 and, in more detail, in Table 1 of the Appendix.

Any period in which growth takes place calls for an additional allowance of iron; such periods include pregnancy, lactation, and childhood from infancy through adolescence. With infants, requirements for iron to support rapid growth are relatively high per unit of body weight because of the small weight, but they are not high quantitatively (see

Table 12–2 RECOMMENDED DAILY IRON ALLOWANCES*

	Age (yrs)	*Iron (mg)*
Children	0–½	10
	½–3	15
	4–10	10
Males	11–18	18
	19 on	10
Females	10–50	18
	51 on	10
	Pregnant	18+
	Lactating	18

*From Food and Nutrition Board 1974.[1] See Appendix Table 1D for FAO recommendations.

Chapter 21). The iron requirements for small growing children are relatively high, as is the requirement for older boys and girls during the growth spurt that occurs in the teen-age period (11 to 18 years). The U.S. recommended allowance of 18 mg per day between the ages of 11 to 18 is designed to permit optimum storage of iron against possible drains on iron reserves, especially in young women because of menstruation, pregnancy, and lactation. The standardization of recommendations for iron intake among different countries is difficult because of the influence of so many factors on the iron requirement, including levels of intake of animal foods (which have iron of high availability) and the level of vitamin C in the diet.

Most countries currently advise iron intakes of about 7 to 10 mg a day for men and 12 mg or higher for women of childbearing age (see Appendix, Table 1C). The FAO/WHO recommendations for women of childbearing age, in countries where intakes of animal foods are less than 10 percent, is set at 28 mg per day.[13]

Iron Content of Foods

Figures for the amount of iron in some typical foods, both in milligrams per 100 gm and in an average serving, are given in Table 12–3 (see also Table 2 of the Appendix for other foods). In many instances, the distribution of iron follows that of other mineral elements, as it is relatively high in foods of low moisture content and low in fresh fruits and vegetables, which contain large amounts of water and fiber. Milk, which is one of the best sources of many other nutrients, is poor in iron, while organ meats, such as liver and the blood-forming organs (spleen and bone marrow, seldom consumed in this country), are unusually rich in iron. Good sources of iron are eggs, lean meats, legumes, nuts, dried fruits, whole grains or enriched cereal foods, and all green, leafy vegetables. Such foods as dark molasses, raisins, and nuts (often featured as rich sources of iron) are used infrequently or in small servings, so that they do not constitute sources of this element as important as some staple foods of lower iron content — such as whole-grain or enriched breads and cereals.

The addition of iron salts to bread, breakfast cereals, flour, and other cereal products in conjunction with the enrichment program has been a considerable help in raising the available iron content of the American diet. Approximately 30 percent of our total iron intake comes from enrichment sources (see Chapter 18). Unfortunately, not all states of the United States have enrichment regulations. Unenriched highly milled cereals or bread, sugar, and fats are either very low or lacking in iron.

The amount of iron in a food can be quite variable, and too much trust should not be put in food composition tables as far as iron content of foods is concerned. The iron content of processed and manufactured foods is extremely variable unless iron is added. The use of iron cooking utensils in food manufacture, as used to be the case with molasses, is a factor, as are iron cooking utensils used in the home.[14] Some water supplies are high in iron, but this is not a dependable source. The student should learn to read food labels and, if in doubt about the iron content of a manufactured food, he should write to the manufacturer.

However, the extent of the body's *need* for iron still remains the *primary* factor that controls the relative amount of the iron content of all types of food in the diet that will be absorbed; this makes differences in degree of utilization of iron from different types of food of less importance. If the margin between the total amounts needed and those furnished by the food intake is small, the relative utilization from all types of food will be "stepped up." If only small amounts of iron are needed for body maintenance, less will be absorbed and much of the food iron will remain unabsorbed to be

Table 12–3 TYPICAL FOODS AS SOURCES OF IRON*

Food	*Size of Serving*	*Iron, in Milligrams* Per Average Serving	Per 100 gm of Food
Liver:			
Lamb, broiled	2 slices (75 gm)	13.4	17.9
Beef, fried	2 slices (75 gm)	6.6	8.8
Chicken, cooked	¼ c (50 gm)	4.3	8.8
Meats (lean or medium fat):			
Beef, round, cooked	1 large hamburger (85 gm)	3.0	3.5
rib roast, cooked	3 slices (100 gm)	2.6	2.6
Pork, chop, cooked	1 medium large chop (80 gm)	2.5	3.1
Lamb, shoulder chop	1 chop, cooked (90 gm)	1.6	1.8
Baked beans, canned with			
pork and molasses	½ c (130 gm)	3.0	2.3
pork and tomato	½ c (130 gm)	2.3	1.8
Fruits, dried (uncooked)			
Apricots	4 halves, (30 gm)	1.7	5.5
Prunes	4–5 medium, (30 gm)	1.2	3.9
Figs	2 small (30 gm)	0.9	3.0
Raisins	2 tbsp (20 gm)	0.6	3.5
Legumes:			
Soy beans, dry	½ c scant, cooked (30 gm dry)	2.5	8.4
Peanut butter	2 tbsp scant (30 gm)	0.6	2.0
Lima beans, fresh	½ c, cooked (80 gm)	2.0	2.5
Peas, fresh, green	½ c, cooked (80 gm)	1.4	1.8
Molasses, med.	1 tbsp (20 gm)	1.2	6.0
Eggs, whole	1 medium (50 gm)	1.2	2.3
Leafy vegetables:			
Spinach	½ c, cooked (90 gm)	2.0	2.2
Beet greens	½ c, cooked (100 gm)	1.9	1.9
Chard	½ c, cooked (100 gm)	1.8	1.8
Kale (leaves only)	½ c, cooked (55 gm)	0.9	1.6
Turnip greens	½ c, cooked (75 gm)	0.8	1.1
Vegetables:			
Potatoes, sweet	1 medium baked (110 gm)	1.0	0.9
white	1 medium baked (100 gm)	0.7	0.7
Broccoli	⅔ c (100 gm)	0.8	0.8
Brussels sprouts	5–6 medium (70 gm)	0.8	1.1
Cauliflower	¾ c, cooked (100 gm)	0.7	0.7
Carrots	⅔ c, diced, cooked (100 gm)	0.6	0.6
String beans	¾ c, cooked (100 gm)	0.6	0.6
Beets	2, 2-in diameter (100 gm)	0.5	0.5
Bread:			
White, enriched	1 slice	0.6	2.5
Whole-wheat	1 slice	0.5	2.3
White, unenriched	1 slice	0.2	0.7
Cereals, whole grain (oats, corn, wheat, rice):	See label on package – range from 0.2 to 0.7 mg unenriched, up to 10 mg enriched, per serving.		
Fresh fruits and fresh vegetables	100 gm serving, mostly	0.3–0.6	
Milk, whole, fluid, cow's	½ pt, or 8 oz glass (244 gm)	0.10	0.04
Human	½ pt, or 8 oz (244 gm)	0.24	0.1

*Most of these data from *Composition of Foods,* Agriculture Handbook No. 8, U.S. Department of Agriculture, 1963. (See also Table 2 of the Appendix for additional values).

discarded in the feces — that is, the degree of availability will be lower for all types of food.

How to Get Recommended Allowance of Iron in the Diet

In Table 12–4 are listed two groups of common foods, in average servings, that furnish 10 mg and 18 mg of iron. These are the daily allowances of iron for men over 18 years of age or children 3 to 10 years of age (10 mg) and for women ages 11 to 50 years and males ages 11 to 18 years (18 mg), respectively. It is apparent that if two or three servings of some relatively iron-rich foods are included, other normal items of the diet that provide minor amounts of iron will make up the desired total. On days when liver is used, the total iron intake will probably be higher than the standard allowance, but the excess can be stored to make up for a day when a slightly less than normal amount is taken. Liver can be ground up and mixed with hamburger to make a very palatable mixture rich in iron.

Because it is important, both for body welfare and for good utilization of iron, that the diet be adequate in all essential nutrients, the groups of foods listed under (1) of Table 12–4 represent a well-balanced diet. If one follows the recommendation to include in the daily diet one pint of milk, one serving of meat, one egg, three or four slices of whole-wheat or enriched bread, one serving of potato, two servings of other vegetables (using colored and leafy vegetables fairly often), and two servings of fruit (one citrus or tomato), these foods alone provide 9 to 12 mg of iron daily. To bring the daily iron intake up to 18 mg requires either more liberal use of meats (liver or other organ meat eaten once a week is good insurance); increased amounts of eggs, green, leafy vegetables, legumes, nuts, or enriched bread and cereals; or the use of a special iron supplement (especially for persons with reduced caloric intakes). The Food and Nutrition Board (1974) states:[1] "It is obvious that, for women of childbearing age, the objective of the RDA . . . cannot be met with respect to iron in the typical American diet. . . . It is possible, however, to increase the iron intake by selecting iron-rich foods whenever possible and by including in the diet foods that are known to increase the absorption of iron present in the diet; for example, meat and citrus fruit. During pregnancy, daily supplements of 30–60 mg. of iron are recommended." This is a noteworthy statement, since it departs from the traditional advice of nutrition educators that all nutrients for all normal persons can be obtained readily from the basic foodstuffs. The advice for these added iron needs is based on good experimental evidence.[1, 15]

Table 12–4 GROUPS OF FOODS THAT FURNISH IRON AT LEVELS OF 10 AND 18 mg

(1)	*Iron mg*	*(2)*	*Iron mg*
Hamburger, 1 average (85 gm)	3.0	Liver, lamb, broiled, 2 slices (75 gm)	13.4
Beet greens, ½ c cooked	1.9	Beans, snap, ¾ c, canned	1.5
Bread, whole-wheat, 3 slices	1.5	Milk, 1 pt	0.2
Egg, 1 medium large	1.2	Dried apricots or prunes, ½ c, cooked	2.1
Potato, 1 medium	0.7	Bread, white, 2 slices	1.2
Beets, 2 small	0.5		
Banana, 1 medium	0.7		
Orange, 1 medium	0.6		
Milk, 1 pt	0.2		
	10.3		18.4

Iron Intakes and Nutritional Status

Failure of the iron content of the diet to be adequate for actual body needs, as evidenced by the occurrence of nutritional anemia, is found frequently in the United States. The amount of iron in a normal American diet averages about 6 mg for every 1000 kcal.[1, 16] This means that women who are restricting themselves to 1500 to 2000 calories per day are apt to receive too little iron. As mentioned previously, iron deficiency anemia is the most common overt nutritional deficiency in the United States[17] (with an incidence of over 15 percent) and in many developing countries. The most vulnerable age groups are infants and young children, young pregnant teen-agers, women of child-bearing age, and older persons on reduced food intakes. Iron deficiency affects rich and poor alike.

When cost limits the amount of meat and eggs used, greater dependence for iron is placed on legumes and cereals, so that the use of whole-grain or enriched cereal products may provide the margin of safety in low-cost diets.

Anemia most frequently results from low stores of iron, which can be caused by inadequate dietary intake, blood loss, or malabsorption of iron. However, there are many other possible causes of anemia, such as deficiency of another nutrient or inability to mobilize stored iron. A new assay for serum ferritin that appears to be a reliable indicator of iron stores has been developed.[18] The estimation of iron stores by this method helps to determine whether inadequate iron intake might be the cause of anemia in an individual or whether there are other complicating factors.

Toxicity of Iron

As with all trace elements, the toxic level of iron is easily reached by taking in sources outside a normal food supply. The safe range with most of the trace elements is within about 10 to 50 times the requirement.

Iron toxicity is known to exist, for example, in certain members of the Bantu tribe in South Africa who have used iron utensils in cooking and the brewing of alcoholic beverages. In the United States, toxicity from the normal iron in foods is unknown except in a rare genetic disease in which iron accumulates.*

Some people find they have very limited tolerance for single doses of highly ionizable forms of iron (such as ferrous sulfate) if eaten in a supplement in amounts much over 250 mg a day, a nontoxic dose. Such a level each day, over long periods of time, could cause accumulation of excessive iron stores in the body.[19]

*Hemochromatosis.

IODINE

Discovery As a Nutrient

Goiter, a condition caused by an enlarged thyroid gland, was known in China as early as 3000 B.C. and was treated effectively by feeding seaweed or burnt sponge to those affected. In 1820 Coindet,[20] a physician in Switzerland, provided evidence that the then newly discovered iodine* (isolated from seaweed by Courtois in 1811) was the curative agent in seaweed and burnt sponge.[3] Though the idea was not universally accepted then, in retrospect it is clear that iodine was one of the first nutrients, if not the first, to be recognized as essential for humans or animals. Vitamins and amino acids were unknown at the time.

Distribution and Role in the Body

Iodine is absorbed in the inorganic form as iodide ions in the upper part of the intestine. It is freely available; even organic forms are well utilized after being released in the intestine. It may also be absorbed through the skin, if applied. Estimates of the total amount in the body range from 15 to 30 mg, about the size of a matchhead. Of this small amount, about three-fifths is concentrated in the thyroid gland and the rest is mostly in the circulating blood. Iodine serves but one purpose in the body — namely, to form an integral part of the thyroid hormones

*Iodine (I_2) is related chemically to the halogens chlorine, bromine, and fluorine. Its name is derived from the Greek word *iodes*, meaning violet color, from the color of the fumes of iodine (which also have a distinctive odor).

*thyroxine** (discovered by Kendall in 1915) and *triiodothyronine** (a more active but less abundant form discovered in 1952). These hormones are manufactured in the thyroid gland from its stored iodine and the amino acid tyrosine, and they are released in small amounts into the blood. Without the presence of iodine, which, of course, must be obtained originally from dietary sources, these two hormones are completely ineffective.

When carried to the tissues, these hormones are quantitatively the most important single factor in determining the *rate* of *basal metabolism*. The thyroid hormones also have other vital roles in health and reproduction, which, from a nutritional viewpoint, are likewise essential roles of dietary iodine (see Chapter 13). Control of the level of the thyroid hormones in the blood is effected by release or suppression of a stimulating hormone from the pituitary gland.

Iodine is supplied to the body by intake of foods or water, in which it is contained in minute amounts. Dietary iodine is absorbed from the alimentary tract, after which approximately 30 percent is removed by the thyroid gland, where most of it is stored as the complex protein *thyroglobulin*. The remainder is excreted in the urine, with minor amounts in the feces.

*Thyroxine is formed by the union of two tyrosine molecules and the substitution of four iodine atoms for four hydrogens. Triiodothyronine is exactly the same except that it carries three, instead of four, iodine atoms in the molecule. Kendall later received the Nobel Prize for his work on this and other hormones.

Iodine Deficiency: Goiter

Simple, or endemic, goiter is an enlargement of the thyroid gland in the neck due to an insufficiency of iodine supply. The gland enlarges in an attempt to compensate for the shortage of iodine, which is an essential ingredient for making its hormones (see Fig. 12–3). This disorder was prevalent for centuries before its cause was recognized. Although others had suspected iodine,[3] interest in the thyroid gland and its relation to iodine was stimulated by the accidental discovery in Germany by Baumann in 1895 that the thyroid gland was especially rich in iodine.[21] This eventually led to final proof that iodine was necessary for goiter prevention and for formation of the thyroid hormones, and was an essential nutrient for humans and animals. Research began in earnest then on finding the mechanism of action of iodine and on correlating the iodine content of water and soil with the incidence of goiter in certain areas.

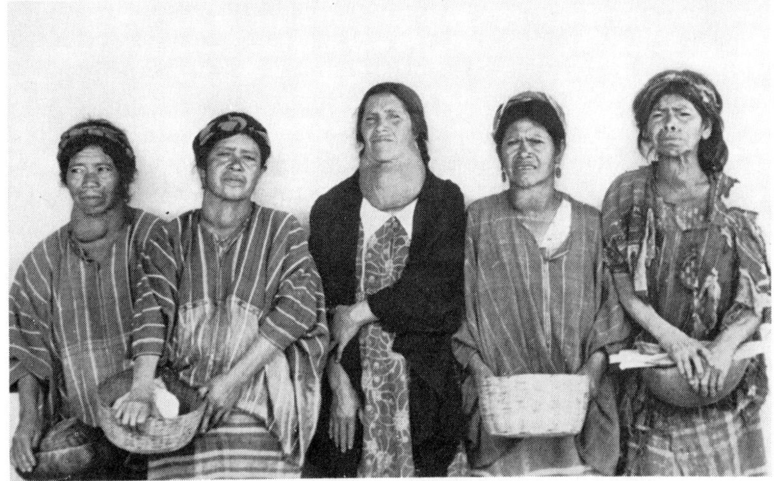

Figure 12–3 A group of women from a goitrous region in Guatemala, an example of the prevalence of simple goiter in many isolated sections of the world today. (Courtesy of Dr. N. S. Scrimshaw and the Institute of Nutrition of Central America and Panama.)

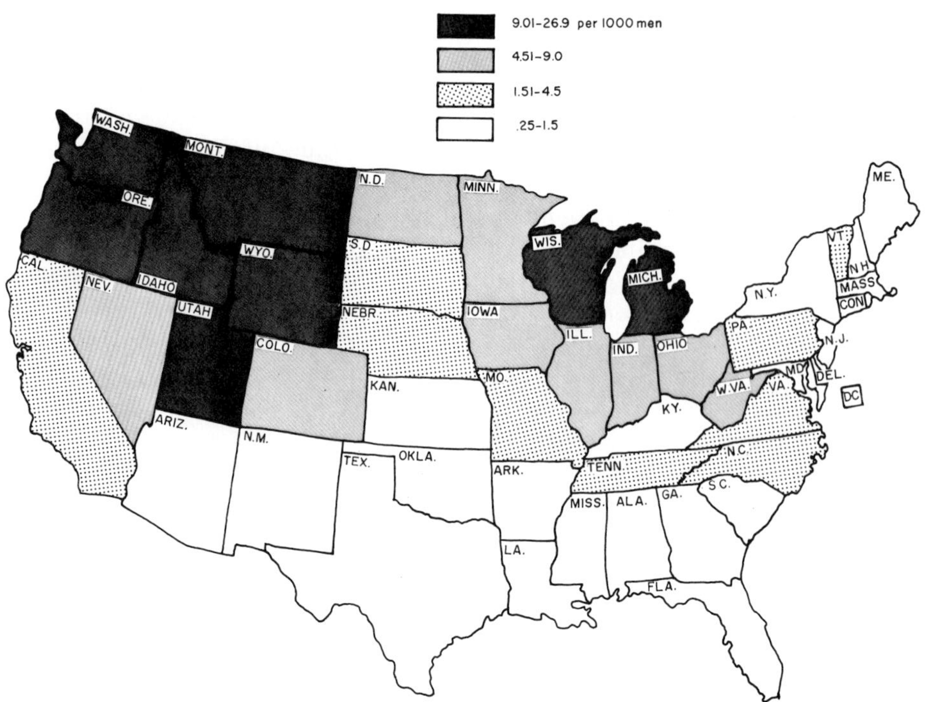

Figure 12–4 A "goiter map" of the then 48 states, showing (in black) the regions where goiter among draftees in 1917–18 was most prevalent. It also occurred fairly commonly in the shaded and dotted states, but was almost totally absent in the states in white. The use of preventive measures (iodine in drinking water and iodized salt) has greatly reduced the incidence of simple goiter, even in the states where it was most prevalent. However, in recent years the incidence in some of these states, plus several states in the South (Texas and Louisiana), has increased somewhat (see text). (From Love and Davenport: *Geographic Distribution of Simple Goiter Among Drafted Men,* 1917–18. U.S. Department of Public Health.)

French, American, and Swiss chemists, in whose countries there was a high incidence of simple goiter, found that in certain isolated mountain valleys, both water and soil are low in iodine content. The inhabitants subsisted almost entirely on products grown in the locality. Salts of iodine became a popular treatment for goiter in these areas for both humans and animals.

Several sets of events around 1917 and 1918 directed the attention of the public and of scientists to the distribution of simple goiter in different parts of the United States (Fig. 12–4). One was the publication of figures on the incidence of goiter among men drafted during World War I, which showed that this disorder was most prevalent in the basin of the Great Lakes and in the Pacific Northwest in the United States and Canada. In areas adjacent to the ocean, where both soil and foods grown on it were relatively iodine-rich and where seafoods were commonly eaten, goiter proved to be almost nonexistent. The second disclosure was that farm animals in goitrous regions showed the same evidence of iodine deficiency as humans, and their tendency to produce stillborn or weak and sickly young was a source of concern and a financial loss to farmers.

During the World War I years, Marine and Kimball,[22, 23] on the basis of evidence accumulated over a period of 6 years, administered small doses of iodine to school children in Akron, Ohio, where mild goiter was common among adolescent girls (females are more subject to goiter than males, and it is most likely to make its appearance at such periods as adolescence and pregnancy). Small doses of potassium iodide were given during two 10 day periods each year to about 800 girls, while about 1800 untreated girls of the same age group served as controls. No goiter developed in the treated group, while 26 percent of the control group developed enlarged thyroids in the same time period. Similar treatment with iodides, undertaken among the school children in three cantons of Switzerland, produced a tremendous decrease in the incidence of adolescent goiter.

In 1918, Hart and Steenbock published results of a study of the "hairless pig malady," a condition in which apparently normal sows gave birth to stillborn young that were nearly hairless and had thick, goitrous necks.[24] This condition was found to be the result of iodine deficiency, and the addition of iodide to the feed enabled the sows to produce normal young. The condition is similar to *endemic cretinism* in severely handicapped and dwarfed children born with underdeveloped thyroids due to a deficiency of iodine in their mothers during the first 3 months of pregnancy or before conception.

These studies and others established without question the practicability of prevention of simple goiter by administration of small quantities of some iodine compound (Fig. 12–5). It was finally decided that iodized salt (refined salt to which sodium or potassium iodide has been added in amounts up to 0.01 percent) offered the best preventive, because salt is a low-cost food that is commonly used by all people. The use of iodized salt (or some other carrier) is now recommended in all localities where simple goiter is endemic, and iodization of salt is required by law in Switzerland, Canada, Colombia, Guatemala, and other countries. In the United States, the iodization of salt is not legally mandatory but is very common, and educational campaigns have wisely encouraged its widespread use. Under a 1972 Food and Drug Aministration regulation, iodized table salt must be labeled, "This salt supplies iodide, a necessary nutrient." Uniodized salt will be labeled, "This salt does not supply iodide, a necessary nutrient."

Because the cause and means of prevention of endemic goiter have thus been well known since 1920 and much progress toward its eradication has been made in certain countries, it is perhaps surprising that goiter is still one of the most prevalent nutritional deficiency diseases in the world. Many millions of persons (200 million has been estimated) are affected today. Much remains to be done in clear-

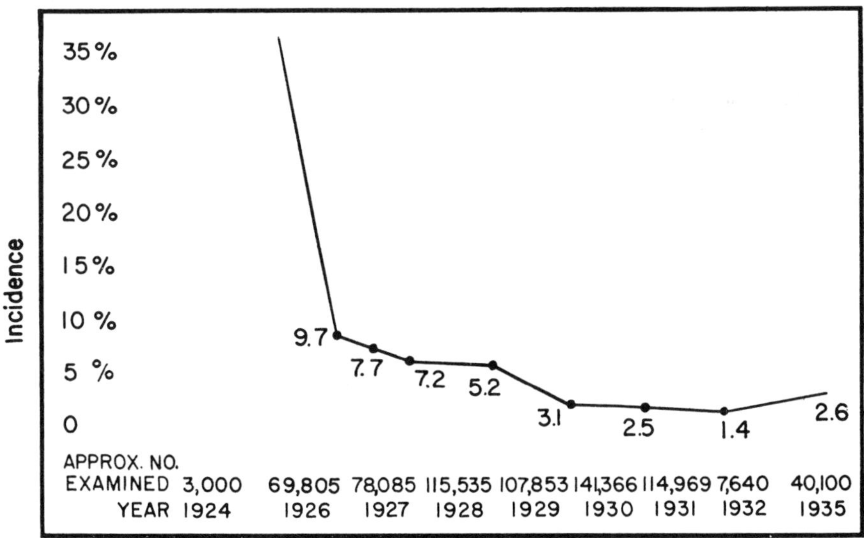

Figure 12–5 The marked decrease in simple goiter among Detroit school children between 1924 and 1935, due to the use of iodized salt. (From Kimball, O. P.: *Journal of American Medical Association*, 1937.)

ing up the last of it even in more advanced countries, and it is still rife in many developing countries and out-of-the-way places, such as isolated valleys of Austria, northern India, South and Central America, and Yugoslavia. There remains much work yet to be done by educational, medical, and public health agencies before its final eradication is accomplished.

It should be stressed that once a goiter has developed in adult life, taking supplementary iodine will not decrease the size of an enlarged thyroid gland. Persons on low-salt or salt-free diets, especially pregnant women, may need some other source of supplementary iodine (prescribed by a physician). Iodized oil, by injection, can serve this purpose in endemic areas.[25]

Mention should be made of the fact that enlarged thyroid glands (goiter) can also be caused by the eating of large amounts of foods such as turnips, cabbage, and rutabaga over long periods of time. Such foods contain natural antithyroid compounds called *goitrogens*, which inhibit the formation of thyroid hormones. The normal use of these foods, as in this country, is in no way harmful. Certain drugs such as thiouracil and several sulfa drugs also have a goitrogenic effect, and there are known inherited defects that can cause goiter.

Iodine Needs and Sources

It is evident that iodides are present in the body and in foods in amounts small enough to be counted as "traces," and naturally the requirement to replace losses in the urine is very small.

Recommended allowances for iodine have been set in the United States at about two times the minimal amount essential to maintain a normal balance in order to ensure a margin of safety. The recommendation for young men (age 19 to 22) is 140 micrograms (0.14 mg) per day; it is 100 micrograms for young women of this same age group.[1] The needs are increased during pregnancy and lactation (see Appendix, Table 1, for the details of needs of other age groups). Iodine intakes at this level have no harmful effects and serve to build up a reserve store of this element in the thyroid gland for use in emergencies. Possibly the smallness of the quantities of iodine required may best be appreciated by considering that the standard allowance of iron for an adult woman for 2 days (36 mg) would weigh about the same as a whole year's allowance (36.5 mg) of iodine. It is truly a "trace" element.

For intakes of iodine to replace losses, man is dependent on the amounts present in foods, soil, and water. Iodine in drinking and cooking water varies widely in different regions; in some areas, such as near the oceans, it is high enough to meet the daily requirement. The iodine content of foods also varies widely, depending chiefly on the iodine content of the soil or that of animal feeds (to which iodide salts are routinely added in most countries). Today, iodine is also in our food supply as a contaminant because of quite widespread use of iodine salts in food processing operations. Because these amounts, stated in *parts per billion* of fresh material, are so small and variable, it seems wiser to confine oneself to general statements about the relative value of different foods as sources of this element.[2]

To put iodine values in food composition tables would be most misleading for reasons explained previously.

In general, marine fish, shellfish, dried seaweed (in countries where it is used), and cod-liver oil are relatively rich in iodine; butter, milk, cheese, and eggs may be good sources when animals have been fed on iodine-rich rations; vegetables grown in soils of at least moderate iodine content are fairly good sources; cereal grains, legumes, and fresh fruits (even from nongoitrous regions) are of low iodine content. Highly refined foods are generally very low in or devoid of iodine, unless it has been added in some way or is present owing to contamination.

Persons living in nongoitrous areas are practically certain to get enough iodine to meet their requirement from water supplies, and from any well-balanced diet — one not too high in cereals and highly refined foods. Those living in goitrous regions may supplement their diet with seafoods and vegetables or other foods shipped in from regions where there is more iodine in the soil. However, by using iodized salt, persons in almost any area may be assured of getting their quota of this element without considering the small and variable amounts provided by the diet.

Nutritional Status

As mentioned, iodine deficiency is rampant throughout many areas of the world in spite of the extremely low amounts needed and the low cost (less than a few cents a year). In the United States, lessons learned in the past are easily forgotten, and nutrition education programs are only beginning to be truly effective. The National Nutrition Survey[17] uncovered significant numbers of American children with goiter due to iodine deficiency — incidences of as high as up to 5 percent in some low-income areas.

In areas of low iodine intake, it would appear logical to require *universal* enrichment of salt with a stable form of iodine (0.5 to 1 part per 10,000), along with new education programs and better labeling of food products. Better regulations also should be established for the use, or misuse, as the case may be, of iodine salts in food manufacturing.

Iodine Toxicity

As with the other trace elements, there is not too great a spread between iodine requirements and detrimental levels. In humans, high levels of 25 to 50 times the recommended levels over long periods of time are known to depress the thyroid in acting as goitrogen. Therapeutic use of iodine and large intakes of kelp (seaweed) in the diet could produce a toxic effect in an estimated 1 to 3 percent of the American population.[26] Treating oneself with compounds of iodide or concentrates of iodine in dried seaweed over long periods is a hazardous procedure.

COPPER

The discovery of copper (Cu) goes back to prehistoric times (8000 B.C., during the Late Stone Age).* Its unexpected essential role as a nutrient for mammals was not discovered, however, until 1928, when Hart and associates[27] found that iron alone was not sufficient to prevent anemia in rats fed a milk diet. They found that a cure could be effected by adding to the food the ash of either lettuce or liver. They noticed the ash had a pale blue color. Suspecting that this color might be due to copper, they fed this element with iron to a deficient rat, and in just a few days' time there was a marked improvement in hemoglobin formation and growth. They were as surprised that copper was effective as we would be today to find a similar effect with, say, such common elements as aluminum, silver, or lead (although copper had been known to be essential for certain marine invertebrates).

Shortly thereafter, in 1931, Josephs[28] provided evidence that copper was more effective than iron alone in overcoming the anemia of milk-fed infants. Though not accepted at first, there is now convincing evidence that copper deficiency can exist in special situations in milk-fed infants.[29] Such deficiencies in infants are more generally complicated with chronic diarrhea or metabolic diseases, while defi-

*The later Bronze Age (3000 to 1000 B.C.) takes its name from the use during this period of bronze — an alloy of copper and tin. The word "copper" is derived from the Latin *cuprum*, a corruption of cyprium, named after the island of Cyprus (which was a source of much copper about 3000 B.C.).

ciencies in adult man are unknown either naturally or experimentally. However, because the copper content of refined foods is not a certain entity, because of the recognition of copper deficiency in infants, and because of the current very high interest in this trace element in human nutrition, it is important to have an understanding of its role in the body and distribution in food.

Distribution in Body and Function

A usual day's intake of copper for an adult is about 2 to 5 mg, most of which is in food as the organic form. About 30 percent of this is absorbed in the upper small intestine or stomach as the inorganic ion, after digestion. A total of 75 to 150 mg of copper is present in the entire human adult body, most of it bound to various essential proteins. Most of the body copper is in blood and muscle, though the brain, heart, liver, eye, hair, and kidney have higher concentrations, suggestive of important functions in these tissues.[2]

In the blood serum most of the copper is present in the protein *ceruloplasmin* (also known as *ferroxidase I*), which is essential for iron utilization.[30, 31] Excess copper is excreted normally through the bile.

Copper is present in several important enzymes,* thus playing a role in many essential reactions in the body, including the synthesis of hemoglobin (or release of iron for this purpose), the metabolism of glucose and release of energy, the formation of phospholipids in the nerve wall, and the formation of connective tissue.

In copper deficiency in animals a variety of symptoms are known to occur besides anemia, including skeletal defects, gray or depigmented hair (see Fig. 12–6), faulty wool or hair structure, degeneration of the nervous system, cardiovascular lesions, and reproductive disorders.[1, 2] Many useful pioneer studies have been made with copper-deficient swine, especially at the University of Utah by Cartwright and Wintrobe. In deficient human infants, low copper levels in the blood ("hypocupremia") and other tissues are observed, as well as other blood and bone disorders.

Elevation of plasma copper has been reported in a number of diseases, including Hodgkin's disease, rheumatoid arthritis, schizophrenia, coronary heart disease, and hyperparathyroidism.[32] The significance of the increase is not yet understood.

Requirement, Food Sources, and Nutritional Status

The Food and Nutrition Board (U.S.)[1] states that "copper intakes of 1.3 and 2 mg/day appear to maintain balance in preadolescent girls and adults, respectively." Most diets provide about 2 mg per day in the United States, a sufficient but not abundant amount.[1] The 1979 RDA is provisionally set, according to Balsley,[33] at a minimum of 2 mg per day for adults. If we compare this amount of copper needed, about 2 mg a day, with the amount in one copper cent, which weighs over 3 gm

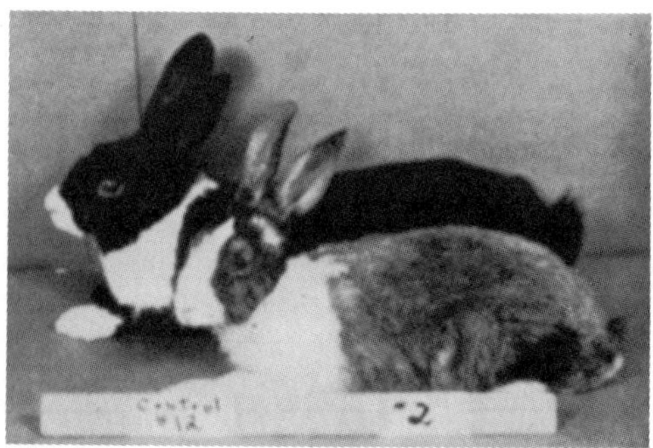

Figure 12–6 The rabbit in the back received sufficient copper in his diet. The rabbit in the foreground, after 6 weeks on a copper deficient diet, displayed smaller size and depigmentation. (From Hunt, C. E., and Carlton, W. W.: J. Nutr., *87*:385, 1965.)

*Copper is present in such enzymes as tyrosinase, monoamine oxidase (essential in elastin formation), and cytochrome-C oxidase. It is also a constituent of the protein erythrocuprein (probably an enzyme) in the red blood cell.

(3000 mg), we see that one cent contains sufficient copper to supply the needs of one person for over 1500 days, or over 4 years. Obviously, if and when the time ever comes when we need to enrich our foods with copper, it will not be expensive. Deficiencies of copper are known in farm animals grazing on copper-deficient soils, so copper is routinely added to most commercial farm rations.

Copper occurs along with other mineral elements in all natural foods. The richest sources are organ meats, shellfish, nuts, dried legumes, and cocoa. Cow's milk is a very poor source of this element, as are many other foods. Human milk contains an adequate amount. The amount of copper in the diet depends on both the choice of foods and the locality in which they are produced.[34, 35] Copper may be added to foods in processing, as in the pasteurization of milk by passing it over copper rollers, or from cooking in copper utensils. Copper levels may be reduced, on the other hand, by the refinement of food. It would be extremely difficult, though, to get an insufficient supply of copper in one's diet when eating a variety of foodstuffs. Natural drinking water often supplies the entire requirement, for example.

Toxicity of Copper

There is a reasonable degree of tolerance for higher levels of food copper than that normally consumed, though the toxic level has not been determined with certainty. Daily intakes of more than 20 to 30 mg over extended periods would be expected to be unsafe. Since copper cooking utensils are rarely used now, there is little danger of toxic intake.[19] Mention should be made of *Wilson's disease,*[36] a rather rare chronic metabolic disease in humans, in which the body has great difficulty in disposing of excess copper; the copper is stored in the liver and other tissues (such as the eyes), finally resulting in toxic concentrations. The level of serum ceruloplasmin is usually very low in this disease. Copper-low diets of "normal foods" have been developed and are used as part of the clinical management of the disease.

MANGANESE

Manganese (Mn) is easily confused with *magnesium* (Mg) (see Chapter 11) because the names are similar, both names being derived centuries ago from the ore "magnesia." Both are essential nutrients, but most of the similarity stops there. This gray metal is the twelfth most abundant element on the earth's crust and a necessary component of plants and animals (as well as the substance added to iron in making steel; hence, it is of great industrial importance).

Inorganic manganese* has been known to be a dietary essential for all higher animals ever since the original discovery in several laboratories (Hart, McCollum, and their associates) in 1931 that it was essential for growth of rats.[37] Later it was shown to be essential for poultry (a deficiency resulted in a tendon and bone disorder), swine, guinea pigs, cattle, and other animals.[2]

Undoubtedly manganese is an essential nutrient for man, even though what signs would identify a deficiency of it have never been determined with certainty. Impaired blood clotting, lowered serum cholesterol, color changes in the hair, and dermatitis have been seen in very limited clinical studies that require confirmation.[38] In any event, the dietary requirement is so low in comparison with the abundant amounts in our environment and in most foods that a deficiency in free-living populations would be quite unlikely.

Manganese has many essential functions in each cell of the body.[2, 3] The highest concentrations in the body are in the

*First recognized as an element in 1774 by a famous Swedish chemist, Carl Wilhelm Scheele, who also discovered chlorine, glycerol, and citric, lactic, and oxalic acids.

pituitary gland, lactating mammary glands, liver, pancreas, kidney, intestinal wall, and bone.

Manganese is an important catalyst and is a cofactor or component of many enzymes in the body.* Because of its relationship to these enzymes, it is needed for synthesis of complex carbohydrates (mucopolysaccharides) in cells, utilization of glucose, lipid synthesis and metabolism, cholesterol synthesis, normal pancreas development, muscle contraction, prevention of skeletal defects, prevention of sterility, and other vital functions. Few elements have as many metabolic functions, though the mechanisms are still quite unknown.

Manganese deficiency has occurred either by simply feeding fowl natural grain and legume diets, or has been induced in several species of animals on manganese-low diets, with symptoms too numerous to itemize.[2, 3] In general, manganese deficiency is associated with failure to grow, interference with sexual processes, and inability to produce normal young.[39] In rabbits, there are deformations of bone. In fowls, a manganese-deficient ration proved to be the chief cause of a disorder called "slipped tendon," resulting in deformed legs, which was a source of economic loss to poultry producers. The addition of small amounts of this element to the ration prevented development of this disease (55 mg per kg of diet is needed by fowl, a relatively high level compared with the normal need of mammals). The brain and nervous system of laboratory animals are particularly susceptible to both manganese deficiency and manganese toxicity.[40]

Adult male humans appear to be in manganese balance with 6 to 8 mg of this element per day, and adult females with 3 to 5 mg (the amount in usual diets).[35, 41] Absorption ranges from only 1 to 20 percent, and, like iron absorption, depends on dietary intake and need. High intakes of iron and of calcium decrease manganese absorption.[2] The human body is said to contain only 12 to 20 mg of manganese.[2]

Manganese is widely distributed in foods of plant and animal origin, especially nuts, vegetables, and fruits,[35, 40] though it is partially lost along with other trace elements in food refining. It is relatively nontoxic. The newly established provisional RDA for adults is tentatively set at 2.5 to 5.0 mg. for adults.[33]

*Manganese is present in such enzymes as *pyruvate carboxylase*, and *superoxide dismutase* (which also contains copper), and is a cofactor in the metabolism of liver arginase, phosphoglucomutase, polymerase (in mucopolysaccharide formation), galactotransferase, acetyl-CoA carboxylase, and others.

ZINC

Interest in the mineral zinc as an essential trace element has increased considerably since the 1960's, when evidence for its need by man was shown,[2, 42] and since the discovery that both animals and humans can become deficient under so-called "natural" conditions when eating foods of plant origin.[2]

Zinc alloys have been known for centuries and since the 13th century as a silver-blue mineral.* It is a constitutent, with copper, of brass. We see zinc around us commonly as the coating of "galvanized" iron and inside flashlight batteries. About 2 gm is present in an adult human body — at least a 200 day supply for nutritional needs.

Its need in the diet of mammals was first proved by Wisconsin nutritionists working with rats in the 1930's.[43] Zinc is now known to be very important in the diet of all animal species studied, including rat, cattle, sheep, dog, pig, mouse, and poultry (see Fig. 12–7).

*Zinc was first isolated as a pure mineral in the 13th century in India and was used to make coins in China in the 15th century. The names of the persons who first discovered zinc and named it are lost in history. The word "zinc" comes from Old High German (zink), Polish, and Greek (*zinn*), from which *zincium*, and old Polish name for zinc ore, was derived.

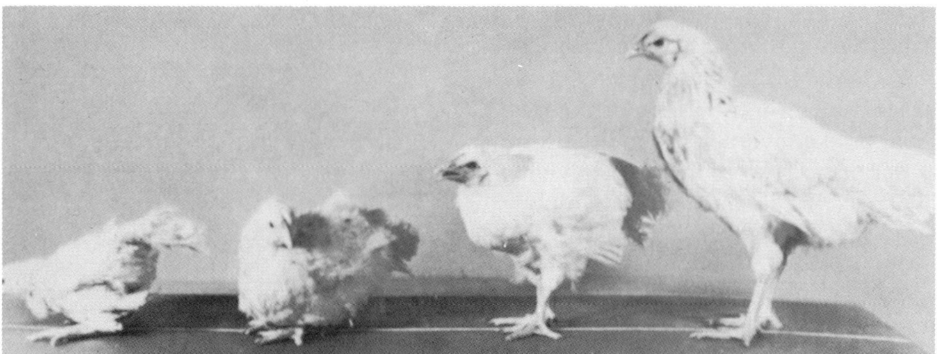

Figure 12–7 These four chickens are all 10 weeks old. From left to right, they were fed increasing amounts of zinc. Note the retarded growth, poor feathering, and difficulty in standing up in the deficient animals. (Courtesy of the American Zinc Institute.)

Distribution in Body and Role

Concentrations of zinc in the human body are highest in the liver, bones, epidermal tissues, prostate gland, testes, sperm cells, hair, nails, eye, and blood, and there is rapid metabolism of it in the pancreas, kidneys, and pituitary gland. In the blood, 75 per cent of the zinc is in the red cells.

Zinc is associated with the hormone *insulin,* which is secreted by the pancreas and involved in carbohydrate metabolism. Two hormones, which are secreted by the anterior pituitary (follicle-stimulating and luteinizing hormones) and which play a role in the female reproductive cycle, have their action enhanced by the presence of zinc.

In enzyme systems, zinc plays an important role as an active component of the enzyme *carbonic anhydrase,* which functions in maintaining equilibrium between carbon dioxide and carbonic acid ($CO_2 + H_2O \rightleftharpoons H_2CO_3$) in tissues and catalyzes the reaction by which hydrogen may be split off from carbonic acid. This reaction not only is important in the transport of carbon dioxide by the blood but also may be involved (by the liberation of hydrogen ions) in the secretion of high concentrations of hydrochloric acid into the gastric juice. Zinc also activates enzymes that function in digestion of proteins by hydrolyzing specific peptide linkages. It is part of alkaline phosphatase, an enzyme essential in bone metabolism and a constituent or activator of a number of other enzymes.[2] It plays an essential role in the formation of RNA and DNA in the synthesis of protein in the cell.

In humans, zinc is essential for normal growth of the genital organs, prevention of anemia, wound healing, general growth of all tissues, and prevention of "dwarfism," or greatly reduced stature.[31, 42]

Zinc Deficiency

In animals, a diet low in zinc, especially one that is also high in calcium or *phytates* (as in whole grains and beans), predisposes to zinc deficiency, symptoms of which may be retarded growth, loss of appetite, skin disorders, many reproduction problems, and abnormal bone metabolism.[2] Zinc-deficient rats have fewer litters, and their offspring are frequently deformed.[44] In zinc-deficient pigs, an increase in zinc intake prevents or cures a disease characterized by roughening of the skin and hair loss, called *parakeratosis,* which formerly caused economic losses.[2] Zinc is now added routinely to commercial poultry and swine diets.

Human zinc deficiency was not recognized until the early 1960's. Some areas in the Middle East have a high incidence of dwarfism with sexual immaturity. After receiving zinc supplements, a group of dwarfs increased in stature and developed secondary sexual characteristics.[45] Recent studies in the United States suggest that some segments of the population have marginal zinc deficiency. School children in the Denver area were found to have low levels of zinc in the hair, accompanied by impaired taste acuity, poor appetite, and suboptimal growth. These symptoms were corrected with increased dietary zinc.[45] In other studies, wound healing and taste acuity were improved with increased zinc intake.[45] Recent studies also show that some cases of acne improved with use of zinc supplements.[46]

Low levels of serum zinc have been found in persons with alcoholic liver diseases or tuberculosis and in women who are pregnant or taking contraceptives, indicative of borderline intakes. It is most likely that other evidence of zinc deficiencies in man will be found as the quality and number of analytical studies improve.

A rare but serious congenital disease of infants, acrodermatitis enteropathica, responds dramatically to zinc therapy, suggesting that a defect in zinc metabolism may be responsible.[47] Zinc (and other trace mineral) deficiency occurs in patients on long-term parenteral nutrition if trace minerals are not added to the fluid.[48]

Requirement and Food Sources

The average American diet supplies about 10 to 15 mg of zinc per day, about half of which is absorbed. This is sufficient to prevent deficiencies, although diets limited only to vegetable sources of protein may be low or inadequate.[1, 2] The latest RDA is 10 mg per day for children 1 to 10 years of age and 15 mg per day for adults.[1] Recommendations for pregnant and lactating women are 20 mg and 25 mg, respectively. (See Table 1A of the Appendix.)

Zinc occurs widely in plant and animal tissues. It is present, therefore, in all natural foods, but it is low in fruits, vegetables, and refined foods (see Table 12–

Table 12–5 APPROXIMATE ZINC CONTENT OF REPRESENTATIVE FOODS*

	mg/100 gm		*mg/100 gm*
Whole grains	1.5–5	Potatoes	0.3
Germ	10–20	Cereal flakes	0.1–0.2
Bran	7–13		
Bread, whole-wheat	2	Bread, white	0.7
Dry legumes	2–5	Vegetables	0.2–0.8
Nuts	2–4	Fruits	0.1–0.3
Muscle meats, fish, fowl	1.5–5	Milk	0.1–0.6
Eggs	1.5		

*Schlettwein-Gsell, D., and Mommsen-Straub, S.: Internat. J. Vit. Res., *40*:659, 1970.[49]

5.[35, 49] Oysters are an unusually rich source of the element.

Zinc absorption varies widely, depending on the level of zinc in the diet, the presence of interfering substances, such as phytate or fiber, and the food eaten.[2] Zinc occurring in animal products is absorbed better than zinc in plants. Therefore, zinc intake should come from a balanced diet containing sufficient animal protein foods. Vegetarians especially need to make sure they take in ample zinc.

Fortunately zinc is not a particularly toxic element, though poisoning is known to occur (presumably from zinc) from drinking acid fruit drink stored in galvanized containers.

FLUORINE

Fluorine (F),* now generally accepted as an essential nutrient for man, is still a most lively topic. One can get very strong reactions from it both in the chemical laboratory or by pointing out the advantages of the fluoridation of public water supplies to those who are opposed to the practice.

Fluorine is a very reactive gas, closely related to the other halogen gases — chlorine, iodine, and bromine. It is widely

*The name is derived from the Latin word *fluere*, meaning to flow — a property of fluorspar, one of its ores, when it is heated. This ore also "fluoresces" (from which the name of the common "fluorescent" lamp comes). Fluorine was first isolated in 1886 by the Frenchman Moissan. The name "fluorine" was first suggested in 1811 by André Marie Ampère, for whom the unit of electric current is named.

distributed in its ion form, fluoride, in natural ores such as fluorspar. It is also present in rock phosphate (a fertilizer that contains 3 to 4 percent fluorine), soil, water, teeth, and bones, and in almost all natural animal and plant foods in small but varying amounts. As with many other trace elements, too large amounts of it have toxic effects.

Discovery in Water Supplies

Interest in the element at first centered on the harmful effects of abnormally high concentrations of fluorine in drinking water in certain areas of the world, since consumption of such waters was shown to be the cause of mottled enamel of teeth (chalky spots that later stain dark brown), which appears in the teeth of children and persists into adult life.[50] In the United States, this tooth disorder was endemic in certain areas in Arizona, Colorado, the Texas Panhandle, and elsewhere. Although disfiguring, this mottling of teeth seemed to do no harm, and later studies indicated that children living in these areas had teeth that were *more resistant to decay* (dental caries) than the teeth of children in areas where drinking water was of lower fluorine content.[2, 3, 51]

Attention that had previously been focused on possible ways of reducing the fluorine concentration in drinking water was now turned to the possible effect of raising the fluorine level in water supplies in which it was low to a point where it might provide protection against dental caries without being harmful. If the fluorine concentration was over about 2 parts per million (2 mg per liter of water), mottling of the enamel of teeth was evident; if it was about 1 part per million, no harmful effects were observed and the incidence of dental decay in children's teeth was markedly reduced by 50 percent or more.

Regulation of the fluorine content of water by addition, or removal, of fluorides in localities where there is a deficiency, or excess, to a range of 0.7 to 1.2 parts per million (allowing for seasonal temperature changes) for prevention of tooth decay is now a fully scientifically accepted, safe, economical, and efficient public health measure for supplying this element.[1, 52] Artifically fluoridated water is now available to over 40 percent of the United States population and to millions in other parts of the world. About nine million additional American citizens and many elsewhere have naturally fluoridated water at about the recommended level (0.7 to 1.2 parts per million). See Chapter 23 for further discussion of the dental aspects of fluoridation.

Role in the Body

There is no known metabolic role in the body for fluorine, although it is known to activate certain enzymes and to inhibit others. All that can be said with certainty is that fluorine is necessary for maximal resistance to dental caries as a structural component of normal teeth.* For this reason, the Food and Nutrition Board, and rightly so, considers fluorine to be an "essential nutrient."[1] Schwarz and Milne report growth retardation in rats kept under special fluorine-low conditions, thus adding preliminary evidence in support of its essential need.† More studies of this sort are needed.

There is much discussion today concerning the possibility that dietary fluorine may also be important for maintenance of strong bone structure in humans and in the prevention, with other minerals, of osteoporosis, or demineralization of the bones (see calcium).[53] While no proven relationship exists, epidemiological evidence strongly suggests that less osteoporosis is found in areas where water supplies have higher levels (4 to 8 ppm) of fluoride.[2]

---

*The form of fluorine in teeth and bones is chiefly *fluorapatile* ($CaF_2 \cdot 3\ Ca_3(PO_4)_2$).

†Schwarz, K. S., and Milne, D. B.: Bioinorganic Chem., *1*:331, 1972.

Fluorine is readily absorbed from the intestine and is distributed widely in the body, with highest concentration in the teeth and bones (where concentrations up to 0.5 percent are possible on a dry basis). The urine is the main route of excretion (about 80 percent of ingested fluorine is excreted in children and up to 98 percent in adults).

Distribution in Food and Requirement

Very few foods contain more than 1 to 2 parts per million of fluorine (unless such foods are raised in a high fluorine environment) and most contain less.[2, 54] Seafood, such as fish eaten with bones, and tea (about 0.2 to 0.3 mg per cup) are among the highest sources. Bone meal, sometimes used as a mineral supplement, is very rich in fluorine (normally 300 to 600 parts per million). A normal day's diet in the United States contains about 0.3 to 0.6 mg of fluorine (as fluorides), not including the amount in drinking water. Including drinking water, a normal intake would be 1 to 2.5 mg per day. The newly established provisional RDA is 1.5 to 4.0 mg per day for adults.[1, 33]

No specific values for food are given here, because the composition of fluorine in plant foods or animal products is dependent largely upon the level in the environment (such as soil, water, and air) or the amount in the feed.[54] Fluorine is not an essential element for plants, so it is not always present in significant amounts in foods from plants.

The most reliable sources of fluorine, therefore, are fluoridated water (at a level of 0.7 to 1.2 parts per million) or fluoridated salt (or other staple food), used in some countries as a means of providing fluorine to children. Sea salt is not a reliable source. Breast milk is very low in fluorine content, though adequate. Fluorine tablets and fluorine toothpastes can serve as reliable, though expensive, sources of this element.

Toxicity

Fluorine has a small safety range — as small as just about any element. However, the range is "wide enough for safe accommodation of normal fluctuations in the fluoride content of foods without risk of inducing the first identifiable indication of an excess — slight mottling of the enamel."[1] Several million Americans live in communities with water levels of natural fluorine from 1.2 to 4 parts per million without any handicap other than slight mottling of the teeth. Their general health is otherwise satisfactory. (See further discussion of this topic in Chapter 23.)

When animals or humans are exposed to levels of fluorine higher than about 6 to 10 parts per million over long periods of time, or when there is environmental contamination, it can result in toxicity (*fluorosis*), manifested by deformed teeth and bones and other toxic symptoms.[2, 55] It has been fully demonstrated that fluorine in drinking water, when present at a level of about 1 part per million, is not harmful to humans or animals, regardless of the amount of water consumed.

COBALT

Cobalt (Co)* is the seventh trace element to be recognized as a dietary essential. In 1935, it was discovered that soils and plants of various areas of Australia, Canada, New York, Florida, and elsewhere where farm animals grazed were very low in cobalt. Sick sheep and cattle grown in these areas responded to additions of cobalt. Without the cobalt they developed progressive anemia, muscular atrophy, listlessness, extreme emaciation, and eventually death (sometimes called wasting disease). About 2 mg of cobalt added

*The name cobalt is thought to have been derived in the 1500's from the German word *Kobold*, meaning goblin or mischievous spirit, from the difficulty found in working with cobalt ores. It was first isolated in 1742 by the Swedish chemist Brandt (though salts of cobalt had been used for centuries for the blue color in decorative glass and pottery).

per kilogram of feed is all that was needed to overcome the deficiency.[2]

In 1948, the important discovery was made that cobalt was an essential structural part of the vitamin B-12 molecule, present at a level of 4 percent by weight (see Chapter 8). Studies since then have shown that the major role of cobalt in the body (if not the only role) is to serve as part of vitamin B-12. When vitamin B-12 was injected into deficient cows and sheep, all symptoms were overcome, whereas injection of equivalent amounts of cobalt had no effect. In other words, cobalt had been effective in much larger levels fed to them or injected (excessive amounts were returned to the gut) because these made it possible for rumen microorganisms to synthesize vitamin B-12. Without cobalt there was no synthesis.

Obviously then, a dietary source of inorganic cobalt is essential for vitamin B-12 production in the gut only by those animals (such as sheep, cattle, goats, deer, horses, guinea pigs, and rabbits) that normally live on plant substances alone and that are not otherwise given a vitamin B-12 source. To some extent, humans also have this ability to synthesize vitamin B-12 from cobalt by microorganisms. This probably explains, in part, why true vegetarians can live many years without vitamin B-12 itself in the diet. Synthesis in the gut is not a sure thing in humans at all, so we generally regard human need of cobalt in terms of the intact vitamin B-12 molecule and not in terms of inorganic cobalt itself.

Physiologically speaking, since no animal can manufacture vitamin B-12 in its tissues (but only in the intestine), the specific need in the body for cobalt is only in the organic form — as vitamin B-12. Inorganic cobalt in the diet, then, serves only indirectly, but this can be very important, nutritionally, for many animals if not for humans. This is somewhat similar to the situation with the mineral *sulfur*, which is a constituent of the amino acids methionine and cystine (see Chapter 5). Inorganic sulfur in the diet serves little, if any, practical purpose except in ruminants, which can make their own methionine and cystine from free sulfur in the rumen.

There is no evidence that humans must ever be concerned about their intake of inorganic cobalt. In other words, a cobalt deficiency has never been described for humans and would be difficult to obtain. The normal day's intake of 150 to 600 mcg of inorganic cobalt is far greater than any possible requirement.[56] Cobalt ions are distributed throughout the body, especially in the liver and heart, and they do not accumulate with age.

Cobalt is present in almost all foods in varying amounts,[2, 56] but since analytical techniques are still uncertain and since we really do not have to worry about it, to present figures would serve no purpose. There appears to be no shortage, and our concern, actually, in human nutrition is about vitamin B-12 and not cobalt. Undue amounts of cobalt in the diet of humans and animal species other than ruminants cause stimulation of bone marrow, with excessive production of red corpuscles (polycythemia) and higher than normal hemoglobin. Toxic reactions from unusually large levels in food have been known; in one study, beer was found to be contaminated with excessive cobalt, resulting in the death of several persons.[57]

MOLYBDENUM

With the discovery in 1953 that *molybdenum* (Mo)* is a component of the essential enzyme *xanthine dehydrogenase* (and later other enzymes), a new era of essential microelement research was ushered in and still continues.

Needs for this element are minute, and human deficiencies are not known. Certain animals (rats, poultry, and sheep) rendered deficient by artifically low levels of

*From the Greek word *molybdos* for lead. Molybdenum was first obtained in pure form in the late 1700's. It is a hard silver-white material used widely in alloys. It is essential for the growth of all higher plants.

molybdenum intake (and often with use of the antagonistic action of other trace elements such as copper or tungsten) produce weak and malformed young.[59] Sulfate intake in animals has a marked effect on molybdenum status. High dietary sulfate inhibits absorption and increases urinary excretion of molybdenum.[2]

Molybdenum is widely distributed in foods in very small amounts. About the only foods known to contain as much as 0.6 part per million are legumes, cereal, organ meats, and yeast.[60] The molybdenum content of foods varies greatly, depending on the soil on which the foods were grown.[2] It is rapidly absorbed in both organic and inorganic forms, and the main route of excretion is the urine.

A normal day's intake is about 0.1 to 0.4 mg, which must be slightly greater than the human requirement (which is still an unknown entity). A deficiency is unlikely to occur under normal conditions.[2] Schroeder and coworkers[60] present evidence that marginal or deficient intakes of molybdenum are a possibility if one were to choose by accident the wrong mixture of low-value foods, emphasizing again the importance of choosing diets containing a variety of traditional foodstuffs. The Food and Nutrition Board provisionally recommends 0.15 to 0.5 mg a day for adults to provide a generous and safe allowance.[33]

Severe molybdenum toxicity (molybdenosis) in animals, particularly cattle, has been seen in many parts of the world where the soil has a high molybdenum content. Symptoms include weight loss, growth retardation, and connective tissue changes.[2] A greater incidence of gout in man has been associated with areas where molybdenum content of soil is high.

SELENIUM

The rapidly evolving story of selenium in nutrition is most fascinating, and only a few highlights can be given here (for further reading, see the references at the end of this chapter and current publications). It now is evident that selenium is just as important a nutrient for man as better known trace elements such as zinc, iron, and copper.

Discovery and Toxicity

The element selenium (Se) was discovered and named by the Swedish chemist Berzelius in 1817.* It is closely related chemically to sulfur but is much less abundant. Animal scientists first became interested in selenium when it was determined in the 1930's[2] that soils and certain plants in parts of western North America and in other parts of the world contained levels of this element that were toxic to farm animals. Grazing animals in such *seleniferous areas* (areas with toxic levels of selenium) developed symptoms of "alkali disease" or "blind staggers" characterized by stiffness and lameness, loss of hair, deformed hoofs, blindness, paralysis, and eventually death. Toxic symptoms not unlike those in animals are also known in humans but include an increased incidence of dental caries as well.

It was with considerable surprise, then, that an element as toxic as, or more so than, mercury and lead (as we know them today) would be found to be nutritionally essential. In the early 1950's Dr. Schwarz and coworkers produced *dietary liver necrosis* — death of liver tissue due to a deficiency — *poor growth*, and *death* in rats[2,61] fed special diets containing torula yeast (which is very low in selenium and vitamin E). Schwarz found that an unidentified water-soluble substance in brewer's yeast and kidney greatly reduced or eliminated the vitamin E need of the rat and appeared to be necessary. Less than 0.5 part per million of selenium, when it was identified as the missing component, was

*Named for the Greek word *selene*, or moon, since selenium was closely associated with the element tellurium, named for the earth. Selenium is important in making photoelectric cells, exposure meters, rectifiers, and photocopying machines. It is also important in the ceramics industry and is often used to produce red glass.

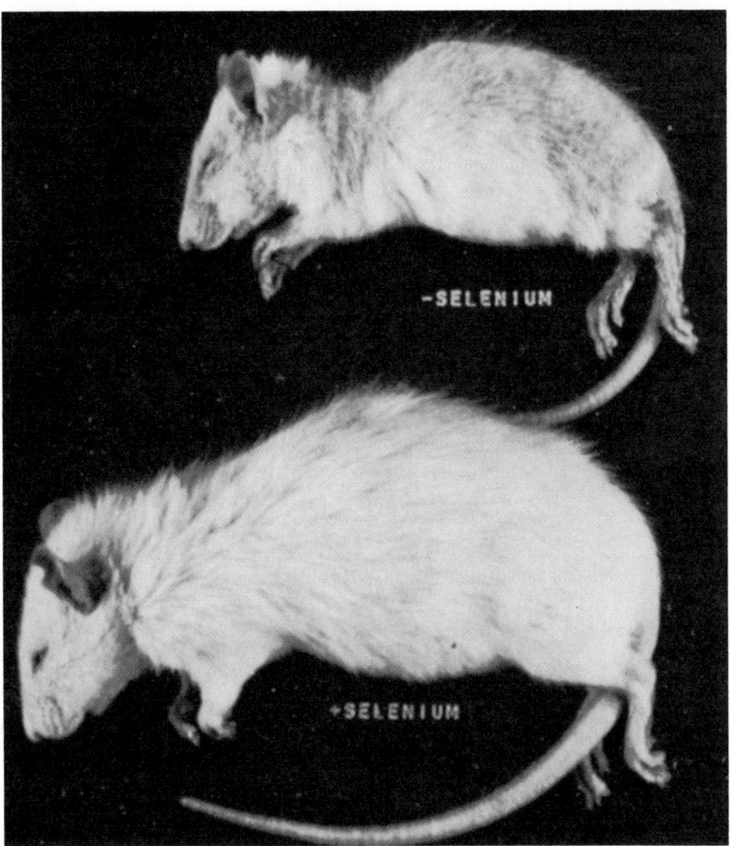

Figure 12–8 Selenium-deficient rat (above) compared with selenium-supplemented rat (below). (From Hurt, H. D., Cary, E. E., and Visek, W. J.: J. Nutr., *101*:761, 1971.)

found to be as effective as 50 parts per million of vitamin E, which it replaced (see Fig. 12–8). Later work has shown that selenium has specific functions in addition to its vitamin E sparing effect (in fact, it now would appear that much of the need for vitamin E is to spare the selenium requirement).

Deficiency Signs in Animals and Function

Besides poor growth and liver necrosis in rats, a wide variety of deficiency signs were found in animals deficient in both selenium and vitamin E. Extensive *striated muscular degeneration,* known widely as *white muscle disease,* or "nutritional muscular dystrophy," occurs in young sheep, cattle, horses, and rabbits under farm conditions. This occurs in many areas of the United States (mainly west of the Rocky Mountains and east of the Mississippi River — see Fig. 12–9) and other parts of the world, such as New Zealand, where soils are deficient in this element. As many as 20 to 30 percent of all lambs in some flocks may be affected, for example. Deficient chicks develop large greenish-blue spots under the skin because of blood leakage from capillaries and soon die. Deficient mice develop damaged hearts. Pigs deficient in selenium and vitamin E develop diseased livers and die suddenly. Selenium, in the absence of much higher amounts of vitamin E (the requirement of which is greatly reduced by selenium), is essential for reproduction in all animals studied. Selenium additions are widely made to livestock in deficient

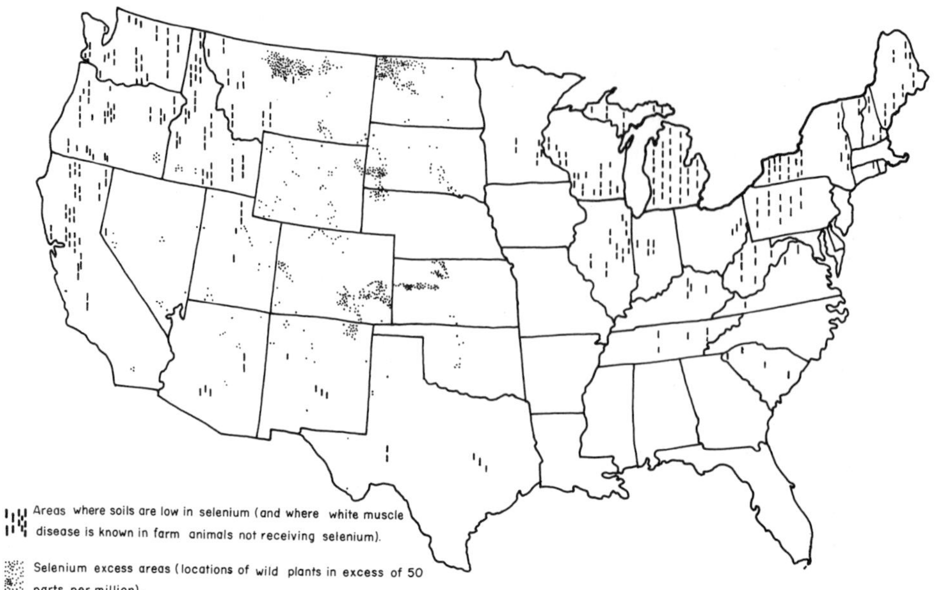

Figure 12–9 Selenium-deficient and selenium-excess areas in the United States (approximate). (Adapted from U.S. government figures. See Muth and Allaway: J. Amer. Vet. Med. Assoc., *142*:1379, 1963; and Kubota, et al.: J. Agric. Food Chem., *15*:448, 1967.)

areas by injection or by the addition of selenium-rich foods to the diet.

Selenium, though closely related to vitamin E in its function, is now known to have a specific essential role of its own in nutrition even when vitamin E is present in the diet.[2, 62] Selenium occurs in animal tissues bound to proteins. Its most important currently known function is as part of the enzyme *glutathione peroxidase.* Each molecule of glutathione peroxidase contains 4 molecules of selenium. The enzyme catalyzes the conversion of H_2O_2 (hydrogen peroxide) to water, and it is a powerful antioxidant protecting cellular membranes. Liver has the highest glutathione peroxidase activity; and erythrocytes, heart muscle, lungs, and kidneys have moderately high activity. The amounts of selenium needed by animals in the diet are exceedingly small, in the range of only 0.05 to 0.5 part per million. This is only about 50 to 500 mcg per kilogram of diet, making it more potent than many of the vitamins. Toxic levels in animal diets start at about 5 to 10 parts per million, which is not much of a margin of safety. Over half of the dietary selenium is absorbed and is excreted in both urine and feces.

Selenium in Food and Nutritional Status of Man

Selenium, probably bound to protein, occurs naturally in all seafood, meat, and those grains raised on selenium-containing soils. Fruits and vegetables are very low in it. Levels in most plants depend quite entirely on the level of selenium in the soil.[2, 63, 64] Variations of over 100-fold are known to occur, so general tables of the selenium content of food are quite useless. The few wild plants* that accumulate the element in selenium-rich soils contain toxic levels (from 0.1 to 1 percent of selenium) for any grazing animals that might consume them.

Considerable losses of selenium can occur in processing, refinement of foods, and cooking.

A person eating a mixed diet of foods of different origins would most likely be getting about 75 to 200 mcg of selenium per day. This amount appears to be more than the amount needed. The provisional current RDA (1979) for adults, allowing an ample margin of safety, is expected to be

*Gray's vetch and woody aster.

50 to 200 mcg per day,[1, 33] which is about equal to the selenium content of American foods. People eating very poor diets in selenium-deficient areas may well have low levels of this element, but this is only a supposition based on animal studies.

Several studies have shown that there are low levels of selenium in the diet or in the blood of severely malnourished children in developing countries,[2, 31, 63, 65] but additional studies are needed to establish specifically the essential nature of this element in man.

Besides the toxic symptoms previously mentioned, selenium has produced tumors in certain strains of rats fed 2 to 3 parts per million over long periods of time (about ten times, or more, the requirement). Other studies have indicated that selenium can protect against tumors in other situations in the rat. Obviously food and drug administrators are being very careful in permitting selenium additions to any feed or food. It would appear, however, that selenium may need to be used eventually in food enrichment programs, unless it is restored to large land areas.

CHROMIUM

Very few persons would have guessed before 1959 that chromium, the mineral most of us know as that which makes the shiny "chrome"-plated bumpers and strips on automobiles, is essential in the diet of mammals, including humans.

Chromium (Cr), originally discovered in 1797,* has been known for many years to be present in food and animal tissues. In 1959, Schwarz and Mertz,[66] then of the U.S. National Institutes of Health, made the important discovery that very small amounts of chromium (only when in the stable trivalent state, as Cr^{3+}) were necessary in the diet for normal metabolism of blood glucose in the rat. Over 47 different elements were tested by Schwarz and Mertz before the specificity of chromium was announced as the *glucose tolerance factor* (GTF), as it was called.

There is now sufficient evidence, both direct and indirect, that supports the inclusion of chromium among the essential trace elements for man. It has a variety of functions, including (1) the stimulation of enzymes involved in glucose and energy metabolism, (2) the stimulation of synthesis of fatty acids and cholesterol in the liver, (3) an involvement in insulin metabolism, and (4) a role as a part of several other enzymes, including one of the protein-digesting enzymes in the intestine.[66] In rats, mice, and monkeys, a deficiency results in decreased growth and increased mortality, as well as decreased rate of glucose removal from the blood. An organic form of chromium, "glucose tolerance factor," has been isolated from brewer's yeast. It contains nicotinic acid, glycine, glutamic acid, and a sulfur-containing amino acid.[67] The practical importance of this factor is still unknown.

Nutritional Status and Requirements

Poorly nourished children in several parts of the Middle East (Turkey and Lebanon, where chromium levels of some soils and water supplies appear to be low) show signs of poor glucose utilization correctable in some instances by the addition to the diet of small amounts of chromium (250 mcg).[68] This was explained on the basis of the role of chromium in insulin metabolism. Similar effects have been seen in a few diabetic adults who apparently were deficient in chromium. Recent indications that chromium may play a role in the prevention of atherosclerosis in humans and cholesterol metabolism in animals are interesting but require confirmation.

The human body contains only a

---

*Discovered by the French chemist Vauquelin (who also isolated the first amino acid) and named from the Greek word *chroma* for color. Most salts of chromium are brightly colored and are used widely as pigments. The red color of the ruby and the green color of the emerald are due to salts of chromium. It is an important component of stainless steel, which has 10 to 18 percent chromium.

small amount of chromium — less than 6 mg[31] — which declines with age. A typical daily intake in the United States usually ranges between 50 and 120 mcg. Absorption varies considerably, depending on the form of chromium. Inorganic chromium compounds are 1 to 3 percent absorbed, while the glucose tolerance factor is 10 to 25 percent absorbed.[2] The newly established provisional RDA for 1979 has been proposed to be 50 to 200 mcg per day for adults.[33]

Food Sources

Good *food sources* of chromium are fats such as corn oil (in which it exists as an impurity) and meats. Fruits, vegetables, seafood, and drinking water are generally poor sources. The amount of chromium in plant foods depends to a large extent on the amount in the soil, although tables of chromium content of representative foods are available[69] (but not to be trusted). Processing and refinement reduce the chromium content of foods considerably. For instance, white sugar contains very little, and white flour has much less than whole wheat. Of significance in considering food sources of chromium are the early studies of Mertz and Schwarz, who produced a chromium deficiency in rats by feeding commercial stock diets of natural feedstuffs.[66] They found that brewer's yeast is a particularly rich source of chromium — hence beer is also a good source.

Chromium is not toxic in the forms and levels found in foods, and excesses are rapidly excreted.

NICKEL

Nickel (Ni)* is included among the essential trace elements largely on the basis of reports of its presence in a serum protein in rabbits and humans (called *nickeloplasmin)*[70] and of its apparent requirement by chickens.

Deficient chickens were said by Nielsen (1970) of the United States Department of Agriculture[2, 71] to have slightly enlarged hocks, thickened legs, bright orange leg color (instead of pale yellow-brown), a dermatitis, and a "less friable liver." Nickel at a level of 3 to 5 mg per kg of diet corrected these minor abnormalities. Deficiencies have also recently been studied in rats, pigs, and goats.[2] Nickel is also known to activate several enzyme systems, although whether this is a specific function is not known. It is present in high levels in ribonucleic acids for reasons that are not yet clear.[2]

Nickel is widely distributed in foods, especially plant foods. (Though required by several microorganisms, nickel has not yet been proven to be needed by plants.) The deficiency in chickens was produced after careful removal of all extra sources of nickel, although corn was one of the ingredients of the diet. A deficiency in man has never been seen and would be unlikely to occur except under unusual conditions. Serum nickel concentration is elevated in humans following myocardial infarction, stroke, and severe burns, but the cause of this increase is not known.[2] A normal diet could supply about 0.3 to 0.6 mg per day, and any requirement for the element must be less than this. No provisional RDA has been given for nickel as yet. Dietary nickel is 1 to 10 per cent absorbed, and most of the absorbed nickel is excreted in the feces.[2]

*Discovered originally in 1751 by Cronstedt and named nickel for "Old Nick," a demon. It is the same nickel that our five-cent piece is named after, and the element has wide use in industry.

VANADIUM

The twelfth trace element needed by higher animals was shown to be *vanadium* (V)* in 1970 and 1971, although its essential nature has been suspected for many

*Vanadium was identified in 1831 by Sefström, of Sweden, who named it after the Norse goddess of beauty, Vanadis (from the beautiful color of its compounds). Earlier studies on it had been made by Del Rio in Mexico. It was not obtained in pure form until 1927. It has many industrial uses, especially in vanadium steel.

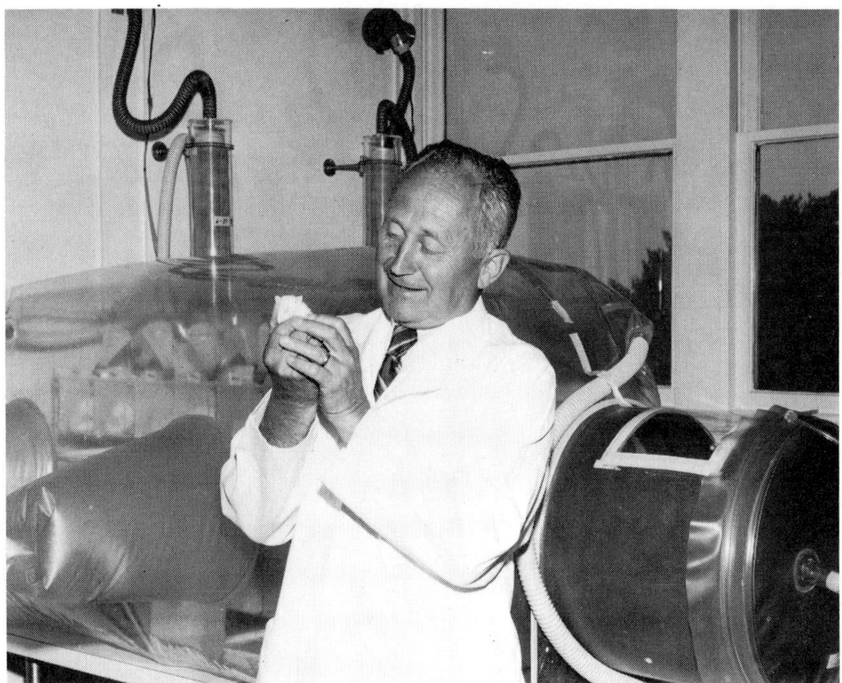

Figure 12–10 The late Dr. Klaus Schwarz, in whose laboratories the growth effects of selenium, chromium, tin, and vanadium were demonstrated. Mineral contamination from the environment was eliminated by use of the isolator shown here.

years. It has long been known to be present throughout the plant and animal kingdoms and to be required by several lower organisms.

Its need by higher animals was amply demonstrated in the laboratory of Dr. Schwarz.[72] (See Fig. 12–10.) The growth of rats raised on special deficient diets in "ultraclean" conditions was increased over 40 percent in a 21 to 28 day period by the addition of 0.25 to 0.5 mg of vanadium (as sodium orthovanadate) per kg of diet. Other effects observed were impaired reproduction, increased packed blood cell volume and iron in blood and bone of rats, and increased hematocrit in chicks.[2] Vanadium is known to be a catalyst in several biological systems and to be present in higher than normal concentrations in teeth.[2]

Earlier preliminary studies in 1970 with chickens (showing reduced growth of feathers), by U.S.D.A. workers Hopkins and Mohr, and with rats, by Purdue University workers, had indicated that vanadium was an essential trace element.[73]

No figure can be given for the vanadium requirement of man, but it would be about in the range of only 0.1 to 0.3 mg per day. Normal diets contain about ten times this amount, so deficiencies would be very rare under usual conditions. The amount of vanadium in our foods and in the environment appears to be considerably lower than the toxic level. Toxic levels in animals (25 ppm) produce growth depression and increased mortality.[2]

SILICON

One of the trace elements most recently shown to be essential for animals (the chick and rat) is silicon (Si). This element, named from the Latin word *silex*, meaning flint, is the most abundant mineral element on the earth's surface. Its most common form is silicon dioxide (SiO_2) or sand from which glass is made. It was originally discovered as an element by Berzelius in 1823.

Dr. Carlisle, nutritionist at the University of California, Los Angeles, reported in 1972 that silicon is needed in microgram amounts for normal growth and bone development in the chick. Silicon has long been known to be required by certain lower forms of life and, apparently, by some plants, but its need by animals was unexpected and constitutes a major nutrition discovery. Silicon deficiency produces growth retardation in chicks and rats, but only in an environment free of trace mineral contamination. It is present in bone in highest concentrations in regions of active growth, which suggests that silicon has a role in bone mineralization and connective tissue synthesis.[74] The high silicon content of connective tissue is due to its presence in mucopolysaccharides (important in connective tissue formation).[2] Silicon is present at the highest level in lymph nodes. High concentrations also occur in the skin, the aorta, the trachea, and the tendons.

Silicon is widely distributed in foods. Because of this, deficiencies in humans (assuming that it is needed) would be virtually impossible on the basis of present knowledge of its distribution.

Silicon in the diet occurs as monosilicic acid, as solid silica, and as a form bound to organic compounds. Human intake has been estimated to be as much as 1 gm a day, which places it in the category of a macromineral. However, little is known about requirements, which are probably well under 1 gm a day. No provisional allowance can be set for silicon because of lack of information. It does not appear to be toxic in the levels usually found in foods.

TWO ELEMENTS POSSIBLY ESSENTIAL

Tin

Tin (Sn) may be included among the essential elements on the basis of the observation in 1970 by Schwarz and coworkers of its growth-promoting effect in deficient rats.[75] By using rats under highly isolated conditions free of contamination with tin, a reduced growth rate was produced within 2 weeks after the start of the experiment. Supplements of tin at levels of about 1 mg per kg of diet increased growth in several different experiments by as much as 30 to 60 percent in only 4 weeks' time.

No studies showing a requirement for tin by man have been made as yet. Tin is widely distributed in foods of animal and plant origin, and a deficiency in man or animals under normal conditions would not be expected to occur. Tin is poorly absorbed and is excreted primarily in the feces.

Tin is not very toxic, and if acid fruit juices or similar products dissolve appreciable amounts of tin from a tin-plated can it is not well-absorbed by man (though the iron might be).[76] A normal tin intake is probably in the range of 1.5 to 5 mg a day, depending on the amount of canned food eaten.[2] The requirement for man is not known but would be expected to be slightly less than 1 mg a day on the basis of the rat studies.

Arsenic

The trace mineral most recently proposed to have an essential role is arsenic. Evidence is not yet conclusive. Neilson demonstrated slower growth and a rough coat in rats fed a diet low in arsenic and maintained in a special trace mineral–free environment.[77] Pigs and poultry also appear to benefit from added dietary arsenic.

Most foods contain less than 0.5 ppm arsenic. Fish and seafoods contain more (2 to 10 ppm). Dietary deficiency appears to be unlikely in humans, if it does prove to be essential.

Arsenic is well known for its toxicity. Acute oral poisoning causes nausea, vomiting, diarrhea, and severe abdominal pains. Chronic exposure to smaller toxic levels produces headache, confusion, convulsions, weakness, and muscular aches.

NONESSENTIAL TRACE ELEMENTS

At least 50 other trace elements are known to be present in plants and animals. Some of these could theoretically be shown to be essential in the diet of higher animals at some time in the future (see Schwarz[75b]), although this is only conjecture at this point. There are small pieces of evidence, such as a requirement by plants or lower organisms, or a catalytic role demonstrated in isolated systems, for a possible future role in nutrition for some elements. For instance, *boron* is known to be required by certain plants, and the element *cadmium* is found associated with zinc in at least one natural protein.[2] These elements are relatively nontoxic in small amounts. They are widely distributed in nature in most plant and animal foods in minute amounts, as are *aluminum, antimony, barium, bromine, gallium, germanium, niobium, rubidium, silver, strontium, titanium,* and *zirconium.*[2] In spite of their widespread occurrence, *there is no evidence as yet that any of these elements plays an essential role in higher animals,* and they must be considered as nonessential elements at this time. Likewise, such elements as *gold, cesium, lead, lithium,* and *mercury* are widely distributed in nature, but this does not prove, or even indicate, any essential function. However, it is well to remember that nickel, selenium, chromium, silicon, and vanadium were listed with these nonessential elements just a few years ago.

TOXICITY AND PICA

Toxicity of Micronutrients at Higher Levels of Intake

It is both interesting and important to call attention to the fact that, although small amounts may be required for body welfare, *any of the trace elements, whether essential or not, are toxic when too large amounts of them are taken into the body.* Sometimes the margin between optimal intake and toxic amounts is not very wide. For example, too large a dose of iodine may overstimulate or inhibit the function of the thyroid gland, or too small an intake results in enlargement of this gland in simple goiter. With fluorine, about three to ten times the amount that provides protection against dental caries will cause mottling of teeth. All the metallic elements are stored in the liver, so that the amount in the body may accumulate to toxic levels. Hence, it is unwise to supplement the diet with high levels of any trace mineral, because all are toxic in sufficient amounts.

Especially of interest today are *mercury, lead,* and *cadmium* because of their presence in toxic amounts in certain segments in the environment.[2] Mercury, though naturally occurring in small amounts, has increased in concentration because of industrial wastes. It has been found to be close to toxic levels in some samples of seafoods. Toxic levels have been known to be reached in isolated instances in Japan and the United States. The highest permissible level in American foods is 0.5 part per million.

Lead has been found in high concentrations in plants and soils near highways owing to discharges of lead from automobile engines. Lead toxicity is a well-known syndrome in children who have chewed on window sills, toys, or other surfaces painted with lead-containing paints. Another source of lead toxicity is lead glazes on dishes. Acid fruit juices should not be kept more than a few hours in any suspected dishes or pitchers; in fact, dishes suspected of having lead glazes should be discarded.

Aluminum toxicity is seen in patients with renal failure who are treated with aluminum compounds to decrease phosphorus levels in plasma.[78] In addition, the concentration of aluminum is increased in a disease of early senility (Alzheimer's disease).[79] Aluminum cooking utensils yield only traces of aluminum, far below levels that might be toxic.

One cannot avoid eating traces of toxic elements, no matter how carefully one attempts to do so, but it does not help to ignore the possibilities and sources of toxicity. We recommend keeping in close touch with, and taking an active interest in, government agencies whose job it is to control levels of toxins in our food and environment.

Pica

Pica (pronounced "pie-ca") is the name for an unnatural craving, most commonly seen in women and young children, to eat laundry starch, clay, ashes, dirt, ice, or similar material. It probably is due, in part, to a natural craving for trace minerals, especially iron. Pica is commonly seen in times of stress such as pregnancy or lactation. It sometimes involves toxic elements such as lead and should be avoided as much as possible. Its cessation can come about only with nutrition education and good eating habits.

QUESTIONS AND PROBLEMS

1. In what special tissue is most of the iron in the body found, and in what special substance in this tissue? What function does it fulfill in this tissue, and what chemical property enables it to carry out this function? How do the smaller amounts of iron located in tissue cells help in oxidation-reduction processes vital to the life of cells?

2. What is the Recommended Dietary Allowance for iron daily for a grown man? A woman? At what periods of life is the need for this element increased, and why? Why is iron sometimes referred to as "the one-way element"? Explain how iron is conserved by the body and how a liberal supply of it in the diet can build up reserve stores that serve to protect the body in times of extra need.

3. What are the symptoms of iron deficiency anemia, and under what conditions may it be caused? Does the existence of anemia necessarily mean that the diet furnished less than normal amounts of iron? Explain reasons for your answer. What other nutritional factors besides iron are important in prevention of anemia?

4. Can the body utilize inorganic and organic iron equally well? In what form or forms is iron most readily absorbed from the intestine? Mention three factors that are favorable and three that are unfavorable to iron absorption. To what extent may the degree of availability and absorption of iron be influenced by the relative need of the body for iron?

5. Why is iodine essential in small amounts for body welfare? In what tissue is this element concentrated, and what is its function there? Can iodine be stored in the body and, if so, where? What is a ductless gland? A hormone? The names of the two iodine-containing hormones of the thyroid gland? The influence of these hormones on body metabolism (tissue oxidations)?

6. Simple goiter is a deficiency disease caused by lack of what element? In what regions is it most prevalent, and why? At what periods of life is it most likely to develop, and why? What public health measure has been used successfully in preventing simple goiter?

7. Name five foods that are relatively rich in iron and three that are relatively rich in iodine. What kinds of food are poor in iron? In iodine?

8. Is copper an essential element? For what special purpose is it necessary? Why does a rat become anemic if kept a long time on a diet consisting only of milk? Why can such an anemia not be cured by giving either iron alone or copper alone? If a baby developed nutritional anemia, would it be of assistance in curing the anemia to give some copper along with some form of iron? Explain why most people are sure of getting enough copper in their food to meet their requirement for this element.

9. Is some form of cobalt essential for humans? For what animals is it essential? What are the symptoms of cobalt deficiency, and how may it be caused? In what

vitamin is cobalt found and why is anemia a prominent symptom in cobalt deficiency in ruminants such as sheep or cattle?

10. Record all the foods you ate on a typical day, with quantities of each, and calculate the amount of iron furnished by this day's diet. Use either Table 12–3 for iron content of foods or tables in the Appendix for nutritive values of foods in average servings. Does the amount of iron in this day's diet come up to the recommended allowance? If not, what changes could be made to furnish more iron?

11. Is fluorine an essential nutrient? In what body tissues is it concentrated? What is the effect of too high an intake of this element, and at what level of fluorine in drinking water do such effects occur? What level of fluorine in water supplies is safe and yet provides protection against tooth decay? Why has fluoridation of public water supplies met opposition in some communities, and is such opposition warranted?

12. Name four trace elements, other than those mentioned in the preceding questions, that are accepted as essential nutrients for man. On what types of evidence is their acceptance as essential based? Can you name two enzymes that contain and presumably are activated by some of these elements? How many of the micronutrients listed in this chapter are beneficial and essential in small quantities but toxic at higher levels of intake? Why may it be unsafe to take tablets or capsules as vitamin-mineral supplements if the kinds and amounts of minerals they contain are not specified in exact terms? Why is it usually unnecessary to take such supplements, if one eats a normal mixed diet?

REFERENCES

General, Iron

1. Food and Nutrition Board: *Recommended Dietary Allowances*. 8th Ed. Washington, D.C., National Research Council, National Academy of Sciences, 1974. (Also see 9th Ed., expected publication date of 1979.
2. Underwood, E. J.: *Trace Elements in Human and Animal Nutrition*. 4th Ed. New York, Academic Press, 1977.
3. McCollum, E. V.: *A History of Nutrition*. Boston, Houghton Mifflin Co., 1957.
4. Boussingault, J. B.: Compt. Rend., *64*:1353, 1867.
5. McCance, R. A., and Widdowson, E. M.: Lancet, *2*:680, 1937.
6. Hahn, P. F., Whipple, G. H., et al.: J. Exper. Med., *70*:443, 1939; Hahn, P. F., et al.: Amer. J. Physiol., *143*:191, 1945; Moore, C. V., Dubach, R., Minnich, V., and Roberts, H. K.: J. Clin. Invest., *23*:755, 1944.
7. Holmberg, C. G., and Laurell, C. B.: Acta Chem. Scand., *1*:944, 1947; Bates, G. W., and Wernicke, J.: J. Biol. Chem., *246*:3679, 1971.
8. Greenberg, G. R., and Wintrobe, M. M.: J. Biol. Chem., *165*:340, 1946.
9. Buckley, R. H.: J. Pediatr., *86*:993, 1975; Strauss, R. G.: Amer. J. Clin. Nutr., *31*:660, 1978.
10. Woodruff, C. W., Latham, C., and McDavid, A.: J. Pediatr., *90*:36, 1977; Coulson, K. M., et al.: Clin. Pediatr., *16*:649, 1977; Barnes, L. A., et al.: Amer. Acad. Pediatr., *58*:765, 1976.
11. Beaton, G. H., et al.: Amer. J. Clin. Nutr., *23*:275, 1970.
12. Leverton, R. M., et al.: J. Amer. Dietet. Assoc., *20*:747, 1944; *24*:480, 1948.
13. FAO/WHO: *Requirements of Ascorbic Acid, Vitamin B_{12}, Folate, and Iron*. WHO Tech. Rpt. Ser. No. 452. Geneva, WHO, 1970.
14. White, H. S.: J. Home Econ., *60*:724, 1968.
15. Pritchard, J. A., and Mason, R. A.: J. A. M. A., *190*:879, 1964.
16. Monsen, E. R., Kuhn, I. N., and Finch, C. A.: Amer. J. Clin. Nutr., *20*:842, 1967.
17. Davis, T. R. A., Gershoff, S. N., and Gamble, D. F.: J. Nutr. Educ., *1* (No. 2, Suppl. 1):40, 1969; U.S. Department of Health, Education and Welfare: *Ten-State Nutrition Survey in the United States, 1968–1970 —Preliminary Report to the Congress, April 1971;* Kelsay, J. L.: J. Nutr., *99*(No. 1, Suppl. 1, Part II):123, 1969; Schaefer, A. E., and Johnson, O. C.: Nutr. Today, *4*:2, 1969.
18. Jacobs, A., and Worwood, M.: N. Engl. J. Med., *292*:951, 1975; Valberg, L. T., et al.: Calif. Med. Assoc. Journal, *114*:417, 1976; Jacobs, A.: Fed. Proc., *36*:2024, 1977.
19. Roe, D. A.: N.Y. State J. Med., *66*:1233, 1966; MacDonald, R. A.: Amer. J. Clin. Nutr., *23*:592, 1970.

Iodine

20. Coindet, J. R.: Ann. chim. phys., *15*:49, 1820.
21. Baumann, E.: Zeit. Physiol. Chem., *21*:319, 1895.
22. Marine, D., and Kimball, O. P.: Arch. Intern. Med., *25*:661, 1920; J. A. M. A., *77*:1068, 1921.
23. Marine, D., and Kimball, O. P.: J. Lab. Clin. Med., *3*:40, 1917 (reprinted in Nutr. Rev., *33*:272, 1975).
24. Hart, E. B., and Steenbock, H.: J. Biol. Chem., *33*:313, 1918.
25. Buttfield, I. H., et al.: Lancet, *2*:767, 1965; Kevany, J., et al.: Amer. J. Public Health, *60*:919, 1970; Amer. J. Clin. Nutr., *22*:1597, 1969.
26. Jubig, W., Carlile, S., and Lagerquist, L.: J. Clin.

Endocrinol. Metab., *44*:379, 1977; J. A. M. A., *233*:10, 1975.

Copper, Manganese

27. Hart, E. B., Steenbock, H., Waddell, J., and Elvehjem, C. A.: J. Biol. Chem., *77*:797, 1928.
28. Josephs, H. W.: Bull. Johns Hopkins Hosp., *49*:246, 1931 (also see Lewis, M. S.: J. A. M. A., *96*:1135, 1931; Usher, S. J., MacDermott, P. N., and Lozinski, E.: Amer. J. Dis. Child., *18*:642, 1935).
29. Sturgeon, P., and Brubaker, C.: Amer. J. Dis. Child., *92*:254, 1956; Cordano, A., Baertl, J. M., and Graham, G. G.: Pediatrics, *34*:324, 1964; Cordano, A., Placko, R. P., and Graham, G. G.: Blood, *28*:280, 1966; Cordano, A., and Graham, G. G.: Pediatrics, *38*:596, 1966; Graham, G. G., and Cordano, A.: Johns Hopkins Med. J., *124*:139, 1969; Holtzman, N. A., et al.: Johns Hopkins Med. J., *126*:34, 1970; Al-Rashid, R. A., and Spangler, J.: N. Engl. J. Med., *285*:841, 1971.
30. Holmberg, C. G., and Laurell, C. B.: Acta Chem. Scand., *2*:550, 1948; Frieden, E.: Nutr. Rev., *28*:87, 1970; Osaki, S., Johnson, D. A., and Frieden, E.: J. Biol. Chem., *246*:3018, 1971.
31. Sandstead, H. H., Burk, R. F., Booth, G. H., Jr., and Darby, W. J.: Current concepts on trace minerals, clinical considerations. Med. Clin. North Amer., *54*:1509, 1970.
32. Bajpayll, D. P.: Ann. Rheum. Dis., *34*:162, 1975; Lancet, *1*:902, 1975; Pfeiffer, C. C., and Bacchi, D.: J. Appl. Nutr., *27*(2):3, 1975; Punsor, S., et al.: J. Chronic Dis., *28*:259, 1975; Malette, L. E., and Henkin, R. I.: Amer. J. Med. Sci., *272*:167, 1976.
33. Balsley, M.: J. Amer. Dietet. Assoc., *71*:149, 1977. (Also see current issues of J. Amer. Dietet. Assoc. and J. Nutr. Ed. for current status of the 1979 RDA's.)
34. Lawler, M. R., and Jelenc, M. A.: J. Amer. Dietet. Assoc., *57*:420, 1970; Hook, L., and Brandt, I. K.: J. Amer. Dietet. Assoc., *49*:202, 1966.
35. Murthy, G. K., and Rhea, U. S.: J. Dairy Sci., *54*:1001, 1971 (milk and infant foods); Meranger, J. C.: Bull. Env. Cont. Tox., *5*:271, 1970 (fruit juices and carbonated beverages); Zook, E. G., and Lehmann, J.: J. Amer. Dietet. Assoc., *52*:225, 1968 (fruits); Gormican, A.: J. Amer. Dietet. Assoc., *56*:397, 1970.
36. Wilkins, R. H., and Brody, I. A.: Arch. Neurol., *25*:179, 1971 (reprint of the original paper by Wilson, S. A. K.: Brain, *34*:295, 1912).
37. Kemmerer, A. R., Elvehjem, C. A., and Hart, E. B.: J. Biol. Chem., *92*:623, 1931; Orent, E. R., and McCollum, E. V.: J. Biol. Chem., *92*:651, 1931 (also see McCarrison, R.: Ind. J. Med. Res., *14*:641, 1927).
38. Leach, R. M., Jr.: In Hoekstra, et al.: *Trace Element Metabolism in Animals—2*. Baltimore, University Park Press, 1974.
39. Hurley, L. S., et al.: J. Nutr., *74*:274, 1971; J. Nutr., *79*:23, 1963; Med. Clin. North Amer., *60*:771, 1976; Plumlee, M. P., et al.: J. Animal Sci., *15*:352, 1956; Rojas, M. A., Dyer, I. A., and Cassatt, W. A.: J. Animal Sci., *24*:664, 1965; Shrader, R. E., and Everson, G. J.: J. Nutr., *94*:269, 1968.
40. Cotzias, G. C., et al.: Med. Clin. North Amer., *60*:729, 1976.
41. Schroeder, H. A., Balassa, J. J., and Tipton, I. H.: J. Chronic Dis., *19*:545, 1966; Schlettwein-Gsell, D., and Mommsen-Straub, S.: Int. J. Vit. Nutr. Res., *41*:268, 1971.

Zinc

42. Prasad, A. S., et al.: J. Lab. Clin. Med., *61*:537, 1963; Prasad, A. S., et al.: Amer. J. Clin. Nutr., *12*:437, 1963; Sandstead, H. H., et al.: Amer. J. Clin. Nutr., *20*:422, 1967; Prasad, A. S.: Amer. J. Clin. Nutr., *20*:648, 1967; Carter, J. P., et al.: Amer. J. Clin. Nutr., *22*:59, 1969.
43. Todd, W. R., Elvehjem, C. A.., and Hart, E. B.: Amer. J. Physiol., *107*:146, 1934; Stirn, F. E., Elvehjem, C. A., and Hart, E. B.: J. Biol. Chem., *109*:347, 1935.
44. Millar, J. J., Fischer, M. I., Elcoate, P. V., and Mawson, C. A.: Can. J. Biochem. Physiol., *36*:557, 1958; Hurley, L. S., and Swenerton, H.: Proc. Soc. Exp. Biol. Med., *123*:692, 1966; Swenerton, H., and Hurley, L. S.: J. Nutr., *95*:8, 1968; Agpar, J.: Amer. J. Physiol., *215*:160, 1968; J. Nutr., *100*:470, 1970.
45. Prasad, et al.: Arch. Intern. Med., *111*:407, 1963; Hambidge, K. M., et al.: Pediatr. Res., *6*:868, 1972; Pories, W. J., et al.: Ann. Surg., *165*:432, 1967; Henkin, R. I., et al.: J. A. M. A., *217*:434, 1971.
46. Michaëlsson, G., Juhlin, L., and Vahlquist, A.: Arch. Dermatol., *113*:31, 1977; Brit. J. Dermatol., *96*:283, 1977.
47. Amador, M., et al.: Lancet, *1*:1379, 1975; Nutr. Rev., *33*:375, 1975.
48. Solomans, N. W., et al.: Gastroenterology, *70*:1022, 1976; Tucker, S. B., et al.: J. A. M. A., *235*:2399, 1976.
49. Schlettwein-Gsell, D., and Mommsen-Straub, S.: Int. J. Vit. Res., *40*:659, 1970; Tusl, J.: J. Assoc. Offic. Analyt. Chem., *53*:1190, 1970. (Also see p. 434 of Prasad, A. S.: *Zinc Metabolism*, listed under supplementary reading at top of p. 310.)

Fluorine, Cobalt, Molybdenum

50. Smith, M. C., Lantz, E. M., and Smith, H. V.: Univ. Ariz. Agric. Exp. Stat. Tech. Bull. 32, 1931; Churchill, H. W.: Ind. Chem. Eng., *23*:996, 1931.
51. Dean, H. T., et al.: Public Health Rep., *56*:761, 1941.
52. McClure, F. J.: *Water Fluoridation*. Washington, D.C., Superintendent of Documents, 1970; McClure, F. J.: *Fluoride Drinking Waters*. Public Health Service Pub. 825. Washington, D.C., Superintendent of Documents, 1962; various authors of papers published in J. Amer. Dent. Assoc., *80*:697–786, 1970; National Academy of Sciences: *The Problem of Providing Optimum Fluoride Intake for Prevention of Dental Caries*. National Research Council Pub. 294. Washington, 1953; British Ministry of Health: *Report on the Five Year Fluoridation Studies in the United Kingdom*, July 3, 1962; Roy. Soc. Health J.,

82:173, 1962. (Also see supplementary reading on fluoridation.)
53. Bernstein, D. S., et al.: J. A. M. A., *198*:499, 1966; Cohn, S. H., Dombrowski, C. S., Hauser, W., and Atkins, H. L.: Amer. J. Clin. Nutr., *24*:20, 1971; Brit. Med. J., *3*:660, 1970 editorial; Faccini, J. M.: Calcif. Tissue Res., *3*:1, 1969; Hegsted, D. M.: J. Amer. Dietet. Assoc., *50*:105, 1967; Iskrant, A. P.: Amer. J. Public Health, *58*:3, 1968.
54. Waldbott, G. L.: Amer. J. Clin. Nutr., *12*:455, 1963; Sengupta, S. R., and Pal., B.: Ind. J. Nutr. Dietet., *8*:66, 1971 (gives content of Indian foods); McClure, F. J.: *Fluorine in Foods: Survey of Recent Data.* Washington, D.C., Superintendent of Documents, 1949.
55. Roholm, K.: *Fluorine Intoxication, A Clinical Hygienic Study.* London, H. K. Lewis and Co., Ltd., 1937; Committee on Animal Nutrition: *The Fluorosis Problem in Livestock Production.* Washington, D.C., National Academy of Sciences, National Research Council, 1955.
56. Schlettwein-Gsell, D., and Mommsen-Straub, S.: Int. J. Vit. Res., *40*:673, 1970; Schroeder, H. A., Nason, A. P., and Tipton, I. H.: J. Chron. Dis., *20*:869, 1967.
57. Kesteloot, H., et al.: Circulation, *37*:854, 1968; Sullivan, J., Parker, M., and Carson, S. B.: J. Lab. Clin. Med., *71*:893, 1968.
58. Richert, D. A., and Westerfeld, W. W.: J. Biol. Chem., *203*:915, 1953; deRenzo, E. C., et al.: J. Amer. Chem. Soc., *75*:753, 1953.
59. Higgins, E. S., Richert, D. A., and Westerfeld, W. W.: J. Nutri., *59*:536, 1956; Reid, B. L., Kurnich, A. A., Svacha, R. L., and Couch, J. R.: Proc. Soc. Exp. Biol. Med., *93*:245, 1956; Leach, R. M., Jr., and Norris, L. C.: Poultry Sci., *36*:1136, 1957; Ellis, W. C., and Pfander, W. H.: J. Animal Sci., *19*:1260, 1960.
60. Schroeder, H. A., Balassa, J. J., and Tipton, I. H.: J. Chronic Dis., *23*:481, 1970; Westerfeld, W. W., and Richert, D. A.: J. Nutr., *51*:85, 1953.

Selenium, Chromium

61. Schwarz, K., and Foltz, C. M.: J. Amer. Chem. Soc., *79*:3292, 1957; for early experiments with selenium deficiency in the chick also see Schwarz, K., Bieri, J. G., Briggs, G. M., and Scott, M. L.: Proc. Soc. Exp. Biol. Med., *95*:621, 1957; Patterson, E. L., Milstrey, R., and Stokstad, E. L. R.: Proc. Soc. Exp. Biol. Med., *95*:617, 1957.
62. Bull, R. C., and Oldfield, J. E.: J. Nutr., *91*:237, 1967; McCoy, K. E. M., and Weswig, P. H.: J. Nutr., *98*:383, 1969; Thompson, J. N., and Scott, M. L.: J. Nutr., *97*:335, 1969 and *100*:797, 1970; Hurt, H. D., Cary, E. E., and Visek, W. J.: J. Nutr., *101*:761, 1971.
63. Schroeder, H. A., Frost, D. V., and Balassa, J. J.: J. Chronic Dis., *23*:227, 1970.
64. deMondragon, M. C., and Jaffe, W. G.: Arch. Lat. Amer. Nutr., *21*:185, 1971; Morris, V. C., and Levander, O. A.: J. Nutr., *100*:1383, 1970.
65. Schwarz, K.: Lancet, *1*:1335, 1965; Majaj, A. S., and Hopkins, L. L., Jr.: Lancet, *2*:593, 1966; Burk, R. F., Pearson, W. N., Wood, R. P., and Viteri, F.: Amer. J. Clin. Nutr., *20*:723, 1967; Levine, R. J., and Olson, R. E.: Proc. Soc. Exp. Biol. Med., *134*:1030, 1970.
66. Schwarz, K., and Mertz, W.: Arch. Biochem. Biophys., *85*:292, 1959; Fed. Proc., *20*:111, 1961; Mertz, W.: Fed. Proc., *26*:186, 1967; Physiol. Rev., *49*:163, 1969.
67. Mertz, W.: Nutr. Rev., *33*:129, 1975.
68. Hopkins, L. L., Jr., Ransome-Kuti, O., and Majaj, A. S.: Amer. J. Clin. Nutr., *21*:203, 1968; Gürson, C. T., and Saner, G.: Amer. J. Clin. Nutr., *24*:1313, 1971.
69. Schlettwein-Gsell, D., and Mommsen-Straub, S.: Int. J. Vit. Res., *41*:116, 1971.

Vanadium, Silicon, and Others

70. Nomoto, S., McNeely, M. D., and Sunderman, F. W., Jr.: Biochem., *10*:1647, 1971.
71. Nielsen, F. H.: Fed. Proc., *29*:696, 1970 (abstract); Nielsen, F. H., in *Newer Trace Elements in Nutrition.* (Ed. by Mertz, W., and Cornatzer, W. E.) New York, Marcel Dekker, Inc., 1971.
72. Schwarz, K., and Milne, D. B.: Science, *174*:426, 1971.
73. Hopkins, L. L., Jr., and Mohr, H. E., in *Newer Trace Elements in Nutrition* Ed. by Mertz, W., and Cornatzer, W. E. New York, Marcel Dekker, Inc., 1971; Fed. Proc., *30*:462, 1971; Strasia, C. A., and Smith, W. H.: J. Animal Sci., *31*:1027, 1970 (abstract).
74. Carlisle, E.: Fed. Proc., *31*:700, 1972 (abstract); J. Nutr., *106*:478, 1976.
75. Schwarz, K., Milne, D. B., and Vinyard, E.: Biochem. Biophys. Res. Commun., *40*:22, 1970; Schwarz, K., in *Newer Trace Elements in Nutrition* Ed. by Mertz, W., and Cornatzer, W. E. New York, Marcel Dekker, Inc., 1971.
76. Calloway, D. H., and McMullen, J. J.: Amer. J. Clin. Nutr., *18*:1, 1966.
77. Neilson, F. H., Givand, S. H., and Myran, D. R.: Fed. Proc., *34*:923, 1975.
78. Dent, C. E., and Winter, C. S.: Brit. Med. J., *1*:551, 1974.
79. Cropper, D. R., Krishnan, S. S., and Quittkal, S.: Grain, *99*(1):67, 1976.

SUPPLEMENTARY READING

Trace Elements — General

Reviews and History

Cuthbertson, D. P.: Human requirements for minerals and trace elements. Ind. J. Nutr. Dietet., *10*:31, 1973.

Hambidge, K. M.: The clinical significance of trace element deficiencies in man. Proc. Nutr. Soc., *33*:249, 1974.

Henkin, R. I.: Trace metals in endocrinology. Med. Clin. North Amer., *60*:779, 1976.

Hoekstra, W. G., Suttie, J. W., Ganther, H. E., and Mertz, W. (eds.): *Trace Element Metabolism in Animals-2.* Baltimore, University Park Press, 1974.

Nielsen, F. H., Sanstead, H. H.: Are nickel, vanadium, silicon, fluorine, and tin essential for man? A review. Amer. J. Clin. Nutr., *27*:515, 1974.

Prasad, A. S. (ed.): *Trace Elements in Human Health and Disease,* Vol. 1, *Zinc and Copper.* Vol. 2, *Essential and Toxic Elements.* New York, Academic Press, 1976.

Reinhold, J. G.: Trace elements — a selective survey. Clin. Chem. *21*:476, 1975.

Schwarz, K.: Recent dietary trace element research, exemplified by tin, fluorine, and silicon. Fed. Proc., *33*:1748, 1974.

Underwood, E. J.: *Trace Elements in Human and Animal Nutrition.* 4th Ed. New York, Academic Press, 1977.

Ulmer, D. D.: Trace elements. N. Engl. J. Med., *297*:318, 1977.

Williams, R. B.: Trace elements and congenital abnormalities. Proc. Nutr. Soc., *36*:25, 1977.

Content and Availability in Foods

Chesters, J. K.: Trace elements: adventitious yet essential dietary ingredients. Proc. Nutr. Soc., *35*:15, 1976.

Davies, N. T., and Nightingale, R.: The effects of phytate on intestinal absorption and secretion of zinc, and whole-body retention of zinc, copper, iron and manganese in rats. Brit. J. Nutr., *34*:243, 1975.

Hauer, E. C., and Kaminski, M. V.: Trace metal profile of parenteral nutrition solutions. Amer. J. Chem. Nutr., *31*:264, 1978.

Thornton, I., and Alloway, B. J.: Geochemical aspects of the soil-plant-animal relationship in the development of trace element deficiency and excess. Proc. Nutr. Soc., *33*:257, 1974.

Walker, M. A., and Page, L.: Nutritive content of college meals. III. Mineral elements. J. Amer. Dietet. Assoc., *70*:260, 1977.

Welch, R. M., and Cary, E. E.: Concentration of chromium, nickel, and vanadium in plant materials. J. Agric. Food Chem., *23*:479, 1975.

Zook, E. G., and Lehmann, J.: Total diet study: content of ten minerals — aluminum, calcium, phosphorus, sodium, potassium, boron, copper, iron, manganese, and magnesium. J. Assoc. Offic. Analyt. Chem., *48*:850, 1965.

Other References

Ainscough, E. W., and Brodie, A. M.: The role of metal ions in proteins and other biological molecules. J. Chem. Educ., 53(3):156, 1976.

Buck, W. B., and Ewan, R. C.: Toxicology and adverse effects of mineral imbalance. Clin. Toxicol., *6*:459, 1973.

Fleming, C. R., Hodges, R. E., and Hurley, L. S.: A prospective study of serum copper and zinc levels in patients receiving total parenteral nutrition. Amer. J. Clin. Nutr., *29*:70, 1976.

Greger, J. L., et al.: Calcium, magnesium, phosphorus, copper, and manganese balance in adolescent females. Amer. J. Clin. Nutr., *31*:117, 1978.

Greger, J. L., et al.: Nutritional status of adolescent girls in regard to zinc, copper, and iron. Amer. J. Clin. Nutr., *31*:269, 1978.

Jacob, R. A., Klevay, L. M., and Logan, G. M.: Hair as a biopsy material. Hair metal as an index of hepatic metal in rats: copper and zinc. Amer. J. Clin. Nutr., *31*:477, 1978.

Jacobson, S., and Wester, P. O.: Balance study of twenty trace elements during total parenteral nutrition in man. Brit. J. Nutr. *37*:107, 1977.

Klevay, L. M.: Coronary heart disease: the zinc/copper hypothesis. Amer. J. Clin. Nutr., *28*:764, 1975.

Levander, O. A.: Selenium and chromium in human nutrition. A review. J. Amer. Dietet. Assoc., *66*:338, 1975.

Mahloudji, M., et al.: Combined zinc and iron compared with iron supplementation of diets of 6- to 12-year old village schoolchildren in southern Iran. Amer. J. Clin. Nutr., *28*:721, 1975.

McKenzie, J. M.: Alteration of the zinc and copper concentration of hair. Amer. J. Clin. Nutr., *31*:470, 1978.

Mertz, W.: The newer essential trace elements, chromium, tin, vanadium, nickel and silicon. Proc. Nutr. Soc., *33*:307, 1974.

Myron, D. R., et al.: Intake of nickel and vanadium by humans. A survey of selected diets. Amer. J. Clin. Nutr., *31*:527, 1978.

Robinson, M. R., McKenzie, J. M., Thomson, C. D., and van Rij, A. L.: Metabolic balance of zinc, copper, cadmium, iron, molybdenum and selenium in young New Zealand women. Brit. J. Nutr., *30*:195, 1973.

Schroeder, H. A., and Nason, A. P.: Interactions of trace metals in mouse and rat tissues: zinc, chromium, copper and manganese with 13 other elements. J. Nutr., *106*:198, 1976.

Widdowson, E. M., Dauncey, J., and Shaw, J. C. L.: Trace elements in foetal and early postnatal development. Proc. Nutr. Soc., *33*:275, 1974.

Iron

(also see refs. 1–19)

Reviews and History

Bannerman, R. M.: Genetic defects in iron transport. Fed. Proc., *35*:2281, 1976.

Bowering, J., Sanchez, A. M., and Irwin, M. I.: A conspectus of research on iron requirements of man. J. Nutr., *106*(7):985, 1976.

Committee on Nutrition of the Mother and Preschool Child, Food and Nutrition Board, National Research Council, National Academy of Sciences: *Iron Nutriture in Adolescence.* DHEW Pub. No. (HSA) 77–5100. Washington, D.C., 1976.

Fairbanks, V. F., Fahey, J. L., and Beutler, E.: *Clinical Disorders of Iron Metabolism.* New York, Grune & Stratton, Inc., 1971.

Gaines, E. G., and Daniel, W. A., Jr.: Dietary iron intakes of adolescents. Relations of sex, race and sex maturity ratings. J. Amer. Dietet. Assoc., *65*:275, 1974.

International Nutritional Anemia Consultive Group: *Guidelines for the Eradication of Iron Deficiency Anemia.* New York, Nutrition Foundation Inc, 1977.

Leibel, R. L.: Behavioral and biochemical correlates of iron deficiency. J. Amer. Dietet. Assoc., *71*:398, 1977.

Pollitt, E., and Leibel, R. L.: Iron deficiency and behavior. J. Pediatr., *88*:372, 1976.

Availability and Absorption

Ashworth, A., Milner, P. F., Waterlow, J. C., and Walker, R. B.: Absorption of iron from maize

(*Zea mays* L.) and soya beans (*Glycine hispida* Max.) in Jamaican infants. Brit. J. Nutr., *29*:269, 1973.

Aung-Than-Batu, Thein-Than, and Thane-Toe: Iron absorption from Southeast Asian rice-based meals. Amer. J. Clin. Nutr., *29*:219, 1976.

Björn-Rasmussen, E., Hallberg, L., and Rossander, L.: Adsorption of "fortification" iron. Bioavailability in man of different samples of reduced Fe and prediction of the effects of Fe fortification. Brit. J. Nutr., *37*:375, 1977. (Also see Amer. J. Clin. Nutr., *25*:317, 1972; *26*:1311, 1973; *29*:772, 1976; *30*:539, 1977.)

Cook, J. D., et al: Absorption of fortification iron in bread. Amer. J. Clin. Nutr., *26*:861, 1973.

Cook, J. D., and Monsen, E. R.: Food iron absorption in human subjects. III. Comparison of the effect of animal proteins on nonheme iron absorption. Amer. J. Clin. Nutr., *29*:859, 1976. (Also see Amer. J. Clin. Nutr., *28*:1289, 1975; *29*:614, 1976; *29*:1142, 1976.)

El-Hawary, M. F. S., El-Shobaki, F. A., Kholeif, T., Sakr, R., and El-Bassoussy, M.: The absorption of iron, with or without supplements of single amino acids and of ascorbic acid, in healthy and Fe-deficient children. Brit. J. Nutr., *33*:351, 1975.

Hazell, T., Ledward, D. A., and Neale, R. J.: Iron availability from meat. Brit. J. Nutr., *39*:631, 1978.

Layrisse, M., Martínez-Torres, C., and González, M.: Measurement of the total daily dietary iron absorption by the extrinsic tag model. Amer. J. Clin. Nutr., *27*:152, 1974. (Also see Amer. J. Clin. Nutr., *25*:401, 1972.)

Martínez-Torres, C., Leets, I., Renzi, M., and Layrisse, M.: Iron absorption by humans from veal liver. J. Nutr., *104*:983, 1974.

Martínez-Torres, C., Renzi, M., and Layrisse, M.: Iron absorption by humans from hemosiderin and ferritin, further studies. J. Nutr., *106*:128, 1976.

Monsen, E. R., et al.: Estimation of available dietary iron. Amer. J. Clin. Nutr., *31*:134, 1978.

Motzok, I., Davies, M. I., Verma, R. S., and Pennell, M. D.: Biological availability of iron from foods and tonics containing various iron supplements. Nutr. Rpt. Internat., *15*:459, 1977.

Narasinga Rao, B. S., Prasad, J. S., and Vijaya Sarathy, C.: An animal model to study iron availability from human diets. Brit. J. Nutr., *37*:451, 1977.

Olszon, E., et al.: Food iron absorption in iron deficiency. Amer. J. Clin. Nutr., *31*:106, 1978.

Senchak, M. M., Howe, J. M., and Clark, H. E.: Iron absorption by adults fed mixtures of rice, milk, and wheat flour. J. Amer. Dietet. Assoc., *62*:272, 1972.

Vaghefi, S. B., Ghassemi, H., and Kaighobadi, K.: Availability of iron in an enrichment mixture for bread. J. Amer. Dietet. Assoc., *64*:275, 1974.

Waddell, J.: Bioavailability of iron sources. Food Prod. Dev., *8*:80, 1974.

Other References

Ashworth, A., and March, Y.: Iron fortification of dried skim milk and maize-soya-bean-milk mixture (CSM): availability of iron in Jamaican infants. Brit. J. Nutr., *30*:577, 1973.

Aung-Than-Batu, U Hla-Pe, Thein-Than, and Khin-Kyi-Nyunt: Iron deficiency in Burmese population groups. Amer. J. Clin. Nutr., *25*:210, 1972.

Cook, J. D., Lipschitz, D. A., Miles, L. E. M., and Finch, C. A.: Serum ferritin as a measure of iron stores in normal subjects. Amer. J. Clin. Nutr., *27*:681, 1974.

Derman, D. P., et al.: Serum ferritin as an index of iron nutrition in rural and urban South African children. Brit. J. Nutr., *39*:383, 1978.

El-Shobaki, F. A., et al.: Iron metabolism in Egyptian infants with protein-calorie deficiency. Brit. J. Nutr., *28*:81, 1972.

Gardner, G. R., et al.: Physical work capacity and metabolic stress in subjects with iron deficiency anemia. Amer. J. Clin. Nutr., *30*:910, 1977.

Goldsmith, G. A.: Iron enrichment of bread and flour. Amer. J. Clin. Nutr., *26*:131, 1973.

Gross, S. J., Stuart, M. J., Swender, P. T., and Oski, F. A.: Malabsorption of iron in children with iron deficiency. J. Pediatr., *88*:795, 1976.

Haghshenass, M., Mahloudji, M., Reinhold, J. G., and Mohammadi, N.: Iron-deficiency anemia in an Iranian population associated with high intakes of iron. Amer. J. Clin. Nutr., *25*:1143, 1972.

Jansen, C., and Horrill, S.: Intakes and serum levels of protein and iron, for 70 elderly women. Amer. J. Clin. Nutr., *30*:1414, 1977.

Koerper, M. A., Dallman, P. R.: Serum iron concentration and transferrin saturation in diagnosis of iron deficiency in children–normal development changes. J. Pediatr., *91*:870, 1977.

Layrisse, M., Martínez-Torres, C., Renzi, M., Velez, R., and Gonzalez, M.: Sugar as a vehicle for iron fortification. Amer. J. Clin. Nutr., *29*:8, 1976.

O'Neal, R. M., *et al.*: The incidence of anemia in residents of Missouri. Amer. J. Clin. Nutr., *29*:1158, 1976.

Shah, B., and Belonje, B.: Liver storage iron in Canadians. Amer. J. Clin. Nutr., *29*:66, 1976.

Strauss, R. G.: Iron deficiency, infections, and immune function: a reassessment. Amer. J. Clin. Nutr., *31*:660, 1978.

Takkunen, H., and Seppänen, R.: Iron deficiency and dietary factors in Finland. Amer. J. Clin. Nutr., *28*:1141, 1975.

Weinberg, E. D.: Iron and susceptibility to infectious disease. Science, *188*:1038, 1975.

Articles in Nutrition Reviews

The ferrous to ferric cycles in iron metabolism (by Frieden, E.). *31*:41, 1973.

The role of transferrin in iron absorption. *31*:131, 1973.

The value of iron fortification of food. *31*:275, 1973.

Serum ferritin and body iron stores. *33*:11, 1975.

Hyperlipemia and iron deficiency. *33*:55, 1975.

The relationship between infection and the iron status of an individual. *33*:103, 1975.

Iron and the regulation of erythropoiesis. *33*:144, 1975.

The relation of iron to blood platelets. *34*:25, 1976.

A specific skeletal muscle dysfunction in iron deficiency. *35*:76, 1977.

Iron and immunocompetence (by Chrandra, R. K.). *34*:129, 1976.

Intestinal malabsorption of iron. *34*:270, 1976.
Physical acceptability and bioavailability of iron fortified food. *34*:298, 1976.
Serum ferritin and early hemochromatosis. *34*:304, 1976.
Mucocutaneous fungal lesions and iron deficiency. *34*:203, 1976.
Iron absorption from breast milk or cow's milk. *35*:203, 1977.
Population screening for iron deficiency. *35*:271, 1977.

Iodine

(also see refs. 19–26)

Reviews and History

Brush, B. E., and Altland, J. K.: Goiter prevention with iodized salt: results of a thirty-year study. J. Clin. Endocrinol. Metab., *12*:1380, 1952.
Follis, R. H.: Patterns of urinary iodine excretion in goitrous and nongoitrous areas. Amer. J. Clin. Nutr., *14*:253, 1964.
Kojima, N., and Brown, H. D.: The effects of iodized salt in processed fruits and vegetables. Food Tech., *9*:103, 1955.
Lowenstein, F. W.: Iodized salt in the prevention of endemic goiter: a world-wide survey of present programs. Amer. J. Public Health, *57*:1815, 1967.
Talbot, J. M., Fisher, K. D., and Carr, F. J.: *A Review of the Significance of Untoward Reactions to Iodine in Foods.* Prepared for Division of Nutrition, Bureau of Foods, FDA, Washington, D.C., 1974.
Wayne, E. J., Koutras, D. A., and Alexander, W. D.: *Clinical Aspects of Iodine Metabolism.* Oxford, Blackwell, 1964.

Other References

Bautista, A., Barker, P. A., Dunn, J. T., and Sanchez, M.: Lack of correlation between thyroid size and body growth in an area of endemic goiter. Amer. J. Clin. Nutr., *31*:275, 1977.
Cullen, R. W., and Oace, S. M.: Iodine: current status. J. Nutr. Ed., *8*:101, 1976.
Fierro-Benitez, R., et al.: The clinical pattern of cretinism as seen in highland Ecuador. Amer. J. Clin. Nutr., *27*:531, 1974.
Ingenbleek, Y., and Beckers, C.: Evidence for intestinal malabsorption of iodine in protein-calorie malnutrition. Amer. J. Clin. Nutr., *26*:1323, 1973.
Iodine and the thyroid (editorial). Brit. Med. J., *2*:1566, 1977.
Karmarkar, M. G., Deo, M. G., Kochupillai, N., and Ramalingaswami, V.: Pathophysiology of Himalayan endemic goiter. Amer. J. Clin. Nutr., *27*:96, 1974.
Kidd, P. S., Trowbridge, F. L., Goldsby, J. B., and Nichaman, M. Z.: Sources of dietary iodine. J. Amer. Dietet. Assoc., *65*:420, 1974.
Koutras, D. A., et al.: Endemic goiter in Greece: nutritional status, growth and skeletal development of goitrous and nongoitrous populations. Amer. J. Clin. Nutr., *26*:1360, 1973.
Stewart, J. C., and Vidor, G. I.: Thyrotoxicosis induced by iodine contamination of food — a common unrecognised condition? Brit. Med. J., *1*:372, 1976.
Thilly, C. H., Delange, F., and Ermans, A. M.: Further investigations of iodine deficiency in the etiology of endemic goiter. Amer. J. Clin. Nutr., *25*:30, 1972.
Trowbridge, F. L., Hand, K. A., and Nichaman, M. Z.: Findings relating to goiter and iodine in the Ten-State Nutrition Survey. Amer. J. Clin. Nutr., *28*:712, 1975.
Trowbridge, F. L., Matovinovic, J., McLaren, G. D., and Nichaman, M. Z.: Iodine and goiter in children. Pediatrics, *56*:82, 1975.
Whitehead, D. C.: Uptake and distribution of iodine in grass and clover plants grown in solution culture. J. Sci. Food Agric., *24*:43, 1973.

Articles in Nutrition Reviews

The etiology of endemic cretinism. *29*:227, 1971.
Endemic goiter and antithyroid agents. *33*:171, 1975.
(Also see reprints of two classic early studies on iodine in *33*:272 and 338, 1975.)

Copper

(also see refs. 27–36)

Reviews and History

Elvehjem, C. A.: The biological significance of copper and its relation to iron metabolism. Physiol. Rev., *15*:471, 1935.
Evans, G. W.: Copper homeostasis in the mammalian system. Physiol. Rev., *53*:535, 1973.
Holtzman, N. A.: Menkes' kinky hair syndrome: a genetic disease involving copper. Fed. Proc., *35*:2276, 1976.
Peisach, J., Aisen, P., and Blumberg, W. E. (eds.): *The Biochemistry of Copper: Proceedings of the Symposium on Copper in Biological Systems.* New York, Academic Press, 1966.
Symposium on Copper Metabolism and Wilson's Disease. (Nine papers), Mayo Clin. Proc., *49*:361, 1974.

Other References

Allen, K. G. D., and Klevay, L. M.: Cholesterolemia and cardiovascular abnormalities in rats caused by copper deficiency. Atherosclerosis, *29*:81, 1978.
Baker, D. E.: Copper: soil, water, plant relationships. Fed. Proc., *33*:1188, 1974.
Butler, L. C., and Daniel, J. M.: Copper metabolism in young women fed two levels of copper and two protein sources. Amer. J. Clin. Nutr., *26*:744, 1973.
Fleming, C. R., Hodges, R. E., and Hurley, L. S.: A prospective study of serum copper and zinc levels in patients receiving total parenteral nutrition. Amer. J. Clin. Nutr., *29*:70, 1976.
Hambidge, K. M.: Increase in hair copper concentration with increasing distance from the scalp. Amer. J. Clin. Nutr., *26*:1212, 1973.

Karpel, J., and Peden, V. H.: Copper deficiency in long-term parenteral nutrition. J. Pediatr., *80*:32, 1972.
Klevay, L. M.: The ratio of zinc to copper of diets in the United States. Nutr. Rpt. Internat., *11*:237, 1975.
Krishnamachari, K. A. V. R.: Some aspects of copper metabolism in pellagra. Amer. J. Clin. Nutr., *27*:108, 1974.
Lei, K. Y.: Cholesterol metabolism in copper-deficient rats. Nutr. Rpt. Internat., *15*:597, 1977.
O'Dell, B. L.: Biochemistry of copper. Med. Clin. North Amer., *60*:687, 1976.
Oster, G., and Salgo, M. P.: The copper intrauterine device and its mode of action. N. Engl. J. Med., *293*:432, 1975.
Pennington, J. T., and Calloway, D. H.: Copper content of foods. Factors affecting reported values. J. Amer. Dietet. Assoc., *63*:143, 1973.
Rucker, R. B., et al.: Effects of nutritional copper deficiency on the biomechanical properties of bone and arterial elastin metabolism in the chick. J. Nutr., *105*:1062, 1975.

Articles in Nutrition Reviews

Menke's kinky hair syndrome. *31*:17, 1973.
Copper toxicity, rats and Wilson's disease. *33*:51, 1975.
The steely-hair syndrome. *33*:189, 1975.
Brain and myocardial lesions in copper-deficient young rats. *33*:306, 1975.
Copper metabolism in patients with liver disease. *35*:136, 1977.
(Also see reprint of 1928 classic paper by Hart, et al. on need for copper in the rat, in Nutr. Rev., *31*:56, 1973.)

Manganese

(also see refs. 37–41)

Reviews and History

Cotzias, G. C.: Manganese in health and disease. Physiol. Rev., *38*:503, 1958.
Schroeder, H. A., Balassa, J. J., and Tipton, I. H.: Essential trace metals in man: manganese. A study in homeostasis. J. Chronic Dis., *19*:545, 1966.
Utter, M. F.: The biochemistry of manganese. Med. Clin. North Amer., *60*:713, 1976.

Other References

Abrams, E., Lassiter, J. W., Miller, W. J., Neathery, M. W., Gentry, R. P., and Scarth, R. D.: Absorption as a factor in manganese homeostasis. J. Animal Sci., *42*(3):630, 1976.
Hurley, L. S.: Trace elements and teratogenesis. Med. Clin. North Amer., *60*:771, 1976.
Hurley, L. S., and Bell, L. T.: Genetic influence on response to dietary manganese deficiency in mice. J. Nutr., *104*:133, 1974.
McLeod, B. E., and Robinson, M. F.: Dietary intake of manganese by New Zealand infants during the first six months of life. Brit. J. Nutr., *27*:229, 1972.
McLeod, B. E., and Robinson, M. F.: Metabolic balance of manganese in young women. Brit. J. Nutr., *27*:221, 1972.

Zinc

(also see refs. 42–49)

Reviews and History

Brewer, G. J., and Prasad, A. S. (eds.): *Zinc Metabolism: Current Aspects in Health and Disease.* New York, Alan R. Liss, Inc., 1977.
Halsted, J. A., Smith, J. C., Jr., and Irwin, M. I.: A conspectus of research on zinc requirements of man. Nutr., *104*:345, 1974.
Hambidge, K. M.: Zinc deficiency in children. In *Trace Element Metabolism in Animals-2* Ed. by Hoekstra, W. G., Suttie, J. W., Ganther, H. E., and Mertz, W. Baltimore, University Park Press, 1974.
Pores, W. J., et al.: *Clinical Application of Zinc Metabolism.* Springfield, Ill., Charles C Thomas, 1974.

Content of Foods and Availability

Brown, E. D., McGuckin, M. A., Wilson, M., and Smith, J. C., Jr.: Zinc in selected hospital diets. Comparison of analysis vs. calculation. J. Amer. Dietet. Assoc., *69*:632, 1976.
Freeland, J. H., and Cousins, R. J.: Zinc content of selected foods. J. Amer. Dietet. Assoc., *68*:526, 1976.
Haeflein, K. A., and Rasmussen, A. I.: Zinc content of selected foods. J. Amer. Dietet. Assoc., *70*:610, 1977.
Ismail-Beigi, F., Faraji, B., and Reinhold, J. G.: Binding of zinc and iron to wheat bread, wheat bran, and their components. Amer. J. Clin. Nutr., *31*:1721, 1978.
Johnson, P. E., and Evans, G. W.: Relative zinc availability in human breast milk, infant formulas, and cow's milk. Amer. J. Clin. Nutr., *31*:416, 1978.
Murphy, E. W., Willis, B. W., and Watt, B. K.: Provisional tables on the zinc content of foods. J. Amer. Dietet. Assoc., *66*:345, 1975.
O'Dell, B. L., Burpo, C. E., and Savage, J. E.: Evaluation of zinc availability in foodstuffs of plant and animal origin. J. Nutr., *102*:653, 1972.
Ter-Sarkissian, N., et al.: High phytic acid in Iranian breads. J. Amer. Dietet. Assoc., *65*:651, 1974.
White, H. S.: Zinc content and the zinc-to-calorie ratio of weighed diets. J. Amer. Dietet. Assoc., *68*:243, 1976.

Other References

Alberts, J. C., Lang, J. A., Reyes, P. S., and Briggs, G. M.: Zinc requirement of the young guinea pig. J. Nutr., *107*:1517, 1977.
Antoniou, L. D., et al.: Reversal of uremic impotance by zinc. Lancet, *2*:895, 1977.
Arakawa, T., et al.: Zinc deficiency in two infants during total parenteral alimentation for diarrhea. Amer. J. Clin. Nutr., *29*:197, 1976.

Davies, N. T., and Williams, R. B.: Zinc balance during pregnancy and lactation. Amer. J. Clin. Nutr., *30*:300, 1977; Evans, G. W.: Answer to Drs. Davies and Williams. Amer. J. Clin. Nutr., *30*:301, 1977.

Greger, J. L., Abernathy, R. P., and Bennett, O. A.: Zinc and nitrogen balance in adolescent females fed varying levels of zinc and soy protein. Amer. J. Clin. Nutr., *31*:112, 1978.

Greger, J. L., and Sciscoe, B. S.: Zinc nutriture of elderly participants in an urban feeding program. J. Amer. Dietet. Assoc., *70*:37, 1977.

Hambidge, K. M.: The role of zinc and other trace metals in pediatric nutrition and health.: Pediatr. Clin. North Amer., *24*:95, 1977.

Hambidge, K. M., et al.: Zinc nutrition of preschool children in the Denver Head Start Program. Amer. J. Clin. Nutr., *29*:734, 1976.

Henkin, R. I., et al.: A double blind study of the effects of zinc sulfate on taste and smell dysfunction. Amer. J. Med. Sci., *272*:285, 1976.

Hess, F. M., King, J. C., and Margen, S.: Zinc excretion in young women on low zinc intakes and oral contraceptive agents. J. Nutr., *107*:1610, 1977.

Hess, F. M., King, J. C., and Margen, S.: Effect of low zinc intake and oral contraceptive agents on nitrogen utilization and clinical findings in young women. J. Nutr., *107*:2219, 1977.

Morrison, S. A., et al.: Zinc deficiency: a cause of abnormal dark adaptation in cirrhotics. Amer. J. Clin. Nutr., *31*:276, 1978.

McBean, L. D., Dove, J. T., Halsted, J. A., and Smith, J. C., Jr.: Zinc concentration in human tissues. Amer. J. Clin. Nutr., *25*:672, 1972.

Osis, D., Kramer, L., Wiatrowski, E., and Spencer, H.: Dietary zinc intake in man. Amer. J. Clin. Nutr., *25*:582, 1972.

Ronaghy, H. A., et al.: Zinc supplementation of malnourished schoolboys in Iran: increased growth and other effects. Amer. J. Clin. Nutr., *27*:112, 1974.

Sandstead, H. H.: Zinc nutrition in the United States. Amer. J. Clin. Nutr., *26*:1251, 1973.

Sandstead, H. H., et al.: Zinc deficiency: effects on brain and behavior of rats and rhesus monkeys. Teratology, *16*:229, 1977.

Schraer, K. K., and Calloway, D. H.: Zinc balance in pregnant teenagers. Nutr. Metabol., *17*:205, 1974.

Solomons, N. W., Rosenfield, J. R. A., and Sandstead, H. H.: Growth retardation and zinc nutrition. Pediatr. Res., *10*:923, 1976.

Walravens, P. A., and Hambidge, K. M.: Growth of infants fed a zinc supplemented formula. Amer. J. Clin. Nutr., *29*:1114, 1976.

Articles in Nutrition Reviews

Growth and zinc deficiency. *31*:145, 1973.

Metabolic changes in acrodermatitis enteropathica. *32*:170, 1974.

Zinc availability in leavened and unleavened bread. *33*:18, 1975.

Zinc deficiency in sickle cell disease. *33*:266, 1975.

Zinc deficiency in pregnant, fetal and young rats. *34*:84, 1976.

Zinc and parturition. *35*:279, 1977.

Zinc deficiency and bone metabolism in rats. *36*:152, 1978.

Zinc deficiency, taste acuity and growth failure. *36*: 213, 1978.

Acrodermatitis Enteropathica, zinc and human milk. *36*:241, 1978.

Fluorine

(also see refs. 50–55)

Reviews and History

Ericsson, Y. (ed.): *Fluorides and Human Health.* WHO Monograph Series No. 59. Geneva, WHO, 1970.

Hodge, H. C., and Smith, F. A.: Fluorides and man. Ann. Rev. Pharmacol., *8*:395, 1968.

Horowitz, H. S.: Fluoride: research on clinical and public health applications. J. Amer. Dent. Assoc., *87*:1013, 1973.

Knutson, J. W.: Water fluoridation after 25 years. J. Amer. Dent. Assoc., *80*:765, 1970.

McClure, F. J.: A review of fluorine and its physiological effects. Physiol. Rev., *13*:277, 1933; *Water Fluoridation: The Search and the Victory.* Washington, D.C., Superintendent of Documents, 1970.

Simons, J. H. (ed.): *Fluorine Chemistry. IV. Biological Properties of Inorganic Fluorides and Effects of Fluorides on Bones and Teeth.* New York, Academic Press, 1965.

Sognnaes, R. F.: Fluoride protection of bones and teeth. Science, *150*:989, 1965.

Other References

Kramer, L., Osis, D., Wiatrowski, E., and Spencer, H.: Dietary fluoride in different areas in the United States. Amer. J. Clin. Nutr., *27*:590, 1974.

Messer, H. H., Armstrong, W. D., and Singer, L.: Influence of fluoride intake on reproduction in mice. J. Nutr., *103*:1319, 1973.

Newbrun, E.: The safety of water fluoridation. J. Amer. Dent. Assoc., *94*:301, 1977.

Osis, D., Kramer, L., Wiatrowski, E., and Spencer, H.: Dietary fluoride intake in man. J. Nutr., *104*:1313, 1974.

Spencer, H., Kramer, L., Wiatrowski, E., and Osis, D.: Magnesium-fluoride interrelationships in man. I. Effect of fluoride on magnesium metabolism. Amer. J. Physiol., *233*:E165, 1977. (Also see J. Nutr., *105*:733, 1975.)

Spencer, H., Kramer, L., Osis, D., and Wiatrowski, E.: Excretion of retained fluoride in man. J. Appl. Physiol., *38*:282, 1975.

Tao, S., and Suttie, J. W.: Evidence for lack of an effect of dietary fluoride level on reproduction in mice. J. Nutr., *106*:1115, 1976.

Taves, D. R.: Fluoridation and mortality due to heart disease. Nature, *272*:361, 1978.

Using fluoride to curb osteoporosis. Med. World News, *15*:58, 1974.

Wolinsky, I., and Guggenheim, K. Y.: The effect of fluoride on the mechanical strength of bone. Baroda J. Nutr., *3*:177, 1976.

Articles in Nutrition Reviews

Prenatal exposure to fluoride. *25*:330, 1967.
Fluoride concentration in enamel and bone. *26*:75, 1968.
Physiological distribution of fluoride. *26*:103, 1968.
Skeletal fluorosis and dietary calcium, vitamin C and protein. *32*:13, 1974.
Genu valgum due to fluoride toxicity. *33*:76, 1975.

Other Essential Trace Elements

Roginski, E. E., and Mertz, W.: A biphasic response of rats to cobalt. J. Nutr., *107*:1537, 1977.
Smith, S. E., and Loosli, J. K.: Cobalt and vitamin B_{12} in ruminant nutrition: a review. J. Dairy Sci., *40*:1215, 1957.
Taylor, A., and Marks, V.: Cobalt—a review. J. Human Nutr. (Britain), *32*:165, 1978.
Thomas, B., Roughan, J. A., and Watters, E. D.: Cobalt, chromium and nickel content of some vegetable foodstuffs. J. Sci. Food Agric., *25*:771, 1974.

Molybdenum

Cohen, H. J., Johnson, J. L., and Rajagopalan, K. V.: Molecular basis of the biological function of molybdenum. Developmental patterns of sulfite oxidase and xanthine oxidase in the rat. Arch. Biochem. Biophys., *164*:440, 1974. (Also see J. Biol. Chem., *249*:5046, 1974.)
Schroeder, H. A., Balassa, J. J., and Tipton, I. H.: Essential trace metals in man: molybdenum. J. Chronic Dis., *23*:481, 1970.
Standish, J. F., Ammerman, C. B., Wallace, H. D., and Combs, G. E.: Effect of high dietary molybdenum and sulfate on plasma copper clearance and tissue minerals in growing swine. J. Animal Sci., *40*:509, 1975.
Suttie, N. F.: Recent studies of the copper-molybdenum antagonism. Proc. Nutr. Soc., *33*:299, 1974.

Selenium

Bieri, J. G., and Ahmad, K.: Selenium content of Bangladeshi rice by chemical and biological assay. J. Agric. Food Chem., *24*:1073, 1976.
Combs, G. F., and Scott, M. L.: Nutritional interrelationships of vitamin E and selenium. Bioscience, *27*:467, 1977.
Ferretti, R. J., and Levander, O. A.: Selenium content of soybean foods. J. Agric. Food Chem., *24*:54, 1976.
Lawrence, R. A, and Burk, R. F.: Species, tissue and subcellular distribution of non–Se-dependent glutathione peroxidase activity. J. Nutr., *108*:211, 1978. (Also see J. Nutr., *108*:981, 1978.)
Levander, O. A.: Selenium and chromium in human nutrition. J. Amer. Dietet. Assoc., *66*:338, 1975.
Lombeck, I., et al.: The selenium state of healthy children. Eur. J. Pediatr., *125*:81, 1977.
McConnell, K. P., Broghamer, W. L., Jr., Blotcky, A. J., and Hurt, O. J.: Selenium levels in human blood and tissues in health and disease. J. Nutr., *105*:1026, 1975.
McKeehan, W. L., Hamilton, W. G., and Ham, R. G.: Selenium is an essential trace nutrient for growth of WI-38 diploid human fibroblasts. Proc. Nat. Acad. Sci., *73*:2023, 1976.
Rotruck, J. T., et al.: Selenium: biochemical role as a component of glutathione peroxidase. Science, *179*:588, 1973.
Sakurai, H., and Tsuchiya, K.: A tentative recommendation for the maximum daily intake of selenium. Environ. Physiol. Biochem., *5*:107, 1975.
Schwarz, K.: Essentiality and metabolic functions of selenium. Med. Clin. North Amer., *60*:745, 1976.
Scott, M. L.: The selenium dilemma (editorial). J. Nutr., *103*:803, 1973.
Shearer, T. R., and Hadjimarkos, D. M.: Geographic distribution of selenium in human milk. Arch. Environ. Health, *30*:230, 1975. (Values given are for the U.S.)
Stadtman, T. C.: Selenium biochemistry. Science, *183*:915, 1974.
Symposium: Biochemical function of selenium and its interrelationships with other trace elements and vitamin E (three review papers). Fed. Proc., *34*:2082, 1975.
Thomson, C. D., Rea, H. M., Doesburg, V. M., and Robinson, M. F.: Selenium concentrations and glutathione peroxidase activities in whole blood of New Zealand residents. Brit. J. Nutr., *37*:457, 1977. (Also see Brit. J. Nutr., *39*:579 and 589, 1978.)
Thompson, J. N., Erdody, P., and Smith, D. C.: Selenium content of food consumed by Canadians. J. Nutr., *105*:274, 1975.
Thorn, J., et al.: Trace nutrients. Selenium in British food. Brit. J. Nutr., *39*:391, 1978.

Chromium

Gürson, C. T., and Saner, G.: Effects of chromium supplementation on growth in marasmic protein-calorie malnutrition. Amer. J. Clin. Nutr., *26*:988, 1973.
Hambidge, K. M.: Chromium nutrition in man. Amer. J. Clin. Nutr., *27*:505, 1974. (Also see Amer. J. Clin. Nutr., *25*:376, 380, 384, 1972.)
Jeejeebhoy, K. N., et al.: Chromium deficiency, glucose intolerance, and neuropathy reversed by chromium supplementation, in a patient receiving long-term parenteral nutrition. Amer. J. Clin. Nutr., *30*:531, 1976.
Levander, O. A.: Selenium and chromium in human nutrition. J. Amer. Dietet. Assoc., *66*:338, 1975.
Liu, V. J. K., and Morris, J. S.: Relative chromium response as an indicator of chromium status. Amer. J. Clin. Nutr., *31*:972, 1978.
Mahalko, J. R, and Bennion, M.: The effect of parity and time between pregnancies on material hair chromium concentration. Amer. J. Clin. Nutr., *29*:1069, 1976.
Mertz, W.: Chromium and its relation to carbohydrate metabolism. Med. Clin. North Amer., *60*:739, 1976.

Mertz, W.: Chromium as a dietary essential for man. In *Trace Element Metabolism in Animals-2*. Ed. by Hoekstra, W. G., Suttie, J. W., Ganther, H. E., and Mertz, W. Baltimore, University Park Press, 1974.

Mertz, W., Toepfer, E. W., Roginski, E. E., and Polansky, M. M.: Present knowledge of the role of chromium. Fed. Proc., *33*:2275, 1974.

Mitman, F. W., Wolf, W. R., Kelsay, J. L., and Prather, E. S.: Urinary chromium levels of nine young women eating freely chosen diets. J. Nutr., *105*:64, 1975.

Pekarek, R. S., et al.: Relationship between serum chromium concentrations and glucose utilization in normal and infected subjects. Diabetes, *24*:350, 1975.

Punsar, S., Wolf, W., Mertz, W., and Karvonen, M. J.: Urinary chromium excretion and atherosclerotic manifestations in two Finnish male populations. Ann. Clin. Res., *9*:79, 1977.

Saner, G., and Gürson, C. T.: Hair chromium concentration in newborns and their mothers. Nutr. Rpt. Internat., *14*:155, 1976. (Also see Nutr. Rpt. Internat., 11, 387, 1975.)

Nickel

Kirchgessner, M., and Schnegg, A.: Malate dehydrogenase and glucose-6-phosphate dehydrogenase activity in livers of Ni-deficient rats. Bioinorganic Chem., *6*:155, 1976.

Nielsen, F. H., and Ollerich, D. A.: Nickel: a new essential trace element. Fed. Proc., *33*:1767, 1974.

Nielsen, F. H., Myron, D. R., Givand, S. H., and Ollerich, D. A.: Nickel deficiency and nickel-rhodium interaction in chicks. J. Nutr., *105*:1607, 1975.

Nielsen, F. H., et al.: Nickel deficiency in rats. J. Nutr., *105*:1620, 1975.

Spears, J. W., Hatfield, E. E., and Forbes, R. M.: Interrelationship between nickel and zinc in the rat. J. Nutr., *108*:307, 1978.

Sunderman, F. W.: A review of the metabolism and toxicology of nickel. Ann. Clin. Lab. Sci., *7*:377, 1977.

Thomas, B., Roughan, J. A., and Watters, E. D.: Cobalt, chromium and nickel content of some vegetable foodstuffs. J. Sci. Food Agric., *25*:771, 1974.

Vanadium

Cantley, L. C., Jr., et al.: Vanadate is a potent (Na, K)-ATPase inhibitor found in ATP derived from muscle. J. Biol. Chem., *252*:7421, 1977.

Curzon, M. E. J., Losee, F. L., Brown, R., and Taylor, H. E.: Vanadium in whole human enamel and its relationship to dental caries. Arch. Oral Biol., *19*:1161, 1974.

Hafez, Y., and Kratzer, F. H.: The effect of dietary vanadium on fatty acid and cholesterol synthesis and turnover in the chick. J. Nutr., *106*:249, 1976.

Hopkins, L., Jr.: Essentiality and function of vanadium. In *Trace Elements in Animals-2*. Ed. by Hoekstra, W. G., Suttie, J. W., Ganther, H. E., and Mertz, W. Baltimore, University Park Press, 1974.

Silicon

Byczkowski, S., and Wrześniowski, K.: Studies on the physiological hair silicon content in men. Toxicology, *5*:123, 1975.

Carlisle, E.: Silicon as an essential element. Fed. Proc., *33*:1758, 1974.

Carlisle, E.: In vivo requirement for silicon in articular cartilage and connective tissue formation in the chick. J. Nutr., *106*:478, 1976.

Chipperfield, B., Chipperfield, J. R., and Bower, N. R.: Silicon and aluminum in heart deaths. Lancet, *1*:755, 1977.

Kennedy, B. M., and Schelstraete, M.: A note on silicon in rice endosperm. Cereal Chem., *52*:854, 1975.

Schwarz, K.: Silicon, fibre, and atherosclerosis. Lancet, *1*:454, 1977.

Articles in Nutrition Reviews

Mercury toxicity reduced by selenium. *31*:25, 1973.

Selenium: an essential element for glutathione peroxidase activity. *31*:289, 1973.

Selenium as a feed additive. *32*:158, 1974.

Cobalt. (by Underwood, E. J.) *33*:65, 1975.

Effects and metabolism of glucose tolerance factor. (by Mertz, W.) *33*:129, 1975.

Studies on selenium. *33*:138, 1975.

Bisulfite toxicity in molybdenum-deficient rats. *33*:185, 1975.

Silicon. (by Carlisle, E. M.) *33*:257, 1975.

Selenium and human health. *34*:347, 1976.

Effect of dietary α-tocopherol in aging rats. *35*:50, 1977.

Vitamin E. *35*:57, 1977.

Biological function of selenium. (by Stadtman, T. C.) *35*:161, 1977.

Possibly Essential Trace Elements

(also see refs. 75–77)

Tin

Hiles, R. A.: Absorption, distribution and excretion of inorganic tin in rats. Toxicol. Appl. Pharmacol., *27*:366, 1974.

Schwarz, K.: Tin as an essential growth factor in rats. In *Newer Trace Elements in Nutrition*. Ed. by Mertz, W., and Cornatzer, W. E. New York, Marcel Dekker, Inc., 1971.

Arsenic

Klevay, L. M.: Pharmacology and toxicology of heavy metals: arsenic. Pharmacol. Ther. (A.), *1*:189, 1976.

Lakso, J. U., and Peoples, S. A.: Methylation of inorganic arsenic by mammals. J. Agric. Food Chem., *23*:674, 1975.

Lunde, G.: Isolation of an organoarsenic compound present in cod liver. J. Sci. Food Agric., *26*:1247, 1975.

Walkiw, O., and Douglas, D. E.: Health food supplements prepared from kelp — a source of elevated urinary arsenic. Clin. Toxicol., *8*:325, 1975.

Nonessential Elements (and Toxicity)

(also see refs. 78 and 79)

Reviews and History

Bremner, I.: Heavy metal toxicities. Q. Rev. Biophys., *7*:75, 1974.

Clarkson, T. W.: Factors involved in heavy metal poisoning. Fed. Proc., *36*:1634, 1977.

Fishbein, L.: Environmental metallic carcinogens: an overview of exposure levels. J. Toxicol. Env. Health, *2*:77, 1976.

Huisingh, D., and Huisingh, J.: Factors influencing the toxicity of heavy metals in food. Ecol. Food Nutr., *3*:263, 1974.

Levander, O. A.: Nutritional factors in relation to heavy metal toxicants. Fed. Proc., *36*:1683, 1977.

Neathery, M. W., and Miller, W. J.: Metabolism and toxicity of cadmium, mercury, and lead in animals: a review. J. Dairy Sci., *58*:1767, 1975.

Other References

Aluminum and Alzheimer. Lancet, *1*:1281, 1976.

Beattie, A. D., et al.: Role of chronic low-level lead exposure in the aetiology of mental retardation. Lancet, *1*:590, 1975.

Cam, J. M., Luck, V. A., Eastwood, J. B., and deWardener, H. E.: The effect of aluminum hydroxide orally on calcium, phosphorus and aluminum metabolism in normal subjects. Clin. Sci. Mol. Med., *51*:407, 1976.

Chatterjee, P., and Gettman, J. H.: Lead poisoning: subculture as a facilitating agent? Amer. J. Clin. Nutr., *25*:324, 1972.

Crapper, D. R., Krishnan, S. S., and Quittkat, S.: Aluminum, neurofibrillary degeneration and Alzheimer's disease. Brain, *99*:67, 1976.

Hutcheson, D. P., Gray, D. H., Venugopal, B., and Luckey, T. D.: Studies of nutritional safety of some heavy metals in mice. J. Nutr., *105*:670, 1975.

Kaehny, W. D., Hegg, A. P., and Alfrey, A. C.: Gastrointestinal absorption of aluminum from aluminum-containing antacids. N. Engl. J. Med., *296*:1389, 1977.

Klauder, D. S., and Petering, H. G.: Anemia of lead intoxication. J. Nutr., *107*:1779, 1977.

Kshirsagar, S. G.: Effect of stable strontium on the tissue alkaline and acid phosphatase activities of the rat: feeding studies. J. Nutr., *106*:1475, 1976.

Lin-Fu, J. S.: Vulnerability of children to lead exposure and toxicity. N. Engl. J. Med., *289*:1229, 1973.

Recker, R. R., Blotcky, A. J., Leffler, J. A., and Rack, E. P.: Evidence for aluminum absorption from the gastrointestinal tract and bone deposition by aluminum carbonate ingestion with normal renal function. J. Lab. Clin. Med., *90*:810, 1977.

Schroeder, H. A., and Mitchener, M.: Life-term studies in rats: effects of aluminum, barium, beryllium, and tungsten. J. Nutr., *105*:421, 1975.

Ziegler, E. E., et al.: Absorption and retention of lead by infants. Pediatr. Res., *12*:29, 1978.

Pica

Bruhn, C. M., and Pangborn, R. M.: Reported incidence of pica among migrant families. J. Amer. Dietet. Assoc., *58*:417, 1971.

Editorial: Clay eating. Lancet, *2*(Sept. 16): 614, 1978.

Halsted, J. A.: Geophagia in man: its nature and nutritional effects. Amer. J. Clin. Nutr., *21*:1384, 1968.

Neumann, H. H.: Pica — symptom or vestigial instinct? Pediatrics, *46*:441, 1970.

Roselle, H. A.: Association of laundry starch and clay ingestion with anemia in New York City. Arch. Intern. Med., *125*:57, 1970.

Vessal, K., Ronaghy, H. A., and Zarabi, M.: Radiological changes in pica. Amer. J. Clin. Nutr., *28*:1095, 1975.

Articles in Nutrition Reviews

Mercury levels in the blood and hair of individuals eating methylmercury-contaminated fish. *31*:53, 1973.

Does lead make children hyperactive? *31*:88, 1973.

Pyridoxine and the anemia of cadmium toxicity. *32*:345, 1974.

Ethanol and lead toxicity. *32*:347, 1974.

Possible aluminum intoxication. *34*:166, 1976.

Recommendations for the prevention of lead poisoning in children. (Committee on Toxicology, National Research Council) *34*:321, 1976.

Lead biopsies of human teeth. *36*:144, 1978.

Calcium and vitamin D intake of lead-burdened children. *36*:212, 1978.

Part 2

Food Intake and Utilization

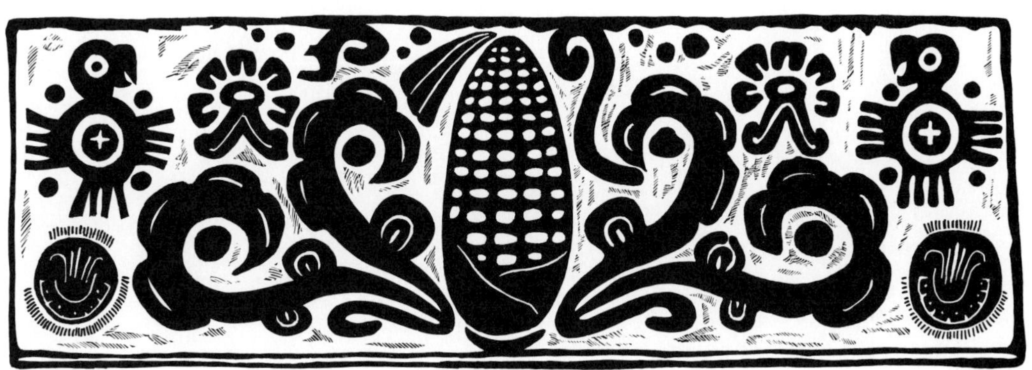

Chapter 13

The Nervous and Endocrine Systems and Regulation of Food Intake

A number of intricate processes work harmoniously to maintain conditions in the body within the narrow range required for health, to provide for the nourishment and repair of cells, and to rid the body of wastes. The activities of organs and tissues are so regulated and integrated that small changes in the internal environment trigger reactions that tend to restore conditions to the prior state, that is, to achieve *homeostasis*. To some extent each cell is self-regulating. We have referred, for example, in Chapter 10, to the fact that sodium is actively pumped out of a cell so that a low level of this mineral is maintained in the intracellular fluid. Somewhat more elaborate processes regulate protein synthesis, as described in Chapter 5. Still more complicated processes are coordinated and regulated by a variety of interactive signals from the two main control systems of the body, the *nervous* and *endocrine* systems.

CHARACTERISTICS OF CONTROL SYSTEMS

Control systems in the body do not keep conditions absolutely constant; rather, it is the changes in conditions that both start and stop the homeostatic processes. A home central heating system can be used to illustrate the principles involved. The typical system consists of a temperature-sensing unit, a control apparatus, and a heating element. Suppose the thermostat is set at 68°F (20°C). On a cold evening, the house gradually loses heat to the outdoor environment, so the inside temperature falls below 68°. The sensing unit detects this change and signals an electrical control system, which activates a gas furnace or electric heater, and heated air is sent into the room. When the sensor detects that the temperature has risen above 68°, it signals the control system, which stops the heating element from generating heated air. Over the course of the evening the cycle repeats many times, and the room temperature is maintained within a narrow range above and below 68°, not precisely at 68°. The key elements of the control system thus are seen to be a *sensor*, a *control*, and a *responder*. The process, a very important one in biological systems, whereby the responder component creates a substance or change in conditions (in our example, heat) that turns off the response, is called *negative feedback or feedback inhibition*.

Many of the body's control systems

are more elaborate than the simple servo-system just described. Many systems have push-pull controls, that is, separate systems for causing increases and decreases in a state. It is as if, in our earlier example, the home thermal system included both a heater and a cooler. This feature increases the spectrum of responses possible; a decrease can be brought about by either turning off the increasor or turning on the decreasor, or both.

Often, two or more central systems are interrelated. The regulation of the composition, volume, and pressure of the fluid in the circulatory system is an example. As noted in Chapter 10, the amount of sodium in the extracellular fluid is carefully regulated. If an increased amount of sodium in the plasma is detected, the body can adjust the level by causing greater excretion of sodium or by retaining water to dilute the sodium. (Which mechanism will be used depends on the extracellular fluid volume and pressure in the circulatory system.) Sometimes there are redundant systems; a second, backup system becomes operative when the primary system is overloaded or fails. This commonly occurs in routing of metabolism along different pathways.

The complete scope of the control systems is the subject of physiology. In this chapter and subsequent sections we shall discuss only a few systems most relevant to nutrition. This chapter introduces the nervous and endocrine systems and describes the physiological processes that regulate food intake and achieve homeostasis of energy balance in normal persons.

THE NERVOUS AND ENDOCRINE CONTROL SYSTEMS

The nervous system both receives signals from within and outside the body and transmits signals that control diverse actions of tissues and organs — muscular contraction, glandular secretions, sexual arousal, and so forth. The brain and spinal cord constitute the *central nervous system* (CNS, Fig. 13–1). The nervous tissue includes both neurons, which are the basic nerve cells, and other cells that support and sustain the neurons (glial cells). The transmission of a signal along a nerve involves changes in electrical potential brought about by the interaction of electrolytes (sodium, potassium, chloride). Communication between nerve cells and between nerve cells and cells of the effector organs is achieved by chemical *neurotransmitters.* One of these neurotransmitters, acetylcholine, is derived from the vitamin choline (choline is obtained as such from the diet, or derived in the body from the amino acids methionine and serine). (See Chapter 8.) The other five known neurotransmitters all are derived from amino acids: serotonin (from tryptophan), gamma-aminobutyric acid (from glutamic acid), and the so-called catecholamines, epinephrine, norepinephrine, and dopamine (all from tyrosine).

The central nervous system is richly supplied with blood and is absolutely dependent on a continuous supply of oxygen and glucose. (The brain has no reserve energy supply and cannot use energy substrates other than glucose until after a period of adaptation, when some capacity to use fat end-products, or ketones, develops. The brain is irreversibly damaged by 3 to 4 minutes of lack of oxygen and glucose.) However, the brain is partially protected from the great variations in types and amounts of some substances present in the blood by a phenomenon called the "blood-brain barrier." The brain and spinal cord are surrounded by the cerebrospinal fluid, which is similar to, but not the same as, plasma. The cerebrospinal fluid is a selective secretion and is richer in sodium and chloride than other extracellular fluids. Some substances do cross the blood-brain barrier and can affect the ongoing processes of transmission and integration, but generally the CNS is responding to signals brought in via the nervous system and effecting changes by internal formation

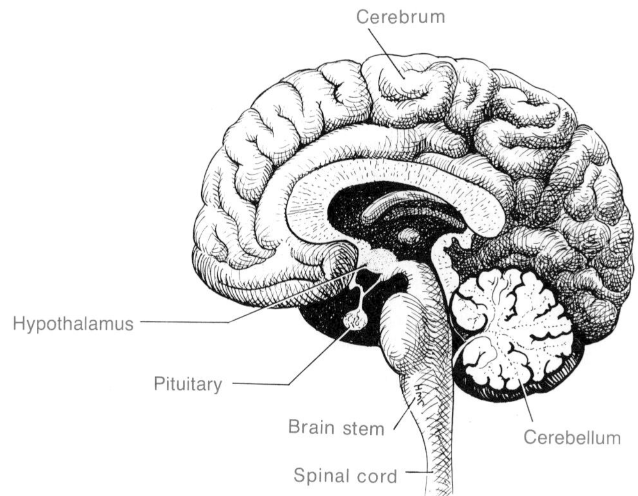

Figure 13–1 The brain has three main divisions: brain stem, cerebellum, and cerebrum. All nerve fibers from the spinal cord pass through the brain stem to the higher brain centers, and nerves that control the muscles of the head and muscles and glands of the abdominal organs arise there. Unconscious coordination of muscle movements is the function of the cerebellum. The hypothalamus, a small area (5 to 6 cm^3) in the base of the cerebrum, is an important integrating center for reflexes that regulate body temperature and control eating and drinking. Note that the hypothalamus is adjacent to and exerts control over the pituitary gland.

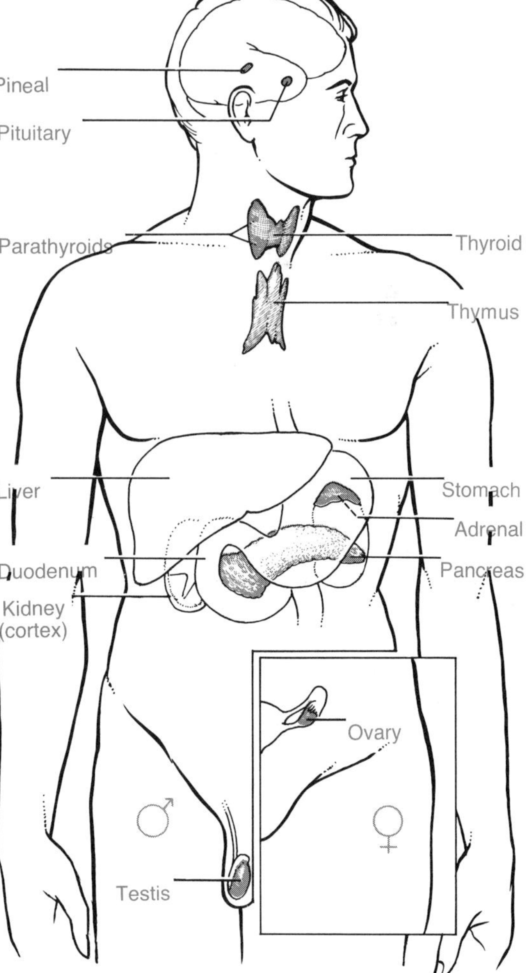

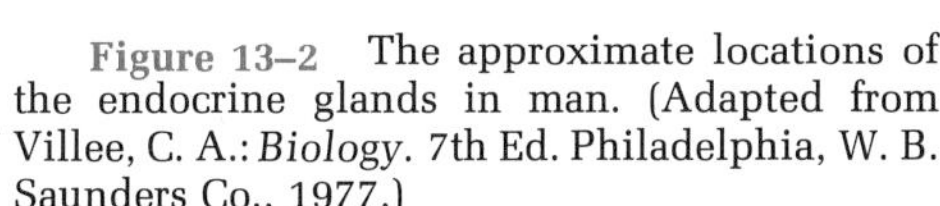
Figure 13–2 The approximate locations of the endocrine glands in man. (Adapted from Villee, C. A.: *Biology*. 7th Ed. Philadelphia, W. B. Saunders Co., 1977.)

Table 13–1 HORMONES AND THEIR MAJOR ACTIONS

Gland/Organ	*Product*	*Target Organ/Action*
Hypothalamus	Hormone releasing/inhibiting hormones	Anterior pituitary. See below.
Anterior pituitary (hypophysis)	Growth hormone (GH, Somatotropin)*,†	Growth; stimulates formation of somatomedin by liver; metabolic effects (↑ protein synthesis, ↓ carbohydrate utilization, ↑ blood sugar, ↑ fat mobilization).
	Thyroid-stimulating hormone (TSH)*	Stimulates thyroid gland to form thyroxine.
	Adrenocorticotropic hormone (ACTH)*	Stimulates adrenal cortex to form cortisol.
	Gonadotropic hormones (FSH, LH)*	Stimulates testes/ovaries to form sex hormones.
	Prolactin*,†	Stimulates breast development and milk production.
	Melanocyte-stimulating hormone*,†	Stimulates production of black pigment by melanocytes.
Posterior pituitary (neurohypophysis)	Oxytocin	Stimulates contraction of uterus; milk ejection.
	Antidiuretic hormone (vasopressin)	↑ Water reabsorption in the kidney; blood pressure.
Thyroid	Thyroxine	↑ Metabolic rate and protein synthesis; inhibits TSH formation.
	Calcitonin	↓ Loss of calcium from bone and ↑ its deposition; lowers calcium in blood.
Parathyroids	Parathormone (PTH)	Mobilizes calcium from bone, ↑ calcium in blood; required for renal hydroxylation of vitamin D; ↑ growth of thymus cells.
Adrenal cortex	Cortisol (hydrocortisone)	↑ Formation of glucose from protein, ↓ carbohydrate utilization, ↑ blood sugar, ↓ body protein, ↑ liver protein; anti-inflammatory; inhibits ACTH formation.
	Aldosterone	↑ Recovery of sodium and chloride and excretion of potassium from the kidney.
	Androgens	Weak male sex hormones (see below).
	Estrogens	Minute amounts only; female sex hormone (see below).
Adrenal medulla	Epinephrine (adrenaline)	↑ Breakdown of muscle (and liver) glycogen, ↑ fat mobilization, ↑ blood flow in heart and skeletal muscle; neurotransmitter.
	Norepinephrine	↑ Constriction of blood vessels; neurotransmitter.
Gonads		
Ovaries	Estrogens	Development of secondary sex characteristics; ↑ (slightly) protein synthesis; closes epiphysis of bones; ↑ sodium and water retention; inhibits FSH and LH formation.
	Progesterone	Prepares uterus for implantation; ↑ breast development; ↓ protein synthesis.
Testes	Testosterone (and other androgens)	Development of adult primary and secondary sex characteristics; ↑ protein formation and bone growth; inhibits FSH and LH formation.
Kidneys	Renin	↑ Constriction of blood vessels, ↑ blood pressure.
	Erythropoietin	Stimulates red blood cell production in bone marrow.
Stomach	Gastrin‡,§	Formation of acid in the stomach, ↑ motility of stomach (antrum), stimulates growth of acid-forming mucosal cells.
	Somatostatin‡	Role of G.I. peptide undetermined but inhibits acid secretion. Hypothalamic counterpart inhibits growth hormone–releasing factor.
Intestine	Secretin¶	Stimulates formation of pancreatic secretion (bicarbonate), ↑ action of CCK; counteracts tropic action of gastrin on stomach mucosa and ↑ tropic action of CCK.
	Cholecystokinin (CCK)§	Stimulates pancreatic secretion (enzymes), ↑ action of secretin, stimulates intestinal and gallbladder motility (emptying), inhibits stomach (fundus) motility, stimulates pancreatic cell growth.
	Enteric glucagon	Physiological role unknown but not equivalent to pancreatic glucagon.
	Gastric inhibitory peptide**	↑ Insulin release by glucose.

Table continued on next page

Table 13–1 HORMONES AND THEIR MAJOR ACTIONS (*Continued*)

Gland/Organ	*Product*	*Target Organ/Action*
Pancreas	Insulin††	↑ Carbohydrate uptake in tissues, ↓ blood sugar, ↑ glycogen storage, potentiates growth hormone, ↑ protein synthesis, ↓ protein degradation.
	Glucagon	↑ Breakdown of liver glycogen and formation of glucose from protein; ↑ blood sugar, stimulates insulin production.
	Somatostatin	See entry under Stomach.
Liver	Somatomedin	Mediates growth hormone action; ↑ growth of bones and connective tissue; ↑ synthesis of RNA and DNA; insulinlike action on muscle and fat cells.
Pineal	Melatonin	↑ Secretion when environmental light decreases (diurnal cycle); inhibits some aspects of gonadal, thyroid, and adrenal function; deactivates the central nervous system.
Thymus	Thymosin	Stimulates development of white blood cells (lymphocytes).

*Secretion regulated by hypothalamic releasing hormone.
†Secretion regulated by hypothalamic inhibiting hormone.
‡Immunoreactive counterparts formed or present in brain tissue.
§Released by protein feeding.
¶Released by acid (HCl).
**Released by fat feeding.
††Released by carbohydrate feeding.

and release of transmitters.

The endocrine system consists of a number of small ductless glands and cells scattered throughout the body (Fig. 13–2). Their chemical products, called *hormones,* are discharged into the blood in very small amounts and exert profound effects on either remote or adjacent body tissues and cells. Many hormones have interrelated or counteractive effects, and their further interaction with the nervous system provides for the translation of external stimuli into signals to which the endocrine glands can respond. When the endocrine glands function normally, the metabolism of the body operates smoothly in all respects. When one or more of the glands become overactive or underactive, the normal equilibrium of the endocrine system is disturbed, leading to more or less grave abnormalities of metabolism, growth, sexual development, or body functioning.

Over 30 hormones have been isolated and studied, and most of them can now be synthesized in the laboratory. (See Table 13–1.) Many are peptides and two are derivatives of amino acids; others are steroids, related to cholesterol. Generally, the peptide hormones exert their action in target cells by combining with a specific membrane receptor, which then activates an enzyme to form a second messenger substance.* The steroidal hormones combine with receptor proteins in the cytoplasm of their target cells and move to the cell nucleus, where synthesis of a specific protein occurs. Thus, although the hormones are carried by the blood to all tissues, only specific cells with the correct receptor apparatus are able to respond to them.

The complex character of hormonal control is well illustrated by the action of the pituitary gland. The pituitary gland (also called the hypophysis), which lies in a groove at the base of the brain, is composed of two distinct parts called the anterior and posterior lobes. The anterior lobe is often referred to as the master gland of the body because it secretes a

*Usually the second messenger is the nucleotide cyclic AMP (cyclic adenosine monophosphate), but insulin and growth hormone act via cyclic GMP (cyclic guanosine monophosphate). (See Chapters 5 and 15.)

group of peptide hormones that have a marked influence on the other endocrine glands and on total body growth. The anterior pituitary hormones are called tropins — a term which indicates that they stimulate activity of other organs or glands. One of these hormones, ACTH, is said to be adrenocorticotropic because it stimulates the adrenal cortex to produce the adrenal steroidal hormones, cortisol and aldosterone (see Table 13–1). The thyrotropic hormone (or thyroid-stimulating hormone, TSH) stimulates the activity of the thyroid gland, and other tropins act on the reproductive glands. Frequently there is feedback regulation of the anterior pituitary by these target endocrine glands, which serves to regulate the amount of the hormone secreted. For instance, a decline in the output of the thyroid hormone *thyroxine* causes the pituitary to secrete thyroid-stimulating hormone, while an increased output of thyroxine suppresses secretion of the thyroid-stimulating hormone by the pituitary (Fig. 13–3). Similar reciprocal relationships exist with respect to the other tropic hormones and the specific organs on which they act.

There is yet another system of regulation built into this central system; it is centered in the *hypothalamus,* a small area at the base of the brain cortex (cerebrum). The hypothalamus produces a number of very small peptides that control the release of the pituitary hormones. These peptide hormones are fairly specific — for example, there is a thyrotropin–releasing hormone (called TRH, or TRF using the original nomenclature, which was "releasing factor"), adrenocorticotropin–releasing hormone (ACTH–RH), and so on — but they may have lesser effects on the release of other pituitary tropic hormones. It is partly by these hypothalamic agents that the endocrine system is brought under neural control.

The anterior pituitary also manufactures *growth hormone* (GH, or somatotropin), which differs from the other tropic hormones in promoting the growth of the general body (somatic) cells. In the presence of somatomedin, a hormone formed in the liver, GH stimulates the growth of both long bones and soft tissues of the body, and thus it is anabolic, promoting retention of nitrogen, potassium and phosphorus. The neural control system

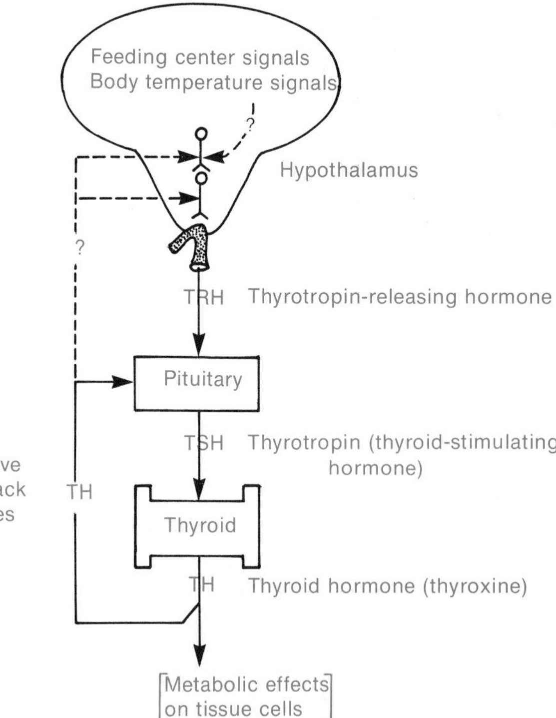

Figure 13–3 Hypothalamic-pituitary-thyroid system for the control of thyroid hormone secretion. Pituitary formation of thyroid-stimulating hormone (TSH) is controlled by two opposing factors: (1) inhibition by the thyroid hormone thyroxine (classical negative feedback) and (2) release by thyrotropin-releasing hormone (TRH). Secretion of TRH is controlled by nerve cells; it has been suggested that formation of TRH may be responsive to the presence of thyroxine or to signals from other centers in the hypothalamus that relate to feeding drive and body temperature regulations, or to both factors. (Adapted from Reichlin, S., et al.: Recent Progr. Horm. Res., *28*:229, 1972.)

for GH also is different. There are two peptides from the hypothalamus that control GH secretion, a releasing factor (SRF) and a release-inhibiting factor, called somatostatin. Hypothalamic inhibitory as well as releasing factors also occur for the pituitary tropins that regulate breast growth (prolactin) and the pigment-producing cells of the body (melanocyte-stimulating hormone). These pituitary hormones all appear to be tonically inhibited by the hypothalamus, acting to prevent unbridled growth.

GH secretion also is responsive to metabolic changes in the body, particularly to levels of glucose and some amino acids in the blood. GH has opposite effects to those of the pancreatic hormone insulin, being one of several agents that promote elevation of blood sugar. Blood sugar regulation and other metabolic effects of the hormones will be discussed in Chapter 15.

In the past the hormones were regarded as each being the discrete product of a particular gland, such as the hormone insulin, which is formed only by cells found in the pancreas. Now we know that several hormonelike substances are formed by cells in more than one location, even though one site may be quantitatively more important than another. Several of the small peptide hormones of the brain (hypothalamus) also are produced by cells located in the gastrointestinal tract, for example. The distinction between the hormones and the substances that transmit messages throughout the nervous system have also become less sharp. Epinephrine (also called adrenaline) is itself a hormone, and some physiologists refer to the neurotransmitter acetylcholine as a "local hormone." The prostaglandins (Chapter 4) and the hydroxylated derivatives of vitamin D (Chapter 7) are other transitional compounds. For our purposes, it is sufficient to understand that the nervous and endocrine systems act jointly to detect and effect changes throughout the body, that these effects often are moderated or mediated by other chemical substances, and that the nervous system is the mechanism by which sights, sounds, odors, ideas, and previous cultural experiences can alter the hormonal outflow and body processes. Nowhere is the interactive nature of these central systems more evident than in the regulation of food intake and the factors that affect or abridge this regulation, to which we now turn.

PHYSIOLOGICAL REGULATION OF FOOD INTAKE[1, 2]

During at least some stage of the life cycle, all animals must eat to live, and all have some mechanism that directs them to take food. Behavior patterns are diverse, but in almost every case some control is exerted over the kind and amount of food that is taken. A remarkably complicated system is necessary for achieving homeostasis of the animal's internal environment. The animal must react behaviorally to present cues about its internal state even though the full metabolic effect of the behavior will occur only after a lapse of time. When in need of food energy, the animal must respond by locating and ingesting foods that will adjust the internal state after a delay due to digestion and absorption, and eating must stop before that state is reached. Similarly, the animal must reject quickly and completely substances that would produce toxic effects at a later time.

In some of the lower forms, food seeking and consuming behavior, presumably in response to a hunger signal, occupy most of their lifetime. Carnivores may eat enormously of a fresh kill and then not eat again for a long period; some insects eat but once between molts. Robins eat during the day, and mice mainly by night. Cats hunt optionally by day or night, depending on the relative abundance of robins and mice, or they may forego hunting in favor of a domestic bill of fare. Country cats are rarely fat, but the indulged household tabby very well may be.

That is to say, basic inherent regulation of food intake exists in all species — regulation as to time of intake and kind and amount of food — but can be abridged by environmental factors and learning.

Hunger and appetite are not synonymous terms. *Hunger* refers to the unpleasant group of sensations that are experienced when there is an urgent need for food. *Appetite,* on the other hand, means a desire for food whether or not the individual is hungry. Hunger is a physiologic condition, and while appetite has physiologic components, it is basically an affective state. *Satiety* refers to the set of conditions that exist when the individual stops eating because his hunger is satisfied, but it is recognized that hunger can be overcome without the food having satisfied the appetite fully. Most of us have taken a bit of sweet or a brandy after our true hunger has been satisfied; we are responding to a learned appetite directed according to the way our culture teaches a meal should be ended.

Regulation of Energy Balance

Most people maintain their weight reasonably well in spite of large day-to-day variations in physical activity and, thus, energy need. A person may sit in an office or classroom for the better part of 5 days a week and then spend almost the entire weekend in active recreation. Or a person may work in heavy construction all week and spend his weekend watching baseball in front of the television set. People do not necessarily eat sufficiently more food on days of increased activity, perhaps even the contrary, yet body weight shifts but little from week to week. Experiments with animals have shown that food intake is regulated each day, approximately according to the day's energy output. Superimposed on the daily regulation is a fine adjustment that corrects for small errors in the daily balance over a longer period of days or weeks. Humans show the same general regulatory pattern except that the daily regulation is less precise than in laboratory animals.

At very low levels of energy output, neither animals nor humans are able to regulate energy balance precisely, with the result that both become fat. Similarly, at very high levels of forced work output, regulation of intake is inadequate to maintain constant body weight. Miraculously, over broad ranges of physical activity and food availability, input and output are nearly balanced. An average adult consumes about a million calories a year. Average Americans gain about 20 pounds between ages 25 and 45, or about 1 pound a year. This yearly fat gain represents about 3600 kcal, which means that the error in balance is less than 0.5 percent of intake, or out of adjustment by only 10 kcal per day. Regulation is 99.5 percent accurate.

Gastrointestinal Factors

Hunger sensations occur simultaneously with contractions of the stomach. These contractions are forceful and recur in groups lasting for varying periods of time from a half-hour to an hour and a half. A common experience is to feel hunger contractions that subside whether or not one eats, only to reappear later in greater intensity unless food is taken. Contractions are inhibited by a number of things, including simply tightening the belt (which probably gives rise to the use of that expression as denoting straitened financial circumstances). Eating food, of course, inhibits the contractions but so does tasting or chewing food without swallowing it, drinking cold water or alcoholic beverages, smoking, or experiencing the emotions of fear or hate. Contractions are enhanced by administration of insulin and inhibited by glucagon, hormones that respectively lower and raise the blood sugar level (Chapter 15). Hunger contractions continue even when the main nerve to the stomach (the vagus nerve) is severed,* but the sensation, the hunger pang, is no longer perceived. Severing the vagus nerve does not stop a person from eating the needed amount of food, so the awareness of hunger contractions is apparently not a necessary feature of food intake regulation.

Animals stop eating long before the full metabolic impact of a meal can be felt, so the gastrointestinal tract must participate in events that lead to cessation of eating. The act of eating and swallowing food is one possibility, but if food is prevented from reaching the stomach (by cutting through the esophagus), animals eat for a longer than normal period of time before stopping, and they begin eating again in a short period of time. If food is placed directly into the stomach by means of a tube (intragastrically), so that the animal does not taste, chew, or swallow the food, some lowering of oral intake occurs, depending on the volume of material administered by tube. In animals, intragastric volumes less than 20 percent of the normal intake are without effect on oral intake, but volumes on the order of 50 percent cause a compensatory reduction of intake. This happens no matter if the material given intragastrically is food or a bulk material without energy value. Young men also are reported to reduce their oral intake of a formula diet only if 40 percent or more of their usual oral energy intake were given intragastrically. Even then they consistently took more total energy (oral plus tube) during the days of combined feeding than when they ate only by mouth. However, when the men were not allowed any food by mouth and were required to administer their own intragastric feedings, they did consume an adequate amount of energy.[3]

Several stimuli are involved in the gastrointestinal contribution to cessation of eating. As the preceding discussion suggests, one is distention or stretch due to the presence of bulk, which triggers neural responses. Nutrient substances cause release of hormones that act to alter secretion in the alimentary tract (Chapter 14) and that also affect other hormonal systems, specifically those of insulin and glucagon. Thus, the gastrointestinal system anticipates and initiates the integrated mechanisms that ultimately stop one from eating.

*This nerve is sometimes cut surgically to stop acid secretion in persons with ulcers.

The Hypothalamus

Attention was focused on a specific portion of the brain as containing a regulatory feeding center when French pathologists observed at autopsy that very obese people had lesions in that area (Fig. 13–1). Because of their anatomic proximity there was some question whether the regulatory center was in the pituitary gland or in the hypothalamus, with which the pituitary is intimately connected. Development of an instrument capable of destroying a minute area in the brain of a living animal made possible experiments which proved that the center is in the hypothalamus. In the early 1940's Heatherington at Chicago and Brobeck at Yale reported that destruction of two small areas located in the central portion of the hypothalamus (the ventromedial portion) caused rats to eat voraciously and become obese. That is, the rats became hyperphagic because the satiety center had been destroyed. Later, Anand and Brobeck discovered that destruction of two areas in the side region of the hypothalamus (the lateral portion) caused just the opposite effect: The rats refused water and food, and some of them starved to death unless forcibly fed. This meant that they had destroyed the center that causes an animal to eat and drink. Mayer and his colleagues at Harvard proved that the failure of animals to eat after destruction of the lateral centers was not due to the failure to take in water, and subsequent research has shown that the eating and drinking centers are separate but quite near each other in the rat. Since then, lesions have been made in chickens, cats, dogs, monkeys, and goats, and all show similar anatomic locations and feeding responses. Electrical stimulation of the feeding and satiety centers causes the reactions that would be expected. Stimulation of the satiety center causes animals to stop eating, and stimulation of the feeding center causes them to eat. Precise location of the drinking center is easier in some animals — the goat, for instance — than others, and stimulation of this area of the hypothalamus causes an animal to drink whether or not it is thirsty, thus disproving an old adage; as Mayer has said, you can now lead a (goat) to water and you can make him drink.

Further study of the hypothalamic centers has shown that the satiety center is dominant in regulating eating behavior. It is thought to act like a brake on the feeding center. The nerve fibers in the hypothalamus have been mapped out and connections found between the two centers. Once the control center was located, further research uncovered the major signals to which it responds. The most enduring concept has been that a signal is generated in response to the utilization of glucose, the so-called glucostatic theory of regulation.

Glucostatic Theory of Regulation

This theory, proposed by Mayer, postulates that there are receptors in the satiety center that are especially sensitive to glucose and are activated according to the rate at which it is being utilized. When food is taken, blood sugar rises and the rate of glucose utilization in the tissues rises. The receptors are stimulated, and the satiety center signals the responses to stop eating. Conversely, some hours later, blood glucose falls, and the receptors detect low utilization rate; the brake is released and eating begins.

An important distinction is that the hypothalamic receptors are responsive to *utilization* of glucose rather than to the level of glucose in the blood. In the disease diabetes, appetite is great even though blood sugar levels are elevated. The normal fuel of the brain is glucose, and the brain is different from most other tissues in the body in that it does not require insulin in order to utilize glucose. With respect to glucose utilization, the hypothalamus behaves in the same way as the other body tissues (muscle, fat, etc.). That is, unlike the rest of the brain, of which it is a part, the hypothalamus is not able to use glucose without insulin. In diabetes, the message would be "food is needed," irrespective of the fact that the blood sugar level is high.

Animals with lesions in the hypothalamus have alterations in behavior other than those relating simply to the amount of food eaten. Rats that have been operated on are less active, have diminished libido, and have altered responses to test situations involving food. They are more encephalized. Placed in a situation in which they must risk a shock to obtain food, they are less responsive to hunger than is the normal animal. The animal with a lesion is also more prone than the normal one to reject food that has an unpleasant taste (for instance, with quinine added to it). Depending on how precisely placed the lesion is, animals may have deranged water intake, as noted earlier, and they may be unable to regulate body temperature adequately.

It is known that the central feeding circuit is integrated with the sympathetic nervous system because injection of the neurotransmitter norepinephrine into the hypothalamus elicits eating in food-satiated animals.* The drinking circuit is part of the parasympathetic system and is triggered by application of another neurotransmitter, acetylcholine. Thus in normal animals, these anatomically overlapping systems react to clearly separate and distinct signals, even though eating and drinking are paired behaviors and are

*The amphetamines, drugs commonly prescribed to suppress appetite, affect the DOPA system, which counterbalances the norepinephrine transmitter. Some psychotropic drugs (chlorpromazine, cyproheptadine) have the opposite effect of increasing food intake, again by affecting the balance among transmitters and allied compounds.

both reactive to changes in the osmolality of body fluids. Also, while the various hormones that affect food intake — primarily insulin and growth hormone and, to a lesser extent, estrogen — affect the blood level and tissue utilization of glucose, so do they influence the level and utilization of amino acids and lipids (Chapter 15). Severe imbalances of amino acids in the diet lead immediately to cessation of eating, and dietary lack of single nutrients usually causes loss of appetite as an early symptom of deficiency. All of this suggests that regulation of the most vital animal processes is even more complex and interrelated than we now appreciate and that there is participation of higher brain centers in all these functions.

Long-Term Regulation of Energy Balance

Little is known about the mechanism whereby the daily small errors in energy regulation are compensated so that body weight remains nearly constant (if that is appropriate), or so that weight is regained after an illness or period of food deprivation. A lipostatic theory of regulation is currently the most accepted. This theory suggests that precise information on the current level of fat stores is relayed from the adipose tissue to the nervous control center. If the stores are filled, the animal is directed to stop eating; but if the stores are low, eating continues past the point at which the satiety center is usually activated. Several observations provide general support for this theory. One is that animals with lesions in the satiety center do not go on gaining indefinitely but stop at some degree of obesity. If the obese lesioned animal is then starved, when food is again available it regains its original obese weight, not some other degree of fatness. Also, when rats are made fat by forced feeding, they subsequently reduce their voluntary food intake until the excess weight is lost. Animals with lesions in the lateral hypothalamus similarly preserve a stable, reduced body weight.

What this adipose tissue sensor might be is unknown. The probability of a humoral substance is suggested by an observation made about animals that are joined surgically so that their blood interchanges but their organs remain separate (parabiotic preparation). If one member of the pair has the satiety center destroyed, it becomes obese; the other member of the pair becomes thin. Presumably this happens because some message is transmitted from the large adipose stores of the fat partner through the blood to the regulatory center of the normal pair member; energy intake of the normal partner is then reduced because excessive fat stores have been sensed. By whatever mechanism, the organism apparently is able to detect whether fat stores are being filled or emptied and to adapt food intake accordingly.

REGULATION OF ESSENTIAL NUTRIENTS

Besides energy regulation, animals somehow must manage to select diets that are nutritionally adequate, or they cannot live and reproduce. Adequacy could be coincidental with satisfaction of energy needs because, in nature, nutrients are not found singly. Food plants and animals are all mixtures of organic compounds and minerals, and animals come to occupy an ecological niche where the food available to them matches their needs for energy and nutrients. However, animals do show specific hunger for isolated nutrients — salt is a familiar example — and to some extent they are able to choose the better of nutritional alternatives. Given a choice of mixed diets that are protein-free or contain an adequate amount of protein, rats eat very little of the poorer one. Rats will also eat a reasonable balance of two diets that have widely different protein qualities, but they do not make very fine discriminations between proteins that are marginally different. When they are required to select among pure foodstuffs (pure protein, pure fat, and sugar), some animals are able to do so, but others within the same strain and age group are unable. There is little information regarding human capability in this respect, but in one brief study men were unable to select a complete mixture of amino acids over one that was lacking a single essential amino acid.[4]

Specific Hunger

Specific hunger refers to the situation in which an animal is deficient in one nutrient and seeks out that specific nutrient. Some specific hunger is thought to be genetically determined in that animals can recognize a substance in which they are deficient and will go to it selectively, even if they have never before been deficient in that nutrient. Salt is thought to be in this class. Other specific hungers are learned, as illustrated in Harris'[5] classic experiments with rats deficient in B vitamins.

The general pattern of experiments was to deprive rats of the vitamin B complex or a single B vitamin, thiamin. The animals were then offered diets flavored with easily recognizable substances that were thought to mask the vitamin odor: Bovril (without B vitamin) or yeast or marmite, both containing B vitamin. The deficient rats reliably learned to select the diets containing the vitamin, but nondeficient rats showed no such preference among the diets. However, if animals made deficient were given a large number of diets (six to ten), only one of which contained the missing vitamin, they were unable to pick the correct one. The rats could be taught to choose the correct diet by giving them a training period when only that diet was given; later, when all the different diets were offered again, the rats would continue to choose the one they had learned contained the vitamin. If the vitamin was then removed from that diet and added to a diet with a different flavor, the rats continued to eat the previously learned, but now deficient, diet. They could be reeducated to accept the new flavor of diet by repeating the process of offering only one choice while they were in a deficient state. This indicates that the ingestion of the vitamin that had been lacking caused some reaction in the animal's body that provided a sufficient cue to establish learning. Additional experiments with pantothenic acid, which does not have a readily identifiable taste or odor (as thiamin does), showed that the rats did not seek out a vitamin per se, but rather a flavor because they were unable to find the vitamin unless a recognizable flavor was added to direct their choice of diet. Thus, the animals sense well-being, but there is nothing innate about vitamin recognition.

Ability to Choose a Balanced Diet

Perhaps nutritional food habits are formed by a comparable learning process. Animals that are deficient in one or more nutrients may try eating something in their environment, and if they feel better according to some internal cue, they learn that this is what animals should eat, and they develop a taste for it. That this mechanism is faulty is well known, because animals will eat things they like that are to their detriment. Animals will founder in a cornfield, birds eat fermented fruit to the point of drunkenness, which shortens their life span if predators are handy, and people seem to prefer sweet, rich foods over the simpler ones, in spite of internal cues that signal satiety and intellectual awareness of too much body fat. Animals, including humans, develop an aversion to foods that are associated with illness and thus learn to avoid toxins.[6] Sensitivity to these is part of the process of gustation, but the aversion will develop in animals even if they are anesthetized at the time of ingestion, indicating that this regulatory process is quite different from usual associative learning. Many toxins have a bitter taste, which probably contributes to the low preference for bitter substances. Certainly, liking for such items as olives and quinine (tonic) water is a learned response.

One famous experiment is usually cited as proof that humans can choose their diet wisely. Davis[7] allowed three newly weaned infants to choose their own diets from among 30 common natural food materials. The choice was restricted to foods thought suitable for infants, and neither mixed dishes nor sweets were offered. Two of the infants were studied for 6 months and the other for a year. At first the babies tried anything in their mouths — inedible plates as well as edible foods — but they became selective and developed definite tastes. Their food preferences were erratic and unpredictable, and their diets were not balanced within a day. Sometimes the babies would indulge in binges, eating many oranges a day for several days and then none, for instance. Some of the babies' choices did suggest specific selection. They ate salt only rarely and obviously did not enjoy it, even crying when they took it, but they did go back for more. Davis regarded her experiment as flawed, in retrospect, because she had limited the possible choices the babies might make to what her knowledge dictated they should have, and she thought the test might otherwise have failed. However, the infants did balance a diet from among 30 options daily, and their health and growth were acceptable by 1928 standards.

In sophisticated man, appetite seems to be a somewhat fickle guide to choosing an adequate diet. Some individuals are always found to have poor intakes in any group of people, in spite of abundant availability of nutritious foods. For this reason, guides are needed to good eating, based on scientific knowledge of nutrient requirements and accumulated human wisdom regarding what constitutes suitable food.

Diet, Nutrition and the Nervous and Endocrine Systems

Selye was probably the first to recognize that malnutrition is a stressor, and it, like other stressful agents, causes characteristic and marked changes in the endocrine system. These changes include enlargement of the adrenal glands and an outpouring of adrenal hormones, and depressed activity of the pituitary, the thyroid, and the gonads. In the classic laboratory-created stress syndrome, early and moderate stress exposure initiates the endocrine changes that alter tissue metabolism and allow the animal to survive in a new, adapted state; if the stress is prolonged or severe, the adaptation fails and the animal succumbs. In addition to this "general adaptation syndrome," a number of more specific alterations are induced by lack of specific nutrients. We have seen, for example, that lack of iodine is particularly damaging to the thyroid and leads to goiter, and that deficiencies of zinc and of vitamin A specifically affect gonadal tissues and the hormones they produce.

In human populations, malnutrition due to inadequacy of total food intake is the most common occurrence, and the affected population is likely also to be exposed simultaneously to a number of other stressors — disease, insufficient and unsanitary water, and inadequate clothing and shelter. Because no two individuals will have had exactly the same experiences up to the time of study, a wide range of neuroendocrine states exists, and we must turn to animal models to determine which changes are due to malnutrition *per se*. The total body of evidence must be reviewed with understanding that malnutrition can affect the nervous and endocrine systems in a variety of ways. Lack of nutrients can result in:

1. Failure to form, renew, or organize endocrine or neural tissue.

2. Reduced capacity of neuroendocrine tissues to form or secrete a product.

3. Reduced responsiveness of target organs or receptors.

4. Altered rates of degradation or excretion of neuroendocrine substances.

Effects of malnutrition will differ according to the age at which it occurs. Tissues undergoing growth, differentiation, and organization will be especially affected in the young. In animals, severe prenatal and postnatal malnutrition alters hypothalamic and pituitary function; growth hormone production is low, and dwarfing results. Brain size and the number of functional neurons are reduced, resulting in altered behavior patterns. Malnourished infants are apathetic and inattentive. If the female is malnourished before and at the time of conception, the hormone needed for implantation may fail and the ovum may be resorbed. In starved adult animals, and in humans in times of famine, a condition of hypopituitarism develops, thyroid function is diminished, estrus ceases, and males become impotent. In the adult, refeeding usually restores full neuroendocrine function; in the young animal, damage may be permanent.

It is now known that diet can have more subtle effects on neuroendocrine function than had been imagined. New techniques have allowed not only identification of the neurotransmitters but also study of the way in which the balance among them is achieved. The right amounts and proportions of these compounds are needed for smooth functioning of most body processes and for healthy emotional and behavioral states. The idea that diet might alter the balance of transmitters formerly was dismissed on the grounds that the blood-brain barrier prevented direct access of most substances to the central nervous system. There is now clear evidence that lack of dietary tryptophan (using a rat diet based on maize corn) results in lowered brain serotonin content and heightened sensitivity to pain; values of both parameters are retored to normal by injection of tryptophan.[8] High levels of tryptophan in the blood reduce brain tyrosine content and DOPA formation; the subject becomes drowsy and drifts off to sleep. Dietary choline level affects choline and acetylcholine content of the brain. These changes may prove to be one way in which the body signals the brain about its nutritional and metabolic state.

Some of these observations have already found medical application, and further unraveling of the puzzle may lead to improved understanding of the way body states affect behavior and how environmental factors, including nutrition and diet, may impact upon the regulatory processes.

QUESTIONS

1. What are the endocrine glands, and what is a hormone? Why has the pituitary been called the "master gland"? Is the hypothalamus a nervous center, an endocrine tissue, or both? How do the pituitary and hypothalamus relate anatomically? How do they relate functionally?

2. What is meant by "homeostasis"? What are the principal components of a control system? What is meant by "feedback regulation"? Give an example of it.

3. For each of the following endocrine glands, tell what influence their hormone or hormones have on metabolism: adrenal cortex, parathyroid, and thyroid. From your knowledge of previous chapters of this book, what nutrients are of special importance to each of these hormones?

4. Over what periods of time is energy balance regulated? Where is the regulatory center located? How was this proved to be the regulatory center? What changes in the body cause the center to be activated? What mechanisms are involved in long-term regulation of energy balance? How does the gastrointestinal tract participate in regulation of energy balance?

5. What is meant by specific hunger? Is specific hunger genetic or learned? Do

human beings have the ability to select an adequate diet? Justify your answer.

6. If you were a nutritionist or a physiologist, what question relating to food intake regulation would you wish to investigate? What factors do you think might affect a person's preference for specific foods, other than the ones discussed in this chapter? What factors might affect his intake of food?

7. List four ways in which malnutrition can affect the hormonal system. What nutrients have particular effects on the nervous system and under what conditions?

REFERENCES

1. Code, C. F. (ed.): Food and water intake. In *Handbook of Physiology,* Section 6, Volume 1. Baltimore, The Williams & Wilkins Co. for Amer. Physiol. Society, 1967.
2. Novin, D., Wyrwicka, W., and Bray, G. A. (eds.): *Hunger: Basic Mechanisms and Clinical Implications.* Raven Press, New York, 1976.
3. Jordan, H.: Voluntary intragastric feeding: oral and gastric contributions to food intake and hunger in man. J. Comp. Physiol. Psychol., *68*:498, 1969.
4. Bowering, J., Margen, S., and Calloway, D. H.: Failure of men to select a balanced amino acid mixture. J. Nutr., *99*:58, 1969.
5. Harris, L. J., Clay, J., Hargreaves, F., and Ward, A.: Appetite and choice of diet. The ability of the vitamin B deficient rat to discriminate between diets containing and lacking the vitamin. Proc. Roy. Soc. Lond., Ser. B., *113*:161, 1933.
6. Garcia, J., Hankins, W. G., and Rusiniak, K. W.: Behavioral regulation of the milieu interne in man and rat. Science, *185*:824, 1974.
7. Davis, C. M.: Self-selection of diet by newly weaned infants. Amer. J. Dis. Child., *36*:651, 1928.
8. Fernstrom, J. D.: Effects of diet on brain neurotransmitters. Metabolism, *26*:207, 1977.

SUPPLEMENTARY READING

Nervous and Endocrine Systems

Arnaud, C., Glorieux, F., and Scriver, C. R.: Serum parathyroid hormone levels in acquired vitamin D deficiency of infancy. Pediatrics, *49*:837, 1972.

Bergström, S., Carlson, L. A., and Weeks, J. R.: The prostaglandins: a family of biologically active lipids. Pharmacol. Rev., *20*:1, 1968.

Butterworth, C. E., Sauberlich, H., et al.: Symposium: Effects of oral contraceptive hormones on nutrient metabolism. Amer. J. Clin. Nutr., *28*:519, 1975.

Catt, K. J.: ABC of endocrinology. Lancet, *1*:763, 1970.

Delange, F., Camus, M., and Ermans, A. M.: Circulating thyroid hormones in endemic goiter. J. Clin. Endocrinol. Metab., *34*:891, 1972.

Freedland, R. A., Murad, S., and Hurvitz, A. I.: Relationship of nutritional and hormonal influences on liver enzyme activity. Fed. Proc., *27*:1217, 1968.

Gill, G. N.: Mechanism of ACTH action. Metabolism, *21*:571, 1972.

Hamwi, G. J., and Tzagournis, M.: Nutrition and diseases of the endocrine glands. Amer. J. Clin. Nutr., *23*:311, 1970.

Jennings, I. W.: *Vitamins in Endocrine Metabolism.* Springfield, Ill., Charles C Thomas, 1970.

Nathanson, J. A.: Cyclic nucleotides and nervous system function. Physiol. Rev., *57*:158, 1977.

Olson, R. E.: Introductory remarks: nutrient, hormone and enzyme interactions. Amer. J. Clin. Nutr., *28*:626, 1975.

Williams, R. H. (ed.): *Textbook of Endocrinology.* 5th Ed. Philadelphia, W. B. Saunders Co., 1974.

Regulation of Food Intake

Baile, C. A.: Control of feed intake and the fat depots. J. Dairy Sci., *54*:564, 1971.

Baumgardt, B. R., et al.: Symposium: Control of feeding and the regulation of energy balance. Fed. Proc., *33*:1139, 1974.

Belbeck, L. W., and Critz, J. B.: Effect of exercise on the plasma concentration of anorexigenic substance in man. Proc. Soc. Exp. Biol. Med., *142*:19, 1973.

Brobeck, J. R.: Nature of satiety signals. Amer. J. Clin. Nutr., *28*:806, 1975.

Cabanac, M., and Duclaux, R.: Specificity of internal signals in producing satiety for taste stimuli. Nature, *227*:966, 1970.

Durnin, J. V. G. A.: "Appetite" and the relationships between expenditure and intake of calories in man. J. Physiol., *156*:294, 1961.

Hoebel, B. G.: Feeding: neural control of intake. Ann. Rev. Physiol., *33*:533, 1971.

Kekwick, A., and Pawan, G. L. S.: Body weight, food and energy. Lancet, *1*:822, 1969.

Koupmans, H. S.: Jejunal signals in hunger satiety. Behav. Biol., *14*:309, 1975.

Leopold, A. C., and Ardrey, R.: Toxic substances in plants and the food habits of early man. Science, *176*:512, 1972.

Lepkovsky, S., et al.: Symposium: Regulation of food intake. Fed. Proc., *32*:1705, 1973.

McCance, R. A., Chairman: Symposium: The regulation of voluntary food intake. Proc. Nutr. Soc., *30*:103, 1971.

Miller, O. N., et al.: Symposium: Metabolic, hormonal and neural regulation of feeding and its relation to obesity. Amer. J. Clin. Nutr., *30*:741, 1977.

Payne, P. R., and Dugdale, A. E.: Mechanisms for the control of body weight. Lancet, *1*:583, 1977.

Pokiros, K. P., Booth, G. and Varltallie, T. B.: Effect of covert nutritive dilution on the spontaneous food intake of obese individuals: a pilot study. Amer. J. Clin. Nutr., 30:1638, 1977.

Spiegel, T. A.: Caloric regulation of food intake in man. J. Comp. Physiol. Psychol., *81*:24, 1973.

Yaksh, T. L., and Myers, R. D.: Neurohumoral substances released from hypothalamus of the monkey during hunger and satiety. Amer. J. Physiol., *222*:503, 1972.

Malnutrition and the Nervous and Endocrine Systems

Brozek, J.: Malnutrition and behavior. J. Amer. Dietet. Assoc., *72*:17, 1978.

Drummond, T.: Immunohistochemical detection of changes in growth hormone cells in rat pituitaries in protein deficiency. Brit. J. Nutr., *33*:11, 1975.

Enwonwu, C. O., and Glover, V.: Alterations in cerebral protein metabolism in the progeny of protein-calorie–deficient rats. J. Nutr., *103*:61, 1973.

Hoeldtke, R. D., and Wurtman, R. J.: Excretion of catecholamines and catecholamine metabolites in kwashiorkor. Amer. J. Clin. Nutr., *26*:205, 1973.

Kajubi, S. K.: The endocrine pancreas after kwashiorkor. Amer. J. Clin. Nutr., *25*:1140, 1972.

Parsons, P. L., Shrader, R. E., and Zeman, F. J.: Adrenal function in young of protein-deprived pregnant rats. J. Nutr., *106*:392, 1976.

Read, M. S.: Malnutrition, hunger, and behavior. I. Malnutrition and learning. J. Amer. Dietet. Assoc., *63*:379, 1973.

Read, M. S.: Malnutrition, hunger, and behavior. II. Hunger, school feeding programs, and behavior. J. Amer. Dietet. Assoc., *63*:386, 1973.

Siassi, F., and Siassi, B.: Differential effects of protein-calorie restriction and subsequent repletion on neuronal and nonneuronal components of cerebral cortex in newborn rats. J. Nutr., *103*:1625, 1973.

Articles in Nutrition Reviews

Food intake and brain temperature. *28*:17, 1970.

"Overnutrition" and brain function. *29*:190, 1971.

Endocrine adaptation to malnutrition. *30*:103, 1972.

Perinatal undernutrition, postnatal growth, and pituitary growth hormone. *30*:141, 1972.

Effect of famine on later mental performance. *31*:140, 1973.

Tryptophan and the brain. *31*:160, 1973.

Hormones, amino acids, and malnutrition. *31*:306, 1973.

Thyroid function in experimental and clinical undernutrition. *33*:88, 1975.

Brain growth in kwashiorkor. *33*:107, 1975.

The endocrinology of adult protein-calorie malnutrition. *33*:299, 1975.

Nutrition, somatomedin and growth. *35*:150, 1977.

The role of the adrenal cortex in the development of marasmus. *35*:204, 1977.

Effect of somatostatin on exocrine pancreatic function. *35*:210, 1977.

Satiety and body weight regulation in parabiotic rats: a case for a humoral satiety factor. *35*:215, 1977.

Gastrin and glucose homeostasis. *35*:232, 1977.

Growth hormone and sex steroid stimulated growth at puberty. *35*:268, 1977.

Pancreatic structure and function in malnourished rats. *36*:25, 1978.

Chapter 14

Digestion and Absorption of Food

DIGESTION

Why Digestion Is Necessary

Digestion, which takes place in a series of organs known collectively as the alimentary tract, is the *process by which food is prepared for absorption* into the body proper. As eaten, most of the food materials are in the form of complex substances, which are either insoluble in water or of such a nature that they cannot cross the membranes that line the digestive organs and cannot be absorbed into the blood.

Moreover, even if the material could get through the intestinal lining and into the blood stream, the *tissues could make no use of most of these complex substances*, for the cells are so constituted that they use in their life processes only simple substances.* Starch and the more complex sugars are all compounds made by linking together simple sugars (Chapter 3); proteins are complex substances formed by linking together amino acids (Chapter 5); fats are made by the combination of fatty acids with the simple substance glycerol (Chapter 4). The process of digestion is chiefly concerned with breaking down these three classes of foodstuffs into simple *sugars, amino acids, fatty acids,* and *glycerol,* which are the forms in which *food materials are usable by the tissues,* either as energy or for tissue building.

*Tissues can use fat if it is injected into the blood stream, but food fat cannot cross the intestinal barrier without first being broken down into simpler substances. When patients are fed parenterally (bypassing the digestive system and administering nutrients by vein, or intravenously), amino acids, rather than proteins, and glucose, rather than disaccharides or starch, must be given; fat must be very finely emulsified and is not well tolerated. The subject of intravenous alimentation is beyond the scope of this book, but references for individual study are included in the supplementary readings at the end of this chapter.

Digestive System

The alimentary or gastrointestinal (GI) tract is best understood if it is considered as organized for its main functions: *motor, secretory*, and *absorptive*. Muscular activity is required for mixing the food mass with digestive juices and for moving partially digested material from one part of the alimentary tract to another. The GI tract and associated organs (the liver, pancreas, and gallbladder — Fig. 14–1) form the important *digestive fluids,* which are responsible for bringing about the chemical breakdown of foodstuffs. These fluids contain enzymes, electrolytes, and emulsifiers needed for the digestive process and for promoting the absorption of the digestion products. The endocrine cells of the digestive organs secrete *hormones* that regulate the motor and secretory ac-

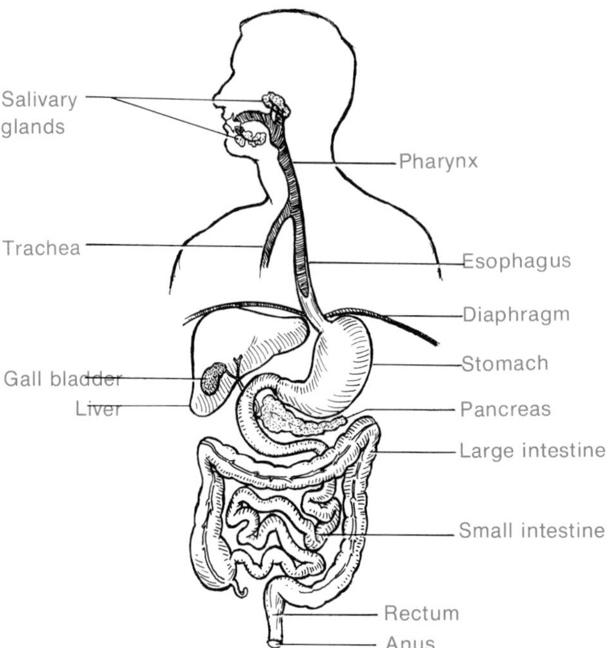

Figure 14–1 Schematic drawing of the digestive system.

tivities of the GI tract itself, and that also participate in blood sugar regulation and the control of food intake (see Chapter 13). All of the available nutrients are finally absorbed and transferred into a rich network of blood and lymphatic vessels (Fig. 14–2).

The structure of the walls of the alimentary canal is essentially similar throughout its whole length — a *mucous membrane* lining the cavity, two coats of *muscular tissue,* one consisting of *circular* and one of *longitudinal* muscle fibers,* and a very thin membrane covering the outside of the tract.

The mucous membrane and its secretion serve to protect and lubricate the more delicate tissues that lie within and below it. The cells of the mucous membrane that lines the digestive tract are constantly renewed, in much the same way as are skin and hair. The lining of the small intestine turns over completely about every 1½ days, which means that this is one of the most rapidly growing tissues of the body. The aged cells are discharged into the digestive tract. These cells (as well as the digestive secretions) are largely recovered in the processes of digestion and absorption, and their constituents are used again by the body just as are nutrients from the diet.

Some of the cells that secrete the digestive enzymes and fluids are located in crypts and glands that lie within the walls of the stomach and intestine; others are located in the pancreas and liver, and their secretions pass through a duct system into the small intestine. Hormone-producing cells are present in the stomach, pancreas, and intestine; the hormones may act locally or be transported by the blood to target tissues elsewhere within and outside the GI tract. The tract also has an extensive network of nerves that both receive and transmit information between the gut and the central nervous system. Motor activity, secretion, and blood flow all are under neural, as well as endocrine, control.

The smooth muscle of the healthy GI tract is never fully relaxed but maintains a steady state of contraction referred to as *tonus.* When the circular muscle fibers

*The stomach has a slightly more complex system of muscular coats, in which there are diagonal as well as circular and longitudinal fibers, so that its movements are more varied than, though generally similar to, the movements of the intestines.

contract, as they do in small, separate segments, they produce a squeezing motion, which presses the contents of the tube closely against its inner wall and churns and mixes the mass in separate segments. When the longitudinal muscle fibers contract, the resulting motion pushes the food mass along the digestive tract. These contractions occur in regular waves that pass along the tract almost always in such a way as to propel the food caudally — that is, from the mouth toward the rectum and its outlet, the anus. Such rhythmical, recurring waves of contraction are referred to as *peristalsis*. Each wave of contraction is preceded by a wave of relaxation, which allows the sequential gut segment to receive the food bolus.

Progress of Food Material Through Digestive Organs

In the *mouth*, food is more or less finely divided by *chewing* and is mixed with saliva, which moistens the food and also produces a chemical action, and with mucus, which assists in lubricating the food for swallowing. The swallowed food mass is carried down the esophagus by peristalsis.

In the *stomach*, swallowed food col-

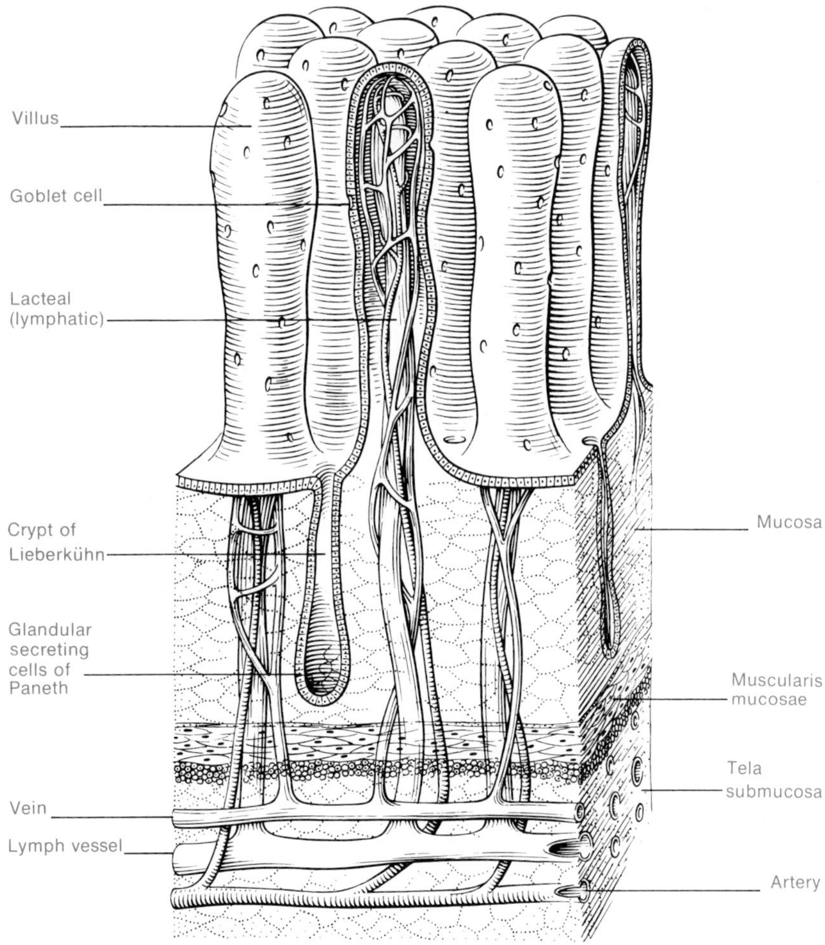

Figure 14–2 Detailed diagram of the absorptive surface of the small intestine, showing the structure of the villi and blood and lymph vessels. Other features of the intestinal wall are indicated by labels at sides of the drawing. The surface epithelial cells of the villi have a characteristic "brush border" of microvilli, which greatly increases the surface area. (From Villee, C. A.: *Biology*, 7th Ed. Philadelphia, W. B. Saunders Co., 1977.)

lects largely in the muscularly inactive upper part (cardiac end), which acts as a reservoir where food may remain for some time before it is gradually pushed along toward the outlet, the pylorus. The portion of the stomach adjoining the pylorus (a circular muscle that guards the opening into the intestine) is muscularly active, and in its wall are situated the glands that secrete the digestive fluid gastric juice. Here the food mass is mixed with gastric juice and churned about until, partly by mechanical means and partly by action of the digestive fluid, it is reduced to a semiliquid state (chyme). From time to time, the pylorus opens and a peristaltic wave sends a gush of the more fluid portion of the stomach contents into the first part of the intestine (duodenum); thus the stomach is gradually emptied. As it empties, the stomach contracts upon itself, so that it is relatively small and usually contains only a little fluid between meals. The rate at which the stomach empties is chiefly dependent on the type of foods that compose the meal. Liquids leave the stomach relatively quickly; concentrated foods are retained longer. In general, carbohydrate-rich foods tend to pass out faster than foods high in protein, and these faster than fatty foods, while mixtures of proteins and fats leave the stomach more slowly than either alone. The average time for the stomach to discharge an ordinary meal is about 3 hours. When the stomach is empty for a long period, strong rhythmical contractions occur, the *hunger contractions*. The inclusion of some fat or fat and protein in a meal delays the onset of these hunger contractions.

Food material that has been passed on from the stomach into the *duodenum* is well mixed with the digestive juices poured in at that point. It is then gradually pushed along into lower portions of the intestine by peristaltic contractions and by further discharges from the stomach. The largest part of the processes of digestion and absorption takes place in the small intestine. These processes are aided by contractions of the intestinal muscles — those of the circular muscle fibers, which divide intestinal segments, thus mixing the contents thoroughly and squeezing them against the intestinal walls; and those of the longitudinal fibers, whose peristaltic movements gradually pass the intestinal contents along toward the opening (ileocecal valve) into the large intestine. By the time the outlet to the large intestine is reached, food material is nearly completely *digested and absorbed*. The length of time required for food material to pass along the small intestine varies with the relative muscular activity of that organ in various persons. Irritating or toxic substances within the intestine, as well as some cathartics, stimulate peristalsis and are the usual cause of diarrhea, a condition in which food residues pass through the intestines so quickly as to be excreted in fluid condition.

The *large intestine* has about twice the diameter of the small intestine but is much shorter and less muscularly active. It acts as a reservoir in which food residues stay for some time and are concentrated by absorption of the large volume of water added in the digestive process. Propulsive motion moves the progressively drier mass into the descending colon and rectum. These propulsive waves are strongest after eating and are enhanced by physical activity. Final evacuation through the anus, an opening guarded by a double ring of circular muscle fibers, is voluntarily controlled in healthy older children and adults and housebroken animals. Food residues and excretory material remain in the colon from 18 to 96 hours, and conditions for bacteria to grow are more favorable here than in any other part of the alimentary tract. Some of these bacteria are beneficial, such as those that manufacture vitamins; others form products that may be absorbed and must be detoxified elsewhere in the body.

Chemical Processes in Digestion

The chemical processes by which foodstuffs are broken down in preparation for absorption and use by the tissues constitute digestion in the narrower, correct use of the term.

In digestion, complex food materials are cleaved into simpler component parts. In the case of very complex substances like proteins and starch, this chemical breakdown takes place gradually, so that a good many intermediate compounds are formed in the process of digestion before the original material is reduced to its simplest components. The long chains of glucose units that constitute starch molecules are gradually broken down by splitting off two sugar groups at a time (maltose molecules), the intermediate compounds being dextrins with smaller-sized molecules. Eventually the dextrins are completely converted to maltose, and the maltose is broken down into the simple sugar, glucose (Fig. 14–3). The very large molecules of proteins are likewise broken down in orderly fashion into those of gradually decreasing size (polypeptides, tripeptides, dipeptides) until they are completely reduced to those amino acids from which they were originally built (as shown diagrammatically in Fig. 14–4).

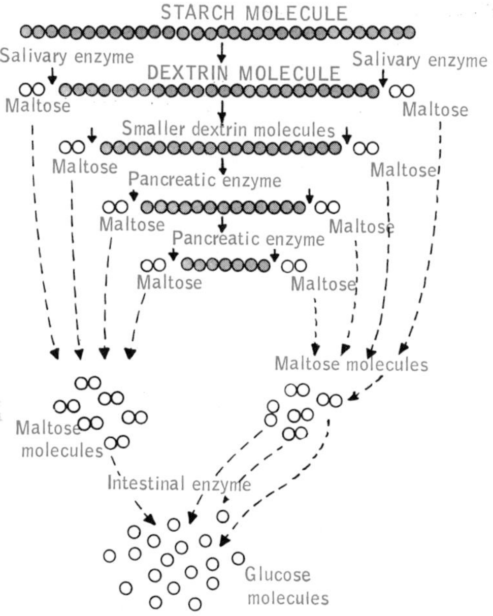

Figure 14–3 Gradual breaking down of large starch molecules by enzymes in digestion. The disaccharide maltose is split off by enzymes in the saliva and pancreatic juice, with smaller and smaller dextrin molecules formed as intermediate products, until the starch has been completely reduced to maltose. An intestinal enzyme then acts on the maltose molecules, splitting them into molecules of the monosaccharide glucose.

Fats, although they have molecules much smaller and simpler than those of starch and protein, are also broken down in a series of steps. The fatty acids are split off one at a time, forming di- and monoglycerides. A good portion of fat is absorbed in the form of monoglycerides; only 40 to 50 percent of the fat is completely broken down into fatty acids and glycerol.

The disaccharides (sucrose, lactose, and maltose) are broken up at a single step into their components — the simple sugars (glucose, fructose, and galactose). The simplest constituents of the diet do not need to be broken down by digestion. This is true of simple sugars, alcohol, and water, which are absorbed in the form in which they are consumed.

The gradual chemical breakdown of proteins and of starch through various intermediate stages until they are finally reduced to their simplest units, and the simpler cleavage of fats and disaccharides into their components during digestion, are summarized in Table 14–1.

Digestive Enzymes

In each instance the splitting of a larger molecule into a number of smaller ones is brought about by means of a chemical reaction with water — a process known as hydrolysis — through the agency of substances called *enzymes*. The same chemical changes take place if proteins, starch, fats, or disaccharides are subjected to prolonged heating with water and acid or alkali in the laboratory. The acid or alkali acts as a catalyst — that is, an agent that speeds up the chemical change merely by its presence. In the body, digestive enzymes bring about these chemical changes more rapidly and at lower temperatures than the catalysts mentioned

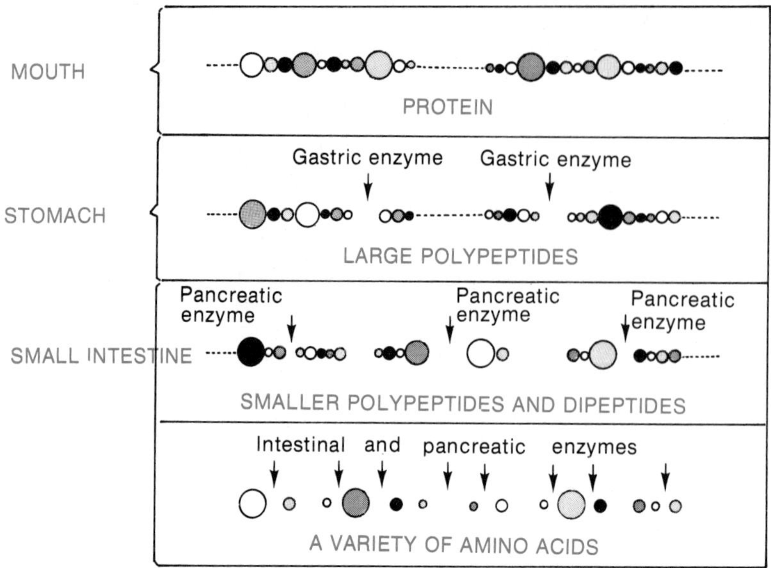

Figure 14–4 Gradual breaking down of the large molecules of protein into their constituent amino acids during digestion, with poly- and dipeptides as intermediate products. The molecules of protein are too large to be represented in this diagram by more than small segments (as indicated by the dotted lines). When digestion is complete, each huge protein molecule is broken down into the different amino acids of which it was composed.

Table 14–1 SUMMARY OF DIGESTION AND ABSORPTION OF THE ENERGY-YIELDING NUTRIENTS

Substrate	*Enzyme Activity*	*Final Products Formed*	*Products Absorbed*
Starch	Salivary amylase (ptyalin)	Dextrins, maltose	
Glycogen	Pancreatic amylase	Maltose	
Disaccharides	Intestinal disaccharidases	Monosaccharides	
Maltose	Maltase	Glucose	In small intestine via blood vessels to liver
Sucrose	Sucrase (invertase)	Glucose and fructose	
Lactose	Lactase	Glucose and galactose	
Monosaccharides			
Hexoses	None		In small intestine via blood vessels to liver
Pentoses			
Protein	Rennin (gastric)	Precipitate of casein	
	Pepsins (gastric)	Polypeptides	
Protein and polypeptides	Trypsin (pancreatic)	Small polypeptides	
	Chymotrypsin (pancreatic)	Small polypeptides	
Polypeptides	Carboxypeptidase (pancreatic)	Amino acid (and peptide residue)	In small intestine via blood vessels to liver
	Aminopeptidase (intestinal)	Amino acid (and peptide residue)	
Dipeptides	Intestinal dipeptidases	Amino acids	
Fats	Salivary lipase	Diglycerides, fatty acids	In small intestine, glycerol and fatty acids of < 10 C atoms via blood to liver; of > 10 C atoms via lymphatics, thoracic duct to blood.
Fats emulsified with bile	Pancreatic lipase	Mono- and diglycerides, fatty acids	
Monoglycerides	Intestinal lipase	Glycerol and fatty acids	
Ethanol	None		In stomach and small intestine via blood to liver and tissues

previously. They do not themselves take part in the chemical processes by which foodstuffs are broken down, but their presence facilitates these processes. Enzymes are catalysts that are formed by living cells,* and the digestive enzymes are formed by the secreting cells of the digestive tract.

Enzymes are typical *proteins,* although of relatively small molecular size. They are formed in the body from the amino acids brought to cells by the blood. Their enzymatic activity is lost if they are exposed to any chemical that renders protein insoluble, or to a degree of heat sufficient to coagulate protein. All enzymes are sensitive to heat and cold; they are destroyed by boiling temperatures, and their activity is suspended by cold. The digestive enzymes all seem to work best at about body temperature (37°C).

Enzymes are *specific* in that each one acts only on a certain type of substance (called a substrate) and brings about only one special chemical reaction. Thus, when a digestive fluid has the ability to act on two or more kinds of foodstuffs, we know that there must be separate enzymes in it for the performance of each of these chemical reactions. Nor are the enzymes in different digestive juices that act on the same kind of foodstuff identical — we know this because they require different working conditions. The enzyme in the gastric juice that acts on protein requires quite a high degree of acidity to be effective, whereas there is a protein-splitting enzyme in the pancreatic juice that works well in either a slightly acid or an alkaline medium. Each of the digestive enzymes has some optimum pH at which it works best and a certain range outside which it will not work at all. Cells located in the stomach secrete strong hydrochloric acid, which after a time acidifies the mixture of saliva and food present, reducing the pH below the optimum for the starch-splitting enzyme present in saliva but optimizing conditions for the action of the proteolytic gastric enzymes. Secretions of the pancreas and intestine are rich in bicarbonate and are therefore alkaline, which neutralizes the acid in the chyme as it leaves the stomach and provides the pH needed for the pancreatic and intestinal enzymes.

In addition to optimum temperature and pH, two other conditions are required for the action of digestive enzymes. One is *surface contact* with the substance acted on, and for this reason intimate mixing of digestive juices with finely divided food material and getting the food material ultimately into solution or colloidal dispersion (as with fats) are important. Also important is the *removal of the products* formed by the reaction. Hence it is only in the small intestine, where the products of digestion are continuously removed by absorption, that conditions are favorable for digestive processes to run to completion.

Enzymes are usually named to indicate the substances on which they act. To this substrate root is added the suffix *-ase,* which indicates that it is an enzyme, and often an adjective is prefixed to show the source of the enzyme. Thus, all protein-splitting enzymes are called *proteases*; fat-splitting enzymes are *lipases* (from the word *lipids,* for fats); and starch-splitting enzymes are *amylases* (from the Latin name *amylum,* for starch). To distinguish between the different enzymes, the starch-splitting enzyme found in saliva is called *salivary amylase* and the one secreted by the pancreas is known as *pancreatic amylase.* Although this system of naming is more descriptive, many enzymes have other names which are well established.

*Enzymes are formed in both plant and animal tissue cells and can facilitate many different types of chemical changes — oxidation, reduction, transfer of some chemical group from one compound to another, splitting off the amino or carboxy radicals, and so on. Practically all chemical reactions in body tissues take place through the action of enzymes. Enzymes and coenzymes, in which various vitamins are incorporated, catalyze the important oxidation-reduction reactions in tissues by means of which foodstuffs yield energy for the body (Chapter 15). Since (as catalysts) they are not used up in the reaction they bring about, a small amount of enzyme can act on a large amount of substance even at high dilutions.

For instance, the salivary amylase is well known by the name of *ptyalin*, while almost everyone is familiar with the names of *pepsin* and *trypsin*, which are respectively gastric and pancreatic proteases (Table 14–1).

Enzymes secreted farther along in the alimentary canal carry on the digestive processes started by those in saliva and gastric juice. Thus, any of the foodstuff that escapes digestion by the action of one enzyme is subjected to digestion by others secreted lower down in the digestive tract, which makes for very efficient utilization.

Fats are insoluble in water, and their digestion is almost entirely dependent on the action of pancreatic lipase (formerly called steapsin). *Bile*, which is formed by the liver and discharged from the gallbladder and liver into the intestine, is important for good digestion of fats, even though it contains no enzymes. Bile acts to emulsify fats and assists in the absorption of the fatty acids formed by digestion so that they are removed from the intestinal contents and digestion goes to completion.

Rennin, contained in the gastric juice, is an enzyme that precipitates milk in solid form (curds). Heat-treated cow's milk and human milk form a finer, more easily digested curd than ordinary cow's milk. Rennin is especially abundant in gastric juice of young animals fed on milk; it is less important in adults.

Secretion of Digestive Fluids

Secretion and motility are stimulated or inhibited by a variety of factors acting in concert. Although all parts of the GI tract are under neural control, the neural component of secretion is more important at the upper levels of the digestive tract, with hormonal agents playing the chief role in the later stages of gastric secretion and secretion at the intestinal level. Control of motility throughout the tract is primarily neural, as is blood flow to and from the gut.

Small amounts of saliva and gastric juice are secreted all the time, but their flow is stimulated when food is present. Factors that stimulate the flow of saliva are chewing, and the taste, sight, smell, or even the thought of food. The latter type of stimulus causes what is known as *psychic secretion*, and the traditional "watering of the mouth" that occurs with odors or thoughts of appetizing food also causes the stomach to secrete more gastric juice in preparation for receiving food. *Appetite* (a psychic factor) thus initiates the secretion of digestive juices. In turn, appetite is influenced, either favorably or unfavorably, by one's state of mind, by companionship, and by the attractiveness of the table service and food, so that all these factors may have an influence on digestion. Fear, anger, worry, other strong emotions, and fatigue all produce undesirable effects on the secretion of gastric juice and have a strong effect on the muscular movements of the alimentary tract.

By far, the strongest stimulus to the secretion of gastric juice results from the presence of food in the stomach; it is mediated by discharge of the vagus nerve and the formation and release of a hormone called *gastrin* in the pyloric glands of the stomach. These agents stimulate the muscular activity of the stomach and the secretion of gastric acid. One of the signals to which the neuroendocrine controls respond is distention of the stomach with food or fluid, and some foods elicit a more copious secretion of gastric juice than others. Meats and meat extract (as in soups made from meat) and dilute alcoholic beverages are thought to have an especially stimulating effect.

The chief stimulus to the secretion of the pancreatic juice and bile comes from the hormones *secretin* and *cholecystokinin*. These are hormones formed in the duodenum in response to substances (acid and the partially digested proteins and fats) present in the chyme discharged from the stomach into the duodenum. Secretin stimulates the formation of pancreatic bicarbonate, the secretion of bile, and the gastric enzyme pepsin. Cholecystokinin stimulates the secretion of pancreatic enzymes, augments the action of secretin, and causes the emptying of stored bile from the gallbladder. The presence of fatty food residues and glucose in the small intestine leads to formation of another hormone, called *gastric inhibitory peptide* (GIP), which, as the name implies, inhibits gastric acid production but also stimulates the production of the hormone insulin. (See Chapter 15.)

Some GI hormones also have tropic action; that is, they stimulate the growth of their target tissues. Gastrin stimulates growth of the gastric mucosa, and cholecystokinin stimulates growth of the exocrine pancreatic tissue. Secretin counteracts the tropic effect of gastrin but augments that of cholecystokinin. When GI hormone secretion is low, as in food deprivation or when patients are fed by vein rather than by mouth, there is thinning or deterioration of these tissues.

Conditions That Affect Digestion

The chief factors that affect digestion may be grouped in the following categories:

1. Nervous or psychological factors
2. General nutritive factors
3. Food factors

Each of these factors acts either *by affecting the motor functions* of the digestive organs, *by exerting an influence on the flow of the digestive juices*, or *by altering the health of the digestive tract itself.* Different conditions exert a favorable or unfavorable influence on digestion, depending on whether they have a stimulating or inhibiting action.

Nervous Factors

Fear, worry, anger, irritation, and stress all exert *unfavorable* influences on secretion and motility. Prolonged tension and suppressed aggression or dependency needs are common in the life experiences of people who develop peptic ulcers. In these persons, emotionality is accompanied by increased acid secretion and gastric blood flow. Others react to fear or sadness with decreased acid production and blood flow.

The reverse conditions exert a *beneficial* influence on digestion through promoting good secretion of digestive fluids and proper muscular activity of the alimentary tract. Peace and quiet, cheerful companionship, appetizing food, and attractive surroundings all favor good digestion.

General Nutritive Factors

Because the lining of the digestive tract is continuously and rapidly being renewed, and because secretions and enzymes are formed constantly and in large volume, the digestive system is particularly susceptible to the effects of poor nutrition. Lack of thiamin is especially likely to be associated with lack of appetite, and diarrhea is one of the typical symptoms of pellagra, a niacin-deficiency disease. Iron deficiency and failure to secrete gastric acid occur together. Protein is needed for formation of digestive enzymes and intestinal cells, as are other vitamins and minerals. Deficiencies of protein and of the B vitamin folacin often result in failure of absorption.

Through these effects on the digestive system, deficiency of one nutrient can impair the utilization of *virtually all* other nutrients. In fact, a person who is in *poor general nutritive condition*, whatever may be its cause, is likely to show the effects of this condition in a *poorly functioning alimentary tract.*

Food Factors

This category includes the factors to which the lay person attributes most of the ills of digestion, but these factors are less important than is usually supposed.

The healthy stomach and intestines can digest any ordinary food or combination of foods without trouble. A few people are unquestionably sensitive to certain foods and are made ill by them, but *food allergy* is not very common and needs to be confirmed by the tests of a physician. The reason many persons experience digestive distress when they eat foods or combinations of foods that they believe will give them trouble is that the apprehension of harm to come is sufficient in itself to alter gastrointestinal motility and blood flow.

Some types of food are digested more slowly than others, and such foods are often spoken of as being "hard to digest." In general, liquids and finely divided foods are those most rapidly handled by the digestive tract. Fats and foods rich in fats (especially mixtures of proteins with fats), foods that are introduced into the stomach in large pieces (and especially in chunks coated with fat), and protein-rich foods that have been made tough in texture by overcooking are digested more slowly but not less completely than other foods.

The *influence of cooking* operates more through making the food palatable and appetizing than through any effect on the nutritive properties or digestibility of the food. Most raw foods are well digested, but starchy foods (especially potatoes) and those that contain tough fiber need thorough cooking in order to rupture the starch granules and to soften the fiber so that the digestive juices can penetrate them. There is seldom more than 5 percent difference between the extent to which raw or poorly cooked foods are ultimately digested and absorbed, and the degree of utilization of the same foods when properly cooked.

Incomplete digestion is likely to result in the formation of *gases* (through bacterial action in the intestine), which may cause pain and distention of the intestines. The diet may be at fault, but the general condition of the individual, nervous or otherwise, is a contributing factor. Some foods, such as legumes, have carbohydrates that are not digested by human enzymes but that are used by bacteria, with formation of gas and other end-products. The intestinal bacteria will attack almost any foodstuff that is not absorbed in the small intestine, so gas formation and, in severe cases, cramping pain and diarrhea always accompany malabsorption. In recent years it has been discovered that many adults and some youngsters have little or no lactase enzyme in the intestine and experience flatulence and softening of stools when they drink *large* amounts of milk or other products containing the milk sugar, lactose. The incidence of this lactase deficiency is higher in American Indian, Asiatic, Mediterranean, and African populations than in Caucasians of northern European extraction. The incidence increases with age and also occurs temporarily or permanently as a result of severe protein malnutrition and of diseases that damage the intestine. People who have this problem can eat cheese without any distress, proving conclusively that sugar absorption is at fault.

Naturally, it is a matter of discretion to take only *small amounts* of the *easily digested foods* if a *digestive upset* or other *illness* has affected the gastrointestinal tract. This is the reason convalescents are given smaller amounts of food at shorter intervals.

ABSORPTION

Absorption is the process by which the products of digestion pass through the lining of the intestine *into the blood* and *lymph.** Simple sugars, amino acids, and short-chain fatty acids are absorbed directly into the blood stream, but the products of fat digestion pass chiefly into the lymph, which is collected through tiny lymph vessels and finally emptied into

*Lymph is a straw-colored fluid that is the intermediary between the blood and the tissues, since the blood is enclosed in blood vessels and does not come directly in contact with the tissue cells.

the blood (via the thoracic duct in the neck).

The *absorption* of food material *takes place almost entirely in the small intestine* and is favored by the fact that the area of the inner surface of this part of the digestive tract is much increased by being formed into tiny projections called *villi* (Fig. 14–2). Each of these villi contains numerous small *blood vessels* and a *lymph space* and is covered with still smaller units (microvilli). Both the blood and lymph are brought very close to the intestinal membrane, and the muscular contractions of the intestine serve to bring its contents into close contact with its wall and to "milk" blood and lymph into and out of the villi. Because chyme is emptied from the stomach gradually and the products of digestion are absorbed as they are formed, the intestine is not overwhelmed with a great surplus of food material to be absorbed at one time.

Anything that makes for either more intimate contact of the intestinal contents with the lining membrane or slower passage of food through the small intestine favors more complete absorption. Incomplete absorption may be the result of an irritated, highly motile intestine that hurries food through too rapidly, of the formation of insoluble compounds in the intestine, or in the case of fat absorption, of lack of bile.

Water-soluble substances can be absorbed by the passive process of diffusion, but in most instances transport is carried out by active or facilitated processes. *Active transport* processes enable absorption of a large amount of nutrient in a much shorter time than would be possible by simple diffusion. In active transport, the absorbing cells perform metabolic work and require energy. Active transport mechanisms have been described for all essential and some nonessential amino acids, for most simple sugars (fructose is an exception), and for some micronutrients. For active transport of sugars and amino acids, sodium is required as well as oxygen, energy sources, and carrier substances within the cell.

The absorption of vitamin B-12 is carried out by a unique process in which *intrinsic factor*, a protein secreted in the stomach, facilitates absorption in the small intestine. Thus, if the glands that produce intrinsic factor are inactive (or if that portion of the stomach is removed surgically), the vitamin B-12 deficiency disease called pernicious anemia develops, even though the diet contains as much vitamin as is normally required (see Chapter 8). Absorption of some nutrients (calcium, for example) depends on the presence of specific carrier substances, usually proteins, in the intestinal wall.

Bile plays an essential role in enabling products of fat digestion and fat-soluble vitamins, which are insoluble in water, to pass through the membrane lining the intestine. Bile salts combine with monoglycerides formed during fat digestion to make compounds that are able to bind with both water and lipids, acting much in the same way as dishwashing detergents, which bind greasy food residues in dishwater. The short-chain fatty acids (10 carbons or fewer) may pass directly into the blood, but those with larger molecules (chains of 16 and 18 or more carbon atoms) pass into the lymph. Fatty acids of intermediate size may enter either system. Rather than being transported in the blood as free fatty acids, however, most fatty acids are re-formed by the cells of the intestine into fats, which are then carried in loose combination with protein.

Normal amounts of mixed food fats are well digested and absorbed by healthy persons. In diseases with associated impairment of lipid digestion and absorption and in experimental studies, differences in the absorbability of various forms have been demonstrated. In general, short-chain fatty acids appear to be better absorbed than those of long-chain length, and unsaturated acids are absorbed better than saturated acids of the same length. Fatty acids may unite with calcium and magnesium ions to form insoluble compounds, resulting in failure to absorb both the mineral and the lipid. This is usually of little significance unless either the diet contains very large amounts of hard fat or absorption is impaired.

Absorption of both calcium and iron (and of some of the other minerals) is adversely affected when the diet includes large amounts of substances that form highly insoluble compounds with these metals. For example, iron and calcium form insoluble salts with phytic acid, which is found in whole-grain cereals; and calcium reacts with oxalic acid found in rhubarb, spinach, and beet tops to form the insoluble calcium oxalate (see Chapter 11). Normally, the diet does not contain enough of these interfering substances to impair nutrition, but these could assume importance if the diet provides only marginal amounts of the nutrients or if absorptive processes are impaired by disease.

Dietary factors can also influence absorption favorably. Iron is more readily absorbed in reduced (ferrous) state than when oxidized (ferric form). Thus, the presence in the diet of factors that promote reduction or prevent oxidation — such as vitamins C and E and antioxidants that are added to fats — favors absorption of iron. Calcium absorption depends on an adequate supply of vitamin D.

Absorption is usually very efficient and complete; the energy nutrients (carbohydrates, fats, and proteins) are about 90 percent digested and absorbed in a mixed diet and under normal conditions. Absorption is less complete when the diet has a very high content of coarse cereal grains, legumes, and other vegetable matter.

Excretion Through the Intestine

The intestinal waste, feces, consists of:

1. *Indigestible, undigested,* and *unabsorbed food residues.*

2. Residues from *digestive secretions, mucus,* and *cell debris* from the lining of the alimentary tract.

3. Small amounts of *material secreted* into the digestive tract.

4. *Bacteria* and the products of their action.

5. *Water.*

The bulk of the feces is made up of water, and food and digestive residues. When the diet has large amounts of animal products and refined cereals, fecal weight is about 100 to 150 gm per day; with coarse diets, fecal weight may be as much as 300 to 400 gm per day. In either case the fecal matter is about 60 to 80 percent water. This reflects the remarkable ability of the intestine to reabsorb water, considering that the daily fluid intake is on the order of 1500 to 2000 ml and that the digestive fluids add up to some 7 *liters* a day. The water content is higher when the fecal material is hurried through the alimentary tract and lower when its excretion is long delayed, owing to further absorption of water in the colon.

Some *mineral salts* (notably salts of calcium and phosphorus) are excreted through the intestinal wall into the lower digestive tract; the main pathway for excretion of excess or unutilized calcium and iron is by way of the intestine. Some of the substances present in bile (e.g., bile salts) are partially reabsorbed and recirculated in the bile; others are degraded in the intestine and excreted in the feces or reabsorbed and excreted in the urine. The *pigment* that gives the feces their brown color is formed from the bile pigment, which in turn comes from hemoglobin. Bile is the major excretory route for cholesterol and is used as a disposal system for some heavy metals and drugs.

About one-tenth to one-third of the feces consists of *bacteria* (both living and dead), and the number excreted per day has been estimated to vary between 50 and 500 billion. The presence of bacteria in the intestinal contents is entirely normal, and some of them may even be beneficial in that they synthesize certain vitamins. (See Chapters 7 and 8.)

Factors Affecting Excretion. We have already discussed some ways in which the nature of the diet affects absorption of specific nutrients and the amount of unabsorbed material passed on to the large intestine; we have also noted the importance of good nutrition in maintaining the health and normal muscular tone of the digestive tract. In healthy persons, almost all the components of a normal diet are nearly completely digested and absorbed, leaving little residue.

The factor that most affects the *volume* of feces passed by normal persons is the amount of *water* retained in the feces. Indigestible substances consumed (chiefly cellulose and other complex carbohydrates) and the growth of intestinal bacteria contribute to *fecal dry matter.* A combination of these influences accounts for the increased bulk of feces formed when the diet contains large quantities of vegetables and fruits, unrefined cereals, and milk, in contrast to large amounts of meat and refined cereals.

About 50 years ago, dietary "roughage" (fiber; see Chapter 3) was considered important for promoting laxation to rid the body of toxins presumed to be formed by the intestinal bacteria (Metchnikoff's theory of autointoxication). With the advent of specific antibiotic therapies, this subject no longer received medical attention, but more recently, interest was reawakened by observations and hypotheses advanced by Burkitt and others to the effect that lack of dietary fiber leads to chronic intestinal disorders, including constipation, inflammation, and cancer.[1] There is no question concerning laxation; the unabsorbed carbohydrates provide a rich substrate for the intestinal bacteria, and some of the end-products of bacterial metabolism stimulate motility. However, there is as yet no direct proof that the diseases in question are caused by lack of fiber or that in its presence the numbers or ratios of intestinal bacteria are altered beneficially, or that mutagenic effects are lessened.[2] Such beneficial effects as have been indicated (reduction of intestinal complaints, lowered serum cholesterol) are associated with administration of sources of pectin and hemicellulose and of cereal brans and gums, but *not* with intake of cellulose. Some caution in the addition of fiber to the diet is needed because of interference with absorption of calcium and the trace elements.

Some foods stimulate intestinal motility in the same way laxative drugs do. Prune juice is especially effective in this respect. Similar but less potent effects are produced by acid fruit juices and cooked pulp of dried fruits. Little information is available concerning the active factors in these foods. Mineral oil softens the feces and is often used as a mild laxative, but its regular use is to be avoided because fat-soluble nutrients are also soluble in mineral oil and are excreted along with this nonabsorbable substance.

Stimuli produced by the presence of feces in the rectum result in the desire and ability to defecate. *Psychic influences,* such as hurry and overanxiety to have a movement daily, have the effect of inhibiting these stimuli and preventing the normal reflex, which causes the colon to contract and expel its contents. Thus, a good many people either have, or think they have, trouble in producing bowel movements with sufficient frequency or regularity. This problem may persist at intervals throughout life, and it is perhaps especially frequent among elderly persons. Constipation can usually be corrected by establishing a regular time for going to the toilet, preferably shortly after breakfast; drinking one or two glasses of water half an hour before breakfast; and increasing consumption of prunes, figs, fibrous vegetables, fruits, unrefined cereals and milk, as well as taking some brisk physical activity.

Diarrhea is another commonly encountered symptom that may be due to many causes: irritant substances or toxins in food, infectious disease, allergy, and so on. Mild, transient cases of diarrhea usually respond favorably to severe restriction of dietary fat, fruits, and vegetables, and to increased consumption of tea in preference to coffee. The loss of fluids and minerals is potentially *very* dangerous, particularly in infants and children.* A physician should be consulted if the condition persists beyond a few hours in infants and more than a few days in adults, or if there are accompanying symptoms such as fever or vomiting.

QUESTIONS

1. What is digestion? Why is it necessary? Describe the alimentary tract and show how it is especially adapted for carrying out the process of digestion.

2. What are the end-products of digestion of proteins, starch, table sugar, and fats? Name the principal digestive fluids that bring about the chemical breakdown of these foodstuffs into their simplest components. Tell where each of these digestive fluids is formed, and give the main functions of each.

3. Chemical changes involved in digestion are brought about or facilitated by the presence of enzymes in the digestive fluids. What is an enzyme? What is meant by saying that enzymes are specific in their action? Name the different enzymes (and substances on which they act) in gastric juice and in pancreatic juice, and those formed in the intestinal mucosa. What is the chemical nature of enzymes, and why is their activity destroyed by boiling? What are the optimum conditions for activity of the enzymes in saliva, in gastric juice, and in the digestive fluids in the intestine?

4. What are the chief factors that stimulate or inhibit the secretion of saliva and gastric juice? Explain the action of hormones in stimulating the flow of the digestive fluids that act on food in the small intestine. What happens to food residues in the large intestine or colon?

5. Describe how absorption of amino acids, simple sugars, and end-products of fat digestion takes place in the intestine. What substances taken in food can be absorbed without being chemically changed in digestion? Explain how bile helps in the digestion and absorption of fats. What substances are found in the residues at the end of the digestive tract — the feces — and what factors alter the consistency and composition of the feces?

6. Discuss the effects that nervous factors, general nutritive condition of the individual, and different types of food eaten have on the relative ease and comfort with which digestion is accomplished; upon the completeness of digestion.

7. What are the main constituents of the feces? Which of these may be described as residues from the contents of the digestive tract? What waste products of metabolism are excreted through the intestine?

*A formula recommended by WHO for emergency oral rehydration is given in Chapter 10, p. 248.

REFERENCES

1. Burkitt, D. P., Walker, A. R. P., and Painter, N. S.: Dietary fiber and disease. J.A.M.A., *229*:1068, 1974.
2. Weininger, J., and Briggs, G. M.: Nutrition update, 1976. J. Nutr. Ed., *8*:172, 1976.

SUPPLEMENTARY READING

Adibi, S. A.: Intestinal phase of protein assimilation in men. Amer. J. Clin. Nutr., *29*:205, 1976.

Barboriak, J. J., and Meade, R. C.: Effect of alcohol on gastric emptying in man. Amer. J. Clin. Nutr., *23*:1151, 1970.

Bayless, T. M. (ed.): Symposium: Structure and function of the gut. Amer. J. Clin. Nutr., *24*:44, 1971.

Booher, L. E., Behan, E., and McMeans, E.: Biological utilizations of unmodified and modified food starches. J. Nutr., *45*:75, 1951.

Calloway, D. H., and Chenoweth, W. L.: Utilization of nutrients in milk- and wheat-based diets by men with adequate and reduced abilities to absorb lactose. I. Energy and nitrogen. Amer. J. Clin. Nutr., *26*:939, 1973.

Castell, D. O.: Diet and the lower esophageal sphincter. Amer. J. Clin. Nutr., *28*:1296, 1975.

Code, C. F. (ed.): Alimentary canal. In *Handbook of Physiology,* Section 6, Vols. II–V. Baltimore, The Williams & Wilkins Co. for Amer. Physiol. Society, 1967–1968.

Cook, G. C.: Effect of systemic infections on glycylglycine absorption rate from the human jejunum in vivo. Brit. J. Nutr., *32*:163, 1974.

Finegold, S. M., et al.: Fecal microbial flora in Seventh Day Adventist populations and control subjects. Amer. J. Clin. Nutr., *30*:1781, 1977.

Floch, M. H. (ed.): Symposium: The exocrine pancreas in human nutrition. Amer. J. Clin. Nutr., *26*:290, 1973.

Floch, M. H. (ed.): Symposium: Diet, bacteria and the colon. Amer. J. Clin. Nutr., *29*:1409, 1976.

Gupta, M. C., Basu, A. K., and Tandon, B. N.: Gastrointestinal protein loss in mild hookworm and roundworm infections. Amer. J. Clin. Nutr., *27*:1386, 1974.

Hazuria, R. S., Sarin, G. S., Srivastava, P. N., Misra, R. C., Bhatt, I. N., and Chuttani, H. K.: Intestinal dipeptidases in primary protein malnutrition. Amer. J. Clin. Nutr., *27*:760, 1974.

Herlihy, P., Stanaszek, W. F., and Covington, T. R.: Total parenteral nutrition. A brief review. J. Amer. Dietet. Assoc., *70*:279, 1977.

Hirschhorn, N., and Denny, K. M.: Oral glucose-electrolyte therapy for diarrhea: a means to maintain or improve nutrition? Amer. J. Clin. Nutr., *28*:189, 1975.

Holdstock, D. J., Misiewocz, J. J., Smith, T., Rowlands, E. N.: Propulsion (mass movements) in the human colon and its relationship to meals and somatic activity. Gut, *11*:91, 1970.

Huang, C. T. L., Gopalakrishna, G. S., and Nichols, B. L.: Fiber, intestinal sterols, and colon cancer. Amer. J. Clin. Nutr., *31*:516, 1978.

Johnson, L. R., Chairman: Symposium: Gastrointestinal hormones: physiological implications. Fed. Proc., *36*:1929, 1977.

Klipstein, F. A., Lipton, S. D., and Schenk, E. A.: Folate deficiency of the intestinal mucosa. Amer. J. Clin. Nutr., *26*:728, 1973.

Kritchevsky, D., and Story, J. A.: Binding of bile salts in vitro by nonnutritive fiber. J. Nutr., *104*:458, 1974.

Lebenthal, E., Antonowicz, I., and Schwachman, H.: Correlation of lactase activity, lactose tolerance, and milk consumption in different age groups. Amer. J. Clin. Nutr., *28*:595, 1975.

MacDonald, I., Chairman: Symposium: Nutrition and enteric disease. Proc. Nutr. Soc., *31*:45, 1972.

Mao, C. C., and Jacobson, E. D.: Intestinal absorption and blood flow. Amer. J. Clin. Nutr., *23*:820, 1970.

McIntyre, N., and Isselbacher, K. J.: Role of the small intestine in cholesterol metabolism. Amer. J. Clin. Nutr., *26*:647, 1973.

Munro, H. N., Chairman: Symposium: Iron absorption and nutrition. Fed. Proc., *36*:2016, 1977.

Nasset, E. S., and Ju, J. S.: Amino acids in gut contents and blood plasma of rats as affected by dietary amino acid imbalance. J. Nutr., *105*:69, 1975.

Ockner, R. K., Pittman, J. P., and Yager, J. L.: Differences in the intestinal absorption of saturated and unsaturated long chain fatty acids. Gastroenterology, *62*:981, 1972.

Paul, D., and Hoskins, L. C.: Effect of oral lactobacillus feedings on fecal lactobacillus counts. Amer. J. Clin. Nutr., *25*:763, 1972.

Rosenberg, I. H., and Scrimshaw, N. S. (eds.): Symposium: Workshop on malabsorption and nutrition. Part I. Amer. J. Clin. Nutr., *25*:1045, 1972.

Rubini, M. E., and Chojnacki: Principles of parenteral therapy. Amer. J. Clin. Nutr., *25*:96, 1972.

Saint-Hilaire, S., Lavers, M. K., Kennedy, J., and Code, C. F.: Gastric acid secretory value of different foods. Gastroenterology, *39*:1, 1960.

Saraya, A. K., Tandon, B. N., Ramachandran, K., and Saikia, B.: Intestinal structure and function in megaloblastic anemia in adults. Amer. J. Clin. Nutr., *24*:622, 1971.

Stephenson, L. S., and Latham, M. C.: Lactose intolerance and milk consumption: the relation of tolerance to symptoms. Amer. J. Clin. Nutr., *27*:296, 1974.

Stephenson, L. S., and Latham, M. C.: Lactose tolerance tests as a predictor of milk tolerance. Amer. J. Clin. Nutr., *28*:86, 1975.

Symposium: Gut microflora and nutrition in the non-ruminant. Proc. Nutr. Soc., *32*:41, 1973.

Walker, A. R. P.: Effect of high crude fiber intake on transit time and the absorption of nutrients in South African Negro schoolchildren. Amer. J. Clin. Nutr., *28*:1161, 1975.

Watts, J. H., et al.: Fecal solids excreted by young men following the ingestion of dairy foods. Amer. J. Dig. Dis., *8*:364, 1963.

Williams, R. D., and Olmstead, W. H.: The manner in which food controls the bulk of the feces. Ann. Intern. Med., *10*:717, 1936.

Articles in Nutrition Reviews

Amino acid, dipeptide, and protein absorption in human beings. *31*:272, 1973.

Oxaluria in patients with ileal dysfunction. *31*:308, 1973.

Diet, intestinal flora and colon cancer. *33*:136, 1975.

Gastric emptying, pancreatic and biliary secretion during digestion. *33*:169, 1975.

Malnutrition, salivary volume and protein concentration. *33*:178, 1975.

Effects of oral and parenteral feeding on pancreatic enzyme content. *33*:187, 1975.

Pharyngeal lipase activity in man. *33*:205, 1975.

Bile acid excretion. *33*:285, 1975.

Total parenteral nutrition. *34*:90, 1976.

Small intestine, stress and adaptation. *34*:107, 1976.

Oral pancreatic supplements to correct pancreatic malabsorption. *35*:190, 1977.

Nutritional significance of lactose intolerance. *36*:133, 1978.

Chapter 15

Metabolism and Excretion

Metabolism is a *general* term to designate all the *chemical changes that occur in living matter in the course of its vital activities.* These changes are of two kinds — anabolic and catabolic. *Anabolism* includes all chemical changes by which the absorbed products of digestion are used to *replace* substances broken down during life processes and to build new tissues in growth. *Catabolism* refers to processes by which nutrients, reserve tissue material, and cellular substances are broken down into chemically simpler compounds with the liberation of energy. In catabolism, energy-yielding nutrient and tissue components are oxidized by a series of biochemical reactions, ultimately yielding carbon dioxide, water, some nitrogen compounds (from protein catabolism), and energy. Part of the energy released by catabolism is used as the source of energy for anabolism, and the remainder is used to accomplish the chemical and physical work of the organism. Heat, used to maintain body temperature, is the final product of this energy expenditure.

Discussion in this chapter is limited to the metabolism of the three main nutritients in food — proteins, carbohydrates, and fats. Much is known about the intermediate compounds formed in the catabolism of these three nutrients, the enzymes and coenzymes involved in bringing about these chemical changes, and the ways in which intermediate products may be built into other substances as needed by the body. This chapter presents a simplified version of this information.

It should be emphasized that the body constituents are in a *dynamic state,* with both diet and body tissues contributing to a common metabolic pool in which the chemical compounds from each source are functionally indistinguishable. Thus, when the fate of glucose is being discussed, for example, it includes both the glucose coming from the diet and that coming from the tissues. It is possible to demonstrate this dynamic state and to measure the size and activity of the common metabolic pool by analyzing the metabolism of compounds containing isotopic elements — such as heavy or radioactive forms of carbon, hydrogen, and nitrogen.

Cells: Functional Units of Metabolism

All living matter is composed of cells and cell products. Metabolism of carbohydrate, fat, and amino acids derived from protein takes place within the cells of the body. The structural components of the cell are important functional elements in this process. (See Fig. 15–1).

Membranes subdivide the cell into compartments and regulate the passage of substances into, out of, and within the

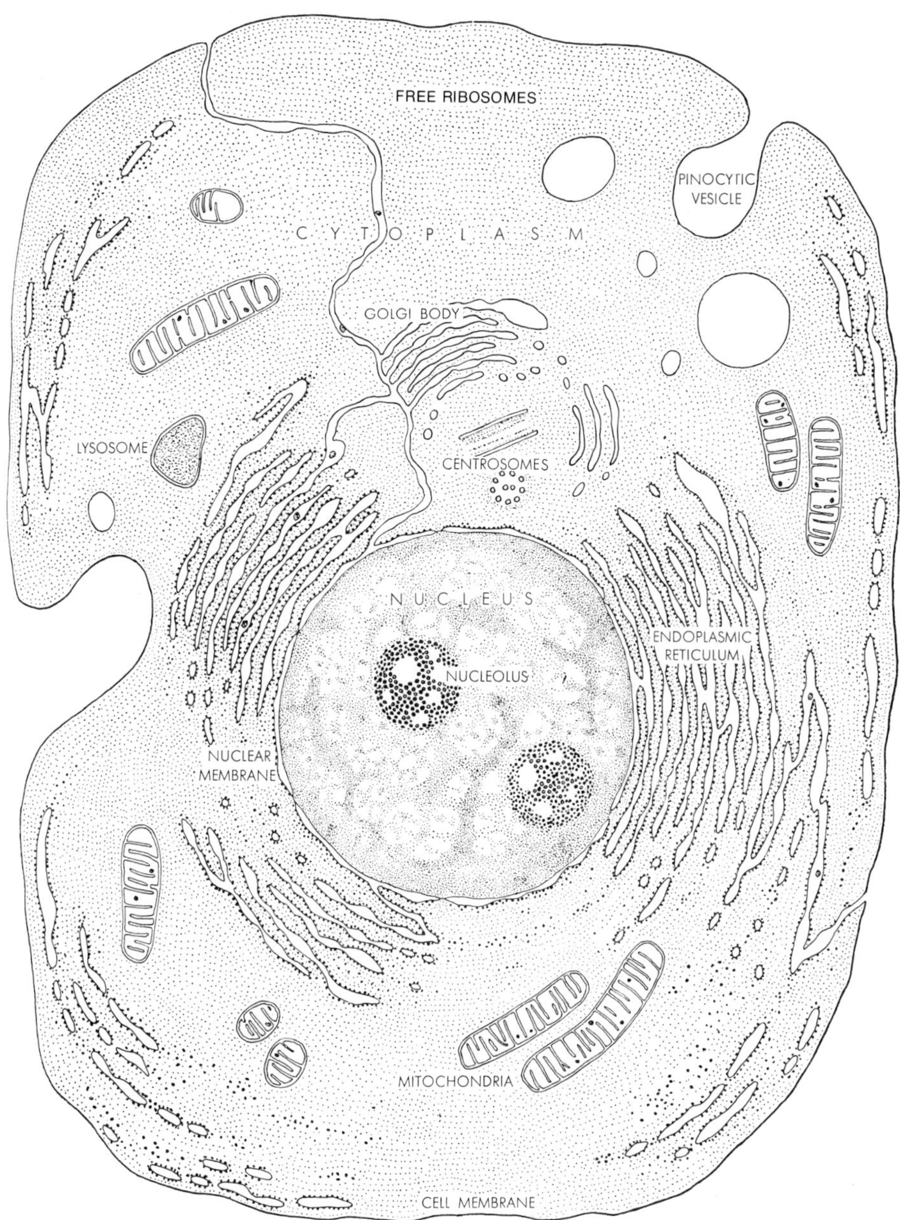

Figure 15–1 A typical cell. Cells are highly variable in structure and function. Within the human body there are many different cell types, such as the striated muscle cell, the smooth muscle cell, the nerve cell, the liver cell, and the sperm cell. However, all cells have certain structural constituents in common, though they may vary in appearance and quantity. These similarities give rise to the concept of the typical cell. (Modified from The Living Cell, by Jean Brachet. Copyright © 1961 by Scientific American, Inc. All rights reserved.)

cell. The membranes include those of the endoplasmic reticulum, the mitochondria, the golgi body, and the lysosomes, as well as those surrounding the nucleus and the cell itself. For example, the cell membrane separates the cell from the external environment and selectively controls the rate of movement of nutrient and waste material into and out of the cell. Generally, large molecules do not pass directly through the cell membrane; however, they may be taken into the cytoplasm by engulfing the molecule in a pinocytic vesicle. The endoplasmic reticulum acts, in part, to transport substances through the cell to the exterior (e.g., the secretion of plasma proteins). All the cell membranes (including those surrounding organelles) are composed of lipid and protein arranged in such a fashion that both water-soluble and lipid-soluble substances can pass through the membranes. Often the membranes contain specific receptor molecules, which permit hormones to act. Enzymes important in mediating such hormone action, as well as those facilitating the transport of nutrients and wastes, are located within the membranes of the cell.

Simply, most cells consist of a *nucleus* and a surrounding *cytoplasm* with its organelles. The *nucleus plays a coordinating role* in the organization and perpetuation of the cell. The deoxyribonucleic acid (DNA) within the nucleus directs the synthesis of all cell proteins by means of messenger ribonucleic acid (RNA), which carries the information to the protein-synthesizing sites in the cytoplasm, the ribosomes. The DNA duplicates itself during cell division so that each cell of an organism obtains identical genetic information in the form of chromosomes containing the DNA. Thus, an intimate link exists between genetic inheritance and the capacity of the cell to synthesize specific proteins, such as enzymes, which will permit specific reactions to occur in the cells. The nucleolus is the site of origin of the ribosomes, which also contain RNA.

In the cytoplasm, the messenger RNA becomes attached to ribosomes. Amino acids are then linked together according to the genetically determined composition of the messenger RNA, and a protein is made. Proteins for intracellular use are made by ribosomes present in the cytoplasm. Some of the ribosomes are attached to the endoplasmic reticulum, and the proteins made by these ribosomes are secreted from the cell. In some cells much of the endoplasmic reticulum is free of ribosomes (smooth endoplasmic reticulum) and is thought to be involved in synthesis of complex lipids (e.g., cholesterol) and glycogen as well as in the detoxification of a variety of compounds. The golgi body stores cell products prior to their secretion and appears to participate in the synthesis of complex carbohydrates (e.g., glycoproteins) for secretion.

The membrane-rich *mitochondria* are the *sites of the final oxidation of nutrients* into carbon dioxide and water with the generation of energy. Approximately 40 percent of the energy released can be used to synthesize the high-energy phosphate bonds of adenosine triphosphate (ATP; see Fig. 15–2). The remainder of the energy is released as heat. The ATP formed provides energy for the anabolic reactions in the cell. The lysosomes of the cell contain, within a membrane, enzymes capable of splitting important complex compounds such as proteins, nucleic acids, and polysaccharides. Disruption of the membrane frees the enzymes, and the cell digests itself. In the body, the death of individual cells and their replacement by means of cell replication occur in the normal course of events.

THE FATE OF ENERGY NUTRIENTS IN THE CELL

The initial phases of carbohydrate, fat, and amino acid catabolism proceed more or less independently of each other to yield identical two- and three-carbon intermediates. From this common metabolic pool of intermediates, carbohydrate, fat, and protein can be synthesized, or the intermediates can be further oxidized to carbon dioxide and hydrogen atoms by the citric acid cycle enzymes. It is the oxidation of the hydrogen atoms to water by a series of enyzmes called the electron transport system that is the primary source of ATP production for the cell (see Fig. 15–3).

Each metabolic reaction is catalyzed by a specific enzyme (a protein that increases the reaction rate). Often cofactors are required for the reactions to proceed.

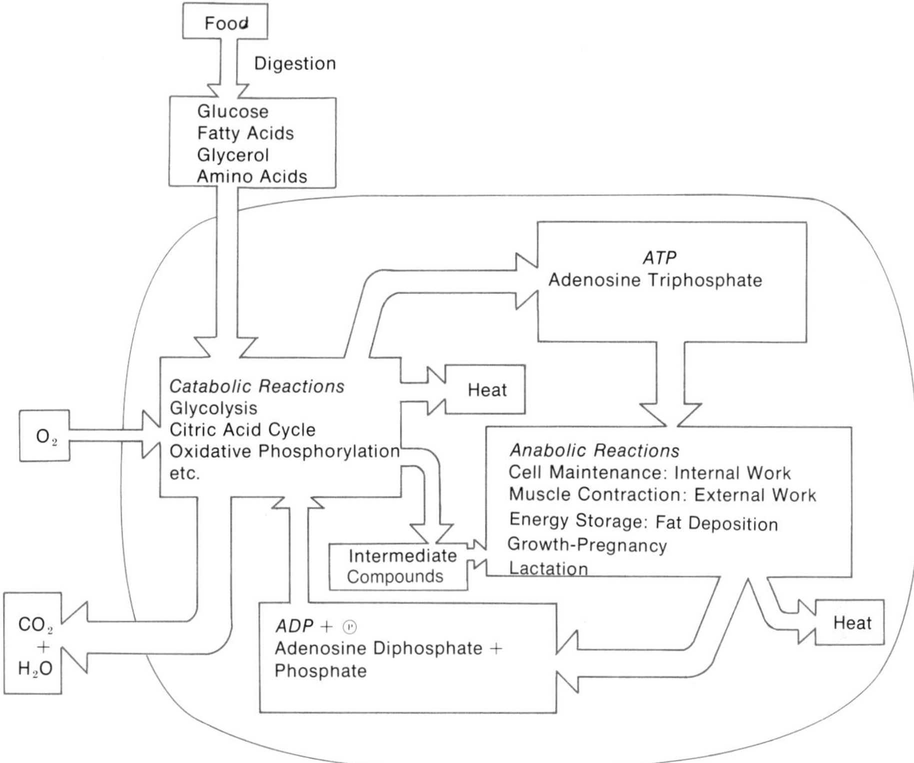

Figure 15–2 Diagrammatic interpretation of the role of adenosine triphosphate (ATP) in the cell. Whenever energy-producing reactions take place, such as the oxidation of glucose to carbon dioxide and water, some of the energy set free goes into forming ATP by the addition of a high-energy phosphate bond to adenosine diphosphate (ADP). The energy for anabolic reactions, whereby simpler groups or compounds are built into larger, more complex molecules, is supplied by the splitting of a high-energy phosphate bond of ATP, leaving ADP plus a free phosphate group. Thus, in the cell ATP acts as a messenger between those reactions that supply energy and those that utilize energy. Heat is a by-product of metabolism; it warms the body but is of no value as a source of internal or external work.

These nonprotein substances are usually common to a number of enzymes. Cofactors frequently contain vitamins, such as pantothenic acid, thiamin, riboflavin, and niacin, as part of their structure. Thus, deficiencies of the vitamins may profoundly change the course of metabolism. Mineral elements, such as iron, copper, and magnesium, are also cofactors for some metabolic enzymes. (See Chapters 8, 11, and 12). The enzymes required for the chemical reactions shown in Figure 15–3 are not necessarily present in all cells. Furthermore, the entry of nutrients into cells and their subsequent metabolism are often regulated by hormones (see Chapter 13).

The Citric Acid Cycle and Oxidative Phosphorylation

The *citric acid cycle* is the *common final oxidative pathway* for the intermediate compounds of carbohydrate, fat, and protein catabolism. It is also known as the tricarboxylic acid cycle or the Krebs cycle (named after the man who first worked it out). The carbon compound to be oxidized as the end-product in all three pathways is acetic acid, which is presented to the citric acid cycle in the form of acetyl-CoA (Fig. 15–3). For example, pyruvic acid from the breakdown of carbohydrates must enter the mitochondria and be converted to acetylcoenzyme A before enter-

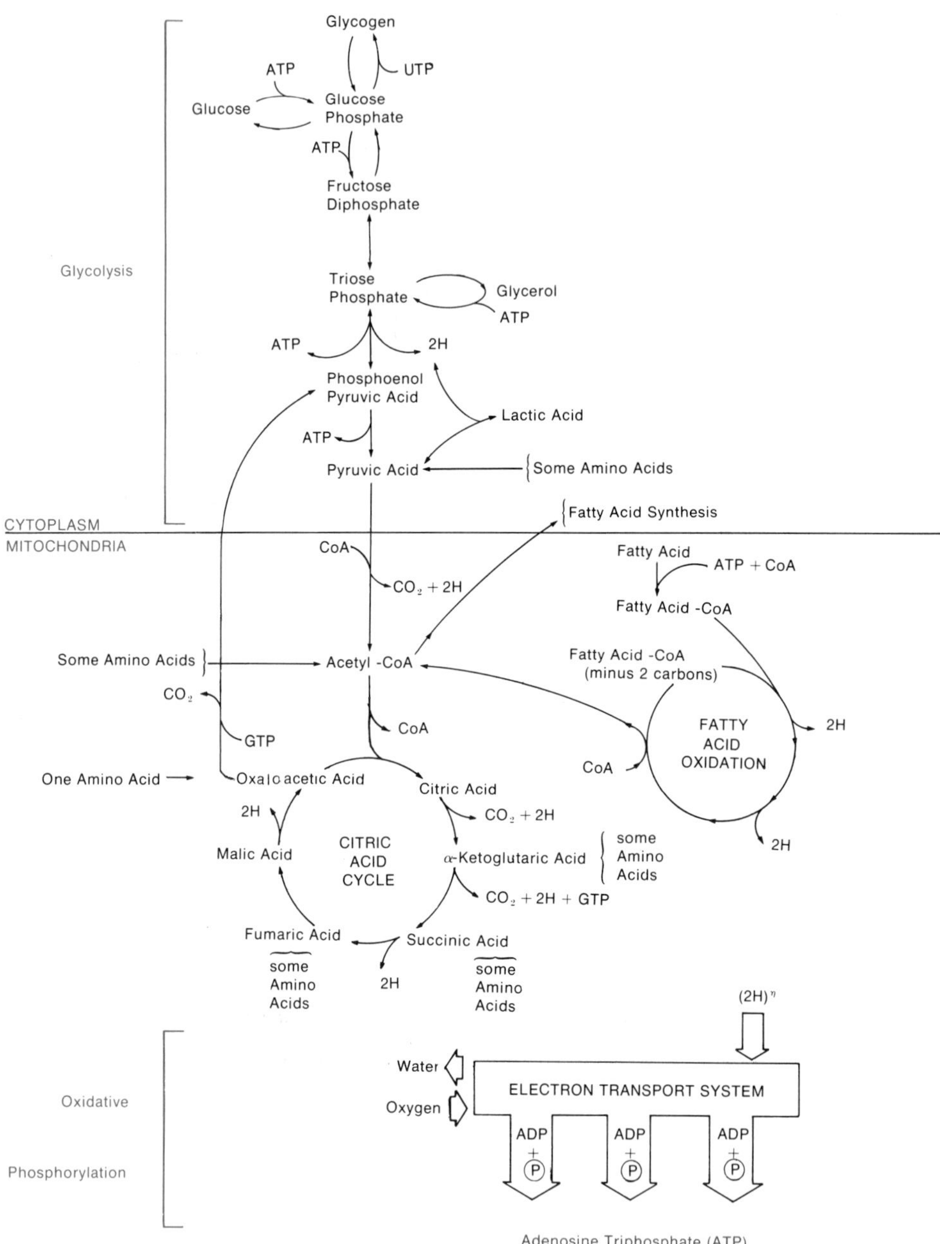

Figure 15–3 This is a simplified illustration of some of the interactions in carbohydrate, fat and protein metabolism. Acetyl-CoA (CoA contains the vitamin pantothenic acid) serves as an important central compound in the metabolism of these nutrients. ATP acts as an intermediary between the energy-producing and the energy-consuming reactions of the cell (See Fig. 15–2; the end-products of the use and the precursors of the synthesis of ATP are not shown in order to simplify the diagram). GTP (guanosine triphosphate) and UTP (uridine triphosphate) are compounds with high-energy phosphate bonds similar to ATP. The hydrogen atoms (2H) produced in metabolism (these are carried by coenzymes containing riboflavin or niacin) are generally oxidized by the electron transport system, which is the major site of ATP production for the cell. Cell compartmentalization of the various sequences of reactions is essential for the life of the cell.

ing the citric acid cycle. The formation of acetyl-CoA from pyruvic acid requires five enzymes and five coenzymes, four of which each contain a different vitamin (pantothenic acid, thiamin, niacin, and riboflavin). The coenzyme A (CoA) contains pantothenic acid as part of its structure. The CoA is released when the two-carbon acetic acid combines with the four-carbon oxaloacetic acid to begin the cycle with the formation of citric acid, a six-carbon compound.

The citric acid cycle is represented in Figure 15–3. The diagram omits a few intermediate substances but includes all steps at which hydrogen atoms, carbon dioxide, or ATP is formed. The reactions by which carbohydrate, glycerol, fatty acids, and amino acids enter the cycle are shown in abbreviated form. The cycle moves only clockwise, starting with citric acid and ending with oxaloacetic acid. Each revolution accomplishes the degradation of one molecule of acetic acid to carbon dioxide and water. At the end, a molecule of oxaloacetic acid is left, free to combine with another acetyl-CoA to form citric acid and start the cycle again.

The hydrogen atoms formed in the citric acid cycle are transported as coenzymes (containing either niacin or riboflavin) to a nearby set of enzymes called the electron transport system. The hydrogen is oxidized to water with oxygen by this system of enzymes. Some of the energy released by the oxidation of a pair of hydrogen atoms can be used to synthesize three high-energy phosphate bonds of ATP. This process is referred to as *oxidative phosphorylation* and is the *major source of the ATP needed* as the driving force *in many anabolic reactions* in cells. The complete set of citric acid cycle enzymes is found in proximity to the electron transport enzymes within the mitochondria of the cell.

Carbohydrates

Glucose is the main product of carbohydrate digestion. Within the tissue cells, the first phase of the breakdown of glucose takes place in the cytoplasm of the cell. This series of ten chemical reactions is known as *glycolysis,** the *anaerobic stage* of carbohydrate catabolism. It consists of the conversion of glycogen (the storage form of glucose in the body) or glucose to pyruvic acid, which under conditions of adequate oxygen is converted to carbon dioxide and water. In anaerobic conditions (limited oxygen supply), the conversion of pyruvic acid to lactic acid is necessary for the regeneration of a niacin-containing coenzyme (NAD), so that glycolysis can continue to produce ATP. (See Fig. 15–3.)

During glycolysis only a small amount of the potential energy of glucose is set free, but it is sufficient to permit a muscle to operate temporarily when oxygen is not brought to it fast enough by the blood. When an adequate oxygen supply is restored, only about a fifth of the accumulated lactic acid is converted into pyruvic acid and then further catabolized by the citric acid cycle; the rest is conserved by resynthesis into glycogen (Fig. 15–4).

The anabolic formation of glucose from the intermediate compounds of metabolism is called *gluconeogenesis*. In addition to lactic acid, the glycerol moiety of fat and some of the amino acid intermediates can be used to make glucose and glycogen in the body (see Fig. 15–3).

These biochemical reactions must be carefully regulated in the body in order to insure the maintenance of an adequate concentration of glucose in the blood. Glucose homeostasis is particularly critical for the brain (central nervous system), which requires a continuous supply of glucose. Most tissues of the body can use

*There are several other pathways through which carbohydrates may pass. The amount of traffic over a given pathway varies, depending on hormonal influences, tissue conditions, and the need for specific intermediate compounds. For example, glucose is oxidized to a variable extent by a shunt pathway in which pentoses are formed (such as ribose needed for building nucleic acids and ATP), as well as a coenzyme (containing niacin) required in several steps of fatty acid and steroid synthesis.

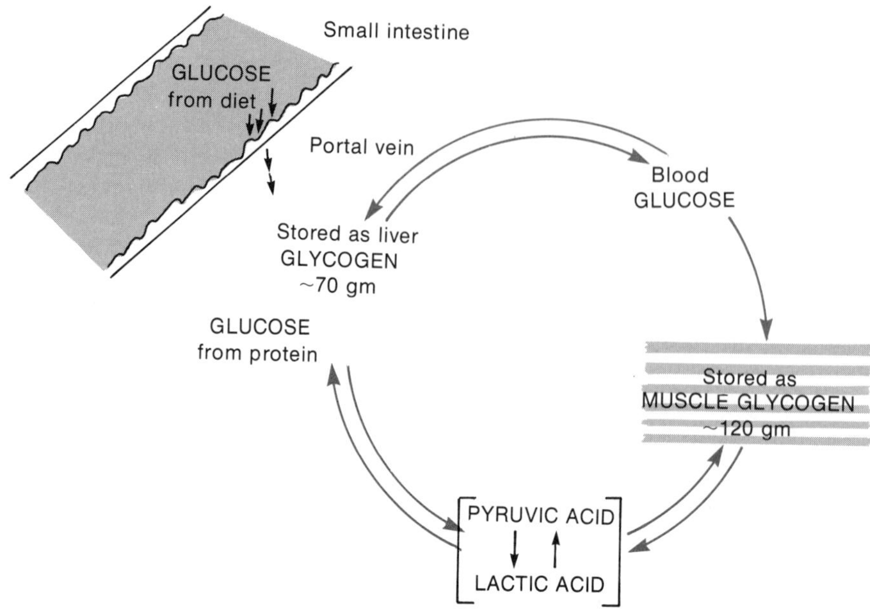

Figure 15–4 General scheme of anaerobic carbohydrate metabolism. This provides for the production of some ATP even though the oxygen supply to the body is limited. When the oxygen supply is adequate, pyruvic acid is oxidized completely via the citric acid cycle to provide energy for metabolism. The lactic acid that is produced during short-term oxygen shortage is largely (80 percent) converted to glycogen on restoration of an adequate oxygen supply.

other energy sources, such as amino acids and fats. However, if the blood glucose supply to the brain falls below a critical concentration, unconsciousness will result; if glucose is not provided, death will follow.

There are a number of ways in which the body obtains and regulates blood glucose. The products of digestion of carbohydrates — chiefly glucose, with smaller amounts of fructose and galactose — are absorbed from the intestine into the blood, which passes directly to the liver. The liver has the ability to remove excess glucose from the blood and to take up and metabolize fructose and galactose (since only glucose is found in significant amounts in the general circulation). Thus, after a meal rich in carbohydrates, a great deal of glucose appears in the portal vein, but the glucose content of the blood in circulation in the rest of the body is only slightly increased and soon returns to its remarkably constant level.

The *liver* is the regulator of the blood sugar and the main storage house for carbohydrate in the body. It takes the simple sugars brought to it from the intestine and combines them to form the more complex and less soluble carbohydrate, *glycogen* (see Chapter 3). This name, meaning "sugar former," was given to this compound because whenever the body needs extra glucose, the glycogen can be reconverted into glucose and released into the blood. In this way, the liver acts as a reservoir to keep the body from being flooded with glucose just after meals and from running short of it at other times. Tissues continually withdraw glucose from the blood for their own uses, and the glycogen in the liver must be reconverted to glucose (glycogenolysis) to maintain blood glucose at the normal level.

The *muscles* also can store glycogen. Even though muscle glycogen can be readily drawn on for the energy needed for muscular work, liver glycogen is the only reservoir from which the glucose of the blood can be replenished. The amount of glycogen in the liver and muscles naturally depends somewhat on whether the supply of carbohydrate (or of energy in other forms) in the diet has been liberal or scanty, but there is an upper limit beyond which no more glycogen is normally stored.

Dietary *carbohydrate* in excess of the relatively small amount that can be converted into glycogen *is stored as fat* in the fatty (adipose) tissues of the body. In the case of a lack of food, the glycogen stores are practically exhausted in 1 to 2 days, after which the body draws largely on its reserves of fat and muscle protein for energy. The limited stores of glycogen in liver and muscles serve as short-interval energy reserves, while the main depots of extra fuel are the fat deposits in various parts of the body.

Blood Sugar Regulation. In healthy individuals, the blood sugar concentration is normally controlled within the range of 70 to 150 mg per 100 ml of blood (sometimes written as 70 to 150 mg%). The concentration of blood glucose is the result of the equilibrium between the rate of entry of glucose into the blood and the rate of glucose uptake by the tissues (removal from the blood). This process is regulated by the available supply of glucose, as previously discussed, and by the homeostatic influence of hormonal regulation (see Chapter 13 for a general discussion of hormonal control).

Insulin has a central role in the regulation of blood glucose. It is produced by the pancreas and is secreted when the blood glucose levels exceed 80 to 100 mg per 100 ml. It increases the rate of glucose uptake by insulin-sensitive tissues, such as adipose (fat) and muscle tissues, thereby reducing the level of blood glucose. *Glucagon* is another hormone secreted by the pancreas (by a different type of cell), but the stimulus for secretion of this hormone is a lowered level of blood glucose. The primary function of glucagon is to promote the breakdown of glycogen into glucose in the liver, thus raising the level of blood glucose. Glucagon acts with insulin to control the extent of the daily fluctuations of blood glucose imposed by the marked changes in glucose supply due to the fasting-feeding cycles within the day. The appropriate hormone is secreted and acts within a few minutes of a change in blood glucose to restore the blood concentration to normal. For example, in a short fast the liver, under the influence of glucagon, is able to release sufficient glucose to supply the brain and to maintain the blood glucose concentration at about 80 mg per 100 ml. Following a meal containing carbohydrates, glucose is absorbed from the intestine, transported to the liver in the portal blood, and overflows to some extent into the general circulation. This rise in blood glucose causes a decrease in glucagon secretion by the pancreas and an increase in insulin secretion, resulting in deposition of glycogen in liver and muscle and an accelerated conversion of glucose to fat in adipose tissue. The blood glucose concentration does not usually increase above 130 mg per 100 ml. During exercise, glucose uptake and utilization by muscle is increased, but the blood glucose levels are maintained in an acceptable range by the action of glucagon released from the pancreas.

Other hormones also influence blood glucose concentrations. Under stress conditions, *epinephrine* is immediately released from the adrenal gland and causes blood sugar to rise by stimulating the breakdown of liver glycogen to glucose. Epinephrine, unlike glucagon, also facilitates conversion of muscle glycogen to lactic acid, which may be converted to glucose in the liver. *Cortisol,* a steroid hormone from the adrenal gland, acts more slowly than epinephrine to depress glucose utilization by muscle, to promote the release of amino acids from the muscle, and to promote gluconeogenesis in the liver (from the deaminated amino acids). All these actions tend to raise blood glucose levels. *Growth hormone,* secreted from the pituitary, blocks insulin action, particularly in the muscle, and as a result raises the blood glucose level. However, growth hormone, unlike cortisol, stimulates the uptake of amino acids by the muscle, thereby promoting anabolism.

Thyroid hormones (thyroxine and triiodothyronine) affect the metabolism of virtually all the tissues of the body. Their net effect is to favor elevation of blood glucose. This appears to be a complex function consisting of action on intestinal absorption and on general metabolism, and of influences on other hormones.

The complexity of the blood glucose–regulating system is apparent. A disturbance in any one of the factors may result in faulty maintenance or adjustment of blood glucose levels. In the disease *diabetes mellitus* there is a deficiency of or insensitivity to insulin, resulting in excessively high blood glucose levels. As muscle and other insulin-sensitive tissues are unable to use this glucose, the body must provide fatty acids to meet the energy needs of these tissues. In the absence of adequate carbohydrate metabolism, fat oxidation is not fully completed, and incompletely oxidized products (ketones) accumulate. In severe diabetes, the combination of elevated blood glucose level and ketones results in a sequence of events leading to coma and death if insulin is not provided. In adults a milder form of diabetes occurs more commonly, usually in association with obesity. Blood sugar levels are high, but ketosis is rare in this type of diabetes; the disease can usually be controlled by reducing body weight to normal, increasing exercise, and avoiding sugar-rich foods.

While many hormones (glucagon, epinephrine, cortisol, growth hormone, thyroid hormones) act to insure adequate blood levels of glucose, insulin is the only hormone preventing excess accumulation of glucose. Thus, it is not surprising that hypoglycemia, the state of having abnormally low blood glucose, is relatively rare. The most common form of hypoglycemia occurs in diabetics who accidentally take too much insulin. In other very rare instances (for example, an insulin-producing pancreatic tumor or severe liver disease) hypoglycemia will be present as one symptom in a constellation of symptoms typical of these diseases. Some few individuals have hypoglycemia that has no evident organic basis. This functional hypoglycemia is diagnosed by a finding of very low blood sugar levels (30 to 40 mg per 100 ml) 3 to 5 hours after administration of a test dose of glucose *and* the simultaneous presence of characteristic symptoms (tremors, etc.). This functional disorder usually responds to simple dietary management, including more frequent, small meals (5 or 6 a day) containing generous amounts of protein-rich foods, and avoidance of free sugars.

Fats

Fats, being insoluble in water, require a special system for transportation in blood, an aqueous medium. Triglycerides, phospholipids, and cholesterol are combined with globulin proteins and carried to the tissues as lipoprotein complexes. Chylomicrons are the largest of the lipoprotein complexes and are basically large fat droplets covered with a very thin protein layer. After a meal rich in fats, plasma becomes turbid from the chylomicrons formed in the intestine, which are taken up by the lymph system and released into the blood; but this extra fat leaves the blood and passes into the tissues within a few hours. The liver is the primary site of synthesis of the other lipoproteins. These particles are the means of fat transport to the tissues from the liver; they are smaller than chylomicrons and contain varying amounts of protein, from 10 to 60 percent of their weight. These lipoproteins are separated into three classes according to their density, which is related to the ratio of fat to protein in the particles. These classes are (beginning with those with the highest fat to protein ratio) very low-density lipoprotein (VLDL), low-density lipoprotein (LDL), and high-density lipoprotein (HDL). While physically distinct, there are many complex metabolic relationships between these lipoprotein classes. Disorders in lipid metabolism will result in changes in the blood concentration of one or more of these lipoprotein classes. A small amount of free fatty acids is always present in the blood and is bound to the albumin protein of the blood for transport from adipose tissue. Free fatty acids are thought to be the most active form of lipids involved in metabolism. Their concentration in the blood is affected by the mobilization of fat from fat depots and by the action of several hormones.

The liver and adipose tissue are the main sites for fat metabolism, but other tissues can also perform the same chemical transformations. Dietary fat is changed into various related fatty substances that the body cells either need for their structure or can readily use for energy production. Thus, some fat may be transformed into phospholipids; saturated fatty acids may be converted to unsaturated ones and vice versa; and fats not characteristic of the animal may be converted into the molecular arrangement needed for storage in the tissues.

Most of the fat ingested is used as *body fuel*. Formerly it was thought that carbohydrate was the main source of energy used by the tissues, but it is now known that fat also performs this function. In fact, it is now known that even the brain and other nervous tissues are not totally dependent on glucose for energy.

The final *end-products of fat oxidation* are the same as those formed by the complete oxidation of glucose — namely, *carbon dioxide* and *water*. The intermediate steps are very different, and the amount of energy liberated is two and one-quarter times as great as would be produced by oxidizing an equal weight of glucose.

Initially, fats must be broken down into glycerol and fatty acids, which follow different chemical paths of catabolism. *Glycerol* is transformed in the cytoplasm of the cell into a triose (three-carbon sugar) phosphate intermediate of glycolysis. The triose phosphate can be used to make glucose, or it can be oxidized to carbon dioxide and water via the citric acid cycle (Fig. 15–3). The *fatty acids*, with their long chains of carbon atoms, are oxidized stepwise into two-carbon fragments in the form of acetyl-CoA, which is then metabolized by the citric acid cycle and the electron transport system in the manner described previously.

The breakdown of fatty acids takes place in the mitochondria of the cell. Initially, a molecule of ATP is required to supply energy to convert the two-carbon units of fatty acid to the coenzyme A intermediate necessary for further catabolism (Fig. 15–4). This reaction is followed sequentially by hydrogen removal (by means of a coenzyme containing riboflavin), addition of water, removal of another hydrogen (with a niacin-containing coenzyme), and finally the addition of another CoA. Acetyl-CoA is split off, and a fatty acid (minus two carbons)-CoA is formed, which then goes through the series of reactions again. For a fatty acid like stearic acid, which has a chain of 18 carbon atoms, this series of reactions would have to be repeated eight times in order to produce the nine two-carbon molecules of acetyl-CoA. The citric acid cycle completely oxidizes acetyl-CoA, so there is no net synthesis of glucose from fatty acid oxidation.

Acetyl-CoA may be used for building other substances, including new fatty acids and cholesterol. As acetyl-CoA is also formed during catabolism of both glucose and amino acids, it is easy to explain how fat can be synthesized from either carbohydrate or protein when these are eaten in excess of the body needs for energy. The deposit of fat in the tissues represents fuel taken in excess of the energy needs of the body, whether it is taken as fat or made from excess carbohydrate or protein.

Although adipose tissue was formerly thought to be rather inert, experiments with fatty acids tagged by containing an isotopic element indicate that there is a more active interchange of fatty acids between these tissues and the blood than was previously supposed. Stored fat can, of course, be withdrawn from adipose tissue and oxidized to provide energy, whenever energy intake is insufficient for current body needs.

Proteins

The products of protein digestion — *amino acids* — are absorbed into the blood and carried to the liver, and the amino acids released from the liver into the blood are taken up rapidly by the other tissues of the body. The amino acids that are absorbed by the tissues following a meal disappear within a few hours.The primary and unique function of amino acids is to provide the components for synthesis of *tissue* proteins (including the important proteins of the blood) as needed for maintenance and *growth,* and to serve as precursors of antibodies, some hormones, and a vitamin. (See Chapter 5.) Normally the body does not store protein, although small reserves of protein are accumulated in the liver and muscles by actual growth of the tissue. These and blood proteins can be used for more essential purposes when protein intake is inadequate.

Experiments with amino acids containing isotopic elements demonstrate that amino acids are very labile compounds capable of being converted one into another and into substances other than tissue proteins. The first step in this conversion is the loss of the nitrogen-containing amino group ($-NH_2$), called *deamination.* Deamination can occur by a reaction in which the amino group is transferred to an acceptor keto-acid

$$R-\underset{\underset{O}{\|}}{C}-COOH$$

to form a new amino acid and leaving a new keto-acid. The enzymes catalyzing these reactions are called transaminases and usually require a vitamin B-6–containing cofactor for activity. This is the way the body makes many of the amino acids described as nonessential, meaning that they do not have to be supplied by protein in the diet because they can be made in the body. The formation of ammonia and a keto-acid from amino acid is another type of deamination. The enyzmes catalyzing these reactions, called amino acid oxidases, generally require riboflavin-containing enzymes for activity. Most deamination occurs in the liver, but the kidneys also have enzymes that can perform this function, if needed.

The keto-acid intermediates of amino acids are *subject to oxidation,* either directly or after transformation into other compounds, depending on the composition of the different amino acids (Fig. 15–3). For instance, the simple amino acid alanine on deamination becomes pyruvic acid, which can readily be oxidized to carbon dioxide and water or used to synthesize glucose. Some amino acids, including alanine, are said to be *glucogenic* because the deaminized fragment may be converted into some intermediate of glucose synthesis. Other amino acids are said to be *ketogenic,* because on deamination compounds that are oxidized like fatty acids are produced. All of the deaminated intermediates can enter the citric acid cycle and be completely oxidized to carbon dioxide and water with ATP production by the electron transport system.

The fate of the *nitrogen-containing* groups split off from the amino acids presents a special metabolic problem. Most of this nitrogen (70 to 90 percent of the nitrogen excreted) is transformed into *urea* in the liver and *excreted in the urine,* since the body is unable to store protein or other nitrogen-containing substances to any considerable extent (except in growth).

The amino acids that are deaminated and then oxidized of course yield energy, but the ones that are built into tissue protein yield no immediate energy to the body. If the diet supplies carbohydrate and fat in too small amounts to meet the body's energy needs and more of the amino acids from protein have to be

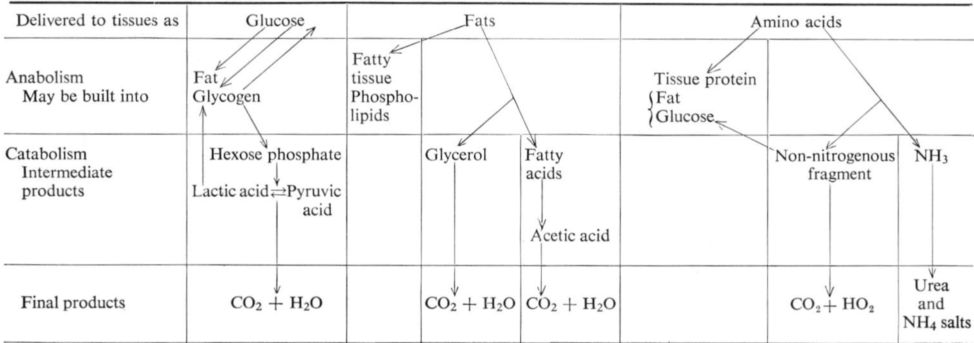

Figure 15–5 Condensed summary of the metabolism of the three energy nutrients—carbohydrates, fats, and proteins.

burned for energy, the quota left for tissue building is reduced. Hence, in growth, pregnancy, or recovery from wasting illness, when it is desirable to build up tissue protein in the body, sufficient food must be eaten so that protein will not be oxidized for energy but can instead be used for tissue protein synthesis.

A simplified summary of metabolism of the three energy nutrients is given in Figure 15–5. This diagram shows graphically that the final products of oxidation of all three are the same — *carbon dioxide and water* — with the exception of those substances formed from the nitrogen split off from the amino acids. If the food supplies energy in excess of body needs, the excess is formed chiefly into glycogen or fat for storage. If the food supplies inadequate energy to meet body needs, the insufficiency is made up by destruction of some body materials —that is, by oxidizing first the stored glycogen, then adipose and muscle tissue, and finally the essential tissue proteins.

Role of the Thyroid Hormones in General Metabolism

In addition to their effect on blood glucose, thyroxine (T_4) and triiodothyronine (T_3) affect the metabolism of virtually all the tissues of the body. Essential for normal rates of protein synthesis and most other metabolic processes, they increase the rates of reactions such that the rate of energy utilization is increased. As little as a single milligram of thyroxine raises basal metabolism 3 percent above normal. Apparently only about one-third of a milligram needs to be released daily from storage in the thyroid into the blood to keep basal metabolism at a normal level. The specific sites of action of these hormones have not been fully elucidated at this time.

The regulation of thyroid hormone synthesis is complex. The pituitary gland synthesizes a protein, thyroid-stimulating hormone (TSH), which is responsible for stimulating the thyroid gland to synthesize and release thyroid hormones. In addition, the hypothalamus in the brain secretes a peptide, thyrotropin-releasing hormone, which has some regulatory effects on the pituitary TSH production. This system is then subject to feedback inhibition by thyroid hormones (discussed in Chapter 13).

T_4 and T_3 are derivatives of the amino acid tyrosine, and have iodine atoms in their structures. They are stored in the thyroid gland as part of a large protein molecule called thyroglobulin, and are slowly liberated into the blood either free or combined with blood proteins.

When the thyroid is markedly underactive and secreting too little hormone, low basal metabolism and sluggish mentality result. A child who is born with the thyroid gland missing or underdeveloped is called a *cretin* and is either a potbellied dwarf or a pudgy, stunted child with limited intelligence. Such a child may usually be made to grow and develop fairly normally by administration of thyroxine. Underactivity of the thyroid in later life results in a condition known as *myxedema,* which is characterized by puffiness of the hands and face and by thick, dry skin. Other symptoms are low basal metabolism, dulling of mental activity, sluggishness of body processes, and a tendency to put on weight. However, the commonly held belief that underactivity of the thyroid gland leads to fatness is erroneous. The greater proportion of weight gained when the thyroid is underactive results from water held because of faulty protein structure in the tissues. Animals in which the thyroid gland is removed actually have a lower percentage of body fat than do normal animals. Basal metabolism may be markedly increased by giving thyroxine, which also improves the other symptoms.

Hyperthyroidism, or overactivity of the thyroid with excessive secretion of thyroxine, is evidenced by an abnormally *high rate of basal metabolism,* emaciation, rapid heartbeat, nervousness, and frequently by protruding eyes. The energy need may be increased to two or three times normal, causing loss of weight in spite of increased consumption of food. The overactive gland usually becomes enlarged, and such a condition is known as toxic or exophthalmic goiter (the latter name because of the eye involvement).

Simple goiter is a nutritional disease, brought about by an insufficient supply of iodine, and is discussed in Chapter 12. The gland enlarges because the pituitary continues to form TSH owing to inadequate feedback inhibition in the absence of sufficient thyroid hormone. Basal metabolism may or may not be affected, depending on how severe the deficiency is, but the symptoms of excessive thyroxine seen in toxic goiters are absent.

EXCRETION

Excretion is the process by which the body rids itself of waste products. True waste products fall into four general categories:

1. Materials that cannot be digested and absorbed.
2. Materials that, although absorbed, cannot be utilized.
3. Materials that are consumed or produced in the body in larger amounts than the body can use or is able to store.
4. The end-products of the metabolism of foodstuffs, chiefly urea (and other nitrogen-containing substances) and carbon dioxide.

Material that has never been absorbed passes out by the intestinal route, as discussed in the previous chapter. Waste products of the second class (absorbed but not utilizable) are relatively uncommon. Examples are the artificial sweetener saccharin and the pentose sugar xylose, which are absorbed and largely excreted unchanged in the urine. The third class of waste products is more common. They are useful to the body up to a certain level (which may vary according to circumstances) but are detrimental if allowed to accumulate. Water might be said to belong to this class, although technically it is not a waste product. Water is consumed in large amounts and is also an end-product of the metabolism of foodstuffs. It is vital to the body welfare, yet the water balance in the body must be maintained. This usually calls for the excretion of a variable amount of excess water mostly through the kidneys but also by way of the skin, lungs, and feces. The excess of water-soluble vitamins, above the limited amounts that are needed or that can be held in the tissues, is also excreted in the urine.

Urea and other nitrogenous substances (end-products of metabolism of protein and other nitrogen-containing substances) leave the body almost entirely through the kidneys. Excess *carbon dioxide* is excreted by the lung and to a limited extent as carbonate in urine.

Under the general heading of excretion it is sometimes helpful to consider all pathways of *ultimate loss* from the body, whether or not the substances removed are of any further utility. Dead cells and hair are constantly being lost from the body surface and, in a less conventional sense, may be thought of as waste products. Sometimes the excretion of one substance causes the unavoidable loss of another — for instance, water vapor (useful substance) is lost with carbon dioxide (waste product) in breathing. Losses of material from the skin generally are secondary to sweating for body heat regulation and do not figure in processes of waste removal for homeostasis. Sweat is almost a filtrate of plasma, and as such it contains electrolytes, urea, amino acids, vitamins, and trace elements; but these substances are not "excreted" in the true sense. The final adjustment made to maintain constancy in the internal environment is the work of the lungs and, above all, the kidneys.

Excretion Through the Lungs

Excess *carbon dioxide* passes into the blood from the tissues and is held in three forms: as dissolved CO_2, as bicarbonate ions (HCO_3^-), and as a form chemically bound to the blood proteins, chiefly hemoglobin. When the blood reaches the lungs, it is brought into contact in the fine capillaries with air in the innumerable small air sacs of the lungs — that is, there is between the blood and air only a double membrane consisting of the very thin walls of the capillary and of the air sac, permitting the free exchange of gases. Carbon dioxide diffuses across these membranes because it is in higher concentration in the blood than in the inspired air.* According to chemical principles requiring a balance among CO_2, HCO_3^-, and carbonic acid (H_2CO_3), additional CO_2 is immediately released from hemoglobin, and so the excess CO_2 is removed. In passing through the lungs the blood loses about one-sixth of its carbon dioxide content in gaseous form to the carbon dioxide–poor air in the lungs, and takes up from inspired air gaseous *oxygen,* which is carried to the tissues in loose chemical combination with the hemoglobin.

The inspired air becomes saturated with *water vapor* while in the lungs, which accounts for the considerable and constant loss of water through the lungs. Small amounts of other volatile substances present in the blood are also found in exhaled air (e.g., alcohol, ammonia, gases formed by intestinal bacteria); and gaseous substances present in inhaled air are absorbed into the blood (e.g., anesthetics, auto fumes).

Frequency of respiration is controlled by the respiratory center in the brain, this center in turn being chiefly affected by the carbon dioxide content of the blood. Thus, after exercise during which the production of carbon dioxide is more rapid, stimulation of the respiratory center causes an increased rate of breathing, with the result that the excess of carbon dioxide is removed from the body through the increased ventilation of the lungs. In ordinary shallow breathing only about one-sixth to one-fifth of the air contained in the lungs is involved, although the whole volume of air is probably fairly efficiently renewed at least twice every minute. Efficient respiration is an important factor in good health and physical fitness.

Excretion by the Kidneys

The kidneys are *perfused by an exceptionally large amount of blood* from which they selectively remove waste products. The kidneys actively secrete other substances to form the final product — urine. Urine is secreted continuously (although more rapidly under certain stimuli), and is collected in the urinary bladder.

---

*Fresh air contains only 0.03 to 0.04 percent of carbon dioxide and about 20 percent of oxygen. The process of *respiration* in animals consists essentially of taking up 4 to 5 percent of oxygen from the inspired air and giving off 3 to 4 percent of carbon dioxide to the expired air.

The functional unit of the kidney is the *nephron,* in which blood enters a tuft, or network, of capillaries called the *glomerulus,* and is filtered through this into the surrounding double-walled, funnel-like *Bowman's capsule,* which leads to a series of collecting tubules. Only water-soluble substances of relatively low molecular weight can pass through the semipermeable membrane of the glomerulus and into the filtrate. These include salts, glucose, amino acids, vitamins, and very limited amounts of simple proteins. Large protein molecules, lipids, and blood cells are retained in the blood stream unless the membrane is injured. It is the task of the cells that line the tubules to reabsorb selectively such useful substances as glucose and amino acids, along with large amounts of water, and to secrete certain other products into the urine, while efficiently removing waste products. Some substances are nearly completely reabsorbed by the tubule when their concentration in the blood plasma is at a normal level. For instance, glucose appears in the urine only when plasma concentration is high, as in diabetes, or when kidney tubular function is impaired. Other substances, such as sodium, potassium, and chloride, are either selectively reabsorbed or secreted, according to body needs. Waste products (such as urea and creatinine) are reabsorbed only slightly or not at all. Both absorption and secretion are active processes requiring energy. That the work of the tubule cells is very great may be appreciated from the fact that the volume of glomerular filtrate is 80 to 100 times larger than the final volume of urine excreted and is of vastly different composition.

Of the products excreted in the urine, *water* is by far the largest in quantity (urine is about 96 percent water). When an unusual amount of water is lost through the skin in hot weather, or during very active exercise, or through the alimentary tract under abnormal conditions (vomiting and diarrhea), the amount excreted by the kidneys is correspondingly less. Likewise, if the water intake is low, water is conserved in the body, and the kidneys secrete a smaller volume of more concentrated urine.

The next most abundant constituents of urine are the *nitrogenous end-products of protein metabolism* (see Chapter 5). One of these alone — *urea* — makes up about half the total solutes of the urine and constitutes the form in which about 80 percent of the nitrogen from metabolized proteins is excreted. Smaller amounts of *uric acid, creatinine,* and *ammonium salts* account for most of the remaining nitrogen in urine. These nitrogenous waste products can be eliminated from the body in significant amounts only through the activity of the kidneys.

Although some *mineral salts* are excreted by the intestine, the bulk of the salts leaves the body in the urine. *Sodium* is excreted largely in the urine. When the kidneys fail to function well, sodium may accumulate in the blood and tissues, holding back sufficient water to dilute salt to normal concentration in the tissues (see Chapter 10), thus causing the edema that often accompanies diseases of the kidneys. The kidney is also the main route for excretion of potassium. *Phosphates* and *sulfates* that appear in the urine come chiefly from the metabolism of proteins.

There are a number of other substances that appear in the urine in only small amounts but that have important physiological implications. Variable and usually minor constituents of the urine include pigments, hormones, vitamins and their derivatives, intermediate metabolic products, and detoxified substances.

Factors That Govern Excretion Through the Kidneys. For purposes of discussion, we may divide the factors that influence urinary excretion into two main groups: (1) physiological factors — hormones, diuretics (substances that stimulate urine flow), and the amount of blood supply to the kidneys; and (2) dietary factors — that is, variations in the kinds and amounts of nutrients ingested, including water. The dietary factors are important, for they may alter the effectiveness of the kidneys in two of its most important roles:

1. Maintaining normal osmotic pressure and the concentration of electrolytes in body tissues and fluids — that is, the internal environment of body cells and organs.

2. Maintaining the acid-base balance of the body.

The pituitary gland secretes a hormone that decreases the volume of urine (an antidiuretic hormone), while the adrenal cortex elaborates hormones that affect mineral metabolism, especially the relative amounts of sodium and potassium excreted in the urine. Just as the respiratory center responds with increased activity to small increases in the carbon dioxide content of the blood, the secretion of these hormones by the pituitary and adrenal glands is triggered by small changes in osmotic pressure and by the composition and volume of body fluids, thus providing rapid response to alterations in amounts of water and salts absorbed into or lost from the body.

The most common *diuretics* are coffee and tea. Both increase urine flow, owing to their content of caffeine (and related substances), which increases the rate of blood flow through the kidneys and alters the transport of salts and water by tubule cells. Another diuretic — alcohol — brings about increased urine flow by depressing the production of pituitary antidiuretic hormone.

A number of dietary factors may affect the *excretion of water* by direct effects on the kidneys. Healthy kidneys can concentrate substances dissolved in urine to a remarkable extent and can handle easily the salts (either ingested as such or arising from protein metabolism) and urea that need to be excreted by a person on a normal, mixed diet. However, there is a limit to the extent of concentration the kidneys can achieve, and if such soluble substances are present in excessive quantities, additional water is required to dilute them to the point where they can be excreted. Normally, drinking more water can supply this need, but if the water supply is limited, the extra water needed is drawn from body fluids or tissues. This is why drinking sea water, which has such a high content of salts, takes water away from the body and thus is damaging to water-deprived castaways. Excretion of the large amounts of urea formed as a result of a very high protein intake may also require extra water. This may become important if water consumption is inadequate, if water loss from other routes is unusually large, or in some diseased states.

It is very generally recognized that drinking large amounts of water results in the excretion of a much increased volume of urine. This urine is very light in color and more dilute than usual in its content of dissolved solids. In other words, the amount of pigment and waste products excreted remains about the same, so that the extra water merely renders the urine more dilute.

The important part that the kidneys play in maintaining the normal level of electrolytes (chiefly ionized mineral salts) in the blood and tissue fluids, which in turn are largely responsible for normal conditions of *osmotic pressure,* should be apparent from much of the previous discussion.* The loss of sodium, potassium, and chloride from the body is regulated almost exclusively by the kidneys. Ordinarily the kidneys have no difficulty in keeping these substances at a normal level in blood and tissues by promptly excreting any excess amounts, and if losses from other routes are excessive (from sweat or diarrhea), urinary excretion may fall to very low values. In this way the constancy of amount of various mineral salts in the blood and extracellular fluids is safeguarded.

The kidneys play an important role in maintenance of body neutrality. The normal pH of blood is 7.35; death occurs within a few hours if pH falls to 7.0 or rises to about 7.7. Any increased level of

*The action of mineral salts in exchange of body fluids and in normal functioning of muscles and nerves was treated in Chapter 10.

acidic ions (chloride, sulfate, or phosphate) in the blood perfusing the kidneys is excreted as salts in the urine, after being balanced with ions of some strong base (sodium, potassium, and, to a much lesser extent, calcium or magnesium). The kidneys are able to conserve these basic elements and eliminate acidic groups, thus regulating the acid-base balance of the body. This is done by exchanging for basic elements hydrogen ions that are secreted by the tubular cells, shifting the form of phosphate eliminated from a more basic to a more acidic salt and forming a more acid urine. Under conditions in which there is a large excess of acidic products to be eliminated, the kidneys can produce ammonium groups to use up hydrogen ion.*

Just as there is a limit to the degree to which soluble substances can be concentrated by the kidney, so there is a limit to the acid-base range within which urine can be excreted. Normally the acid-base balance of the diet is well within the functional range of the kidney. The chief acidic products of the diet are sulfates and phosphates formed in the process of protein metabolism. The organic acids found in most fruits and vegetables do not yield acid residues because they are oxidized in metabolism to carbon dioxide and water and are accompanied in the foods by large amounts of potassium and other basic elements. However, if very large amounts of organic acid (such as the 5 to 10 gm doses of ascorbic acid taken indiscriminately to counteract the common cold) are consumed, the urine will become acidic and extra minerals will be required for neutralization. The most frequently encountered instance in which large amounts of acidic substances must be excreted is when fat is incompletely oxidized in the body and acidic intermediate products of its metabolism (ketone bodies) accumulate, as in starvation and diabetes. Ingestion of extremely high-fat, low-carbohydrate diets has this same effect. Under these conditions, basic elements (chiefly sodium and potassium) are required for their neutralization, and thus they are lost from the body.

*In the kidney, H^+ is substituted for Na^+ by the following reaction:

$$H_2CO_3 + Na_2HPO_4 \rightarrow NaH_2PO_4 + NaHCO_3$$

Base may be conserved by formation of ammonium ion, as symbolized by the following overall equation:

$$2\ NH_3 \text{ (from amino acids)} + 2\ H_2CO_3 + Na_2HPO_4 \rightarrow (NH_4)_2HPO_4 + 2\ NaHCO_3$$

In both cases the H ion comes from a coupled shift of carbonic acid to bicarbonate.

QUESTIONS

1. Define metabolism. Why is digestion not included in metabolism? What happens when the intake of energy is in excess of body needs? When it is inadequate for body needs?

2. Describe the metabolism of carbohydrate, covering the following points: the form in which it is absorbed from the intestine into the blood, the form in which it is carried in the blood to the tissues, the role of the liver in carbohydrate metabolism, the fate of glucose in the tissues (both that needed to supply energy and that in excess of immediate needs), and the final products of carbohydrate metabolism. How is blood sugar level regulated? What causes hyperglycemia? Hypoglycemia?

3. Describe the metabolism of fats, covering the same general points listed in Question 2 for carbohydrate metabolism. Describe the chemical changes that amino acids undergo in the tissues, including the fate of both the nitrogenous and the nonnitrogenous parts of the molecule. What are the chief end-products of the metabolism of the three fuel foodstuffs?

4. What common pathway do all three foodstuffs follow in the final stages of oxidation to carbon dioxide and water? Why is this route called a cycle? Why the citric or carboxylic acid cycle? What makes acetylcoenzyme A such an important intermediate compound in the cycle? What are the advantages of having a common pool of lower metabolites from all three foodstuffs?

5. What two products of metabolism are excreted through the lungs? When a man exercises, there is increased energy expenditure and hence increased production of carbon dioxide. How is this sudden excess of carbon dioxide excreted?

6. What is the chief substance excreted through the skin? What other substances are present in perspiration?

7. What waste products are excreted through the kidneys? In a normal person, what conditions cause an increased or a decreased output of each of the following in the urine — water, urea, sodium chloride, phosphates, and ammonium salts? Is urine normally acid or alkaline, and what may cause its reaction to vary?

SUPPLEMENTARY READING

Alleyne, G. A. O., Trust, P. M., Flores, H., and Robinson, H.: Glucose tolerance and insulin sensitivity in malnourished children. Brit. J. Nutr., *27*:585, 1972.

Aoki, T. T., Muller, W. A., Brennan, M. F., and Cahill, G. F. Jr.: Metabolic effects of glucose in brief and prolonged fasted man. Amer. J. Clin. Nutr., *28*:507, 1975.

Berdanier, C. D. (ed.): Carbohydrate Metabolism: Regulation and Physiological Role. New York, Halsted Press, Div. of John Wiley & Sons, Inc., 1976.

Berlin, R. D., et al.: The cell surface. N. Engl. J. Med., *292*:515, 1975.

Black, A. L., and Kaneko, J. J., Chairmen: Symposium: Energy metabolism and its regulation. Fed. Proc., *29*:1522, 1970.

Broquist, H. P.: Amino acid metabolism. Nutr. Rev., *34*:289, 1976.

Carmel, N., Konijn, A. M., Kaufmann, N. A., and Guggenheim, K.: Effects of carbohydrate-free diets on the insulin-carbohydrate relationships in rats. J. Nutr., *105*:1141, 1975.

Dallman, P. R., Spirito, R. A., and Siimes, M. A.: Diurnal patterns of DNA synthesis in the rat: modification by diet and feeding schedule. J. Nutr., *104*:1234, 1974.

Danowski, T. S., Nolan, S., and Stephan, T.: Hypoglycemia. World Rev. Nutr. Dietet., *22*:288, 1975.

Edelman, I. S.: Thyroid thermogenesis. N. Engl. J. Med., *290*:1303, 1974.

Eisenstein, A. B. (ed.): Gluconeogenesis: a Symposium. Amer. J. Clin. Nutr., *23*:971, 1970.

Felig, P., et al.: Symposium: Managing diabetes. Postgrad. Med., *59*:113, 1976.

Flatt, J-P., and Blackburn, G. L.: The metabolic fuel regulatory system: implications for protein-sparing therapies during caloric deprivation and disease. Amer. J. Clin. Nutr., *27*:175, 1974.

Hofeldt, F. D., Dippe, S., and Forsham, P. H.: Diagnosis and classification of reactive hypoglycemia based on hormonal changes in response to oral and intravenous glucose administration. Amer. J. Clin. Nutr., *25*:1193, 1972.

Hultman, E., and Nilsson, L. H.: Factors influencing carbohydrate metabolism in man. Nutr. Metab., *18* (Suppl. 1):45, 1975.

Kelsay, J. L., et al.: The effect of kind of carbohydrate in the diet and use of oral contraceptives on metabolism of young women. Amer. J. Clin. Nutr., *30*:216, 1977.

Krebs, H. A.: The history of the tricarboxylic acid cycle. Perspect. Biol. Med., *14*:154, 1970.

Lech, J. J., Chairman: Symposium: Control of endogenous triglyceride synthesis in adipose tissue and muscle. Fed. Proc., *36*:1984, 1977.

Lennarz, W. J.: Lipid metabolism. Ann. Rev. Biochem., *39*:359, 1970.

Long, C. L., et al.: Whole body protein synthesis and catabolism in septic man. Amer. J. Clin. Nutr., *30*:1340, 1977.

Mann, M. D., Becker, D. J., Pimstone, B. L., and Hansen, J. D. L.: Potassium supplementation, serum immunoreactive insulin concentrations and glucose tolerance in protein-energy malnutrition. Brit. J. Nutr., *33*:55, 1975.

McCracken, K. J.: Effect of feeding pattern on the energy metabolism of rats given low-protein diets. Brit. J. Nutr., *33*:277, 1975.

Palade, G.: Intracellular aspects of the process of protein synthesis. Science, *189*:347, 1975.

Pike, R. L., and Brown, M. L.: The cell. In *Nutrition: An Integrated Approach.* 2nd Ed. New York, John Wiley & Sons, Inc., 1975.

Pirola, R. C., and Lieber, C. S.: Hypothesis: energy wastage in alcoholism and drug abuse: possible role of hepatic microsomal enzymes. Amer. J. Clin. Nutr., *29*:90, 1976.

Shambaugh, G. E.: Urea biosynthesis. IV. Normal and abnormal regulation. Amer. J. Clin. Nutr., *31*: 126, 1978.

Sherwin, R. S., et al.: Hyperglucagonemia and blood glucose regulation in normal, obese and diabetic subjects. N. Engl. J. Med., *294*:455, 1976.

West, K. M.: Prevention and therapy of diabetes mellitus. Nutr. Rev., *33*:193, 1975.

Symposium: Protein metabolism and hormones. Proc. Nutr. Soc., *31*:171, 1972.

Symposium: The influence of amino acid supply on polynucleotide and protein metabolism. Proc. Nutr. Soc., *31*:249, 1972.

Articles in Nutrition Reviews

Thyroid hormones and fetal growth. *31*:67, 1973.

The time course of changes in carbohydrate and lipid metabolism. *31*:222, 1973.

Metabolic effects of glucocorticoids in man. *32*:301, 1974.

Lipolysis, aging and hormones. *32*:312, 1974.

Insulin in hypertriglyceridemia. *33*:199, 1975.

Bihormonal control of ketogenesis. *33*:347, 1975.

Potassium depletion and impaired insulin release in protein-energy malnutrition. *34*:16, 1976.

Insulin receptors, insulin resistance, diabetes and obesity. *34*:145, 1976.

Fever and amino acid metabolism. *34*:267, 1976.

Adaptive responses of amino acid degrading enzymes to variation of amino acid protein intake. *34*:343, 1976.

Implications of the cellular transport step for amino acid metabolism. *35*:129, 1977.

Part 3

Foods As Sources of Nutrients and Nonnutrients

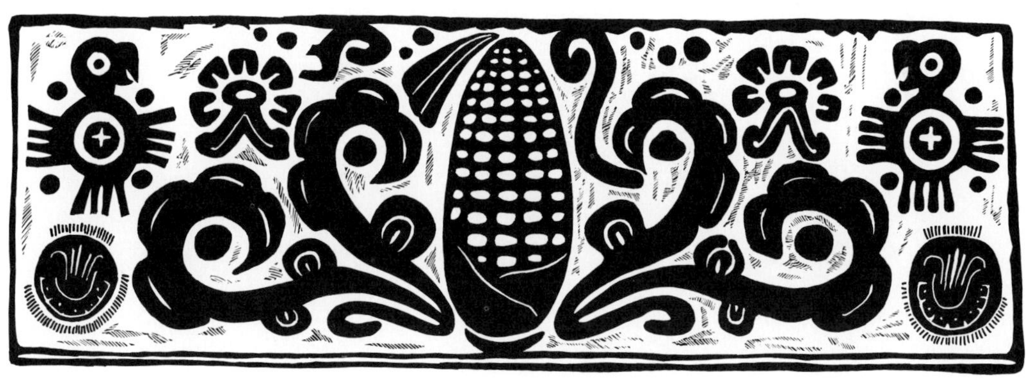

Chapter 16

Food Habits and Beliefs

Food is one of the basic needs of existence. In every society that has been studied, food plays a central part in people's beliefs about life and health, and is included in some fashion in sacred rituals. Joy is celebrated in feasts, for which — whether it is an American Thanksgiving dinner, European country wedding or tribal feast — special, more expensive foods are obtained and prepared. Ritual overeating may be practiced at such times. There is scarcely a group that does not express hospitality to a guest through an offer of food or drink, and through such customs a whole etiquette may evolve into a tradition.

The importance of food to life is recognized by its use in nonfood ways, especially among pretechnological peoples, in magical rites, in divination, and in matrimonial rites.* Among the Monssay of Chad, for example, a groom prepares his bride's first meal in his home, thereby rendering harmless future meals prepared by her.[1] Women guests at a Malay wedding are given hard-boiled eggs dyed red and formed into flowers, as a symbol of fertility. Guests at an American wedding throw rice at the departing bride and groom in a similar gesture. A form of punishment in or out of prisons has been reduction of food to bread and water. Mothers sometimes withhold sweet desserts from a child for some infraction of their rules. Political or spiritual leaders go on hunger strikes to make a point or force an issue.

Food is a powerful force in society. It may truly be said that, while culture forms the diet, the food of a people also molds the kind of culture in which it is eaten (Fig. 16–1). Nutrition is just one expression of this force.

Among primitive people, omission of "forbidden foods" (usually foods of animal origin) contributes to inadequate diets. It is not uncommon for women and children to develop protein malnutrition and experience premature aging and early death.[2]

Food habits and beliefs about properties and qualities of foods have a profound influence on nutritional status through their effect on the selection of diet by the individual or groups who hold them. A classic case in point is the deficiency disease pellagra, discussed more fully in Chapter 8. It was highly prevalent among poorer people in the southern United States in the early years of this century, when diets consisted of maize cornmeal, molasses, fatback, some greens, and very little meat or other foods of animal origin. This diet was chosen from what was economically and culturally available.

*In traditional societies, religious authorities offer the first fruits to the divinities. Food, "the gift of God," is charged with power; it is sacred and cannot be consumed without ritual. This is one of the reasons why meals are generally eaten respectfully, and often in silence, in rural societies. See DeGarine, I.: The socio-cultural aspects of nutrition. Ecol. Food Nutr., 1:142, 1972.

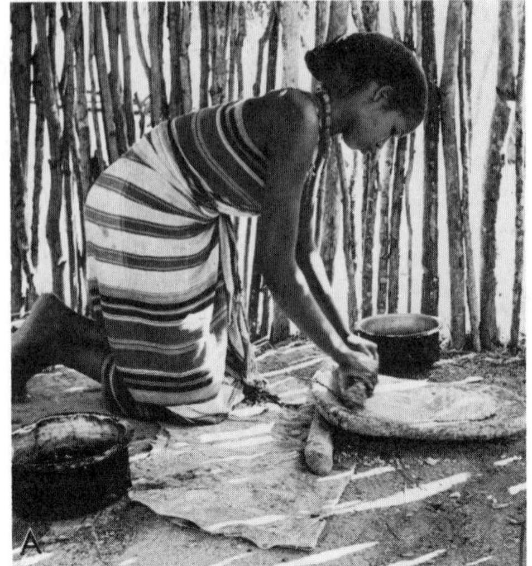

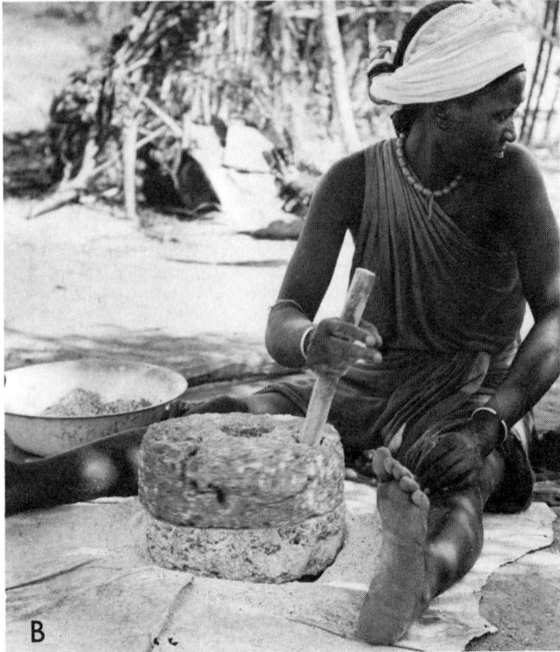

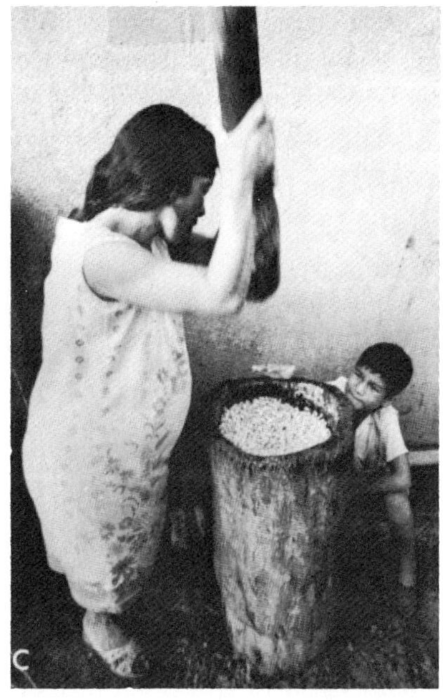

Figure 16–1 Traditional methods of preparing food grains often occupy many hours of a woman's workday. Rural women need improved facilities to relieve the drudgery of their daily lives and to allow them to participate as full and equal members of society. (**A** and **B** from World Health, Aug. 1976; courtesy of WHO. **C** from Kaiser Aluminum News, *26*:26, 1968; courtesy of Kaiser Aluminum & Chemical Corporation.)

Among corn eaters in Latin America, however, pellagra does not exist, despite low animal protein intakes. This is due to the cultural practice of soaking corn with limestone before grinding and making it into the flat-bread, tortilla. Laboratory research[3] showed that this indigenous practice, arrived at empirically, made the previously chemically bound niacin in the corn available to the people.

Food beliefs and food practices of different population groups have long been observed and documented by anthropologists and ethnographers, but the effect of these attitudes on nutritional status has been studied relatively little until recent years. Ogbeide[2] studied 12 ethnic groups in Mid-West Nigeria, each with stringent taboos affecting children, pregnant women, and mothers. Milk, meat, and eggs were common foods forbidden to children and lactating mothers.

One such study[4] demonstrated that Malay women's beliefs prohibiting foods considered "cold" or "cooling" to the body in the 40 days following childbirth resulted in deficiency, as measured in the blood, of folacin, vitamin A, and carotene. The foods defined as "cold" included nearly all fruits and vegetables. The women were afraid that if they ate them, air would enter their bodies and damage the tissues, causing them to bleed.

Food habits tend to persist among people entering another social group after other cultural differences are erased. Nutritionists and social scientists would like to know what causes changes in selection of types of foods people eat, and whether and how such changes might be directed. A good deal of research has been applied to these problems, which center on habits involving choice of foods to eat. Food *habits* are often the result of economic pressures. *Taboos* function as a code for human conduct. Religious groups utilize taboos; the Hindus, for example, are forbidden to eat the sacred cow. *Beliefs* about food and its properties, are often more subtle and are resistant to efforts at alteration. Beliefs about food are usually woven into the fabric of a society or group; they are an integral part of the culture. They can, however, change with other aspects of a culture and may only be temporary. Taboos, on the other hand, are far more restrictive, controlled, and rigid. To learn the reasons behind food belief, we must often study the whole structure of the society for an explanation of their role.[5] This kind of research has not been done so widely as have studies about food habits and their change.

NUTRITION AS A PART OF CULTURE

Eating is one of the fundamentals, essential to all life. But even for a Robinson Crusoe or a dedicated misanthrope, eating is done in a cultural setting. The ways of the group determine who is served first, who shall get which portions of which foods offered, what utensils shall be used, and how much may be eaten—Thais, for example, are reared to believe it is greedy to take more than the smallest morsel of the foods served with rice. In most American and European households, families eat together around a table, each from his own plate. Asians have separate bowls of rice and help themselves to side dishes with fingers, chopsticks, or spoons, often sitting or squatting on the floor (Fig. 16–2). Certain African groups share from a communal pot and eat with their fingers. The choicest food is offered to a guest or eaten by the men of the household. In many societies, women eat apart from or at a later time than the men. Children, too, often come at the end of the line of distribution of cooked food, with nutritional implications for reduction in availability and variety of foods and nutrients. And if father won't eat leftovers, a thrifty housewife often warms them over for herself, lowering their vitamin content in the process.

The culture or society defines a meal with regard to both time and content. We would not call the usual coffee break, or the hot dog, potato chips, and popcorn eaten at a game, a meal. However, to a host of Britons and many other peoples, tea is a meal, small or large, that precedes (evening) dinner and consists of a cup or more of hot tea and cakes or sandwiches. Tea, accompanied by fruit or bread, precedes breakfast in some countries. Western people like to complete a meal by serving a sweet dessert. Continental Europeans prefer cheese and fruit. Many Americans prefer to start their day with cereal and fruit. In other parts of the world as far apart as South America and Southeast Asia, fruit is never eaten save as a snack food, picked from the trees in passing or brought home from market for immediate consumption.

Just as we buy jars and cans of foods especially prepared for babies, other cultures define certain foods as "children's foods." Often these are fruits. There are also people who restrict consumption of some foods to women only or prohibit them to girls who have not yet reached maturity.

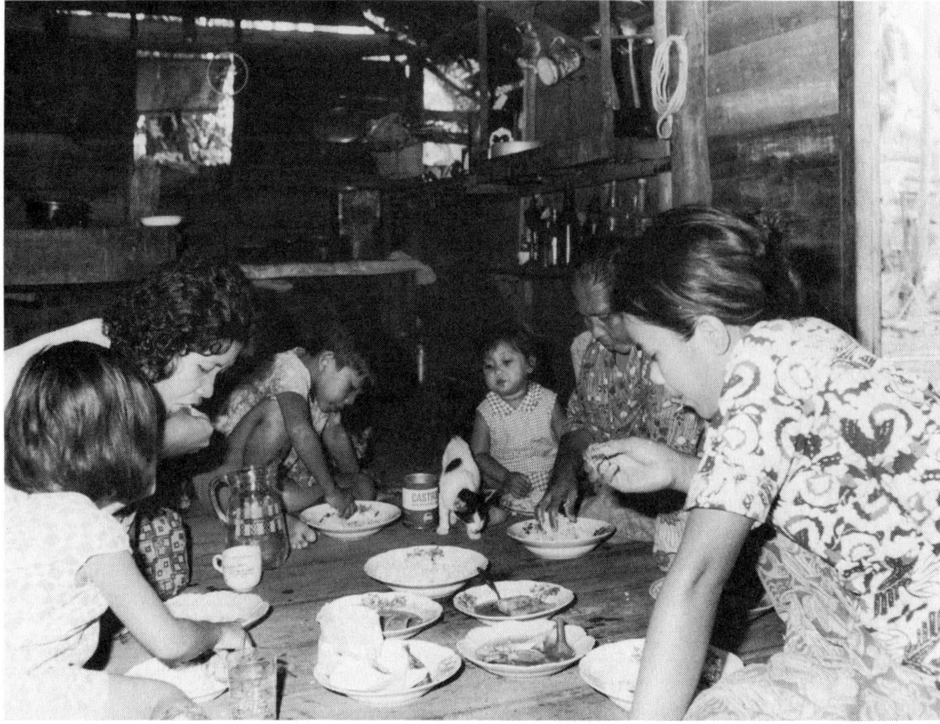

Figure 16–2 Eating customs differ throughout the world, and what is considered good form in one culture may be unacceptable in another. Even within a culture, accepted modes may vary from one social group to another. In this Malay family, the traditional food service of the fishing village is used, in which each member serves himself from communal bowls placed on the floor and eats his own food with fingers. (Courtesy of Dr. C. Wilson, University of California.)

Most cultures have a staple food that they believe is fundamental to existence. Around this food, beliefs, rituals, and traditions have sprung up. Jelliffe[6] has called them "cultural superfoods." Thus, to that large portion of the world that subsists on rice, a meal is usually defined as a time when rice is taken. A morning meal of other foods is considered a snack. For many Asians, a customary greeting is, "Have you taken rice?" If the answer is affirmative, it is considered that all is well with the speaker. Food is thought to play a part in preventing and curing diseases, especially among the Chinese from rural communities.[7] The Indians of the Americas revered the maize corn, and much of their cultural activities related to its cultivation and propagation. Rice among Malays is imbued with a spirit that is both respected and perpetuated through rituals. We ourselves speak of our basic staple, bread, as "the staff of life," while also admitting "man does not live by bread alone."

DIET PATTERNS — HOW THEY COME ABOUT

Despite the coast-to-coast distribution of certain restaurant companies selling hamburgers and soft drinks, and of national food store chains, there are still regional as well as ethnic differences in the kinds of foods eaten in this country. New England has its baked beans, codfish cakes, and lobsters on Saturday night. Southerners like cornmeal, whether served as spoonbread or hush puppies, a "mess" of greens, and other components now classed as "soul food." Black-eyed peas are not readily available in all markets outside the South, and one finds more tacos, enchiladas, and refried beans in areas where there are large concentrations of Mexican-Americans. An order for fried eggs for breakfast in the South will be served with hominy grits. In New England and parts of the Midwest, the plate will include fried potatoes instead.

The reasons for these differences are several. Some components of diets are chosen on the basis of local availability of foods, what grows well, or what is easily obtained. Now that we have refrigerated storage and transport countrywide, our theoretical choice is very large indeed. Newly developed franchises of fast-food restaurants have introduced consumers to ethnic foods as well as changed their dietary habits. Out-of-season foods and scarce gourmet items can be ours at any time, provided we are only able and willing to pay the price. But this situation is relatively new, and diet habits, once established, tend to persist. Current diets thus reflect to some extent what was available at periods in the past.

It should be noted that the groups of people studied thus far never eat all the potential edible commodities available to it. For various cultural or other reasons, some things are still not defined as food, though they may safely be eaten. In Europe, the Jerusalem artichoke, a tuber, is used as cattle feed. In the United States it is considered a delicacy.

It is probable that taste, physiological reactions subsequent to eating a particular item (whether a food was toxic or not), and local climatic, environmental, and economic conditions determined what foods made up the diet of pretechnological man. Traditional diets with which people have lived satisfactorily for long periods, and which have been studied for their nutritive value, have been shown to meet the known requirements of the population. Thus, empirical trial and error over time produced a diet suited to the individual from potential foods he was free to choose. (The Chuave of New Guinea, for instance, relish the insect, which is a rich protein source. One hundred grams of fried termites are approximately 561 kcal.)[8]

Effects of Storage Conditions

Foods that could be kept well for long periods under prevailing living conditions would be selected for storage for later consumption in areas where food could not be raised the year round. Many American farm families used to have root cellars to keep carrots, onions, potatoes, turnips, and other food for winter consumption. The Eskimo still uses the permanently frozen ground as his storage area for berries and similar foods. Africans, South Americans, and some Southeast Asians who depend upon tapioca (cassava or manioc) roots as a carbohydrate source often leave them in the ground until the need for them arises. Grains traditionally have been kept in large, dry containers, such as elevators in the American midwest. Asians dry fish or make fermented fish products for later consumption. In a like way, South Americans dry beef, and cheese and other milk products are altered for longer useful nutrient life.

There have always been some people who do not store any food. Thus New Guineans eat all their fish catch at once. One of the functions of feasts among traditional people when an animal or animals are killed is probably the very practical one of disposing of all the meat while it is still in excellent condition so far as nutrient content and taste are concerned. Such activities, when observed by technologically oriented people, may have provided the basis for the long-held view of eating patterns of traditional peoples as "a feast or a famine."

Effect of Other Factors

Different national groups who have settled our country brought with them many different cuisines that have persisted, the recipes being adapted in accordance with local availability of crops. However, other forces have had far more profound influence on the American diet in the last generation. We are all aware that advertising in newspapers, magazines, radio, and television, and food industry innovations such as convenience foods, frozen specialties and frozen complete dinners, "instant" drinks, and "instant" almost everything else edible have introduced new foods and new ways of eating. The U.S. Department of Agriculture, which regularly keeps track of these things, has found that the foods we are now buying or being persuaded to buy provide fewer nutrients than the National Research Council recommends. The U.S. Department of Agriculture 1965–66 Household Consumption Survey showed that diets meeting these recommended daily nutrient intakes dropped from 60 percent of those studied in 1955 to 50 percent in 1965. In the same time, diets considered "poor," that is, meeting less than two-thirds of the recommended dietary allowances, rose from 15 to 20 percent of the families studied.

Parrish has presented the reasons for these changes.[9] Most could be considered cultural as well as nutritional. Families now raise only a little of their own food compared with 30 years ago, and prepare much less food at home. Snacking has increased as a general food habit, and people prefer their snacks to be convenience foods. More meals are eaten away from home, and more people are skipping meals. Prices of individual food items have changed over time. At the time of Parrish's report (1971), the prices of eggs and chicken had dropped 7 to 10 percent and those of fruits and vegetables had risen 22 to 50 percent higher than they were 10 years earlier. It is not hard to see why families have been buying less of the latter. Finally, Parrish cites present preferences for convenience foods, which are particularly low in vitamins A and C.

From 1972 to 1974, the U.S. Department of Labor studied the food and alcohol expenditures of 63,000 families. Single people and families with two wage earners spent most of their food dollar on restaurant food (food away from home). Single parents with one child spent the most on food. They had an appreciably higher cost, also, as 20 percent of their food money was spent on restaurant food too.*

*How consumers divide their food and alcohol spending. Weekly Digest, 85:8, March 18, 1978.

People are increasingly following dietary and health food fads. Mass media has changed people's viewpoints of beauty and health. Before World War II, when the United States was a more rural society, obesity was considered healthy. Today, many people, teen-agers especially, skip meals to attain slimness, a sign of beauty. In doing so, they ignore and misuse food of high nutrient value.

Whoever goes out to obtain the foods and prepare them for the family's consumption is usually the final arbiter of what is served at family meals. This is true whether all foods are bought from the nearest supermarket, selected at a peasant village market, gathered in the fields, or carried on the head of a tribeswoman. Children may act as friendly persuaders, with more or less success, depending on the leniency of the mother or the culture. The personal preferences of the male household head are also usually considered. It is the homemaker who decides what foods will enter the home. For this reason, efforts in nutrition education are primarily directed to homemakers.

In this country, as indicated by Parrish's report, the cultural patterns of eating have been changed drastically by changes in economic patterns. More mothers have full-time jobs outside the home. Much less time is spent on meal preparation at home. More meals are eaten out, including children's lunches at school. Margaret Mead, commenting on the North American diet pattern in 1943,[10] remarked, ". . . father presides over meat and fish, the mother over milk, vegetables, fruit juices and liver, while adolescents . . . demonstrate their independence by refusing to eat what is good for them." Perhaps only the description of the teenager is as true and applicable today as it was a quarter of a century ago.

FOOD CULTS

While the quality of the diet of the average present-day American concerns nutritionists, we do still have a wide potential choice of foods from which to select all the nutrient sources we need, using our knowledge of nutrition and a little intelligent thought. However, a number of subgroups or cults with widely different diets from the norm have sprung up among us. Most of these people have little basic nutritional information. These groups, in attempting to attain perfection through a "natural" diet, have many proscriptions and taboos. Some of them are good; we could all learn from some of their simplifications of diet. However, the zeal with which these people have limited their potential food choices has also eliminated some needed nutrients. Erhard has described some of these food cults, from personal observations and study.[11]

All those studied were Caucasians, and all were vegetarians. Diet is the focus of their philosophy and their living habits. Some of them will eat milk, cheese, and eggs; some omit eggs; others, vegans or pure vegetarians, spurn all animal foods, including seafoods, eggs, and dairy products. Those who follow Zen Buddhism are influenced by the Chinese philosophy of *yin* and *yang*, and try to achieve a balance between the two by adjusting amounts of *yin* foods (relaxing ones) and *yang* foods (activating ones), eaten together. Meat is too *yang* and hence is discouraged, though not strictly prohibited. Fruitarians (who eat only raw or dried fruits, nuts, honey, and olive oil), and others who eat only organic foods observe fasts as part of their regimen. One group observed an "acid fast" by drinking only citrus or tomato juice one day a week to "clean out the system." These people treat all diseases by herbs, special adaptations of allowed foods, and proprietary vitamin preparations. Those who condemn animal products need to plan very carefully to obtain enough nutrients from the foods they allow themselves to eat (see Chapter 19). Erhard found that, all too often, they do not have the knowledge to do so.

Another subgroup whose food habits are often deleterious to nutritional status are dieters (see Chapter 24). The faulty food habits that led to overweight in the first place are frequently replaced by others that may shed pounds and deplete nutrient stores at the same time.

FOOD BELIEFS — PREFERENCES AND AVERSIONS

The folklore of food of the United States population has been studied far less than it has for many other cultures. Examination of food beliefs and rituals is the province of the social scientist, ethnographer, anthropologist, or psychologist rather than the nutritionist. Thus, although we have a large body of published material on food habits that is potentially relevant to nutritional status — what people eat in different cultural groups in this country, how prepared and when — we have far less written information on what American people believe about foods. What is available is chiefly part of studies by anthropologists of various ethnic groups in specific localities. Most ethnographical studies — descriptions of the lives and customs of a particular population group — include a section on usual diet and beliefs and rituals concerning foods.

Though they have not yet been compiled in a readily available resource, there is, however, a body of food ideology in the culture of the United States. Consider, for example, the long-held belief that fish is brain food — or that eating red meat is strengthening, especially for athletes. Cannibalism arose originally, it is said,[12] because man wanted to destroy the ghost of his killed enemy or relative, and acquire his courage. Although the views in the two last sentences are not too far apart, not eating our fellow humans is Western man's foremost taboo. If consumed together, fish and ice cream were once believed by many Americans to cause "ptomaine" poisoning. Some Americans of the Jewish faith still practice the religious ritual of separating dairy and meat prod-

Table 16–1 REFUTING ERRONEOUS IDEAS ABOUT FOODS

Fallacies	*Facts*
About certain foods Onions—cure a cold. Fish—is a brain food. Celery—is a nerve tonic. Oysters—increase sexual potency.	Foods in the same food group are more or less interchangeable, and the different tissues take up whatever nutritive elements they need from the blood stream, to which common reservoir of body-building materials all foods have contributed when they were absorbed after digestion. Special foods do not build special tissues.
Lemons—aid digestion. Oranges—cause acid stomach.	Acid fruits are supposed by some to be a cure for dyspepsia and by others to cause acid stomach. The stomach secretes a digestive fluid that contains hydrochloric acid, which is many times more strongly acid than lemons. If we did not have an acid stomach, conditions would be very abnormal and unfavorable for digestion.
Meats—necessary to build muscle and red blood. —extra amounts needed for muscular work. —poison the system.	Meats, especially organ meats, are excellent sources of iron, protein, and B vitamins, which are important for regeneration of red blood cells and plasma proteins. However, other foods, such as eggs and leafy vegetables, also furnish these nutrients. The energy for muscular work comes mostly from oxidation of carbohydrate and fat. If meats are inspected (free of bacteria and spoilage), kept refrigerated, and well cooked, they have no harmful effects.
Combinations of foods Some food combinations are to be feared or shunned (fish and ice cream, tomatoes and milk).	Fear of certain foods or food combinations is psychologically bad and may lead to one-sided diets that do not provide essential nutrients in adequate quantity. When eaten in moderate amounts and under proper conditions, there are no foods that are incompatible. Selection of foods from all food groups, in the suggested number and size of servings, furnishes a better balanced diet, and thus one that is better for building health.
Nature cults Foods should be eaten in their natural state, mostly raw.	It is good to eat some foods raw, but others (such as whole grains and meats) are usually cooked to soften fiber, develop flavor, and promote their digestibility. If properly cooked, the loss of minerals and vitamins is moderate. Enzymes present in raw foods are proteins, and are destroyed during digestion, so they do not have systemic effects as is claimed.
Natural sugars, such as honey and raw sugar, are better for one than refined sugar.	Although one may enjoy honey or raw sugar for the traces of impurities which give them flavor, they are no better as body fuel than refined sugar (cane or beet). The small amounts of minerals and vitamins in the unrefined products do not add appreciably to the whole day's quota, which must be furnished chiefly by other types of food.
Opposition to use of Iodized salt	Adding small amounts of iodide to refined sea salt is simply replacing the iodine lost in the refining process. Use of iodized salt has proved a safe and effective way of preventing simple goiter in regions where both the water and soil are iodine-poor.
Fluoridated water	Addition of fluorine compounds to city water supplies in areas where water has less than normal amounts of this element represents regulating the naturally low fluorine content to a level that is entirely safe but sufficient to effectively reduce dental caries.

Table continued on opposite page

ucts. Some fallacious food beliefs held by many people in the United States are presented with refutations, in Table 16–1.

Food Fads and Health Foods

There seem always to have been superstitions and false theories about food in this country. It is possible that the present ideas are echoes of the food beliefs of our more traditional forefathers.[13, 14] Some of these current beliefs or fads are exploited by "health food" manufacturers and quack "doctors" at considerable profit to themselves. Fad foods are big business. It has been estimated that at least 10 million

Table 16-1 REFUTING ERRONEOUS IDEAS ABOUT FOODS (*Continued*)

Fallacies	*Facts*
Pasteurized milk	Pasteurization of milk gives important protection against harmful bacteria and does insignificant damage to the nutrients in milk, except for some loss of vitamin C. The normal content of this vitamin in milk is too low and undependable to be counted on in the diet, so that it must be supplemented anyway by one or more rich sources of this vitamin.
Highly milled grains—should never be used.	Either whole or highly milled grains are good sources of energy and furnish some protein. However, the removal of the embryo and outer coats of the grain in milling involves loss of a relatively large proportion of the original content of higher-quality protein, of minerals, B vitamins, and all the vitamin E (in the embryo). Whole-grain products tend not to keep as well in storage, and thus the highly milled products are favored by millers and bakers. If bread and cereals made with highly milled grain are used, they should be of the "enriched" variety—with several B complex vitamins and iron added to replace amounts lost in milling, and other rich sources of the missing nutrients must be included in the diet. Although whole grains have a higher content of minerals and vitamins, bread and cereals made either from the whole grains or from highly milled ones, when enriched, are good food.
Devitalization by overprocessing The American food supply is devitalized by overprocessing.	Some processes do result in lowered nutrient content. Commercial firms take care to protect food flavor, color, and texture. This requires use of techniques that coincidentally tend to conserve nutrients better than home preservation does. Factories for canning or quick-freezing are located in the midst of areas where special crops are produced. Foods are canned in sealed tins from which air has been evacuated before the sterilization process. Dehydrated foods are processed at relatively low temperatures, under conditions (such as in vacuum) in which water is lost quickly. Special packaging also helps conserve vitamin content of foods before they reach the consumer.
Food additives are poisons.	Substances added to foods must pass rigid tests that the foods themselves were never required to do, and the probability is that most are safer than some substances in casual food use (cassava, nutmeg, etc.). Some common additives are nutrients (vitamin C to prevent browning and carotene to provide color).
Vitamin and mineral concentrates —are needed by most persons.	The Federal Food and Drug Administration has stated: "According to the subclinical deficiency myth, anyone who has 'that tired feeling, or an ache or pain in almost any part of the body, is probably suffering a 'subclinical deficiency' and needs to supplement his diet with some concoction. . . . Of course, no normal person can go through even a small part of his life without experiencing some of these symptoms. There is no basis for believing that they are usually due to subclinical deficiencies."

people spend well over half a billion dollars a year on special foods, food supplements, and "health" lectures or literature. Many persons who are without adequate scientific nutrition information can be readily persuaded to try fad foods, especially if their purveyor makes exciting promises and tells a likely story that jibes with the individual's own folklore. Many of these health foods sell for higher prices than regular foods. Many Americans believe, for example, that certain foods, such as oysters and mushrooms, are aphrodisiacs. People believe that raw sugar, wheat germ, honey, and alfalfa sprouts have health-giving properties superior to those of the ordinary wholesome food in the grocery stores.

Some food fads may do little harm except to relieve one of money that might be spent more profitably. If the special diet is administered at a sanatorium, improvement in health may also be induced by baths, outdoor life, and more exercise. Often a fake diet — composed of "cancer-preventing" foods, for instance — may give a false sense of security or hope of relief to a person suffering from a disease or disorder for which it promises a "sure cure," thus causing him to forego consulting a doctor for proper diagnosis and treatment. The quack will claim success in curing diseases for which medicine has yet to find a cure. Patients who suffer from severe and chronic disease conditions not only fail to obtain relief but also may delay seeing a doctor until it is too late.

The food quacks of today probably take the place of the medicine man of traditional cultures and of the vendors of patent medicines in the United States of an earlier era.

Food Aversions

We are all familiar with some religious fiats concerning foods. Most prevalent are those of the Hindus, the Muslims, and the Jews, who have stringent dietary rules forbidding consumption of a wide variety of protein sources. Roman Catholics used to substitute fish for other flesh foods in order to fast on Friday. Many Western people would feel they were committing cannibalism if they were to eat either dog or horse meat. They would perhaps experience a physical revulsion at the idea of dining off their animal friends. Yet dog is relished by some Africans, and the Chinese have long considered dog flesh a delicacy. Horse meat was reintroduced at times of scarcity in Europe in the eighteenth and nineteenth centuries, and is still eaten in some Western countries and by some Western peoples to this day. Indeed, it has been a popular menu item at the Harvard Club in Boston for many years! During the food shortages of World War II it is probable that many people in the United States ate horse meat without being aware of it.

Many theories have been put forth to explain the Biblical food prohibitions against shellfish and the meat of pigs and other animals that do not chew the cud or cleave the hoof, first presented to the Israelites in Leviticus 11:27. Douglas suggests that these prohibitions may have been only an attempt by the priests to restrict animals eaten to those meeting their definition of perfection as part of the worship and sacrifice in the Temple, rather than a codification of the dangers of eating undercooked pork.[15]

There are foods classed by different groups as unfit for human consumption, despite their being as nutritious as the usual dietary components. Efforts to introduce sorghum to one country were futile because the people considered it donkey food. Recommendations to add sweet potatoes to the rations of troops of another country deficient in vitamin A were rejected because sweet potatoes were usual food for swine. Maize corn has been grown in Europe for centuries, but except for Eastern Europe and the Iberian peninsula it is used as animal feed. Its fairly recent introduction to Southeast Asian countries for this latter purpose has had a reverse side influence: It is sold by shops and sidewalk vendors, boiled on the cob, as a snack food.

Chicken used to be a food reserved for special occasions in the United States. When chicken rearing moved from the back yard to big batteries of broiler and egg factories, prices went down and chicken became one of our best meat buys. However, chicken and their eggs are avoided by some social groups. They have been traditionally important in divination for many societies, both the eggs and the entrails and bones of the chicken.

Folk Medicine: "Hot" or "Cold" Foods

Food beliefs and all traditional medical systems are rather closely entwined. This is particularly true of the Ayurvedic (traditional Hindu) and Chinese medical systems. This fact is being demonstrated repeatedly in a new discipline called medical anthropology. A few generations ago the arrival of spring was the signal for a dose of "sulfur and molasses" or for eating a boiled-up mess of dandelion greens. Some people still "feed a cold and starve a fever." Folk medicine survives among subgroups or in out-of-the-way areas in our own country. Not so many years ago a Vermont doctor made a bit of money selling honey and vinegar as a twentieth century cure-all, and even published a book about it.

Latin Americans, including Mexicans who have emigrated to our country, ascribe to most foods an assumed physiological "heating" or "cooling" effect. These beliefs about innate characteristics of food that can be transferred to those eating them are found throughout a large part of the world. Latin Americans obtained them from the colonizing Spaniards, who in turn probably received them from the Moors. They were spread by the Arabs along with Islam to Southeast Asia, including Indonesia, the Philippines, and the Malay Peninsula. Mainland Chinese hold similar beliefs.[16] The ultimate origin of these beliefs that foods are of themselves "cold" or "hot" is not yet known with certainty. We find an echo of it in our own saying "cool as a cucumber." These categorizations have nothing to do with temperatures of the foods, nor does "hot" mean the peppery hotness of red chilis. Even today, spicy foods are popular in many warm climates of the world.

To most persons holding these views, other things besides foods, including illnesses, have "hot" or "cold" properties. The assignment of the quality of "hot" or "cold" is not, however, consistent from one population group to another, or even among the people within the group who have these beliefs. Thus, some societies will define an illness as "hot" and try to bring the body into balance by treating it with food or medicine having "cooling" properties, or vice versa. Some cultural groups try to "balance" the diet by setting "hot" foods against "cold" ones at the same meal. This practice is observed by the Chinese and many Latin Americans. For centuries, the Chinese have held a special place for food in their lives, even before the knowledge of nutrients. Many Chinese believe ginger root, a "hot food," strengthens their heart muscles. Seaweed, white turnips, and bean sprouts, all "cold foods," are believed responsible for frequent urination, low blood pressure, and shortness of breath.[7] Others, like Malays, allow only people culturally defined as quite healthy to eat "cold" foods. Clark, while studying a Mexican community in California, found that women who wish to conceive, as well as those who have just given birth, must avoid "cold" foods, with fruit juices, tomatoes, and most vegetables being regarded as "too cold" for the stomach.[17] Pork, ordinarily defined by most people in the community as "hot," is also to be avoided by the woman who is lying in. If she eats them, she will get varicose veins of the leg. Like the Malay woman,[4] the Mexican women in this California community observed the dietary proscriptions against "cold" foods for 40 days. Those more tradition-oriented continued them until the child was weaned, which at the time of the research was anywhere from 6 to 8 weeks to a year or 18 months.

Food Choices of Special Groups

We have numerous subgroups in the United States with their own distinctive diets and cuisines, not yet wholly altered by contact with supermarkets and advertising. Puerto Ricans, Seventh-Day Adventists, Amish, American Indians, health food advocates, and Southern Negroes are all peoples who for various cultural reasons (such as religion, economics, or habitual choice) eat differently. Though their food habits may be known, little study has been made of their beliefs about food and its properties, to see how far they may deviate from present-day scientific knowledge, or what effect their beliefs may have upon nutrient intakes of the groups in question. Much more needs to be done in this area.

It should be emphasized that food beliefs and practices that differ from our own are not all deleterious. Problems arise with such diets when they are changed in some ways by the groups who eat them coming in contact with other types of foods that seem more desirable but are not balanced nutritionally.

Lee[18] has described an extreme example of nutritional adaptation to a rather harsh environment in his study of the Bushmen of the Kalahari Desert. Their diet consists solely of edible items available in the area. They have various reserve foods used in emergencies when climatic conditions interfere with the usual food supply. The diet is nutritionally adequate, and they do not suffer in periods of shortage of their usual staple, a local nut.

Prestige Value of Foods

One other aspect of beliefs about food that can influence nutrient intake is the relative status that certain foods are accorded. Sometimes prestige is attached to scarce, high-priced items, making them sought after. We can think immediately of white flour and white bread, which replaced natural "black" bread in Europe in the last century. These same products have been considered prestigious and hence have been much sought after when introduced to peoples in developing regions of the globe, despite higher prices than those of the indigenous foods for which they substituted. The same has been true for polished white rice, sweetened canned condensed milk, biscuits (sweet cookies), and other foods once reserved for the upper social strata. Sometimes low-status foods are good nutrient sources, and their consumption ought to be encouraged rather than looked down on. During the 1800's beans had a higher status than today. Beans were used as coinage, as well as for a rich source of protein. Gold miners valued beans at 100 dollars a pound. Subsequently, food merchants were richer than miners. Many cultures consider local indigenous greens "emergency" or "poor folks" foods, and although they may eat them, they are most reluctant to allow outsiders to know of it. The Indians of the high Andes of South America have low regard for the local grain *quinoa,* which grows only in this region, despite its being one of their staples. Chemical examination has shown it to be high in protein, calcium, phosphorus, iron, and niacin content.[19] Seacoast Southeast Asians who dry their surplus fish catch for times of scarcity consider dried fish far less desirable than fresh.

CHANGING FOOD HABITS

Authorities agree that food habits are one of the most difficult things to try to change. Especially in countries where problems of malnutrition have reached serious proportions, government authorities would like to know how to alter traditional patterns of feeding that nutritionists have shown to be deleterious, or how to introduce new, more nutritious foods. But food habits do change spontaneously, all the time, and new foods are constantly being introduced. The potato, maize corn, chocolate, cassava, tomato, and cashew are just a few foods that were taken by the Spanish conquerors of the New World back to Europe, from which they have spread worldwide. Latter-day conquerors of a different sort have caused refined flour and sugar and cola and other soft drinks to be available in nearly every corner of the globe.

The problems that changing food habits present are indeed complex, and there do not appear to be any simple answers, although knowledge has progressed beyond an earlier attitude that people would change their "bad" food habits if only they were told how to do so. During the Second World War, the U.S. National Research Council established a Committee on Food Habits, which examined some of the cultural and psychological aspects of eating and made some concrete suggestions for improving diets.[10, 20] The Committee was created, among other reasons, to help encourage consumption of less familiar foods among the population at home when much that was customary had been diverted for troop feeding abroad.[21] Diet improvements included introduction of substitutes resembling familiar foods, and enrichment. Research supported by the Committee showed the importance of emotional and cultural components of attitudes about food in choice of diet.

New foods may be accepted if they resemble some already-liked item in taste or texture. Foods already eaten by leaders or other prestigious persons, or foods with a money value, are also more likely to be incorporated into diets. It is far more difficult to eradicate undesirable food habits. It also seems likely that, once people have begun to change, it would be futile to try to hold them back to the more traditional way of eating that they are trying to abandon. When attempts are made to change food habits, it has always to be remembered that what is really being changed is part of the culture. When changes in the culture go along with the changes in food practices in ways that help reinforce and encourage the latter, both have a better chance of success.

Burgess and Dean[19] have emphasized that food habits learned very early in life in a pleasurable home environment are most resistant and difficult to change. Other workers have found that the food habits of some people do change more readily when they move to a very different cultural setting. At present there are no formulas that would permit prediction in advance about whether or not a particular habit or group of attitudes will respond to efforts to guide or direct changes.

Because an individual's choices of food are affected by so many variables, such as climate, availability, religion, emotions, taste, economics, local agricultural practices, and traditions, many factors must be studied and considered before attempts at change are made. Many disciplines are combining to contribute further to knowledge about this area. Much still remains to be done.

QUESTIONS AND PROBLEMS

1. Make a list of any prejudices that you may have against the eating of certain foods or combinations of foods. Are these prejudices warranted in the light of facts? Are you inclined to indulge in certain well-liked foods or classes of food to the exclusion of other food groups that are needed for proper nutrition? Have you any dietary fads or fancies?

2. Talk with several other persons, and make a list of any superstitions about food, prejudices against or in favor of certain foods, or practice of dietary fads, which you may find among these people. Which of these may have some basis in fact and which are not based on reason? Give reasons for your conclusions.

3. Discuss reasons — physical, economic, psychological, or emotional — why persons develop and persist in faulty food habits or go along with food fads. Make suggestions on ways to induce such persons to alter their food habits.

REFERENCES

1. DeGarine, I.: The socio-cultural aspects of nutrition. Ecol. Food Nutr., *1*:143, 1972.
2. Ogbeide, O.: Nutritional hazards of food taboos and preferences in Mid-West Nigeria. Amer. J. Clin. Nutr., *27*:213, 1974.
3. Laguna, J., and Carpenter, K. J.: Raw versus processed corn in niacin-deficient diets. J. Nutr., *45*:21, 1951.
4. Wilson, C. S.: Food beliefs affect nutritional status of Malay fisherfolk. J. Nutr. Educ., *2*:96, 1971.
5. Katona-Apte, J.: The socio-cultural aspects of food avoidance in a low-income population in Tarnilnad, South India. Environ. Child Health, *23*:83, 1977.
6. Jelliffe, D. B.: *The Assessment of the Nutritional Status of the Community.* WHO Monograph Series No. 53. Geneva, World Health Organization, 1966.
7. Chang, B.: Some dietary beliefs in Chinese Folk Culture. J. Amer. Dietet. Assoc., *65*:436, 1974.
8. Rochow, V. B.: Edible insects in three different ethnic groups of Papua and New Guinea. Amer. J. Clin. Nutr., *26*:673, 1973.
9. Parrish, J. B.: Implications of changing food habits for nutrition educators. J. Nutr. Educ., *2*:140, 1971.
10. Mead, M.: *The Problem of Changing Food Habits.* Washington, D.C., National Academy of Sciences–National Research Council Bulletin 108, 1943.
11. Erhard, D.: Nutrition education for the "now" generation. J. Nutr. Educ., *2*:135, 1971.
12. Wagner, P. M.: Food as ritual. In *Food and Civi-*

lization, A Symposium. Springfield, Ill., Charles C Thomas, 1966.
13. Deutsch, R. M.: Who's to blame for nutrition nonsense? Today's Health, May, 1967, p. 66.
14. Stare, F. J., and Nelson, P.: Don't fall for fads. Family Health, *2*:41, 1970.
15. Douglas, M.: *Purity and Danger. An Analysis of Concepts of Pollution and Taboo.* Harmondsworth, England, Penguin, 1970.
16. Hart, D. V.: *Bisayan Filipino and Malayan Humoral Pathologies: Folk Medicine and Ethnohistory in Southeast Asia.* Data Paper No. 76. Ithaca, New York, Southeast Asia Program, Cornell University, 1969.
17. Clark, M.: *Health in the Mexican-American Culture.* Berkeley, University of California Press, 1970.
18. Lee, R. B., and DeVore, I. (eds.): *Man, The Hunter.* Chicago, Aldine, 1968.
19. Burgess, A., and Dean, R. F. A.: *Malnutrition and Food Habits.* New York, Macmillan, 1962.
20. National Research Council: *Manual for the Study of Food Habits.* Washington, D.C., National Academy of Sciences–National Research Council Bulletin 111, 1945.
21. Mead, M.: *Food Habits Research: Problems of the 1960's.* Washington, D.C., National Academy of Sciences–National Research Council Publication 1225, 1964.

SUPPLEMENTARY READING

General, History, and Reviews

Blix, G. (ed.): *Food Cultism and Nutrition Quakery.* Symposia of the Swedish Nutrition Foundation VIII, 1970.

Barrett, S., and Knight, G.: *The Health Robbers.* Philadelphia, George F. Stickley Co., 1976.

Caliendo, M. A., and Sanjur, D.: The dietary status of preschool children: an ecological approach. J. Nutr. Ed., *10*:69, 1978.

Church, M., and Doughty, J.: Value of traditional food practices in nutrition educatioin. J. Hum. Nutr., *30*:9, 1976.

Deutsch, R. M.: *The Nuts Among the Berries.* Rev. Ed. Menlo Park, Calif., Bull Publishing Co., 1977.

Famine symposium. (7 papers) Ecol. Food Nutr., *7*: 1–57, 1978.

Garn, S. M., and Clark, D. C.: Economics and fatness. Ecol. Food Nutr., *3*:19, 1974.

Grivetti, L. E.: Food habit research: a review of approaches and methods. J. Nutr. Ed., *5*:204, 1973.

Grivetti, L. E., and Pangborn, R. M.: Origin of selected Old Testament dietary prohibitions. An evaluative review. J. Amer. Dietet. Assoc., *65*:634, 1974.

Hertzler, A. A., and Owen, C.: Sociologic study of food habits — a review. J. Amer. Dietet. Assoc., *69*:377, 1976.

Kallen, D. J.: Malnutrition, learning and behavior. Ecol. Food Nutr., *2*:133, 1973.

Lowenberg, M. E.: The development of food patterns. J. Amer. Dietet. Assoc., *65*:262, 1974.

Oddy, D. J.: Food in nineteenth century England: nutrition in the first urban society. Proc. Nutr. Soc., *29*:150, 1970.

Phillips, D. E., Bass, M. A., and Yetley, E.: Use of food and nutrition knowledge by mothers of preschool children. J. Nutr. Ed., *10*:73, 1978.

Renner, H. D.: *The Origin of Food Habits.* London, Faber and Faber, 1944.

Robson, J. R. K.: Changing food habits in developing countries. Ecol. Food Nutr., *6*:187, 1977.

Simoons, F. J.: The determinants of dairying and milk use in the Old World: ecological, physiological, and cultural. Ecol. Food Nutr., *2*:83, 1973.

Symposium: Flavor and culture (five papers). Food Tech., *29*:34–51, 1975.

Symposium: Sense of taste and nutrition (6 papers). Amer. J. Clin. Nutr., *31*:1057–1104, 1978.

Todhunter, E. N.: Food habits, food faddism, and nutrition. World Rev. Nutr. Dietet., *16*:286, 1973.

Wilson, C. S.: Food habits: a selected annotated bibliography. A handbook of references. J. Nutr. Ed., 5(1):Supplement 1, Jan. 1973.

Yudkin, J., and McKenzie, J. C. (eds.): *Changing Food Habits.* London, MacGibbon and Kee, 1964.

(Also see current issues of the journal Ecology of Food and Nutrition. The address is provided at the end of Chapter 1.)

Foods — Attitudes, and Taboos

International

Bolton, J. M.: Food taboos among the Orang Asli in West Malaysia: a potential nutritional hazard. Amer. J. Clin. Nutr., *25*:789, 1972.

Coe, J. C.: Food habits in Chile: a report of an anthropological study in four neighborhoods in Santiago. J. Applied Nutr. *28*:30, 1976.

Ernster, M.: Investigation of dietary changes in the Gezira, Sudan. Ecol. Food Nutr., *5*:217, 1976.

Geissler, C., Calloway, D. H., and Margen, S.: Lactation and pregnancy in Iran. 1. Social and economic aspects. Amer. J. Clin. Nutr., *31*:160, 1978.

Hsu, L. C.: Nutrition from China to the west art-science quality of nutrition. Ecol. Food Nutr., *3*:303, 1974.

Hunt, S.: The food habits of Asian immigrants. Part I, Nutr. Food Sci., *43*:2, 1976; Part II, Nutr. Food Sci., *44*:15, 1976.

Jansen, G. R., Jansen, N. B., Shigetomi, C. T., and Harper, J. M.: Effect of income and geographic region on the nutritional value of diets in Brazil. Amer. J. Clin. Nutr., *30*:955, 1977.

Knutsson, K. E., and Selinus, R.: Fasting in Ethiopia. An anthropological and nutritional study. Amer. J. Clin. Nutr., *23*:956, 1970.

Omololu, A.: Changing food habits in Africa. Ecol. Food Nutr., *1*:165, 1972.

Robson, J. R. K., and Wadsworth, G. R.: The health

and nutritional status of primitive populations. Ecol. Food Nutr., *6*:187, 1977.

Sakr, A. H.: Fasting in Islam. J. Amer. Dietet. Assoc., *67*:17, 1975.

Simoons, F. J.: The purificatory role of the five products of the cow in Hinduism. Ecol. Food Nutr., *3*:21, 1974; Rejection of fish as human food in Africa: a problem in history and ecology. *3*:89, 1974; Fish as forbidden food: the case of India. *3*:185, 1974.

Wilson, C. S.: Food taboos of childbirth: the Malay example. Ecol. Food Nutr., *2*:267, 1973.

Woolfe, J. A., Wheeler, E. F., Van Dyke, W., and Orraca-Tetteh, R.: The value of the Ghanian traditional diet in relation to the energy needs of young children. Ecol. Food Nutr., *6*:175, 1977.

North America

Bremer, M., and Weatherholtz, W. M.: Nutrition attitudes in a university community. J. Nutr. Ed., *7*:60, 1975.

Brittin, H. C., and Zinn, D. W.: Meat-buying practices of Caucasians, Mexican-Americans, and Negroes. J. Amer. Dietet. Assoc., *71*:623, 1977.

Calloway, D. H., and Gibbs, J. C.: Food patterns and food assistance programs in the Cocopah Indian community. Ecol. Food Nutr., *5*:183, 1976 (a study of pantothenic and other vitamins at risk).

Cosper, B. A., and Wakefield, L. M.: Food choices of women: personal, attitudinal, and motivational factors. J. Amer. Dietet. Assoc., *66*:152, 1975.

Dilling, L. A., Ellestao-Sayed, J., Coodin, F. J., and Haworth, J. C.: Growth and nutrition of preschool Indian children in Manitoba: 1. Vitamin D deficiency. Can. J. Pub. Health, *69*:248, 1978.

Duyff, R. L., Sanjur, D., and Nelson, H. Y.: Food behavior and related factors of Puerto Rican–American teenagers. J. Nutr. Ed., *7*:99, 1975.

Inano, M., and Pringle, D. J.: Dietary survey of low-income, rural families in Iowa and North Carolina. II. Family distribution of dietary adequacy. J. Amer. Dietet. Assoc., *66*:361, 1975.

Jakobovits, C., et al.: Eating habits and nutrient intakes of college women over a thirty-year period. J. Amer. Dietet. Assoc., *71*:405, 1977.

Kaufman, N. A., Posnaski, R., and Guggenheim, K.: Eating habits and opinions of teenagers on nutrition and obesity. J. Amer. Dietet. Assoc., *66*:264, 1975.

Kight, M. A., et al.: Nutritional influences of Mexican-American foods in Arizona. J. Amer. Dietet. Assoc., *55*:557, 1969.

Kuhnlein, H. V., and Calloway, D. H.: Contemporary Hopi food intake patterns. Ecol. Food Nutr., *6*:159, 1977.

Lewis, J. S., and Glaspy, M. F.: Food habits and nutrient intakes of Filipino women in Los Angeles. J. Amer. Dietet. Assoc., *67*:122, 1975.

Myres, A. W., and Kroetsch, D.: Influence of family income on food consumption patterns and nutrient intake in Canada. Can. J. Pub. Health, *69*: 208, 1978.

Natow, A. B., Heslin, J. A., and Raven, B. C.: Integrating the Jewish Dietary Laws into a dietetics program. Kasruth in a dietetics curriculum. J. Amer. Dietet. Assoc., *67*:13, 1975.

Prothro, J., Mickles, M., and Tolbert, B.: Nutritional status of a population sample in Macon County, Alabama. Amer. J. Clin. Nutr., *29*:94, 1976.

Sims, L. S., and Morris, P. M.: Nutritional status of preschoolers. J. Amer. Dietet. Assoc., *64*:492, 1974.

Wenkam, N. S., and Wolff, R. J.: A half century of changing food habits among Japanese in Hawaii. J. Amer. Dietet. Assoc., *57*:29, 1970.

Food Faddism

American Academy of Pediatrics, Committee on Nutrition; Nutritional aspects of vegetarianism, health foods, and fad diets. Pediatrics, *59*:460, 1977.

Calvert, G. P., and Calvert, S. W.: Intellectual convictions of "health" food consumers. J. Nutr. Ed., *7*:95, 1975.

Dwyer, J. T., et al.: Preschoolers on alternate life-style diets. Associations between size and dietary indexes with diets limited in types of animal foods. J. Amer. Dietet. Assoc., *72*:264, 1978.

Dwyer, J. T., et al.: The new vegetarians: the natural high? J. Amer. Dietet. Assoc., *65*:529, 1974.

Jukes, T. H.: Mutiny on the Bounty. Nature, *261*:92, 1976.

Khan, P., and Adams, G.: Food faddism, a new religion? Food Prod. Dev., April 1976, p. 40.

McBean, L. D., and Speckmann, E. W.: Food faddism: a challenge to nutritionists and dietitians, Amer. J. Clin. Nutr., *27*:1071, 1974.

Rhee, K. S., and Stubbs, A. C.: Health food users in two Texas cities. Nutritonal and socioeconomic implications. J. Amer. Dietet. Assoc., *68*:542, 1976.

Robson, J. R. K.: Food faddism. Symposium on nutrition in pediatrics. Pediat. Clin. North Amer., *24*: 189, 1977.

Schafer, R., and Yetley, E. A.: Social psychology of food faddism. Speculations on health food behavior. J. Amer. Dietet. Assoc., *66*:129, 1975.

Sherlock, P., and Rothschild, E. O.: Scurvy produced by a Zen macrobiotic diet. J.A.M.A., *199*:794, 1967.

Sims, L. S.: Food related value-orientations. Attitudes, and beliefs of vegetarians and non-vegetarians. Ecol. Food Nutr., *7*:23, 1978.

Smith, E. B.: A guide to good eating the vegetarian way. J. Nutr. Ed., *7*:109, 1975.

Other Readings on Food and Culture

Barlow, D. H., and Tillotson, J. L.: Behavioral science and nutrition: a new perspective. J. Amer. Dietet. Assoc., *72*:368, 1978. (Also see p. 378.)

Food — economic and labeling violations. FDA Consumer, *8*(9):40, 1974.

Greecher, C. P., and Shannon, B.: Impact of fast food

meals on nutrient intake of two groups. J. Amer. Dietet. Assoc., *70*:368, 1977.

Heenan, J.: Myths of vitamins. FDA Consumer, *8*:4, 1974.

Krondl, M. M., and Lau, D.: Food habit modification. Can. J. Pub. Health, *69*:39, 1978.

Malo-Juvera, D., and Boykin, L.: La Marqueta: a food habits learning experience. J. Nutr. Ed., *7*:58, 1975.

Nobmann, E. D., and Adams, S.: Survey of changes in food habits during pregnancy. Pub. Health Rpt., *85*:1121, 1970.

Schafer, R. B.: Factors affecting food behavior and the quality of husbands' and wives' diets. J. Amer. Dietet. Assoc., *72*:138, 1978.

Schafer, R. B., and Bohlen, J. M.: Exchange of conjugal power in the control of family food consumption. Home Econ. Res. J., *6*:131, 1977.

Schwartz, N. E., and Barr, S. I.: Mothers—their attitudes and practices in perinatal nutrition. J. Nutr. Ed., *9*:169, 1977.

Seshadri, S., and Harrill, I.: Nutrient intake of college students from India in the United States. Nutr. Rpt. Internat., *3*:159, 1971.

Wang, V. L.: Changing nutritional behavior by aides in two programs. J. Nutr. Ed., *9*:109, 1977.

Weathersbee, P. S., Olsen, L. K., and Lodge, J. R.: Selected beverage consumption patterns among Mormon and non-Mormon populations from the same geographic location. Amer. J. Clin. Nutr., *30*:1162, 1977.

Articles in *Nutrition Reviews*

Stuff on which quackery thrives? *32*:316, 1974.

Chinese herbal medicines. *32*:317, 1974.

Changing patterns of food consumption in Britain (by Hollingsworth, D.). *32*:353, 1974.

Cultural practices and anemia in Nigeria. *34*:269, 1976.

The unripe Akee — forbidden fruit. *34*:349, 1976.

Nutritional aspects of vegetarianism, health foods, and fad diets. *35*:153, 1977.

(Also see Supplement 1, July 1974, pp. 1–67, with 17 papers on food faddism and taboos.)

Chapter 17

Food: From the Producer to the Consumer

In the preceding chapters, the individual nutrients and their functions and fate in the body have been studied. In nature these nutrients are the chemical structures that compose almost all of the plant, animal, or human body. Though food is made up of chemicals, most of which are nutrients, it would be foolish to attempt to live solely on mixtures of synthetic or purified nutrients. Commonly available foodstuffs are our preferred sources of required nutrients for social, nutritional, and economic, as well as practical, reasons. Food, while serving as a vehicle for bringing people their nutrients, also fulfills the important need for variety, sensory pleasure, and social identification (see Chapter 16).

This chapter deals briefly with the channels through which nutrients travel from the farm to reach your body. These channels include food production and processing, and the distribution of food to the retail store, restaurant, fast-food outlet, or home kitchen (see Fig. 17–1). The chapter also describes in some detail the most common foodstuffs available to us in North America and tells how one may stretch the food dollar without sacrificing good nutrition. For the student who wishes to pursue these topics further, additional reading suggestions are given at the end of the chapter. (Also see the remaining chapters for advice on personal food choices.)

TO THE MARKET FROM THE FARM

Plant material is the source of most food, either directly or indirectly. Farmers and ranchers raise crops, breed fish and poultry, and herd cattle. This food ultimately leaves the farm in the form of plants, seeds, fruits, milk, eggs, or meat. The farmer's first concern is to produce, at a profit, the food that will be purchased in the marketplace by the consumer. This is the major factor in the choice of foods the farmer will produce.

For most of the world's population, either food must be produced at home or a household member must go to a marketplace — or a combination of these two. At its simplest, a market can be someone sitting by a roadside selling surplus food they have raised to passing neighbors.

Food on an American breakfast table is a result of a very complex market system. It might include a melon grown in Texas, toast made from wheat grown in Kansas and made into bread in a nearby city bakery, coffee from Latin America, sugar grown in Louisiana or Hawaii and

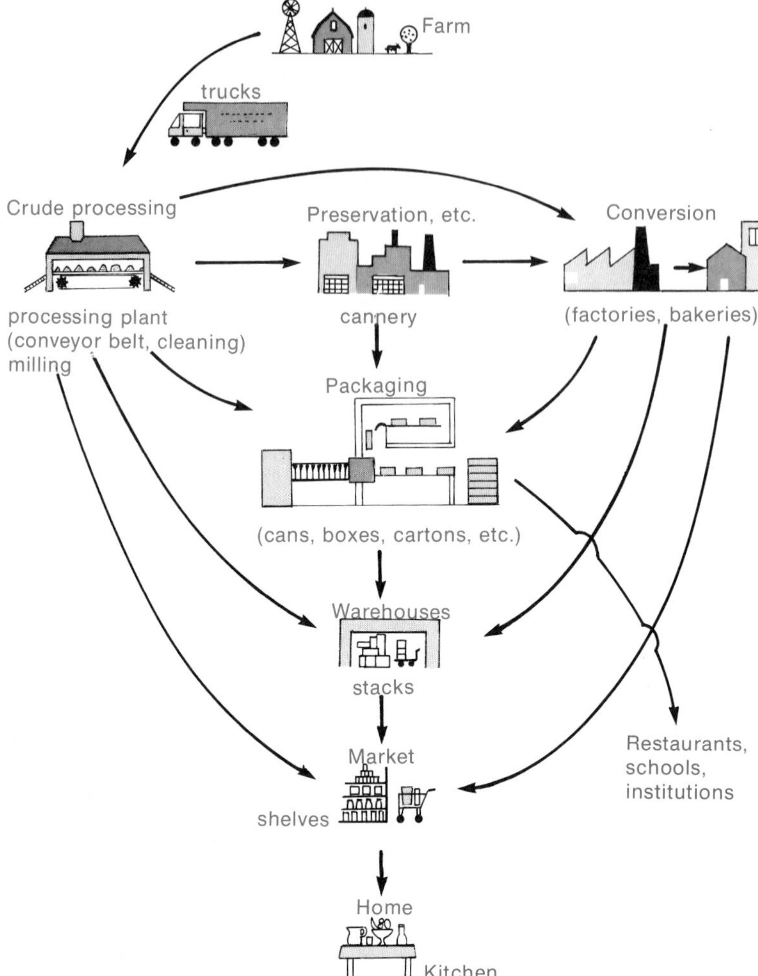

Figure 17–1 Diagram of food channels from farm to consumer.

refined in California or Boston, and marmalade made in Scotland from bitter oranges grown in Spain. All this food reaches the consumer through a long chain of middlemen — food brokers, food industries, shippers, and truckers — until the food reaches the shops or supermarkets where it is bought and brought home to serve.

The existence of markets and the middlemen who supply them means that some kind of organization has taken place in the production of food. This is as important to an abundant food supply as is climate, soil fertility, and other geographic conditions.

Improvements in technology and transportation have long since made many products available worldwide on a year-round basis for much of the technically advanced world, and in more cosmopolitan centers of developing countries. Income permitting, one can buy fresh strawberries in winter, French truffles in New York, American turkey in Singapore, and frozen peas in a host of cities in between. Despite our highly complex marketing system, which depends on a sophisticated food technology industry along with a large and highly developed and integrated network of transportation, the modern market still can be reduced to the same fundamental components as the earliest and most primitive market. Ultimately there is a producer — a farmer, herder, or fisherman — and a consumer. They interact, though many intermediates stand between them. This interaction of consumer and producer influences what the middleman offers for sale. In a free market economy, consumers want products and producers seek profit; thus, whether a food appears in a market depends on what price the consumer is willing to pay and on what the middleman has to offer.

A producer will be discouraged from raising crops that cannot be readily sold or easily processed. In many agricultural communities, including here in the United States, it has often been more profitable to raise nonfood crops for cash — tobacco, cotton, flax, trees, and so on.

Development of Efficient Agriculture

In the United States and a number of other Western countries today, agriculture has become so highly specialized that one farmer can feed about 45 other people.* The converse of this situation still holds in many parts of the developing world, where up to 70 percent or more of the adult population work in agriculture in order to feed the population. In many parts of the world, especially in warm climates, one finds peasants using primitive methods of agriculture employed by their ancestors, such as wooden plows, water wheels used for irrigation that are turned by camels or manpower, and primitive methods of threshing.

In pre-Columbian North America, food was obtained by hunting and gathering, or by subsistence agriculture. With European colonization, a prosperous economy developed in which the farm homes and small towns were mostly self-sufficient in food supplies and crafts needed for making other necessities of life — such as cloth, soap, tools, and household utensils. Industrialization and the resultant migration to cities came somewhat later in the United States than in Europe, but it developed from the early 1800's, with increasing rapidity during the 50 years between 1880 and 1930.

With high emigration rates and the popularity then of large families, the population of the United States increased rapidly, making it necessary to use all available land for farming purposes. In the past 60 years, with the opening of foreign markets for our surplus foods because of famines, wars, droughts, and population pressures, there has been a great incentive to increase food production. Because land is in short supply, this has been done largely by increasing the yield per acre through application of scientific agriculture. This developed primarily as a result of our well-known system of *land-grant colleges* and their efficient agriculture experimental and extension programs throughout the 50 states. Agricultural efficiency has been increased by crop rotation, fertilization of soils, improved farm machinery, better strains of seeds, better pesticides, irrigation, improved ecological measures (such as biological control of pests and soil conservation), as well as improved breeds of animals and more efficient production of meats, eggs, and milk.

In the United States, fewer farmers produce more food on less land. Former farm or pasture land is being subdivided for housing developments near larger population centers, converted to parks or golf courses, or paved over for highways.

Food travels to markets around the world in many ways as there are types of transportation. Whether by refrigerated trailer trucks, box cars, freighters, planes, horses, camels, donkeys, bicycles, or canoes, transportation is vital for marketing of fresh food, even if it must be carried on foot. Highway systems, paved all-weather roads, ports, and suitably dredged water-

*However, many middlemen are necessary to accomplish this feat. Some furnish the equipment, supplies, and research that allow one farmer to grow enough for 45 people. Others are shippers, processors, inspectors, wholesalers, and retailers who facilitate distribution of the food.

ways are thus important contributors to improvements in marketing.

Most of the food on America's tables comes from the farmer by way of various processors for canning, freezing, drying, packaging, or other types of food preparation such as the making of biscuits, noodles, bread, cakes, sauces, and condiments. Then, through other middlemen, it reaches wholesalers, including food chain warehouses, from which it is shipped again to retail stores and supermarkets.

METHODS OF PROCESSING AND PRESERVING FOOD

Even food that we buy in its "natural" state, such as eggs, fresh fruits, and vegetables, is usually routed through various middlemen and undergoes processing such as cleaning, sorting, and packaging. Inedible portions of the food, such as husks and pods, are removed. Naturally occurring toxins are inactivated. Filth and impurities such as twigs, pebbles, and dirt are washed out. Other processing operations are performed to preserve food products so that they can remain free of microbial spoilage, rancidity, flavor loss, destruction by enzymes present in the food, and other types of deterioration over the period of time necessary for transportation and storage. Such processing helps ensure digestible, safe, and clean products. The following six sections outline the major types of basic food processing procedures in use today before food is even packaged, stored, or brought to the marketplace. Some of these date back to ancient times.

Milling

Grains are milled to flour by removing the bran and germ of the kernel and crushing the endosperm. The products are separated by a series of sifters and rollers. The degree of milling will vary with the grade of flour desired. In the United States about 30 percent of the wheat kernel, mainly the bran and the germ, is removed to make our common white flour (see Table 17–1). Thus, about 70 percent of the wheat is recovered as white flour — which is called in the trade an "extraction rate" of 70 percent. White flour keeps better over long periods than does ground whole wheat, since most of the germ and bran is removed. Federal standards at present prevent us from having an intermediate grade of flour of about 80 to 85 percent extraction rate. Such a flour would be nutritionally superior to our present white flour.

Most white flours in the country have had bleaching and maturing agents added to them, although the white color develops naturally to a great extent in storage.

Heating and Canning

Canning has probably contributed more than any other form of food processing to the maintenance of an adequate food supply throughout the year. The industry had its beginning in the United States in 1819, but gained in volume

Table 17–1 LOSSES OF NUTRIENTS IN THE REFINING OF WHEAT*

Nutrient	*Wheat* *mcg/gm*	*White Flour* *mcg/gm*	*Loss in Refining* %
Thiamin	3.5	0.8	77.1
Riboflavin	1.5	0.3	80.0
Niacin	50	9.5	80.8
Vitamin B-6	1.7	0.5	71.8
Pantothenic acid	10	5	50.0
Folacin	0.3	0.1	66.7
α-Tocopherol	16	2.2	86.3
Choline	1089	767	29.5
Manganese	46	6.5	85.8
Iron	43	10.5	75.6
Zinc	35	7.8	77.7
	%	%	
Calcium	0.045	0.018	60.0
Phosphorus	0.433	0.126	70.9
Magnesium	0.183	0.028	84.7
Potassium	0.454	0.105	77.0

*Adapted from Schroeder, H. A.: Amer. J. Clin. Nutr., *24*:562, 1971.

steadily after the introduction of steam pressure processing in sealed tins in 1874. Under steam pressure, processing is accomplished at higher temperatures and in a much shorter time, and results in a better quality product. The high temperature is important to inactivate microbes that may produce toxins in the sealed can. For many foods (including some that have been concentrated by removal of water), the sealed can offers the most convenient method for transportation and storage without refrigeration. Pasteurization is another process employing heat.

A new process known as *aseptic canning*, in which food is canned under aseptic conditions—in which levels of bacteria are kept as low as possible during canning, allows certain foods to be canned with much less heat than is otherwise necessary.

Heating of food can result in the loss of the amino acid lysine and reduce the vitamin B content of some foods, but it will not affect food minerals. Some foods may be improved nutritionally by heating because of the destruction of certain inhibitors naturally present in food (such as the trypsin inhibitors in various legumes).

Dehydration

Dehydration (removal of most or all of the water) is still one of the best ways of preserving foods and reducing transportation costs. It is a time-honored method of food preservation, and technological advances have made possible products of much-improved quality at lower cost. New methods include quick drying at lower temperatures under vacuum or reduced pressure, with controlled temperature and fans for removal of the water vapor. If the product is in liquid form, it may be blown in small droplets into a heated chamber, where it dries almost instantly to a fine powder. The resulting product has excellent keeping qualities and can later be "reconstituted" by the addition of water. This process has given us the very useful dried milk, which is the least expensive and most transportable form of milk solids. Other products made by spray-drying are cream substitutes for use in coffee, citrus products, other fruit beverages, and instant coffee, all of which are ready for use merely by adding suitable amounts of water.

Partial dehydration, as in condensed or evaporated milks, has long been in use. Foods may be dehydrated by being cut in thin slices that are passed on a conveyor belt through an oven, or they may be finely mashed and placed on a perforated tray or mat. A current of heated air is blown up through the perforations. Such processes have been successfully used in drying fruits (for use in prepared cereals), vegetables (for casserole dishes), and soup mixes. Fatty foods are not suitable for drying, since drying may reduce the stability of the fat components and lead to rancidity.

Dehydrated foods, precooked or raw, have been developed for activities that require lightweight foods (for individual carrying or air drop) that keep without refrigeration over long periods and can be reconstituted with the mere addition of water (hot or cold, as the food requires). With special packaging, such foods can be readily adapted for space travel.

Freezing

Frozen foods first came into wide use some years ago, when deep-freeze refrigerator compartments and separate units for quantity storage became available in the home. Meats, fish, and vegetables are the foods most commonly preserved by this process. The variety and quality of frozen foods continue to improve, and one can purchase them in packages of quantities to suit the size of the family. Because of their excellent flavor and the saving of labor in preparation, frozen vegetables are strong competitors with the fresh varieties. Frozen fruits retain their fresh flavor and nutritive value better than canned fruits. Such items are especially valuable for variety in the diet during the seasons when fresh fruits and vegetables are scarce or high in price.

Most frozen foods must constantly be kept refrigerated in storage, in transport, and finally in the grocer's display counter, all of which adds to their cost. Those frozen foods that sell in very large volume are competitive in price with fresh products, or they may even be cheaper (e.g., frozen, concentrated orange juice usually is cheaper than fresh orange juice). Other frozen foods that entail considerable labor in preparation and expense in packaging and refrigeration tend to be luxury items, which the consumer may buy, regardless of cost, in order to save time and labor in preparing meals.

Freeze-Drying

Foods may be frozen raw or precooked and may be partially dehydrated either before or after the freezing process. In the latter process (known as freeze-drying), raw food is quickly frozen, then passed into a special vacuum chamber, where the moisture is removed from the food by sublimation — that is, ice crystals go directly into the vapor state without passing through the liquid state. Freeze-dried foods have a spongy texture but retain their shape and flavor, require no refrigeration in storage, and can be reconstituted readily by placing in warm water. The reconstituted product looks and tastes very much like its fresh counterpart. Many products, including instant coffee, onions, chives, and vegetables, are freeze-dried.

Radiation

Radiation preservation is being tested as a means to decrease product spoilage by bombarding the product with ionizing radiation. In the United States, the Atomic Energy Commission and the Food and Drug Administration are involved in long-term studies to determine the nutritional losses and safety of this method. The most practical use of radiation processing today is administration of low dosages to destroy insects that infest cereals and to inhibit sprouting of onions and potatoes, but even these applications are not used commercially in the United States at present.

In summary, preservation by the methods just described, along with adequate packaging and storage procedures, allows for the transport of a selection of foods to areas of the country or of the world that do not have a continuous supply of local food. Although processing may decrease nutrient content of the food, the loss may be made up by including several different sources in the diet. Also, it should be kept in mind that a major loss in vitamin and mineral contents of foods often occurs during final preparation in the home or establishment just prior to eating.

COST AND DEMAND

Our food supplies on the whole are less expensive today than they would be without present preservation methods. But in some cases, services built into a product add to the price the consumer pays for the food. The advertising necessary to sell products and to make consumers aware of the availability of new products also adds to the price. The 12 largest corporate food organizations spent $1.3 billion dollars in advertising in 1976. This is an average of about 5 percent of their sales.[1] For each dollar the consumer spends in the market for farm foods, the farmer receives about 34 cents.[2] The farmer's share varies with the product (see Fig. 17–2 and Table 17–2).

Many marketing factors affect the cost of food (see Fig. 17–3). Foods that are scarce or out of season are often relatively higher priced. Those that are staples, have good storage life, and are in constant demand are cheaper. Choice cuts of meat are

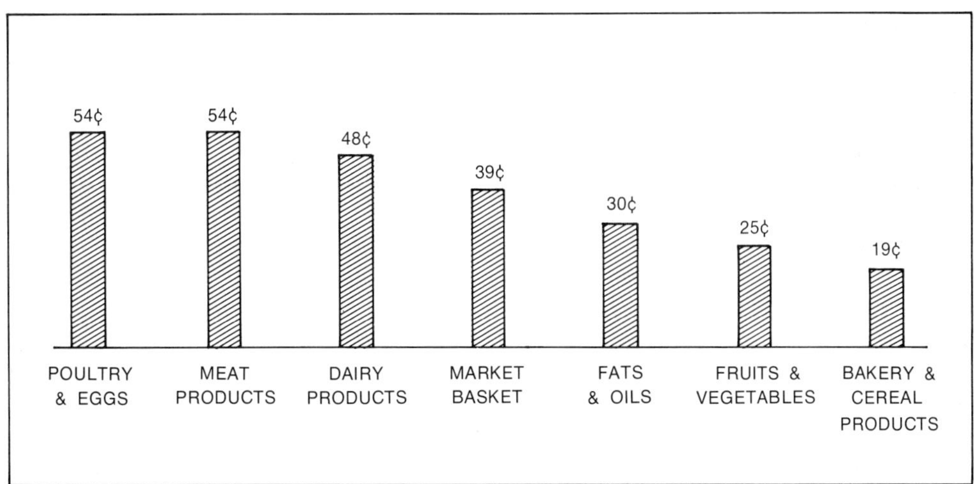

Figure 17–2 The U.S. farmer's share of the consumer's dollar spent on food varies with the product and the costs of processing, marketing, and so on. (From U.S.D.A. Economic Research Service. Published in 1971 Handbook of Agricultural Charts, Agriculture Handbook No. 423, U.S.D.A.)

higher priced because the amount of them is small in proportion to the whole carcass.

The cost of transportation and of getting the food to the consumer in good condition must be added to the total. Lettuce from Georgia or peaches and apples from Oregon often cost more in New York City than the same foods locally produced. Precooked and fancily packaged foods (especially in small portions) are usually more expensive. Advertised brands are no assurance of a higher quality than brands produced by smaller firms that do not advertise widely. "Cash and carry" groceries may sell at lower prices than the same items purchased at stores that make deliveries or extend credit. Large chain stores often package and market their own "house brands" of staple foods at econom-

Table 17–2 WHAT THE FOOD DOLLAR BUYS OF FARM FOODS IN THE UNITED STATES*

Product	*Percent of Consumer Dollar Spent for Domestic Farm Foods*	*Percent of Total Farm Value of U.S. Foods Consumed in U.S.*
Beef	18.2	24.5
Pork	10.0	12.3
Other red meats	1.3	1.0
Fluid milk and cream	7.0	10.3
Other dairy products	7.9	9.5
Poultry	4.8	7.0
Eggs	2.5	4.6
Fresh fruits	3.8	3.3
Fresh vegetables	6.2	5.6
Processed fruits	3.1	2.2
Processed vegetables	7.3	4.1
Grain mill products	3.5	1.8
Bakery products	10.2	4.0
Fats and oils	3.7	3.2
Other foods	10.5	6.5

*From Weekly Digest, Oct. 29, 1977. Percentages are based on 1976 figures (though they vary little from year to year).

ical prices. Many stores offer special bargain days for certain foods they wish to "move" in quantity or for "loss leader" items, which can serve to draw people into their stores.

In spite of increased costs and rapidly growing inflation rates, the food budget of most American families is still only a relatively small part of their disposable income — about 17 percent for the average family. Low-income families spend up to about 40 percent for food and sometimes more.*

Because it is impossible to tell how much foods will cost at any given time, it is imperative that a discussion of food costs should be on a *relative cost basis.* Even if the general level of prices goes up or down, certain *kinds* or *classes* of food are always less expensive than others. We also have to take into account what return in nutritive essentials is obtained by equal amounts of money spent for different types of food.

Items on the grocery shelf generally appear in response to consumer *demand.* But in modern marketing, this "demand" is often created. Usually a new product is devised, promoted through advertising campaigns, and then put to the test of consumer *acceptance.* For example, the change in preference from home preparation of cakes from basic ingredients to the use of mixes has come about primarily as a result of convenience coupled with advertising. Consumers are constantly being urged to try new products. Those the consumer likes and continues to buy survive. The others join the several thousand new food products doomed to failure each year. It is the consumer's vote in the marketplace, influenced by advertising, that determines the long-term success of any food product or new convenience. This is why we need educated consumers to distinguish the nutritionally sound products from those with little or no nutritional value.

*This average figure excludes alcoholic beverages, which when included would add significantly to some food budgets. Also, the percentage of income spent on food varies widely according to area of the country, number in the family, and income level.

PURCHASING, AND CONTRIBUTIONS OF, COMMON FOODS

The objective of production and marketing processes is to bring food to the consumer. Wise buying of groceries calls for budgeting the income and planning nutritious, appealing meals within the limits of purchasing power. Even when money is not scarce, good planning is essential to ensure the purchase of foods that make up a nutritious diet.

To facilitate wise practices in purchasing food, it is useful to consider food grouped according to similar composition. Since 1956, most nutrition educators in the United States have been using the U.S.D.A. "Basic Four Food Groups" plan, which provides a nutritious diet and encourages the use of foods from each of the following basic groups: *milk, meat or equivalent, fruits and vegetables,* and *grains.* These broad categories were designated on the basis of the nutrient composition of the foods within that group. For example, foods in the "meat group —such as beef, pork, poultry, eggs, fish, beans, legumes and nuts — are considered together because they all supply significant amounts of protein, minerals, and vitamins. The milk group also provides protein but is considered separately because its distinguishing feature is that it is a primary source of calcium, as well as of other important minerals and vitamins.

Milk and Milk Products

Milk is especially important in the diet for its outstanding contributions of (1) *high-quality protein,* (2) *calcium,* (3) *riboflavin,* and (4) *vitamin D.* In addition, it provides some of practically all other essential nutrients in well-balanced amounts and in easily assimilated forms.

The chief *proteins* in milk are casein and lactalbumin. Together they form an

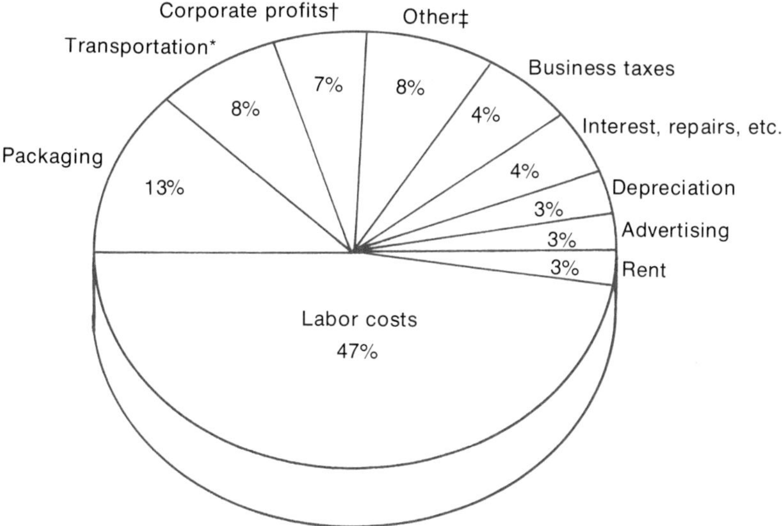

Figure 17–3 Breakdown of food marketing costs. These marketing costs reflect about 65 percent of total food costs. (Redrawn from Agricultural Outlook, Oct. 1977.)

Key: *, intercity rail and truck; †, before taxes; ‡, includes such costs as utilities, fuel, promotion, local for-hire transportation, and insurance.

excellent mixture of amino acids. Milk proteins supplement the amino acids found in grains and are a fairly economical source of protein. Only cereals and dried legumes furnish protein at less cost, and their proteins are not of as high a biological value as those of milk or eggs.

In most American dietaries, milk and its products are usually the mainstay for calcium and riboflavin. No other common food approaches them for richness in *calcium,* and it is difficult to plan a diet that provides the recommended allowance of this element without use of a moderate amount of milk products. Two cups (1 pint) of milk furnishes 66 per cent of the total daily calcium allowance for an adult.* The quantities of milk that provide total recommended daily allowances of calcium for specific periods of life are:

3 cups — full calcium allowance for child 2 to 6 years.

4 cups — full calcium allowance for child 6 to 12 years.

5 cups — full calcium allowance for a teen-ager 12 to 18 years and for pregnant or lactating woman.

6 cups — full calcium allowance for pregnant or lactating young (teen-age) woman.

Along with calcium, milk provides high levels of *phosphorus* needed for building strong bones and teeth, and together these two mineral elements are present in a ratio to each other that favors excellent utilization.

Milk's contribution of *riboflavin* is almost as outstanding as that of calcium. In a recent survey of American diets, the food group of milk, cheese, and ice cream accounted for 13 percent of the average food expenditure, while it furnished 75 percent of the calcium and 39 per cent of the riboflavin (see Table 17–3 and Fig. 17–4). Because these two nutrients are among those most likely to be supplied in less than optimal quantities, liberal use of milk in the diet, whenever possible, is a wise procedure.

*When milk and milk products are not a traditional part of the diet, or if one does not wish to consume so much milk, the needed calcium can be obtained from other sources, such as soft fish bones, added lime water or ashes, certain leafy vegetables, and sesame seeds (with hulls) — see Table 11–3.

Table 17–3 APPROXIMATE SOURCES OF NUTRIENTS IN THE AVERAGE UNITED STATES DIET*

Food Groups	Food energy	Protein	Fat	Carbohydrate	Calcium	Phosphorus	Iron	Magnesium	Vitamin A Value	Thiamin	Riboflavin	Niacin	Vitamin B-6	Vitamin B-12	Ascorbic Acid
								PERCENT							
Meat (including pork fat cuts) poultry, and fish	20.0	42.6	34.1	0.1	4.0	28.5	30.9	14.1	22.4	25.9	24.3	45.2	47.4	70.5	1.1
Eggs	1.8	4.8	2.7	.1	2.2	5.0	4.7	1.2	5.5	2.0	4.5	.1	1.8	7.9	0
Dairy products, excluding butter	11.1	22.0	12.5	6.7	74.6	35.0	2.5	21.7	13.0	8.6	39.0	1.4	10.6	20.1	3.9
Fats and oils, including butter	18.1	.2	43.3	(†)	0.4	0.2	0	.4	8.3	0	1.0	0	(†)	0	0
Citrus fruits	.9	.5	.1	2.0	1.0	.7	.8	2.3	1.6	2.7	.5	.8	1.2	0	27.4
Other fruits	2.1	.6	.3	4.6	1.2	1.1	3.3	3.9	5.5	1.7	1.5	1.6	5.6	0	11.6
Potatoes and sweet potatoes	2.9	2.3	.1	5.4	1.0	3.6	4.3	7.2	5.2	4.9	1.4	6.3	8.9	0	15.0
Dark green and deep yellow vegetables	.2	.4	(†)	.5	1.5	.6	1.5	2.0	20.2	.8	1.0	.6	1.7	0	8.8
Other vegetables, including tomatoes	2.5	3.2	.4	4.8	4.9	4.9	8.9	10.5	15.8	6.3	4.3	5.7	9.3	0	28.6
Dry beans and peas, nuts, soy flour, and grits	3.1	5.4	3.8	2.1	2.9	6.1	6.3	11.9	(†)	5.3	1.8	6.8	4.3	0	(†)
Flour and cereal products	19.2	17.6	1.3	34.7	3.4	12.2	27.9	17.9	.4	41.6	21.0	27.9	8.9	1.5	0.0
Sugars and other sweeteners	17.3	(†)	0	38.5	2.2	.5	6.8	.2	0	(†)	(†)	(†)	(†)	0	(†)
Miscellaneous‡	.7	.4	1.2	.5	.8	1.6	2.2	6.7	2.2	.1	.6	3.5	.1	0	3.6

*From *National Food Review.* Washington, D. C., U.S. Department of Agriculture, Jan. 1978. Percentages were derived from nutrient data that include quantities of iron, thiamin, and riboflavin added to flour and cereal products; quantities of vitamin A value added to margarine and milk of all types; and quantities of vitamin C added to fruit juices and drinks.

†Less than 0.05 percent.

‡Chocolate liquor equivalent of cocoa beans.

§Components may not add to total due to rounding.

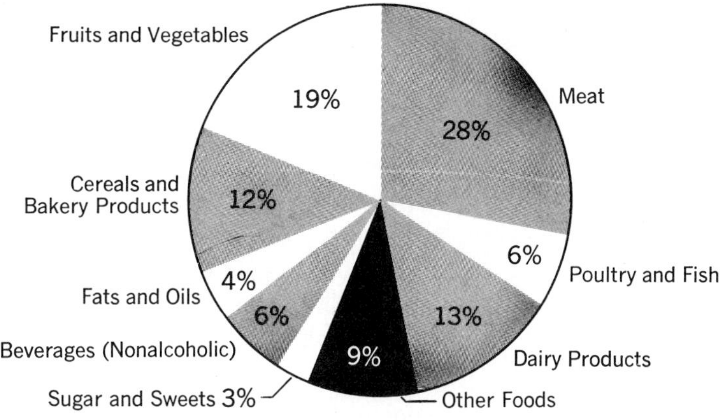

Figure 17–4 The average American family divides its food dollar according to this pattern (weight of food on fresh market basis). (From *Grocery Industry Barometer*. Washington, D.C., Grocery Manufacturers of America, Inc., 1970. Based on "Food Consumption of Households in the U.S.," Spring 1965, Agricultural Research Service, U.S.D.A.)

Milk is a dilute food — 87 percent water. Whole milk's 13 percent of solids is fairly evenly distributed between proteins, fat, and milk sugar (lactose). These nutrients supply considerable energy (630 kcal per quart). Skim milk is about 0.1 percent or less fat, compared with 3.5 percent of fat in whole milk. The product known as "2 percent milk" contains 2 percent fat. Through homogenization, the fat (and the vitamin A it carries) is dispersed in a finely divided or emulsified condition, which favors its digestion and absorption. People on low-fat diets can benefit from the nutrients in milk by drinking fortified skim milk.

The function of milk in nature is to serve as the sole food for young animals, and milk contains all the vitamins and minerals needed for this prupose. Both *carotene* and *vitamin A* are found in the fat globules, varying somewhat with the feed of the cow, and variable amounts of vitamin D are also present. In the United States, milk is generally fortified with 400 IU of vitamin D per quart. The water-soluble vitamins are carried in the whey. Milk contains only about one-sixth as much thiamin as riboflavin, but all the B vitamins are present, including B-12. The value of milk as a source of niacin is augmented by the amino acid tryptophan in its proteins. Although fresh milk contains moderate amounts of vitamin C, much of this may be lost in handling, storage, and pasteurization, so it is not to be depended on for this vitamin. The content of iron and copper in milk is rather low, but what iron is present is well assimilated.

Per capita milk production and consumption in this country have been declining since 1945. Between 1957–59 and 1971, consumption dropped 24 percent.[3] Nearly half the milk produced is used in the manufacture of dairy products (butter, canned milks, cheese, and ice cream).

Many people prefer to consume at least part of their milk allowance in the form of milk products rather than as fluid milk. These products all share the nutritive properties of milk, in greater or lesser degree.

Cream. Light cream has only slightly less protein than fresh milk and six times its fat content. Heavy cream contains about ten times as much fat as whole fresh milk. The content of protein, calcium, and riboflavin decreases as the fat content increases.

Processed Milks. In all these products, much of the water or fat, or both, is removed. Water is evaporated in a partial vacuum at fairly low temperatures, with little resultant loss of vitamins other than vitamin C, except in the production of dry skim milk, in which vitamin A is removed along with the fat in processing.

Condensed milks keep because of added sugar (about 50 percent of final product).
Evaporated milk keeps because they are sterilized in the can — no sugar is added, but half the water is removed.
Dried skim milk powders keep because of low water content (only 3.5 percent) and because fat has been removed.
Filled milks may be fresh, dried, condensed, or evaporated. They contain the nonfat milk solids, but with nondairy fat substituted for the butterfat.

Canned milks meet the need for a concentrated preserved milk that is economical to transport. Evaporated milk is used in infant feeding because its curd is softer and finer in comparison with that formed by raw milk. Condensed milk is a good substitute for cream in coffee and will keep for long periods in an opened can if properly refrigerated. Dried milk powders are used often in commercial bakeries, as well as in home cooking. Dried skim milk is the cheapest form in which to purchase milk; it may be reconstituted or used dry in cooking processes. Dried milk in which much of the fat has been retained has a creamier taste and a higher energy value and usually has some antioxidant added to insure keeping quality. The use of dried milk powder (or granules) in breads, cream sauces, casseroles, and soups is an excellent way to reinforce the diet with protein, calcium, and riboflavin.

Filled milk* has the same protein and other nutrients as whole fresh milk, and the number of calories per serving is the same. If the fat that replaces the butterfat is high in polyunsaturates, filled milk can be used as a component of fat-modified diets; but filled milk cannot be used if coconut oil, which has a greater saturated fat content than butterfat, is substituted. The source of fat should be mentioned on the label.

Cheeses. Cheeses vary considerably in water content (hard and soft cheeses) and fat content. They contain all of the casein and fat of the milk from which they were made, but usually some of the lactalbumin and calcium are lost in the whey that separates from the curd used for the cheese. In ripened cheeses, the protein has been partially digested and rendered more soluble by bacterial action. American (cheddar) cheese is a hard cheese (37 percent water), so it is a concentrated source of all milk solids. Cottage cheese (as made from skim milk) is low in fat and high in protein, but has only about one-eighth of the calcium content of American (cheddar) cheese. Cream cheese differs from other soft cheeses in having more fat and less protein.

Ice Cream. Ice cream is a popular form in which to take part of one's milk quota. Ice creams vary widely in composition, depending on substances added. Most "ice milks" contain about 4 to 5 percent fat, and regular ice creams from 10 to 16 percent fat (the "richer" the ice cream, the greater the amount of fat). Most ice creams are, in effect, a frozen mixture of milk and cream with some added table sugar (about 16 percent of the final product on a weight basis — or about 1⅔ tablespoons of sucrose per cup of final product) plus various flavors, fruits, stabilizers, and often egg. Ice cream, before freezing, contains about 63 percent water and has up to 100 percent air beaten into it during the freezing process. This improves the texture and taste for many people.

Fermented Milks. Fermented milks may be made from either fat-free milk (buttermilk) or whole milk (koumiss, yogurt, acidophilus milk, etc.). They are made by fermentation with various strains of bacilli that convert the lactose to lactic acid or alcohol. Because much of the lactose has been split in its manufacture, fer-

*Filled milk, by this name, is illegal in some states in the United States on the basis that it is no longer "milk." In other states, such as California, the legal name is "imitation milk," a term that in most other places describes a product that looks like milk but has few of its nutritional properties.

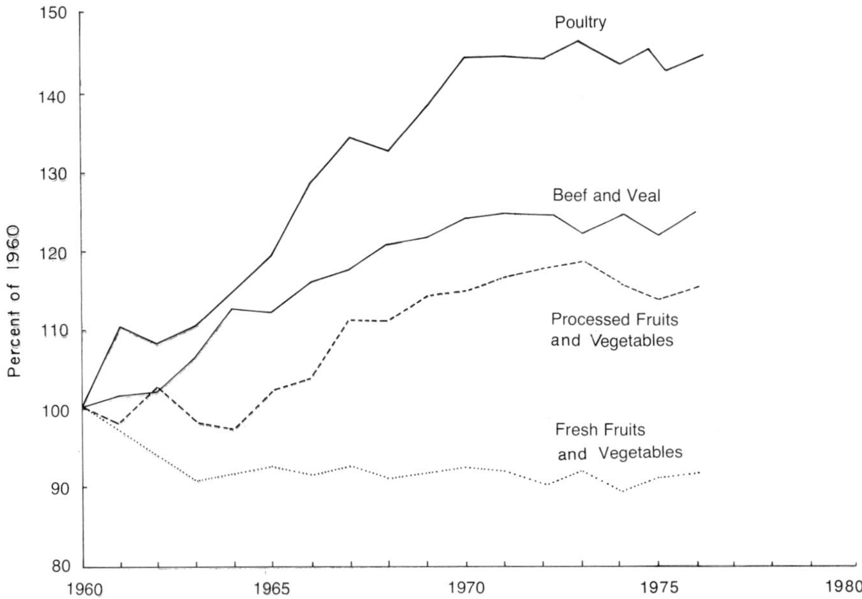

Figure 17–5 Poultry consumption has increased rapidly in the United States in the past 20 years. Americans are also buying more beef and veal. Processed fruit and vegetable sales are increasing, while sales of fresh fruits and vegetables are decreasing. (Adapted from data in the Handbook of Agricultural Charts, U.S.D.A.)

mented milks are often used by persons who have difficulty digesting this sugar.

Meats and Other Protein Foods

The outstanding contributions of these foods to the diet are (1) *high-quality protein* in concentrated form, (2) *B vitamins*, especially vitamins B-6, B-12, and niacin, and (3) *iron* and other trace elements. The proteins of meat are somewhat similar to those of milk and eggs in their amino acid make-up and, therefore, in the efficiency with which they supplement those of the cereal grains and some other vegetable proteins.

Meats, Fish, and Poultry. Meats are well-liked foods and give the feeling of satiety. They are usually consumed in larger amounts if the economic level permits and have come to be associated psychologically with prosperity and with a higher standard of living. Their need in the diet can be entirely met by the use of milk, cheese, and eggs. Judicious use of legume seeds (beans) in the diet of vegetarians (see Chapter 19) is acceptable if vitamin B-12 needs are satisfied.

An average American buys about 250 pounds of meat, fish, and poultry per year. This is an average of 11 oz per day per person[3] (though nearly one-half of this is bone, skin, and unconsumed fat). Average expenditure for this food group amounts to about 36 cents of every dollar spent for food (see Fig. 17–4). Consumption of meat and poultry is increasing in the United States (see Fig. 17–5).

Meat is an excellent food, containing good protein in concentrated form, but it should not be consumed to the extent that other protective foods, rich in minerals and vitamins, are excluded. It takes only 1½ pints of milk or three eggs to provide approximately as much protein as an average (3½ oz) serving of meat. One medium-sized serving of meat daily is a great help in securing an adequate protein intake. One should not lose sight of the fact that the same amount of meat may be purchased for less money if the cheaper cuts are chosen and cooked in an appetizing manner.

The composition of flesh of all animals (mammals, birds, fish, or shellfish) is essentially the same. The difference in composition of flesh from different portions of the same animal is sometimes greater than the usual variation in flesh of different animals. Variations in composition are due chiefly to differences in *water* or *fat* content. These are largely dependent on the species — for example, fish is usually higher in moisture content than beef or lamb; salmon is relatively high in fat, compared with cod or flounder; and pork is often richer in fat than many other meats. The fat content varies in different cuts of meat and according to previous feeding. Fat that is in layers surrounding the lean portion is usually discarded and should not be counted in the caloric value of the meat eaten. Fat may also be lost in drippings during cooking.

There are some variations in mineral elements and vitamins. Pork is richer in thiamin than other muscle meats. Fatty fish (e.g., canned salmon) has a good content of vitamin D. The glandular organs, such as liver and kidneys, are especially rich in vitamin A, the B vitamins, and iron. All lean meats are good sources of phosphorus. Marine fish and shellfish are good sources of iodine, which is a scarce element in most foods.

Eggs. The general composition of eggs is roughly three-fourths water, one-eighth protein, and one-eighth fat. The protein is about equally divided between the white and the yolk, but all the fat, as well as the mineral elements and vitamins (except riboflavin), is in the yolk. The proteins of eggs are as efficient for promoting growth and supplementing deficient vegetable proteins as are those of milk, and egg fat, like milk fat, is finely divided or emulsified, making it easily and fully digested.

Egg yolk (like milk) serves as food for young, growing animals and contains practically all the essential minerals and vitamins, some in higher concentration than others. It is rich in phosphorus, iron, and vitamin A plus carotene; it is a fair source of the B vitamins. Eggs are completely lacking in ascorbic acid.

The ease of digestion of eggs and their high content of tissue-building nutrients make them a valuable food for growing children or convalescents. They are especially useful in cookery where they serve the purposes of thickening (as in custards) or stiffening and lightening texture (as in batters and doughs).

Eggs are a rich source of dietary cholesterol (about 270 mg per egg), which is a cause of much conflicting dietary advice. We believe that one or two eggs per day are nutritionally very useful in most people's diets. There are some persons who have difficulty handling cholesterol in the diet, probably less than 5 percent of the American population. Such persons can generally be identified by physicians on the basis of lipid analysis of the blood or other tests or symptoms.

Legumes and Nuts. Legumes are plants with root nodules, containing bacteria that can "fix" nitrogen—hence their seeds, grown in pods, are high in protein. Nuts, although technically hard-shelled fruits, are similar to dry legume seeds in composition. This food group resembles the grains more than any other group, but is characterized by having almost twice as much protein as grains. The dried legumes (beans, grams, peas, lentils, and cowpeas), with their low moisture content, are as much as 60 percent carbohydrate (starch) and 22 percent protein — figures that may be misleading because in the state in which we eat them, as fresh or cooked, their protein content ranges from only about 6 to 8 percent.

Although they are often classed as "meat substitutes," an average serving of a legume furnishes probably only about one-third as much protein as an average (3½ oz or 100 gm) serving of meat. The quality of their proteins tends to be inferior to that of animal foods, except for the proteins of the peanut and soybean, which are of good biological value. However, legume proteins do supplement in a satisfactory manner the proteins of cereal grains. This is particularly true of the proteins of peanuts ("groundnuts"), soybeans, and peas, when combined with wheat. The addition of small amounts of peanut or soybean flour improves the nutritive quality of white (wheat) bread.

The digestibility of legumes is improved by cooking. Dried legumes and soybeans require long, slow cooking, and the undigestible carbohydrates in beans may lead to intestinal fermentation and flatulence. Dried legumes have considerable use in thick soups (purées) and canned bean products (pork and beans, beans with tomato sauce, chili con carne, etc.). In the southern sections of the United States, cowpeas and chickpeas are well liked and widely used.

Nuts also have a relatively high protein content (7 to 18 percent), but, instead of being rich in starch as are legumes, they have high fat content (roughly 50 to 70 percent). Soybeans and peanuts are high in both protein and fat, being more like nuts in this respect than like legumes. Being low in water and high in fat, nuts have a relatively high energy value, and they are apt to be avoided by calorie-conscious individuals. The proteins of nuts are usually deficient in one or more of the essential amino acids but excellently supplement other proteins. In a survey by the U.S. Department of Agriculture, dried legumes and nuts accounted for only 1 percent of the food money, and for this outlay they furnished 5 percent of the protein, 6 percent of the iron, and 5 percent of the thiamin of the total diet (see Table 17–3).

In the discussion of food sources of mineral elements and B complex vitamins, it may be recalled that legumes (especially dried) and nuts rank high in the list of such sources. They are excellent sources of *phosphorus, iron,* and *thiamin* and are fair sources of calcium and riboflavin. Unfortunately, they are practically entirely *lacking in vitamins A, C, and B–12.*

Peanuts and peanut butter enjoy wide popularity (especially with children and teen-agers). If consumed in sufficient quantity, they can reinforce the dietary protein, calcium, iron, and thiamin for which the requirement is high during periods of growth.

Vegetables and Fruits

Fruits and vegetables are of value in the diet for their fiber and as carriers of mineral elements and vitamins. Increasing the quantity and variety of fruits and vegetables in the diet usually improves its quality.

We are dependent almost entirely on fruits and vegetables for *vitamin C,* and all of them contain some of this vitamin, especially if eaten raw. Canned fruits have smaller amounts of vitamin C, and in dried fruits it has been almost completely destroyed. Dried fruits are rich in mineral elements, especially iron in apricots, peaches, prunes, and raisins. Most fruits are poor in vitamin A value; exceptions are apricots, yellow peaches, prunes, avocados, and cantaloupe. Fresh fruits have a low percentage of the B complex vitamins and the mineral elements.

Potatoes and Sweet Potatoes. White potatoes and sweet potatoes are not related botanically, but both are bland foods, furnish energy at low cost, and are high in carbohydrate. The white potato has 17 percent starch, while the carbohydrate content of the sweet potato (26 percent) includes 5 to 8 percent simple sugar. Because they are approximately three-fourths water, their mineral and vitamin content does not look impressive, but when eaten in quantity, they may make considerable contribution to safeguard the diet in these respects. These two foods furnish iron and thiamin but are low in calcium. The valuable contribution of vitamin C that potatoes make to the diet has been noted under the discussion of scurvy prevention. Retention of their mineral and vitamin content requires care in cooking procedures. The protein of potatoes, although low in amount, is of good nutritive value. White potatoes have almost no vitamin A value; but sweet potatoes have a total vitamin A activity value of 600 to 10,000 IU per 100 gm, varying with the depth of color in different varieties, with the main variety having a value around 8000 IU. If sweet potatoes were commonly used, they would bolster the intake of vitamin A activity.

Green and Yellow Vegetables. Green and yellow vegetables are grouped together because they contain *carotenes* and the provitamins A, and constitute our vegetable sources of this vitamin. They may be subdivided into the leafy vegetables, other green vegetables, and yellow vegetables, because of differences in their contributions to the diet of nutrients other than vitamin A activity.

LEAFY VEGETABLES. Leaves are the most active parts of a plant, the chemical laboratories in which (with the aid of sunlight and chlorophyll) are built various substances necessary for the life of the plant. Hence, they are richer in mineral elements and vitamins than are other parts of the plant. They are especially rich in *calcium* and *iron*, in *provitamins A*, *ascorbic acid (C)*, and *riboflavin* with a good content of other B vitamins. They supplement grain products, especially in regard to calcium and vitamin A value. The calcium in a few leafy vegetables is at least partially nonabsorbable, because it is bound in insoluble combination with oxalic acid, but these vegetables nevertheless are valuable sources of iron and many vitamins. Leafy vegetables with bound calcium include spinach, chard, sorrel, parsley, and beet greens. In other leafy vegetables, the calcium is in forms available to the body. Both in calcium and in vitamin A value, they rank next to milk as important sources. The vitamin C level is so high in broccoli, Brussels sprouts, collards, kale, mustard greens, and turnip greens (100 to 190 mg per 100 gm) that, if cooked for a short time in small amounts of water, these vegetables will still be richer in vitamin C than citrus fruits. Their iron content, fairly well utilized, is a valuable contribution to the diet. Their energy and protein values are negligible.

The greener the leaf, the richer it is in vitamins and minerals. The blanched inner leaves of lettuce, cabbage, or celery are no richer in mineral salts and vitamins than are the stalks or roots of some other plants used as food.

OTHER GREEN VEGETABLES. These are usually stalks, stems, or green pods. Young shoots (such as green asparagus tips) are high in vitamin A value and similar in other composition to green leaves. Broccoli and cauliflower (which consist of flowerets with some leaves) contain only slightly less of certain minerals and vitamins than leafy vegetables do. Green string beans and peppers represent pod vegetables, which are intermediate between the green leaves and roots in minerals and vitamins. Loose leaf lettuce and cabbage rank much lower in vitamin A value than do vegetables with dark green leaves. Head lettuce (iceberg), along with blanched celery and asparagus, has little vitamin A value.

YELLOW VEGETABLES. This category includes fleshy roots (carrots, sweet potatoes, and rutabagas), fruit parts of plants (pumpkin, winter squash, cantaloupe, and other yellow fruits), and yellow corn. The vitamin A value varies with the depth of yellow color, but in deep-colored varieties, it is of almost the same magnitude as that of dark green leaves. These vegetables contribute relatively small amounts of the other vitamins and mineral elements, although if consumed in quantity they may be counted on to supply some of these nutrients.

Citrus Fruits and Tomatoes. These are grouped together as relatively rich sources of vitamin C, and they are reasonably inexpensive and well enough liked to be consumed in quantity. They also hold their vitamin C content well on cooking or canning. Grapefruit, lemons, and oranges have higher vitamin C contents (40 to 50 mg per 100 gm) than do tomatoes (23 mg). Other than their vitamin C content, citrus fruits contain about 10 percent readily assimilable sugar along with some calcium and thiamin. Tomatoes have considerable vitamin A activity, about 900 IU (150 RE) per 100 gm.

In planning an adequate diet, it should be remembered that there are other foods whose vitamin C content equals or exceeds that of citrus fruits and tomatoes. We have previously called attention to such green vegetables as broccoli, kale, turnip greens, and sweet green peppers for high vitamin C value. Green peppers contain vitamin C in the same magnitude (70 to 90 mg per 100 gm, cooked), while fresh strawberries and raw cabbage contain amounts (59 and 47 mg per 100 gm, respectively) comparable to that in citrus fruits. If one of these foods is used in the day's meals, it would not be necessary to include citrus fruit or tomatoes.

Bread and Cereal Group

This group includes the cereal grains and all foods that consist wholly or largely of grain in some form. This includes breads, pasta, ready-to-eat and cooked cereals, pastry, and anything with flour or cornstarch.

The importance of this food group in the diet is that it furnishes *food energy* and *protein* at relatively low cost and at the same time makes worthwhile contributions of minerals and vitamins, especially when used in quantity. This holds true, however, only if the grains have not been subjected to a high degree of milling in which part of the protein and most of the minerals and vitamins have been removed. For this reason, the bread and cereals should be preferably whole-grain, or enriched or restored. Although whole grains make a many-sided contribution in regard to vitamins and minerals, perhaps the nutrients most missed when enriched products are not used are iron and thiamin, because these are furnished in rather low amounts by the milk group and by most fruits and vegetables.

Cereal grains are seeds of grasses. From the beginning of agriculture, all peoples have relied chiefly on grains for their food supply. They are easily cultivated and stored and can be rather simply made into palatable, wholesome, economical foods. Grains are usually crushed into a fine meal or flour and made into bread, which is often leavened by yeast. Bread has been for centuries literally "the staff of life" of many nations, especially of Europe and America.

The principal grains are *rice, wheat, rye, barley, oats,* and *corn (maize)*. Rice, grown in moist tropical or semitropical climates, is consumed more than any of the grains because of its very important place in the diet of the populous countries of the East. Wheat comes next in total amount produced and consumed, largely because its higher content of gluten (a protein) makes it the preferred grain for making yeast breads. Rye is grown in northern climates, and rye bread is commonly used in Germany and the Scandinavian countries. Barley thrives in more arid sections. In the United States, it is used as pearl barley in soups and as barley flour for infant foods. Oats must be combined with another cereal (usually wheat) if used in making bread. In Scotland and Sweden oats are consumed chiefly in the form of oatcakes, or scones, and cooked oatmeal (porridge). Cooked oatmeal is a breakfast food also common to Americans. In amount produced, corn is the main grain product of the United States, but most of it is used for feeding animals. Only 10 to 15 percent of the corn crop is used for human consumption, and much of this is used for the manufacture of corn syrup (glucose) and corn starch, rather than being consumed directly as hominy grits or corn meal (chiefly in the southern part of the United States). In Central and South American countries, as well as in parts of Africa and the Near East, corn is the chief grain used in the diet.

Milling and Enrichment

For human food, all grains are usually *milled*. The extent of this milling process

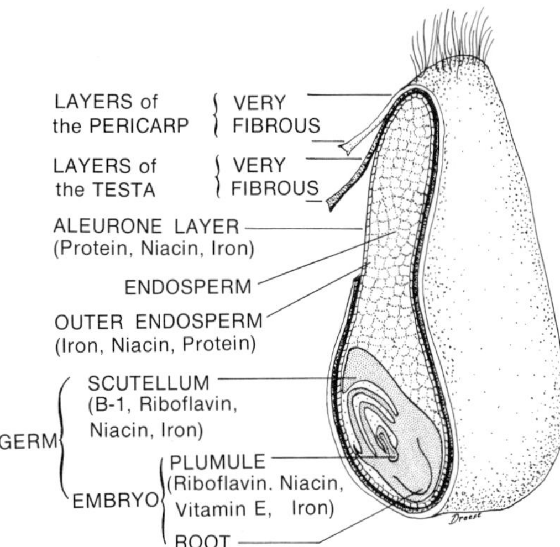

Figure 17–6 The distribution of nutrients in the wheat grain. (Courtesy of Sir J. Drummond, Dr. T. Moran, and *The Lancet.*)

determines how much of the original nutrients in the whole grain are left for human consumption. The reason for this is clear once one understands the distribution of the various constituents in the cereal grains (Fig. 17–6). Each kernel consists of (1) the outer husks, or bran; (2) the brownish outer part of the kernel, or aleurone layer; (3) the inner main portion, or endosperm; and (4) the small germ (embryo) at one end of the kernel. Most of the vitamins and minerals, and much of the protein, are in the aleurone layer and germ. The inner part of the kernel consists chiefly of starch, with some protein.

The outer bran is usually removed to leave a finer flour. Bran is mostly cellulose and hemicelluloses and is now quite widely used to increase the fiber content of the American diet. The germ is also often removed in milling to improve the keeping qualities of the product. If, in addition, most of the aleurone layer is removed, as in milling of a high degree, very little of the original vitamin and mineral content of the grain is left. Thus, about 75 percent of the thiamin and a large part of the protein, iron, other B complex vitamins, and many minerals are lost in the process of making white wheat flour.[4] Much of the same situation occurs when rice or corn is highly milled. The by-products (containing the germ and outer coats of the grain) are generally used for animal feed. (See Table 17–1).

The legal standards of enrichment bring the levels of thiamin, riboflavin, niacin, and iron approximately up to the levels found in whole-wheat bread; but other B complex vitamins and minerals other than iron are also removed by much milling, and they are not replaced. Nevertheless, the enrichment program has considerably increased the amount of the three added vitamins and iron in the American diet, varying in individual cases with the quantities of bread and cereal products that one eats. Families that depend more heavily on these carbohydrate foods benefit most. For average families at all income levels, it has been estimated that the percentage of the total nutrient in the diet added by enrichment of cereals is: thiamin, 40 percent; riboflavin, 15 percent; niacin, 20 percent; and iron, 25 percent (see page 423). It costs less than one-tenth of 1 cent to enrich a loaf of bread.[5]

But even with widespread enrichment, surveys have shown below adequate iron intakes for women and low or deficient hemoglobin levels for children and the elderly, especially from low-income groups. This phenomenon exists partly because the consumption of enriched flour and bread has decreased, while consumption of non-enriched foods has increased. In the last decade, per capita consumption of bread products has dropped 6 percent, while consumption of other baked goods rose 67 per cent.[6]

Other means, besides the official enrichment of white flour or the use of whole-grain products, may be used to increase the amount of thiamin, riboflavin, niacin, and iron contained in bread and cereal foods. Peanut butter, soy grits, and dried skim milk are all excellent sources of thiamin; any of these may be incorporated in home-baked breads, muffins, or cookies. Baking companies sometimes improve the nutritive quality of bread by adding dried skim milk, dried brewer's yeast,* or wheat germ. (See pages 422 to 424 for more on enrichment.)

Other Contributions of Grains

All grain products (highly milled or otherwise) are characterized nutritionally by their high content of starch (nearly 70 to 80 percent) and moderate content of protein (ranging from 7.5 to 14 percent). Hence they serve as *economical sources of energy* and of some *protein*. The protein content is somewhat higher and of better quality if only the coarsest bran has been discarded and some outer coats and the embryo are retained. Grain products are readily handled in large amounts by the digestive tract and make for favorable texture of food residues.

Nutrients that grains *do not supply* in any considerable amounts are calcium and vitamins A (except for yellow corn) and C, if the grain products are unenriched. Also, to be satisfactory for growth and reproduction needs, the proteins in grains need to be supplemented (to a moderate extent) by some protein richer in the essential amino acids lysine and tryptophan. Milk or some other animal protein would meet this need. There are now available many breads that have been improved in their calcium and protein content by incorporating in the dough one or more of the following: milk solids (at a 4 to 6 percent level), soybean or peanut flour, wheat germ, or dried yeast. Of course the supplementation may be accomplished by foods taken separately.

In various surveys of American dietary habits, grain products are found to account for about 10 percent of the total cost of food, and for this outlay they contribute 19 percent of the total energy value and 18 percent of the protein of the diet (see Table 17–3 and Fig. 17–4). The per capita consumption of bread has decreased in the United States in recent years, but there is still wide use of grains in such foods as breakfast cereals, macaroni and similar products, crackers, cookies, and so on.

*Brewer's yeast is eight to ten times richer in thiamin than is baker's yeast. It should be dried and ground to kill the living yeast cells if used as a dietary source of thiamin.

Foods Outside the Basic Four

Although the American diet is based on the traditional "four food groups," several other foods not assigned a specific group are consumed in large amounts. These foods provide variety, convenience, palatability, and alternate sources of energy and nutrients. The problem of possible excessive use, or misuse, of these foods is discussed in other chapters.

Fats and Oils. Fats are essential in the diet to provide linoleic acid, which the body cannot manufacture (see Chapter 4). Fats also provide a concentrated source of fuel, improve the flavor and satiety value of food, and contain the fat-soluble vitamins. Regarding their energy value, weight for weight all pure fats are alike, whether solid, fluid, or of animal or vegetable origin. Butter and margarine are good sources of vitamin A (and, if enriched, of vitamin D). Most vegetable oils contribute vitamin E and abundant amounts of the essential unsaturated fatty acid that is characteristic of low-melting-point fats.

It is generally stated that in order to assure a well-balanced diet, not more than 25 to 35 percent of the fuel value of the diet should come from fats. The Select Committee on Nutrition and Human Need of the U.S. Senate has suggested a reduction of overall fat consumption from the average U.S. consumption of 40 to 45 percent to about 30 percent of energy intake. In Oriental diets, fats often furnish no more than 10 percent of the calories.

While the consumption of fat has been steadily increasing in the United States (see Fig. 17–7), there has been a definite shift from the use of animal fats to the use of vegetable fats. This has resulted in an increased intake of polyunsaturated fatty

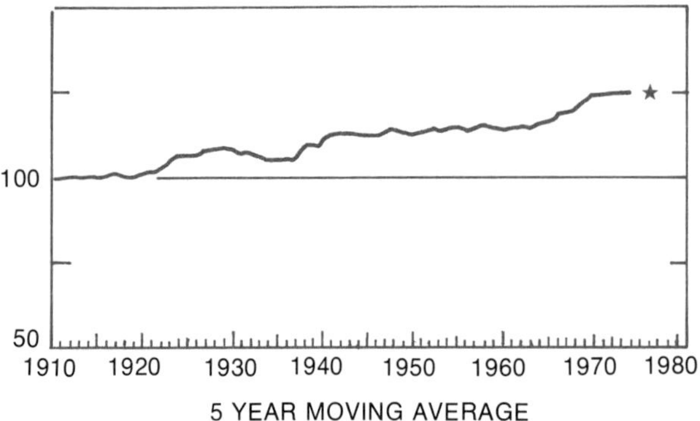

Figure 17–7 Fat consumption has been steadily increasing in the United States. The symbol * indicates preliminary estimate. (From Handbook of Agricultural Charts, Agricultural Handbook No. 504, U.S. Department of Agriculture, 1976.)

acids and a decreased intake of saturated fat in the American diet.[7]

Fats vary widely in cost, and economic considerations may cause people to alter the amount or kinds of fats consumed. Relatively inexpensive fats, such as lard and salt pork, may provide for low-cost energy sources. Olive oil is now so expensive that people make use of refined cottonseed, peanut, or corn oil instead for salad dressings. The popular demand for margarine as a substitute for butter has given rise to its fortification with vitamin A up to the average level of butter. Most margarines are now made from vegetable oils (by hydrogenation) and contain a considerable proportion of linoleic acid. Hydrogenation, partial or complete, may reduce the level of linoleic acid, depending on the extent of the process. Many fat products, like margarine, have unhydrogenated oils added to the hardened oil to provide this nutrient and give the desired texture.

Sugar and Concentrated Sweets. These foods furnish *energy* in relatively inexpensive, readily digested, and quickly available form; they also are useful for *flavor* and have some satiety value. They are completely *devoid of protein, minerals, and vitamins.* Except as an energy source, they are not considered nutritious foods.

We use sugar chiefly as refiined cane sugar or beet sugar (sucrose). Corn syrup, a concentrated solution of glucose, and often fructose manufactured from glucose, is widely used in making candies, jams, and bakery products. Sugar consumption in the United States has increased 10 percent in the past decade and now amounts to more than an average of 100 pounds per person yearly, or about ¼ pound each day for every person in the country. This includes sugar consumed in candies, syrups, jams, and jellies, as well as that used on the table and in cooking. Our annual candy bill is over two billion dollars. We spend over nine billion dollars a year on soft drinks in the United States, which are made solely from carbonated water, sugar, and flavoring. This buys about 30 gallons of soda drinks per year for an average American (see Table 17–4). Our soft drink intake surpasses our intake of alcoholic beverages, tea, juices, and milk, Since soft drink consumption is increasing while that of coffee is decreasing, soft drinks are now our number one national beverage.

Sugar is one of the cheaper forms in which to buy energy, although the price of sugar has increased considerably in recent years. The content of essential nutrients in sugar, syrups, and honey is negligible. Hence, we recommend that not more than 5 to 10 percent of the energy intake come from sugar and other concentrated sweets, about half of the current contribution (16.4 percent).

Figure 17–8 shows what a large pro-

Table 17-4 SOFT DRINK SALES, PER CAPITA CONSUMPTION, AND AMOUNTS AND VALUE OF SUGAR USED IN THEIR MANUFACTURE, 1960 TO 1975*

Year	*Sales ($ Millions)*	*Per Capita Soft Drink Consumption* 16 oz	Gal	*Per Capita Sugar Consumption (lb)*	*Value of Sugar ($ Millions)*
1960	$1857	109	13.6	11.3	188
1965	3195	154	19.2	15.2	274
1970	5016	193	24.1	19.2	420
1975	9426	221	27.6	21.5	1218

*From Sugar and Sweetener Report, Vol. 1, No. 8, Sept. 1976. Washington, D.C., Economic Research Service, U.S. Department of Agriculture.

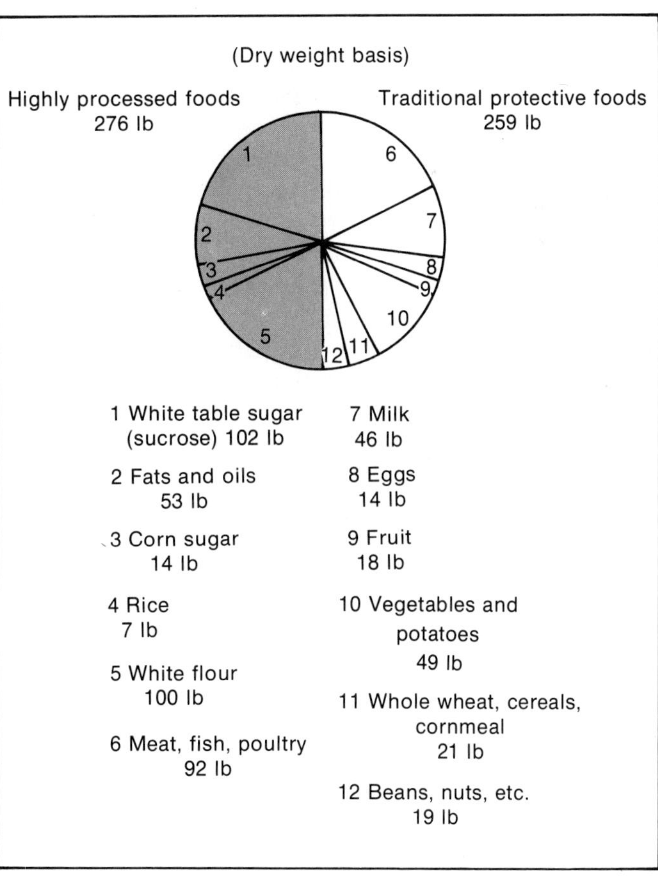

Figure 17-8 Comparison of intakes of highly processed vs. protective foods in the United States. On a dry weight basis, the average American consumption of highly processed foods exceeds the consumption of traditional foods—most of which are processed very little comparatively. (From the 1972 *Britannica Yearbook of Science and the Future,* p. 252.)

portion of the diet (on a dry basis) is made up of sugars and other refined foods.

Other Foods. Coffee, tea, and alcohol (in various forms), commonly consumed in many countries, share the characteristic of having significant drug action. They are carriers of small amounts of nutrients, and alcohol provides metabolizable energy (though no argument can be made for distilled spirits, nutritionally speaking). Some spices and condiments also provide nutrients in small amounts.

CONVENIENCE FOODS

Part of the change to a middleman system of marketing has involved the altering of food by the middlemen to make their product appealing to the consumer. This has led to probably the most important change in American dietary habits over the past several decades: the great shift from more conventional types of food to so-called "convenience" foods. Examples of these foods include meal-in-one dishes; mixes for soups, dressings, sauces, and desserts; frozen entrées; and minute rice, instant mashed potatoes, and precooked cereals. These foods, either processed from natural foods or created *de novo,* have increased the quantity and variety of foods available in this country. Some new products are of questionable nutritional value — for example, imitation milk. Some processed foods, such as quick-frozen vegetables, are essentially equivalent nutritionally to their fresh counterparts. However, some foods lose a large proportion of their nutrients through refining (see Table 17–1) or exposure to water, heat, light, or oxygen during processing (refer to Chapters 7 through 12 for effects on specific nutrients). The extent of the loss depends on the food, the degree of processing, and the food particle size. If these foods are the exclusive source of the lost nutrient, there is cause for concern. However, if other foods of the mixed diet can provide these nutrients, the advantages of processing may outweigh the disadvantages. For example, a small loss of vitamin C from milk during pasteurization is not so important, because milk is a poor source of vitamin C anyway. A population that depends on potatoes for vitamin C, though, will not get enough of the nutrient from dehydrated potato flakes.

The *advantages* of by-passing some of the more tedious processes in the preparation and cooking of foods are evident, and many foods that formerly were made in the home are now almost entirely commercially produced—for example, making bread, baking beans, and making pickles, jams, and jellies. The wide variety of ready-to-cook frozen vegetables also relieves the homemaker of labor, and as purchased, they are free from waste. The convenience of buying certain specially prepared foods under certain circumstances may well be worth the price; sometimes it may not—facts that people must decide for themselves.

Not all convenience foods are more expensive than their home-prepared equivalents. In general, meat products, bakery goods, and desserts are more expensive as convenience items, but some fruit and vegetables cost less when frozen or canned than when fresh. The cost of time saved and the quality of the product has to be considered in deciding whether the fresh or processed product is a better buy.

A few *precautions* should be mentioned for the benefit of those who are inclined to be heavy users of specially prepared and precooked foods. While most Americans enjoy sufficient intakes of most nutrients, those citizens with borderline intakes of one or more nutrients cannot afford to trade nutrients for convenience. Also, there is still need for meal planning to make sure that the family receives the recommended number of servings of the four food groups to insure an adequate intake of all nutrients each day. A hastily assembled dinner, with no previous planning, may not supplement the other two meals of the day properly.

The so-called fast-food restaurants are spreading rapidly and gaining popularity. The same precautions just stated about convenience foods apply here. The most important point to remember is that all the nutrients come only from a diet that varies and complements itself from meal to meal.

Increasing numbers of Americans are eating *manufactured* or *fabricated foods.* These sometimes resemble, and are substituted for, traditional foods. For example, imitation milk might replace whole milk as a *food* in the diet, but its *nutrient* content does not compare favorably with whole milk's. Imitation milk, consisting of water, sugar, vegetable fat, emulsifiers, stabilizers, and a source of protein (casein or soy), is nutritionally inferior to milk.[8]

Similarly, coffee whiteners, whipped toppings, breakfast drinks, desserts, and meat substitutes may imitate the appearance, but not the nutrient content, of the foods they replace. These foods are gaining in popularity for a number of reasons: (1) They are convenient, requiring minimum storage and preparation. (2) They are attractive. Formulated topping holds up better during transportation than does whipped cream. (3) They fill specific needs; for example, vegetarians use textured vegetable protein rather than meat. The Council on Foods and Nutrition of the American Medical Association has stated that "The composition of an imitation or a new food becomes especially important when it contributes 10 percent or more of the recommended daily intake of any essential nutrient, including calories. The imitation or fabricated food should contain on a caloric basis at least the variety and the amounts of the important nutrients contained in the food which it replaces.[9]

Total dependence on fabricated products would not be wise nutritional practice (nor would total dependence on *any* single food item). We do not know enough about the composition of natural foods or the nutritional requirements of man to manufacture a food entirely from pure chemicals.

The consumer must depend on informative nutrient and ingredient labeling to know what substances are in a fabricated food. Labeling becomes more critical when a product appears to be one thing but actually is something different. Consumers who for years have depended on certain foods to provide particular nutrients naturally assume that substitute foods will provide the same nutrients, which they often do not.

PLANNING THE BUDGET

The exact nature of the food budget depends on a number of factors, among which are:

1. Overall income and eligibility for food stamps or commodities.
2. The availability of free or low-cost school food service programs.
3. The number of members in the family and their food habits.
4. Where the family lives and how conveniently located the shopping areas are.
5. The amount of food produced or preserved at home.
6. Special dietary needs, as in pregnancy and disease states.

What Proportion of the Income Should Be Spent for Food? In general, the *less the income, the greater the proportion of it that must be spent for food in order to secure a nutritionally adequate diet.* While the "average" American spends 17 percent of his disposable income on food, an American family at a low income level may have to spend over half of their total income for food in order to obtain a "*minimum-cost adequate diet.*" At very low income levels, even the most necessary expenditures for clothing and housing may rob a food budget that is

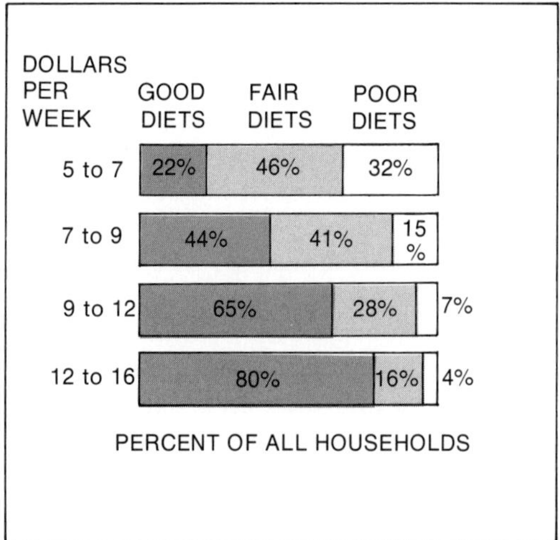

Figure 17–9 Relationship of income and quality of diets by money value of food per person in a week, 1965–66. Low-income families have a greater proportion of poor diets than high-income families, because lack of money makes it difficult to buy the required nutrients. Having money does not ensure proper selection of nutrients, however, as can be seen from the percentage of poor diets in the upper-income groups. (Redrawn from Community Nutrition Institute Weekly Report, 2:6, August 3, 1972.)

already low, making it inadequate to maintain health over long periods. A mass of statistics proves that among such families are higher death rates (especially among young children and pregnant women), more sickness and absences from work or school, and smaller relative growth of children than are found in families at higher income levels. In the 1965 dietary survey of United States households, a greater proportion of low-income families' diets, compared with high-income families' diets, were rated "poor" (see Fig. 17–9). However, the low-income families squeezed out a better nutritional return for each dollar spent. In most states, low-income families can participate in the United States Department of Agriculture's food stamp, commodity, or school food programs, all of which stretch the food dollar and help these families meet their nutritional requirements.

As the income level rises, the family may purchase a more "liberal diet." The student of nutrition recognizes, of course, that this does not mean more liberal in terms of calories, since overconsumption of calories carries a penalty. It does imply that certain foods of relatively higher cost having nutritional value may be provided more easily. These foods include the so-called "protective foods" — milk, eggs, fruits, vegetables, and probably either more or higher-cost meats. The greater freedom of choice insures a better diet nutritionally *only if wisely exercised,* for the higher-cost foods are not necessarily those best for health. A so-called "luxury consumption" of meats, rich foods, alcohol, and sweets does not insure health, and many cases of malnutrition still occur in families in which there is plenty of money for food. However, there is certainly less chance of malnutrition and its resultant ill health when the money spent for food is liberal than when it is scarce.

The *size of a family* is also a determinant of the food budget. It is obvious that it costs more to feed four persons than one or two. A family of two adults usually has the most leeway on the amount to be spent for food, while the larger family, especially if there are several growing children, must spend not only a larger amount but also a greater proportion of its income for food. Young children and rapidly growing teen-agers need a larger allowance of certain foods that are relatively more expensive (such as fresh whole milk, meat, and eggs for good quality protein; and fruits and vegetables for minerals and vitamins). In certain sections of the country, such as the North Atlantic, Midwestern, and Pacific Coast states, the cost of living is higher than in other parts. City food costs vary more than in small towns, and when one lives on a farm and can produce part of the family food supply, the money spent for food is naturally less. If the food is produced locally and the homemaker has the time, equipment, and storage facilities, then home freezing, canning, drying, or other methods of preserving foods plentiful only in certain seasons may prove economical in the long run.

Efficient Buying and Preparation of Food. Efficient buying and preparation of food are the most satisfactory means of all to reduce food costs, because they *involve no diminution in the variety, attractiveness, or nutritive value* of the menu. By merely "stopping the leaks," enough saving may be effected to provide a better diet at less cost. Waste can occur in the course of buying, storing, preparing, or serving foods. Sometimes one's carelessness enriches food merchants or allows nutrients to be thrown away in cooking water or disappear in an overflowing garbage pail.

Considerable money savings can be effected by *thrifty marketing*. Some suggestions for efficient food buying practices are discussed in Table 17–5. In general, buying in larger quantities, watching for special bargains on certain foods, going to the market to select perishable foods that are of good quality, and selecting less expensive types or brands of food when these are suitable all result in lowering the food bill. One should plan to use some of the cheaper cuts of meat as often as feasible, for they are just as nutritious as more expensive ones and may be made very palatable if properly cooked. Plan to use the organ meats, fish, or legumes or cheese in place of meat occasionally. Also, smaller amounts of meat may be "extended" by combining with a starchy food, such as bread crumbs, noodles, or rice.

Table 17–6 gives suggestions of inexpensive food sources of various nutrients, helpful in connection with the information in Table 17–5.

Read package labels to know what you are paying for. Ingredients are listed in descending order of amount present. Look for the total contents in canned foods. Often a can with twice the quantity does not cost very much more than the smaller one. With fruits and vegetables, higher price is usually based on appearance, and those of lower quality and price may well be suited for one's use, such as small, tart apples for applesauce.

Waste in the kitchen may occur in many ways. Some of the chief ones are: (1) discarding portions of food that have nutritive value (vegetable trimmings, meat trimmings, cooking water, liquid from canned vegetables) and that are suitable for cooking; (2) burning foods or carelessly scraping them from cooking utensils in serving; (3) failure to utilize leftover foods properly; (4) wasting food at the table by taking individual portions that are too large or, in one way or another, rendering what is not eaten unfit to serve again; and (5) spoilage of food through improper care in storage.

Some rules for minimizing the loss of nutrients in home storage and preparation are:

1. Store perishables in a cool, dark place; buy no more than can be used.
2. Prepare perishables shortly before serving.
3. Save the water used in cooking vegetables, and use it for soup stock.
4. Cook vegetables in a small amount of water, or steam them until just tender. To shorten cooking time, add the vegetables to boiling water.
5. Leave on skins of vegetables, if clean.

Planning the menu ahead will help insure more efficient marketing. Keep in mind family food habits, preferences, and needs, and design meals that you know will be enjoyed. The nutrients in food and the food in the market are of no value to you and your family if the food you buy and prepare is not eaten (also see Chapter 19).

Nutrients must travel a long road before they reach the body. Food, which carries the nutrients, must be grown or raised on the farm, and then distributed, processed, and marketed through complex economic channels. It must then be bought at a store and prepared into appetizing meals. At every link of the chain, the nutrients in the food are subject to extinction or reduction. Careful processing, handling, and preparation of food, with an awareness of the instability and value of the nutrients within, can help insure that the money spent on food buys the nutrients necessary for a healthy life.

Table 17-5 THE ECONOMY OF SUBSTITUTING CHEAPER FOODS IN THE SAME FOOD GROUP

Grain products – Even in this relatively inexpensive food group some foods are cheaper than others.
Corn and *rice* are usually cheaper than wheat.
The processed, fancy *ready-to-serve cereals* are relatively expensive.
Uncooked cereals bought in large quantity are usually cheaper than in small packages.
Oatmeal and *whole-wheat cereals* give especially good value because of their higher content of protein, mineral salts, and B complex vitamins.
Homemade *breadstuffs* are cheaper than some bakery products, and plain breads are cheaper than those with special flavor appeal. Crackers, sweet buns, cake, cookies, and doughnuts are expensive when purchased at the store.

Sweets – *Sugar* is one of the cheapest fuel foods but should not furnish more than 5 to 10 percent of total calories.
Granulated white sugar and *brown* sugar are cheapest; *powdered* sugar, *loaf* sugar, and *maple* sugar are considerably more expensive.
Molasses, corn syrup, and *cane* syrups are inexpensive; blended syrups are of moderate cost; maple syrup and strained honey are expensive. Molasses and open-kettle sugar-cane syrup have a *mineral content* especially valuable in a low-cost diet.
Jellies, jams, marmalades, and preserves are relatively expensive, but may be useful to make bread and other inexpensive starchy foods more acceptable. Homemade jams and jellies are least expensive.
Candy, except for simple hard candies, is an expensive form of sweets.

Fats – *Meat fats, vegetable shortening* (from cottonseed, corn, or peanut oils), and *margarines* are relatively inexpensive; *butter* and *cream* are relatively expensive. *Butter* and *olive oil* are the most expensive fats.

Protein-rich foods – Cereal grains and legumes are the cheapest sources of protein, but should not be the only protein-bearing foods in the diet. Nuts are an excellent source, but except for peanuts and peanut butter, are now high-cost foods. American (cheddar) cheese, milk (dried milk is one of the cheapest sources of complete protein), and *fresh* or *canned fish* provide excellent quality protein at moderate cost. Eggs are a more economical protein source than most cuts of meat. Meats, fish or shellfish, and poultry are usually the most expensive of the protein-rich foods.

Flesh foods – Within this group cost levels differ greatly. Certain *fatty meats* may be relatively inexpensive, next come the *cheaper cuts* of red meats and the less expensive *fish,* next the more *tender cuts* of lean meats and cuts that involve considerable waste, along with the more expensive forms of seafood such as shellfish. *Poultry* is usually moderately priced the year round. *Dried or canned fish* may offer good protein at low cost; canned *salmon* is valuable for vitamins A and D, and costs less than fresh salmon. *Frozen fish* are of excellent quality and have little waste.

Fruits – *Dried fruits* (raisins, dates, figs, apricots, prunes, peaches, and apples), an excellent source of minerals and some vitamins, were formerly inexpensive but have recently become high-cost. Any of them that are relatively inexpensive (e.g., prunes) should be used in the low-cost dietary. *Canned* or frozen *fruits* are usually less expensive than fresh, but they may not be when a fresh fruit is in season and plentiful. Of the *fresh fruits, apples, bananas* and *oranges* are apt to be the least expensive, though some of the others may be relatively cheap at the height of their season. The *citrus fruits* and *tomatoes* are especially valuable for their vitamin C content. Canned or frozen orange and grapefruit juices are usually the least expensive sources of vitamin C. Most expensive are the less common fruits and fresh fruits which are out of season.

Vegetables – *Potatoes* and the *root vegetables* are usually the least expensive.
Cabbage and some of the other *leafy vegetables* in their season are relatively inexpensive.
Leafy, green and *yellow vegetables* have the highest vitamin A value.
Dried legumes are relatively inexpensive. *Canned vegetables* are often moderately priced, and *canned tomatoes* are especially useful for adding flavor and vitamins to a low-cost diet.
Frozen vegetables (and fruits) afford variety in moderate-cost diets. They have the full nutritive value of fresh vegetables without having any of the waste.
Most *fresh vegetables* (especially the succulent ones) are at least fairly expensive, except at the height of their season.
The *less frequently used vegetables* and those that are out of season are the most expensive of all.

Table 17-6 INEXPENSIVE SOURCES OF VARIOUS NUTRIENTS

Nutrients	*Food Sources*
Energy	Fats, oils, flour, cereals, breads, potatoes, sugar, dried beans or peas, and peanut butter.
Protein	Dried beans or peas, peanut butter, whole-grain cereals or breads, milk (especially dried skim milk), cheaper cheeses, eggs, poultry, and less expensive meats and fish.
Calcium	Milk (especially dried skim milk), ice milk (dessert), cheese, dark green, leafy vegetables, whole-grain products, and legumes.
Iron	Dried beans or peas, liver, whole-grain or enriched breads or cereals, dark green, leafy vegetables, eggs, less expensive meats, potatoes and sweet potatoes, and prunes.
Vitamin A	Dark green and deep yellow vegetables, liver, fortified margarine, canned tomatoes, prunes, and less expensive cheeses.
Vitamin C	Canned or frozen citrus fruit juices, canned tomatoes, raw cabbage, some dark green, leafy vegetables, and potatoes.
Thiamin	Dried legumes, whole-grain or enriched bread and cereals, liver, inexpensive cuts of pork, and potatoes.
Riboflavin	Milk, ice milk (dessert), cheese, whole-grain or enriched breads, eggs, dried legumes, and dark green, leafy vegetables.
Niacin	Dried beans or peas, peanuts or peanut butter, whole-grain and enriched cereal products, meat, poultry, fish, and some dark green, leafy vegetables.

QUESTIONS AND PROBLEMS

1. What types of food supply and level of civilization are characteristic of the following different stages of development in a country or region?
   a. Tribal organization, hunting, primitive agriculture, or herding of animals as main occupations.
   b. Larger area under central government, most people engaged in agriculture, and agricultural methods still primitive.
   c. Smaller proportion of people engaged in agriculture, with more working in industries or other pursuits.
   d. High degree of industrialization, more efficient agriculture which produces more food with labor of fewer people, and rise of cities and large towns.

2. What motivated the development of so many new, processed foods since 1945? Name five methods of food preservation or processing that are now commonly used and two food products prepared by each type of processing. To what extent has the introduction of "convenience foods" changed our food habits and the consumption of different food groups? What are the advantages and disadvantages of extensive use of ready-to-serve and precooked foods?

3. Name four factors that influence the cost of foods. Name four factors, other than food prices, that affect the amount a family must spend to be adequately fed.

4. In respect to what nutrients does milk make an outstanding contribution to the diet? What other nutrients does it furnish in lesser amounts? Is it low or lacking in any essential nutrients, and if so which ones? In respect to what nutrients does it supplement the grains? The legumes? Lean muscle meats? Name some of the milk products that may, at least in part, be substituted for fresh whole milk in the diet. What is the least expensive product in which one can buy milk solids?

5. For what reasons are meats, fish, poultry meat, and eggs especially valuable in the diet? In regard to the essential nutrients that they provide, how do lean meats resemble and how do they differ from milk? How do eggs differ from meats and from milk in these respects? From the point of view of cost to the national resources, which of these types of food is most costly and which is most economical to produce — grains, milk, eggs, beef? Is this reflected in their market cost?

6. Are legumes and nuts good sources of protein? Inexpensive sources? Do any or all of them furnish protein mixtures that are complete in terms of essential amino acid content? Which ones are especially good for supplementing the proteins of wheat? Why? Are legumes and nuts "alternates" or complete "substitutes" for meats in the diet? Explain why. What mineral elements and vitamins are found in good quantities in legumes and nuts?

7. For what vitamin are we almost entirely dependent upon fruits and vegetables? For what other reasons are these classes of foods needed in the diet? What are the special contributions made to nutrition by each of the following subgroups: potatoes and sweet potatoes? green and yellow vegetables? leafy vegetables? citrus fruit and tomatoes?

8. What are the chief contributions of grains and their products (bread, breakfast cereals, etc.) to the diet? In what nutrients are they rich and in which ones are they lacking? In what ways nutritionally do highly milled grains differ from whole grains, and why? Is enriched white bread nutritionally equivalent to bread made from whole grain?

9. Of what value are fats and sugar in the diet? What are their shortcomings as foods? To how great an extent may they safely be included in the diet? What dangers may be associated with too high a consumption of fats and concentrated sweets?

10. Give three principal ways in which economies in the food budget may be effected. Which are especially useful for families of low income, moderate income, and high income? Why?

11. Tell in what respects the following factors affect the type of meals planned:

a. Size of family and occupation and habits of family members.
b. Individual likes and dislikes of family members, regional or racial food habits.
c. Age difference of family members.
d. Cost and availability of different foods.
e. Storage facilities available in the home.

12. Calculate the grams of protein yielded by 1 dollar's worth each of legumes, milk, eggs, chicken, and wholewheat bread using today's prices. How many calories would a dollar's worth of each of these foods provide?

REFERENCES

1. Weekly Digest,* Sept. 10, 1977.
2. Weekly Digest,* Oct. 15, 1977, p. 8.
3. Economic Research Service: National Food Situation. Washington, D.C., U.S. Department of Agriculture. Nov. 1971.
4. *National Academy of Sciences: Proposed Fortification Policy for Cereal Grain Products.* Washington, D.C., National Academy of Sciences, 1974.
5. Harris, R. S.: J. Agric. Food Chem., *16*:149, 1968.
6. Senti, F. R.: Cereal Science Today, *16*:92, 1971.
7. Friend, B.: Amer. J. Clin. Nutr., *20*:907, 1967: also see current issues of the National Food Review of the U.S. Department of Agriculture for more recent figures.
8. Council on Foods and Nutrition: J.A.M.A., *208*: 1686, 1969.
9. Council on Foods and Nutrition: J.A.M.A., *205*: 160, 1968.

SUPPLEMENTARY READINGS

Reviews, Books, and General

American Medical Association: *Nutrients in Processed Foods.* Acton, Mass., Publishing Sciences Group, Inc., 1974.

---

*Weekly Digest is published by the American Institute of Food Distribution, Inc., P.O. Box 523, Fair Lawn, N.J. 07410.

American Medical Association, Council on Foods and Nutrition: Improvement on the nutritive quality of foods: general policies. J.A.M.A., *225*:1116, 1973.

Borgstrom, G.: *Principles of Food Science.* The Macmillan Co., New York, 1968.

Friend, B.: Nutritive value of the United States per capita food supply. Amer. J. Clin. Nutr., *27*:1, 1974.

Harris, R. S., and Karmas, E.: *Nutritional Evaluation of Food Processing.* 2nd Ed. Westport, Conn., Avi Publishing Co., Inc., 1975.

Hertzler, A. A., and Anderson, H. L.: Food guides in the United States. J. Amer. Dietet. Assoc., *64*:19, 1974.

Hertzler, A. A., and Hoover, L. W.: Development of food tables and use with computers. Review of nutrient data bases. J. Amer. Dietet. Assoc., *70*:20, 1977.

Institute of Food Technologists: Nutritional improvement debate: supplementation of foods vs. nutrition education. Food Tech., *28*:55, July, 1974.

McWilliams, M.: *Food Fundamentals.* New York, John Wiley & Sons, Inc., 1966.

Meyers, L. D., and Jansen, G. R.: A nutrient approach in the fifth grade. J. Nutr. Ed., *9*:127, 1977.

Oltjen, R. R., and Dinius, D. A.: Production practices that alter the composition of foods of animal origin. J. Anim. Sci., *41*:703, 1975.

Popkin, B. M., and Latham, M. C.: The limitations and dangers of commerciogenic nutritious foods. Amer. J. Clin. Nutr., *26*:1015, 1973.

Sebrell, W. H., Haggerty, J. J., and the editors of Life: *Food and Nutrition.* New York, Time, Inc., 1967.

White, P. L., Fletcher, D. C. (eds.): *Nutrients in Processed Foods: Fats and Carbohydrates.* Acton, Mass., Publishing Sciences Group, Inc., 1975.

White, P. L., and Fletcher, D. C. (eds.): *Nutrients in Processed Foods: Protein.* Acton, Mass., Publishing Sciences Group, Inc., 1974.

Food Processing and Storage, and Nutrient Losses

Binkerd, E. F.: The luxury of new product development. Food Tech., *29*:26, Sept. 1975.

Braskaram, C., and Sadasivan, G.: Effects of feeding irradiated wheat to malnourished children. Amer. J. Clin. Nutr., *28*:130, 1975.

Burger, I. H., et al.: Symposium: The Effect of Processing on the Nutritive Value of Food. Proc. Nutr. Soc., *32*:1, 1973. (Also see p. 9, 17, 23, 31.)

Chichester, C. O.: *Nutrition in food processing.* World Rev. Nutr. Dietet., *16*:318, 1973.

Fennema, O.: The U.S. frozen food industry: 1776–1976. Food Tech., *30*:56, June 1976.

Food and Agriculture Organization of the United Nations: Wholesomeness of irradiated food. Rome, FAO, 1977.

Fulton, L., and Davis, C.: Cooking chicken and turkey from the frozen and thawed states. J. Amer. Dietet. Assoc., *64*:605, 1974.

Fulton, L., and Davis, C.: Cooking frozen and thawed roasts. Beef, pork, and lamb cuts. J. Amer. Dietet. Assoc., *67*:227, 1975.

Head, M. K.: Nutrient losses in institutional food handling. J. Amer. Dietet. Assoc., *65*:423, 1974.

Head, M. K., and Giesbrecht, F. G.: Effects of storage and handling on vitamins in fresh lima beans. J. Amer. Dietet. Assoc., *69*:640, 1976.

Hopkins, H.: Canless canning with food pouches. FDA Consumer, *11*:24, Nov. 1977.

Knight, S., and Winterfeldt, E. A.: Nutrient quality and acceptability of mechanically deboned meat. J. Amer. Dietet. Assoc., *71*:501, 1977.

Korschgen, B. M., Baldwin, R. E., and Snider, S.: Quality factors in beef, pork, and lamb cooked by microwaves. J. Amer. Dietet. Assoc., *69*:635, 1976.

National Dairy Council: The role of processing in extending the food supply. Dairy Council Dig., *48*:19, 1977.

Ream, E. E., et al.: Tenderness of beef roasts. Microwave vs. conventional cooking methods. J. Amer. Dietet. Assoc., *65*:155, 1974.

Symposium on current studies on the chemistry of food irradiation (7 papers) J. Agric. Food Chem., *26*:1, 1978.

Fabricated Foods, Soy Protein, and New Foods

Childs, M. T., and Ostrander, J.: Egg substitutes: chemical and biologic evaluations. J. Amer. Dietet. Assoc., 68:229, 1976.

Cross, H. R., et al.: Effect of fat and textured soy protein content on consumer acceptance of ground beef. J. Food Sci., *40*:1331, 1975.

Heidelbaugh, N. D., et al.: Clinical nutrition applications of space food technology. J. Amer. Dietet. Assoc., *62*:383, 1973.

Kies, C., Fox., H. M., and Nelson, L.: Triticale, soy-TVP, and millet based diets as protein suppliers for human adults. J. Food Sci., *40*:90, 1975.

Lipinsky, E. S., and Litchfield, J. H.: Single-cell protein in perspective. Food Tech., *28*:16, May 1974.

Nielsen, L. M., and Carlin, A. F.: Frozen, precooked beef and beef-soy loaves. Eating quality, fat and thiamin content. J. Amer. Dietet. Assoc., *65*:35, 1974.

Ostrander, J., et al.: Egg substitutes: use and preference — with and without nutritional information. J. Amer. Dietet. Assoc., *70*:267, 1977.

Stadler, C. R., et al.: Skylab menu development. J. Amer. Dietet. Assoc., *62*:390, 1973.

Stephenson, M. G.: Textured plant protein products: new choices for consumers. FDA Consumer, *9*:18, April 1975.

Zezulka, A. Y., and Calloway, D. H.: Nitrogen retention in men fed varying levels of amino acids from soy protein with or without added L-methionine. J. Nutr., *106*:212, 1976.

Basic Foods

Augustin, J.: Variations in the nutritional composition of fresh potatoes. J. Food Sci., *40*:1295, 1975.

Benson, E. M., et al.: Wild edible plants of the Pacific Northwest. Nutritive values. J. Amer. Dietet. Assoc., *62*:143, 1973.

Carpenter, K. J.: High-cereal diets for man. Proc. Nutr. Soc., *36*:149, 1977.

Cereals today and tomorrow (symposium proceedings). Proc. Nutr. Soc., *36*:121, 1977.

Edwards, C. H., et al.: Utilization of wheat by adult man: excretion of vitamins and minerals. Amer. J. Clin. Nutr., *24*:547, 1971.

Edwards, C. H., et al.: Utilization of wheat by adult man: nitrogen metabolism, plasma amino acids and lipids. Amer. J. Clin. Nutr., *24*:181, 1971.

Hellendoorn, E. W.: Beneficial physiologic action of beans. J. Amer. Dietet. Assoc., *69*:248, 1976.

Matthews, R. H., Weihrauch, J. L., and Watt, B. K.: Nutrient content of wheat and rice: present knowledge, problems, and needed research. Cereal Foods World, *20*:348, 1975.

Matthews, R. H., and Workman, M. Y.: Nutrient composition of selected wheat products. Cereal Chem., *54*:1115, 1978.

Nystrom, P. J., Ostrander, J. G., and Martinsen, C. S.: Cheese products: protein, moisture, fat, and acceptance. J. Amer. Dietet. Assoc., *65*:40, 1974.

Skelton, M. M., and Marr, C. W.; Ascorbic acid content, pH, and acceptability of tomatoes processed by different home canning methods. Home Econ.

Watson, K., and Kilgore, L.: Fat, moisture, and protein in "ground beef" and ground chuck. J. Amer. Dietet. Assoc., *65*:545, 1974.

Wong, N. P., LaCroix, D. E., and Alford, J. A.: Mineral contents of dairy products. I. Milk and milk products and II. Cheeses. J. Amer. Dietet. Assoc., *72*:288, and *72*:608, 1978.

Yogurt, Consumer Reports, *43*:7, 1978.

Food Purchasing and Budgeting

Big savings in small packages. Consumer Reports, *42*:315, 1978.

Block, C. E., and Kellerman, B. J.: Food shopping efficiency among the rural poor: an exploratory inquiry. Home Econ. Res. J., *5*:255, 1977.

Bornmann, P. G.: Food retailers help teach food buying. J. Nutr. Educ., *5*:21, 1973.

Harrison, G. G., Rathje, W. L., and Hughes, W. W.: Food waste behavior in an urban population. J. Nutr. Educ., *7*:13, 1975.

Moore, J. L., and Wendt, P. F.: Nutrition labeling — a summary and evaluation. J. Nutr. Educ., *5*:121, 1973.

U.S. Department of Agriculture: *Buying Food—a Guide for Calculating Amounts to Buy and Comparing Costs in Household Quantities.* U.S.D.A. Home Econ. Res. Rpt. No. 42. Washington, D.C., Government Printing Office, 1978.

U.S. Department of Agriculture: *How to Buy Food. Lesson Aids for Teachers.* Agriculture Handbook No. 443. Washington, D.C., Government Printing Office, 1975.

Verma, S., Tucker, D., and Gassie, E. W.: Testing consumers for knowledge of beef concepts. Home Econ. Res. J., *5*:263, 1977.

Government Publications

The following titles are but a few of the Federal publications available. For an up-to-date listing, see current lists of bulletins available from the United States Department of Agriculture, and the Department of Health, Education, and Welfare. These are often available from local country agricultural extension or public health offices, or may be purchased from the Superintendent of Documents, Government Printing Office, Washington, D. C., 20402.

Conserving the Nutritive Values in Foods. Home and Garden Bulletin No. 90.

Family Food Budgeting for Good Meals and Good Nutrition. Home and Garden Bulletin No. 94.

Money-Saving Main Dishes. Home and Garden Bulletin No. 43.

Vegetables in Family Meals: a Guide for Consumers. Home and Garden Bulletin No. 105.

Your Money's Worth in Foods. Home and Garden Bulletin No. 183.

Also (from the U.S. Department of Agriculture) see recent quarterly copies of:
Demand and Price Situation
Fats and Oils Situation
National Food Review — U.S.D.A.
Sugar and Sweetener Report
Vegetable Situation

Community Nutrition Institute publishes a weekly report of nutrition-related policy-making in Washington, D.C. The Institute is located at 1146 19th St., N.W., Washington, D.C. 20036. This is a private agency.

Articles in **Nutrition Reviews**

An index of food quality. (by Hansen R. G.) *31*:1, 1973.

Nutritional quality and food product development. *31*:226, 1973.

The value of iron fortification of food. *31*:275, 1973.

General policies in regard to improvement of nutritive quality of foods. *31*:324, 1973.

Resurvey of the nutrient content of canned foods. *32*:27, 1974.

Genetic improvement of cereals. (by Mertz, E. T.) *32*:129, 1974.

Problems in iron enrichment and fortification of foods. *33*:46, 1975.

The effects of food processing on nutritional values. *33*:123, 1975.

Milk intolerances. (by Woodruff, C. W.) *34*:33, 1976.

Nutritive consequences of replacing meat protein in sausages. *35*:111, 1977.

Lactoferrin and bacterial growth. *36*:22, 1978.

Nutritional implications of the Maillard reaction. *36*:28, 1978.

Chapter 18

Food: Nonnutrients, Enrichment, and Labels

As the list of unfamiliar ingredients on a package grows longer so does the concern of the consumer. After all, how many people are able to recognize most chemical names and associate them with their function and safety? Chemical pollutants in our environment, industrial chemical accidents, and the emergence of newly recognized carcinogens, mutagens, and teratogens has sensitized the public to regard all "chemicals" as potentially hazardous. It may be recognized by some informed consumers that all foods are naturally made up of chemicals, but many persons remain perplexed about which of the added and already present chemicals may contribute to adverse health.

In this chapter the functions of food additives will be discussed, as well as the safety of food additives and naturally occurring nonnutrients. A brief look at food labeling will demonstrate what one can learn by carefully reading such labels.

FOOD ADDITIVES

The use of food additives has been traced to ancient times. Ancient Egyptians used food coloring made from vegetables and insects, while the Romans preserved fruit in honey and considered it a delicacy. Marco Polo and other voyagers sought food additives in the form of precious spices. Salting foods to preserve them was common in the Middle Ages, especially in the northern areas to insure a supply of food throughout the hard winter. Today food additives are routinely used, so that even a meal made from "scratch" in the home contains food additives in the form of spices and herbs added to enhance color and flavor, and leavening to make bread rise.

What Are Food Additives?

Many substances may be considered food additives, but for our purposes food additives will be defined as *small amounts of substances intentionally added to a food for a specific effect or substances that are reasonably expected to become part of the food during processing or packaging.* By this definition *direct* additives include substances used commonly at home, such as vanilla and garlic, as well as ingredients added during industrial processing, such as propyl gallate and citric acid, which are used as antioxidants. Such a definition excludes, quite arbitrarily, added substances that provide a major caloric contribution to the food, such as sugar, corn syrup, unmodified starch, oils, and fats in the forms of shortening, butter, or margarine.

We see that in addition to *direct* additives, which are intentionally added to foods for technical effects, there are *indirect* additives, which inadvertently become part of a food during the handling of the food. Examples of indirect additives are lubricants from processing machinery, plastics and butylated hydroxyanisole (BHA), which, through packaging, become part of the food, and minerals from cooking vessels. Indirect additives such as these are present in such tiny amounts that they are generally negligible. In terms of our definition, it is estimated that there are about 3000 direct additives and 10,000 indirect additives.[1]

Food additives may be pure or impure, products of nature or synthesized in factories. Spices are examples of impure naturally occurring food additives. Calcium propionate, which is naturally found in Swiss cheese, sodium benzoate, which is a natural part of cranberry juice, and many vitamins are examples of pure chemicals that are added to foods but that are also found to occur naturally in foods. Pure chemical substances synthesized but not found in nature include the coal tar dyes, such as FD&C Yellow No. 5.

Food additives were first legally defined in the United States in 1958. This official definition excludes pesticide residues and food colors, which are regulated by separate amendments, and substances that are *generally recognized as safe (GRAS)*. A list of GRAS substances was established in 1958 as a result of a major regulatory amendment, the 1958 Food Additives Amendment, and represents substances that generally were in use prior to 1958 and whose safety was widely accepted by a surveyed sector of the scientific community. This list is the result of a legislative point in time and does not guarantee safety of these additives. (Saccharin and cyclamate are examples of GRAS substances that were removed from the list owing to questionable safety.) Examples of the 600 to 700 GRAS substances are listed in Table 18–1.

Why Use Food Additives?

There are technical, practical (timesaving), and economic reasons — some essential, some not — for using food additives. *Technical* uses of additives enable the manufacturer to achieve an aesthetically pleasing product with an increased shelf life and to supplement the nutritional value of the product. They also allow the manufacturer to "improve" various food properties. Technical uses of food additives include the following:

1. Preservatives *prevent spoilage and wastage* of food by extending its keeping

Table 18–1 A SAMPLING OF GRAS LIST SUBSTANCES*

Substance	*Common Purpose(s)*
Methyl and propyl parabens	Antimicrobial agents
Sorbitol˙	Nutritive sweetener
Gelatin	Thickener
Locust bean gum	Stabilizer and thickener
Garlic and garlic oil	Flavoring agents
Propyl gallate	Antioxidant (preservative)
Sulfuric acid	pH control agent
Calcium sulfate (plaster of paris, gypsum, anhydrite)	14 uses, including anticaking agent, dough conditioner, and nutrient supplement
Benzoic acid	Antimicrobial agent
Dill, cloves, mustard	Flavoring agents

*Subject to change pending the review of all GRAS substances.

quality. This is a valuable use of food additives, especially since food conservation is of vital concern today.

2. *Aesthetic value* is bestowed upon foods by the addition of colors, flavors, emulsifiers, stabilizers and thickeners, and acid-base adjusters. These add not only to eye appeal but also to the texture or "mouth feel." Aesthetic value is, perhaps, the most important function of food additives from the standpoint of the food industry since it has a large bearing on sales. For this reason, more attention is often given to these aspects rather than to nutritional value.

3. Nutrients are added to food to *improve or maintain preprocessing nutritional value.* This important use of food additives has virtually wiped out the occurrence of such nutritional diseases as goiter due to soils poor in iodine, and pellagra, which was chiefly a result of loss of niacin during the refining of grains. Nutrient supplementation is discussed in a later section of this chapter.

4. Maturing agents and agents that promote antifoaming, firming, hardening, drying, crisping, antisticking, anticaking, and whipping *"improve" various characteristics of a food* and enable the manufacturer to produce a uniform product. For example, such food additives allow salt to pour freely and improve the baking characteristics of wheat flour.

A *practical* reason for buying foods with additives is the convenience these foods lend to food preparation. The lifestyle in more developed countries has changed rapidly during this century, and now individuals generally prefer to spend less time preparing food and devote more time to other activities. The difference between preparation of some "convenience" foods versus fresh foods may be overestimated, since preparation of fresh produce and many dishes made from scratch need not be time-consuming. Some convenience foods may also be more expensive, however, this is an acceptable trade-off for many consumers. Other consumers, because of beliefs, whether right or wrong, would prefer to do without most food additives, even at the cost of inconvenience and the possibility of higher prices.

Economically speaking, food additives generally either help cut production costs for the manufacturer or aid in generating sales. For instance, preservatives make possible fewer deliveries to the store and less wastage. This saving to the manufacturer also often results in a lower product price to the consumer. By enabling a pleasing product to be marketed, food additives increase food product revenues.

Apart from the nutrients themselves and preservatives, most food additives have little or no valid nutritional significance.* One exception is carotene, a food coloring that has vitamin A value. It may be argued that food additives may entice a person to eat a food, thus indirectly supplying some nutrition to the individual. The indirect nutritional value, however, depends on whether the individual is enticed to eat wholesome foods or foods lacking in essential nutrients. The technical necessity of some food additives is also questionable. Butylated hydroxytoluene (BHT), for example, is added to the oil of some brands of fried food products such as potato chips, while other brands successfully market their product without this or any other preservative.

Amounts of Food Additives Consumed

The consumption of food additives is on the rise, accompanying the increased production of convenience foods, snack foods, and vitamin-supplemented foods. The amount of food additives consumed by the average American per year is an elusive figure that is difficult to determine because of lack of a uniform definition of additives and lack of accurate quantitative production and consumption data. An es-

*In addition to decreasing spoilage, BHT and other antioxidants may preserve vitamins A, E, and C.

timate was made by the President's Science Advisory Committee in 1973, based on the amount of food additives purchased by industry.[1] On this basis, slightly more than 9 pounds of food additives were ingested per capita, excluding salt, dextrose, corn syrup, added fat, and sucrose. Of these 9 pounds, 7½ to 8 are accounted for by 32 of the most commonly used chemicals, including flavoring agents such as mustard, pepper, and monosodium glutamate; gases for carbonating beverages; nutrient supplements such as calcium salts and sodium caseinate; and 18 agents for leavening and the control of pH. The remaining 1½ to 2 pounds is made up of all the rest of the food additives.

Adolescent and adult males and females eat the least amount of food additives when calculated as milligrams of food additives eaten per kilogram of body weight. This was the conclusion of a study that looked at the consumption patterns of 163 food additives.[2] Infants generally consumed the most food additives when viewed in this manner; thus food additives pose a greater risk for this group, which is more vulnerable to the toxicity of many compounds. The Joint FAO/WHO* Expert Committee on Food Additives recommends that infants less than 12 weeks of age have food with no additives, since their protective and detoxifying mechanisms may not be well developed.[3]

*Food and Agriculture Organization and World Health Organization of the United Nations.

Fortification and Enrichment

Nutrients may be added to foods to *restore* those lost in food processing, such as the vitamin C added to instant mashed potatoes. *Fortification* is the addition of nutrients to foods that may be replacing former common sources of certain nutrients (such as vitamin C in fruit drinks), or the enhancement of the nutritional and economic value of a product (such as vitamins added to snack bars). *Enrichment* is a legal term in the United States referring, for example, to the FDA program that requires thiamin, riboflavin, niacin, and iron to be added back to refined cereals (see Table 18–2). Fortification, enrichment, and restoration are terms often used interchangeably, and meanings attached to them may vary from country to country.

Nutrients may also be added to foods for preservation rather than for improvement of nutrient composition. For example, ascorbic acid (as an antioxidant) can prolong the shelf life of products to which it is added.

Food enrichment is carried out as a public health measure. Sometimes a population or members of a subgroup are deficient in a nutrient. They may suffer gross deficiency symptoms (as goiter in iodine deficiency) or exhibit biochemical signs

Table 18–2 COMPARISON OF THREE B VITAMINS AND IRON IN POUND LOAVES OF WHEAT BREAD*

Wheat Bread	*Thiamin mg*	*Riboflavin mg*	*Niacin mg*	*Iron mg*
Unenriched	0.40	0.36	5.6	3.2
Enriched†	1.1–1.8	0.7–1.6	10–15	8.0–12.5
Whole-wheat	1.17	0.56	12.9	10.4

*From Bread Standards, Code of Federal Regulations, U. S. Food and Drug Administration, Title 21, Chapter 1, Section 17, April 22, 1964; and U. S. Department of Agriculture: *Handbook 8*.

†Enriched bread may also contain added calcium salts (including milk solids) in such quantity that each pound of the finished bread contains not less than 300 mg and not more than 800 mg of calcium. Higher levels of enrichment were proposed in 1972.

of deficiency (as low hemoglobin levels in iron deficiency). A change in a population's food habits may eliminate a source of vital nutrients. With enrichment programs, diets can be nutritionally improved without interfering with food habits. This is important, it can be argued, because people are generally averse to changing their habits. When habits do change, fortification may help keep the population's nutrient intake at an acceptable level. For example, with the increasing use of margarine in preference to butter in this country, it became necessary to fortify margarine with the vitamin A found in butter.

Persons responsible for the quality of our food supply need to respect eating habits and preferences, be they culturally or individually determined. Food is viewed in many ways, only one of which is its role as a vehicle for nutrients. All of our nutrient requirements cannot be insured with any enrichment program unless the diet is properly chosen. Hence, it would seem that a more appropriate long-term goal is the provision of sound nutrition education so that populations will wisely change to more healthful eating habits.

When wholesome food adequate for a balanced diet is available, it may be difficult to see the reason for fortification. This is especially true when "unwholesome" vehicles such as sugar are chosen for fortification. Such vehicles as sugar, however, have served as expedient means of reducing some nutritional deficiencies such as that of vitamin A but should be viewed as only short-term stopgap measures.

A potentially great problem with enrichment is the danger of its mushrooming from a stopgap measure to the major means of coping with malnutrition. It could well stifle efforts of nations to implement long-range agricultural and nutritional improvement programs. There is the danger that an expedient fortification program will give a false sense of security when conducted at the expense of slower but more farsighted measures. Nutrients come from food, and it is impractical to provide them through fortification alone.

Aside from these advantages and disadvantages of enrichment, there are some practical problems with long-term fortification programs. As people's eating habits change, so do their nutrient intakes. Constantly adjusting enrichment levels to meet changing trends is cumbersome; not to do so, however, would defeat the public health objective of enrichment. In the United States, bread enrichment standards were established over 35 years ago to provide thiamin, riboflavin, niacin, and iron because the population was deficient in these nutrients. But with

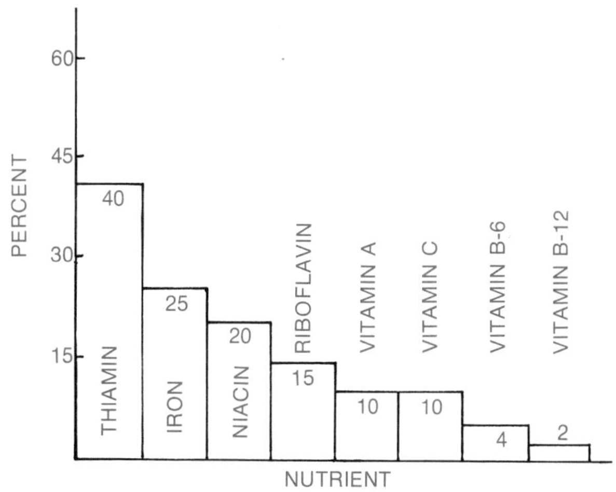

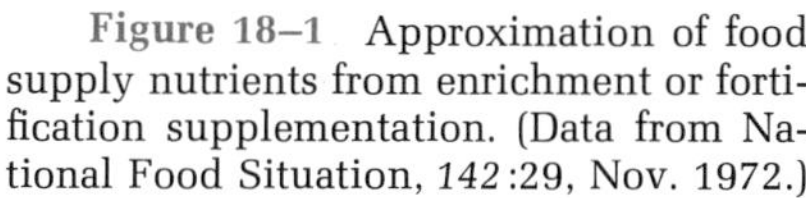
Figure 18–1 Approximation of food supply nutrients from enrichment or fortification supplementation. (Data from National Food Situation, *142*:29, Nov. 1972.)

today's decreased bread consumption, the population is not receiving the amounts of these nutrients from bread, as planned. Also, additional nutrients have been shown to be low in our diets, namely calcium and folic acid. Our needs change, but fortification levels often do not change as quickly, owing to a lag in legislation.

The idea of fortifying a food to make it self-sufficient presents another problem. No food but human milk for the infant is the "perfect" food, and even that needs supplementation for infants after several months (see Chapter 21). Each food needs to be complemented by different types of foods to make an adequate diet. According to what we now know about nutrition, dependence on one so-called complete food would be unwise.

The addition of three or four vitamins to foods with low nutritional value may cause the consumer to rationalize that it is legitimate to eat them in sizeable quantities, since they are obtaining some added nutrients by doing so. The high-caloric and less nutritive aspects of the food may offset this benefit, however, and may prevent the consumer from eating sources of other needed nutrients not included in the fortification. Another problem for the consumer is industry's manipulation of food fortification for economic benefit without true concern for the consumer's health. Advertisements and articles in food technology and food product journals speak of the benefits of "new markets" and increased sales of foods that result from food fortification. Advertisements in 1978, for example, claim the cost of adding one-third of the U.S. RDA of vitamins A, D, E, thiamin, riboflavin, niacin, B-6, and B-12 per serving is less than one-tenth of a penny; however, the price increase added to the product because of fortification is usually proportionally much higher.

Technical Considerations. Once enrichment is deemed necessary, decisions must be made concerning which foods should carry the nutrient in question. This determined, in part, by who constitutes the target group. The food consumption habits of those in this group must be known, so that the food supplying the nutrient will be consumed in sufficient quantity to make a contribution to the diet.

A second technical consideration is the chemical form in which the nutrient is added. The nutrient should be in a utilizable form and should not change the appearance, flavor, odor, or keeping qualities of the food. For example, food technologists had to contend with the unfamiliar yellow color that riboflavin imparted to rice. Adding the fat-soluble vitamins A and D to nonfat milk also posed a challenging technical problem. In order to keep bread volume high in protein-fortified loaves, dough conditioners and emulsifiers have been added along with the protein.

The manner in which food will be prepared must also be considered. Coating rice with water-soluble vitamins, when the rice is cooked in water that is then discarded, does not increase the nutrient intake of the population. A more useful method of fortification of rice is the addition of a white rice-shaped vitamin-mineral preparation in a ratio of 1 to 200 rice grains.

Nutrients found to be low in the diet of a population can be added to almost any product that is used widely. Staples such as wheat, rice, and corn have served as vehicles for niacin, riboflavin, thiamin, iron, calcium, and vitamin D. Vitamin D was first added to milk in the United States in 1929, and since 1924, salt has been fortified with iodine in the United States.

Regulation of Food Additives

In the latter half of the nineteenth century, adulteration of food through the addition of harmful food additives in the United States was not uncommon. A sampling of candy in Boston in 1880 revealed 46 per cent containing one or more toxic

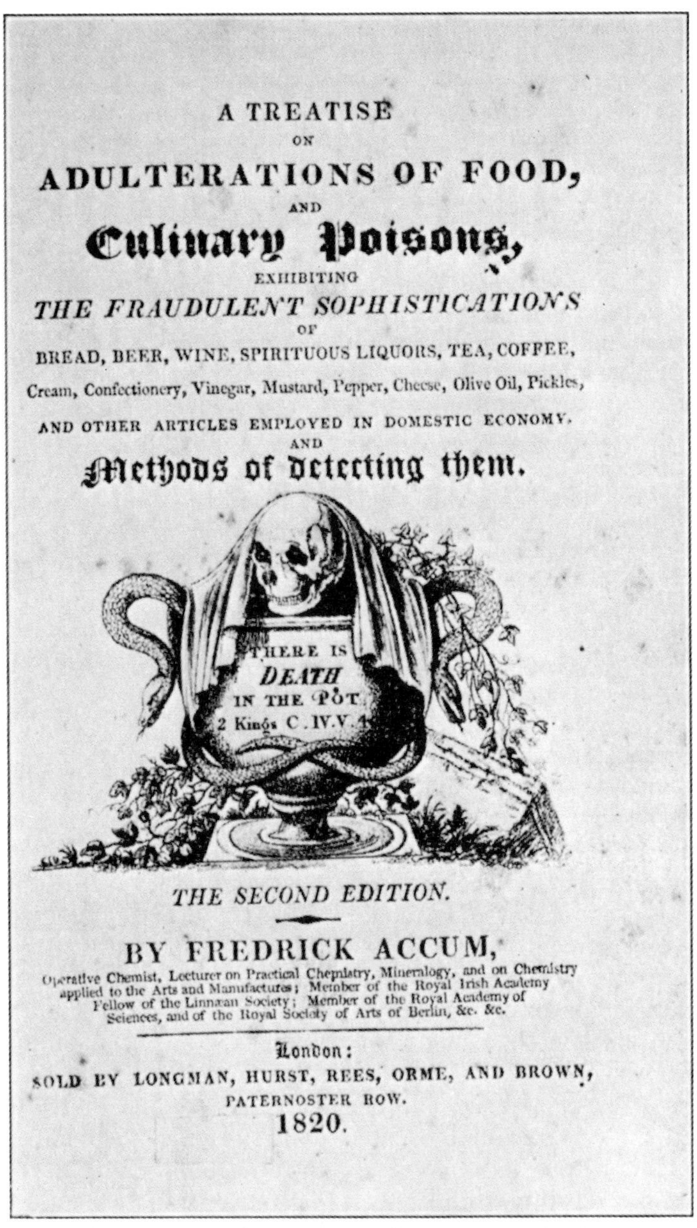

A TREATISE
ON
ADULTERATIONS OF FOOD,
AND
Culinary Poisons,
EXHIBITING
THE FRAUDULENT SOPHISTICATIONS
OF
BREAD, BEER, WINE, SPIRITUOUS LIQUORS, TEA, COFFEE,
Cream, Confectionery, Vinegar, Mustard, Pepper, Cheese, Olive Oil, Pickles,
AND OTHER ARTICLES EMPLOYED IN DOMESTIC ECONOMY.
AND
Methods of detecting them.

THE SECOND EDITION.

BY FREDRICK ACCUM,
Operative Chemist, Lecturer on Practical Chemistry, Mineralogy, and on Chemistry applied to the Arts and Manufactures; Member of the Royal Irish Academy Fellow of the Linnæan Society; Member of the Royal Academy of Sciences, and of the Royal Society of Arts of Berlin, &c. &c.

London:
SOLD BY LONGMAN, HURST, REES, ORME, AND BROWN,
PATERNOSTER ROW.
1820.

Figure 18–2 Prior to their regulation, food additives often constituted food adulteration. *Fredrick* Accum was a pioneer in exposing food adulteration in England. Authorship of this book led to the loss of his business and his friends. (From Chemistry, *46* (5):16, 1973.)

mineral pigments, chiefly lead chromate.[4] Cheese was colored with mercury (HgS) and red lead (Pb_3O_4) compounds. No federal laws governing food additives existed at this time.

Adulteration was a deep concern of Dr. Harvey Wiley, a chemist for the U.S. Department of Agriculture from 1883 to 1930, whose influence helped bring about the legislation of the Federal Pure Food and Drugs Act of 1906. This act prohibited the adulteration of foods and was followed in 1938 by the U.S. Federal Food, Drug, and Cosmetic Act, which included further provisions against adulteration and also required the certification of coal tar dyes. Later, three amendments to this act shifted the burden of proof for safety of food additives, pesticide residues, and food colors to industry before their use could be approved. Thus, it was not until the U.S. 1958 Food Additives Amendment that a manufacturer had to prove the safety of an additive to the FDA *before* its use in food, rather than the FDA proving that an additive was unsafe *after* it had already been added to foods.

The 1958 Food Additives Amendment also includes a provision known as the *Delaney Clause.* This clause states that "No additive shall be deemed to be safe if it is found to induce cancer when ingested by man or animals, or if it is found, after tests which are appropriate for the evaluation of the safety of food additives, to induce cancer in man or animals." This has become a controversial clause, since some scientists feel there is a "no risk" level of ingestion of carcinogens; hence, they feel the clause interferes with the exercise of scientific judgment. Others feel that a low risk of cancer is outweighed by the benefits of some food additives. Still to be proven, however, is whether in fact carcinogenic substances have a no-effect ingestion level or merely present a lower risk when eaten in trace amounts. For this reason, other scientists prefer the clause as it is stated, based on the unknown rather than on our present knowledge, which is incomplete.

The regulation of additives and colors in food for interstate commerce in the United States falls under the jurisdiction of the Federal Drug Administration, while the regulation of pesticide residues, which remain on agricultural produce in interstate shipment, is controlled by the Environmental Protection Agency. International food standards, including those concerning food additives, are in part regulated by the Codex Alimentarius Commission, a joint FAO/WHO commission. The Commission was set up to protect the consumer against health risks and fraud and to facilitate international trade. Over 99 countries have become members of the Commission, and over two-thirds of them are developing countries.

Safety of Food Additives

A chemical cannot be judged for safety on the basis of whether it is naturally occurring or artificially synthesized. There are many naturally occurring toxins and carcinogens, just as there are safe synthesized food additives. In addition, most consumers are not familiar with chemical names, so that reading a chemical name on the label does not tell them if it is natural or artificial, safe or toxic. Background information is needed for each substance before such judgments may be made.

In most developed countries, at least, food additives must now go through a rigorous testing procedure for safety before they will be approved. This was not true prior to 1958 in the United States and was not required for GRAS substances. Even since 1958, methodology and testing procedures have continually improved; thus we have imposed stricter regulations. Owing to this stricter regulation, the number of new food additives (excluding flavors) approved by the FDA dropped from an average of 29 per year in the 1960's to an average of 2 per year during the first half of the 1970's. In addition, consumer alarm over the banning of cyclamates in the United States and the recent suspected safety of some other food additives has led to a review of the safety of GRAS substances, regulated food additives, and food colors.

Before being approved in the United States, a prospective additive must undergo safety testing, which "generally follows the procedures established in recent publications of the National Academy of Sciences–National Research Council, though use of other procedures will not render a food additive petition unapprovable."[5]

Most often, the prospective additive goes through acute, subacute, and chronic (2 year) oral toxicity tests in at least two species of animals (usually rats and dogs), both male and female, to take into account interspecies and sex differences. Evaluations of possible reproductive, teratogenic, and mutagenic effects are made through multigeneration studies. Also, evaluations are made of possible subtle, long-term effects including cancer (with lifetime studies). In some cases psychopharmacological or behavioral effects are evaluated. Investigations also elucidate the metabolic pathway of the additive and a practical method for determining the quantity of the additive in food.[6]

In addition, an additive will not be approved by the FDA unless it has been shown to give the intended effect at the proposed level of use. Generally, the amount approved for addition to foods includes a margin of safety of at least 100 times less than the highest level that caused no toxic effects in animal studies.

There will always be problems involved with testing a compound for its safety. Direct extrapolation of data from animal experiments to humans is not possible, and investigators may not recognize subtle effects from feeding studies. Behavioral effects are particularly difficult to assess in animals. Interpretation of data is often not clear cut, and, owing to human error, experimental procedures may not always be optimal. Industry has been known to influence the interpretation of some experiments, and the lobbying of industries and consumer groups may decide whether a substance is banned or not, even when scientific evidence is inconclusive for such a decision. Subjective evaluation plays a large part in such decision-making, since inconclusive data and lack of scientific agreement often prevail.

It is important to weigh the biological risks against the benefits of each food additive and of the use of food additives in general. This includes looking at how the use of an additive may affect the total food, energy, and environmental system. For instance, if deleting a food additive results in abandonment of one processing method for a new method that increases the amount of carcinogenic air pollutants, is it more of a risk to eat the food additive or to breathe the pollutants? Ideally, it would be best to eliminate both sources, but we are not often given this choice.

A potential problem in the use of food additives may not be the safety of the food additives themselves, but rather the nutritional safety of the fabricated foods that food additives make possible. These foods do not usually supply all of the vital known and unknown micronutrients and often contain high levels of sugar and fat. With the increasing consumption of fabricated foods, the possibility of diluted, imbalanced, and less nutritious diets may become a greater concern.

Only a few examples of some of the problems of using specific food additives are given here. The three examples chosen — food colors, saccharin, and nitrites — are among the most controversial today.

Food Colors

Food colors restore color lost in processing to a product or add color to a food to make it more acceptable and attractive. Consumers associate color with quality and freshness of a food product. During processing, natural pigments often undergo color changes. For example, the chlorophylls in vegetables may turn from green to an olive-brown pigment (pheophytin), owing to a chemical reaction between chlorophyll and acids liberated during heating. You may have noticed this when cooking broccoli, spinach, or green beans. In commercial canning, calcium or magnesium hydroxide may be added to neutralize these acids and thus prevent a large color change in green vegetables.

On a nutritional level most food colors are not justified, unless one assumes that wholesome foods without the added color would not otherwise be eaten. The bulk of food colors are used in baked goods, soft drinks, ice cream, sherbets, dairy products, and candy and confections. Thus, they may entice the consumer to buy some rather less wholesome as well as nutritious foods.

According to the 1938 Federal Food, Drug, and Cosmetic Act, no substance can be added to a food to "make it appear better or of greater value than it is" or it shall be considered adulterated.[7] Federal law also specifies that color cannot be added to foods if it promotes consumer deception by concealing inferiority or by leading a consumer to believe that a product has more of an ingredient than it actually contains (for example, yellow coloring in egg bread). One might question whether or not the addition of many food colors is, by Federal definition, adulteration, since it often lends an attractiveness not inherent in the product, and thus may make the product "appear better or of greater value than it is."

The safety of artificial food colors has been questioned in recent years. Iceland and Norway completely ban the use of synthetic food dyes. It was not until the mid-nineteenth century that artificial colors from coal tar dyes were developed and added to foods, and at the turn of the century about 80 different coal tar or synthetic dyes were used as food additives. This number decreased to 19 coal tar dyes approved for use by the Food and Drug Administration in 1951[7] and continued to decrease to 9 such dyes in 1978, 2 of which have very restricted use.

Since 1938 all FD&C synthetic dyes require certification of purity by the Federal government before they may be used in foods. This test for purity insures against harmful contaminants but does not guarantee the safety of the dye itself. In the early 1950's two instances of human toxicity from food colors occurred when children ate colored Halloween popcorn and candy that gave them diarrhea. This gave rise to additional toxicity testing and reevaluation of artificial colors. The FDA is again reviewing pertinent toxicity studies of the FD&C colors.

The toxicity of naturally occurring food dyes such as beet juice, turmeric, and carrot oils has been less rigorously tested than that of the artificial dyes. Their centuries of use without apparent harm (which may not always be a correct assessment) plus results of known toxicity tests on these compounds has led to their addition to foods according to the Good Manufacturing Practice Code of the Federal government, but without official certification. Only about 10 per cent of food coloring comes from naturally occurring dyes, since the synthetic dyes are generally much more stable.[8]

Nitrates, Nitrites, and Nitrosamines

Inorganic salts of nitrate and nitrite have been used to cure meats for centuries.* Originally, nitrate was an impurity in the salts used to cure meats. Nitrite is responsible for the characteristic color and flavor of cured meats, such as bacon, ham, and salami, in addition to inhibiting the growth of *Clostridium botulinum* and other bacteria. *C. botulinum* produces a potent toxin that causes botulism poisoning when ingested.

Nitrates may be converted to nitrites by bacteria in the mouth and intestines, and in plants. It has been found in laboratories that nitrite may combine with secondary and tertiary amines found in the diet, usually in the presence of acid, to form nitrosamines. Over 75 per cent of the nitrosamines tested have been found to be highly carcinogenic in test animals; thus there is concern that nitrosamines present in food before ingestion or the possible formation of nitrosamines in our bodies may be contributing to the incidence of cancer.

Nitrosamines have been found in some cured meats prepared for ingestion, primarily in bacon, as well as in tobacco

*Potassium nitrate is also known as saltpeter.

smoke, cheese, fish, milk, mushrooms, alcoholic beverages, flour, and animal feed.[9] The U.S. Department of Agriculture analyzed 25 samples of bacon that had been cooked by consumers in their normal manner and found 1 to 39 ppb of two different nitrosamines in the samples, with 10 samples having more than 10 ppb.[10] Some scientists estimate 10 ppb nitrosamines to be a safe level of ingestion; however, the U.S. Department of Agriculture has called for not more than 5 ppb nitrosamines in bacon that has been cooked, an essentially zero tolerance, since this is virtually the lowest level at which nitrosamines may be reliably detected.

It is known that the presence of ascorbic acid in the food and in the diet seems to protect against the formation of carcinogenic nitrosamines. Thus, the use of ascorbic acid during the curing process at a high enough level may prevent nitrosamine formation in cured meats, and such processing methods are under study. The removal of nitrites and nitrates from bacon would eliminate this source of nitrosamines in our diet. The risk of botulism poisoning from such an action is thought to be negligible by some, while others fear an increase in deaths from this toxin.

Our major dietary source of nitrates and nitrites is not cured meats. Nitrates occur in leafy and root vegetables, with consistently high levels in celery, beets, spinach, and lettuce; and they also occur in drinking water.* Our major source of nitrite is our saliva, in which residing bacteria in our mouths convert nitrate to nitrite. Thus, a potential but unconfirmed risk of formation of nitrosamines from salivary nitrite and amines in our foods has always existed. Some scientists feel that the concentrated amounts of nitrites (and possibly nitrosamines) introduced to the body when eating cured foods presents a greater hazard than the constant dilute amount contributed by saliva. However, recent Danish and Canadian studies on feeding cured meats to rats concluded that there was no increase in the cancer rate in animals of the experimental versus the control group.[11] It is still as yet unresolved whether nitrites in moderate amounts in our food are a significant health hazard.

* The level of nitrate in drinking water in the United States is restricted to 45 ppm; however, some well waters have been known to contain more than 200 ppm.

Saccharin

Saccharin, discovered in 1879, is the only artifical sweetener presently allowed on the market in the United States. Molecule per molecule, saccharin is 300 times sweeter than sucrose. It is added to "diet" soft drinks (the main source of saccharin consumption) and other diet foods, chewable vitamins, gum, toothpaste, and children's drugs. Diabetics have used saccharin for more than 80 years.

The safety of saccharin is being questioned because its consumption has been associated with an increase in bladder cancer in studies in which saccharin was fed to rats at a level of 5 per cent of the diet. Some questions were raised in the two studies about whether this was due to the saccharin or a contaminant, orthotoluenesulfonamide (OTS); however, a later two generation study conducted by the Health Protection Branch of the Canadian government with virtually no contaminant also showed an increased incidence of bladder tumors in the experimental group as compared with the controls when saccharin constituted 5 percent of the diet.[12] These studies have been criticized because the level of saccharin fed to the rats is equivalent to a person drinking hundreds of diet soft drinks each day. In toxicity and cancer studies, high levels need to be fed to the animals in order to obtain meaningful statistics using a relatively small number of animals. The alternative, feeding a low level of the additive and detecting rates of cancer as low as 1 in 10,000, would involve feeding so many animals that it would not be technically and monetarily feasible. However, one must also be aware of the possibility of such large doses overwhelming the protective mechanisms that would normally detoxify the compound at lower levels.

Whether saccharin poses a risk at the levels presently ingested is unknown. In 1977 the FDA proposed a ban on the use of saccharin in food, and in November of that year an 18 month moratorium was placed on this ban. In the meantime, the FDA is conducting a 1.375 million dollar epidemiological study on the role of saccharin and other variables in bladder cancer.

The benefits as well as the risks of saccharin are debatable. It has not been shown that diet soft drinks and other saccharin-containing foods have aided in the reduction of obesity. Diabetics are able to control their intake of calories and carbohydrates with or without saccharin. The removal of saccharin has become an emotional and hotly debated subject that is complicated by the lack of an acceptable substitute.

NATURALLY OCCURRING NONNUTRIENTS IN FOODS

Thousands of chemicals occurring naturally in plants and animals have no known nutritional value to humans. The common potato alone has hundreds of identified compounds that have no recognized human nutritional significance. Nonnutrients, encompassing many categories of chemicals, serve no useful normal functional purpose and may or may not pose a threat to the body. Some even may be antinutrients, such as avidin in raw egg whites (see Chapter 8) and thiaminases found in some raw fish, bracken fern, and blueberries. Some are plant pigments, such as chlorophyll. Some nonnutrients in food are mycotoxins, metabolites produced by fungi, including the toxins in poisonous mushrooms such as *Amanita phalloides*, the "death cup."

Other naturally occurring compounds in food produce pharmacological effects and are used as drugs, such as reserpine, a tranquilizer, from the *Rauwolfia serpentina* plant. The roots of this plant have a long history of use in India for several conditions including mental disorder. Other compounds naturally present in food may inhibit enzymes, interfere with the central nervous system, give hallucinogenic effects, or promote goiter. Some have the capacity to increase blood pressure or cause cancer. Safrole, a natural component of sassafras, was used as a food additive to flavor root beer until it was reported to produce cancer in laboratory animals. Glycyrrhizic acid, a component of licorice, may cause electrolyte imbalance if ingested daily in large enough quantities. Pressor amines, compounds found in fermented foods such as cheese, wine, and salami, as well as in bananas and avocados, when eaten with some prescribed tranquilizers may lead to an increase in blood pressure.

Thus, in some cases the consumption of certain naturally occurring nonnutrients may have adverse effects ranging from mild discomfort to serious consequences. In fact, many common natural components of food probably would never be allowed as food additives, since they would fail our strict safety regulations. In addition, many naturally occurring substances, if allowed as food additives, would not be permitted in foods at the levels found naturally. As you will recall, the margin of safety for the level to which food additives may be added to foods is about 100 times less than the highest level that produced no adverse effects on subjects in animal studies. The margin of safety for many naturally occurring toxicants, however, is less than that permitted for food additives.* For exam-

*A lower margin of safety is not, in itself, necessarily hazardous, but depends on the conditions of ingestion. This disparity between the levels of some naturally occurring substances and those of permitted food additives points up the strictness of regulations concerning food additives.

Table 18–3 EXAMPLES OF NATURALLY OCCURRING TOXINS, THEIR SOURCES AND TOXIC ACTIONS

Nonnutrient	*Food Source*	*Mode of Action*
Safrole	Sassafras, mace, nutmeg	Carcinogen
Myristicin	Nutmeg, dill, parsley	Hallucinogen
Methylmercury	Swordfish, tuna	Neurotoxin
Cyanogenic glycosides	Fruit seeds, cassava, legumes	Cyanide poisoning
Solanine	Potato shoots and skin	Acetylcholinesterase inhibitor
Aflatoxin	Mold-contaminated farm products	Carcinogen, liver toxin
Avidin	Raw egg whites	Biotin antagonist
Goitrogens	Brussels sprouts, broccoli, kale, soybeans	Promote goiter
Carototoxin	Carrots	Nerve poison
Benzo(a)pyrene	Smoked and charcoal-broiled meats	Carcinogen
Thiaminase	Bracken fern, raw clams and mussels, tea	Thiamin deficiency
Ergot alkaloids	*Claviceps purpurea*–infested grain	Gangrenous syndrome, CNS syndrome
Glycyrrhizic acid	Licorice plant	Hypertension
Genistein (estrogen)	Soybeans	Decreased weight and reproductive failure in rats
Amanitans	Amanita mushrooms	Liver and kidney damage
Tetrodotoxin	Liver and sex organs of puffer fish	Respiratory paralysis

ple, the margin of safety for goitrogenic (goiter-promoting) substances is estimated as less than ten.[13] It should also be noted that the margin of safety for some naturally occurring nutrients in our diet is much lower than 100. The margin of safety for sodium is estimated at less than 5; for iron, zinc, copper, and fluorine at 5 to 10; and for vitamins A and D at 25 to 40 for adults.[13]

It is hypothesized that early humans discovered which foods were toxic by trial and error; thus foods associated with ill effects that occurred soon after ingestion were avoided. This procedure exposed foods that produce short-term toxic effects but revealed very little about long-term effects of eating nonnutrients. Humans also discovered that some foods containing toxic substances could be prepared in ways that would detoxify or remove such substances. American Indians leached poisons out of acorns, and in Africa and South America cassava is prepared by a water-soaking and fermentation process that releases hydrogen cyanide from the compound *linamarin* before the cassava is eaten. In addition, merely the usual heat used in cooking will inactivate many natural toxins, such as the *thiaminase* in fish; the *avidin* in egg; and the *enzyme inhibitors, hemagglutinins,* and *goitrogens* in legumes and other plants. Thus, staying clear of some foodstuffs and methods of food preparation has allowed humans to avoid the toxic effects of many natural nonnutrients. (See Table 18–3)

In more recent times, new strains of plants have been developed so that the content of toxic substances is lessened. Thus, lima beans in the United States have a low content of *cyanogenic glycosides* (hydrogen cyanide–releasing substances); and *gossypol*, a toxic substance present in cottonseed, has largely been eliminated. Caution must always be exercised with genetic manipulation, however, since changing the proportion of a plant component may result in the increase of another hazardous component or creation of an undesirable balance of nutrients in the plant. An example of plant breeding that led to a mixture of both desirable and undesirable qualities was the development of a potato that had excellent chipping and browning properties. Unfortunately, this newly developed strain also contained high levels of *solanine*, an acetylcholinesterase inhibitor, and could not be permitted on the market by federal regulations.

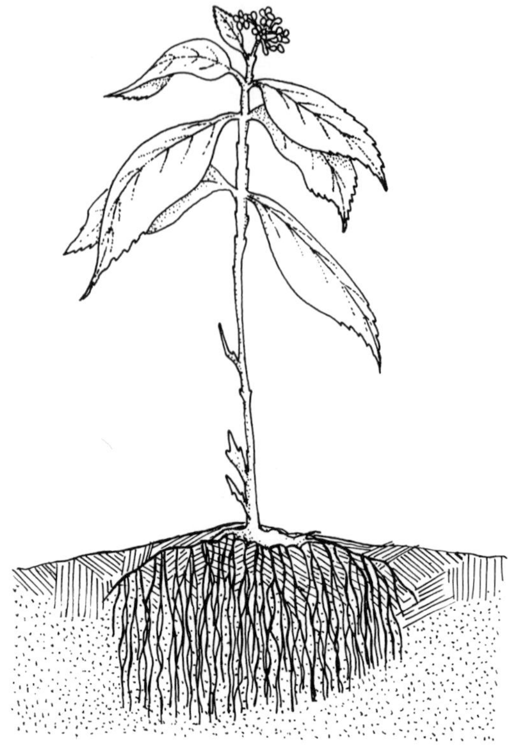

Figure 18–3 Some naturally occurring nonnutrients serve as therapeutic drugs. The root of the Rauwolfia plant is a source of reserpine, a tranquilizer. The root has been used in India for centuries to treat many diseases, including mental disorders.

Is There a Hazard Involved In Ingesting Naturally Occurring Toxicants?

All substances have an intrinsic *toxicity*; that is, if they are ingested at a certain level for a specified length of time, adverse effects will result. Even water is toxic if taken in excess quantities. However, humans can ingest small amounts of many substances of varying toxicity with no ill effects because of the remarkable detoxifying and defense mechanisms in the body. It is when the body's mechanisms become overwhelmed that we see most of the obvious toxic reactions. Therefore, the *hazard* of eating naturally occurring toxins is a relative phenomenon, depending on the context in which the food is eaten. Conditions of ingesting a food or naturally occurring toxin that might pose a hazard to the consumer (including amount, pattern, and interactions with other compounds in the diet) are more important to consider than the intrinsic toxicity of a compound.

On a worldwide basis, toxins in food that result from microorganisms and naturally occurring components of food have contributed the greatest number of food-related injuries to man. Inadvertent or accidental contaminants of both natural and manmade toxicants have contributed a lesser amount to food-related injuries, while food additives, agricultural chemicals, and chemicals produced in food during food processing reportedly have not led to adverse effects on human health when used according to good manufacturing and agricultural practices and when their intake is not grossly excessive.[13]

Range livestock in many areas of the world routinely ingest variable amounts of poisonous plants, resulting in symptoms ranging from no observable signs to moderate toxicoses to death. It is estimated that tens of thousands of livestock deaths occur yearly in the Western United States from toxic plant ingestion while perhaps five times as many animals suffer moderate toxicoses.[14] In addition, it has been discovered that many congenital deformations in livestock previously assumed to be of genetic origin are produced by plant teratogens. Problems with domestic animals occur also, since underprocessed feed may contain hazardous levels of natural toxicants. For instance, raw soybean meal is known to contain a pancreas-stimulating factor, a trypsin inhibitor, goitrogenic substances, saponins, estrogenic factors, hemagglutinins, and anticlotting factors. Upon heating, however, which is now common practice for animal feeds, many of these potentially hazardous substances are inactivated.

You may wonder how you can safely eat any foods, given the large number of naturally occurring toxins. Although many potentially harmful substances occur in our diet, usually no significant threat is posed. As previously mentioned, methods of preparation and breeding have helped to minimize the hazard. Additionally, proper storage of food reduces the hazard from microbial toxins, and the fact that many substances are present in such minute amounts, relative to their toxic level, insures safety. Notably, the interaction between substances in foods often reduces risk, or at least does not contribute to it. The toxicity of most chemicals is not additive, and interactions of some trace minerals are known to reduce the toxicity of other trace minerals. An example of the latter is the protective effect of zinc against cadmium toxicity. Also, the widespread distribution of food throughout the world has helped to eliminate hazards deriving from local geochemical imbalances in the environment.

Circumstances do occur, however, in which naturally occurring substances in the diet do pose a threat. Certain foods usually avoided owing to their toxicity may accidentally or unavoidably be eaten, as has occurred in the misidentification of mushrooms and other plants. Also, foods generally avoided may be eaten in times of famine. *Lathyrism*, a neurological disorder involving weakness and paralysis of the lower limbs, has occurred periodically in parts of India and is associated with the consumption of a chickling vetch pea, *Lathyrus sativus*, during times of famine.

Ingestion of poisonous seafood and food containing sufficient bacterial or fungal toxins will also lead to ill health, as will overconsumption of a food that is not hazardous when eaten in "normal" quantities. Other conditions influencing the danger of ingesting certain foods include malnutrition, allergies, inborn errors of metabolism, and disease states. Thus, some people may not be able to tolerate lactose, and some may develop hemolytic anemia from the ingestion of cooked faba beans (*Vicia faba*) owing to a genetic predisposition.

A diverse and varied diet is the best way to eliminate any problems that arise from ingesting naturally occurring nonnutrients. This includes avoiding prolonged "fad" diets that involve an excess intake of any one food or an unbalanced food consumption.

A few examples of naturally occurring toxins are briefly discussed in the remainder of this section to illustrate their diverse nature and common occurrence in our food supply. Bacterial toxins are not discussed; however, one should note that bacteria are natural inhabitants of all external surfaces, including soil, air, water, plants, and even our skin, mouths, and gastrointestinal tracts. Thus, some bacteria are usually present in all our foodstuffs. It is the amount and type of microbes that determine whether beneficial or ill effects result from their presence.

Aflatoxins

One of the most potent liver carcinogens known is *aflatoxin* B_1, one of a group of *mycotoxins* (fungal metabolites) collectively known as *aflatoxins*. *Aspergillus flavus* contamination of foodstuffs including peanuts and corn appears to be the main source of aflatoxins. Wheat, rice, jowar, cottonseed, and grain sorghum also support the growth of *A. flavus*, as well as any food product in which the proper growing conditions prevail. Tropical areas with their high humidity and warm ambient temperatures favor the growth of *A. flavus*. Recently, there has been concern that unusual mold appearing on bread, cheese, jam, and other food products may signal danger of aflatoxin contamination, and caution should be exercised regarding their ingestion.[15]

Aflatoxins were unknown until 1960–61, when an epidemic of turkey pullet deaths occurred in England. The unknown cause was dubbed "Turkey X Disease." Similar occurrences among ducklings, chicks, swine, and calves followed. The culprit was traced to moldy, aflatoxin-containing peanut meal used as feed.

No direct evidence of carcinogenesis in humans due to ingestion of aflatoxins has been established; however, close associations have been noted. In Southeast Asia and parts of Africa, analyses of diets led to estimation of an aflatoxin intake from 8 ng per kg to more than 300 ng per kg of body weight per day. These intakes corresponded to estimated incidences of liver cancer of 5 to 25 per 100,000 population per year.[16] Other factors such as parasitic disease and malnutrition may be playing a part in this carcinogenesis, so that no cause-and-effect relationship of aflatoxin and liver cancer may be drawn from this data. Other studies have associated the intake of aflatoxins with Indian childhood cirrhosis[17] and, in Thai children, with a disease analogous to Reye's syndrome, which involves encephalopathy and fatty degeneration of the viscera.[18]

The susceptibility to carcinogenesis from aflatoxin consumption in animals is so different among species that it is difficult to apply such data to humans. Animal studies have shown that aflatoxins may also be responsible for other carcinomas, notably bowel and renal. It has also been shown in animal studies that diet composition, including levels of vitamin A, protein, and lipotrophs, may influence aflatoxin toxicity.

The removal of all aflatoxin-containing foods from the diet would greatly decrease the available food supply, resulting in malnutrition or starvation in some regions of the world. In the United States, corn (thought to be the greatest source of aflatoxin in the United States) and peanut products with more than 20 ppb aflatoxins are illegal for interstate commerce, and fluid milk products with more than 0.5 ppb aflatoxin M_1 are not permitted by the FDA to be used in the manufacture of other dairy products.[19] As yet, we do not know the hazard to humans, but the possibility exists that this unavoidable contaminant in the world food supply contributes to the occurrence of cancer.

Paralytic Shellfish Poisoning

At certain times of the year, a red or reddish-brown coloration of sea water may occur, a phenomenon known as "red tide." This red tide is caused by proliferation of dinoflagellates, an algae which can be toxic or nontoxic. Dinoflagellates are concentrated in the flesh of filter-feeding bivalve mollusks, such as mussels, clams, oysters, and scallops. If, perchance, the concentrated dinoflagellates are the poisonous *Gonyaulax catenella* (on the Pacific coast of the United States) or *Gonyaulax tamarensis* (on the New England coast) and the seafood is ingested, numbness and progressive paralysis of the mouth, lips, face, and extremities, and nausea, vomiting, and diarrhea may occur. In severe cases, repiratory paralysis leads to death, usually within 12 hours of ingestion. Saxitoxin, the cause, is a heat-stable neurotoxin, so cooking does not eliminate or reduce its danger. Such poisonings usually occur at latitudes above 30 degrees N and below 30 degrees S and lack of a red coloration of the sea does not insure safety from the toxin.

Solanine

Solanine, a naturally occurring toxin and pesticide found in potatoes and tomato leaves, is an inhibitor of acetylcholinesterase, an enzyme needed for proper nerve transmission. In humans an oral dose of 2.8 mg per kg (about 200 mg total) has led to drowsiness and itchiness behind the neck. Greater consumption has resulted in vomiting and diarrhea.

Potatoes are not allowed on the market if they contain an excess of 200 ppm solanine, and bought fresh from the store, they usually contain less than 100 ppm solanine. When potatoes are stored (even in dark places), their solanine content increases, being concentrated mainly in the shoots and to a lesser extent in the skin. About 4.5 pounds of whole potatoes with 100 ppm solanine would have to be eaten at one sitting to produce the initial effects.

Caffeine

The amount of caffeine in about two 5 ounce cups of coffee (about 200 mg) has a pharmacological effect. At this level it is known to stimulate the central nervous system, decrease fatigue, have a diuretic effect on the kidneys, increase heart rate, dilate blood vessels, and perhaps elevate levels of free fatty acids and glucose in the plasma. About 1 gram of caffeine will lead to insomnia, nervousness, and nausea. Larger amounts will lead to convulsions and respiratory failure, with a lethal dose estimated at more than 10 grams (about 100 cups of coffee). Caffeine is found in coffee, tea, cocoa, cola, and many drugs.

Caffeine has been proposed as a mutagen and a teratogen (a cause of birth defects). This is an important consideration because caffeine crosses the placenta, and the blood concentration found in the fetus is the same as that in the mother. Also, caffeine can move freely into human ovaries and testes, so that it would have a chance to cause mutations at crucial sites.

Studies that use extremely large amounts of caffeine have shown caffeine to cause chromosome damage in nonmammalian systems — bacteria, plants, fruit flies — and even in a mammalian cell culture. But when caffeine was used in the cell culture at a concentration equivalent to that consumed by a heavy coffee drinker, no increase in chromosomal abnormalities was shown. Two mouse and rat studies — in which an amount of caffeine equivalent to that in 3 to 95 cups of coffee per day was administered — did not reveal any significant mutagenic or teratogenic effects; however, one study showed a decrease in litter size and fetal weights and an increase in fetal resorption.[20] Some *in vitro* studies have demonstrated caffeine to enhance cell mutation rates by inhibiting the DNA repair system. However, *in vivo* studies have not supported an effect of caffeine to increase mutagenic activities of x-rays or other mutagens in mice.[21]

Caffeine appears to be a weak mutagen in at least some nonmammalian systems; however, its significance to the human population is still unknown. Retrospective studies of women and their caffeine intake during pregnancy have shown no association between caffeine and birth defects. It has been suggested that humans may be protected from ill effects of caffeine because of their rapid metabolism of this chemical.

FOOD LABELING

Food labeling ideally aids the consumer in making informed choices while shopping. In the United States, food labeling is a vehicle for both nutrition education and for revealing product information.

In the United States, food labels are required to list (1) the name of the product, (2) the name and place of business of the manufacturer, packer, or distributor, and (3) the net contents or net weight (Fig.

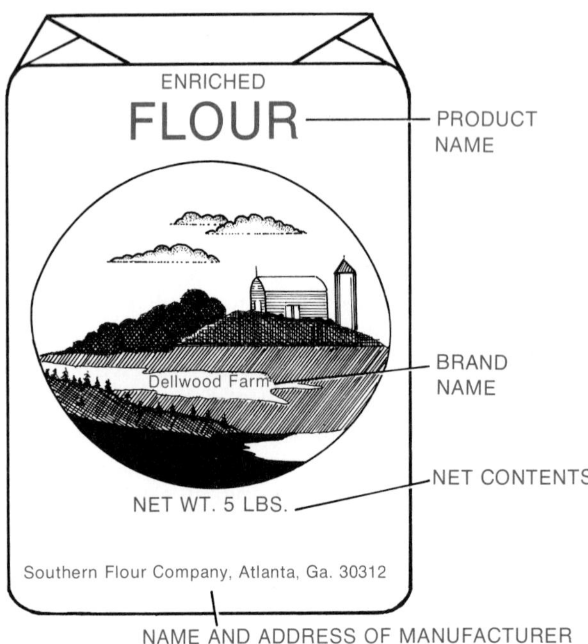

Figure 18–4 Food label with product name, net contents, and name and address of the manufacturer. Ingredients are not listed, since enriched flour is a standardized product.

18–4). The net weight includes the liquid in which canned products are packed.

Most food labels in this country also require a listing of the ingredients in order of descending weight. Fats or oils now must be listed by their common or usual name (for example, coconut oil) rather than by a generalized name such as vegetable oil. At present, colors and flavors do not have to be listed by name but may simply be listed as "color" or "flavor," and the label must indicate if they are artificial. Federal law does not require the listing of coloring agents added to butter, cheese, and ice cream.

Over 200 foods have a *standard of identity*, which is a standard "recipe" specifying limits of mandatory ingredients in a food. The standards also allow for optional ingredients. The mandatory ingredients of a food with a standard of identity need not be listed on the label; however, optional ingredients must be listed. All of the ingredients in some standardized foods have been designated as optional and, therefore, these particular foods require full ingredient labeling. Margarine, ice cream, peanut butter, jelly, soda water, macaroni and noodle products, and mayonnaise are examples of foods with standards of identity.

When the standards of identities were devised in the 1930's, it was still not uncommon to prepare such foods at home. Therefore, purchasers anticipated the presence of certain familiar ingredients in these foods that they purchased. The standards of identity insured that products would contain the expected ingredients in appropriate proportions. The FDA is now considering requiring foods with standards of identity to list all ingredients, since consumers are now often out of touch with what goes into many of these products.

Food labels of some 300 food products may bear a *USDA grade* (for example, USDA Grade A), which is voluntary but widely used, since the grade affects the price of these products. Products that may carry this grade include meats, eggs, and fresh, canned, and frozen fruits and vegetables. These grades are not based on the nutritional value of the food but primarily on appearance or texture, or both. The grade on milk and milk products is based on FDA recommended sanitation standards for the production and processing of these products.

Food labels may also include "*open dating*," which indicates any one of the following: (1) the date when the product was packaged or processed, or the "pack date," such as appears on fresh meats in some markets; (2) the last day on which a retail store may offer a food for sale (which still allows for a reasonable time for product use before spoilage occurs), or the "pull date," which may appear on milk and refrigerated dough products; (3) the "use by" or "quality assurance date," after which the quality of a food has passed its peak but the product still may be used, which may appear on flour packages; or (4) the "expiration date," which denotes the last day a product should be used. This last is used, for example, on yeast and baby formula. Although these dates are potentially useful to the consumer, there is confusion about which meaning is to be attributed to a date on the product. No standardized format exists to indicate the meaning of the date or to specify the location of dates on the product.

CANNED FRUIT

NUTRITION INFORMATION

(PER SERVING)

SERVING SIZE = ½ CUP

SERVINGS PER CONTAINER = 4

CALORIES 120

PROTEIN .... 0 GRAM

CARBOHYDRATE ... 30 GRAMS

FAT .... 0 GRAM

PERCENTAGE OF U.S. RECOMMENDED DAILY ALLOWANCES (U.S. RDA)

VITAMIN C 2

THIAMINE 2

IRON 4

CONTAINS LESS THAN 2% OF U.S. RDA OF PROTEIN, VITAMIN A, RIBOFLAVIN, NIACIN, AND CALCIUM

Figure 18–5 A nutritional label panel containing the minimum information allowed.

Nutritional Labeling and the "U. S. RDA's"

If a food is fortified with a nutrient or if a nutritional claim such as "low in cholesterol" is made for the food, then nutrient labeling is required; otherwise, nutritional labeling is voluntary. Nutrition labeling must include information specifying per serving size (Fig. 18–5): the amount of protein, carbohydrate, and fat in grams; the number of calories; and the percent of the U.S. RDA (United States Recommended Daily Allowances) fulfilled by seven vitamins and minerals. Information for 12 other vitamins and minerals and for cholesterol, fatty acids, and sodium content is optional.

U.S. RDA's are the Food and Drug Administration's simplified version of the Recommended Dietary Allowances set by the Food and Nutrition Board in 1968. The U.S. RDA's (Table 18–4) usually represent the highest recommendation for a nutrient for nonpregnant and nonlactating females and males above 4 years of age. Therefore, the U.S. RDA's actually may overestimate nutrient recommendations for some age and sex groups according to the Food and Nutrition Board RDA's, so that consumption of less than 100 percent of the U.S. RDA does not necessarily result in a deficient diet. (This is also true for eating less than 100 percent of the Food and Nutrition Board RDA's.) Also, eating 100 percent of the U.S. RDA for the seven listed vitamins and minerals does not insure an adequate diet, since these seven are just a few of the more than 40 nutrients essential to humans. In addition, the consumer should be conscious of the serving size for which the percent of U.S. RDA's are listed. The serving size may be much smaller or larger than that which you nor-

Table 18–4 U.S. RDA's*

	Used for Conventional Food or "Special Dietary Foods"	*Used for "Special Dietary Foods" Only*	
	ADULTS AND CHILDREN 4 OR MORE YEARS OF AGE	INFANTS AND CHILDREN UNDER 4 YEARS OF AGE	PREGNANT OR LACTATING WOMEN
	*Nutrients That Must Be Declared on Label**		
Protein†	45 gm "high quality protein" 65 gm "proteins in general"		
Vitamin A	5000 IU	2500 IU	8000 IU
Vitamin C (ascorbic acid)	60 mg	40 mg	60 mg
Thiamin (vitamin B-1)	1.5 mg	0.7 mg	1.7 mg
Riboflavin (vitamin B-2)	1.7 mg	0.8 mg	2.0 mg
Niacin	20 mg	9 mg	20 mg
Calcium	1.0 gm	0.8 gm	1.3 gm
Iron	18 mg	10 mg	18 mg
	Nutrients That May Be Declared on Label		
Vitamin D	400 IU	400 IU	400 IU
Vitamin E	30 IU	10 IU	30 IU
Vitamin B-6	2.0 mg	0.7 mg	2.5 mg
Folic acid (folacin)	0.4 mg	0.2 mg	0.8 mg
Vitamin B-12	6 μg	3 μg	8 μg
Phosphorus	1.0 gm	0.8 μg	1.3 gm
Iodine	150 μg	70 μg	150 μg
Magnesium	400 mg	200 mg	450 mg
Zinc	15 mg	8 mg	15 mg
Copper‡	2 mg	1 mg	2 mg
Biotin‡	0.3 mg	0.15 mg	0.3 mg
Pantothenic acid‡	10 mg	5 mg	10 mg

*These figures are utilized for label information on any food that is enriched to provide more than 50 percent of the RDA of any given nutrient, plus any food that is said to be a special dietary food. If the dietary food is for young children or pregnant or lactating women, RDA's from the appropriate columns are used. (From the Food and Drug Administration, USDHEW.)

†"High quality protein" is defined as having a protein efficiency ratio (PER) equal to or greater than that of casein (a milk protein). "Proteins in general" are those with a PER less than that of casein. Proteins with a PER less than 20 percent that of casein are considered "not a significant source of protein" and may not be expressed on the label.

‡As of this writing, there are no Food and Nutrition Board RDA's for copper, biotin, and pantothenic acid. These are proposed new values.

mally eat, and therefore you would be eating either less or more of the U.S. RDA values listed on the label.

U.S. RDA's should be used to compare one food with another for nutrient density (to relate the ratio of nutrients to calories or the ratio of nutrients to weight of the product), to learn which foods are good sources of the different nutrients, and as a guideline for eating a balanced diet—but not as the last word on an optimum diet plan.

Importance of Information and Clarity

No one claims that present labeling regulations allow for as much product information as is desirable or that the format is without confusion. The FDA is at present considering changes in labeling with the hope that consumers will benefit from a more pertinent and informative format. One such proposal is the listing of both net weight (which includes liquid and solids) and drained weight of canned fruits and vegetables, so that the consumer will know the amounts of liquids and solids for which they are paying.

Another consideration is the listing of food colors by individual names, since a small portion of the population may be allergic to specific food colorings. It has been claimed, for example, that 47,000 to 94,000 persons in the United States may be allergic to FD & C Yellow No. 5, or tartrazine.[22] This estimate is based on the number of people who are allergic to aspirin, since these same people are often allergic to tartrazine. Many consumer groups would like to see the use of special symbols on labels that would indicate the presence of artificial colors or other food additives that may be of importance to consumers for other health reasons as well as allergies.

Nutrition labeling is being sought for nearly 100 percent of the food on the market. This would greatly increase the amount of nutritional information available to the consumer, but it is not without its drawbacks. Nutritional labeling would be especially difficult for fresh agricultural products, since the nutrient content varies with strain, weather, storage conditions, and a host of other variables. In respect to nutrient content, nutrient labeling favors fabricated foods to which precise amounts of nutrients can be added. Also, in fabricated foods more of the specific nutrients identified in nutritional labeling may be added to make the product appear more nutritious than natural products, often unjustifiably so. Furthermore, nutritional labeling may be more difficult for small companies that have no laboratories to analyze their products for nutrient content, whereas such facilities are often present in larger companies.

The U.S. government is proposing voluntary nutritional quality guidelines for certain classes of foods such as frozen dinners, breakfast cereals, and meat replacements. These guidelines would indicate appropriate levels and ranges of nutrients that should occur in these products. A guideline for frozen heat-and-serve dinners has already been established. A product that meets these guidelines may include on its label a statement that the contents abide by the U.S. Government's stipulated nutritional guidelines for that class of food. In our opinion, guidelines should take into account trace elements and vitamins lost during processing, and fiber, as well as proportions and types of protein, fat, and carbohydrates. Guidelines not encompassing such a wide range of considerations may instill a false confidence in the consumer, who may feel that the statement of compliance with federal guidelines insures that the product is completely healthful and nutritious.

QUESTIONS AND PROBLEMS

1. What is the difference between a GRAS substance and a regulated food additive (as legally defined in the United States)? Give examples of each.
2. List at least four considerations you would make before approving the fortification of a widely used candy with iron and folic acid. Which considerations are technical and which are nontechnical?
3. What arguments would you use to support the Delaney clause? To refute it?
4. What is the difference between the hazard and the toxicity of a compound? Under what conditions might the consumption of a naturally occurring toxin be hazardous? In general, does eating naturally occurring toxins in your diet pose a great threat? Explain.
5. Locate the following on a food label: (a) name and place of business of the manufacturer, packer, or distributor; (b) net contents or net weight; (c) list of ingredients; (d) nutritional information (is this information required or voluntary for this label?); (e) open dating. What other information is given on the label?
6. List the differences between the U.S. RDA's and the Food and Nutrition Board RDA's for your sex and age using the tables in the Appendix of this book.
7. Give examples of five foods you eat that are enriched. Estimate what percent of your total daily intake of these particular vitamins and minerals is supplied by these enriched foods.

REFERENCES

1. Middlekauff, R. D.: Food Tech., *28*:42, May 1974.
2. Murphy, C. M., and Armbruster, G.: Human Ecology (Cornell), *3*:19, Winter 1973.

3. Joint FAO/WHO Expert Committee on Food Additives: 15th Report. WHO Tech. Rpt. Ser. No. 488. Rome, FAO, 1972.
4. Damon, G. E., and Janssen, W. F.: FDA Consumer, *7*:15, July/Aug. 1973.
5. Food Drug Cosmetic Law Reports, Food Additives, ¶ 56,053, Commerce Clearing House, Inc., Chicago, 1977.
6. Food Protection Committee, National Research Council: *Evaluating the Safety of Food Chemicals*. Washington, D. C., National Academy of Sciences, 1970.
7. MacKinney, G., and Little, A. C.: World Rev. Nutr. Dietet., *14*:85, 1972.
8. *Food Additives: What They Are, How They Are Used*. Washington, D. C., Manufacturing Chemists' Assoc. Inc., 1971.
9. McGlashen, N. D., et al.: Lancet, *2*:1017, 1968.
10. Wasserman, A. E., Pensabene, J. W., and Piotrowski, E. G.: J. Food Sci., *43*:276, 1978.
11. Food Chemical News, *19*:18, Apr. 11, 1977.
12. Health Protection Branch, National Health and Welfare Dept. Canada, 1977; Division of Toxicology, U.S. FDA, May 15, 1973; Tisdel, M. O. et al.: In Inglett, G. (ed.): Westport, Conn., Avi Publishing Co., Inc., p. 145, 1974.
13. Institute of Food Technologists' Expert Panel on Food Safety and Nutrition: J. Food Sci., *40*:215, 1975.
14. Keeler, R. F.: Lloydia, *38*:56, 1975.
15. Food Chemical News, *19*:13, Feb. 6, 1978.
16. Crampton, R. F., and Charlesworth, F. A.: Brit. Med. Bull., *31*:209, 1975.
17. Amla, I., et al.: Amer. J. Clin. Nutr., *24*:609, 1971.
18. Munro, I. C.: Clin. Toxicol., *9*:647, 1976.
19. Food Chemical News, *19*:37, Jan. 9, 1978.
20. Gilbert, E. F., and Pistey, W. R.: J. Reprod. Fertil. *34*:495, 1973; Fujii, T., and Nishimura, H.: Toxicol. Appl. Pharmacol., *22*:449, 1972; Thayer, P. S., and Kensler, C. J.: Toxic Appl. Pharmacol., *25*:169, 1973.
21. Thayer, P. S., and Kensler, C. J.: Toxic Appl. Pharmacol., *25*:157, 1973; Donovan, P. J., and DiPaolo, J. A.: Cancer Res., *34*:2720, 1974; Epstein, S. S., Bass, W., Arnold, E., and Bishop, Y.: Food. Cosmet. Toxic., *8*:381, 1970.
22. HEW News, U.S. Dept. of Health, Education, and Welfare, Feb. 3, 1977.

SUPPLEMENTARY READING

Food Additives

General

Damon, G. E.: Primer on food additives. FDA Consumer, *7*:10, May 1973.
Filer, L. J., Jr.: Patterns of Consumption of Food Additives. Food Tech., *30*:62, July 1976.
Food additives: an industry view. FDA Consumer, *11*:6, Dec. 1977/Jan. 1978.
Furia, T. E. (ed.): *Handbook of Food Additives*. 2nd Ed. Cleveland, Chemical Rubber Co., 1972.
General Foods: Today's Food and Additives. White Plains, N. Y., General Foods Corporation, 1976.
Harper, A. E.: Nutritional regulations and legislation — past developments, future implications. J. Amer. Dietet. Assoc., *71*:601, 1977.
Jukes, T. H.: Food additives. N. Engl. J. Med., *297*:427, 1977.
Larkin, T.: Exploring food additives. FDA Consumer, *10*:4, June 1976.
Mayer, J.: Experts are divided about food additives. Family Health/Today's Health, *8*:36, July 1976.
National Dairy Council; Microconstituents and food safety. Dairy Council Dig., *49*:1, Jan.-Feb. 1978.
Sapeika, N.: Food additives. World Rev. Nutr. Dietet., *16*:334, 1973.

Food Colors

Boffey, P. M.: Color additives: botched experiment leads to banning of Red Dye No. 2. Science, *191*:450, 1976; and Color additives: is successor to Red Dye No. 2 any safer? Science, *191*:832, 1976.
Collins, T. F. X., et al.: Teratological evaluation of FD&C Red No. 2 — a collaborative government-industry study. I. Introduction, experimental material, and procedures. J. Toxicol. Environ. Health, *1*:851, 1976 (see also pp. 857, 863, 867, 875 for related papers).
Drake, J. J.: Food colours — harmless aesthetics or epicurean luxuries? Toxicology, *5*:3, 1975.
Ershoff, B. H.: Effects of diet on growth and survival of rats fed toxic levels of tartrazine (FD&C Yellow No. 5) and Sunset Yellow FCF (FD&C Yellow No. 6). J. Nutr., *107*:822, 1977.
Hopkins, H.: Countdown on color additives. FDA Consumer, *10*:5, Nov. 1976; see also Corwin, E., and Pines, W. L.: *10*:18, Apr. 1976.
Little, A. C., and Mackinney, G.: The color of foods. World Rev. Nutr. Dietet., *14*:59, 1972.
Philip, T.: Utilization of plant pigments as food colorants. Food Prod. Dev., *9*:50, Apr. 1975.
Radomski, J. L.: Toxicology of food colors. Ann. Rev. Pharmacol., *14*:127, 1974.
Zlotlow, M. J., and Settipane, G. A.: Allergic potential of food additives: a report of a case of tartrazine sensitivity without aspirin intolerance. Amer. J. Clin. Nutr., *30*:1023, 1977; see also Lockey, S. D.: Ann. Allergy, *38*:206, 1977.

Monosodium Glutamate

Oser, B. L., Morgareidge, K., and Carson, S.: Monosodium glutamate studies in four species of neonatal and infant animals. Food Cosmet. Toxicol., *13*:7, 1975.
Pizzi, W. J., Barnhart, J. E., and Fanslow, D. J.: Monosodium glutamate administration to the newborn reduces reproductive ability in female and male mice. Science, *196*:452, 1977.
Reif-Lehrer, L.: A questionnnaire study of the prevalence of Chinese restaurant syndrome. Fed. Proc. *36*:1617, 1977; Possible significance of adverse reactions to glutamate in humans. Fed. Proc., *35*:2205, 1976.
Stegink, L. D., et al.: Monosodium glutamate metabolism in the neonatal monkey. Amer. J. Physiol., *229*:246, 1975.

Hyperactivity (Hyperkinesis)

Conners, C. K., et al.: Food additives and hyperkinesis: a controlled double-blind experiment. Pediatr., *58*:154, 1976.

Margen, S.: Why your child is hyperactive. J. Nutr. Educ., *7*:79, Apr./June 1975.

Wender, E. H.: Food additives and hyperkinesis. Amer. J. Dis. Child., *131*:1204, 1977.

Nitrates, Nitrites, and Nitrosamines

Binkerd, E. F., and Kolari, O. E.: The history and use of nitrate and nitrite in the curing of meat. Food Cosmet. Toxicol., *13*:655, 1975.

Frantz, C. N., and Malling, H. V.: Factors affecting metabolism and mutagenicity of dimethylnitrosamine and diethylnitrosamine. Cancer Res., *35*:2307, 1975.

Marquardt, H., Rufino, F., and Weisburger, J. H.: Mutagenic activity of nitrite-treated foods: human stomach cancer may be related to dietary factors. Science, *196*:1000, 1977.

Ridder, W. E., and Oehme, F. W.: Nitrates as an environmental, animal, and human hazard. Clin. Toxicol., *7*:145, 1974.

Sen, N. P., Donaldson, B., Charbonneau, C., and Miles, W. F.: Effect of additives on the formation of nitrosamines in meat curing mixtures containing spices and nitrite. J. Agr. Food Chem., *22*:1125, 1974; see also Newmark, H. L., et al.: Food Tech., *28*:28, May 1974.

Shirley, R. L.: Nutritional and physiological effects of nitrates, nitrites, and nitrosamines. Bioscience, *25*:789, 1975.

Tannenbaum, S. R., Weisman, M., and Fett, D.: The effect of nitrate intake on nitrite formation in human saliva. Food Cosmet. Toxicol., *14*:549, 1976.

White, J. W., Jr.: Relative significance of dietary sources of nitrate and nitrite. J. Agric. Food Chem., *23*:886, 1975; see also Heisler, E. G., et al.: *22*:1029, 1974; Walker, R.: J. Sci. Food Agric., *26*:1735, 1975.

Wild, A.: Nitrate in drinking water: health hazard unlikely. Nature, *268*:197, July 21, 1977.

Food Safety and Benefit/Risk Evaluation

Commoner, B.: When there is an established risk, how do we judge the benefits? Food Prod. Dev., *11*:15, May 1977; see also Schmidt, A. M.: *9*:78, Feb. 1975.

Day, H. G.: Food safety — then and now. J. Amer. Dietet. Assoc., *69*:229, 1976.

Hallstrom, C. H., Johnson, H. G., and Mayer, W. J.: A food scientist's guide to food regulatory information. Food Tech., *32*:72, Oct. 1978.

Institute of Food Technologists' Expert Panel on Food Safety and Nutrition: The risk/benefit concept as applied to food. Food Tech., *38*:51, Mar. 1978.

Joint FAO/WHO Expert Committee on Food Additives: *Evaluation of Certain Food Additives, 20th Report.* Rome, Food and Agriculture Organization of the United Nations, 1976.

Jukes, T. H.: How safe is our food supply? Arch. Intern. Med., *138*:772, 1978.

Mantel, N., and Schneiderman, M. A.: Estimating "safe" levels, a hazardous undertaking. Cancer Res., *35*:1379, 1975.

Rucker, M. H., Tom, P. Y., and York, G. K.: Food safety — what do the experts say? J. Nutr. Educ., *9*:158, 1977.

Symposium: Benefit/risk: consideration of direct food additives (5 papers). Food Tech., *32*:54, Aug. 1978.

Saccharin

Isselbacher, K. J., and Cole, P.: Saccharin — the bitter sweet. N. Engl. J. Med., *296*:1348, 1977.

Kessler, I. I., and Clark, J. P.: Saccharin, cyclamates, and human bladder cancer. J.A.M.A., *240*:349, 1978.

Pines, W. L., and Glick, N.: The saccharin ban. FDA Consumer, *11*:10, May 1977.

Rhein, R. W., Jr., and Marion, L.: *The Saccharin Controversy, A Guide for Consumers.* New York, Monarch Press, 1977.

Saccharin: Where do we go from here? FDA Consumer, *12*:16, Apr. 1978.

Wightman, N.: Saccharin — are there alternatives? J. Nutr. Educ., *9*:106, 1977.

Fortification and Enrichment

Austin, J. E.: Cereal fortification reconsidered. Cereal Foods World, *23*(5):229, 1978.

Council on Foods and Nutrition: Improvement of the nutritive quality of foods. J.A.M.A., *225*:1116, 1973.

Disler, P. B., et al.: Studies on the fortification of cane sugar with iron and ascorbic acid. Brit. J. Nutr., *34*:141, 1975; see also Viteri, F. E., García-Ibañez, R., and Torún, B.: Amer. J. Clin. Nutr., *31*:961, 1978.

Dymsza, H. A., et al.: Supplementation of foods vs. nutrition education. Food Tech., *28*:55, July 1974.

el Lozy, M., Kerr, G. R., and Stare, F. J.: Lysine supplementation of wheat products. Amer. J. Clin. Nutr., *28*:672, 1975; see also Graham, G. G., et al.: *24*:200, 1971; Vaghefi, S. B., Makdani, D. D., and Mickelsen, O.: *27*:1231, 1974; and Pereira, S. M., et al.: Brit. J. Nutr., *30*:241, 1973.

Graham, D. M., and Hertzler, A. A.: Why enrich or fortify foods? J. Nutr. Educ., *9*:166, 1977.

Layrisse, M., Martinez-Torres, C., and Renzi, M.: Sugar as a vehicle for iron fortification. Amer. J. Clin. Nutr., *29*:274, 1976; see also Layrisse, M., et al.: *29*:8, 1976; Layrisse, M., and Martinez-Torres, C.: *30*:1166, 1977.

Mertz, W.: Effective fortification programs demand knowledge of human requirements and nutrient interactions. Food Prod. Dev., *11*:62, July/Aug. 1977; and Fortification of foods with vitamins and minerals. Ann. N.Y. Acad. Sci., *300*:151, 1977.

National Research Council, Food and Nutrition Board: *Proposed Fortification Policy for Cereal-Grain Products.* Washington, D. C., National Academy of Sciences, 1974.

Olsson, K. S., Heedman, P. A., and Staugard, F.: Preclinical hemochromatosis in a population on a high–iron-fortified diet. J.A.M.A., *239*:1999, 1978.

Other References — Food Additives

Artman, N. R.: Safety of emulsifiers in fats and oils. J. Amer. Oil. Chem. Soc., *52*:49, Feb. 1975.

Food Chemical News (Louis Rothschild, Jr., ed., Suite 400, Wyatt Building, 777–14th St., N.W., Washington, D. C., 20005) published weekly, is an up-to-date source of information on several aspects of food additives and naturally occurring nonnutrients.

Institute of Food Technologists' Expert Panel on Food Safety and Nutrition: Carrageenan. J. Food Sci., *38*:367, 1973.

Interview with M. F. Jacobson: Food regulation: a consumer advocate's view. FDA Consumer, *11*:5, May 1977.

Jacobson, M.: The real problem with food additives. Nutr. Action, *3*:10, Aug. 1976.

Peringian, L., Shier, N., and Leavitt, R. A.: Consumer beliefs concerning intentional and unintentional additives in health food breads: chlorinated hydrocarbon pesticide residues. J. Food Protection, *41*:160, 1978.

Articles in Nutrition Reviews

The use of chemicals in food production, processing, storage and distribution. *31*:191, 1973.

Nitrosamines and cancer. *33*:19, 1975.

Sulfites as food additives. *34*:58, 1976.

Diet and hyperactivity: any connection? *34*:151, 1976.

Misuse in foods of useful chemicals (by Johnson, P. E.). *35*:225, 1977.

Proposed nutritional guidelines for utilization of industrially produced nutrients (by Darby, W. J., and Hambraeus, L.). *36*:65, 1978.

Naturally Occurring Nonnutrients

General

Committee on Food Protection, Food and Nutrition Board, National Research Council: *Toxicants Occurring Naturally in Foods*. 2nd ed. Washington D.C., National Academy of Sciences, 1973.

Coon, J. M.: Natural toxicants in foods. J. Amer. Dietet. Assoc., *67*:213, 1975.

Gross, R. L., and Newberne, P. M.: Naturally occurring toxic substances in foods. Clin. Pharmacol. Therap., *22*:680, 1977.

Hall, R. L.: Safe at the plate. (Article about naturally occuring toxins in our diet.) Nutr. Today, *12*:6, Nov./Dec. 1977.

Larkin, T.: Natural poisons in food. FDA Consumer, *9*:5, Oct. 1975.

Mickelsen, O., and Yang, M. G.: Naturally occurring toxicants in foods. Fed. Proc., *25*(I):104, 1966.

Symposium on Natural Food Toxicants (20 papers). J. Agric. Food Chem., *17*:413, 1969.

Symposium: Safety in man's food (6 papers). Proc. Nutr. Soc., *36*:85, 1977.

Aflatoxin

Alfin-Slater, R. B., et al.: Dietary factors and aflatoxin toxicity: 1. Comparison of the effect of two diets supplemented with aflatoxin B_1 upon two different strains of rats. J. Amer. Oil Chem. Soc., *52*:266, 1975.

Kumar, G. V., and Sampath, S. R.: Aflatoxins: their nature and biological effects. Ind. J. Nutr. Dietet., *8*:85, 1971.

Ward, J. M., Sontag, J. M., Weisburger, E. K., and Brown, C. A.: Effect of lifetime exposure to aflatoxin B_1 in rats. J. Natl. Cancer Inst., *55*:107, 1975.

Caffeine and Coffee

Headaches and coffee. Brit. Med. J., *2*:284, July 30, 1977; Caffeine, coffee, and cancer. Brit. Med. J., *1*:1031, May 1, 1976.

Heyden, S., et al.: Coffee consumption and mortality. Arch. Int. Med., *138*:1472, 1978.

Punke, H. H.: Caffeine in America's food and drug habits. J. Sch. Health, *44*:551, 1974.

Shorofsky, M. A., and Lamm, R. N.: Caffeine-withdrawal headache and fasting. N. Y. State J. Med., *77*:217, 1977.

Simon, D., Yen., S., and Cole, P.: Coffee drinking and cancer of the lower urinary tract. J. Natl. Cancer Inst., *54*:587, 1975.

Stephenson, P. E.: Physiologic and psychotropic effects of caffeine on man. A review. J. Amer. Dietet. Assoc., *71*:240, 1977.

Ufberg, R. M.: Commentary. (A review article on caffeine and possible deleterious effects.) J. Home Econ., *69*:2, Mar. 1977.

Other References — Naturally Occurring Nonnutrients

Epstein, M. T., Espiner, E. A., Donald, R. A., and Hughes, H.: Effect of eating liquorice on the renin-angiotensin aldosterone axis in normal subjects. Brit. Med. J., *1*:488, Feb. 19, 1977.

Hughes, J. M., and Merson, M. H.: Fish and shellfish poisoning. N. Engl. J. Med., *295*:1117, 1976; see also Foo, L. Y.: J. Sci. Food Agric., *27*:807, 1976; Harsanyi, Y. L.: FDA Consumer, *7*:22, July/Aug. 1973.

Jain, R. C., and Vyas, C. R.: Garlic in alloxan-induced diabetic rabbits. Amer. J. Clin. Nutr., *28*:684, 1975.

Jamalian, J.: Favism-inducing toxins in broad beans (*Vicia faba*). Determination of vicine content and investigation of other non-protein nitrogenous compounds in different broad bean cultivars. J. Sci. Food Agric., *29*:136, 1978; see also Marquardt, R. R., Ward, A. T., Campbell, L. D., and Cansfield, P. E.: J. Nutr., *107*:1313, 1977; Ward, A. T., Marquardt, R. R., and Campbell, L. D.: J. Nutr., *107*:1325, 1977.

Lehmann, P.: Food and drug interactions. FDA Consumer, *12*:20, Mar. 1978.

Liener, I. E.: Toxic factors associated with legume proteins. Ind. J. Nutr. Dietet., *10*:303, 1973.

Valyasevi, A., and Dhanamitta, S.: Studies of bladder stone disease in Thailand. XVII. Effect of ex-

ogenous source of oxalate on crystalluria. Amer. J. Clin. Nutr., *27*:877, 1974.
Vimokesant, S., et al.: Food habits causing thiamine deficiency in humans. (Article on the consumption of foods with antithiamine factors.) J. Nutr. Sci. Vitaminol., *22*(Suppl.):1, 1976.
Welch, R. M., House, W. A., and Van Campen, D.: Effects of oxalic acid on availability of zinc from spinach leaves and zinc sulfate to rats. J. Nutr., *107*:929, 1977.
Wislocki, P. G., et al.: Carcinogenic and mutagenic activities of safrole, 1′-hydroxysafrole, and some known or possible metabolites. Cancer Res., *37*:1883, 1977.

Articles in Nutrition Reviews

Toxicity of mold-damaged sweet potatoes (by Wilson, B. J.). *31*:73, 1973.
Possible mechanism of action of neurotoxin from *Lathyrus sativus*. *31*:282, 1973.
Patulin, a carcinogenic mycotoxin found in cider. *32*:55, 1974.
Phthalates in food. *32*:126, 1974.
Toxicants occurring naturally in foods. (by Strong, F. M.). *32*:225, 1974.
Natural food toxicants — a perspective (by Coon, J. M.). *32*:321, 1974.
Chemical preservatives for prevention of mycotoxin production. *34*:31, 1976.
Epidemic of hepatitis in man due to aflatoxicosis. *34*:45, 1976.
Coffee drinking and peptic ulcer. *34*:167, 1976.
Lathyrism in the rat. (by Geiger, B. J., Steenbock, H., and Parsons, H. T.). *34*:240, 1976. (A reprint of part of J. Nutr., *6*:427, 1933.)
Aflatoxin and oral contraceptives. *35*:110, 1977.
Safeguarding our food (by Ward, A. G.), *35*:116, 1977.
Caffeine — its identity, dietary sources, intake and biological effect (by Graham, D. M.). *36*:97, 1978. (Also see letter of Jacobson, M: *36*:231, 1978.)

Food Labels

General

Babcock, M. J., and Murphy, M. M.: Two nutritional labeling systems. J. Amer. Dietet. Assoc., *62*:155, 1973.
Food and Drug Administration: *We Want You to Know About Labels on Foods*. Washington, D. C., Dept. of Health, Education, and Welfare Pub. No. (FDA) 75–2008, 1973; see also *We Want You to Know About Nutrition Labels on Food*. Washington, D. C., Dept. of Health, Education and Welfare Pub. No. (FDA) 74–2039, 1974.
Hopkins, H.: Getting specific about fats and oils. FDA Consumer, *10*:13, Mar. 1976; see also Toward more nutrition labeling. FDA Consumer, *11*:22, Oct. 1977.
Johnson, O. C.: The Food and Drug Administration and Labeling. J. Amer. Dietet. Assoc., *64*:471, 1974.
Kennedy, D.: Better regulation through labeling. FDA Consumer, *12*:12, Feb. 1978; see also Stephenson, M.: *9*:13, Oct. 1975; anon.: *10*:4, Feb. 1976.
Morrison, M.: A consumer's guide to food labels. FDA Consumer, *11*:4, June 1977.
National Dairy Council: Food labeling. Dairy Council Dig. *45*:1, Mar./Apr. 1974.
Peterkin, B.: The RDA or U.S. RDA? J. Nutr. Educ., *9*:10, Jan./Mar. 1977.
Ross, M. L.: What's happening to food labeling? J. Amer. Dietet. Assoc., *64*:262, 1974.

Articles in Nutrition Reviews

Nutrition labeling. *30*:247, 1972.
Nutrition labeling. *31*:36, 1973.
Nutrition labeling — II. *31*:133, 1973.
Nutrition labeling. *32*:251, 1974.

Part 4

Applied Nutrition

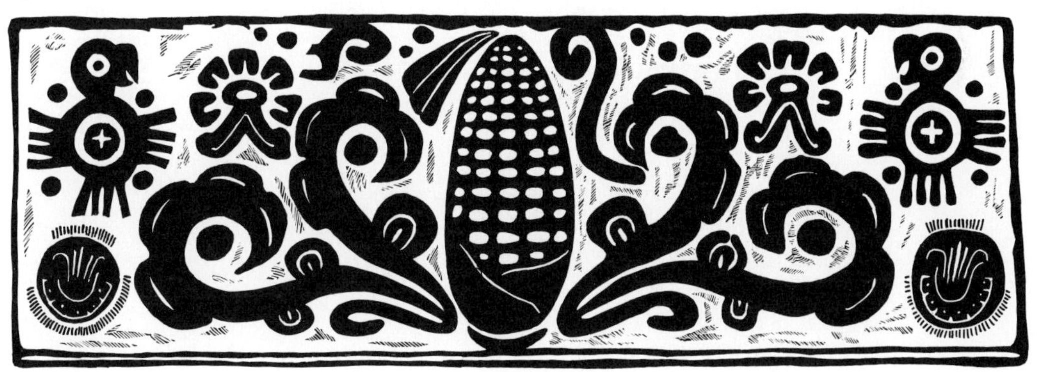

Chapter 19

Adequate Diets for Healthy People

JUDGING NUTRITIONAL ADEQUACY

We usually detect malnutrition by certain outward signs that are the effects produced by that condition. It would seem to be an easy matter to tell whether or not a person is well nourished, and it is true that to the trained eye such differences in nutritional condition seem obvious and are quickly noted. However, it must be remembered that there are all degrees of malnutrition and that the average individual is not apt to look at himself or his own child with unprejudiced eyes. Lacking a real awareness of what a healthy child should be, the parent often assumes that the child is all right. For this reason, a list of some of the more striking characteristics of the well-nourished individual, contrasted with those usually found in undernourished individuals, is given in Table 19–1.

There are physical signs of deficiency of protein, vitamins, and some minerals. If adequately trained, a physician will look for these signs in a patient. An examiner

Table 19–1 CHARACTERISTICS OF GOOD NUTRITION AND POOR NUTRITION*

Good Nutrition	*Poor Nutrition*
About average *height* for age	Body undersized or poorly developed
About average *weight* for height	Thin (more than 10 percent underweight) or fat and flabby (more than 10 percent overweight)
Good layer of *subcutaneous fat*	Subcutaneous fat lacking or in excess
Muscles well developed and firm	Muscles small; pot belly
Skin turgid and of healthy color	Skin pale, sallow, or rough (hyperkeratosis); edema; seborrhea; dermatitis
Gums firm and *mucous membranes* of mouth reddish pink	Mucous membranes pale; tongue abnormally red or smooth; lesions at corners of mouth; gums swollen or bleeding
Hair smooth and glossy	Hair rough and without luster; thin; easily plucked
Eyes clear, good night vision	Angular lesions of eyelids; reddened or thickened, opaque conjunctivae; night blindness
Legs straight	Bowed legs; knock-knees; beaded ribs
Appetite good	Appetite poor; diminished taste acuity
General health excellent	Susceptible to infections; lack of endurance and vigor
Good-natured and full of life	Irritable, overactive; or phlegmatic, listless, unable to concentrate

*A number of these signs are nonspecific; that is, they may relate to more than one nutrient and to other conditions of health besides nutritional state. Taken in conjunction with a good history, however, they provide a reasonable index of nutritional state.

will evaluate the quality of the skin and hair as well as observe the eyes for inflammation about the cornea that may be the result of riboflavin deficiency, and for Bitot's spots and evidence of difficulty in seeing in dim light, indicative of vitamin A deficiency. The mucous membranes of the mouth and the tongue will be examined for signs that indicate a lack of niacin or riboflavin. Inquiries concerning appetite, and tests of nerve reflexes provide clues to deficiency of thiamin. The presence of an enlarged thyroid gland suggests iodine deficiency. Unsatisfactory bone development indicates lack of vitamin D or calcium, or both. Sometimes the hand and wrist are radiographed to see whether ossification has been or is taking place satisfactorily. Much can be learned from simple anthropometric measures such as height, weight, arm and head circumferences, and skinfold thickness (a measure of fatness).

The visible signs of severe or longstanding malnutrition, then, are easily noted, but more refined tests are needed to detect milder grades of malnutrition.* Examination of the blood cells and chemical analyses of the blood may be made to determine the presence of nutritional anemia or unacceptably low levels of certain vitamins and minerals. A so-called "loading" test may be performed in which a test dose of a vitamin is administered, after which its excretion in the urine is measured. Excretion of an abnormally small proportion of the vitamin given indicates that it has been taken up by the blood and tissues, which had too low a supply resulting from previous lack of that vitamin in the diet. The albumin content and ratios of amino acids in the plasma are commonly used indexes of protein nutrition. Other tests measure metabolic functions, enzyme activities, and the like.

Conditions of nutrition vary in different sections of a country and at different economic levels. The estimation of the amount of malnutrition that exists in a country depends on the standards set for good nutrition. If only those who are actually examined and found to be markedly underweight or those who show gross signs of poor physical condition are classified as malnourished, the numbers may be reassuringly few. At the other extreme, if everyone in whom chemical tests show that the body is not saturated with certain vitamins is classed as undernourished, a lot of apparently healthy people will be included and the numbers will be alarmingly large. Estimates based on food availability and consumption at the national levels are of little value because the figures do not take into account uneven distribution of food among people, or even losses of nutrients that occur in the period between production and consumption. When surveys are made of foods consumed by individuals (dietary records) and the results are judged by comparison with the yardstick of recommended allowances for the U.S. National Research Council's Food and Nutrition Board, the conclusions still may be misleading, for reasons now to be discussed.

Use of Recommended Allowances

Obviously, there are wide variations in energy requirements, according to sex, age, size, and especially the amount of physical activity. The protein requirement also varies with the amount of lean body tissue and the need to build new tissues. The recommended energy and protein allowances are given in terms of average or reference adults and are meant to be adapted to individual needs. Criteria for adjusting the mineral and vitamin allowances are not usually indicated, except for the obvious scaling of some of the vitamin B allowances for energy expenditure. However, we know there are differences between individuals in the efficiency with which they utilize these nutrients,

*Standard values used to determine nutritional state (i.e., below-normal levels of hemoglobin, etc.) will be found in the Appendix, Table 14.

so that some function well on smaller amounts while others require larger amounts to meet body needs.

The U.S. National Research Council's Recommended Dietary Allowance (RDA)[1] for all nutrients, except energy, are based on the average requirement plus two standard deviations (about 30 percent) above the average need, if these figures are known.* The RDA's are placed at a high level with the idea that this covers the needs of even those with especially high requirements. For energy, the average figure is used as the RDA because both over- and under-consumption present problems, in contrast to the nutrients, modest excesses of which are harmless.

Allowances set for the United Kingdom are also intended to be "sufficient or more than sufficient for the nutritional needs of practically all healthy persons in a population."[2] Canadian standards are "considered adequate . . . to meet the physiological needs of practically all healthy persons . . . [and] exceed the minimum requirements of most individuals."[3]

Because we know that the majority of the population have their nutritional requirements met by lesser amounts than the U.S. RDA's, it is a mistake to assume that anyone whose intake falls below these levels is necessarily getting an inadequate diet. All that this comparison can indicate is the degree of risk of inadequacy at a given intake; the further below the RDA the intake falls, the greater becomes the chance that an individual's needs are not met.† Furthermore, the body has some ability to adjust to somewhat lower levels of various nutrients. Adults have been maintained satisfactorily over long periods on as little as 40 gm of protein, 400 to 600 mg of calcium, and only a few milligrams of iron per day. However, a generous supply of nutrients is unquestionably needed by pregnant and lactating women and by children.

For the world population as a whole, the World Health Organization (WHO) and Food and Agricultural Organization (FAO) have established somewhat lower standards than the U.S. Food and Nutrition Board. For example, the international calcium allowance is 400 to 500 mg per day in contrast to the U.S. allowance of 800 mg. FAO/WHO standards, however, conform to the expectation of smaller body size and a limited degree of adaptation to habitually lower intakes.

Many nutritionists in this country believe that a substantial amount of protein, minerals, and vitamins over the minimum required levels will promote better health for all individuals of our varied population. However, this is by no means proved. Recommended allowances are revised as new information comes to light, and diets judged adequate or below standard on the basis of 1958 figures may be rated differently when measured against present allowances. (For instance, 12 mg of iron daily was recommended for adult women in 1958, 15 mg in 1963, and 19 mg in 1974.) A person whose diet meets the lower British standard for vitamin C might be judged poorly nourished if the U.S. Food and Nutrition Board allowances were used as the standard. Thus, final evaluation of the nutritional status of an *individual* must be determined by the condition of the person consuming the diet, not by comparison of calculated nutrient intake against standards intended for population groups and not necessarily applicable to an individual whose needs may vary from the norm.

Recommended allowances are intended to be a help in planning well-balanced diets for *groups of people.* They should not be regarded as a rigid standard that the diet must meet every single day. Slight shortages or surpluses cancel out from day to day. However, over a span of several days the diet should conform to accepted nutritional standards. The RDA

*Average daily requirements of many nutrients have not been established. For these nutrients, RDA's are based on customary intakes of apparently healthy people, evaluated in light of requirements of other animals.

†For additional discussion of this point, see Chapter 25.

should be met to prevent any continued shortage of protein, minerals, or vitamins. The energy intake must be adjusted to individual needs, for even a slight excess, if long continued, leads to overweight.

Occurrence of Malnutrition

Malnutrition is most apt to occur in infants and growing children, and the proper nutrition of our children is a matter of great concern. Surveys of school children in poverty areas have indicated that symptoms of undernutrition may be found in 15 to 25 percent of the children observed.

Taking households as a whole (both adults and children), the 1965 dietary surveys of the Department of Agriculture indicated that the nutritive value of diets had been declining rather than improving in the previous 10 or 15 years.[4] About one-fifth of the diets provided less than two-thirds of the RDA for one or more nutrients and were rated "poor." Even in households with incomes over 10,000 dollars, more than one-third of the diets were below the RDA in one or more nutrients.

More recent surveys of the U.S. population[5, 6] and the Canadian National Nutrition Survey[7] have evaluated nutrient intakes from food eaten in one 24 hour period as recalled by the respondents. Even if the information is accurate (that is, people remember correctly, serving sizes are properly estimated, food preparation practices are taken into account, etc.), such data have limited value. A single day may not be indicative of an individual's habitual intake. Nutritional status is governed by the quality of foods eaten over time, individual requirements, and environmental factors. However, data for population groups do indicate the range of foods eaten and the overall quality of customary diets of that population. In all surveys, a large number of substandard intakes were recorded, particularly among pregnant women, the aged, and ethnic minorities. When the total food energy intakes were low, the diets were low in a number of essential nutrients, the amounts of most of which would have been corrected by larger intakes of the same variety of foods (Table 19–2). Nutrients commonly at risk irrespective of energy intake were calcium, iron, vitamin A, and vitamin C. None of the surveys has examined dietary intakes of other trace elements (zinc, copper, iodine), several of the B complex vitamins (folacin, vitamin B-6, pantothenic acid), or fat-soluble vitamins other than vitamin A. Failure to include these nutrients is due to the more recent recognition of their deficiency

Table 19–2 MEAN 24 HOUR ENERGY INTAKES AND NUTRIENT INTAKE PER 1000 KCAL OF FOOD EATEN BY POOR PEOPLE AGED 60 YEARS AND OVER, U.S. TEN-STATE NUTRITION SURVEY, COMPARED WITH RECOMMENDED DIETARY ALLOWANCES.[5,*]

		Intake of Males				*Intake of Females*		
Nutrient	*NRC RDA*	White	Black	Spanish-American	*NRC RDA*	White	Black	Spanish-American
Energy, kcal	2400	1937	1508	1812	1800	1442	1174	1623
per 1000 kcal								
Protein, gm	23	40	43	43	26	40	41	42
Calcium, mg	333	449	358	255	444	433	416	361
Iron, mg	4	6	7	8	6	7	7	7
Vitamin A, IU	2083	2652	3334	1851	2222	2630	4997	2120
Vitamin C, mg	19	30	37	28	25	46	52	47

*Note that the *quality* (nutrients per 1000 kcal) of food selected generally met nutritional standards, except for calcium in diets of black men and Spanish-Americans of both sexes. If people had eaten *enough* of this same mixture of foods, nutrient intakes would have been satisfactory. Intakes of about three-fourths of the population were below the RDA for energy. Similar findings were recorded in the 1971–72 HANES survey,[6] and persons with incomes below the poverty level had lower energy intakes than did those living above poverty.

states and the lack of adequate information on their presence in foods.

The underlying causes of faulty nutrition in children have been stated to be *poverty, disease,* and *lack of home control.* These are the home or community conditions responsible for the factors that cause undernutrition. Left to their own discretion, inadequately informed and motivated, children often spend their lunch money on "soda pop," French-fried potatoes, and sweets (or spend it for other purposes entirely), in preference to a more adequate but less socially acceptable school or home-packed lunch. Disorganized households in which full meals are rarely prepared and the family does not eat together provide no protection against poor eating behavior outside the home and offer no guidance in food selection by parental example.

If one doesn't have the means to obtain or the money to buy enough food or the more expensive but essential foods such as milk, fruits, and vegetables, it is impossible to prevent undernutrition.

PLANNING THE FAMILY DIET

It would be an almost impossible task to calculate and balance the diet with respect to 40 or more nutrients every day (not to mention flavor, cost, and availability considerations) without access to sophisticated computer programs. For this reason, one needs some general rule or set of rules that assure adequacy if followed in planning the diet.

The most commonly accepted plan is one sponsored many years ago by the Home Economics Research Division of the U.S. Department of Agriculture,[8] and one that most children have been taught in elementary school, the "Basic Four Food Groups." This plan specifies the inclusion in the diet each day of definite amounts of foods from each of four food groups — milk, meat, cereals, vegetables and fruit — in a basal or foundation diet. The basal diet, listed below, is intended to provide practically the full allowances of all nutritive essentials except energy. (The basic plan provides about 1200 kcal.)

Food group	*Servings per day*
MILK 1 c milk, yogurt, *or* Calcium Equivalent (1½ oz, or 45 gm cheddar cheese; 1 c pudding; 1¾ c ice cream; 2 c cottage cheese)	3 for child 4 for adolescent 2 for adult
MEAT 2 oz cooked, lean meat, fish, poultry, *or* Protein Equivalent (2 eggs; 2 oz, or 60 gm cheddar cheese; ½ c cottage cheese; 1 c dried beans or peas; 4 tbsp peanut butter; 2 oz nuts)	2
FRUIT-VEGETABLE ½ c cooked or juice 1 c raw	4, including 1 from vitamin C group 1 from vitamin A group
GRAIN, whole-grain or enriched 1 slice bread; 1 tortilla; 1 c ready-to-eat cereal; ½ c cooked cereal, rice, pasta, grits	4

Weakness of the Basic Four Food Groups Plan

This simple plan based on four food groups is by no means foolproof even for populations whose preferred style of eating fits the categories specified. It is quite easy to defeat the system by consistently making poorer choices within the group alternatives, by skimping on serving sizes, and by cooking or processing a food in such a way that its nutrient content is substantially lowered. This latter problem becomes increasingly important with the development of substitute foods that mimic but do not match the original.

Any simplified eating plan is based on the assumptions that (1) there are a *few key nutrients* that *must be monitored* out of the more than 40 possible; and (2) the *nutrients not being monitored inevitably follow* in the variety of foods selected for

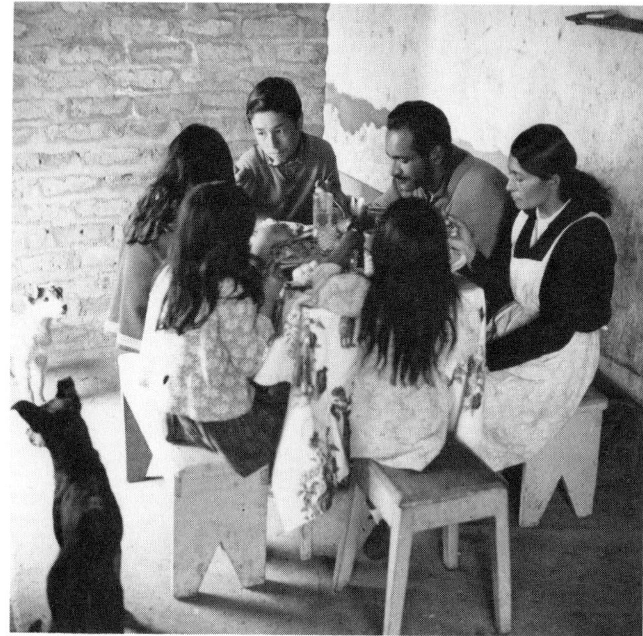

Figure 19–1 Family diet — eating well. A pleasant and healthy diet, not necessarily an expensive one, is one of the most satisfying and stimulating activities of family life. It contributes to the physical, mental and social well-being of all members of the family. (Courtesy of WHO/P. Almasy.)

the key or index nutrients. The Basic Four has oversimplified the indices. For example, legumes are accepted alternatives in the protein-index "Meat" Group of the Basic Four food plan. Almost the only thing all these foods have in common is protein of good quality. Meats contain vitamin B-12 and beans do not; most legumes are rich in folacin and most meats are only fair. Even the "meats" are not alike; marine fish provide iodine, but cattle and poultry flesh contribute very little of this nutrient. The consequences of these differences in composition depend upon all the other choices one makes. The absence of vitamin B-12 from the "Meat" Group alternative is irrelevant if the person selects the Milk Group as specified. The iodine in fish is of no importance to the inlander who uses iodized salt. On the other hand, a person who is allergic to milk or one who wishes to forego all animal food might carefully provide for his calcium needs elsewhere (remembering that calcium is the key nutrient in the Milk Group), but conclude by having a diet deficient in vitamin B-12. Similarly, the person who has no marine food, whose native soil is low in iodine, and who does not use iodized or sea salt may develop a goiter.

Substitute foods are even more likely to defeat an index system. Vitamin C–fortified, orange-flavored sugar is a far cry from a fresh orange, in terms of both vitamin and, especially, mineral content. Again, the consequences of its use will vary. The impact will be minimal if all the rest of the diet is of high quality; the juice substitute might be an improvement if it replaced a sugared drink without any vitamins at all or if the diet were lacking in vitamin C and nothing else. In a poor-quality diet, the substitution could be the final poor choice that changes a diet from marginal to deficient.

In time, food technologists will probably be able to develop substitute foods that more nearly match the natural counterpart, provided that nutritionists are well able to give advice about which nutrients to add and in what amounts. Unfortunately, knowledge is not this far advanced. Several of the B vitamins were scarcely recognized at the time the original legislation on enrichment of refined cereals was drafted, and they are not, to this date, restored in milled grains and their products. We are rapidly expanding our knowledge of trace minerals but have not yet proved the essentiality of some of them for man, and for only a few can we say how much is needed. As you have learned in earlier chapters, in some instances the risk of too much is as great as the hazard of too little of a nutrient, and the balance between some of them is critical. Under these circumstances, food fabrication is difficult and carries a high nutritional risk.

We cannot plan for what we do not recognize or know to be essential. This has been a weakness in all food plans proposed thus far. The Basic Four made no certain provision for, among other nutrients, vitamin E, folacin, magnesium, or zinc — and with reason. When the plan was devised, there was no adequate information on the amount that should be included in the diet of all age groups, nor was there knowledge of the distribution of these nutrients in foods. The situation is not a great deal improved today in regard to two of those four nutrients, and we have added new ones to the list.

Dietary Goals

In the decades since the Basic Four Food Groups Guide was developed, not only have nutrition knowledge and food supply intake patterns changed, but so have life-styles and health conditions. People are less active physically and obesity is common; they die far more often from heart disease and cancer than from infectious diseases, the scourge of earlier generations. In 1976 and 1977 the U.S. Senate Select Committee on Nutrition and Human Needs considered the evidence linking health states and dietary intakes of the American public, and on the basis of this study and the testimony of experts, the Committee elaborated a set of "U.S. Dietary Goals." Although these Goals do not provide a menu or food selection guide, they do suggest changes in eating habits intended to reduce the risk of the most common degenerative diseases. In brief, the Goals recommend the following:

1. Avoidance of overweight.
2. Increased consumption of complex carbohydrates (starches) and naturally occurring sugars (to a level of at least 48 percent of total energy intake).
3. Reduced intake of refined and processed sugars (to about 10 percent of total energy intake).
4. Reduced intake of fat (not to exceed 30 percent of total energy intake).
5. Reduced intake of saturated fat (to less than 10 percent of total energy intake).
6. Reduced cholesterol consumption (to about 300 mg per day).
7. Limited intake of sodium (to about 5 gm per day of salt, NaCl).

There has been lively scientific debate over the exact levels of substances specified in the Goals, but the recommendations have been widely supported in principle. The changes suggested are most appropriate for those at significant risk of the diseases cited (especially mature male adults), but the recommendations are not harmful to anyone and would probably be beneficial for all. Unfortunately, there is little hope of the average consumer being able to meet these Goals unless he or she is exceptionally well-informed as to composition of foods, and is able to store and accumulate the needed information from each meal and snack as the day wears on. For the Goals to be effective, they must be linked to a simple food guide.

The only reasonable alternative to some sort of scientifically designed plan of family feeding is reliance on the accumulated wisdom of a cultural group whose children grow well, who reproduce successfully, and who live to a spry old age, environmental conditions permitting. Some primitive groups have met these criteria, and their diets must have been adequate if the traditional patterns were followed *exactly*. Often some seemingly minor component of the diet or some method of food preparation was absolutely essential for adequacy of the total diet. Consumption of the stomach contents and all the organs and soft bones of fish and aquatic mammals provided the calcium and vitamin C needed in the primitive Eskimo diet, as one example. The common experience is that introduction of sophisticated diets has worked to the disadvantage of primitive peoples who cling to some of the old practices and adopt only some of the new, showing the importance of adherence to *all* the old traditions without picking and choosing among them. (Sometimes this primitive wisdom is not so wise as it should be, and a native practice or taboo interferes with good nutrition. See Chapter 16.)

What the Basic Four attempts to do is combine scientific knowledge with Western cultural wisdom and, faulted though it is, there is not now an equally simple, equally workable alternative plan for Western food patterns. Our goal, then, will be to add to the scientific basis of the Four Food Groups, making finer discriminations among the group alternatives based on newer knowledge of nutrients and the foods in which they occur.

Selection of foods within groups to meet the U.S. Dietary Goals will be considered as will ways to modify the Basic Four Food Groups Plan to suit other preferred patterns of eating. The one rule to be emphasized is that *the family diet should include a wide variety of natural foods chosen from among a number of food classes.*

Basic Four Food Groups Foundation Diet

Table 19–3 presents an evaluation of some of the nutrients provided by a conventional American Basic Four Plan diet compared with the total amounts specified as the recommended allowance. The nutrients tabulated are the well-studied ones around which the Basic Four Food Groups plan was designed. The foundation diet is intended to be supplemented by other foods but does in itself provide almost enough of most of the listed nutrients to meet the recommended allowances, except for energy, iron for women, and thiamin for men. (Although 30 percent low for men in preformed niacin, it probably meets the need for this vitamin by synthesis from tryptophan in the protein.) The foundation diet furnishes only about 1200 kcal, so supplementary food is needed for energy—for the man a considerable amount, 1500 kcal, and for the woman perhaps 800 kcal. The final quality of the diet will depend heavily on the food choices made to provide the extra energy.

To understand this better, let us consider a typical American menu that might be devised from the foods listed in Table 19–3. The menu given in Table 19–4 allows for a lunch carried from home and includes more servings from the Vegetable-Fruit Group than the plan demands. Listed below this are the foods typically added to the foundation diet. Except for larger servings of some of the basic foods, most of the usual supplements add little in the way of essential nutrients. It is small wonder, then, that iron deficiency is a common finding in women and girls, who are likely to forego the increased portions of ordinary foods to "save calories" for desserts and sweets. Men, with their higher energy requirements, are able to eat both larger servings and high-energy foods having little other nutritive value and so may be better nourished than women.

Even the man's nutritional status may still be in jeopardy with this diet. Table 19–5 compares the content of lesser-studied nutrients in the typical menu plan with the allowances for them. With the exception of phosphorus, in which the

Table 19–3 WELL-KNOWN NUTRIENTS IN A DIET PLANNED ACCORDING TO THE BASIC FOUR FOOD GROUPS.*

Adult Plan	*Grams*	*Approximate Measure*	*Energy (kcal)*	*Protein (gm)*	*Calcium (mg)*	*Iron (mg)*	*Vitamin A (IU)*	*Thiamin (mg)*	*Riboflavin (mg)*	*Niacin (mg)*	*Vitamin C (mg)*
Milk Group, 2 servings											
Milk	488	2 glasses (1 pt)	330	17	570	0.4	740	0.14	0.82	0.4	4
Meat Group†, 2 servings											
Meat, fish, or poultry	100	1 avg. serving, cooked, lean only	295	24	11	2.2	178	0.16	0.21	6.0	2
Egg	50	1 medium	80	6.5	27	1.2	590	0.06	0.15	0.1	0
Vegetable and Fruit Group, 4 or more servings											
Vegetables:											
Deep green or yellow‡	100	½ c cooked	29	2.0	5	1.1	3900	0.07	0.11	0.6	29
Potato	100	1 medium, baked	93	2.6	9	0.7	Trace	0.10	0.04	1.7	20
Other§	100	½ c cooked	42	2.1	22	0.8	220	0.07	0.06	0.7	13
Fruits:											
Citrus or tomato¶	185	6 oz juice	55	1.1	20	0.7	519	0.09	0.04	0.7	50
Other**	100	1 avg. serving	75	0.7	13	0.7	550	0.04	0.05	0.5	11
Cereal Group, 4 or more servings											
Bread, white, enriched	70	3 slices	180	6.0	57	1.8	Trace	0.18	0.15	1.8	Trace
Cereal, whole-grain or enriched	30 dry wt.	⅔ c flakes	70	1.8	5	0.6	Trace	0.09	0.03	0.6	0
Total nutrients in foundation diet			1250	64	740	10.2	6700	1.00	1.66	13.1	130
Recommended allowances:										Niacin Equivalents†† (mg)	
Man, 70 kg, moderately active, 23–50 yrs.			2700	56	800	10	5000	1.4	1.6	18	45
Woman, 58 kg, moderately active 23–50 yrs.			2000	46	800	18	4000	1.0	1.2	13	45

*Solid boxes indicate that 25 percent or more of the daily need of that nutrient is expected to be derived from that food group; dashed boxes indicate an expectation of 10 to 25 percent of the nutrient from that group.[8] Compositional data are all from reference 9.

†Average of the ten 100 gm servings of lean, edible portion of meats, including beef, lamb, pork, poultry, and fish.

‡Average of ten 100 gm servings, one each of asparagus, broccoli, Brussels sprouts, carrots, green snap beans, green lettuce and romaine, spinach, yellow (winter) squash, and sweet potato.

§Other vegetables: average of ten 100 gm servings of beets, cauliflower, celery, corn, green peas, lima beans, onions, summer squash, turnips, and zucchini.

¶Daily average based on three servings of orange juice, two servings of grapefruit juice, three servings of tomato juice, and two servings of fresh raw tomatoes.

**Other fruits: daily average based on one average serving each of fresh apple, banana, peach, pear; one serving each of canned applesauce, apricots, peaches, and pineapple, plus one serving of dried or stewed prunes.

††Includes niacin as such and from tryptophan conversion.

Table 19–4 TYPICAL AMERICAN MENU FOR THE BASIC FOUR FOOD GROUPS DIET IN TABLE 19–3

Breakfast	*Carried Lunch*	*Dinner*	*Snacks*
		Foundation Diet, 1200 kcal	
Small glass of orange juice Corn flakes with milk	Egg sandwich on white bread Raw tomato	Small chicken breast Baked potato Yellow summer squash Pickled green beans Hot bread or roll	Raw apple and cheese
		Typical Supplement, 800–1500 kcal	
Coffee, tea, or chocolate Larger serving of juice Sugar for coffee, cereal Cream in lieu of milk Toast, butter, jam	Coffee or tea Butter and/or mayonnaise on sandwich Cookies Potato chips Soft drink	Larger serving of chicken Butter for potato, roll, and squash Sweet dessert Coffee or tea Alcoholic beverages Sugar in coffee More rolls and butter	Coffee or tea Sugar in coffee Soft drink or alcoholic beverages Candy

diet is disproportionately high, this menu provides one-half to two-thirds, or less, of the recommended allowances. For some of the nutrients tabulated, especially folacin and zinc, the compositional data are not as reliable as one would like, but the discrepancies between content and recommended intake are so sizable that this does not negate the conclusions that must be drawn. Either the Basic Four Food Groups plan diet is marginal to inadequate *as commonly followed*, or allowances are unrealistically high, or both.

The extra foods listed in Table 19–4 (e.g., 5 tsp sugar, 5 tsp butter, 1 tbsp jam, 4 cookies, 20 potato chips, 6 oz cola, 1/2 c ice cream, 2 glasses wine, 1 oz mints) would provide about 125 gm refined sugar, and 45 gm fat. In the total diet 13 percent of energy would be derived from protein, 30 percent from fat and 57 percent from carbohydrate, with 23 percent coming from refined sugar. Without knowing the composition of fat used in the processed foods, the amounts of saturated and polyunsaturated fatty acids cannot be calculated, but these would be not less than 14 percent of energy from saturated forms and not more than 8 percent from the polyunsaturates. The diet fails to meet the specified Goals.

An Improved Basic Four Food Plan

How might these defects be rectified? In part, the missing nutrients can be added by selecting different foods from within the categories and taking larger servings of some of them. Others are best handled by adding more servings or different types of foods.

Had liver been chosen instead of chicken, the contribution of one serving from the Meat Group would have been: iron, 8.8 mg; zinc, 5.1 mg; vitamin A, 53,400 IU; thiamin, 0.26 mg; riboflavin 4.19 mg; niacin, 16.5 mg; ascorbic acid, 27 mg; vitamin E, 1.62 IU; free folacin, 82 mcg; vitamin B-6, 0.8 mg; vitamin B-12, 80 mcg; and pantothenic acid, 7.7 mg. (Amounts of the other nutrients tabulated would not differ appreciably, but there would be major added contributions of copper, molybdenum, manganese, and all other substances that are stored in the liver.) The *difference* in iron yields a 12 percent improvement in the *daily average*

Table 19–5 LESSER-STUDIED NUTRIENTS* IN A MENU BASED ON PATTERN OF FOUR FOOD GROUPS IN TABLE 19–4

Food	*Grams*	*Phosphorus (mg)*	*Sodium (mg)*	*Potassium (mg)*	*Magnesium (mg)*	*Zinc (mg)*	*Vitamin E (IU)*	*Free Folacin (mcg)*	*Vitamin B-6 (mg)*	*Vitamin B-12 (mcg)*	*Pantothenic acid (mg)*
Milk Group											
Milk	244	227	122	352	32	1.0	0.1	12	0.10	1.0	0.83
Cheddar Cheese	30	143	210	25	14	0.9	0.1	<1	0.02	0.3	0.15
Meat Group											
Chicken	100	257	78	381	20	1.8	0.4	4	0.30	0.4	0.90
Egg	50	102	61	64	6	0.7	0.2	25	0.06	1.0	0.80
Vegetable and Fruit Group											
Green beans	100	32	1	152	20	0.3	0.1	7	0.07	0	0.14
Summer squash	100	25	1	141	16	0.2	<0.1	2	0.06	0	0.17
Potato	100	65	4	503	20	0.2	<0.1	12	0.09	0	0.25
Tomato, raw	100	18	3	227	10	0.2	1.0	18	0.10	0	0.25
Orange juice, fresh	100	16	1	186	10	<0.1	<0.1	35	0.03	0	0.16
Apple, raw	100	10	1	110	8	<0.1	0.31	3	0.03	0	0.10
Cereal Group											
Bread, enriched, white	70	68	355†	73	15	0.5	0.1	8	0.03	trace‡	0.30
Corn flakes	30	14	300†	36	5	0.1	<0.1	4	0.02	0	0.06
TOTAL		977	1137†	2250	176	6	~3	130	~1	3	4
Recommended allowance											
Men		800	§	§	350	15	15	200¶	2	3	¶
Women		800	§	§	300	15	12	200¶	2	3	¶

*Compositional data for these nutrients (except for phosphorus and potassium) are not as reliable as one would wish and are tabulated only to indicate the order of magnitude of a nutrient. Methods are poor for the vitamins and minerals vary by a factor of 10 to 100, depending on soil composition and processing contaminants. Entries for minerals except zinc are from reference 9; vitamin B-6, B-12, and pantothenic acid from reference 10; vitamin E from reference 11. Folacin values are from reference 12 and various literature sources as compiled in unpublished tables of S. Cohenour and J. King, University of California, Berkeley; values in parentheses are for the raw food. Zinc data are from a published review: Schlettwein-Gsell, D., and Mommsen-Straub, S., Internat. J. Vit. Forschung, *40*:659, 1970 (in German), and from USDA tables.

†Sodium added to these cereal products in manufacture. Other foods would have salt added in cooking. The expected daily total would be about 5 gm of sodium, with these additions and use of salted butter or margarine.

‡Vitamin B-12 due to added milk in recipe.

§Recommended daily allowances of these have not been established. The probable need is about 10 mg of pantothenic acid.
Potassium need is on the order of 2.5 gm a day, and a ratio of about 1:1 of sodium to potassium and of calcium to phosphorous is desirable.

¶WHO recommendation for *free* folacin; NRC RDA is 400 mg *total* folacin.

intake if the liver were eaten only once weekly. Vitamin A content would meet the full allowance for 10 days. Liver would add a 2-week supply of vitamin B-12 and a full 2-day allotment of riboflavin. Half of a daily allowance of folacin, vitamin B-6, and ascorbic acid would be provided. Its high content of ascorbic acid makes liver almost unique among animal foods. (Fish roe is also high in vitamin C, and breast milk, while not high in this nutrient, contains enough to meet all the needs of an infant.

Not everyone will eat liver, liver sausage, or paté de foie gras, and a great improvement can be made in the diet from a few simple changes that are perhaps easier to practice on a day-to-day basis. (Considering the relative amounts of muscle and liver in a carcass, it is evident that the whole population could not have liver every week in any case.) Substitution of whole-grain cereals for refined milled ones—in our example, three slices of whole-wheat bread and a serving of oatmeal instead of enriched white bread and corn flakes—would increase the magnesium contribution from the Cereal Group fivefold and triple the amount of folacin, vitamin B-6, and pantothenate derived from this group. Vitamin E content is ten times higher in the whole grains. Note that potato is quite a good food and contributes nutrients that suggest it could well be classified with the Cereal Group with vitamin C as a bonus.

Another key change is to include larger and more frequent servings of dark green, leafy vegetables. Products such as mustard and turnip greens, kale, dandelion greens, and collards all have about one-third more of all the essential nutrients than do the substitutes presently allowed (other green and yellow vegetables). A 100 gm serving of mustard or other greens meets almost the entire daily allowance of ascorbic acid and vitamin E. Addition of a generous serving of a *raw* leafy green, such as romaine, cos, or leaf lettuce, will go far toward guaranteeing the adequacy of folacin in the diet. These vegetables also contribute a large amount of calcium with relatively little phosphorus, a direction in which we wish to improve the diet. Many of the greens are as good a source of calcium as is milk on a gram-for-gram basis. Fruits are generally more expensive than vegetables as a source of vitamins A and C, for which we rely on the Vegetable-Fruit Group, and many are lower in content of B vitamins. Note, however, that fresh or frozen orange juice contributes folacin, and so do bananas.

It is worth considering addition of a third serving of food from the Meat Group every day and for this serving, choosing frequently fish (for iodine and other trace minerals) and dry beans or nuts (for more thiamin and folacin). This change would have the effect of increasing the spectrum of foods and thereby increasing the probability of including the nutrients we know very little about today. Meats, but not the alternative legumes or nuts, are the only recognized good source of zinc habitually included in the American diet. Fish, legumes, and nuts would also improve the ratio of saturated to polyunsaturated fatty acids in the diet.

The Milk Group contributes most of the calcium in the typical American diet and makes good contributions of protein and B vitamins. Since calcium is the key nutrient in this group, cheese is an accepted substitute for milk. However, the bulk of the water-soluble nutrients present in milk are lost in the whey, so cheese compares unfavorably with milk with respect to all the B vitamins, magnesium, and potassium. Owing to the lactose present, some persons experience intestinal gas or softening of the stools when they drink milk (Chapters 3 and 14). Cheese, which lacks the offending sugar, will be a good source of calcium for them. Lactose-intolerant persons may also be able to tolerate traditional yogurt or soured milk, in which lactose content is reduced by the action of bacteria, but most commercial yogurt has extra milk solids added for body and still has nearly as much lactose as normal fluid milk when the desired level of acidity is reached. Other calcium sources do exist, of course. The dark leafy greens are one (excepting those that are high in oxalic acid, Chapter 11), and they provide as much riboflavin as does cheese. Fish bones eaten in sardines, smelt, salmon, or dried fishes are another. Another source commonly used in the Near and Middle East is whole sesame seed or sesame seed paste, the tahini of Egyptian cookery and a basic ingredient in the Oriental candy halvah. The plant sources of calcium are lacking in vitamin B-12, which will need to be added from other sources.

To raise the vitamin E content of the diet, it is necessary to turn to another food group, fats and oils. A few foods such as peanuts and soybeans are high in vitamin E, and oil expressed from these foods is a still more concentrated source of this fat-soluble vitamin. Peanuts contain about 7 mg of alpha-tocopherol per 100 gm of nuts or 14 mg per 100 gm of crude fat. Potato chips, because they are fried in vegetable oil, have about the same concentration of this vitamin as do peanuts. Salad oils and mayonnaise made from vegetable oil have 5 to 40 mg of vitamin E per 100 gm, depending on which oil is used. The amount taken with a salad, about one tablespoon (15 gm), would provide about 1 to 6 mg of vitamin E. Margarines have about 13 mg of vitamin E per 100 gm and butter only 1 mg. Vegetable oils (except coconut) and margarines and salad dressings made from them would augment the intake of polyunsaturated fatty acids. (See Chapter 4 for composition.)

Vitamin D is not found in popular American foods in significant amounts, except for fatty marine fish (Chapter 7). Vitamin D adequacy is assured by the use of fortified milk and exposure to sunlight. Iodine nutrition has been approached in the same way, by selection of salt fortified with iodine if marine foods are not eaten regularly. It is difficult today to give clear advice about this issue because more iodine is creeping into our food supply than was formerly the case. Much of the common cheaper white bread is made by a continuous dough process that uses iodate as a dough conditioner; another potential source is iodine-containing antiseptics used to cleanse commercial food equipment. We know little about the trace minerals, and their concentrations in foods will surely depend on the soil conditions where the vegetables and fruits, cereals, and legumes are grown and on the processes through which the food has passed.

After the needs for essential fatty acids and vitamin E are met, which can be accomplished with one or two tablespoons of oil, there is no nutritional reason to add more energy in the form of fat. There is no nutritional basis for use of sugar and alcohol except as alternative energy sources. How much of fats, sugars, and alcohol the diet can tolerate depends on how well the other items are selected and prepared in the home and how much energy the individual needs. A reasonable plan is to take at least the first 1600 kcal (6700 kJ) from wholesome basic foods to provide a margin of safety for variation in food composition and preparatory losses.

Sweet desserts containing milk (puddings or ice cream) or milk and eggs (custard-filled pastries, cakes) or fruits and nuts (compote, fruit pastries) have some nutritional advantages over those that are mainly whipped cream or sugar. If sugar is added, brown sugar is a slightly better choice than white. Honey has only very small amounts of essential nutrients, and its physiological properties are not superior to those of other sugars. A diet that included not more than 1 tbsp jam or 3 tsp sugar and one small serving of a dessert or sweet would meet the Dietary Goal for most adults.

If alcohol is used, beer is the best choice, because it contains appreciable amounts of B vitamins and minerals; wine is second choice. Distilled spirits are the poorest possible choice in terms of nutritive value.

Other Dietary Components

Some foods usually classed as nonnutritive substances are included in diets the world over. Tea is the favored beverage throughout the Orient and in the British Isles, while coffee and cocoa are more widely used in Europe and the Americas. These beverages do contain minerals because they are extracts of plant materials, but the steps through which they are processed leaves them without significant amounts of vitamins, except for some niacin in coffee (about 0.5 mg in a 6 ounce cup). All three beverages add 10 to 20 mg of magnesium per cup of fluid and 45 to 65 mg of potassium. Tea makes a significant contribution of fluoride (0.3 to 0.5 mg per cup). By themselves they yield no energy, but each *level* teaspoon of sugar used with them adds 16 kcal (67 kJ) and each tablespoon of light cream about 32 kcal (134 kJ). Dry cream substitutes may contain some cream or only a substitute fat, usually coconut oil, which has a higher percentage of saturated fatty acids than does milk fat; the other usual ingredients are isolated milk protein (casein) or nonfat milk solids, corn syrup solids, and chemical additives. At equal "whiteness" in the beverage, cream substitutes may have negligibly lower energy yield than does light cream. Cocoa powder may be mixed with water or milk, and the total nutritional content of the beverage will vary accordingly. These contributions from beverages are not trivial in view of the large amount taken in the day. A not uncommon intake of five servings of beverage would add about 100 mg of magnesium, a nutrient in which diets tend to be low, plus whatever minerals are present in the local water.

Coffee, tea, and cocoa all contain a related group of stimulants, the one highest in concentration in each being caffeine, theophylline, and theobromine, respectively. Caffeine is added to most cola-flavored beverages. Caffeine is the most active of the three compounds and when taken in excess may cause sleeplessness. It has also been reported to increase the levels of glucose[13] and fatty acids[14] in the blood, particularly of persons with diminished or diabeticlike tolerance for glucose. Caffeine is a weak diuretic (Chapter 15). Tea also contains tannins that have astringent properties, and it has enough thiaminase (thiamin-splitting) activity to be of concern if the diet is marginal in this vitamin.[15] All these beverages are taken without apparent untoward side effects in most healthy people, but tea is usually much better tolerated than coffee when there are digestive upsets. Herbal teas have been less well studied, but several are known to contain pharmacologically active compounds;[16] some caution regarding them is warranted, since there is not as yet even the test of long cultural use to help prove their safety.

Herbs, spices, and condiments are plant material and do contain nutrients; the significance of these depends on the amounts used. Chili peppers are high in vitamins C and A, and enough chili is used to make a real difference in Spanish-American and Oriental cookery. Kimchee, a Korean condiment, is also a rich source of vitamin C. Dried kelp and other seaweeds used in Asiatic cookery are high in calcium, magnesium, iodine, and other minerals found in sea water.

Other substances quite casually added in cookery or preserving foods can make important differences in the diet. About half of the folacin in home-baked bread comes from yeast added for leavening,[17] and the yeast and other bread ingredients add more B vitamins, an array of minerals, and some protein. Baking powders add substantial amounts of sodium (potassium tartrate type is an exception) and usually phosphate or sulfate and calcium, but no vitamins. All but about ½ gm of the sodium present in the diet is there because it has been added as salt or one of the other sodium-containing compounds used in preserving or cooking the food, such as sodium nitrite in corning beef, brine for pickles, salt in butter, monosodium glutamate (MSG), and soy sauce in cooking.

Effects of Cooking on Nutritive Values

Some foods can be eaten raw, but most require cooking to improve their digestibility and to insure food safety. Providing that sanitary methods of fertilization and watering are practiced (unprocessed fecal matter harbors bacteria, amebae, and other parasites), most vegetables and fruits can be eaten raw after thorough washing in clean water. Potatoes, cereals, and legumes all should be cooked in order to improve digestibility of the starch; the legumes should be cooked to destroy antidigestive and potentially toxic materials as well. Meats, fish, and poultry can be eaten raw but are better cooked if there is the least question of parasitic, bacterial, or viral infections. Fish, pork, and beef muscle may carry parasites that may be killed during prolonged storage at home freezer temperatures; but for absolute certainty of kill, the muscle should reach an internal temperature of 180° F (82.2° C). Mollusks pick up hepatitis virus from infected water, and poultry and eggs are subject to salmonella infection. Milk must be pasteurized for safety, and this has little effect on nutritive values.

If foods are to be cooked in water, loss of water-soluble nutrients will be lessened if the food is left in large pieces and cooked quickly in a small amount of water. However, traditional Chinese and Japanese cookery sets another excellent example, in which vegetables are stir-fried for a short period of time and all the juices are included in the final product. Another way of coping with the problem of loss of nutrients in cooking water, especially good for coarse vegetables that require a fairly long period of cooking, such as collards and other greens, is to use the cooking water as a soup or soup base. "Pot liquor" from greens is a standard item of diet in the rural southern part of the United States; and in northern Chinese cookery, small bits of food are cooked in broth at the table, and the cooking broth is eaten last, as a soup.

Dry heat is also detrimental to many vitamins, and there is some damage to protein if such treatment is excessive. Well-controlled roasting, broiling, and frying, according to the directions in any good cookery text, will cause only modest losses. Again, juices should be salvaged and used in soup and gravy stock, but unless energy needs are large, it is prudent to skim off and discard the rendered fat.

Some nutrients are susceptible to oxidation, but this is more a problem in commercial food processing than in home preparation. However, unsaturated fatty acids and vitamin E do deteriorate when oils are opened to the air and the products become rancid. Even in frozen storage, prepared foods lose much of their vitamin E content through oxidative changes that continue to occur at these low temperatures. Little vitamin E or unsaturated fatty acid is lost in deep-fat frying in fresh oil, but there is substantial loss of vitamin content on storage.[11] When fats are heated to very high temperatures (250° C) or when oils are reused for long periods of time, damaged and potentially toxic products are formed.[18] Thus both palatability and nutritional considerations dictate that only fresh fats should be used in food preparation.

The only common home food preparation in the United States that involves fermentation with microorganisms is yeast leavening of doughs, to which we have referred earlier. Various bacterial and mold processes are employed quite commonly in Africa and Asia, such as manufacture of oggi from cassava, kefir and yogurt from milk, and tempeh from soybeans. Microorganisms are able to synthesize many nutrients that man requires in the diet, but some have a definite requirement for vitamins that are essential to man. For this reason it is difficult to guess what the net effect of a fermentation process will be in terms of vitamin and amino acid content of the food. Generally, food processing organisms add more vitamins than they use up in their growth, and some bacteria and molds, but not yeast, even make the "animal" vitamin, B-12.[19]

Dill pickles are often cited as a good source of iron (about 1 mg per large pickle), which seems odd because cucumbers are not a good source of iron. The extra iron in pickles was present adventitiously, as a contaminant from processing in metal equipment that is no longer much used by commercial food processors. Pickles packed at home in earthenware crocks would not have much iron either. Unintentionally, we used to add iron in the home by slowly cooking foods such as tomato sauces or greens in iron pots. Also, we made extensive use of foods packed in tinned containers that often took up tin and iron by corrosion of the can on long-term storage.* With the introduction of frozen and ready-to-eat foods, and aluminum, stainless steel, and Teflon-coated pots and pans, these beneficial additions of iron have been lost. Zinc is also taken up from galvanized containers,* and such contamination may account in part for the high concentration of zinc in maple syrup. The mineral content of household water depends not only on the composition of the main water supply, but also upon the kinds of pipes and softening systems through which it flows.

The food that finally reaches the table reflects a host of factors: soil, water, harvesting, processing, transportation, and storage, as well as personal selection and home preparation. No amount of care in the household can make up for damage that has occurred in other steps of the food distribution chain. These other factors are discussed in Chapter 17.

*Zinc and probably tin are essential nutrients, but both are toxic at high levels. For this reason storage of acid products in open tinned or galvanized containers is very hazardous. Poisoning has occurred from party punches made ahead and stored in metal pails.

Vegetarian Diets

A diet that avoids animal flesh but that does include milk and eggs poses no serious nutritional problems.[20] One simply changes the source from which protein is derived by adding more cheese, eggs, milk, dry beans, peas, and nuts. A reasonable menu plan might have an eggnog (1 egg + 1 cup milk; 14 gm protein); a peanut butter (2 tbsp) sandwich and a glass of milk (20 gm protein); and 1 cup cooked lentils and 1 oz cheese (23 gm protein) in addition to the needed amounts of fruits and vegetables, cereals, oils, and other energy sources. Some caution will be required in selection of iron- and zinc-rich alternative foods, and generous intakes of these trace elements are required because they are not well absorbed from vegetable foods. (Chapter 12).

Nutritional planning becomes virtually impossible if all animal products are eliminated from the diet, especially for people accustomed to Western styles of food preparation. Such a diet has no vitamin B-12 and a limited spectrum of calcium sources in addition to the problem areas just mentioned. Traditional cultures that have maintained themselves on strict vegetarian diets have found a source of vitamin B-12 because this is a universal requirement of man. Some possibilities for synthesis may be found in microbial processes applied to foods and unintentional contamination with animal matter, such as insects or their eggs, or with soil microorganisms. There is perhaps some intestinal synthesis of this vitamin, but it is not certain enough to be relied upon, for ample evidence of vitamin B-12 deficiency has been found in strict vegans.[21]

Vitamin Supplements

Vitamin pills will not be needed by people who regularly eat a good diet, except under very unusual conditions. A person who has been well-nourished in the past will have ample reserves of vitamins in the liver and other tissues that will carry him through the ordinary minor illnesses and occasional periods of dietary indiscretion. Supplements will be needed if intestinal absorption is impaired by disease and sometimes during and after prolonged illness.

If a daily supplement is to be taken, it should contain the same balance of water-soluble vitamins as one would wish to have in the regular diet, that is, *all* of the vitamin B complex and ascorbic acid in amounts suggested in the recommended daily allowances. Only for therapeutic purposes and under competent medical advice should a pharmaceutical vitamin preparation be taken that exceeds the recommended allowances.

The fat-soluble vitamins must be treated cautiously, for vitamins D and A are toxic at high dosages (Chapter 7). If the diet includes vitamin D–fortified milk, as it should, then no other supplement of this vitamin should be taken by normal persons. Quite commonly vitamins D and A are added to products such as ready-to-eat cereals, flavoring agents for milk, and "instant" meals, so there is some risk of increasing the intake unduly.

If a person suspects that his diet may not be adequate, his best procedure is to improve the diet, because if vitamins are low, chances are that minerals will be inadequate also. At the present stage of knowledge, we know of no sensible way to prepare an all-round mineral supplement. However, a modest, well-balanced vitamin supplement will do no harm unless the practice of taking it tempts one to ignore the necessity for choosing foods wisely.

Meal Spacing

The times at which meals are eaten and the intervals between them are usually determined by the convenience of the family and the accepted pattern of a culture. All patterns have been utilized, from a very large number of very small meals (a nibbling pattern) to a single large meal daily. The body's metabolic machinery adapts to any habitual pattern so that we are able to cope with a flood of nutrients at one time and maintain critical functions in the intervals, or vice versa. However, in both human studies and animal experiments, a pattern of frequent small meals leads to more satisfactory levels of blood lipids and deposition of more lean and less fat in the body than if one or two large meals are eaten daily.[22]

Other investigations of the effect of omitting meals have centered on (1) the maintenance of blood sugar level as a physiological parameter indicating homeostasis, or (2) the efficiency with which some mental or physical work is performed. Studies of American youth and older persons accustomed to eating three or more meals a day have shown that blood sugar begins to fall about 2½ to 3 hours after breakfast, with the fall occurring somewhat later if protein-rich foods are included in the meal;[23, 24] blood sugar continues to fall unless a second meal is given about that time.[25] There was evidence of lessened efficiency that coincided with the blood sugar changes.[24] However, these subjects were not habituated to skipping meals and so were ill-adapted to this pattern of eating. Recently, a simple test of reaction time was carried out in college students who habitually eat or skip breakfast; breakfast eaters performed less well when breakfast was omitted, but those who skipped breakfast performed equally well with or without breakfast.[26]

People do seem to prefer a nibbling pattern, at least early in life. Infants eat at 2 to 3 hour intervals for the first days or weeks of life and only gradually are accustomed to long periods of sleep between bouts of eating. We think that a three-meals-a-day pattern is set ultimately, but this is not quite true. Most people have two or three main meals a day interspersed with two to four small ones (morning and afternoon coffee or tea, snacks in the evening, the odd bit of fruit or candy, etc.). In the United States Ten-State Survey of low-income populations, the diet histories indicated that both black and white youths 12 to 16 years of age consumed about 20 to 25 percent of their total daily energy intake as between-meal snacks and beverages; the value was 13 to 16 percent for Hispanic teenagers.[5]

The pattern of large infrequent meals is customary in countries where food is in short supply and obesity is infrequent. In richer parts of the world, a larger number of small meals, five or six a day, seem to be preferred and physiologically desirable. However, nibbling is a good practice only if all the food forms part of a well-balanced diet. A midmorning small meal of juice or milk is an asset, but one of a doughnut and black coffee is probably not. Table 19–6 indicates one way in which an American pattern of food consumption can be adapted to a frequent meal schedule without sacrificing nutritional value.

Equally important is the need to arrange mealtimes, at whatever frequency, so that the family or living group eat together at least once and preferably twice a day. Disorganization in the household and lack of commensality contribute heavily toward development and practice of the poor food habits that lead to poor nutritional status.

Table 19–6 MENU PLAN FOR INCREASED MEAL FREQUENCY*

Meal 1	Egg or cheese Whole-grain bread
Meal 2	Fresh or dried fruit Milk
Meal 3	Vegetable or cream-type soup Green salad with vegetable oil–vinegar dressing
Meal 4	Fish, meat, or nut butter sandwich Milk, fruit or vegetable juice
Meal 5	Meat, fish, poultry, or cheese Potato or whole-grain cereal product Leafy, green vegetable Other vegetables
Meal 6	Fruit Yogurt or ice cream

*Condiments, beverages, and more servings of cereals, fruits, vegetables, fats, and oils to be added as needed to meet energy requirements.

NUTRITION DURING ADOLESCENCE

At about 10 to 12 years of age, well-nourished girls enter the period of *pubescence*, which culminates with attainment of reproductive capacity at about age 13 to 14 years.[27] Comparable changes occur about 2 years later in boys. Both sexes experience a spurt in growth with the onset of puberty; because the change occurs earlier in girls, between ages 10 and 13 years girls are taller and heavier than boys. Growth of boys then overtakes that of girls, and males are on the average taller and heavier than females during adolescence and adulthood. Growth continues — at a slower rate — however, during the period of *adolescence*, which is from ages 13 to 17 years in girls and 15 to 21 years in boys. The onset of puberty is delayed about 2 years in underfed populations, but the pubescent growth spurt, a phenomenon peculiar to man in contrast to other animal species, allows a final opportunity for catch-up body growth if enough food is available then.[28]

Body composition also changes with puberty.[27] During the pubescent growth spurt and adolescence, boys, under the influence of the anabolic male sex hormones, gain proportionately more lean tissue than fat, develop a heavier skeleton, and increase their pool of red blood cells. Mineralization of the skeleton is also completed at this time in girls, but the female sex hormones promote the deposition of proportionately more fat than lean tissue, and the red blood cell pool of females remains lower than that of males throughout adolescence and adulthood. For these reasons, boys need more energy and more of the body-building nutrients than girls do during pubescence and adolescence, but needs for both sexes are increased during this period.

The U. S. recommended dietary allowances for boys and girls aged 11 to 14 years are quite similar except for energy, for which the RDA is 2400 kcal (10.0 mega joules, or MJ) for girls and 2800 kcal (11.7 MJ) for boys. The reasons for this difference are that the girls' pubescent growth spurt will have ended at the midpoint age (13 years), whereas the boys' growth spurt is beginning, and that after puberty, many girls tend to reduce their customary levels of physical activity, while boys remain active. At ages 15 to 18 years, the disparity between usual activity patterns remains, and some boys are completing the accelerated growth phase; the RDA for energy at this age is 2100 kcal (8.8 MJ) for young women and 3000 kcal (12.6 MJ) for young men. Allowances for protein drop from 1 gm per kg body weight at ages 11 to 14 to the mature allowance of 0.8 gm per kg at ages 19 to 22 years. During the pubescent and adolescent periods, the RDA's for calcium and phosphorus are increased to 1200 mg per day, and 18 mg of iron per day is suggested for both sexes.

Canadian boys and girls engaged in their usual school activities are thought to require 2800 and 2200 kcal, respectively, between ages 13 and 15 years.[3] Between 16 and 18 years of age, girls reach adult size and are thought to become less active, whereas boys continue to grow and engage in very active sports. The Canadian allowances for this age span are 3200 kcal for boys, which is 107 percent of the adult men's value; and 2100 kcal for girls, which is the same as the adult women's allowance. Protein, mineral, and vitamin intakes are adjusted upward for girls at the appropriate earlier age of 10 years and lowered to mature values at age 16; for boys, the increase occurs at age 13 and lasts until age 19.

Adolescence is a time of great physical, biological, and emotional adjustment. The teen-ager may exhibit immature judgment and uncertain behavior. The demand for independence may lead to abandonment of dietary practices taught in the family and acceptance of fad diets and food patterns decreed by the peer group. School, work, and social activities take teen-agers away from home a great deal, with the result that food habits, frequently not good before, become even poorer. Young people living continuously on diets providing suboptimal amounts of nutrients are in poor condition to withstand the stresses and strains of their hectic life, let alone prepare their bodies for later productive career work and reproduction.

Dietary studies in the United States consistently show that intakes of calcium, iron, and vitamin A, and sometimes riboflavin and vitamin C, may fall far short of the probable needs of many teen-agers.[5, 6] Energy intakes of low-income white girls and low-income black boys and girls often were substandard, which coincides with findings of reduced growth in these groups. An Australian survey found that 16- to 19-year-old youths who were employed had poorer dietary intakes than those who remained in school, particularly the girls. The diets of only 3 percent of employed 16-year-old girls and 33 percent of the boys met Australian standards for all of eight nutrients tabulated.[29] The Canadian National Nutrition Survey[7] also found the diets of teen-agers commonly to be substandard with respect to iron; calcium; vitamins A, D, and C; and riboflavin. The situation was worse for Eskimos and Indians than for the rest of the population, but some diets were at risk levels in all groups.

Usually, boys offer less of a problem than girls because their appetite is excellent and their energy need is so large they can afford to eat more. Girls of this age frequently have a capricious appetite, preferring sweets and highly flavored foods; and if they develop an obsession about remaining slender, it is difficult to get them to take all the protective foods they need. The less food eaten, the more important it is to make all of it count. Foods with "empty calories" (i.e., little or no minerals or vitamins but plenty of energy) often replace foods with important nutrients. Fast-food establishments often become an important feature of the social scene, and a combination of limited spending money and teen subculture style may lead to selection of foods high in sugar and fat rather than of those with more needed protein, minerals, and vitamins. A soft drink and an order of "fries" or "chips" is relatively cheap and satisfying.

The family meal pattern is satisfactory for the teen-ager, with an increase in the size of servings, if needed to provide additional calcium, iron, and energy. However, teen-agers are often not at home for some of the family meals, which places on them the responsibility of knowing how to select nutritious foods away from home.

Because snacks account for one-fourth of the teen-ager's energy intake, these items should make a proportional contribution of nutrients. If attractive, nutritious snacks are available at home, the teen-ager is able to select what he wants and still get food that contributes to his daily nutritional requirement. Even when eating away from home, there are many nutritious snacks available. Suggested snacks that make a contribution to the health of teenagers include:

Fresh fruits
Fruit juices
Dried fruits
Cheese
Milk beverages
Ice cream
Peanut butter, nuts
Whole-grain crackers
Fresh vegetable pieces
Fruit-and-nut breads
Leftover meats or sausages

Many young people are troubled by acne, a skin condition ascribed to effects of sex hormones on the sebaceous glands. There is no proved association of this disorder with nutritional deficiency or with specific foods, but physicians often suggest elimination of cola beverages and chocolate from the diet and reduction of fat intake. The net effect of such instruction, if followed, would be to reduce the amount of poor-quality foods and increase the intake of other good foods to keep energy intake constant. Such an improved diet could benefit overall health, irrespective of its relevance to the skin disorder.

Obesity is a common finding in teen-agers. Most studies[30] report a prevalence on the order of 15 percent of high school students, as judged by body weight and anthropometric measurements. A key factor in juvenile obesity is inactivity (Chapter 22), and the problem is better prevented or treated by increased energy expenditure than by food restriction at a stressful time of life. Participation in sports is recommended strongly for this reason and for establishing habits that promote life-long health.

NUTRITION OF OLDER ADULTS

A marked change in life-style often occurs at about 65 years of age or with retirement from business. Changes in activity patterns are apt to be much more profound and abrupt for employed men than for women, who often continue with household tasks much as in earlier life. The bodily condition known as "old age" invariably develops sooner or later, but it is not simply the inevitable result of living a certain number of years. The rate of aging is affected by inheritance, nutrition, and other environmental factors. In animals, it is possible to show that aging may be postponed by the right dietary regimen. Epidemiological evidence for humans suggests that a poor diet or careless living habits may bring on premature senility. Some people are "older" in body at 50 years of age than others are at 80. Those who succeed in retaining their youthful vigor in the later years of life are usually not inactive people but, on the contrary, are those who are active mentally and physically.

The process of aging has been described in terms of thermodynamic principles, indicating that aging relates to energetics of the biological system.[31] Currently held concepts suggest that aging begins early in life and that procedures to alter the rate of decline need to begin equally early. However, most people are little concerned about aging until they themselves reach the middle years of life, when processes are well under way. Evidence from human populations is always epidemiological

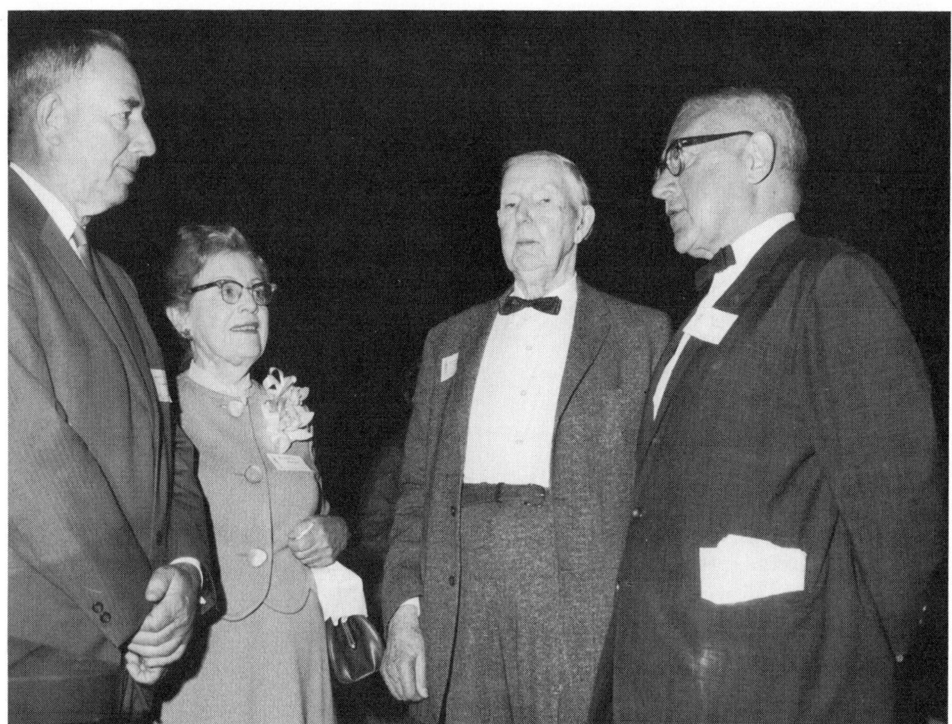

Figure 19–2 Old age need not be a period of isolation and boredom. Shown in this photograph are four famous nutritionists whose active careers extended well past the usual period of diminished productivity. At the time this picture was taken their ages were (left to right): W. H. Griffith 70; Agnes Fay Morgan, 81; E. V. McCollum, 89; Paul György, 72. (Photo courtesy of Ralph N. Smith, A.E.S., University of California, Berkeley.)

and retrospective because the life span of an investigator is no longer than the subject he needs to examine. Thus, animal systems provide our only model for research into methods to interrupt the processes of senile change. Current nutritional research[32] relates to hypotheses that aging is due to oxidative changes that can be modified by increased dosages of vitamin E and other antioxidants; and that delayed growth and maturation rate brought about by restriction of dietary energy early in life leads to a longer life span, or conversely, that overfeeding, with accelerated rates of growth and accumulation of adipose tissue, shortens it. There is no adequate proof for the antioxidant theory to date. Investigators found that rats receiving a lower energy intake in the early postweaning period lived longer than those that were liberally fed. However, there is no evidence that the same results would be true for humans, for in parts of the world where food intake is chronically low, average life span is shorter than in richer countries with more generous food supplies but also better public health practices. A diet that provides energy in *excess* of human needs, resulting in overweight, is definitely known to be associated with an increased incidence of heart and circulatory diseases, diabetes, and earlier mortality (Chapter 24). When the overweight person reduces to normal or even slightly below normal weight, the risk of heart disease decreases. In many cases, adult diabetes may also be controlled simply by reducing body weight to normal, together with moderate restrictions of dietary carbohydrate and judicious exercise.

A long-standing faulty diet may also be associated with osteoporosis, another disorder commonly seen in aged individuals. This disorder, in which there is thinning of the skeleton and lack of bone matrix, occurs especially frequently in old women, and it may lead to spontaneous fracture of the spinal column and loss of height. The principal causes of osteoporosis are thought to be inactivity, lack of hormones, and decreased ability to absorb calcium from the intestine, coupled with chronic low intake of calcium and vitamin D.[33]

In the later years of life, the ability of the body to handle food is diminished. First, the loss of teeth frequently results in inability to masticate hard or coarse foods. Inadequately chewed foods may cause digestive discomfort, while the omission of all coarse foods from the diet may lead to a diet of poorer quality. Blood flow to the alimentary tract, secretion of digestive juices, particularly gastric acid, and intestinal absorption are diminished. There are fewer active cells in the body, and various organs and tissues are either less active or less able to do extra work. The oxidative processes by which foods are utilized in the tissues go on more slowly and sometimes less completely, while the excretion of excessive waste products is more difficult.

Nutritional needs of the older person differ from those of the younger adult, but not to the extent of a sparse and abstemious diet.[34] The idea of such a diet for later life has gone out of style, and for good reason. The same nutritive essentials (energy, protein, minerals, and vitamins) are required in adequate quantities to nourish the body throughout life, and an insufficiency of any of them does harm at any age.

The most significant change in the diets of aging persons is that energy nutrients are needed in smaller quantities, so that principal curtailment should be in the intake of foods that supply only or chiefly energy. The energy requirement of older adults is materially reduced for two reasons:

1. Less energy is used in muscular activity.

2. The basal metabolism is lowered.

It is estimated that the resting metabolic rate between ages 60 and 70 years is about 10 percent less than formerly, 20 percent less from 70 to 90, and about 25 percent less after 90 years of age. Thus, a man of average weight and in middle life requires about 1600 to 1700 kcal per day for maintenance when at rest. Requirements of the same man for maintenance alone at 60 to 70 years would be about 1440 to 1530 kcal, and at 70 to 80 years, 1280 to 1360 kcal. These differences in energy needs may be at least partially accounted for by changes in body composition during aging—an increased percentage of fat and a lesser amount of lean muscle tissue in the body.[25]

Few men in their seventies do enough muscular work to raise their total energy requirement to more than 2400 kcal a day. Small, aged women may have surprisingly low energy needs, but the average need between ages 50 and 70 is about 1800 kcal. It is thus apparent that the total amount of food — especially foods of high caloric value—should be somewhat curtailed after 60 years (slightly so even at 40 to 60 years of age), and considerably reduced after 70. A Baltimore study[36] of 252 men, age 20 to 99 years and from upper income groups, found that energy intake declined from about 2700 kcal for ages 20 to 44, to 2300 kcal for ages 55 to 74 and 2100 kcal over age 75. Body weight was 74 kg for ages 20 to 34, 77 to 78 kg for ages 35 to 74, and only 71 kg for men who lived beyond that age. If the weight factor is taken into account, the sharpest drop in energy intake occurred at about age 60. Over the total age range, energy intake fell by 12.4 kcal per day per year, and the decrease in measured basal metabolism was 5.23 kcal per day per year. The remainder would be due to diminished activity and altered body composition.

Another variation in the needs of older adults compared with those of younger persons may be in protein requirement. Some studies have indicated that the requirement for essential amino acids is higher in men over 50 years of age than in younger adult males,[37] but in other studies no such age difference was apparent.[38, 39] In no case is there any suggestion of a decreased protein requirement with increasing age.

Surveys of the diets of old people have indicated inadequate nutrient intakes. Studies in Britain, Australia, New Zealand, Canada, and the United States all concur in finding inadequate intakes of energy, protein, vitamins C and D, calcium, and iron. Although old people living alone are often in reduced financial circumstances, partially disabled, and without sufficient motivation to prepare foods for their solitary meals, residence in a care center does not guarantee an adequate intake of nutrients.[40, 41, 42] A small group of women in an Australian hostel[40] had unsatisfactory levels of vitamin C in the blood even though the diet was calculated to contain enough of this nutrient; analysis of the food as served showed that 99 percent of the vitamin C had been lost because of poor institutional food practices. Food transported to old people in their homes ("Meals on Wheels") is also prepared in quantity and held warm for some time in the trucks, leading to loss of vitamin C and other heat-sensitive vitamins, thiamin and folacin. Unacceptable blood levels of thiamin[43] and folacin[44] have been found frequently in old people, in addition to ascorbic acid, as noted previously.

In planning diets for the aged person, all aspects of limited functional capability should be considered. Meals should be evenly spaced, with perhaps smaller amounts of food taken at more frequent intervals in view of diminished digestive and absorptive capacity. Adjustment of energy intake to achieve desirable body weight will relieve the strain imposed on the heart and on arthritic joints and an osteoporotic skeleton. The following physical conditions may impair the physical capability to ingest an adequate diet unless it is suitably prepared:

1. Crippling joint disease
2. Muscular tremor
3. Poor vision
4. Missing teeth, badly fitting dentures
5. Reduced senses of smell and taste
6. Difficulties in swallowing

Many workers in the field of geriatrics believe that lack of useful work or ways in which to fill their leisure hours and isolation from other people are the two most prominent factors that lead older people to take an inadequate amount of food. Other factors that have been found to influence food consumption of this group are:

1. Social situation
2. Income
3. Cooking and refrigeration facilities
4. Food faddism
5. Long-standing erroneous concepts of good nutrition.

Planning a diet that is not too high in energy value, yet that at the same time furnishes plenty of high-quality protein, minerals, and vitamins may at times be difficult. The daily food intake should consist mainly of milk, meats, eggs, whole-grain bread or cereals, vegetables, and fruits, with restricted amounts of concentrated sweets and fats. Some raw fruits and vegetables should be included because of the question of nutrient loss in holding food for service. If the old person cannot chew these, fresh juices can be made from them. At this age in life, vitamin supplements may be advantageous, but at least one study[45] indicated that old people who took supplements regularly were the least likely to need them, having otherwise good diets. Because constipation is a common complaint, addition of bran to the diet may be recommended, but some caution is needed. Studies have shown that addition of 10 to 20 gm of unprocessed bran to the diet of old people significantly lowers levels of ionized calcium and iron in the blood, and these levels often are already abnormally low in the elderly.[46] It would be safer to increase bran intake only to the extent of substituting whole-grain cereals and breads for refined products.

Foods included in the menu should be chosen from well-liked foods and presented in attractive, appetizing forms. Many old people have little to anticipate with pleasure in the day except their meals. They should not be deprived of this simple enjoyment by arbitrary insistence on fixed rules of food selection.

A word may be in order concerning the place of mild stimulants such as tea and coffee or the moderate use of alcoholic beverages. Most elderly persons experience comfort and cheer from hot drinks, and hot coffee or tea slightly stimulates the motility of the digestive tract. Their stimulating effect may be welcome to those whose bodily processes are slow. They also help to keep up fluid intake. Except in certain abnormal conditions, there is no reason to forbid their use. Much the same may be said of alcoholic beverages. Alcohol dilates the capillary blood vessels and thus may improve circulation temporarily. The abuse of alcoholic beverages by some persons should not rule out their proper uses by others.

QUESTIONS AND PROBLEMS

1. Plan a day's menu using the tables of Nutritive Values of Foods in the Appendix (pp. A.10 to A.28) and, as far as possible. foods that you commonly use. Estimate how much of each essential nutrient is furnished by the foods in your menus. Compare the total with the recommended daily allowance of needs for one of your sex, body weight, and degree of physical activity. What changes would be needed to adapt this diet for a boy of 16? A woman of 70?

2. Consult Table 19–3, which gives the nutritive evaluation of the foundation diet; determine for each of the individual nutrients listed what proportion of the total values for nutrients in the basal diet comes from certain classes of foods? What are the strengths and weaknesses of the Basic Four Food Groups pattern of menu planning? How may adequacy of lesser-studied vitamins and minerals be assured?

3. Outline briefly the types of dietary pattern characteristic of the following countries — Italy, India, China, and Ethiopia. In each case, what nutrients might be provided in insufficient amounts and what foods are in use or could be used to reinforce the diet in respect to those nutrients?

4. If the diet does not furnish the full amount of the allowance recommended by the United States Food and Nutrition Board (National Academy of Sciences), does it necessarily indicate that a person will suffer a deficiency of the nutritive essential that is provided in less than this quantity? Explain your answer. Why may an intake of certain nutrients in excess of the nutrients needed by the body be desirable, and if so, under what circumstances?

5. What are the main factors affecting the physiological aging process? How is nutrition related to the problem of aging? What are the most common causes of death after 55 years of age, and how may they be related to nutritional status? When should a diet for retarding the aging process begin? What special dietary factors may influence health in the later years of life?

6. According to the Food and Nutrition Board, how much should the total caloric intake of a 60-year-old man be reduced below that recommended for him at 30 years of age? Are protein needs of older people also reduced? What is the evidence?

7. What factors in the social environment of elderly people tend to prevent the consumption of a balanced diet even if finances are adequate? Plan a day's menu for a bedridden 85-year-old man with artificial teeth. How could the foods be adapted to suit his special disabilities or be given in part as between-meal nourishment?

REFERENCES

1. Food and Nutrition Board: *Recommended Dietary Allowances.* 8th Ed. Washington, D.C., National Research Council, National Academy of Sciences, 1974.
2. *Recommended Intakes of Nutrients for the United Kingdom.* Rpt. on Public Health and Medical Subjects, No. 120, London, 1969.
3. Dept. of National Health and Welfare: *Dietary Standard for Canada.* Ottawa, 1975.

4. U.S. Dept. of Agriculture: *Dietary Levels of Households in the United States.* Spring 1965. *Household Food Consumption Survey 1965–66.* Rpt. No. 6, Agric. Res. Serv., 1969.
5. U.S. Dept. of Health, Education, and Welfare: *Ten-State Nutrition Survey, 1968–1970.* Vol. V, Dietary. Dept. of Health, Education, and Welfare Pub. No. (HSM) 72–8133, 1972.
6. U.S. Dept. of Health, Education, and Welfare: *Preliminary Findings of the First Health and Nutrition Examination Survey, United States, 1971–72: Dietary Intake and Biochemical Findings.* Dept. of Health, Education, and Welfare Pub. No. (HRH) 74–1219–1, 1974.
7. Sabry, Z. I.: *Nutrition Canada: National Survey.* Information Canada, Cat. No. H58–36, 1973.
8. Page, L., and Phippard, E. F.: *Essentials of Nutrition.* Home Econ. Res. Rpt. No. 3. Washington, D.C., Government Printing Office, 1957.
9. Watt, B. K., and Merrill, A. L.: *Composition of Foods: Raw, Processed and Prepared.* Agricultural Handbook No. 8. Washington, D.C., U.S. Dept. of Agriculture, 1963.
10. Orr, M. L.: *Pantothenic Acid, Vitamin B_6 and Vitamin B_{12} in Foods.* Home Econ. Res. Rpt. No. 36. Washington, D.C., U.S. Dept. of Agriculture, 1969.
11. Bunnell, R. H., Keating, J., Quaresimo, A., and Parman, G. K.: Alpha-tocopherol content of foods. Amer. J. Clin. Nutr., *17*:1, 1965.
12. Pennington, J.: *Dietary Nutrient Guide.* Westport, Conn. Avi Publishing Co., Inc., 1976.
13. Jankelson, O. M., Beaser, S. B., Howard, F. M., and Mayer, J.: Effect of coffee on glucose tolerance and circulating insulin in men with maturity-onset diabetes. Lancet, *1*:527, 1967.
14. Bellet, S., Kershbaum, A., and Finck, E. M.: The response of free fatty acids to coffee and caffeine. Metabolism, *17*:702, 1968.
15. Vimokesant, S. L., et al.: Effect of tea consumption on thiamin status in man. Nutr. Rpt. Internat., *9*:371, 1974.
16. Siegel, R. K.: Herbal intoxication: psychoactive effects from herbal cigarettes, tea and capsules. J.A.M.A., *236*:473, 1976; Segelman, A. B., et al.: Sassafras and herb tea: potential health hazards. J.A.M.A., *236*:477, 1976.
17. Butterfield, S., and Calloway, D. H.: Folacin in wheat and selected foods. J. Amer. Dietet. Assoc., *60*:310, 1972.
18. Nolan, G. A., Alexander, J. C., and Artman, N. R.: Long-term rat feeding study with used frying fats. J. Nutr., *93*:337, 1967.
19. vanVeen, A. G., and Steinkraus, K. H.: Nutritive value and wholesomeness of fermented foods. J. Agric. Food Chem., *18*:576, 1970.
20. Register, U. D., and Sonnenberg, L. M.: The vegetarian diet. J. Amer. Dietet. Assoc., *62*:253, 1973.
21. Kirtha, A. N., and Ellis, F. R.: Investigation into the causation of the electroencephalogram abnormality in vegans. Pl. Fds. Hum. Nutr., *2*:53, 1971.
22. Fabry, P.: Metabolic consequences of the pattern of food intake. In Code, C. F. (ed.): *Handbook of Physiology,* Section 6. Baltimore, The Williams & Wilkins Co. for Amer. Physiol. Soc., 1967.
23. Thornton, R., and Horvath, S. M.: Blood sugar levels after eating and after omitting breakfast. Studies with teen-agers and young adults. J. Amer. Dietet. Assoc., *47*:474, 1965.
24. Tuttle, W. W., et al.: Effect on school boys of omitting breakfast. Physiologic responses, attitudes, and scholastic attainments. J. Amer. Dietet. Assoc., *30*:674, 1954.
25. Thornton, R. H., and Horvath, S. M.: Blood glucose as influenced by either one or two meals. J. Amer. Dietet. Assoc., *52*:214, 1968.
26. Gordon, H. F.: The Effects of Breakfast on the Performance of Young Adults During the Morning Hours. M. S. Thesis, University of California, Berkeley, 1975.
27. Cheek, D. B.: *Human Growth.* Philadelphia, Lea & Febiger, 1968.
28. McKigney, J. I., and Munro, H. N. (eds.): *Nutrient Requirements in Adolescence.* Cambridge, Mass., MIT Press, 1975.
29. McNaughton, J. W., and Cahn, A. J.: A study of the food intake and activity of a group of urban adolescents. Brit. J. Nutr., *24*:331, 1970.
30. Huenemann, R. L., et al.: *Teenage Nutrition and Physique.* Springfield, Ill., Charles C Thomas, 1974.
31. Calloway, N. O.: The senescent sequences of normal processes. J. Amer. Geriatr. Soc., *14*:1048, 1966.
32. Watkin, D. M. (ed.): Symposium: Nutrition and aging. Amer. J. Clin. Nutr., *25*:809, 1972.
33. Nordin, B. E. C.: Clinical significance and pathogenesis of osteoporosis. Brit. Med. J., *1*:571, 1971.
34. Mayer, J. (ed.): Symposium: Aging and nutrition. Geriatrics, *29*:57, 1974.
35. Forbes, G. B., and Reina, J. C.: Adult lean body mass declines with age: some longitudinal observations. Metabolism, *19*:653, 1970.
36. McGandy, R. B., et al.: Nutrient intakes and energy expenditures in men of different ages. J. Gerontol., *21*:581, 1966.
37. Tuttle, S. G., et al.: Further observations on the amino acid requirements of older men. II. Methionine and lysine. Amer. J. Clin. Nutr., *16*:229, 1965.
38. Watts, J. H., et al.: Nitrogen balances of men over 65 fed the FAO and milk patterns of essential amino acids. J. Gerontol., *19*:370, 1964.
39. Young, V. R., et. al.: In *Nutrition and Aging.* Edited by M. Winick, New York, John Wiley & Sons, 1976.
40. Woodhill, J. M., Nobile, S. R. V., and Perkins, K. W.: Dietary surveys of small groups of elderly people: eight women living in a hostel. Food Nutr. Notes Rev., *27*:51, 1970.
41. Corless, D., et al.: Vitamin D status in long-stay geriatric patients. Lancet, *1*:1404, 1975.
42. Justice, C. L., Howe, J. M., and Clark, H. E.: Dietary intakes and nutritional status of elderly patients. J. Amer. Dietet. Assoc., *65*:639, 1974.
43. Griffiths, L. L., et al.: Thiamine and ascorbic acid levels in the elderly. Gerontol. Clin. (Basel), *9*:1, 1967.
44. Girdwood, R. H.: Folate depletion in old age. Amer. J. Clin. Nutr., *22*:234, 1969.
45. Steinkamp, R. C., Cohen, M. L., and Walsh, H. E.:

Resurvey of an aging population—fourteen year follow-up. J. Amer. Dietet. Assoc., *46*:103, 1965.

SUPPLEMENTARY READING

Allen, D. E., Patterson, Z. J., and Warren, G. L.: Nutrition, family commensality, and academic performance among high school youth. J. Home Econ., *62*:333, 1970.
American Academy of Pediatrics: Nutritional aspects of vegetarianism, health foods and fad diets. Pediatrics, *59*:460, 1977.
Barboriak, J. J., et al.: Alcohol and nutrient intake of elderly men. J. Amer. Diet. Assoc., *72*:469, 1978.
Bebb, H. T., et al.: Calorie and nutrient contribution of alcoholic beverages to the usual diets of 155 adults. Amer. J. Clin. Nutr., *24*:1042, 1971.
Brown, P. T., and Bergan, J. G.: The dietary status of "new" vegetarians. J. Amer. Dietet. Assoc., *67*:455, 1975.
Ellis, F. R., Holesh, S., and Ellis, J. W.: Incidence of osteoporosis in vegetarians and omnivores. Amer. J. Clin. Nutr., *25*:555, 1972.
Frankle, R. T., and Huessenstamm, F. K.: Food zealotry and youth. Amer. J. Pub. Health, *64*:11, 1974.
Garn, S. M., Clark, D. C., and Guire, K. E.: Husband-wife similarities in hemoglobin levels. Ecol. Food Nutr., *5*:47, 1976.
Gershoff, S. N., et al.: Studies of the elderly in Boston. I. The effects of iron fortification on moderately anemic people. Amer. J. Clin. Nutr., *30*:226, 1977.
Grotkowski, M. L., and Sims, L. S.: Nutrition knowledge, attitudes and dietary practices of the elderly. J. Amer. Dietet. Assoc., *72*:499, 1978.
Hardinge, M. G., and Crooks, H.: Non-flesh dietaries. III. Adequate and inadequate. J. Amer. Dietet. Assoc., *45*:537, 1964.
Hegsted, D. M.: Dietary standards. J. Amer. Dietet. Assoc., *66*:13, 1975; Nutr. Rev., *36*:33, 1978.
Hegsted, D. M.: Protein needs and possible modifications of the American diet. J. Amer. Dietet. Assoc., *68*:317, 1976.
Hertzler, A. A., and Anderson, H. L.: Food guides in the United States. J. Amer. Dietet. Assoc., *64*:19, 1974.
Isom, P.: Nutritive value and cost of "fast food" meals. Family Econ. Rev., Fall, 1976, p. 10.
Jansen, G. R., et al.: Menu evaluation—a nutrient approach for consumers. J. Nutr. Ed., *9*:162, 1977.
King, J. C., et al.: Evaluation and modification of the basic four food guide. J. Nutr. Ed., *10*:27, 1978.
Madden, J. P., Goodman, S. J., and Guthrie, H. A.: Validity of the 24-hour recall. J. Amer. Dietet. Assoc., *68*:143, 1976.
Marrs, D. C.: Milk drinking by the elderly of three races. J. Amer. Dietet. Assoc., *72*:495, 1978.
Moore, M. C., et al.: Dietary-atherosclerosis study on deceased persons. Relation of eating pattern to raised coronary lesions. J. Amer. Dietet. Assoc., *67*:22, 1975; Relation of selected dietary components to raised coronary lesions. J. Amer. Dietet. Assoc., *68*:216, 1976.
Munro, H. N.: How well recommended are the Recommended Dietary Allowances? J. Amer. Dietet. Assoc., *71*:490, 1977.
Murphy, E. W., Marsh, A. C., and Willis, B. W.: Nutrient content of spices and herbs. J. Amer. Dietet. Assoc., *72*:174, 1978.
Ohlson, M. A., and Harper, L. J.: Longitudinal studies of food intake and weight of women from ages 18 to 56 years. J. Amer. Dietet. Assoc., *69*:626, 1976.
Pao, E. M., and Burk, M. C.: A computer-assisted approach to meal patterning. J. Amer. Dietet. Assoc., *65*:144, 1974.
Peterkin, B. B., Kerr, R. L., and Shore, C. J.: Diets that meet the dietary goals. J. Nutr. Ed., *10*:15, 1978.
Prothro, J., Mickles, M., and Tolbert, B.: Nutritional states of a population sample in Macon County, Georgia. Amer. J. Clin. Nutr., *29*:94, 1976.
Rockstein, M., and Sussman, M. L. (eds.): *Nutrition, Longevity and Aging*. New York, Academic Press, 1976.
Rose, C. S., et al.: Age differences in vitamin B-6 status of 617 men. Amer. J. Clin. Nutr., *29*:847, 1976.
Ross, M. H.: Dietary behavior and longevity. Nutr. Rev., *35*:257, 1977.
Symposium: Nutrition in hospitals. Proc. Nutr. Soc., *37*:65, 1978.

Articles in Nutrition Reviews

Availability of vitamins and minerals in tablet form. *24*:101, 1966.
Nutrition and metabolic bone disease in the elderly. *25*:71, 1967.
Effects of caffeine in man. *28*:38, 1970.
Diet and coronary heart disease. A statement of the Food and Nutrition Board, National Academy of Sciences, National Research Council, and the Council on Foods and Nutrition, American Medical Association. *30*:223, 1972.
Growth after adolescence. *31*:314, 1973.
Plasma lipids and lipoproteins in vegetarians. *33*:285, 1975.
Coffee drinking and peptic ulcer disease. *34*:167, 1976.
Prevention of coronary heart disease. *34*:220, 1976.
Plant foods and atherosclerosis. *35*:148, 1977.

Chapter 20

Nutrition During Pregnancy and Lactation

For pregnant and nursing mothers, diet is of extra importance because the mother is nourishing the child through her own body, either in the uterus before birth or through the milk she secretes for the baby. Although both are entirely normal physiological processes, they do subject the body to special strain. The nutrients needed for the child must be furnished in the mother's food; they may be drawn to some extent from her own tissues, but with the result that the mother is depleted and the infant is not adequately nourished. Pregnancy in teen-age girls presents a situation of particular stress, because the needs of the developing infant are superimposed on the mother's own needs for adequate growth and development. Maternal and infant complications occur about twice as frequently among early teen-age mothers as among mature women. Pregnancy hazards are also greater in American nonwhite populations than in white, and in women from lower socioeconomic groups.[1]

A young woman who has good food habits and is well nourished when she becomes pregnant has little cause for concern. She will need to alter her diet only by increasing intake of some of the foods she is accustomed to eating. Unfortunately, too many young women have not formed good food habits and thus enter pregnancy in a poorly nourished condition. Any borderline deficiency may become apparent at this time. If previous intake of iron or folacin has been low, anemia may develop during pregnancy, because of the extra demands of the fetus. In goitrous regions, pregnancy is one of the situations in which latent iodine deficiency is likely to be manifested by enlargement of the thyroid gland.

Nutritional Status of Women of Child-Bearing Age

In the United States, the prevalence of adolescent females (ages 11 to 16 years) with nutrient intakes below standards increases with age, and those in the lowest socioeconomic group tend to have lower nutrient intakes than others.[2] Obesity is common in young women, although less so than among older women. Being fat or being anxious about keeping slim leads to chronic self-imposed dieting that may further lower body stores of essential nutrients. Fat women are at least as likely to be poorly nourished as slender women. In the United States, this is especially true in poverty groups. A combination of being unemployed, having no access to recreational sports, and operating on a limited food budget easily leads to consumption of too much cheap, filling food of poor nutritive value. Just when a woman needs to be well nourished, at the time of conception, she is quite likely to be in a poor or marginal state. From the moment of fertilization to the time when the placenta is fully developed, at about 8 weeks, the embryo receives its nutrition mainly from nutrients present in the uterine tissues and secretions. Thus, the prior nutritional status of the mother, as reflected in these tissues, is especially important during this early period, when most of the organs are being formed in the fetus.

After menarche, monthly blood loss increases the need for iron. Iron lost in menstrual flow averages 15 to 30 mg., or 0.5 to 1.0 mg per day over the monthly cycle. Because only 10 to 20 percent of dietary iron is absorbed, iron intake should be increased by 5 to 10 mg per day after menarche, yet older girls and women usually take less iron in the diet than do boys and men. Folacin status is also unsatisfactory in many women, including those who are affluent.[3] This important B vitamin is low in many diets and is very commonly omitted from vitamin pills, so the frequency of folacin deficiency is perhaps not surprising. Diets of people living in poverty and those of people eating little or no animal foods are low or deficient in vitamin B-12. Thus, anemia and undesirably low iron stores are common in women on a worldwide basis (Fig. 20–1). The situation becomes worse during pregnancy when the maternal blood volume must expand and the placenta must be supplied to support the fetus.

In all age and economic groups, dietary histories indicate unsatisfactory intakes of calcium, iron, and vitamin A, and often of B vitamins, vitamin C, and iodine. It is likely that intake of the lesser known nutrients, such as zinc and copper, is also low, but this point has not been well studied. Previous use of oral contraceptive pills may have increased the need for vitamin B-6 and, in some cases, folacin; or the presence of an intrauterine contraceptive device may have led to large monthly losses of blood. Normal or increased needs coupled with poor diets lead inevitably to an undesirable state of nutrition.

Effect of Malnutrition on the Outcome of Pregnancy

An undernourished mother may still be able to produce a healthy child, though there is evidence that a larger percentage of babies in poor condition are born to groups of mothers who were in poor nutritional condition. Illustrative evidence that the nutritional condition of the mother during pregnancy frequently influences not only her own health but also the well-being of her child comes from investigations in Canada[4, 5] and the United States,[6] among others.[1] In each case, pregnant women from low-income groups were studied during the later months of pregnancy, and for some time after birth of the children. At the Boston Lying-In Hospital, 216 women attending the prenatal clinic were classified according to whether their diets were considered good, fair, or poor. No attempt was made to influence the diet, and records were kept of condition of mother and baby at and after delivery. Mothers in the poorest diet group had more complications and difficult types of delivery; moreover, all the stillborn babies and all but one of those who were premature or died soon after birth were born to mothers in this group. Conversely, a higher proportion of babies whose condition was rated at birth as superior or good were born to mothers who had had good or excellent diets during pregnancy (see Fig. 20–2). In the Toronto studies, the women in one group, whose diets were poor, received supplementary food. Those in another group had self-chosen diets but were trained in food selection. Those in the third group were given neither food nor instruction and served as controls. Those who received supplementary food had better health, both before and after delivery, fewer com-

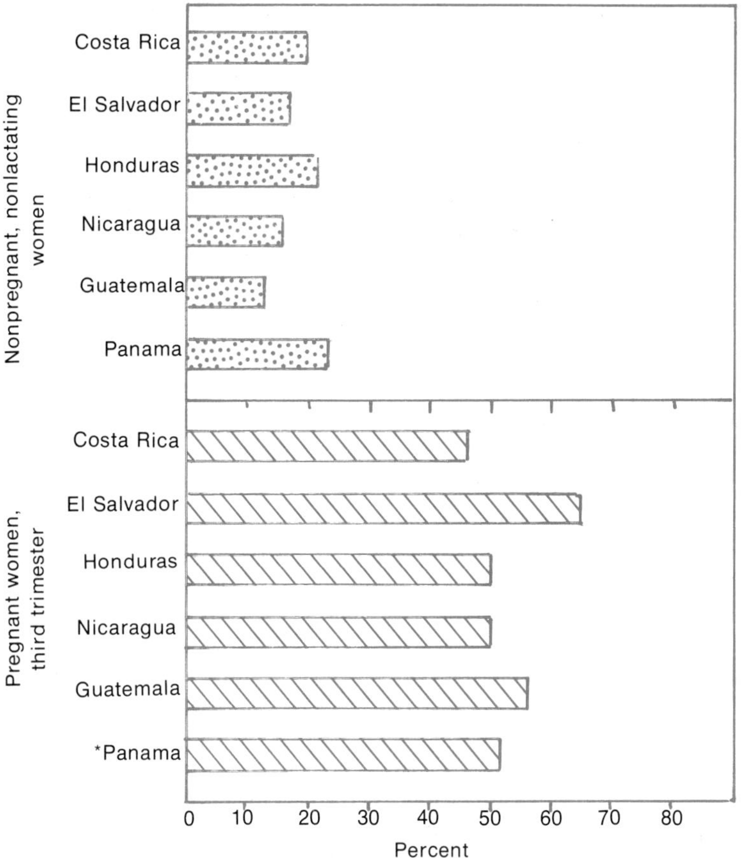

Figure 20–1 Percent of pregnant women with deficient transferrin saturation (< 15 percent), in Central America and Panama (1965–1966). (From Arroyave, G.: Nutrition in pregnancy. Arch. Latinoam. Nutricion. *26*:129, 1976.)

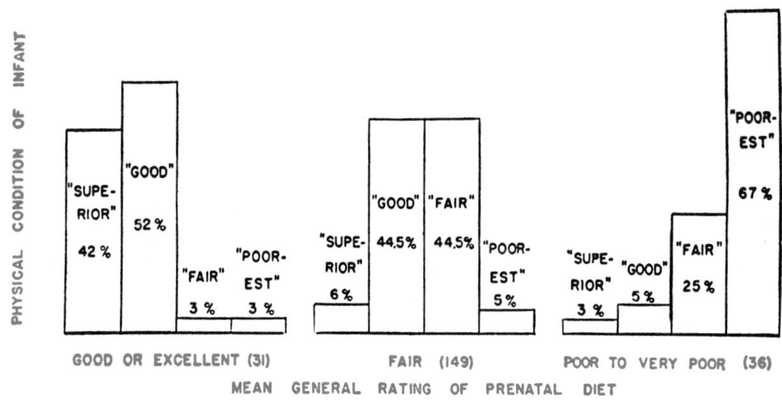

Figure 20–2 Influence of nutrition on condition of the infant during pregnancy, at birth, and in the first two weeks of life. Note the high relative proportion of infants in superior or good physical condition born to mothers whose diet was rated as good or excellent, and the relatively large numbers of babies in fair or poorest condition in the group of mothers whose diet was rated as poor to very poor. (Courtesy of B. S. Burke and the *Journal of Nutrition.*)

plications at delivery, and fewer miscarriages, stillbirths, or premature deliveries, than the mothers who ate poor diets during pregnancy. More recently, Higgins,[5] working with a low-income population at the Montreal Diet Dispensary, has confirmed and extended these observations. The women enrolled there are given dietary advice, encouragement, and food assistance if needed, and they have an average increase of 500 kcal (to 2800 kcal per day) and 30 gm of protein (to 100 gm per day) in the daily diet. Superior birth weights are achieved, and obstetrical performance is better than the average of the hospital in which they are delivered and the province of Quebec as a whole. Beneficial effects of food supplements have also been reported from India[7] and Guatemala.[8] These studies offer evidence of a direct relationship between quality of the prenatal diet and welfare of both mother and child.

Studies made in Europe following severe food restriction during the war years show disasters in reproduction — premature births, stillborn infants, infants below normal weight, and high neonatal death rate. In the Netherlands, food available to pregnant women provided on the average 1925 kcal and 61 gm of protein in 1944; by the spring of 1945, these allowances had fallen to 800 kcal and 35 gm of protein. About 50 percent of women become infertile, and there is an indication that the women who became pregnant were the better nourished. Birth weights of infants were decreased, but rose after relief feeding.[9] The situation was much worse during the siege of Leningrad, where the principal food available was rye bread of very poor quality. The total daily allowance for a working man was 300 to 350 gm of bread. At the height of the seige, the stillbirth rate rose to 56 percent, and the incidence of prematurity was 40 percent. Birth weights were low and infant mortality was high. These women were stressed in many ways, but poor nutrition is thought to have been a dominant factor in the poor outcomes of pregnancy. Ample supportive evidence is available from animal studies in which poor diets were consumed during pregancy.[1] Not only do restricted laboratory and farm animals bear undersized young, but under severe conditions there is permanent stunting of growth and poor intellectual development.

Protein appears to be particulary important in animal studies. Human experience is more difficult to evaluate because when protein intake is low, the diet is also low in energy and usually lacking in other nutrients. In the United States, Dieckman[11] showed that there was an increased incidence of abortion when mothers were on a low-protein intake and, on the positive side, that the number of infants born in excellent condition increased steadily as the protein intake of the mothers was on a progressively higher level. Burke and her associates also found a positive relationship between maternal protein intake (up to 90 gm per day) and infant weight, length, and physical well-being.[12] Adequate energy intake is important, to guarantee that protein is well utilized, and little benefit would be anticipated from adding protein to diets without correction of a limiting energy deficit first. Usually what is needed is a greater total intake of nutritious foods.

Other investigators have failed to find a relationship between the nutrient content of self-selected diets and the quality of pregnancy.[13-15] In some studies the entire population appears to have been reasonably well-nourished, so differences due to minor variations in diet would not have been expected. The diet was poor in one Indian study, which has led to the totally unsupported suggestion that when diets have been poor for generations, adaptive mechanisms may be developed that make for more efficient utilization of nutrients.[15]

In experimental animals, deficiency of specific nutrients at specific stages of fetal development causes malformation or loss of the fetus (see Chapters 5, 7, 8, and 12). Although there is no reason to believe that the same influences could not be manifest in the human fetus, such clear-cut effects have not been demonstrated in population studies. However, birth of deformed infants has occurred following the administration of folacin antagonists to pregnant women with cancer,[16] similar to the experiences in laboratory animals (see Chapter 8). This evidence is sufficiently persuasive to emphasize that *pregnant women should adhere to a well-balanced diet composed of a wide variety of foods.*

Pregnancy is also a time to avoid nonnutritious substances in foods and to forego the use of tobacco and drugs. A characteristic pattern of malformation (small head size, subnormal mentality, facial abnormalities, growth deficiency) has been reported with increasing frequency in babies born to women who drink heavily,[17] and smoking is associated with low birth weights.

PREGNANCY

How the Child is Nourished

There is no direct connection, either nervous or circulatory, between the mother and the fetus, but interchange between the blood streams of mother and child takes place through the placenta (Fig. 20–3). This is a vascular organ on the inner surface of the uterus, in which the blood from the mother and the fetus are brought closely together so that interchange of constituents from one to the other is possible. Thus, the fetal blood takes up nutrients in the simple forms in which they are carried in the mother's blood and carries them to the fetus (through the umbilical cord), where they are built into the more complex substances needed to form the organs, muscles, and other tissues of the child.

Different Stages of Pregnancy

During the first trimester of pregnancy, the daily need of materials for the growth of the fetus is so small as to be practically negligible, but the maternal tissues begin to undergo changes that impose some demands. The mother should eat just what any women should who wishes to preserve or build up her health and vitality. However, this is the period during which many women experience nausea or digestive disturbances. Nausea in early pregnancy is due usually to adjustments in establishing relationships between the fetus and the mother, not primarily due to misfunctioning of the digestive tract itself, and it should soon disappear. Food may be better tolerated in smaller meals at shorter intervals. Eating a few salted crackers before rising may help and certainly will do no harm. If vomiting is severe and prolonged, medical attention is advisable. In spite of optimistic claims, there is no clear evidence that administration of vitamins alleviates the nausea of early pregnancy in the well-nourished patient. In fact, some vitamin-mineral supplements are not well tolerated, and *if prescribed,* these should be taken with, or immediately after, meals.

By the beginning of the *second trimester of pregnancy,* the appetite and digestive abilities of the mother should be normal. The National Research Council recommends increased allowances for almost all the essential nutrients during pregnancy. These recommended allowances, as well as those of the Canadian Department of National Health and Welfare, are found in Table 20–1, contrasted with those of a young, moderately active nonpregnant woman. Some of the extra nutrients allowed are for the building of tissues in the child, and some are intended for the protection of the mother's own tissues. In the early part of pregnancy, the fetus gains hardly more than 1 gm of weight per day. Maternal tissues are growing during this time. The uterus and breasts enlarge, the placenta and amniotic fluid are formed, and the maternal blood volume expands. During the second trimester, the mother stores a substantial amount of fat, which provides a safety factor for the fetus

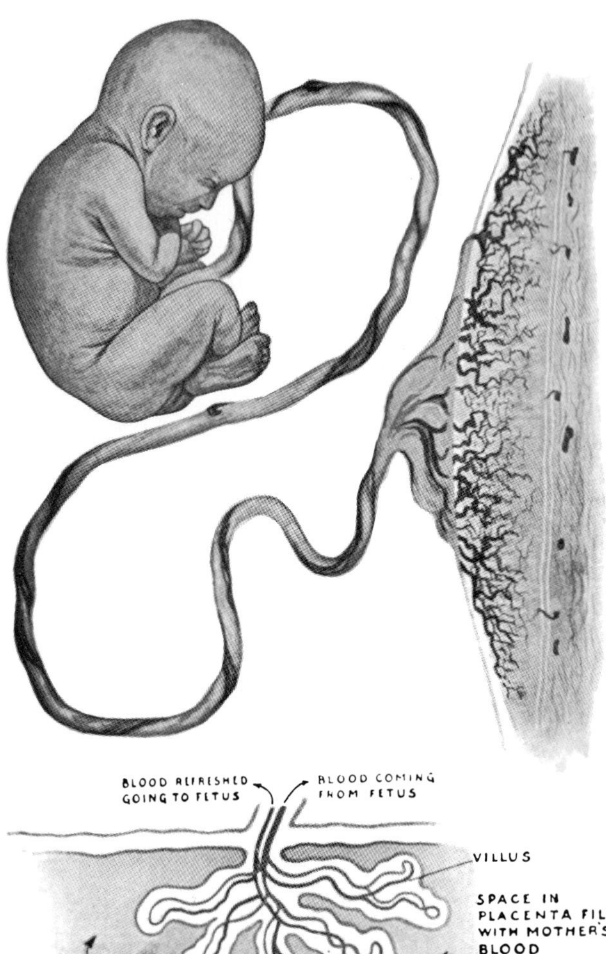

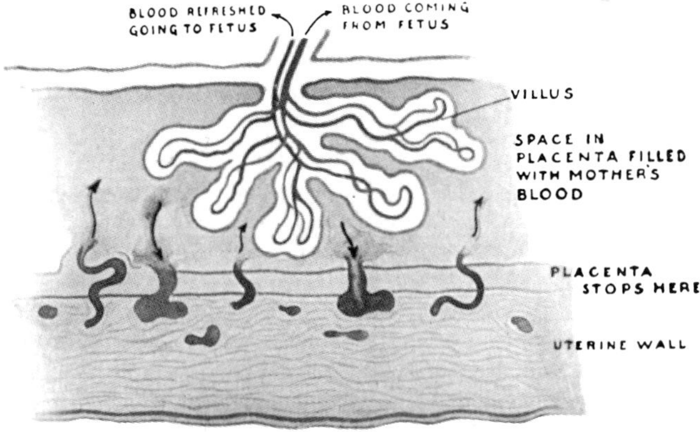

Figure 20–3 Diagram showing relations of maternal and fetal circulations. **Top,** The fetus is connected by the umbilical cord to the placenta, which in turn is attached to the wall of the uterus. **Bottom,** Detail of the fetal and maternal blood vessels in the placenta, with small vessels from and to the fetus immersed in a space filled with the mother's blood. (From Davis and Sheckler: *DeLee's Obstetrics for Nurses.*)

against possible maternal food deprivation and constitutes a physiological reserve energy supply for lactation later. By the sixth month the fetus is gaining about 10 gm daily, but about half the total weight increase of the fetus during gestation occurs in the last 2 months. Therefore, during the final months of pregnancy it is especially important that the diet be unusually rich in all the nutritive factors needed for the growing child. The extra energy needs should be met in the form of foods that also provide high-quality proteins, minerals, and vitamins.

The extra energy allowance suggested by the NRC is not large (300 kcal or 1.26 MJ per day). The energy value of new tissue formed in pregnancy is about 50,000 kcal, of which a substantial portion is maternal fat. The basal metabolic rate is increased, owing to the energy requirement of fetal and supporting tissues and the added burden on the maternal heart and lungs (Table 20–2). The total energy cost of a pregnancy is about 80,000 kcal of metabolizable energy, or 285 kcal per day for the 280 days of gestation. The FAO/WHO and United States standards

Table 20–1 DIETARY ALLOWANCES FOR WOMEN*

	United States			*Canada*		
Nutritive Factors	Nonpregnant (58 kg)	During Pregnancy	During Lactation	Nonpregnant (56 kg)	During Pregnancy	During Lactation
Energy, kcal	2000	2300	2500	2100	2400	2600
Protein, gm	46	76	66	41	61	65
Calcium, gm	0.8	1.2	1.2	0.7	1.2	1.2
Phosphorus, gm	0.8	1.2	1.2	0.7	1.2	1.2
Magnesium, mg	300	450	450	250	275	325
Iodine, mcg	100	125	150	110	125	135
Iron, mg	18	18	18	14	15	15
Zinc, mg	15	20	25	9	12	16
Vitamin A, IU	4000	5000	6000	4400†	4900†	6600†
Thiamin, mg	1.0	1.3	1.3	1.1	1.3	1.5
Riboflavin, mg	1.2	1.5	1.7	1.3	1.6	1.9
Niacin (equivalent) mg	13	15	17	14	16	21
Folacin, mg	0.4	0.8	0.6	0.20‡	0.25‡	0.25‡
Vitamin B-6, mg	2.0	2.5	2.5	1.5	2.0	2.1
Vitamin B-12, mcg	3	4	4	3.0	4.0	3.5
Vitamin C, mg	45	60	80	30	50	60
Vitamin D, IU	–	400	400	100	100	100
Vitamin E, IU	12	15	15	6.6	7.7	8.8

*U.S. National Research Council: *Recommended Dietary Allowances*. 8th Ed., 1974; Canadian Dept. of National Health and Welfare: *Dietary Standard* for Canada, 1975.

†Canadian Standard for vitamin A is given as retinol equivalents (RE): 800 for nonpregnant women, with 100 added during pregnancy and 400 during lactation. The composition of the Canadian diet (Table 9 of the publication) indicates an approximate equivalence of 5.47 IU per RE. For further discussion of equivalency, See Chapter 7.

‡Free folacin.

Table 20–2 ENERGY COST OF VARIOUS ACTIVITIES DURING PREGNANCY AND POSTPARTUM*

Activity	*Energy Cost*†			
	20–28 Weeks	29–36 Weeks	37–40 Weeks	Post-partum
Mature women:		←*calories/kg/min*→		
basal metabolic rate	15	15	15	12
quiet sitting	17	17	17	15
quiet standing	19	19	19	18
work involving upper torso	–	–	28	–
walking, 3.0 mph, 0° grade	64	67	62	61
bicycling, 300 kpm.	61	62	62	61
personal care, eating, child care, child feeding	26	26	26	26
typing and office work	29	29	29	26
driving car	32	32	32	29
housecleaning	46	46	46	46
gardening	64	64	–	–
shopping	–	–	–	62
swimming	–	91	–	–
			Last Trimester	***Postpartum***
Teen-agers:				
basal metabolic rate			16	16
knitting			20	20
combing hair			24	22
cooking			28	26
dishwashing			28	23
sweeping			44	43
climbing stairs			44	60
making beds			48	47
walking stairs with load			73	85

*From Blackburn, M. W., and Calloway, D. H.: J. Amer. Dietet. Assoc., *69*:29, 1976.

†Note that the values are given in small calories. To convert to kcal, divide by 1000. For example, the basal rate of a reference woman who weighs 70 kg (58 kg nonpregnant + 12 kg gain) at 37 to 40 weeks is (15 × 60 × 24) (70) ÷ 1000, or 1512 kcal/day.

allow for this full amount. Previously, the National Research Council RDA was set lower on the basis of the observation that women in the later months of pregnancy are often not very active physically. However, the RDA for nonpregnant women assumes that there is only light activity, and it is now recognized that pregnant women cannot be appreciably less active in ordinary households. If the woman is active, and she should be to maintain fitness, her needs will be great because of the higher energy cost of moving a heavier, awkward body mass. Many women continue working and exercising much as before pregnancy until very near term, and their needs consequently will be large. The additional energy allowance should be adjusted to the needs of the individual, so that the energy costs of building new tissues, of higher metabolic rate (in the fetus), and of physical workload are met. In a University of California study, mature women were found to require 2300 kcal per day in midpregnancy, but about 2500–2600 kcal per day in the last 10 weeks.[18] Women in active occupations or with young children in the household had higher needs of 40–45 kcal per kg of pregnant body weight, in contrast to the minimum 36 kcal per kg recommended by the NRC. Pregnancies involving twins also impose much greater demands.

A normal and desirable weight gain during the 40 weeks of pregnancy is 24 to 28 pounds (12.5 kg) (Fig. 20–4). Maternal

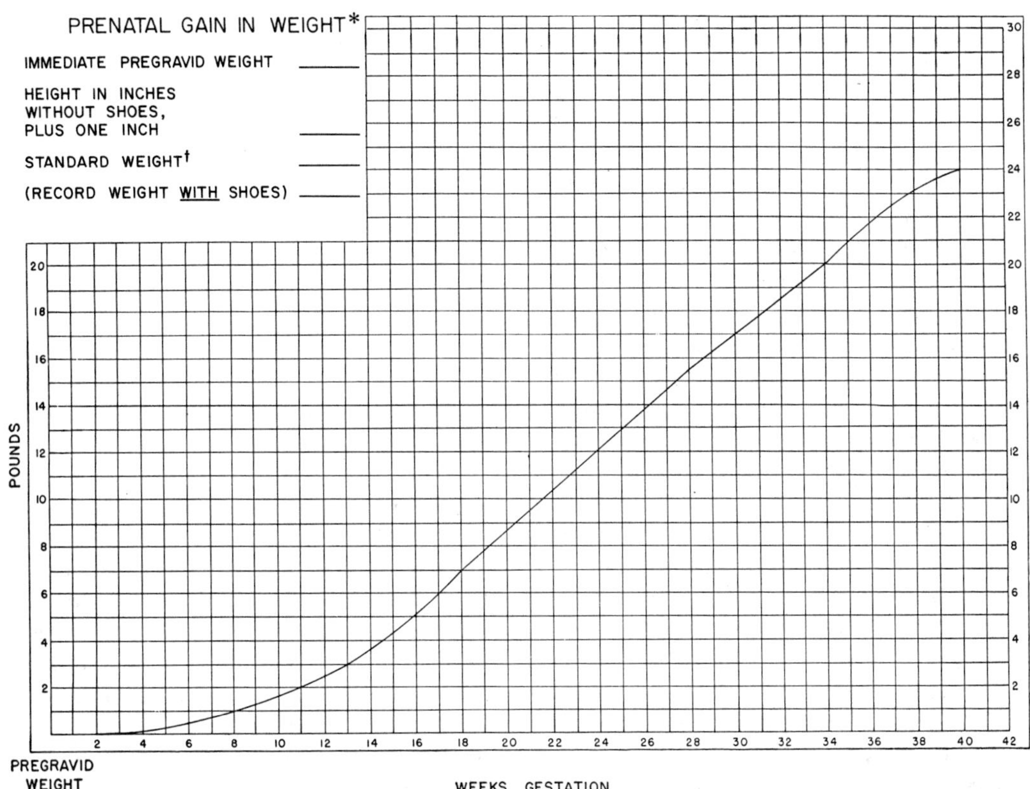

Figure 20–4 Desirable prenatal gain in weight.

*Reprinted with permission from Lull, C., and Kimbrough, R.: *Clinical Obstetrics.* Philadelphia, J. B. Lippincott Company, 1953.

†From Metropolitan Life Insurance Company Actuarial Tables, 1959, and adjusted to comply with instructions appearing on the Gain in Weight Grid, namely: height in inches without shoes plus 1 inch to establish a standard for heels. Standard weights are:

4′-10″ = 104	5′- 5″ = 128
4′-11″ = 107	5′- 6″ = 132
5′- 0″ = 110	5′- 7″ = 136
5′- 1″ = 113	5′- 8″ = 140
5′- 2″ = 116	5′- 9″ = 144
5′- 3″ = 118	5′-10″ = 148
5′- 4″ = 123	5′-11″ = 152

Women should be weighed with shoes as normally worn. The weights are for medium body build and, except for extreme body build deviations, these figures should be used.

For example, a woman whose height, measured without shoes, is 5 feet 4 inches would have 1 inch added; therefore, her standard weight for height would be 128 pounds.

Ranges are not acceptable in estimating standard weight, since this is an objective observation and represents the midpoint. This midpoint must be used for recording purposes.

For women under 25, 1 pound should be deducted for each year.

complications are more frequently associated with marked over- or underweight at the time of conception and with wide deviation from normal *rate* of weight gain during pregnancy. Some studies have suggested an increased incidence of toxemia* in obese pregnant women, but others have not. Large early weight gain has also been regarded as a bad omen of maternal complications. This fear has led to excessive concern with weight gain, especially in the obese woman. With family planning, the obese woman can lose weight prior to pregnancy, but while she is pregnant she should *not* attempt to correct the preexisting condition. If there is a tendency to excessive weight gain, it is far wiser to increase physical activity than to restrict food intake.

Many slender women will need to gain more than the average 25 pounds. A study of 10,000 births showed that higher maternal weight gain was related to higher birth weight, a lower incidence of prematurity, and better growth and performance during the infant's first year of life.[19] The key consideration is that healthy tissue be formed at a smooth progressive rate, irrespective of the total gain, and that the mother's health remain good. Some suggest that the weight gain may be spaced at about 4, 10, and 10 pounds in each of three trimesters, but healthy women vary widely in this regard. Women carrying twins will gain about twice as much as those with single babies.

A Healthy Diet During Pregnancy

The nutritive needs during pregnancy are best met by a simple, wholesome diet, the basis of which is cheese, milk, eggs, meat, legumes, nuts, whole grains, vegetables, especially the dark green, leafy ones, and fruits. If the diet consumed before pregnancy was adequate, only simple modification is required to meet all additional nutrient allowances. Addition of two glasses of milk or cheese equivalent, one egg or larger amounts of fish, poultry, or legumes and one serving of dark green, leafy vegetables, with frequent substitution of fruit for rich dessert and organ meats for other meat, fish, or poultry, is sufficient. In general, the more fruits and vegetables eaten the better, because these foods help to ensure the surplus of vitamins and minerals that is so very advantageous, without appreciably increasing energy intake.

The nutritional recommendations for pregnancy that are most difficult to meet are those for iron, zinc, folacin, and calcium. A diet that meets the allowances for these four nutrients *from food sources* will provide much more protein than the specified RDA and will meet other requirements, as well. The daily diet during pregnancy should be built around the following foods, in regard to types and amounts of foods daily:

Milk: 1 quart of whole or skimmed milk or yogurt.

Milk powder or canned milk may be substituted either as beverage or in cooking: 1½ oz (45 gm) of cheddar cheese may be substituted for one glass of milk. Alternative sources of calcium are discussed in the preceding chapter.

Meat: Eight oz (250 mg) cooked weight of meat, fish, or poultry. Weekly use of liver is desirable. Eggs, cheese, dry legumes (beans, peas, lentils), and nuts may be substituted with cautions as noted in the preceding chapter.

Vegetables and Fruits: Four large servings.

At least one serving should be a dark green, leafy vegetable. One serving should be a vegetable or fruit high in vitamin C content, such as green or red peppers, a citrus variety of fruit (orange, lemon, lime, grapefruit), papaya, melon, cabbage, or tomato.

Breads and cereals: Four slices of whole-grain bread.

Cereal, ½ to ⅔ cooked, may be substituted

*Toxemia usually refers to a condition of blood poisoning that results from growth of microorganisms in the tissues or blood or from the absorption of noxious materials from food and water, or both. Toxemia of pregnancy differs and is a disorder of unidentified cause that is characterized by high blood pressure, protein in the urine, edema, headache, visual disturbances, and, in severe cases, convulsions and death.

for one slice of bread. Potatoes and whole-grain or enriched rice, corn meal, macaroni, spaghetti, barley, or wheat (bulgur) may also be used. Ready-to-eat cereal should be made from whole grain or have added bran or germ. Additional servings from this food group should be taken as required to meet energy needs.

Fat: 2 tbsp of butter, margarine, or vegetable oil. If whole milk or milk products are used, 1 tbsp of vegetable oil may be sufficient, depending on energy needs.

Vitamin D: 400 IU from fortified milk or dietary supplement.

Fluid whole milk, canned evaporated milk, and some dry and skimmed milks are fortified with vitamin D at the level of 400 IU per quart. Some milk powder is not fortified, nor are cheese and ice cream. Package labels specify the addition of vitamin D.

Iodine: Iodized salt should be used in cooking and at the table. The normal intake of salt should be maintained throughout pregnancy.

It is difficult to assure adequate intakes of calcium and iron if a strict vegetarian ("vegan") diet is followed during pregnancy, and there is the further complication of the relatively poor absorption of iron, zinc, and possibly other trace elements from plant sources. Such diets are lacking in vitamin B-12, and supplementation is *mandatory* to prevent damage to the central nervous system of the infant. A more liberal vegetarian diet that includes milk and eggs and perhaps fish can meet the RDA if good selections are made from the food groups listed. The woman should supplement these foods to furnish energy sufficient for her individual needs and desired weight gain, either by taking more of some foods just listed or other foods of her choice. The *energy needs vary* with weight and especially with degree of activitiy, so the calorie allowance should be estimated individually, then increased in the second trimester of pregnancy by about 300 kcal. A moderately active 58 kg woman (as listed in first column of Table 20–1) who needs 2000 kcal normally should have 2300 kcal or more in the latter part of pregnancy. But an active woman whose ordinary daily energy need is about 2400 kcal requires at least 2700 kcal in late pregnancy. Also, a woman who begins pregnancy in an undernourished condition may need a more liberal energy allowance in order to gain some weight. Teenagers must add the pregnancy allowance to the higher energy values recommended for nonpregnant girls of the same level of maturity.

A woman who is overweight when she becomes pregnant will need to keep her physical activity level high, or increase it, in order not to add to her obesity. The diet should not be too restrictive, i.e., not below 36 kcal per kg of ideal pregnant body weight. Foods containing large amounts of sugar, starch, and fats should be the ones eliminated, rather than the more nutritious foods; skim milk, for example, may be substituted for whole milk.

Enough energy must be supplied so that there will be no need to burn protein merely as fuel. Obviously, all the essential amino acids are required for fetal growth, so it is advisable that about half the protein in the diet should be from foods of animal origin (milk, meats, eggs).

Extra *calcium* for the mother during pregnancy (and lactation) goes far toward insuring teeth of good quality and well-calcified bones in the child. The teeth of the child are formed and in large part calcified during the latter half of fetal life and the first few months after birth. About 20 gm of calcium is present in the body of a full-term infant, which means that the mother must supply 80 mg of *absorbed* calcium every day of pregnancy. If the diet is adequate, calcium is also stored in the maternal skeleton during pregnancy, another physiological adaptation to the needs of lactation.

If the mother's diet is rich in *iron* and *copper* during pregnancy, the child will be born with a liver well stored with these trace elements, often a reserve sufficient to last through the months when it will be fed chiefly milk — a food of low iron and copper content. The newborn infant has about 0.2 to 0.3 gm of iron in his body, and another 0.5 gm is present in the placenta and extramaternal tissues. The average woman has about 0.3 gm of storage iron, and another 150 mg will be spared because she is not menstruating. This is only about half the amount needed even if maternal stores were to be totally depleted. Unless the diet is rich in iron, the baby will be born without a good iron reserve, and the woman will become anemic. In accordance with our present state of knowledge, routine supplementation of the diet with salts of trace elements other than iron is not recommended. We know that the *balance* of trace elements is important, not just the amount of each one, and information regarding many of the micronutrients is quite incomplete. The safest course is to eat well. However, supplementary iron is often prescribed, and if it is, a supplement of 15 mg per day should be ample. A folacin supplement may also be needed; 0.3 to 0.4 mg will meet the additional allowance for pregnancy.

Women are sometimes advised to restrict their salt intake when their weight gain is judged excessive and they are accumulating tissue fluid. Some gain in blood volume, and other extracellular fluid is perfectly normal under the hormonal influences of pregnancy. Salt is a dietary essential, and neither maternal nor fetal tissues can be maintained satisfactorily without it.[20-22] The association of sodium, edema, and hypertension (Chapter 10) led to the practice of salt restriction as a medical measure in threatened toxemia, but a careful study by Robinson[22] of over 2000 women showed that there were fewer complications in the group instructed to take more salt than in the one told to restrict it.

If digestion is upset or if there is difficulty in taking enough food, the regular meals may be reduced in size and extra nourishment given between meals in the form of easily tolerated foods, such as milk, eggnog, malted milk, cereal gruels, crackers, fruit, or fruit juice. If preferred, much of the milk may be taken in dishes, such as cream soups and custards. Meals may easily be made to fit into the family schedule, if foods for the family are wisely chosen — that is, planned to be of high nutritive value and cooked simply.

The extra allowances of all the essential nutrients recommended for pregnancy are a protection for both mother and child. They provide an abundance of building materials for growth and development of the infant without any need to deplete the stores of these substances in the mother's body; and in the baby they help to build reserves of such nutrients as can be stored before birth.

LACTATION

Most Nutritive Requirements of Nursing Mother Higher Than for Pregnant Woman

During lactation, there is increased need for energy, protein, minerals, and vitamins: (1) to cover the amounts secreted in the milk for nourishment of the infant, (2) to cover the cost of secreting the milk, and (3) to protect the mother's body (Table 20–1). Energy requirement varies with the amount of milk produced, and intake must be regulated to the individual woman. A woman who is meeting all the needs of a 5 kg infant (11 pounds) must secrete about 850 ml of milk, providing about 600 kcal daily. Human milk is produced with about 80 percent efficiency, so the requirement for lactation is about 750 kcal per day. If the woman has gained properly during pregnancy, about one-third of the extra need can be met from body fat reserves over a 100 day period of lactation. Thus, the RDA is an extra 500 kcal. If the period of lactation extends beyond 3 months, as it should ideally, then energy intake should be increased to the full amount required.

These recommendations accord with the experience of lactating women. A study[23] compared Scottish women who were breast-feeding their infants with those who gave bottle feedings, in terms of energy intake, physical activity level, and loss of body fat. Energy intakes of the two groups were 2716 and 2125 kcal, respectively; both were losing weight and the lactating women negligibly more. Energy available for milk formation was 618 kcal per day, and the calculated energy content of milk was 597 kcal. Body weights of lactating and nonlactating women have been found to be the same 8 to 12 weeks postpartum in recent studies[18, 24] but reported energy intakes of the lactating women were higher by 600 to 900 kcal per day. Thus, an adequate fat reserve is a real benefit during the first few weeks post partum when a mother is physically active and short on sleep and her food intake does not keep up with her needs. Body weight will be normalized without need for special effort at slimming, and the woman who carries through the whole of the reproductive cycle should not become fatter with each pregnancy. There is evidence that lactation performance can be maintained in spite of what appear to be inadequate intakes of energy,[25] sufficient to support low normal infant weights. However, the diet always should be of good quality to prevent depletion of the maternal lean tissues and to guarantee adequate content of vitamins and trace minerals in the milk.

Human milk contains about 12 gm of protein per liter. In arriving at the recommended allowance of an additional 20 gm of protein per day during lactation, the National Research Council has assumed that the dietary protein is of lower quality than milk protein so that conversion is not 100 percent efficient, and that milk production may exceed 1 liter per day. Successful lactation is achieved on lower protein intakes, but there is no clear evidence that this is not detrimental to the mother. The essential amino acids incorporated in milk proteins must be furnished liberally, so it is advisable to obtain the extra protein allowance from high-quality sources. The lipid composition of breast milk is affected by diet, and the milk will be richer in essential fatty acids if the maternal diet contains a liberal amount of polyunsaturated fats.[26]

Because milk is so high in calcium and phosphorus content, its secretion makes great demands for these mineral elements. If a mother increases her own milk intake by the amount she is providing to her child (an additional 1 pint to 1 quart daily), she will meet the high calcium needs, as well as the need for some other nutrients. Nursing mothers are often found to be in negative calcium and phosphorus balance. This causes a drain on the mother's body, but it does not affect milk secretion. The vitamin content of human milk, especially the water-soluble vitamins, is largely dependent on the vitamin intake of the mother. Lactation, like pregnancy, is a period when borderline nutritional status may develop into frank deficiency. Allowances recommended for vitamins are about 50 percent more than those for nonpregnant women. Relatively little iron is secreted in milk (0.5 to 1.0 mg per day), and lactating women usually do not menstruate, so there is no added allowance for iron in lactation. Vitamin D (400 IU) in supplementary form is needed to ensure good utilization of calcium and phosphorus. The high allowances of various nutrients recommended during lactation may be seen by consulting Table 20–1.

Diet for Nursing Mothers

Recommendations for the diet in the nursing period are almost identical with those given for pregnancy, except that the need for almost all nutritive essentials is greater during lactation, especially as the infant grows and takes larger quantities of milk. The *quality* of the diet required remains essentially the same — a diet contaning liberal amounts of milk, eggs, fruits, and vegetables to furnish the extra protein, mineral salts, and vitamins needed.

Milk is the best food for protecting

the mother's bones and teeth against any drain on calcium and phosphorus reserves to supply these elements in her milk. At least 1 quart of milk should be taken daily, or its equivalent in cheese or yogurt. If a woman cannot or will not use dairy products, then alternative calcium sources must be included. It is a good thing to take supplementary nourishment just before nursing the baby in the middle of the morning and afternoon, and at bedtime. It is essential to have a plentiful intake of **fluids** (2 to 3 quarts from all sources) to provide the water in the milk secreted, in addition to that needed by the mother. Fruit and vegetable juices are useful to give added fluids, as well as vitamins and minerals.

Many constituents other than nutrients are passed into milk. Excessive use of alcohol and artificially sweetened products is to be avoided during nursing periods for this reason. Drugs, including those sold without prescription, such as aspirin, laxatives, and sedatives, pass into the milk and should be taken only on the advice of a physician. Oral contraceptive agents are thought to affect lactation adversely, but injected preparations have been used with no detected detriment.[27]

Technique of Breast-feeding

During the latter weeks of pregnancy, the mother should use extra care in cleansing the nipples, preferably without soap, and massage them as needed to assure protractility. The breasts should be mechanically supported by a well-fitting garment. Following delivery, the infant should be offered breast feeding as early and at as frequent intervals as possible, using both breasts. It is important that the infant receive the first flow (colostrum), as it contains much of the immune substances. The infant should not be given supplementary feedings because they decrease the appetite and vigor of sucking. If there is difficulty in the beginning, boiled water should be given from a spoon. When lactation is established, the baby should be suckled from alternate breasts at each feeding, or from both breasts if milk flow is light.

Advantages of Breast-Feeding

In addition to the warmth, closeness, and emotional satisfaction of breast-feeding for both mother and child, human milk for human infants is clearly superior to other kinds of milk (see Fig. 20–5).

Breast milk provides immune substances made by the mother that help the infant to resist infection during the early months of life, and use of breast milk favors the development of desirable strains of bacteria in the intestinal tract of the newborn. Furthermore, human milk is specially adapted for providing all nutrients needed in the right proportions for the rate of growth normal for infants and in forms easily handled by the baby's digestive tract. Cow's milk is designed for the calf, which should double its birth weight in about a third of the time that it takes an infant to do so. Therefore, cow's milk is more concentrated in certain building materials. The relative composition of human milk and cow's milk is shown in Table 20–3.

Cow's milk contains about three times as much protein per 100 gm as human milk does and is much more concentrated in calcium and phosphorus, while human milk is higher in sugar content. When cow's milk is modified for infant feeding, the protein and inorganic substances are reduced by dilution, and sugar (lactose, cane sugar, or corn syrup) is added to increase the energy value. Such modification makes it suitable for infant feeding but simultaneously dilutes its vitamin and trace mineral content and still does not provide various nutrients in the same relative proportions as in human milk. However, cow's milk formulas, as well as diets based on goat's or mare's milk, have been used successfully for infant feeding for years. When breast-

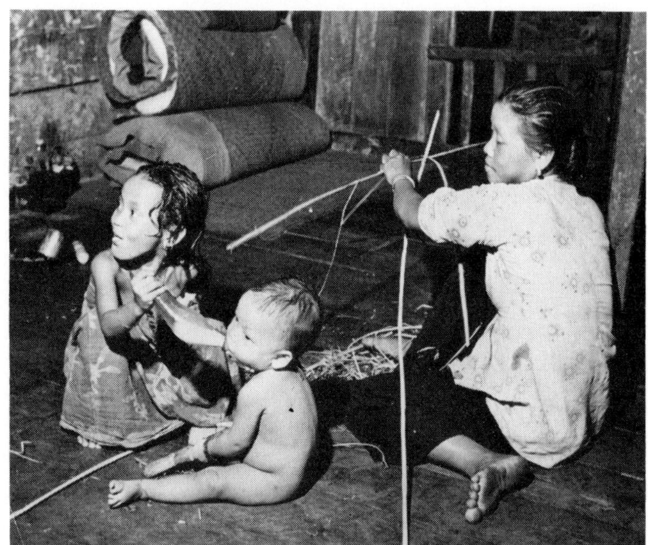

Figure 20–5 Hazards of bottle feeding. The alarming decline in breast-feeding among the low socio-economic urban communities in recent years and its replacement by bottle-feeding with unsatisfactory milk substitutes, prepared and given in the most unhygienic manner, have produced serious health problems. The incidence of malnutrition and gastroenteritis has jumped during the early months of infancy.

The feeding bottle is indeed a dangerous instrument in low socio-economic communities and should be avoided. For supplementary feeding of breast-fed babies the cup and spoon can and should be used. (From *Guide to Family Health,* WHO, 1976.)

feeding is not feasible, pediatricians recommend formulas suited to the infant.

Human milk forms a much finer and more flocculent curd in the stomach than does cow's milk; moreover, cow's milk is liable to become contaminated with bacteria during its handling and storage. Even when boiled cow's milk is given, great care must be taken to have all utensils sterilized and to store the bottles of formula in a cold place. All these difficulties are done away with when the baby is nursed by the mother. The milk is given directly from producer to consumer; the child may take as much as desired, and there is no chance that the formula will not be readily handled by the child's digestive tract.

Table 20–3 NUTRIENTS IN HUMAN AND COW'S MILK*

Nutrient	*Human*	*Cow*
	per 100 grams of milk	
Energy, kcal	77.0	65.0
Protein, gm	1.1	3.5
Fat, gm	4.0	3.5
Carbohydrate, gm	9.5	4.9
Calcium, mg	33.0	118.0
Phosphorus, mg	14.0	93.0
Iron, mg	0.1	Trace
Vitamin C, mg	5.0	1.0

*From Watt, B. K., and Merrill, A. L.: *Composition of Foods.* Agriculture Handbook No. 8 Dec. 1963, p. 39.

Most mothers can nurse their babies adequately, and the advantages certainly warrant serious effort to do so, at least for the first 3 to 6 months of the child's life.

To insure good milk flow, dietary practices should be sound throughout pregnancy, as well as after the birth of the child. Successful nursing demands a quiet, contented life, in which food is intelligently chosen and sunshine, exercise, fresh air, and mental diversion are provided. Anxiety and fatigue are unfavorable to milk production. Breast-feeding should be a happy and rewarding experience for both mother and child.

QUESTIONS AND PROBLEMS

1. Discuss the special problems and energy needs of the different periods of pregnancy. Do the needs for protein, mineral elements, and vitamins differ in early and late pregnancy, and if so, how?

2. By what selection of food groups could the higher energy need of the later months of pregnancy be satisfied and at the same time a diet rich in good quality protein, mineral elements, and vitamins be provided? What food groups should be prominent in the diet during pregnancy?

3. How much weight should be gained in a pregnancy involving a single

child? With twins? What tissues are formed in pregnancy? Is a reserve of body fat advantageous or disadvantageous? Why?

4. Compare the allowances for each of the nutritive factors in late pregnancy with those for a woman who is nursing a baby (see Table 20–1). In what respects do the requirements in lactation differ from those in pregnancy, and why? Why are more calories, protein, calcium, phosphorus, and vitamins needed than are passed on to the baby in the mother's milk? Why do so many women become overweight when nursing a child? What factors in the diet, if taken in plentiful amounts, favor milk secretion? What environmental factors tend to suppress milk secretion?

5. Plan a day's meals for a women in the last 2 months of pregnancy. Calculate the energy and protein in this diet, and compare with the allowances given in Table 20–1 to see if the diet is adequate in these respects. Can you make any suggestions regarding how it might be altered to provide more liberal intake of mineral elements and vitamins? Does the woman need some vitamin D supplement, and why?

6. Plan a day's diet for a nursing mother, and calculate the amount of calcium and vitamin A supplied to see if they are adequate. For meeting the calcium allowance, why are calcium pills not an adequate dietary supplement to use in place of milk? If the diet needs to be improved in these respects, what changes would you suggest?

REFERENCES

1. Committee on Maternal Nutrition, Food and Nutrition Board: *Maternal Nutrition and the Course of Pregnancy.* Washington, D. C., NAS/NRC, 1970.
2. U.S. Dept. of Health, Education, and Welfare: *Ten-State Nutrition Survey, 1968–1970.* Dept. of Health, Education and Welfare Pub. No. (HSM) 72–8133, 1972.
3. Avery, B., and Ledger, W. J.: Folic acid metabolism in well-nourished pregnant women. Obstet. Gynecol., *35*:616, 1970.
4. Ebbs, J. H., Tisdall, F. F., and Scott, W. A.: The influence of prenatal diet on the mother and child. J. Nutr., *22*:515, 1941.
5. Higgins, A. C.: Nutritional status and the outcome of pregnancy. J. Can. Dietet. Assoc., *37*:17, 1976.
6. Burke, B. S. Beal, V. A., Kirkwood, S. B., and Stuart, H. C.: The influence of nutrition during pregnancy upon the condition of the infant at birth. J. Nutr., *25*:569, 1943.
7. Devadas, R. P., Shenbagavalli, P. N., and Vijayalaskshmi, R.: The impact of an applied nutrition programme on the nutritional status of selected expectant women. Ind. J. Nutr. Dietet., *7*:293, 1970.
8. Lechtig, A., et al.: Arch. Latinoam. Nutricion, *2*:101, 117, 1972. (Reviewed in Nutr. Rev., *31*:45, 1973.)
9. Smith. C. A.: The effect of wartime starvation in Holland upon pregnancy and its product. Amer. J. Obstet. Gynecol., *53*:599, 1947; Stein, Z., Susser, M., Saenger, G., and Marolla, F.: *Famine and Human Development: The Dutch Hunger Winter of 1944/45.* New York, Oxford Univ. Press, 1975.
10. Antonov, A. N.: Children born during the siege of Leningrad in 1942. J. Pediatr., *30*:250, 1947.
11. Dieckman, W. J., et al.: Observation on protein intake and the health of mother and baby. I. Clinical and laboratory findings. II. Food intake. J. Amer. Dietet. Assoc., *27*:1046, 1951.
12. Burke, B. S., Harding, V. V., and Stuart, H. C.: Nutrition studies during pregnancy. IV. Relation of protein content of mother's diet during pregnancy to birth length, birth weight, and condition of infant at birth. J. Pediatr., *23*:506, 1943.
13. Thomson, A. M.: Diet in pregnancy. III. Diet in relation to course and outcome of pregnancy. Brit. J. Nutr., *13*:509, 1959.
14. McGanity, W. J., et al.: The Vanderbilt cooperative study of maternal and infant nutrition. VI. Relationship of obstetric performance to nutrition. Amer. J. Obstet. Gynecol., *67*:501, 1954.
15. Bagchi, K., and Bose, A. K.: Effect of low nutrient intake during pregnancy on obstetrical performance and offspring. Amer. J. Clin. Nutr., *11*:586, 1962.
16. Thiersch, J. B.: *Ciba Foundation Symposium on Congential Malformations.* London, 1960, pp. 152–154.
17. Hanson, J. W., Jones, K. L., and Smith, W. D.: Fetal alcohol syndrome: experience with 41 patients. J.A.M.A., *235*:1458, 1976.
18. Blackburn, M. W., and Calloway, D. H.: Energy expenditure and consumption of mature, pregnant, and lactating women, J. Amer. Dietet. Assoc., *69*:29, 1976.
19. Singer, J. E., Westphal, M., and Niswander, K.: Relationship of weight gain during pregnancy to birth weight and infant growth and development in the first year of life. Obstet. Gynecol., *31*:417, 1968.
20. Kirksey, A., and Pike, R. L.: Some effects of high and low sodium intakes during pregnancy in the rat. I. Food consumption, weight gain, reproductive performance, electrolyte balances, plasma total protein and protein fractions in normal pregnancy. J. Nutr., *77*:33, 1962.
21. Palomaki, J. F., and Lindheimer, M. D.: Sodium

depletion simulating deterioration in a toxemic pregnancy. N Engl. J. Med., *282*:88, 1970.

22. Robinson, M.: Salt in pregnancy. Lancet, *1*:178, 1958.
23. Thomson, A. M., Hytten, F. E., and Billewicz, W. Z.: The energy cost of human lactation. Brit. J. Nutr., *24*:565, 1970.
24. Naismith, D. J., and Ritchie, C. D.: The effect of breast-feeding and artificial feeding on body weights, skinfold measurements and food intakes of forty-two primiparous women. Proc. Nutr. Soc., *34*:116A, 1975.
25. Gopalan, C., and Belavady, B.: Nutrition and lactation. Fed. Proc., *20*:177, 1961.
26. Potter, J. M., and Nestel, P. J.: The effects of dietary fatty acids and cholesterol on the milk lipids of lactating women and the plasma cholesterol of breast-fed infants. Amer. J. Clin. Nutr., *29*:54, 1976; Hansen, A. E., et al.: Influence of diet on blood serum lipids in pregnant women and newborn infants. Amer. J. Clin. Nutr., *15*:11, 1964.
27. Pincus, G.: *Control of Fertility*. New York, Academic Press, 1965; Karin, M., et al.: Injected progestogen and lactation. Brit. Med. J., *1*:200, 1971.

SUPPLEMENTARY READING

Adams, S. O., Barr, G. D., and Huenemann, R. L.: Effect of nutritional supplementation on the outcome of pregnancy. J. Amer. Dietet. Assoc., *72*: 144, 1978.

Aitken, F. C., and Hytten, F. E.: Infant feeding: comparison of breast and artificial feeding. Nutr. Abstr. Rev., *104*:341, 1960.

Allen, L. H., and Zeman, F. J.: Influence of increased postnatal nutrient intake on kidney cellular development in progeny of protein-deficient rats. J. Nutr., *103*:929, 1973.

Baker, H., et al.: Vitamin profile of 174 mothers and newborns at parturition. Amer. J. Clin. Nutr., *28*:59, 1975.

Baumslag, N., Edelstein, T., and Metz, J.: Reduction of incidence of prematurity by folic acid supplementation in pregnancy. Brit. Med., J., *1*:16, 1970.

Beal, V. A.: Nutritional studies during pregnancy. J. Amer. Dietet. Assoc., *58*:312, 1971.

Bonnar, J., Goldberg, A., and Smith, J. A.: Do pregnant women take their iron? Lancet, *1*:457, 1969.

Bowering, J., ėt al.: Role of EFNEP aides in improving diets of pregnant women. J. Nutr. Ed., *8*:111, 1976.

Brin. M.: Abnormal tryptophan metabolism in pregnancy and with the oral contraceptive pill. II. Relative levels of vitamin B6-vitamers in cord and maternal blood. Amer. J. Clin. Nutr., *24*:704, 1971.

Bruhn, C. M., and Pangborn, R. M.: Reported incidence of pica among migrant families. J. Amer. Dietet. Assoc., *58*:417, 1971.

Cantile, G. S. D., DeLeeuw, N. K. M., and Lowenstein, L.: Iron and folate nutrition in a group of private obstetrical patients. Amer. J. Clin. Nutr., *24*:637, 1971.

Chopra, J. G.: Effect of steroid contraceptives on lactation. Amer. J. Clin. Nutr., *25*:1202, 1972.

Delgado, H., et al.: Nutrition, lactation and postpartum amenorrhea. Amer. J. Clin. Nutr., *31*:322, 1978.

Dirige, O. V., et al.: Apoenzyme activities of erythrocyte transketolase, glutathione reductase and glutamic-pyruvic transaminase during pregnancy. Amer. J. Clin. Nutr., *31*:202, 1978.

Felig, P.: Maternal and fetal fuel homeostatis in human pregnancy. Amer. J. Clin. Nutr., *26*:998, 1973.

Gebre-Medhim, M., and Gobezie, A.: Dietary intake in the third trimester of pregnancy and birth weight of offspring among nonrprivileged and privileged women. Amer. J. Clin. Nutr., *28*:1322, 1975.

Hytten, F. E., and Leitch, I.: *The Physiology of Human Pregnancy*. 2nd Ed. Philadelphia, J. B. Lippincott Company, 1971.

Jeans, P. C.: Incidence of prematurity in relation to maternal nutrition. J. Amer. Dietet. Assoc., *31*:576, 1955.

Jelliffe, D. B., and Jelliffe, E. F. P. (eds.): Symposium: The uniqueness of human milk. Amer. J. Clin. Nutr., *24*:968, 1971.

Johnston, F. E., and Beller, A.: Anthropometric evaluation of the body composition of black, white, and Puerto Rican newborns. Amer. J. Clin. Nutr., *29*:61, 1976.

King, J. C., Calloway, D. H., and Margen, S.: Nitrogen retention, total body 40K and weight gain in teenage pregnant girls. J. Nutr., *103*:772, 1973.

Lamptey, M. S., and Walter, B. L.: Learning behavior and brain lipid composition in rats subjected to essential fatty acid deficiency during gestation, lactation and growth. J. Nutr., *108*:358, 1978.

Lechtig, A., et al.: Influence of maternal nutrition on birth weight. Amer. J. Clin. Nutr., *28*:1223, 1975.

Lindheimer, M. D., and Katz, A. I.: Sodium and diuretics in pregnancy. N. Engl. J. Med., *288*:891, 1973.

Lonnerdal, B., Forsum, E., and Hambraeus, L.: A longitudinal study of the protein, nitrogen, and lactose contents of human milk from Swedish well-nourished mothers. Amer. J. Clin. Nutr., *29*:1127, 1976.

Macy, I. G.: *Physiological Adaptation and Nutritional Status During and After Pregnancy*. Detroit, Children's Fund of Michigan, 1954.

Mahalko, J. R., and Bennion, M.: The effect of parity and time between pregnancies on maternal hair chromium concentration. Amer. J. Clin. Nutr., *29*:1069, 1976.

Metz, J.: Folate deficiency conditioned by lactation. Amer. J. Clin. Nutr., *23*:843, 1970.

Morse, E. H., et al.: Comparison of the nutritional status of pregnant adolescents with adult pregnant women. I. Biochemical findings. Amer. J. Clin. Nutr., *28*:1000, 1975; II. Anthropometric and dietary findings. Amer. J. Clin. Nutr., *28*:1422, 1975.

Moscovitch, L. F., and Cooper, B. A.: Folate content of diets in pregnancy: comparison of diets collected at home and diets prepared from dietary records. Amer. J. Clin. Nutr., *26*:707, 1973.

Moyer, E. C., et al.: *Nutritional Status of Mothers and Their Infants.* Detroit, Children's Fund of Michigan, 1954.

Oldham, H., and Sheft, B.: Effect of caloric intake on nitrogen utilization during pregnancy. J. Amer. Dietet. Assoc., *27*:847, 1951.

Paige, D. M., Bayless, T. M., and Graham, G. G.: Pregnancy and lactose intolerance. Amer. J. Clin. Nutr., *26*:238, 1973.

Pike, R. L., and Gursky, D. S.: Further evidence of deleterious effects produced by sodium restriction during pregnancy. Amer. J. Clin. Nutr., *23*:883, 1970.

Raman, L., et al.: Effect of calcium supplementation to undernourished mothers during pregnancy on the bone density of the neonates. Amer. J. Clin. Nutr., *31*:466, 1978.

Riopelle, A. J., Hill, C. W., and Li, S-C.: Protein deprivation in primates. V. Fetal mortality and neonatal status of infant monkeys born of deprived mothers. Amer. J. Clin. Nutr., *28*:989, 1975.

Singleton, N. C., Lewis, H., and Parker, J. J.: The diet of pregnant teenagers. J. Home Econ., *68*:43, 1976.

Smithells, R. W., et al.: Maternal nutrition in early pregnancy. Brit. J. Nutr., *38*:497, 1977.

Symposium on breast feeding. J. Human Nutr., *30*:223, 1976.

Thomson, A. M., and Billewitz, W. A.: Nutritional status, maternal physique and reproductive efficiency. Proc. Nutr. Soc., *22*:55, 1963.

Tracy, T., and Miller, G. L.: Obstetric problems of the massively obese. Obstet. Gynecol., *33*:204, 1969.

Widdowson, E. M., and Cowen, J.: The effect of protein deficiency and calorie deficiency on the reproduction of rats. Brit. J. Nutr., *27*:85, 1972.

World Health Organization: Nutrition in pregnancy and lactation. WHO Tech. Rpt. Ser. No. 302. Geneva, 1965.

Articles in Nutrition Reviews

Prenatal exposure to fluoride. *25*:330, 1967.

Diet and mammary gland growth in the pregnant rat. *27*:152, 1969.

Longitudinal studies of diet in pregnancy. *30*:38, 1972.

Smoking, pregnancy, and development of the offspring. *31*:143, 1973.

The caloric cost of pregnancy. *31*:177, 1973.

Maternal nutrition and fetal growth. *32*:241, 1974.

Metabolic adaptation to pregnancy. *32*:270, 1974.

Lactation and composition of milk in undernourished women. *33*:42, 1975.

Vitamin levels at term and in the neonate. *33*:298, 1975.

Iron supplementation for gestational anemia. *33*:332, 1975.

Requirement of vitamin B-6 during pregnancy. *34*:15, 1976.

The influence of maternal food supplements on birthweight in Guatemala. *34*:169, 1976.

Commentary on breast feeding and infant formulas, including proposed standards for formulas. *34*:248, 1976.

Maternal leukocyte enzymes in human fetal malnutrition. *34*:272, 1976.

Influence of intrauterine nutritional status on the development of obesity in later life. *35*:100, 1977.

Chapter 21

Nutrition in Infancy and Childhood

It is essential that infants and children receive a good diet to insure that they grow and develop normally. All body tissues as they form, including the cells of the brain, must receive minimal levels of each nutrient so that each child's full physical and intellectual potential may be reached. This need begins at the moment of conception, continues throughout pregnancy (see Chapter 20), and is no less important after the baby is born.

This chapter will center on the nutritional needs of children from infancy through the early school years. Knowledge of the "basics" of childhood nutrition allows parents to make informed choices regarding healthy diets for these children. In addition, anyone concerned with day-to-day care of children inside or outside the home (teachers, nurses, day-care staff, etc.) needs to be competent in the area of proper nutrition for the young growing child (see Fig. 21–1).

FEEDING OF THE INFANT AND CHILD — GENERAL CONSIDERATIONS

Growth

The normal infant's rate of growth in the first year is truly remarkable (see Fig. 21–2). The birth weight is doubled by age 4 to 6 months and tripled by the age of 1

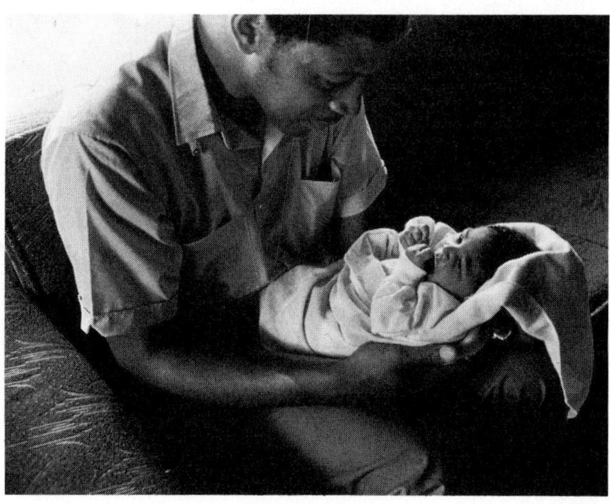

Figure 21–1 Good nutrition along with loving nurture from his parents will help this baby grow and develop to his full potential. (From Livingston, S. K.: J. Nutr. Ed., 3:18, 1971. Courtesy of the National Dairy Council.)

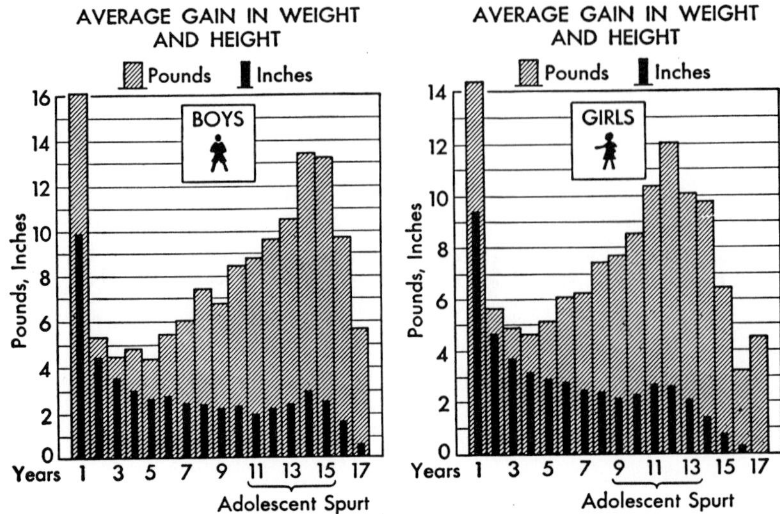

Figure 21–2 Growth increment graphs for boys and girls. (Courtesy of the Metropolitan Life Insurance Co.)

year. If the rate of weight gain of the first 6 months (doubling every 6 months) were to continue, the child would weigh about 7000 pounds, or 3.5 tons, by his or her fifth birthday! Instead, of course, the average weight by 5 years of age is a more reasonable 40 to 42 pounds, and, with a relatively steady growth in the early school years, reaches approximately 70 pounds by 10 years of age.

The average birth weight in the United States is 7 pounds, 8 ounces (3400 gm). Babies commonly lose 5 to 10 percent of their body weight in the first 24 to 48 hours, owing to water loss. Full-term babies can be expected to regain their birth weight by 10 to 14 days. See Table 21–1 for average weight gains for 3 month periods during the first year of life.

Growth records of the infant and child are important indicators of nutritional and general health. Growth patterns of individual children can be recorded on *growth charts*. See Figure 21–3 for nationally used growth charts for children of the United States.[1]

Undernutrition is one reason for impaired physical growth,* and growth increases are seen when nutrition is improved. Perhaps the best example is the increase in height by nearly 3 inches (6 to 7 cm) noted in post-war (Second World War) Japanese children when their heights were compared with pre-war Japanese average heights. This growth increase is attributed to an improvement in nutritional intake.[2] There is also a phenomenon of "catch-up growth"[3] seen in certain individual children who have been malnourished and then are rehabilitated. The growth rates of these children increase when nutrition is improved.

In addition to energy needs for growth, the child has ongoing basal metabolic needs and energy needs of physical

Table 21–1 GROWTH DURING INFANCY

Age	*Weight Gain per Week*
Birth–3 mo	200 gm (6–7 oz)
4–6 mo	140 gm (5 oz)
7–9 mo	85 gm (3 oz)
10–12 mo	70 mg (2½ oz)

*Average weight gain during the first year. Note the normal decrease in the *rate* of weight gain by the end of the first year.

*Metabolic conditions and other factors that affect intake, absorption, or utilization of nutrients also can affect growth. Examples would include certain chronic diseases, such as cystic fibrosis, and drugs or medications that may temporarily depress appetite, such as those used for certain types of hyperactivity.[4]

activity (see Fig. 21–4). The satisfaction of these needs is critical to the child's present and future health and development, and it is for this reason that an understanding of proper infant and child feeding is of particular interest and importance.

Feeding the Low Birth Weight Infant

One of the most vital basic reflexes the healthy newborn is endowed with at birth is the natural sucking reflex for obtaining food. Infants who are born prematurely may not have this sucking reflex developed fully and perfectly; many need specialized care in order to insure that their calorie and nutrient needs are met in a manner that is safe for them. Infants under 5.5 pounds (2500 gm) are considered "low birth weight" babies and are generally given special medical attention, since these are the infants that account for over 70 percent of all infant deaths in the United States.[5] These low birth weight babies may be small owing to either (1) prematurity or (2) inadequate growth during the gestational period because of maternal malnutrition (see Chapter 20) or placental insufficiency. Babies in this second category, born at term, yet underweight, are called "small for dates" infants; the effects of the early stunting of growth tend to persist into later years when these individuals are often found to have a shorter than average height.[6].

An important consideration in feeding the small infant is the more limited capacity of their physiologically immature kidney to excrete a solute load. For the premature infant especially, attention must be given to a safe osmotic level of feedings.

Milk, the Infant's Primary Food

Presently in the United States, there is a resurgence of interest in breast-feeding as the preferred method of infant feeding. Just a few years ago only 20 percent of all infants leaving hospital nurseries were breast-fed, whereas a recent survey (1977) showed that now, in many areas, fully half of infants are started on the breast.[7] For those who use substitute milk preparations, commercially prepared formulas have been more popular than evaporated milk formulas since the early 1960's (see Fig. 21–5). This popularity is due mainly to the ease and convenience of using the newer commercial formulas. The standard evaporated milk formulas are actually more economical than are commercial formulas, but in the past few years the remarkable success of the "ready-to-feed" formulas is another example of how the consumer is often willing to pay more for convenience (see Table 21–2).

Breast milk has been the most readily available and natural food for infants from the beginning of mankind; however, feeding bottles for infants have been found in archeological excavations of the Nile Basin.[8] Historically, artificial feeding of infants (that is, with animal milk or concocted formula rather than with breast milk) had very poor results. It has been estimated that artificially fed babies in the period of the Industrial Revolution, before any of the important bacteriological studies of Pasteur and Koch, had a mortality rate at least three times as high as breast-fed babies. Unfortunately, even today, in the less developed regions of the world, an increase in the practice of bottle feeding can result in an *increased* infant sickness and death rate. This tragic situation may occur when there is (1) a lack of adequate sanitary preparation of bottles and milk substitutes and (2) an inadequate nutritional content of the milk substitutes when prepared in inappropriate fashion (for example, by overdilution) because of misunderstanding or poverty. There is also a danger of using too little water to dilute the milk product; the infant may become dangerously depleted of water.

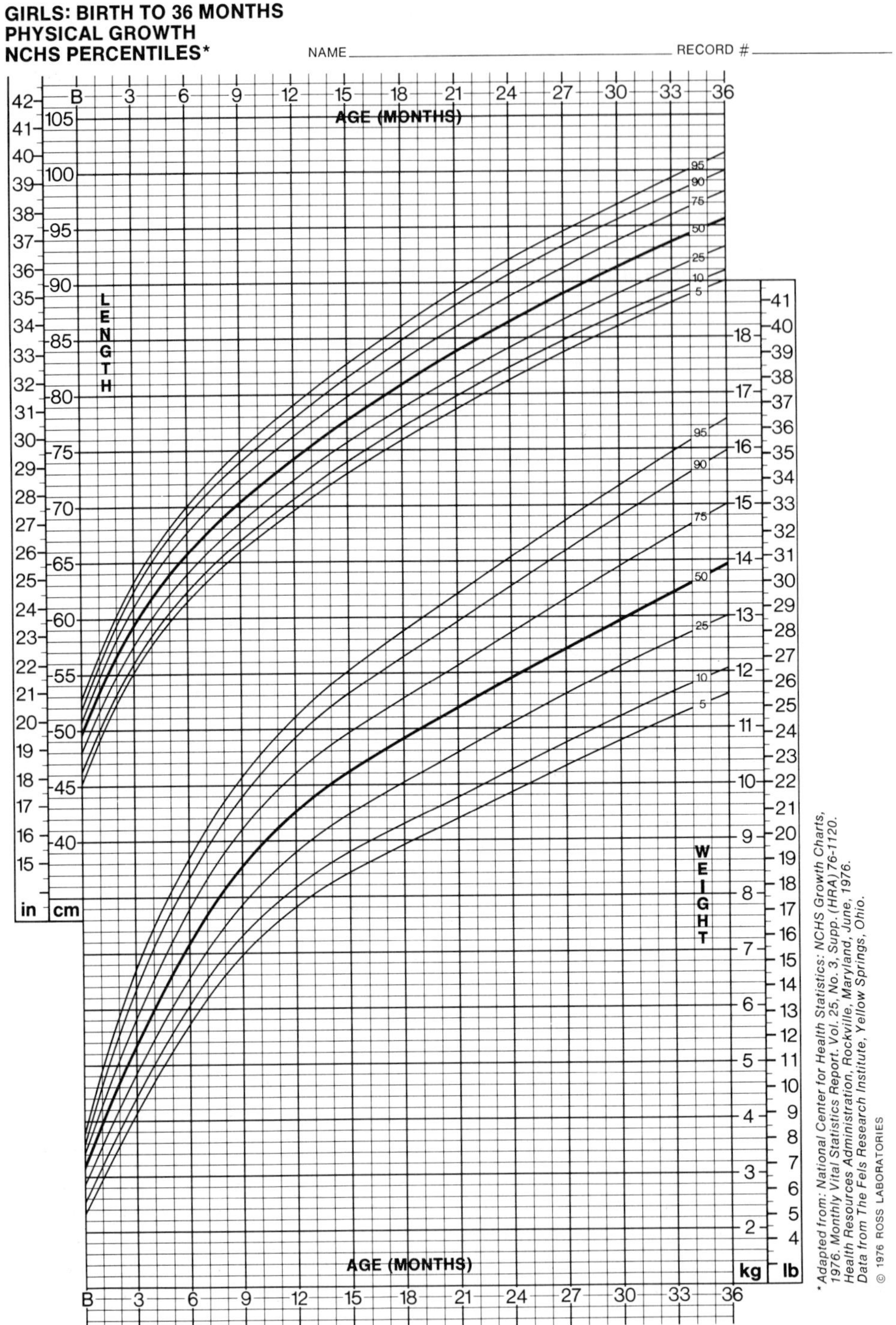

Figure 21–3 NCHS Growth Charts — from the National Center for Health Statistics: NCHS Growth Charts, 1976.[1] Growth charts such as these are based on growth records of large samples of normal, growing children. The 50 percentile line is the average weight or length for children at any given age. A weight plotted on the 75 percentile line, for example, means that 74 percent of normal children are *below* that weight. The 5th and 95th percentiles represent unusual although not necessarily abnormal weights and lengths. There are similar charts showing head circumference for age, and weight for length, which are generally used in conjunction with the charts pictured.

BOYS: BIRTH TO 36 MONTHS
PHYSICAL GROWTH
NCHS PERCENTILES*

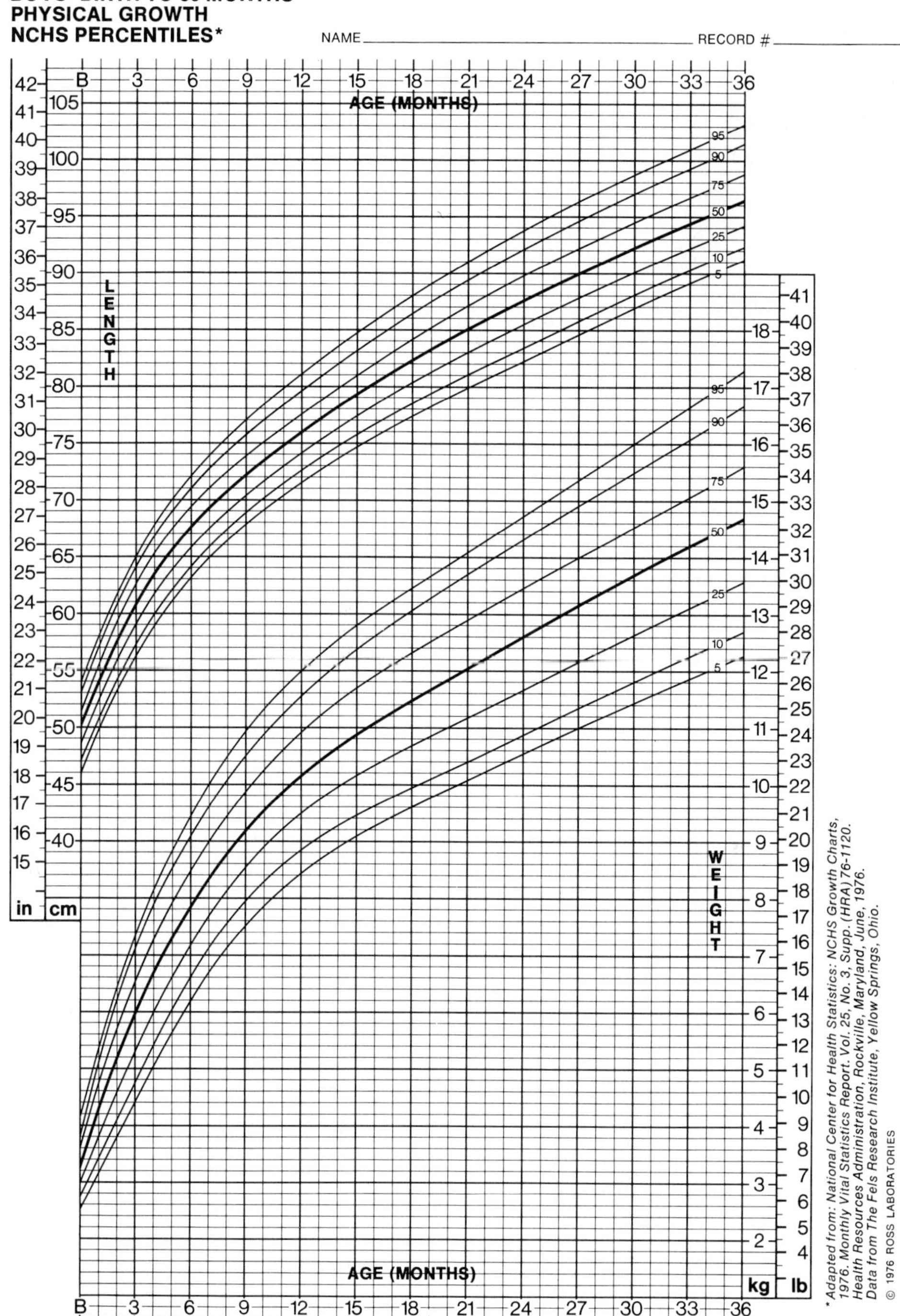

Figure 21–3

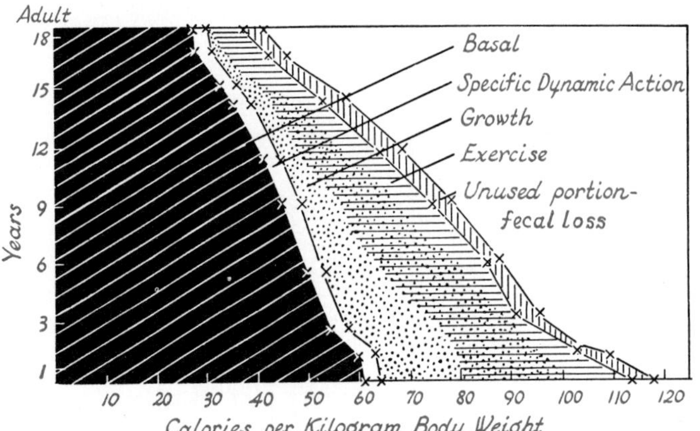

Figure 21–4 Energy expenditure in children: Total daily expenditure of calories per kilogram with approximate distribution among individual factors in relation to age (see also Chapter 2). (From Vaughan, V. C., and McKay, R. J.: *Nelson Textbook of Pediatrics.* 10th Ed. Philadelphia, W. B. Saunders Company, 1975.)

Benefits of Human Milk

Today there is a wealth of scientific evidence to indicate that giving human milk is the best way to feed the infant during the first year of life. Human milk is the "reference standard" against which all other infant feeding practices are judged. An increasing number of official health agencies and organizations have published policy statements recommending breast-feeding.[10]

A sensible alternative to breast-feeding exists, if necessary, in the form of commercially available iron-fortified infant formulas (see Table 21–3). However, certain advantages of breast-feeding have not been duplicated in any of these formulas. One advantage is the protection offered by human milk against infections, specifically certain infantile gastrointestinal infections.[11, 12] There is also evidence of a decreased incidence of respiratory disease in breast-fed babies.[12] Babies fed breast milk are also less likely to develop constipation and certain common infant allergies, and are more likely to be able to self-regulate their intake needs successfully.[13] In addition, many mothers feel that breast-feeding promotes an exceptionally close and harmonious relationship with their child (see Fig. 21–6).

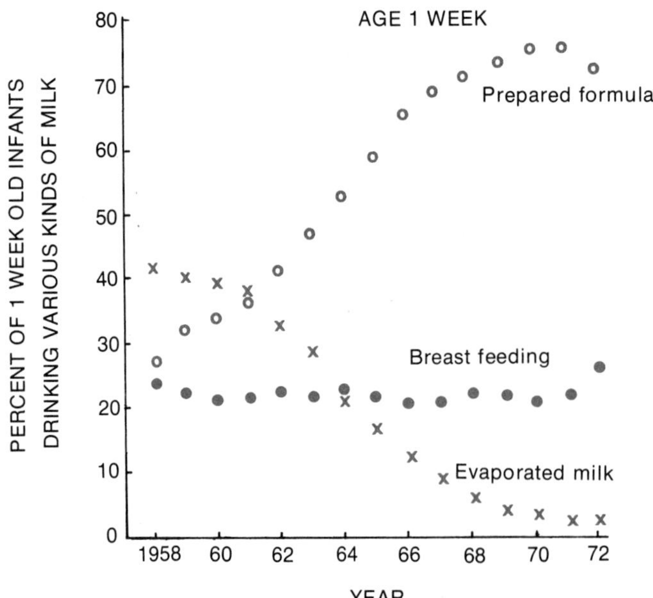

Figure 21–5 Use of the different kinds of milk in infant feeding (1 week old infants) from 1958 to 1972 in the United States. Over the past two decades, the use of evaporated milk for infant feeding has declined significantly while the use of prepared infant formulas has risen. The trend toward breast-feeding in the 1970's is seen in its early stages in this chart. (Adapted from Fomon, S.: *Infant Nutrition.* 2nd Ed. Philadelphia, W. B. Saunders Company, 1975.)

Table 21–2 ECONOMY IN INFANT FEEDING: RELATIVE COSTS OF DIFFERENT MILKS*

Feeding	*Food Cost (in Dollars) per Ounce Fed*	*Estimated Food Cost (in Dollars) for First Year of Life*
Evaporated milk–corn syrup (Karo) formula	.0142	133
Lactation: low-cost foods†	.0165	153
Lactation: moderate-cost foods	.0180	167
Commercial formula		
Concentrated formula		
Enfamil	.0242	227
Similac	.0235	220
Advance (formula for older infants)	.0234	220
Powdered form		
Enfamil	.0263	247
Similac	.0252	237
Ready-to-serve form‡		
Enfamil	.0294	276
Similac	.0288	271
Advance (formula for older infants)	.0278	261

*Boston, June 1976. Adapted from Lamm, E., Delaney, J., and Dwyer, J.: Economy in the feeding of infants. Pediatr. Clin. North Amer., *24*:71, 1977.

Calculations are based on approximately 800 ml of milk a day, or from 9400 to 9700 oz a year. Dietary supplements and solid foods are not included in these calculations. It may be seen that the cost of evaporated milk is approximate to or slightly lower than breast milk, and that breast milk costs 25 percent less than concentrated milk and 40 percent less than ready-to-serve formulas. Whole milk is not included in the chart, as it is not a recommended milk for early infant feeding.

†This item refers to costs of foods chosen for the lactating woman's diet. Lower cost estimates have been reported in some cases.

‡For comparison, strained foods costs 10 to 15 percent more per oz than this most expensive type of milk formula.

Many of the recent policy statements concerning breast-feeding recommend that it be continued for at least the first 4 to 6 months of infancy.* At present it is estimated that only 5 percent of 6-month-old infants are breast-fed.[14]

Volume of Milk Intake

The total volume of milk required varies from infant to infant, with an average intake of about 3 ounces per pound (or 175 to 200 ml per kg) of body weight in the first weeks of life, reduced to 1½ or 2 ounces per pound in the later months of infancy. (A premature baby may need up to 4 to 5 ounces per pound; feeding of low birth weight infants is a specialized topic[15] not covered here.) Milk intake will vary with such factors as individual appetite, growth rate, body size, and the amount of solids and of other liquids taken. Most infants over a few weeks of age will consume about 1 quart (946 ml) of milk a day, with a standard deviation of intake of approximately 25 percent. Daily milk intake per kilogram of body weight is shown in Figure 21–7.

The frequency of breast- or bottle-feedings begins at about seven to ten times a day and gradually decreases to five to six times a day at 2 months, by which time many infants will be content to sleep throughout the night. There is no virtue in fixing rigid feeding times, as most infants will develop their own fairly regular feeding times.

*An organization of mothers willing to assist new mothers who wish to breast-feed is the La Leche League International, 9616 Minneapolis Ave., Franklin Park, Illinois 60131.

Table 21–3. A SAMPLE OF THE VARIETY OF MILK FORMULAS*

			Examples of:		
	Mature Human Milk	*Cow's Milk, Fresh, Whole*	MODIFIED INFANT FORMULA, BASED ON COW'S MILK	SOY-BASED FORMULA	HYDROLYZED PROTEIN FORMULA
Calories/100 ml	75	66	67	67	67
Linoleic acid as percent of fatty acids	10.6	2.1	‡	‡	‡
Gm/100 ml of:					
Protein	1.1	3.5	1.5	2.5	2.2
Carbohydrate	6.8–7.2	4.8	7.0	6.8	8.5
Fat	4.5	3.7	3.7	3.4	2.6
Water	87	87	87	87	87
Calcium: phosphorus ratio (mg/liter)	340:140	1170:920	550:440	800:630	1000:700
Vitamins/liter					
A, IU	1898	1025–1690	1700	2100	1500
C, mg	43	11	55	50	50
D, IU	22	14–33	400	400	400
Thiamin, mg	0.16	0.44	0.4	0.5	0.46
Riboflavin, mg	0.36	1.75	0.6	1	1.8
B-6, mg	0.1	0.64	0.3	0.4	0.5
B-12, mcg	0.3	4	1.5	2	4.5
Pantothenic acid, mg	1.8	3.4	2	2.5	3.2
Niacin, mg	1.5	0.94	7	7	4
Folacin, mcg	52	55	50	100	50
K, mcg	15	60	35	90	18
E, mg/IU	1.8 mg	0.4 mg	8.5 IU	9 IU	10 IU
Iron, mg	0.5	0.5	1.4 (with iron—8–12 mg)	8–12	12

*Adapted from Fomon[9] and manufacturers' data.
†400 IU when fortified.
‡Present, but amount not available.

Starting on Solids

After the infant has been on its "milk only" diet for a few months, the next natural step is to consider when and how to introduce foods other than milk.* In the early 1970's, approximately 90 percent of all infants in the United States were started on solids at 3 months of age or less. (Breast-fed babies tend to be introduced to solids at later dates than bottle-fed babies.) However, it is actually not until the baby reaches 5 or 6 months of age that nutritional needs increase to a point at which they are not entirely met by milk alone. In fact, the latest medical and nutritional recommendations regarding the addition of solid foods to the infant diet state that the introduction of foods supplementing milk is best begun at around 4 to 6 months of age.[9, 10]

Traditionally, the 3- or 4-month-old infant was fed strained baby foods until the first teeth arrived at about 5 to 10 months of age; then "junior" foods, characterized by their soft, chewable consistency, were begun. An alternative is to begin puréed table foods at around the middle of the first year. This is why a blender is a useful and practical addition to a household with a growing infant. Most fresh vegetables and fruits, as well

*There is no common term for this step in infant feeding in the English language. In French the word *ablactation* ("from milk") can be used for the period in which solids are started, and in German there is the word *Beikost,* which is used by Fomon to describe foods other than milk.[9]

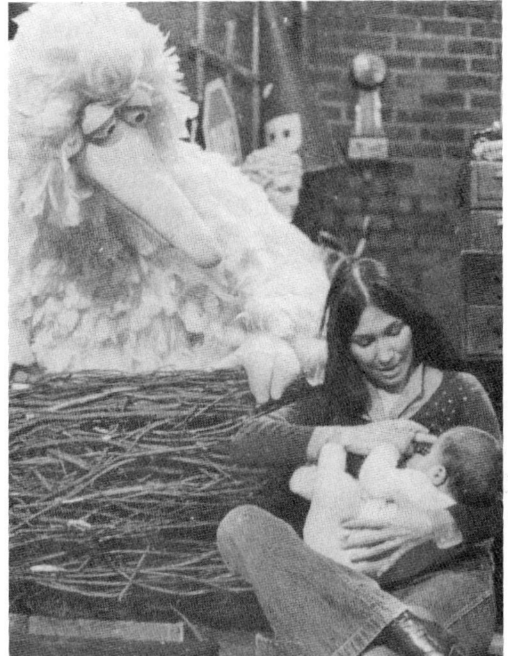

Figure 21–6 Breast-feeding as a normal and natural infant feeding method is receiving increased nationwide attention. For example, singer Buffy Sainte-Marie and her young child Dakota Starblanket have appeared in several Sesame Street programs, the popular preschool series produced by the Children's Television Workshop. (Courtesy of La Leche League.)

as meats, may be ground or blended to the consistency enjoyed by the infant. For many families, this may be the preferred way of preparing all of the infant's meals. This method assures a greater variety of foods earlier in the child's life as well as enabling the family to know exactly what the infant is receiving.

Improved labeling of commercial infant foods also allows more complete knowledge of ingredients. It is interesting to note that owing to consumer interest in more "natural" baby food products, many more infant foods are being prepared without added sugar or salt.

Caloric Distribution of Infant Diets

Studies on the diets of infants in the United States show that by 4 months, about 20 to 30 percent of calories come from foods other than milk or formula, and by 12 months, 60 to 70 percent of the total caloric intake is from foods other than milk.[9] The typical selection of strained foods fed to infants contains approximately 80 percent of calories as carbohydrates. They are generally low in fat content, and the amount of protein depends largely on the presence of meat. Water makes up from 70 to 90 percent of the composition of most varieties of prepared strained and junior foods.

The distribution of calories in milk is shown in Table 21–4. From this table, it is clear how markedly different cow's milk,

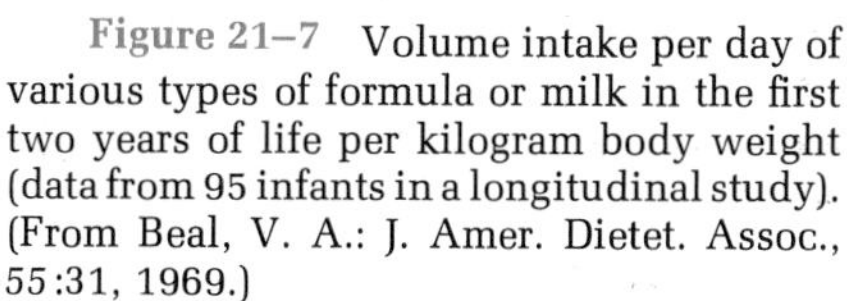

Figure 21–7 Volume intake per day of various types of formula or milk in the first two years of life per kilogram body weight (data from 95 infants in a longitudinal study). (From Beal, V. A.: J. Amer. Dietet. Assoc., 55:31, 1969.)

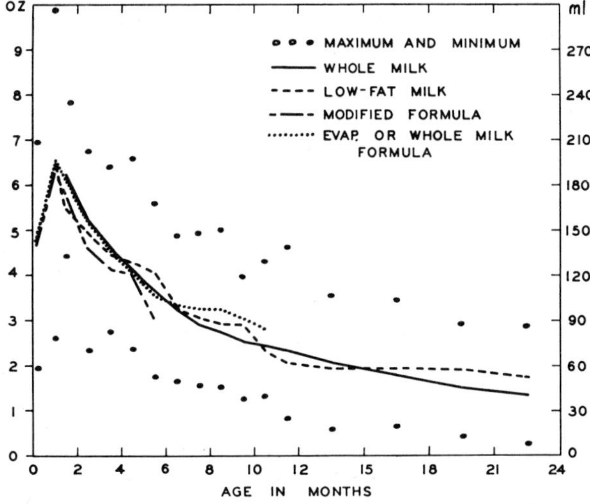

Table 21–4 CALORIC DISTRIBUTION IN VARIOUS TYPES OF MILK*

Type of Milk	*Percent of Total Calories*		
	PROTEIN	FAT	CARBOHYDRATE
Human milk	6–7	56	38
Commercial formulas (standard)	9–13	47–48	40–43
Cow's milk			
Whole milk	22	48	30
Low-fat (2%)	28	31	41
Skim	40	3	57

*The difference in the proportion of protein content found in human milk (and in formulas manufactured to simulate human milk) and that found in cow's milk is clearly seen here. The level found in human milk and in formulas is considered to be the safest level for the young infant.

and skimmed milk in particular, is from human milk and commercial formulas. In fact, the feeding of skim milk to infants results in diets that are calorically inadequate for growth and are undesirably low in fat and undesirably high in protein. It is also deficient in iron, ascorbic acid, and essential fatty acids, and it has no role in the diet of a normal, healthy infant.

Feeding the Toddler and the Preschool Child

At around 8 months to a year, the infant may begin to use a cup rather than the bottle or breast. By this time he or she should be taking, in addition to milk, a varied diet including cereal, cooked and mashed vegetables, puréed meats, fruit juices, and fruit. The child of this age will also enjoy chewing on bread and toast products. More solid, chewy foods direct from the table (whole pieces of meat or hard, raw vegetables) should not be introduced until after 12 months of age, as there is a danger of choking.*

During the second year of life, the child should complete the transition to the cup and to table foods. He or she should be drinking 3 cups of milk a day and, again, eating a balanced diet with products from all four food groups (see Chapters 17 and 20). The mother will often complain about her child "losing its appetite" during this year; but when the normal decline in the child's rate of growth after the first 12 months is understood, it will be clear that his decreased appetite has a physiological basis. In fact, this has been termed the *physiologic anorexia* (anorexia means loss of appetite) of the 1-year-old, and mothers should be reassured that this is normal. The child should continue to be offered a balanced diet suitable for his or her age, with an emphasis on easily self-fed foods ("finger foods"), because this is a time at which the child is developing a sense of independence. Some examples of protein-rich "finger foods" are peanut butter on crackers, celery sticks, bread strips, cheese squares, and hard-boiled eggs. These may be offered as midmorning or midafternoon snacks, as the toddler and preschooler will often adapt more easily to smaller amounts of food offered five or six times a day than to a strict regimen of three large meals each day. A useful "rule of thumb" regarding minimal serving sizes for preschoolers is " one tablespoonful for each year of age" of each separate food served.

A common complaint about preschool children is that they won't eat vegetables (see Table 21–5). In this case, one can attempt to encourage the use of a variety of vegetables — such as cherry tomatoes, carrots, zucchini, and green beans — that can be easily picked up by the child.

*Snack foods such as nuts and popcorn should never be fed to toddlers; food inhaled into the trachea and lung can have serious consequences.

Table 21–5 CONCERNS OF MOTHERS REGARDING EATING BEHAVIOR OF PRESCHOOL CHILDREN*

	Age Group	
Concerns	1–2 YR (% OF 497 SUBJECTS)	2–3 YR (% OF 551 SUBJECTS)
1. Chooses limited variety	35.9	40.3
2. Dawdles with food	30.0	36.8
3. Eats too little fruits and vegetables	22.6	27.2
4. Eats too many sweets	6.2	26.3
5. Eats too little meat	26.4	22.3
6. Eats too little food	14.3	21.6
7. Drinks too little milk	13.7	20.1
8. Drinks too much milk	11.9	10.0
9. Eats too much food	4.4	2.7

*Adapted from Eppright, E. S., et al.: Eating behavior of preschool children. J. Nutr. Ed., *1*: Issue No. I, 16, 1969.

Table 21–6 RECOMMENDED FOOD INTAKE FOR GOOD NUTRITION ACCORDING TO FOOD GROUPS AND THE AVERAGE SIZE OF SERVINGS AT DIFFERENT AGE LEVELS*

Food Group	*Servings per Day*	*Average Size of Servings*			
		1 YR	2–3 YR	4–5 YR	6–9 YR
Milk and cheese 1.5 oz cheese = 1 c milk) (c = 1 cup – 8 oz or 240 gm)	4	½ c	½–¾ c	¾ c	¾–1 c
Meat group (protein foods)	3 or more				
Egg		1	1	1	1
Lean meat, fish, poultry (liver once a week)		2 tbsp	2 tbsp	4 tbsp	2–3 oz (4–6 tbsp)
Peanut butter			1 tbsp	2 tbsp	2–3 tbsp
Fruits and vegetables	At least 4, including:				
Vitamin C source (citrus fruits, berries, tomato, cabbage, cantalope)	1 or more (twice as much tomato as citrus)	⅓ c citrus	½ c	½ c	1 medium orange
Vitamin A source (green† or yellow fruits and vegetables)	1 or more	2 tbsp	3 tbsp	4 tbsp (¼ c)	¼ c
Other vegetables (potato and legumes, etc.) or	2	2 tbsp	3 tbsp	4 tbsp (¼ c)	⅓ c
Other fruits (apple, banana, etc.)		¼ c	⅓ c	½ c	1 medium
Cereals (whole-grain or enriched)	At least 4				
Bread		½ slice	1 slice	1½ slices	1– slices
Ready-to-eat cereals		½ oz	¾ oz	1 oz	1 oz
Cooked cereals (including macaroni, spaghetti, rice, etc.)		¼ c	⅓ c	½ c	½ c
Fats and carbohydrates	To meet caloric needs				
Butter, margarine, mayonnaise, oils: 1 tbsp = 100 calories (kcal)		1 tbsp	1 tbsp	1 tbsp	2 tbsp
Desserts and sweets: 100-calorie portions as follows: ⅓ c pudding or ice cream 2–3 cookies, 1 oz cake, 1½ oz pie, 2 tbsp jelly, jam, honey, sugar		1 portion	1½ portions	1½ portions	3 portions

*Adapted from Vaughan, V. C., III, and McKay, R. J.: *Nelson Textbook of Pediatrics.* 10th Ed. Philadelphia, W. B. Saunders Co., 1975, p. 159.

†Green, leafy vegetables should be eaten every day because of their folic acid content. See text.

Table 21–7 NUTRIENT VALUES OF THE DIETS PRESENTED IN TABLE 21–6

Age	*Calories*†	*Protein (gm)*	*Calcium (gm)*	*Iron (mg)*	*Vitamin A (IU)*	*Thiamin*‡ *(mg)*	*Riboflavin*‡ *(mg)*	*Niacin*‡ *(mg)*	*Ascorbic Acid (mg)*	*Vitamin D (IU)*
1 yr	1020	42	0.6	5.4	2325	0.47	1.0	3.4	40	300
2–3 yr	1320	48	0.8	6.1	3225	0.64	1.0	7.3	51	400
4–5 yr	1720	67	1.0	8.4	4270	0.85	1.5	11.7	60	500
6–9 yr	2130	76	1.1	11.4	5140	1.2	2.0	19.3	88	600

*Adapted from Vaughan, V. C., III, and McKay, R. J.: *Nelson Textbook of Pediatrics.* 10th Ed. Philadelphia, W. B. Saunders, Co., 1975, p. 160.

†Selections from fats and carbohydrate group included for caloric values, but not for other nutrients. Calorie = large calorie = kcal = Cal. (See text.)

‡Based on the following: thiamin, 0.4 mg/1000 calories; riboflavin, 0.025 mg/gm of protein; niacin, 6.6 mg/1000 calories.

Familiarity with food helps to increase its acceptance; so even if once refused, a new food should be reoffered at a later time. Considerations of food attractiveness and periods of enjoyment and comfort related to eating times are also important.

In the preschool years the child continues to strive to assert his new feelings of individuality and independence, resulting in possible "power struggles" at mealtimes. Consistency, adaptability, and creativity on the part of the parents should continue to insure that the child receives the nutritional intake required for his activity and growth needs. For recommended servings and their nutrient values and for menu suggestions, see Tables 21–6, 21–7, and 21–8.

Nutrition of the School-Age Child

The healthy, active school-age child generally has fewer feeding problems than the toddler or preschooler. The child going to school needs a nutritious breakfast to start the day, a complete lunch that satisfies approximately one-third of the

Table 21–8 PRACTICAL MENU SUGGESTIONS FOR CHILDREN AT VARIOUS AGES

1–2 yr	*3–6 yr*	*7–12 yr*
Breakfast	*Breakfast*	*Breakfast*
Orange juice Oatmeal with milk Whole wheat toast Milk to drink	Orange juice Bran flakes with milk Whole-wheat toast Milk to drink	Banana Omelette – plain Toast Milk to drink
Midmorning	*Midmorning*	*Midmorning*
Juice	Raisins	Apple
Lunch	*Lunch*	*Lunch*
Egg, soft poached Mashed potato Peas Zwieback Milk to drink Rice pudding	Egg salad sandwich with lettuce Milk to drink Plain, crisp cookies (1–2) Custard pudding	Vegetable soup with rice Peanut butter and jelly sandwich Milk Fresh peaches
Midafternoon	*Midafternoon*	*Midafternoon*
Milk Crackers with soft cheese spread	Juice Apple and cheese wedges	1–2 molasses cookies Fruit juice or milk
Dinner	*Dinner*	*Dinner*
Fish sticks Spinach or carrots Bread and butter Applesauce Milk	Hamburger with tomato and lettuce Squash Toast and butter Milk Stewed prunes Carrots and celery	Broiled chicken Baked potato Carrots and peas Shredded raw cabbage salad Bread and butter Milk Orange wedges

A meal plan for a child for a day should be based on a knowledge of the "Basic 4" (Chapters 17, 19). For example: *Breakfast:* milk group, 1; fruit-vegetable group, 1; bread-cereal group, 2. *Lunch:* meat-protein group, 1; bread-cereal group, 1; milk group, 1; vegetable-fruit group, 1. *Dinner:* meat-protein group, 1; milk group, 1; vegetable-fruit group, 2; bread-cereal group, 1. Additional servings may easily be added as midmorning or midafternoon snacks.

daily nutritional requirements (see Table 21–8) and a satisfying third meal at the end of the day. Snacks are also a way of life with schoolchildren, and are popular for their energy needs. Midmorning and midafternoon nutritious snacks are appropriate. Attractively presented food and an enjoyable eating environment are just as appropriate for school-age children as for preschool children. The normal, healthy child will naturally increase his or her intake if good nutrition habits are encouraged.

The elementary school child's growth rate is slower than the rate during infancy or adolescence. However, meeting nutrition needs continues to be critical to the development of the child during this time.

NUTRITIONAL REQUIREMENTS OF INFANTS AND CHILDREN

With regard to infants and children, needs for most types of nutrients are proportionately (per unit of size) higher than the needs of an adult. This applies to the need for water protein, vitamins, and minerals. The relative requirement for energy is also greater in the child. For example, the newborn requires about 100 to 120 kcal per kg of body weight, while the average young adult needs 35 to 40 kcal per kg.

Recommended Dietary Allowances (RDA's)

The RDA's for infants are derived from estimated intakes of breast-fed babies, with an additional safety factor added for infants fed on cow's milk formulas. Thus, for the breast-fed baby, the optimal intake of nutrients is by definition less than the RDA. See Table 1A., Appendix, for the complete RDA chart by age group.

Protein

Protein allowances in this age group are in the range of 2 to 4 gm per kg of body weight per day. Breast milk provides approximately 2 gm of protein per kg of the child's weight per day, and countless infants have thrived on this level of protein intake for the first 5 to 6 months of life. Most popular commercial formulas have followed the general composition of breast milk, but with a slightly higher protein content (see Table 21–3).

Carbohydrates

The usable carbohydrates in children's diets, as in those of adults, are sugars and starches* (see Chapter 3). As with adults, diets compatible with good health in children can contain varying quantities of carbohydrates, so there is not a definite RDA allowance set. However, carbohydrates do make an essential contribution to meeting energy requirements of infants and children and in this way are extremely important. If insufficient carbohydrate is ingested to meet daily energy needs, the body must break down a certain portion of dietary and body protein to meet these needs.

In the newborn, the most usual carbohydrates ingested are lactose (from milk), glucose, and sucrose. Nearly all infants (with a few exceptions — for example, those with a specific enzyme defect) can digest and absorb these sugars adequately, unless they are given in high concentrations, when diarrhea is likely to occur.

The infant is considered able to break down starches in the diet to glucose by the age of 1 month. The carbohydrate in-

*Since natural starches in foods tend to undergo changes that both shorten shelf life and may reduce digestibility, manufactured foods often contain *modified starches*, which may supply 10 to 30 percent of the energy of strained and junior dinners, desserts, and fruits. They are essentially "empty calories," for they supply no nutritional value other than energy.

take of the infant is important for both energy requirements and maintenance of the plasma glucose level (important because of the need of brain cells to utilize glucose). The latter consideration is especially vital in the case of the premature baby, whose liver glycogen stores at birth are incomplete and may be inadequate to maintain proper blood glucose levels for the first 24 to 48 hours of life unless glucose is given.

During the first weeks of life, the caloric supply of certain milk formulas (specifically, evaporated milk formulas) needs to be supplemented with extra carbohydrate, commonly in the form of 2 to 4 gm (½ to 1 tsp) corn syrup per feeding.

Fats

Fats contribute about half the energy requirement of the infant who is fed on milk alone. Infant formulas should provide at least 15 percent of the total calories as fat in order to meet the energy needs of infants.

The essential fatty acid, linoleic acid, is important in promoting optimal health in infants. Without it, poor growth and a severe skin rash will result.[16] Great quantities of linoleic acid are found in corn oil, cottonseed oil, soybean oil, and whole-grain cereals. The minimal recommended level of linoleic acid is from 1 to 3 percent of the total amount of calories. Human milk contains 6 to 9 percent of calories as linoleic acid. Skim milk contains only traces of this important fatty acid, and this is one of the reasons it should not be used as an infant food.

Distribution of Calories in the Diet

The distribution of calories in the infant's and child's diet does not differ markedly from that recommended for the adult. Protein should provide at least 7 percent of calories, or growth needs will not be met. A general guideline would be that 7 to 15 percent of total calories come from protein, 35 to 55 percent from fat, and the remainder (about 30 to 60 percent) from carbohydrate.[9]

Vitamins

Growing, active children have a special need, relatively higher than adults, for a complete supply of the known vitamins. These vitamins can usually be supplied in a balanced, varied diet, but there are certain periods when vitamin supplements may be advisable, such as in infancy. Other possible periods when vitamin supplements may be indicated are (1) when the toddler is going through his or her stage of "physiologic anorexia," (2) in times of illness and other periods of possible limited food intake, and (3) in specific disease entities requiring specific vitamins as part of the treatment.

Table 1A in the Appendix gives details of vitamin requirements of infants and children. *Vitamin A* needs are estimated from the amount in human milk. (See Chapter 7, p. 128, for more information on Vitamin A.)

In normal full-term infants, intakes of as little as 100 IU a day of *vitamin D* have prevented rickets. Premature infants are more prone to develop rickets because of their rapid growth rate. Therefore, vitamin D supplementation is recommended early for these small infants. The recommended level of 400 IU is intended to prevent rachitic symptoms in all babies, small or of normal size. This is also the level recommended for growing children and adults. Sunlight (certain ultraviolet wavelengths) is an alternative way to meet the need for vitamin D, through conversion of 7-dehydrocholesterol in the skin to vitamin D_3.* An infant wearing the normal amount of clothes would probably receive an antirachitic dose of sunlight in approximately a 30 to 60 minute exposure each day.

---

*Reasonable caution should be exercised in exposing small infants to sunlight in order to prevent sunburn.

Vitamin D in the mother's diet does not get passed on in breast milk to a significant extent. This is also the case with cow's milk and is the reason that commercial cow's milk is supplemented with this vitamin. Breast-fed infants should receive supplemental vitamin D unless safe exposure to sunlight is assured *every* day as just described. There have been recent cases of rickets reported in the United States that resulted from not giving this vitamin.[17] Vitamin D is now a routine supplement in all commercial infant formulas, including evaporated milk. It is not, however, found in all brands of nonfat dry milk.

The adverse effects of excess quantities of vitamins A and D cannot be overemphasized. An infant who repeatedly receives more than 1800 to 3000 IU of vitamin D per day is in danger of toxicity, which may lead to hypercalcemia and other complications. Thus, the RDA of 400 IU of vitamin D should not be consistently or significantly exceeded. This is sometimes a difficult task, because of the multiplicity of vitamin D–fortified foods. Vitamin A may be toxic if an infant is given dosages of 18,500 IU per day for 1 to 3 months.

Human milk is rich in *vitamin E*, cow's milk is relatively low, and commercial formulas are supplemented with this vitamin. Supplementation has been advised for premature infants because of negligible placental transfer of this vitamin. A syndrome that includes megaloblastic anemia and rash has been described in growing prematures. This syndrome is correlated with low vitamin E levels and disappears with the administration of supplemental vitamin E.[18] A vitamin E toxicity syndrome has not been described.

Because of low values of plasma clotting factors, the newborn infant has a chance of abnormal bleeding in the first few days of life. Thus *vitamin K*, important in attaining the normal levels of prothrombin and other clotting factors, is usually given by injection to newborns (0.5 mg of an aqueous preparation). Adding vitamin K supplements to expectant mothers' diets during the last month to help raise the newborn's level of vitamin K has also been recommended as a possible prenatal preventive measure.[9]

The recommended daily allowance of *vitamin C*, 35 mg, is found in 850 ml of breast milk of well-nourished mothers. The vitamin C content of cow's milk is about one-fifth this amount, and, in addition, treatment of cow's milk for infant use (boiling, evaporation, drying) contributes to the destruction of this relatively unstable vitamin. Thus, most infant formulas are fortified with vitamin C.

Often, pediatricians will recommend that the infant avoid citrus fruits and juices up to the age of a year or so in order to prevent the development of possible allergic reactions to these foods. In these cases, supplemental vitamin C should be given in the form of vitamin drops if the infant is taken off prepared formulas or breast milk and started on regular milk.

All the B vitamins are present in milk formulas or breast milk in sufficient amounts to meet the recommended daily allowances for infants and toddlers who are on a normal milk intake. A diet with B complex vitamins in excess of the requirements is not considered hazardous, because excess amounts, if not over reasonable levels, will be excreted in the urine.

Generally, B vitamin deficiency states in infants and small children are rare in the United States. However, intakes of B-12 and folic acid deserve special attention. *Vitamin B-12* is not found in any plant source, unlike the rest of the B complex vitamins. Therefore, a pregnant woman who is on a strict "macrobiotic" diet or on a vegetarian diet and who does not have an intake of milk or eggs (which are, along with meat and fish, the only food sources of this vitamin) may give birth to an infant with a low vitamin B-12 level. Such infants are at high risk for developing a deficiency state that includes megaloblastic anemia.

Folacin is found both in meats and in

green, leafy vegetables as well as in most milk. However, it is present only in insignificant amounts in goat's milk, which is occasionally used as the primary milk in an allergy-prone infant or child (although commercially prepared, fortified, nonallergenic formulas are replacing it in most cases).* Thus any infant on goat's milk as a primary food should receive folacin supplementation at the recommended level of 50 mcg per day to prevent the deficiency state characterized by megaloblastic anemia. Also, it has been shown that strained baby foods that have been commercially prepared contain significantly lower amounts of this vitamin than do fresh vegetables.

Minerals

The infant's diet must include all the minerals essential for normal metabolism and growth. The major minerals needed by the infant occur in generous amounts in human milk, cow's milk–based formulas, and many other foods common in the infant's diet. (For a review of each mineral and its specific role, see Chapters 10, 11, and 12.) However, iron and fluorine are low in both human and cow's milk. Calcium and phosphorus are particularly important for skeletal growth, as well as for normal body physiology. The requirements for sodium, potassium, and chloride are particularly important to consider in the care and management of sick and dehydrated infants; this is a specialized topic and is not covered here.

Calcium and Phosphorus. Calcium makes up 1.5 to 2 percent of the adult's body weight, with 99 percent being present in bones and teeth; thus it is extremely important in the growth and development of these structures in children. During increased periods of growth, such as in infancy, the calcium absorption rate is higher than when the growth rate slows. Vitamin D, of course, is necessary for this absorption. The advisable intake for calcium is set at twice the calculated requirement of a breast-fed baby, because calcium absorption may be different in infants given nourishment other than human milk.

Usually, the allowance for calcium approximately equals the phosphate allowance, except in the young infant, in whom an excessive phosphate intake may contribute to hypocalcemic tetany. (Human milk contains approximately twice as much calcium as phosphorus.) In older infants, the phosphate allowance may be increased to 80 percent of the calcium allowance, which is the proportion of these minerals found in cow's milk.

A child who is not receiving his required intake of calcium and phosphorus (found primarily in milk and milk products) will still continue to grow, but the mineralization of bones and teeth will not be optimal (see also Chapter 11).

Iron. The importance of this mineral in the diet of infants and children has long been recognized. Recently, definite recommendations have been made to insure that youngsters will be protected from the anemia that results from lack of iron in the diet.*

The anemia of iron deficiency, if present, usually begins to appear at age 6 to 12 months. Up to 6 months of age, the full-term infant's iron stores, which were deposited in fetal life, are generally adequate for body needs (e.g., for the production of hemoglobin). After that age, body stores must be resupplied by the diet to insure proper blood formation. The highest incidence of iron-deficiency anemia in children is in those under 36 months of

*A quantitative listing of all vitamins found in different infant formulas is found in Fomon.[9]

*It has recently been found that iron deficiency may have an adverse effect on learning. Preliminary reports suggest that iron deficiency may have a detrimental effect on alertness, attention span, and the learning process even when the anemia is not severe.[19]

age, and those most often affected are children of low-income families (see Fig. 21–8).

The usual hemoglobin level at birth is high, at 16 to 18 gm per 100 ml of blood, and falls normally to a level of 10 to 11 gm when the child is 3 to 4 months of age. The level of hemoglobin should be maintained thereafter at 11 gm or better. Additional dietary iron is now recommended for formula-fed infants during the early months of infancy so that iron stores will not be depleted in 6 months. Supplemental iron should be added no later than the fourth month for full-term babies and no later than the second month for prematures[20] and should continue at least through the first year. The use of iron-fortified infant formulas has been shown to decrease significantly the incidence of iron-deficiency anemia in later infancy. Milk formulas fortified with iron cost little or no more than nonfortified formulas.

The daily requirement for iron in infancy, according to Fomon,[9] is at least 6 mg a day beginning at birth, or 8 mg a day if supplements are begun at 3 months of age. This requirement can best be met in the formula-fed infant by (1) an iron-supplemented formula or (2) iron drops. Iron-fortified infant cereal may be useful

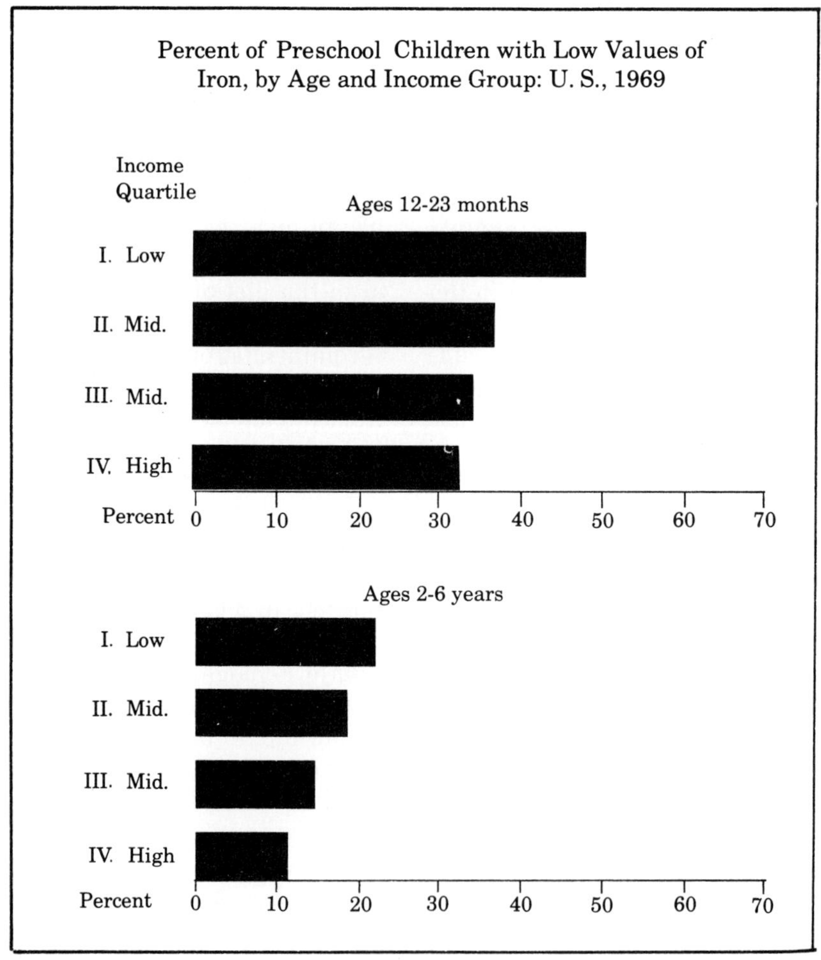

Figure 21–8 An example of the findings of poorer nutrition, here with serum iron values as an indicator, of preschool children in low-income families when compared with children of the same age in families with higher incomes. (From *Profiles of Children: 1970 White House Conference on Children,* p. 66. Washington, D.C., U.S. Government Printing Office.)

in later months.* (Another method of calculating iron recommendations is by body weight, and these recommendations are 1 mg per kg per day for term infants and 2 mg per kg per day for low birth weight infants.) During the preschool years, through age 3, the recommended allowance is set at 15 mg a day, which decreases to 10 mg a day during the years 4 to 10.

Recent evidence regarding absorption of iron in the breast-fed baby has shown that the relatively small amount of iron in breast milk is very efficiently absorbed by the infant,[21] and that breast-fed babies may be less likely to develop anemia than those fed cow's milk. Fresh cow's milk can cause microscopic blood loss in the infant's gastrointestinal system,[22] which then adds to the problem of deficient iron stores in the young child. This is one of the many reasons why the use of fresh cow's milk in the young infant's diet is not recommended.

Strained, prepared infant foods have generally not provided generous amounts of iron for infants' diets. Most prepared infants' dinners, for example, contain less than 1 mg of iron per 100 gm of food.

For more detailed remarks on iron requirements, functions, absorption, and metabolism, see Chapter 12.

Fluorine. This element is particularly important in early infancy and childhood because of its role in the prevention of dental caries. (See also Chapter 23.)

If there is fluoridation of the water supply at approximately 1 part per million, the baby whose powdered formula is made with that water will receive the recommended fluoride intake per day, and the infant receiving equal parts water and formula will also receive the recommended fluorine. However, if the infant is on "ready-to-serve" formula or is breast-fed,† he or she may not take in sufficient quantities of water to provide the necessary fluoride, and thus may need a supplemental dosage. (Supplemental fluoride preparations are available only on prescription.) Baby foods, which usually are composed of 70 to 80 percent water, may have varying quantities of fluoride.

Zinc. Serum levels of zinc have been found to be low in certain recent studies of otherwise normal children, particularly preschoolers, in some areas of the country.[23] Zinc levels appear to be lower in children from low-income groups than in those from middle-income groups. The effects of zinc deficiency are discussed in more detail in Chapter 12 and include growth retardation and loss of appetite.

Measures to prevent zinc deficiency, which include breast-feeding and an adequate intake of animal protein, are wise in infancy and early childhood. Such measures are also likely to be beneficial in respect to other trace elements, knowledge of which is more limited at this time.

NUTRITIONAL STATUS

What is the current status of nutritional health of children in the United States today? To what extent are the nutritional requirements listed previously being met? Data on the existence of specific nutritional problems in the population are essential for the planning of programs to improve nutritional health. Indices used to assess nutritional status in children include: (1) anthropometry with growth charting, (2) dietary history, (3) clinical assessment, and (4) laboratory studies, with x-ray when needed.

Anthropometrical ("man measures") measurements include weight, height, head circumference, fatfold, and upper arm circumference.

A dietary history should be at least of 24 hour duration.

Laboratory studies may consist of biochemical determination of any specific

*Iron added to cereals should be in the form of reduced iron of very small particle size, or as ferrous sulfate, in order to be efficiently absorbed.

†Beast milk contains less than 0.03 ppm of fluoride, regardless of the mother's fluoride intake. Cow's milk contains slightly more, but still not nearly enough to meet the infant's requirement.

nutrient being studied or of tests related to functions of the nutrients. An example of the latter is measuring blood level (hematocrit or hemoglobin) as a method of screening for iron deficiency. The physical exam notes any clinical signs of malnutrition such as cheilosis (seen in riboflavin deficiency) and Bitot spots (vitamin A deficiency). X-rays may be used in confirming cases of rickets or scurvy.

Recent National surveys to assess nutritional status of children in the United States are the following:

1. Preschool Nutrition Survey (1968–1970):[24] 3400 children, 1 to 6 years of age.

2. Ten-State Nutrition Survey (1968–1970):[25] 3700 children, 1 to 6 years of age.

3. Health and Nutrition Examination Survey (1971–1974):[26] 1500 children under 6 years of age.

Selected findings of these surveys are as follows:

1. The overall nutritional status of infants and young children in the United States appeared to be reasonably good.

2. Nutritional status correlates directly with socioeconomic status.

3. Poorer children have a smaller physical size.

4. Iron deficiency is the major nutrient deficiency disorder among children (see Fig. 21–8).

5. From 9 to 11 percent of children up to 1 year old were classified as obese, as were 6 to 8 percent of those 2 to 4 years old. The fatter children tended to be from families of middle and upper middle income.

6. Similarly, children's intakes of nutrients tended to increase with an increase in family income. This association was greatest for vitamin C.

7. Protein intake was an average of one and one-half to two times greater than the RDA's. There was no biochemical evidence of protein deficiency.

8. Twenty-five to 40 percent of preschoolers regularly received vitamin supplements. Unacceptably low levels of vitamin A were found in 30 to 50 percent of Spanish-American children and in 10 percent of black children compared with 1.5 percent of white children.

9. Ten to 15 percent of children had borderline or low ascorbic acid intakes.

10. Between 20 and 30 percent of black children and 10 to 15 percent of white children had levels of calcium below half the RDA.

11. Between 20 and 30 percent of children had iron intakes below 5 mg a day. (About half of all infants, to 2 years of age, in one survey were not receiving the minimum daily requirement of iron.) Anemia was found in 7 to 12 percent of all children studied and was most common in 1- to 2-year-olds of the lowest income groups.*

SPECIAL CONCERNS IN INFANT AND CHILDHOOD FEEDING

Food Allergies

Food allergies are often a subject of concern to parents attempting to give their children a complete and balanced diet. Allergies caused by foods are not as common as inhalant (pollen, etc.) allergies; however, they do occur more frequently in infants and young children than in adults. The infant has a greater tendency to absorb unaltered protein in the gastrointestinal tract and thus to have a greater potential for setting up antigen-antibody reactions, which constitute the allergic response.

Milk Allergy. This has also been termed milk sensitivity, or milk intolerance. Milk intolerance is a term best reserved for the rare condition resulting from a congenital deficiency of lactase, the enzyme that digests the milk sugar (lactose). It is not based on an antigen-

*Results of regional and more specialized nutritional status surveys are summarized in a recent article by Owen, G., and Lippman, G.: Nutritional status U.S.A. Pediatr. Clin. North Amer., *24*:214, 1977.

antibody reaction and thus is not a true allergy. Cow's milk is probably the most common food allergen in the United States. Estimates of the incidence of cow's milk allergy in the population range from 0.3 to 3 percent. It tends to run in families, and an infant who has an allergy to milk may also be allergic to other common food allergens, such as citrus fruits or egg whites.

Cow's milk allergy in susceptible infants is commonly manifested by frequent loose stools, respiratory symptoms, or allergic skin reactions, usually eczema, or any of these. Other signs may include asthma, headache, tension, fatigue, and possibly hyperactivity. More serious problems, such as shock (cardiovascular collapse), may rarely occur. The symptom may occur as early as 2 to 4 weeks of age, or later during the preschool years. Symptoms will begin in a susceptible breast-fed child soon after the first cow's milk feedings are given.

It may sometimes be necessary to eliminate cow's milk and milk products from the diet. Excellent cow's milk substitutes that provide essentially all nutrients normally found in milk are available. They also usually contain vitamin and mineral supplementation.* It has been shown that the growth of infants given these milk substitutes is no different from the growth of infants given breast milk. However, the older child may refuse the milk substitutes, and in these cases care must be taken that a proper diet is selected. For example, supplemental calcium may be necessary in such instances.

Heat treatment of cow's milk (as well as dried and evaporated milk preparations) or substitution of milk of another species (e.g., goat's milk) is sometimes helpful in decreasing allergic symptoms, but is not completely satisfactory because of some cross-reactive milk proteins.

Other Food Allergies. Additional foods that are common offenders as food allergens are chocolate and cola (the kola nut family), corn, eggs, the pea family (chiefly peanuts), citrus fruits, tomatoes, wheat and other small grains, cinnamon, and certain artificial food colors.*

Mothers of small infants who have a family history of allergy are often advised by their pediatricians to avoid, at least in the first few months, foods such as those just listed that may frequently cause allergies at early ages. It is recommended by some authorities that children who have parents with significant allergy problems would be better off without cow's milk or dairy products in the first 6 months.

There are two types of allergic reactions to foods. One is immediate, with the rapid occurrence of symptoms, and may be seen after the ingestion of fish, other seafood, eggs, or nuts. The other, a more common type, is a delayed response that may occur hours or days after the allergenic food (commonly wheat, milk, corn, oranges, or chocolate) is eaten. Examples of possible allergic responses are listed in Table 21–9.

A child who is suspected of having a food allergy should be on a trial period of elimination of the food for 1 to 3 weeks to see if symptoms will clear. Then a "challenge" (reintroduction) of the suspected food may be made, on the advice of the physician, to see if symptoms recur. In this way the diagnosis of food allergy can be made. Treatment consists of avoidance of the identified food or foods. A child with a known food allergy will require special menu planning to allow for a balanced, palatable, and enjoyable diet.

Vegetarian Diets for Children

Can a child be fed successfully on a vegetarian diet? The answer is a qualified yes. It is true that a diet excluding meat

---

*Examples include formulas based on hydrolyzed casein, strained homogenized lamb product, and soybean (a food that is not entirely free of the possibility of causing allergic responses itself).

*Food colors such as amaranth (red dye) and tartrazine (yellow dye) have been shown to cause allergic responses in susceptible individuals.[27]

Table 21–9 ADVERSE REACTIONS ATTRIBUTED TO FOOD ALLERGY*

Systemic: Shock, malaise, fever, failure to grow
Gastrointestinal: Stomatitis, colic, abdominal pain, flatulence, diarrhea, malabsorption, colitis
Central nervous system: Headache, irratability, hyperactivity, tension and fatigue
Muscular: Leg pains
Respiratory: Hay fever, asthma
Skin: Hives, eczema, other skin rashes
Ear: Serous otitis media

*Adapted from Vaughan, V. C., III, and McKay, R. J.: *Nelson Textbook of Pediatrics.* 10th Ed. Philadelphia, W. B. Saunders Co., 1975, p. 519.

protein will allow for adequate growth and development of a child, *provided* it is based on sound nutritional knowledge. There are different types of vegetarian diets, ranging from those that allow eggs and milk as well as fruits, cereal products, varied vegetables, and legumes and nuts, to diets that include primarily cereals and water. (See also Chapter 19.) The first type mentioned (the lacto-ovo-vegetarian type) would be expected to provide for complete nutritional needs *if* the following criteria are met:

1. The protein sources are complemented (that is, come from correct combinations of legumes, grains, and vegetables) in order to supply the essential amino acids, all of which are not found in any *one* vegetarian food.
2. There is an adequate supply of folacin and zinc (sometimes low in these diets).
3. A form of iodized salt is used.
4. The diet does in fact include allowances of milk, cheese, and eggs. (These foods are important because they would be the sole source of vitamin B-12 in this meatless diet, and they also help supply important amino acids, minerals such as calcium and iron, and other vitamins such as vitamin A.)

Vegetarian diets other than this carefully selected lacto-ovo-vegetarian type would not generally be advised for children. To try to raise infants and children without some form of milk or its complete equivalent, such as soy milk substitute, is very difficult and nutritionally unwise.

Failure to Thrive

This is a general term used by pediatricians and others to describe any infant who fails to attain his minimal expected gains in growth and development. It is a problem that requires expert diagnostic study and therapeutic steps. The most common cause is some form of failure to receive adequate nurture and nutrition to meet bodily needs, a process that may even start, as mentioned previously, before birth.

The failure may be at the level of food intake, or there may be a problem in digestion, assimilation, metabolism, or utilization of food. Most instances of failure to thrive in the United States have been identified as resulting from psychosocial circumstances that adversely affect the intake, absorption, or utilization of food. Emotional deprivation and physical neglect and abuse, including withholding of food, are found to be commonly associated.

Organic illnesses may also result in failure to thrive. Examples of diseases that may limit growth include the celiac syndrome (intestinal mucosal hypersensitivity to wheat protein), cystic fibrosis (a complex disease that includes a malabsorption state), galactosemia, and disaccharide deficiency.

There are innumerable other causes, but the problem of inadequate food should not be overlooked. Proper nutritional therapy and rehabilitation are of prime importance for these infants.

Pica and Lead Poisoning in Children

"Pica" is a term used to designate the tendency to eat substances (paper, plaster, paint, laundry starch, dirt) that usually are considered inedible. (See also Chapter 12.) An association of pica and zinc deficiency has been observed in at least one recent report.[28]

Pica is practiced by the child who eats, for example, the peeling paint of windowsills. There can be at least one serious complication associated with this type of behavior. If the substances ingested (paint, plaster, etc.) contain *lead*, lead poisoning may result.

Overnutrition in Infancy and Childhood

Obesity, in children as well as in adults, is very hard to resolve successfully. Prevention is far easier than cure, and is dependent upon early detection of children who are exhibiting an excess rate of weight gain, as well as early identification of factors in the infant or child or in his or her environment that may predispose to obesity.

Overweight in children can result from increased lean body mass, adipose tissue, or both. Skinfold measurements are an important adjunct to the classic measurements of graphing of children's weight and height for their age. Skinfold measurement helps differentiate children who are overweight owing to increased muscle mass from those in the early stages of obesity who need preventive interventions.

Factors considered valuable in the prediction of later obesity include the following:

1. Family history of obesity
2. Weight at 4 to 7 years of age
3. Weight during infancy
4. Birth weight (and weight/height ratio)

Family history of obesity is probably at present the best predictor of later obesity in an infant or child. It has been shown that with one obese parent, there is a 40 percent chance that the child will be overweight, and with two obese parents, the risk increases to the range of 70 to 80 percent.[29] Similar risks have also been demonstrated in children who have been adopted by obese parents;[30] thus, the definite increased incidence of obesity in children with obese parents either may be a result of a genetic disturbance or may simply reflect the family's eating habits (or a combination of both).

The predictive value of early weight history of a child has been the subject of conflicting reports and opinions. Conclusions of different studies include the following.[30, 31, 32]

1. In a group of overweight infants, only 20 percent were overweight at 6 to 9 years of age.
2. For those children overweight later in childhood, 80 percent will remain overweight later in life.
3. Only 10 percent of obesity observed in children at 10 years of age in a Swedish community could have been predicted from observations of weight gain during infancy.
4. On the other hand, a British report showed that infants who gained weight rapidly in infancy did attain a greater height and weight at the age of 6 years.
5. A recent report in the United States showed that newborns who had a high weight/height ratio (were very stocky for their height) as a group tended toward a normal weight by age 7 years, but that a statistically larger percentage of these infants were heavy at 7 years old than were newborns of normal weight. The number of slender newborns who became obese by 7 years was very low. Nearly all children who were overweight by 4 years of age remained heavy at 7 years of age.

Thus it appears that all overweight babies are not marked for a later bout with obesity, but it is slightly more likely for them than for slender infants. Childhood (rather than infantile) obesity has a more definite correlation with adult obesity; one can state with some certainty that if a child is overweight at age 7 years, it is likely he or she will always have a weight problem.

Theories regarding increased numbers of fat (adipose) cells in cases of infantile obesity have been put forth,[33] and although there are inherent difficulties in cell counting techniques, it does appear that the earlier the onset of obesity, the greater the number of adipose cells. Yet correlation of number of fat cells with later obesity is uncertain.

The issue of energy expenditure is also relevant; obese infants and children are often less active than their slimmer companions. Lack of activity with resultant low calorie expenditure may cause obesity in some children whose intakes of food are not unusual. There is no doubt that a vigorous activity program has an important part in the prevention, as well as the treatment, of obesity.

What are some practical recommendations for weight control in overweight children? First, it should be realized that weight *loss* is not a goal for children; rather, the goal is a weight that is kept relatively constant while linear growth continues normally. Total calories should not drop below 1200 to 1400 a day, or growth requirements may be compromised.

A balanced, varied diet should be maintained. Family meals may have to be altered to include fewer foods with excess calories, such as fried foods, gravy, fatty meats, and rich desserts. Carbohydrate snacking between meals should be eliminated, with more nutritious snacks substituted. Parents should learn to recognize the child's cues for satiation and not feed them beyond that point.

The use of food for nonnutritive reasons should be explored with parents, and decreased if possible. Nonnutritive uses of food (rewards for desired behavior, comforting of a frustrated child, etc.) teach children to rely on food to compensate for emotional and social difficulties. This pattern may continue throughout a lifetime if begun early in childhood.

TABLE 21–10 SUGGESTED MEASURES FOR THE PREVENTION OF OVERWEIGHT PROBLEMS IN CHILDREN

1. Breast-feed if possible, and introduce other foods at 4 to 6 months of age.
2. Recognize when the infant or child is satisfied with a meal (the feeding) and STOP there.
3. Try not to use food as a reward, or its withholding as a punishment.
4. Encourage an energetic program of physical activity for all children.
5. Children with overweight parents should have special attention given to the development of good eating and exercise habits, since they are at much higher risk for becoming overweight.

As they grow older, children will begin to make their own decisions about food choices and thus need explanation and support from family regarding a reasonable diet, as well as a systematic program of physical activity.

The problem of overweight is much better prevented early, and suggestions for prevention are summarized in Table 21–10. (Also see Chapter 24.)

Early Prevention of Heart Disease

In the United States, heart disease is the number one cause of mortality in adults. There is growing realization among health professionals that the prevention of heart disease begins in childhood. Nutritionally related risk factors for heart disease include:

1. Level of cholesterol in the blood (high cholesterol levels are associated with increased incidence of atherosclerotic heart disease).

2. Intake of salt in the diet (increased salt intake has been associated with increased incidence of high blood pressure — an important cause of heart disease).

There are several other factors that also have been reported to be associated with the development of heart disease, such as smoking, lack of exercise, family history of heart disease, personality type, and the disease diabetes.

It is agreed by nutritional and pediatric experts that there is no evidence to support sweeping changes in diet to attempt to lower cholesterol levels in normal children.[34] Care should be taken, of course, to use reasonable, not excessive, amounts of fat and calories in the diet.

It is also generally agreed that for children (and adults) with *familial hyperlipoproteinemia** (a genetic condition affecting from 1 in 150 to 300 children) diets *should* be restricted in total fat, saturated fatty acids, and cholesterol. These genetic conditions put affected children at very high risk for early heart attacks, and a modified diet is part of the treatment of the disorder. (Drugs are often used as well to lower the dangerously high cholesterol level.)

With regard to the potential risk factor of high salt intake for later cardiovascular disturbances, it was pointed out in Chapter 10 that the average American diet does include an excess of salt. Young children do not generally enjoy highly salted foods; the liking for salty foods is considered to be an acquired taste. Therefore, it is reasonable to avoid the addition of salt to infants' and children's foods. Infant food manufacturers, for example, have decreased considerably (or stopped) the addition of salt to prepared baby foods.

Dental Caries Prevention

Dental disease is probably the most prevalent disorder found in routine health exams of children in the United States today. See Chapter 23 for a complete discussion of nutritional preventive measures, which include, briefly, (1) decreasing the amount of sugary foods eaten by children, especially sticky, sugary foods eaten between meals and (2) insuring a proper intake of fluorine.

*The hyperlipoproteinemias are a class of inherited disorders in which the serum lipoproteins are elevated, associated with elevations of cholesterol or triglycerides, or both.

Food in Special Conditions

As important as proper feeding is to children who are well, it becomes critical in times of special needs such as illness, as well as during rapid growth periods.

The importance of prenatal nutrition is discussed in the preceding chapter. After delivery, the full-term, normal infant is ready to suck and feed normally, but the low birth weight or sick infant may need special nutritional attention.

Disease treatments that also call for specialized nutritional knowledge include those for illnesses in which the body lacks certain enzymes required for proper digestion and metabolism of ingested foods. Foods must be carefully selected in these cases to avoid the illness symptoms that arise often only when the unacceptable food is eaten. Examples of disease states in children for which special nutritional expertise is needed include phenylketonuria (PKU), galactosemia, hyperlipidemia, food allergies, lactose intolerance, disaccharidase deficiencies, and chronic diarrheas. Individuals with these conditions should be under the supervision of their physicians.

INFANT AND CHILD MALNUTRITION IN DEVELOPING COUNTRIES

The discussion has focused so far on the nutritional needs and practices of children of the United States. Many countries around the world, often those with very low per capita incomes and high population growth rates, have problems of infant feeding not even touched upon here. The infant and childhood mortality rates in these countries are generally high — for the most part as a result of the combined effects of malnutrition, infection (see Fig. 21–9), poor economic conditions, and lack of accurate information about nutrition and health.

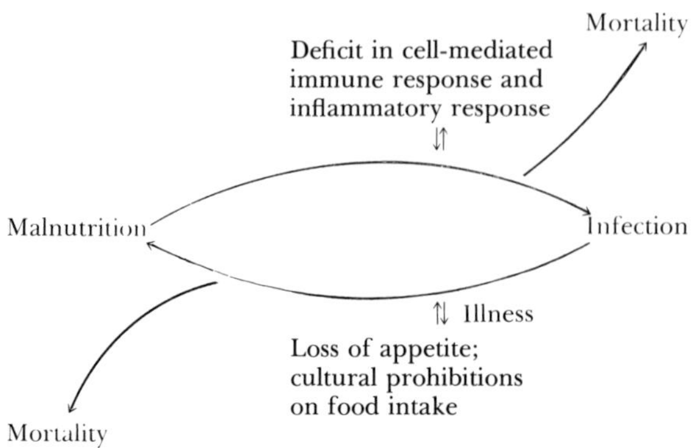

Figure 21–9 The "vicious cycle" of malnutrition and infection, which leads to high mortality in infants and preschool children in developing countries.

Most critical to the development of symptoms of malnutrition in most areas is currently an overall insufficiency of calories.[35] Thus an increasing prevalence of marasmus compared with kwashiorkor (see Chapter 5) has been noted worldwide. Significant protein-energy malnutrition results from maldistribution of food within a family as well as from overall food shortages.

Some specific examples of problems that contribute to childhood malnutrition around the world are:

1. Sudden weaning from the breast of a toddler at the arrival of a new baby demanding all the mother's breast milk. This toddler is then deprived of this already minimal supply of his only high nutrient food, with other portions of his typical weaning diet consisting of foods high in mainly carbohydrate content. This train of events is particularly common in the causation of kwashiorkor.

2. Lack of sufficient supplemental foods for the breast-fed baby after about 6 months of age.

3. Traditional, unscientific customs, such as those demanding that the few high nutrient foods available go first (and often, only) to the adult males of the tribe and family. In some areas, cultural food taboos effectively deny certain protein-rich foods, such as eggs, to pregnant women and young children.

The increasing practice of bottle-feeding, considered to be the "modern method" in some underdeveloped areas, is also a subject of serious concern. The advantages of breast-feeding in these areas are very high, both because of the inherent advantages of human milk and because the facilities for safe, sterile preparation and storage of bottle formulas are limited. (In fact, the infant is lucky if there is actually milk in the bottle; in one location, rice water was given because it resembled the European pictures of bottled formulas!) Halting the decline in breast-feeding in developing countries is a current objective of most international health organizations. Statistics have shown that when breast-feeding declines in these countries, infant death rates stay high or even increase.*

It is clear that childhood nutrition is a very real and high priority concern in many parts of the world (see Fig. 21–10). Childhood undernutrition is not, unfortunately, completely unknown even in the

*Aggressive advertising of bottled formulas in developing countries has recently come under attack by various consumer groups and health professionals.

generally more advantaged United States. This is particularly true in economically deprived areas.

MALNUTRITION DURING INFANCY AND LATER INTELLECTUAL CAPACITY

There is at present no conclusive evidence that malnutrition in infancy causes permanent mental retardation. In animals, a causal relationship has been demonstrated between early malnutrition and body size, brain growth, and brain content of protein, DNA, and RNA. In humans, it has been noted that infants and children within the United States living below the poverty level have unexpectedly small head circumferences, which may be taken as presumptive evidence for diminished brain volumes.[36] These observed physical changes in themselves, however, cannot be assumed to be a direct cause of behavioral changes.

In humans, severe malnutrition usually exists in conjunction with other adverse conditions such as poverty, low levels of education, and inadequate health care. Thus, there is extreme difficulty in pinpointing specific effects of nutritional deficiency alone.

Studies in which infants, after suffering an early severe nutritional insult, were returned to middle-class, enriching environments with adequate nutrition as well as adequate developmental stimulation, identified no permanent defects in intellectual functioning on later follow-up.[37] Studies such as these are leading to the tentative conclusion that certain developmental effects of early, limited periods of malnutrition may be reversible with optimal therapeutic conditions.

A child recovering from early malnutrition should be fed well, not only with nutritious food, but also with social and intellectual stimulation. Conversely, the deleterious effects of early malnutrition will be greatest when, even after nutritional rehabilitation, the child continues to live in an environment in which both

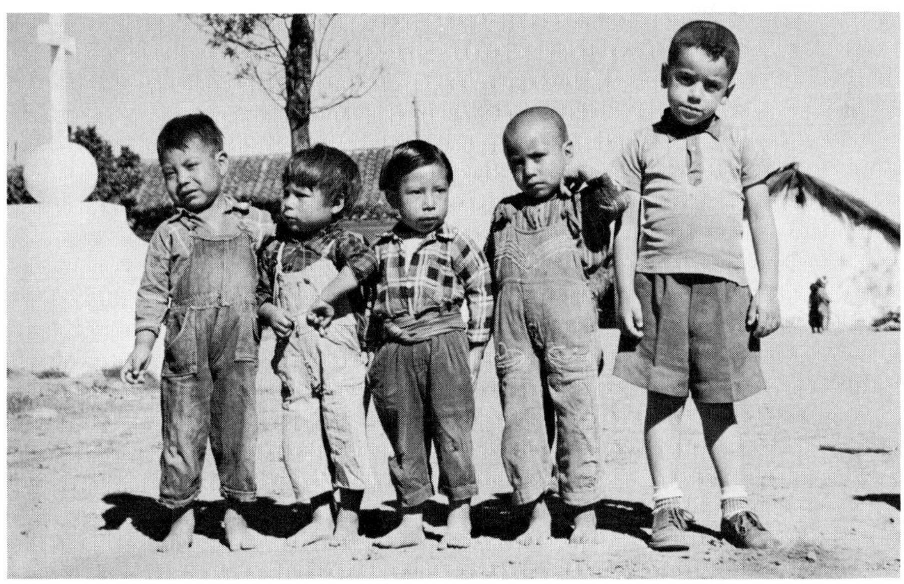

Figure 21–10 Marked difference in growth and general nutritive condition of Guatemalan boys 4 to 5 years of age, contrasting village children reared on the native diet (corn and beans as chief food staples) with a boy of same age group from a professional man's family, in which the diet was superior. The latter boy (at right) is of normal height and weight for this age group; the others show stunted growth and other evidence of poor nutrition. Supplementing the poor diets to meet nutritive needs results in better growth and condition, but tissue damages caused by early deprivation may persist into later life. (Courtesy of Dr. Miguel A. Guzman, Institute of Nutrition for Central America and Panama.)

social and nutritional circumstances are inadequate for his optimal growth and development.

PROGRAMS FOR IMPROVING CHILDHOOD NUTRITION IN THE UNITED STATES

WIC Program*

The objective of this program is to insure optimal nutrition for pregnant women and for children up to 5 years old who otherwise might not be able to meet their nutritional requirements. Vouchers are given, and women can buy milk, eggs, cheese, cereals, and other nutritious food products for themselves and their children.

Evaluations of this program have demonstrated nutritional and health benefits to participating women and children.

School Food Programs

An understanding of school programs is important to parents and teachers who influence the child's eating habits.

Planning the school lunch menu is a challenge for the nutritionist, who must take into consideration government specifications, cost limitations, physical set-up of the school kitchen, cultural and racial background of the children, inclusion of a wide variety of foods, and, most importantly, acceptance of the meal by the children.

The National School Lunch Act was passed in 1946 "to safeguard the health and well-being of the nation's children and to encourage the domestic consumption of nutritious agricultural commodities and other food, by assisting the states through grants-in-aid and other means, in providing an adequate supply of foods and other facilities for the establishment, maintenance, operation, and expansion of nonprofit school lunch programs."

The current National School Lunch Program is based on the original act, and a number of amendments have been added to the original legislation. For example, in 1970, an amendment stipulated that every needy American schoolchild should be given a free or reduced price meal. Also, in 1973 the School Breakfast Program became available to all schools wishing to apply.

As a guideline to insure nutritional adequacy in school food service, the "Type A" pattern is followed by all schools participating in the National School Lunch Program. The lunch pattern is designed to allow flexibility to provide children with a wide variety of foods and to allow consideration of their regional, cultural, ethnic, and special dietary needs and food practices in menu planning.

The Type A lunch must provide one-third of the RDA and meet the following requirements:

1. *Milk*: include the following: 1 of fluid, fresh nonfat milk, low-fat milk, whole milk, or buttermilk.
2. *A protein-rich food*: 2 oz of meat, poultry, fish, or cheese; ½ c of cooked dried beans or peas; or 4 tbsp of peanut butter.
3. *Vegetables and fruits*: ¾ c of at least two types of vegetables or fruits.
4. *Bread*: one slice of whole-grain or enriched bread.
5. *Butter or fortified margarine*: at least 1 tsp as a spread or in preparation of other foods.

Menu planners are advised to include the following in each day's menu:

1. Several foods that are good sources of iron.
2. A good fruit or vegetable source of carotene.
3. At least one raw food each day.
4. A food high in vitamin C content.

*Women, Infants, and Children (WIC), a supplemental feeding program, began in 1972. It is administered by the USDA on the Federal level and by health departments on the state and local levels.

At present, the USDA has proposed very significant changes in these recommended meal patterns. Proposed regulations, expected to be started by 1979, would:

1. Establish minimum food patterns for five age groups that would reduce portion sizes for children age 8 years and under while offering more food to students age 12 years and over (they may request smaller portion sizes).

2. Include a recommendation to "keep fat, sugar, and salt at a moderate level;" change bread requirement from a daily to a weekly requirement and allow enriched or wholegrain rice, macaroni, or noodle products as a bread alternate.

3. Require schools to involve students in their school food service program through activities such as menu planning, enhancement of the eating environment, program promotion, and related student-community support activities.

Children whose families may have difficulty in purchasing school lunch on a daily basis are entitled to subsidized or free lunches. In some areas, there are also school breakfast programs, preschool feeding programs, and summer feeding programs.

Nutrition Education of Children

The elementary grades are an important time to emphasize nutrition education in the classroom. The school lunch can ideally be used as a "learning laboratory" for classroom instruction. An imaginative approach, with field trips, cooking activities, games, use of audiovisual materials, and involvement of children in evaluating and planning their own eating habits can promote an effective nutrition education program.

The subject can be reinforced throughout the school year by integrating nutrition education with other subject areas. For example, in a social studies unit, different cultural food habits can be explored. Also, names of different varieties of foods may be introduced in spelling or mathematics lessons.

CONCLUSION

More study, research, and experience will be required before we know the final answers to many still unresolved questions and problems of infant and childhood nutrition. Above all, however, there is a real need for *application* of nutritional knowledge already gathered to help insure optimal health and development for all the world's infants and children — from children in your own neighborhood to those in the farthest lands.

QUESTIONS AND PROBLEMS

1. By what age will the newborn infant normally double its birth weight? Triple it?
2. List three advantages of breast milk as an infant food.
3. What is an average daily milk intake for a 6-month-old child weighing 15 pounds (7 kg)?
4. By what age should the infant be on a diet that includes meats and other solids?
5. What are advisable dietary supplements for a 3-month-old infant who is breast-fed? For one who is fed an evaporated milk formula?
6. Name three foods that might be suspected if a 9-month-old infant begins to develop signs of allergy.
7. What would you advise a vegetarian mother who asks you about the adequacy of the "vegetarian" diet that she feeds her 2-year-old?
8. Prepare a day's sample menu (including snacks) for a day-care center taking care of 3-to 5-year-olds, open from 7 A.M. to 6 P.M.
9. What are three methods used to determine a child's nutritional status?
10. What would you say is the major

nutritional problem of children in the United States today? In the developing countries? Discuss your choices.

REFERENCES

1. National Center for Health Statistics: NCHS Growth Charts, 1976. Monthly Vital Statistics Report, Vol. 25, No. 3, Supp. (HRA) 76–1120.
2. Mitchell, H. S.: Nutrition in relation to stature. J. Amer. Dietet. Assoc., *40*:521, 1962.
3. Prader, A., Tanner, J. M., and Von Harnack, G. A.: Catch-up growth following illness or starvation. J. Pediatr., *62*:646, 1963.
4. Safer, D., Allen, R., and Barr, E.: Growth rebound after termination of stimulant drugs. J. Pediatr., *86*:113, 1975.
5. U.S. Dep. of Health, Education, and Welfare: *Little Babies: Born Too Soon, Born Too Small.* Dept. of Health, Education, and Welfare Pub. No. (NIH) 77–1079, 1977.
6. Postnatal growth of small-for-dates babies. Nutr. Rev., *31*:51, 1973.
7. Personal communication with La Leche League International, Chicago, Ill., 1977.
8. Wood, A. L.: The history of artificial feeding of infants. J. Amer. Dietet. Assoc., *31*:474, 1955.
9. Fomon, S. J.: *Infant Nutrition.* 2nd Ed. Philadelphia, W. B. Saunders Co., 1974.
10. Committee on Nutrition, American Academy of Pediatrics: Commentary on breast-feeding and infant formulas, including proposed standard for formulas. Pediatr., *57*:278, 1976; Corporation of Professional Dieticians of Quebec: Position paper on infant feeding. J. Can. Dietet. Assoc., *38*:193, 1977; Maternal and Child Health Branch, California Dept. of Health: Breast Feeding — Its Role in Infant Growth and Development. 1977; Resolution of the 27th World Health Assembly (1974): Infant nutrition and breast-feeding. Cajanus, *7*:120, 1974.
11. Goldman, A. S., and Smith, C. W.: Host-resistant factors in human milk. J. Pediatr., *82*:1082, 1973.
12. Gerrard, J.: Breast feeding: second thoughts. Pediatr., *54*:757, 1974.
13. Ounsted, M., and Sleigh, G.: The infant's self-regulation of food intake and weight gain. Lancet, *1*:1393, 1975.
14. Fomon, S.: What are infants fed in the U.S.? Pediatr., *56*:350, 1975.
15. Feeding the baby of low birth weight. Nutr. Rev., *31*:14, 1973.
16. Hansen, A. E., et al.: Influence of diet on blood serum lipids in pregnant women and newborn infants. Amer. J. Clin. Nutr., *15*:11, 1964.
17. O'Connor, P.: Vitamin D deficiency rickets in two breast fed infants who were not receiving vitamin D supplementation. Clin. Pediatr., *16*:361, 1977.
18. Dallman, P. R.: Iron, vitamin E and folate in the preterm infant. J. Pediatr., *85*:742, 1974.
19. Smith, N. J., and Rios, E.: Iron metabolism and iron deficiency in infancy and childhood. Adv. Pediatr., *21*:239, 1975.
20. Committee on Nutrition, American Academy of Pediatrics: Iron supplementation for infants. Pediatr., *58*:765, 1976.
21. McMillan, J. A., Landaw, S. A., and Oski, F. A.: Iron sufficiency in breast fed infants and the availability of iron from human milk. Pediatr., *58*:686, 1976.
22. Woodruff, C. W., Wright, S. W., and Wright, R. P.: The role of fresh cow's milk in iron deficiency. Amer. J. Dis. Child., *124*:26, 1972.
23. Hambidge, K. M., Walravens, P. A., Brown, R. M., et al.: Zinc nutrition of preschool children in the Denver Head Start Program. Amer. J. Clin. Nutr., *29*:734, 1976.
24. Owen, G.: A study of the nutritional status of preschool children in the U.S. 1968–1970. Pediatr., *53*:11, 1974 (Supplement).
25. Dept. of Health, Education, and Welfare: *Ten-State Nutrition Survey 1968–1970.* Dept. of Health, Education, and Welfare Pub. No. (HSM) 72–8132, 1972.
26. Dept. of Health, Education, and Welfare: *Preliminary Findings of the First Health and Nutrition Examination Survey, U.S. 1971–1972.* Dept. of Health, Education, and Welfare Pub. No. (HRA) 74–1219–1, 1975.
27. Speer, F.: Food allergy: the 10 common offenders. A.F.P., *13*:106, 1976.
28. Hambidge, K. M.: The role of zinc and other trace metals in pediatric nutrition and health. Pediatr. Clin. N. Amer., *24*:95, 1977.
29. Bruch, H.: *Eating Disorders.* New York, Basic Books, Inc., 1973, p. 26.
30. Weil, W. B., Jr.: Current controversies in childhood obesity. J. Pediatr., *91*:175, 1977.
31. Charney, E., Goodman, H. C., McBride, M., Lyon, B., and Pratt, R.: Childhood antecedents of adult obesity. Do chubby infants become obese adults? N. Engl. J. Med., *295*:6, 1976.
32. Pipes, P.: *Nutrition in Infancy and Childhood.* St. Louis, C. V. Mosby, 1977, Chapter 9.
33. Dobbing, J.: Fat cells in childhood obesity. Lancet, *1*:224, 1975.
34. Committee on Nutrition, American Academy of Pediatrics: Childhood diet and coronary heart disease. Pediatr., *49*:305, 1972.
35. McLaren, D. S., and Burman, D.: *Textbook of Pediatric Nutrition.* New York. Churchill Livingstone, 1976, Chapter 6.
36. CNI (Community Nutrition Institute) Weekly Report, Jan. 15, 1976.
37. Stein, Z.: Nutrition and mental performance. Science, *178*:708, 1972.

SUPPLEMENTARY READING

General, History, and Reviews

(also see ref. 1–37)

Aykroyd, W. R.: Nutrition and mortality in infancy and early childhood: past and present relationships. Amer. J. Clin. Nutr., *24*:480, 1971.

Beal, Virginia: Nutrition in children. In Wallace, H.,

Gold, E., and Lis, E.: *Maternal and Child Health Practice.* Springfield, Ill., Charles C Thomas, 1973.

Committee on Nutrition, American Academy of Pediatrics: Salt intake and eating patterns of infants and children in relation to blood pressure. Pediatr., *53*:115, 1974.

Committee on Nutrition, American Academy of Pediatrics: Nutritional needs of low birth-weight infants. Pediatr., *60*:519, 1977.

Cravioto, J., and Delicardie, F. R.: Nutrition in early childhood. Food Nutr., *2*:2, 1976.

Fredrickson, D. S. (ed.): Symposium: Factors in childhood that influence the development of atherosclerosis and hypertension. Amer. J. Clin. Nutr., *25*:222, 1972.

Hill, L. F.: Infant feeding: historical and current. Pediatr. Clin. N. Amer., *14*:255, 1967.

Jelliffe, D. B.: *Childhood Nutrition in the Developing Countries. WHO,* Geneva, 1968.

Jelliffe, D. B., and Jelliffe, E. F. P.: A bookshelf of nutrition programs for pre-school children — a recent selected bibliography. Amer. J. Pub. Health, *62*:469, 1972.

Jelliffe, D. B., and Jelliffe, E. F. P.: *Human Milk in the Modern World.* Oxford, Oxford University Press 1978.

Jensen, R. G., Hagerty, M. M., and McMahon, K. E.: Lipids of human milk and infant formulas. A review. Amer. J. Clin. Nutr., *31*:990, 1978.

Lambert-Lagacé, L.: *Feeding Your Child.* Cambridge, Ontario, Hobitex Books, Collier-Macmillan Canada, 1976.

Martin, E. A.: *Roberts' Nutrition Work with Children.* Chicago, University of Chicago Press, 1954.

Martin, H. P.: Nutrition: its relationship to children's physical, mental, and emotional development. Amer. J. Clin. Nutr., *26*:766, 1973.

Neumann, C. G., and Jelliffe, D. B. (eds.): Symposium: Nutrition in pediatrics. Pediatr. Clin. North Amer., *24*:1, 1977.

Read, M. S., and Felson, D.: *Malnutrition, Learning and Behavior.* National Institute of Child Health and Human Development, Dept. of Health, Education, and Welfare Pub. No. (NIH) 76–1036, April 1976.

Spady, Donald W.: Infant Nutrition. J. Can. Dietet. Assoc., *38*:34, 1977.

Vahlquist, Bo: A Two-Century Perspective of Some Major Nutritional Deficiency Diseases in Childhood. Acta Pediatr. Scand., *64*:161, 1975.

Winick, M.: *Childhood Obesity.* New York, John Wiley & Sons, 1975.

Nutrition and Growth

Adrianzen, T. B., Baertl, J. M., and Graham, G. G.: Growth of children from extremely poor families. Amer. J. Clin. Nutr., *26*:926, 1973.

Dugdale, A. E., Chen, S. T., and Hewitt, G.: Patterns of growth and nutrition in childhood. Amer. J. Clin. Nutr., *23*:2180, 1970.

Ferris, A. G., et al.: Diets in the first six months of infants in Western Massachusetts. Part I. Energy-yielding nutrients. J. Amer. Dietet. Assoc., *72*:155, 1978: Part II. Semi-solid foods. J. Amer. Dietet. Assoc., *72*:160, 1978.

Frisancho, A. R.: Triceps skinfold and upper arm muscle size norms for assessment of nutritional status. Amer. J. Clin. Nutr., *27*:1052, 1974.

Garn, S. M.: Malnutrition and skeletal development in the preschool child. In *Pre-School Child Malnutrition, Primary Deterrent to Human Progress.* Pub. No. 1282. Washington, D.C., National Academy of Sciences, National Research Council, 1966.

Gopalan, C., et al.: Effect of calorie supplementation on growth of undernourished children. Amer. J. Clin. Nutr., *26*:563, 1973.

Graham, G. G.: Environmental factors affecting the growth of children. Amer. J. Clin. Nutr., *25*:1184, 1972.

Habicht, J., et al.: Height and weight standards for preschool children. How relevant are ethnic differences in growth potential? Lancet, *1*:611, 1974.

Hamill, P. V., and Moore, W. M.: Contemporary growth charts: needs, construction and application. Public Health Currents, Special Issue, Ross Laboratories, 1976.

Hansen, J. D. L., et al.: What does nutritional growth retardation imply? Pediatr., *47*:299, 1971.

Holliday, M. A.: Metabolic rate and organ size during growth from infancy to maturity and during late gestation and early infancy. Pediatr., *47*:169, 1971.

Kagan, B. M., et al.: Body composition of premature infants: relation to nutrition. Amer. J. Clin. Nutr., *25*:1153, 1972.

Knapp, J., et al.: Growth and nitrogen balance in infants fed cereal proteins. Amer. J. Clin. Nutr., *26*:586, 1973.

Lowrey, G. H.: *Growth and Development of Children.* Chicago, Yearbook Medical Publishers, 1973.

MacLean, W. C., Jr., and Graham, G. G.: Growth and nitrogen retention of children consuming all of the day's protein intake in one meal. Amer. J. Clin. Nutr., *29*:78, 1976.

Neumann, C. G., and Alpaugh, M.: Birthweight doubling time: a fresh look. Pediatr. *57*:469, 1976.

Rueda-Williamson, R., and Rose, H. E.: Growth and nutrition of infants: the influence of diet and other factors on growth. Pediatr., *30*:639, 1962.

Tanner, J. M.: The evaluation of physical growth and development. In Holzel, A., and Tizard, J. P. M. (eds.): *Modern Trends in Pediatrics.* London, Butterworth & Co., Ltd., 1958.

Woodruff, C.: Nutritional aspects of metabolism of growth and development. J.A.M.A., *196*:214, 1966.

Youlton, R., et al.: Serum growth hormone and growth activity in children and adolescents with present or past malnutrition. Amer. J. Clin. Nutr., *25*:1179, 1972.

Nutritional Status

Adebonojo, F. O., and Strahs, S.: Vitamin nutriture in black, urban, day care children. Amer. J. Clin. Nutr., *27*:559, 1974.

American Academy of Pediatrics: The Ten-State Nutrition Survey: a pediatric perspective. Pediatr., *51(6)*:1095, 1973.

Black, A. E., Billewicz, W. Z., and Thomson, A. M.: The diets of preschool children in Newcastle upon Tyne, 1968–71. Brit. J. Nutr., *35*:105, 1976.

Caliendo, M. A., et al.: Nutritional status of preschool children. An ecologic analysis. J. Amer. Dietet. Assoc., *71*:20, 1977.

Cook, R. A., et al.: Nutritional status of Head Start and nursery school children. I. Food intake and anthropometric measurements. J. Amer. Dietet. Assoc., *68*:120, 1976.

Cook, R. A., Hurlburt, R. A., and Radke, F. H.: Nutritional status of Head Start and nursery school children. II. Biochemical measurements. J. Amer. Dietet. Assoc., *68*:127, 1976.

Driskell, J. A., and Price, C. S.: Nutritional status of preschoolers from low-income Alabama families. J. Amer. Dietet. Assoc., *65*:280, 1974.

Frank, G. C., et al.: Adapting the 24-hour recall for epidemiologic studies of school children. J. Amer. Dietet. Assoc., *71*:26, 1977.

Frank, G. C., et al.: Dietary studies of rural school children in a cardiovascular survey. J. Amer. Dietet. Assoc., *71*:31, 1977.

Futrell, M. F., Kilgore, L. T., and Windham, F.: Nutritional status of black preschool children in Mississippi. Influence of income, mother's education, and food programs. J. Amer. Dietet. Assoc., *66*:22, 1975.

Garn, S. M., and Clark, D. C.: Nutrition, growth, development and maturation: findings from the Ten-State Nutrition Survey, 1968–1970. Pediatr., *56*:306, 1975.

Guthrie, H. A.: Nutritional status measures as predictors of nutritional risk in preschool children. Amer. J. Clin. Nutr., *29*:1048, 1976.

Guthrie, H. A., and Guthrie, G. M.: Factor analysis of nutritional status data from Ten-State Nutrition Surveys. Amer. J. Clin. Nutr., *29*:1238, 1976.

Guthrie, H. A., Owen, G. M., and Guthrie, G. M.: Factor analysis of measures of nutritional status of preschool children. Amer. J. Clin. Nutr., *26*:497, 1973.

Jelliffe, D. B., and Jelliffe, E. F. P.: Nutrition programs for preschool children. Amer. J. Clin. Nutr., *25*:595, 1972.

Jenicek, M., and Demirjian, A.: Triceps and subscapular skinfold thickness in French-Canadian school-age children in Montreal. Amer. J. Clin. Nutr., *25*:576, 1972.

Kafatos, A. G., and Zee, P.: Nutritional benefits from federal food assistance — survey of preschool black children from low-income families in Memphis. Amer. J. Dis. Child., *131*:265, 1977.

Marktl, W., and Rudas, B.: Screening for risks of cardiovascular disease in children. A preliminary report. Brit. J. Nutr., *35*:223, 1976.

Rao, K. V., and Rao, N. P.: Association of growth status and the incidence of nutrition deficiency signs. Amer. J. Clin. Nutr., *28*:209, 1975.

Ruffin, M., Calloway, D. H., and Margen, S.: Nutritional status of preschool children of Marin County welfare recipients. Amer. J. Clin. Nutr., *25*:74, 1972.

Sigulem, D. M., et al.: Plasma and urine ribonuclease as a measure of nutritional status in children. Amer. J. Clin. Nutr., *26*:793, 1973.

Sims, L. S., and Morris, P. M.: Nutritional status of preschoolers. An ecologic perspective. J. Amer. Dietet. Assoc., *64*:592, 1974.

Infant Feeding, General*

Addy, D. P.: Infant feeding: a current view. Brit. Med. J., *1*:1268, 1976.

Anderson, T. A., and Fomon, S. J.: Commercially prepared strained and junior foods for infants. J. Amer. Dietet. Assoc., *58*:520, 1971.

Beyer, N. R., and Morris, P. M.: Food attitudes and snacking patterns of young children. J. Nutr. Educ., *6*:131, 1974.

Bowering, J., et al.: Influence of a nutrition education program (EFNEP) on infant nutrition in East Harlem. J. Amer. Dietet. Assoc., *72*:392, 1978.

Brown, A. M., and Matheny, A. P., Jr.: Feeding problems and preschool intelligence scores: a study using the co-twin method. Amer. J. Clin. Nutr., *24*:1207, 1971.

Cowell, C., et al.: Survey of infant feeding practices. Amer. J. Pub. Health, *63*:138, 1973.

Davies, D. P.: Infant's self-regulation of food intake. Lancet, *2*:366, 1975.

Davies, D. P., et al.: Effects of solid foods on growth of bottle-fed infants in first three months of life. Brit. Med. J., *2*:7, 1977.

Fomon, S. J.: Skim milk in infant feeding. J. Amer. Dietet. Assoc., *63*:156, 1973.

Friedman, G., and Goldberg, S. J.: Concurrent and subsequent serum cholesterols of breast- and formula-fed infants. Amer. J. Clin. Nutr., *28*:42, 1975.

Herbert-Jackson, E., Cross, M. Z., and Risley, T. R.: Milk types and temperature — What will young children drink? J. Nutr. Ed., *9*:76, 1977.

Hodgson, P. A., et al.: Comparison of serum cholesterol in children fed high, moderate, or low cholesterol milk diets during neonatal period. Metabolism, *25*:739, 1976.

Hofacker, R., and Brenner, N.: Vegetable parade persuades children to try new foods. J. Nutr. Ed., *8*:21, 1976.

Ireton, C. L., Guthrie, H. A.: Modification of vegetable-eating behavior in preschool children. J. Nutr. Ed., *4*:100, 1972.

Jelliffe, D. B.: World trends in infant feeding. Amer. J. Clin. Nutr., *29(11)*:1227, 1976.

Maslansky, E., et al.: Survey of infant feeding practices. Amer. J. Pub. Health, *64*:780, 1974.

Mathews, R. H., and Norkman, M. Y.: Nutrient content of selected baby foods. J. Amer. Dietet. Assoc., *72*:27, 1978.

Mayer, J.: Baby foods: a new look at old formulas. Family Health, *8*:38, 1976.

Raiha, N. C., et al.: Milk protein quantity and quality in low-birthweight infants: I. Metabolic responses and effects on growth. Pediatr., *57*:659, 1976.

Rickard, K., and Gresham, E.: Nutritional considerations for the newborn requiring intensive care. J. Amer. Dietet. Assoc., *66*:592, 1975.

---

*Including milk substitutes.

Smith, B. A. M.: Feeding overstrength cow's milk to babies. Brit. Med. J., *4*:741, 1974.
Spady, D. W.: Infant nutrition. J. Can. Dietet. Assoc., *38*:34, 1977.
Tomarelli, R. M.: Osmolality, osmolarity, and renal solute load of infant formulas. J. Pediatr., *88*:454, 1976.
Wade, N.: Bottle-feeding: adverse effects of a western technology. Science, *184*:45, 1974.
Willis, A. T., et al.: Breast milk substitute: a bacteriological study. Brit. Med. J., *4*:67, 1973.
Woodruff, C. W.: The science of infant nutrition and the art of infant feeding. J.A.M.A., *240*:657, 1978.

Various Committee Reports and Miscellaneous

Are baby foods good enough for babies? Consumer Reports, *40*:528, 1975.
Citizen's Committee on Infant Nutrition: White paper of infant feeding practices. Center for Science in the Public Interest, 1974.
Committee on Nutrition, American Academy of Pediatrics: Should milk drinking by children be discouraged? Pediatr., *53*:576, 1974.
Current concepts in infant nutrition. Dairy Council Dig., *47*:6, 1976.
Feeding the newborn: Comparative problems in animals and man (symposium proceedings). Proc. Nutr. Soc., *33*:79, 1974.

Articles in Nutrition Reviews

Modified food starches for use in infant foods. *29*:55, 1971.
Infant protein needs provided by a soy-based formula. *32*:42, 1974.
The effect of a breast milk substitute on stool flora. *32*:136, 1974.
Should milk drinking by children be discouraged? *32*:363, 1974.
Oral feeding versus TPN in low birthweight infants. *33*:270, 1975.

Breast-Feeding

Brown, R. E.: Breast-feeding in modern times. Amer. J. Clin. Nutr., *26*:556, 1973.
Chavez, A., Martinez, C., and Bourges, H.: Role of lactation in the nutrition of low socio-economic groups. Ecol. Food Nutr., *4*:159, 1975.
Eastham, E., et al.: Further decline of breast-feeding. Brit. Med. J., *1*:305, 1976.
Fomon, S.: Human milk and the small premature infant. Amer. J. Dis. Child., *131*:463, 1977.
Hadjimarkos, D. M., and Shearer, T. R.: Selenium in mature human milk. Amer. J. Clin. Nutr., *26*:583, 1973.
Hirschman, C., and Sweet, J.: Social background and breastfeeding among American mothers. Soc. Biol. *21*:39, 1974.
Jelliffe, D. B., and Jelliffe, E. F. P.: Nutrition and human milk. Postgrad. Med., *60*:153, 1976.
Jelliffe, D. B., and Jelliffe, E. F. P.: Breast is best: modern meanings. N. Engl. J. Med., *297*:912, 1977.
Jelliffe, D. B., and Jelliffe, E. F. P.: The volume and composition of human milk in poorly nourished communities. Amer. J. Clin. Nutr., *31*:492, 1978.
Jonsson, V., et al.: Chlorohydrocarbon pesticide residues in human milk in Greater St. Louis, Miss., 1977. Amer. J. Clin. Nutr., *30*:1106, 1977.
Pitt, J.: Breast milk leukocytes. Pediatr., *58*:769, 1976.
Stoliar, O. A., et al.: Secretory IgA against enterotoxins in breast-milk. Lancet, *1*:1258, 1976.
Turner, R. W. D.: Breast is best for coronary protection (letter). Lancet, *2*:693, 1976.
Wheeler, E. F.: Food intake and rate of weight gain in two healthy breast-fed infants. Amer. J. Clin. Nutr., *26*:631, 1973.

Committee Reports and Miscellaneous

Breast-feeding: A commentary of the Canadian Pediatric Society and the American Academy of Pediatrics. Pediatr., *62*:591, 1978.
Breast-feeding is best (editorial). Lancet, *2*:1029, 1974.
Breast Feeding (symposium). J. Human Nutr., *30*:223, 1976.
Breast milk for all (editorial). N. Engl. J. Med., *297*:939, 1977.
Is Breast-feeding best for babies? Consumers Reports, *42*:152, March, 1977.

Articles in Nutrition Reviews

To breast feed or not? *30*:112, 1972.
Lactoferrin — a bacteriostatic protein in human milk. *30*:225, 1972.
Commentary on breast-feeding and infant formulas, including proposed standards for formulas. *34*: 248, 1976.
Insecticides in breast milk. *35*:72, 1977.
The role of milk leukocytes in protection from necrotizing enterocolitis. *36*:190, 1978.
Immunological aspects of human milk (by Chandra, R. K.). *36*:265, 1978.

Food and Nutrient Requirements, General

Cuthbertson, W. F.: Essential fatty acid requirements in infancy. Amer. J. Clin. Nutr., *29*:559, 1976.
DeVizia, B., et al.: Digestibility of starches in infants and children. J. Pediatr., *86*:50, 1975.
Fomon, S. J., et al.: Requirements for protein and amino acids in early infancy: studies with soy-isolate formula. Acta Pediatr. Scand., *62*:33, 1973.
Jelliffe, D. B., Ifekwunigwe, A. E., and Jelliffe, E. F. P.: Recommended dietary allowances for infants. Ecol. Food Nutr., *4*:53, 1975.
MacLean, W. C., Jr., and Graham, G. G.: Growth and nitrogen retention of children consuming all of the day's protein intake in one meal. Amer. J. Clin. Nutr., *29*:78, 1976.

Articles in Nutrition Reviews

The influence of dietary fat on the composition of the body fat of infants. *33*:236, 1975.
Protein quality of high protein wheats for young children. *34*:263, 1976.

Total parenteral nutrition in infants and children. *35*:6, 1977.
Dietary protein intake and fat absorption in children. *36*:75, 1978.
Intestinal development affected by prenatal protein deprivation. *36*:191, 1978.

Vitamins

(Also see refs. 9, 17, and 18)

Alvarado, J., et al.: Vitamin B-12 absorption in protein-calorie malnourished children and during recovery: influence of protein depletion and of diarrhea. Amer. J. Clin. Nutr., *26*:595, 1973.
Davis, K. C.: Vitamin E: adequacy of baby diets. Amer. J. Clin. Nutr., *25*:933, 1972.
Davis, K. C.: Vitamin E content of selected baby foods. J. Food Sci., *38*:442, 1973.
Jusko, W. J., et al.: Riboflavin absorption and excretion in the neonate. Pediatr., *45*:945, 1970.
Lakdawala, D. R., and Widdowson, E. M.: Vitamin-D in human milk. Lancet, *1*:167, 1977.
Lampkin, B. C., and Saunders, E. F.: Nutritional vitamin B-12 deficiency in an infant. J. Pediatr., *75*:1053, 1969.
O'Connor, P.: Vitamin D–deficiency rickets in two breast-fed infants who were not receiving vitamin D supplementation. Clin. Pediatr., *16*:361, 1977.
Vobecky, J. S., et al.: Vitamin E and C levels in infants during the first year of life. Amer. J. Clin. Nutr., *29*:766, 1976.
Williams, M. L., et al.: Role of dietary iron and fat on vitamin E deficiency anemia of infancy. N. Engl. J. Med., *292*:887, 1975.

Articles in Nutrition Reviews

Vitamin E therapy in premature babies. *33*:206, 1975. Neonatal calcium homeostasis, vitamin D and parathyroid function. *34*:112, 1976.

Minerals

(Also see refs. 9 and 19 to 23)

Arakawa, T., et al.: Zinc deficiency in two infants during total parenteral alimentation for diarrhea. Amer. J. Clin. Nutr., *29*:197, 1976.
Ashkenazi, A., et al.: The syndrome of neonatal copper deficiency. Pediatr., *52*:525, 1973.
Committee on Nutrition, American Academy of Pediatrics: Zinc. Pediatr., *62*:408, 1978.
Dollman, P. R.: Iron, vitamin E and folate in the preterm infant. J. Pediatr., *85*:742, 1974.
Hambidge, K. M., et al.: Zinc nutrition of preschool children in the Denver Head Start program. Amer. J. Clin. Nutr., *29*:734, 1976.
Johnson, C. C., and Futrell, M. F.: Anemia in black preschool children in Mississippi. Dietary and hematologic findings. J. Amer. Dietet. Assoc., *65*:536, 1974.
Kerr, C. M., Jr., *et al.*: Sodium concentration of homemade baby foods. Pediatr., *62*:331, 1978.
Margo, G., et al.: Anemia in urban underprivileged children. Iron, folate, and vitamin B-12 nutrition. Amer. J. Clin. Nutr., *30*:947, 1977.
Meiners, C. R., et al.: The relationship of zinc to protein utilization in the preadolescent child. Amer. J. Clin. Nutr., *30*:879, 1977.
Momcilovic, B., et al.: Bioavailability of zinc in milk and soy protein–based infant formulas. J. Nutr., *106*:913, 1976.
Picciano, M. F., and Guthrie, H. A.: Copper, iron, and zinc contents of mature human milk. Amer. J. Clin. Nutr., *29*:242, 1976.
Rios, E., et al.: The absorption of iron as supplements in infant cereal and infant formulas. Pediatr., *55*:686, 1975.
Wilson, J. F., Lahey, M. E., and Heiner, D. C.: Studies on iron metabolism. V. Further observations on cow's milk–induced gastrointestinal bleeding in infants with iron-deficiency anemia. J. Pediatr., *84*:335, 1974.

Committee Reports and Miscellaneous

Committee on Nutrition, American Academy of Pediatrics: Salt intake and eating patterns of infants and children in relation to blood pressure. Pediatr., *53*:115, 1974.
Committee on Nutrition, American Academy of Pediatrics: Iron supplementation for infants. Pediatr., *58*:765, 1976.
Neonatal calcium, magnesium, and phosphorus homeostasis (editorial). Lancet, *1*:155, 1974.

Articles in Nutrition Reviews

Salt in infant foods. *29*:27, 1971.
Absorption of trace elements during the neonatal period. *30*:258, 1972.
Fresh cow's milk and iron deficiency in infants. *31*:318, 1973.
Renal handling of salt by preterm infants. *33*:105, 1975.

Overnutrition and Obesity in Children

(Also see refs. 29 to 31)

Coates, T. O., and Thoresen, C. E.: Treating obesity in children and adolescents: A review. A.J.P.H., *68*:143, 1978.
Crawford, P. B., et al.: An obesity index for six-month-old children. Amer. J. Clin. Nutr., *27*:706, 1974.
Crawford, P. B., Hankin, J. H., and Huenermann, R. L.: Environmental factors associated with preschool obesity. III. Dietary intakes, eating patterns, and anthropometric measurements. J. Amer. Dietet. Assoc., *72*:589, 1978.
DeSwiet, M., Fayers, P., and Cooper, L.: Effect of feeding habit on weight in infancy. Lancet, *1*:892, 1977.
Fisch, R. O., Bilek, M. K., and Ulstrom, R.: Obesity and leanness at birth and their relationship to body habitus in later childhood. Pediatr., *56*:521, 1975.
Frank, G. C., Berenson, G. S., and Webber, L. S.: Dietary studies and the relationship of diet to cardiovascular disease risk factor variables in 10-year-old children—the Bogalusa study. Amer. J. Clin. Nutr., *31*:328, 1978.
Huenemann, R. L.: Environmental factors associated with preschool obesity. I and II. Obesity and food practices of children at successive age levels. J. Amer. Dietet. Assoc., *64*:480, 488, 1974.

Mann, G. V.: The influence of obesity on health. N. Engl. J. Med., *291*:226, 1974.
Neumann, C. G.: Obesity in pediatric practice: obesity in the preschool and school-age child. Pediatr. Clin. North Amer., *24*:117, 1977.
Ravelli, G., Stein, Z. A., and Susser, M. W.: Obesity in young men after famine exposure in utero and early infancy. N. Engl. J. Med., *295*:1, 1976.
Stunkard, A.: Influence of social class on obesity and thinness in children. J.A.M.A., *221*:579, 1972.
Taitz, L. S.: Overfeeding in infancy. Proc. Nutr. Soc., *33*:113, 1974.
Winick, M.: Childhood obesity. Amer. J. Clin. Nutr., *29*:124, 1976.

Articles in Nutrition Reviews

Infantile obesity and respiratory infections. *29*:112, 1971.
Nutrition evaluation of preschool children. *30*:34, 1972.
Overfeeding in the first year of life. *31*:4, 116, 1973.
Catch-up growth in celiac disease. *31*:13, 1973.
Postnatal growth of small-for-dates babies. *31*:51, 1973.
The growth of children given stimulant drugs. *31*:91, 1973.
Selected body measurements of children 6–11 years. *31*:230, 1973.
Calorie supplementation and growth of pre-school children. *32*:141, 1974.
Comparison of body weights and lengths or heights of groups of children. *32*:284, 1974.
Growth of the human brain. *33*:6, 1975.
Infant body composition by skinfold measurements. *33*:7, 1975.
Will a fat baby become a fat child? *35*:138, 1977.
Infant feeding, somatic growth, and obesity. *35*:235, 1977.
Special report of the Food and Nutrition Board: Fetal and Infant Nutrition and Susceptibility to Obesity. *36*:122, 1978.

Special Topics

(Also see refs. 1 to 37)

Food Allergy

Eastham, E. J., and Walter, W. A.: Effect of cow's milk on the gastrointestinal tract. Pediatr., *60*:477, 1977.
Feeney, M. C.: Nutritional and dietary management of food allergies in children. Amer. J. Clin. Nutr., *22*:103, 1969.
Johnstone, D. E., and Dutton, A. M.: Dietary prophylaxis of allergic disease in children. N. Engl. J. Med., *274*:715, 1966.
Lebenthal, E.: Cow's milk protein allergy. Pediatr. Clin. North Amer., *22*:827, 1975.
Little, B.: *Recipes for Allergies.* New York, Vantage Press, Inc., 1968.
Mortimer, E. Z.: Anaphylaxis following ingestion of soybean. J. Pediatr., *58*:90, 1961.
Rowe, A. H., and Rowe, A.: *Food Allergy, Its Manifestations and Control and the Elimination Diets: A Compendium.* Springfield, Ill., Charles C Thomas, 1972.
Speer, F.: Management of food allergy. In Speer, F., and Dockhorn, R. J.: *Allergy and Immunology in Children.* Springfield, Ill., Charles C Thomas, 1973.

Failure to Thrive

Lozoff, B.: Kwashiokor in Cleveland. Amer. J. Dis. Child., *129*:710, 1975.
Smith, C. A., and Berenberg, W.: The concept of failure to thrive. Pediatr., *46*:661, 1970.

Vegetarianism

Committee on Nutrition, American Academy of Pediatrics: Nutritional aspects of vegetarianism, health foods, and fad diets. Pediatr., *59*:460, 1977.
Shull, M., et al.: Velocities of growth in vegetarian preschool children. Pediatr., *60*:410, 1977.
Vyhmeister, I., Register, U. D., and Sonnenberg, L.: Safe vegetarian diets for children. Pediatr. Clin. North Amer., *24*:203, 1977.

Malnutrition and Infection

Buckley, R. H.: Iron deficiency anemia: its relationship to infection susceptibility and host defense. J. Pediatr., *86*:993, 1975.
Chandra, R. K.: Immunocompetence in low-birth-weight infants after intrauterine malnutrition. Lancet, *2*:1393, 1974.
Committee on International Nutrition Programs, Food and Nutrition Board: *Immune Response of the Malnourished Child.* Washington, D.C., The National Research Council, 1976.
James, J. W.: Longitudinal study of the morbidity of diarrheal and respiratory infections in malnourished children. Amer. J. Clin. Nutr., *25*:690, 1972.
James, W. P. T., Drasar, B. S., and Miller, C.: Physiological mechanism and pathogenesis of weanling diarrhea. Amer. J. Clin. Nutr., *25*:564, 1972.
Neumann, C. G., et al.: Immunologic responses in malnourished children. Amer. J. Clin. Nutr., *28*:89, 1975.
Suskind, R., et al.: Immunoglobulins and antibody response in children with protein-calorie malnutrition. Amer. J. Clin. Nutr., *29*:836, 1976.
Weinberg, E. D.: Iron and susceptibility to infectious disease. Science, *184*:952, 1974.
Whitehead, R. G.: Infection and the development of kwashiokor and marasmus in Africa. Amer. J. Clin. Nutr., *30*:1281, 1977.

Malnutrition and Mental Development

Barnes, R. H.: Dual role of environmental deprivation and malnutrition in retarding intellectual development. Amer. J. Clin. Nutr., *29*:912, 1976.
Dobbing, J.: Nutrition and brain development. In *Present Knowledge in Nutrition.* Washington, D.C., The Nutrition Foundation, 1976.
Lloyd-Still, J. D., et al.: Intellectual development after severe malnutrition in infancy. Pediatr., *54*:306, 1974.

Nutrition in critical periods of development (editorial). Lancet, *2*:229, 1977.
Stoch, M. B., and Smythe, P. M.: 15-year developmental study on effects of severe undernutrition during infancy on subsequent physical growth and intellectual functioning. Arch. Dis. Child., *51*:327, 1976.
Winick, M.: *Malnutrition and Brain Development.* New York, Oxford Univ. Press, Inc., 1976.

Malnutrition in Developing Countries

Aykroyd, W. R.: Nutrition and mortality in infancy and early childhood: past and present relationships. Amer. J. Clin. Nutr., *24*:480, 1971.
Berg, A.: *The Nutrition Factor.* Washington, D.C., The Brookings Institute, 1973.
Greiner, T.: Regulation and education: strategies for solving the bottle feeding problem. Cornell International Nutrition Monograph Series, No. 4, 1977.
György, P., Devadas, R. P., and Chandrasekhar, U.: Calories in the treatment of PCM. Ind. J. Nutr. Dietet., *10*:252, 1973.
Icaza, S. J.: The nutritionist caring for malnourished children. J. Amer. Dietet. Assoc., *63*:130, 1973.
Jackson, R. L.: Longterm consequences of suboptimal nutritional practices in early life: some important benefits of breast feeding. Pediatr. Clin. North Amer., *24*:63, 1977.
Mata, L. J., and Behar, M.: Malnutrition and infection in a typical rural Guatemalan village: lessons for the planning of preventive measures. Ecol. Food Nutr., *4*:41, 1975.
Pollitt, E.: Behavior of infant in causation of nutritional marasmus. Amer. J. Clin. Nutr., *26*:264, 1973.

Nutrition in School-Age Children

deGroot, I., et al.: Lipids in schoolchildren 6 to 17 years of age. Pediatr., *60*:437, 1977.
Frey, A. L., et al.: Comparison of Type A and nutrient standard menus for school lunch. I. Development of the nutrient standard method (NSM). J. Amer. Dietet. Assoc., *66*:242, 1975.
Guthrie, H. A.: Effect of a flavored milk option in a school lunch program. J. Amer. Dietet. Assoc., *71*:35, 1977.
Harper, J. M., et al.: Comparison of Type A and nutrient standard menus for school lunch. II. Management aspects and acceptability. J. Amer. Dietet. Assoc., *66*:249, 1975.
Head, M. K., and Weeks, R. J.: Major nutrients in the Type A lunch. II. Amounts consumed by students. J. Amer. Dietet. Assoc., *67*:356, 1975.
Head, M. K., and Weeks, R. J.: Conventional vs. formulated foods in school lunches. I. Comparison of student's food and nutrient intakes. J. Amer. Dietet. Assoc., *71*:116, 1977.
Jansen, G. R., et al.: Comparison of Type A and nutrient standard menus for school lunch. III. Nutritive content of menus and acceptability. J. Amer. Dietet. Assoc., *66*:254, 1975.
Karp, R. J., et al.: The school health service as a means of entry into the inner-city family for the identification of malnourished children. Amer. J. Clin. Nutr., *29*:216, 1976.
Paige, D. M., Cordano, A., and Huang, H.: Nutritional supplementation of disadvantaged elementary school children. Pediatr., *58*:607, 1976.

Nutrition Education

Baker, M. J.: Influence of nutrition education on fourth and fifth graders. J. Nutr. Ed., *4*:55, 1972.
Bell, C. G., and Lamb, M. W.: Nutrition education and dietary behavior of fifth graders. J. Nutr. Ed., *5*:196, 1973.
Blakeway, S. F., and Knickrehm, M. E.: Nutrition education in the Little Rock school lunch program. J. Amer. Dietet. Assoc., *72*:389, 1978.
Boysen, S. C., and Ahrens, R. A.: Nutrition instruction and lunch surveys with second graders. J. Nutr. Ed., *4*:172, 1972.
Chethik, B. B.: Volunteers teach nutrition to teachers and students. J. Nutr. Ed., *6*:133, 1974.
Cooper, B., and Philip, M.: Evaluation of nutrition education in everyday teaching environment. J. Nutr. Ed., *6*:99, 1974.
Garton, N. B., and Bass, M. A.: Food preferences and nutrition knowledge of deaf children. J. Nutr. Ed., *6*:60, 1974.
Harrill, I., Smith, C., and Gangever, J. A.: Food acceptance and nutrient intake of preschool children. J. Nutr. Ed., *4*:103, 1972.
Head, M. K.: A nutrition education program at three grade levels. J. Nutr. Ed., *6*:56, 1974.
Johnson, M. J., and Butler, J. L.: Where is nutrition education in U.S. public schools? J. Nutr. Ed., *7*:20, 1975.
Juhas, L.: Nutrition education in day care programs. A new challenge to our profession. J. Amer. Dietet. Assoc., *63*:134, 1973.
Musgrave, K. O., and Thorbury, M. E.: Nutrition education at Indian schools. J. Nutr. Ed., *6*:137, 1974.
Peck, E. B.: Nutrition education specialists. J. Nutr. Ed., *8*:11, 1976.
Wang, M., and Dwyer, J. T.: Reaching Chinese-American children with nutrition education. J. Nutr. Ed., *7*:145, 1975.

Articles in Nutrition Reviews

Gastrointestinal milk allergy in infants. *27*:7, 1969.
Cellular growth in infantile malnutrition. *29*:6, 1971.
Early malnutrition and behavior. *30*:12, 1972.
Commerciogenic malnutrition? *30*:199, 1972.
Cellular immunity and malnutrition. *30*:253, 1972.
Nutrition and the body's defense mechanism. *31*:115, 1973.
Eating between meals — a nutrition problem among teenagers? (by Thomas, J. A., and Call, D. L.) *31*:137, 1973.
Effect of famine on later mental performance. *31*:140, 1973.
U.S. adolescent's growth analyzed. *31*:167, 1973.
Infantile malnutrition and malabsorption. *31*:321, 1973.
The national school lunch program in 1973: some accomplishments and failures (by Lukaczer, M.) *31*:385, 1973.
Comment on the above (by Hekman, E.). *31*:389, 1973.
Effects of the diet on brain neurotransmitters. *32*:193, 1974.
Breast feeding and avoidance of food antigens in the prevention and management of allergic diseases. *36*:181, 1978.

Chapter 22

Nutrition, Physical Work, and Athletics

Sound nutrition and a sensible program of physical activity are two of the chief requirements for health. Most people are aware of the need for a good diet, whether or not they have one, but few people seem to realize how important exercise is to their general well-being. Exercise is a dominant variable in energy balance (total energy expenditure). Energy intake is not adequately regulated to prevent obesity unless enough physical work is done (Chapter 13).

Even a modest but diligently followed program of training has been shown to alter the body composition of sedentary middle-aged men. In one study the men were required to walk only 40 minutes at a speed of 4 to 5 miles per hour four times a week, and yet their weight and body fat were somewhat reduced and their cardiovascular fitness was significantly improved.[1] Measurements of old men showed that among those in the eighth decade of life the ones who were most active had the highest amount of lean body tissue and their muscle strength was equal to that of inactive men who were 10 years younger.[2] Physical activity (defined as any amount of habitual running) was also shown to be equivalent to a difference of 10 years of age as regards parameters of physical fitness in middle-aged men.[3] Fitness is also related in a desirable way to a number of factors associated with risk of heart disease. Inactivity is associated with loss of bone substance (osteoporosis), and the epidemiology of hip fracture suggests that hard physical work throughout life protects against it.[4]

It has been suggested that lack of physical activity and sports in childhood leads to underdeveloped abdominal muscles and weak connective tissue sheaths that then contribute to chronic low back pain in women after pregnancy.[5] Women often restrict physical activity owing to the old-fashioned notion that menses are made difficult by vigorous movement. In most women fitness is slightly reduced 2 to 6 days before the onset of menstruation,[6] yet women athletes perform superbly throughout the menstrual cycle. The last months of pregnancy place a great burden on the maternal circulation. When the mother does physical work, her muscles compete with the placenta for blood, and if her heart is small it may not adequately cope with the double burden. Pregnant women with small hearts have an increased risk of premature delivery.[6] One way to assure good development of the musculature and the cardiovascular system is by a program of regular physical exercise throughout life, for women as well as for men.

Psychologists also point out beneficial effects of physical activity. Exercise is said to be an outlet for unconsumed accumulated energy and so reduces "free floating tension" and channels aggresion outward. Fretfulness, restlessness and insomnia are outcomes ascribed to failure to relieve tension by physical activity.[7]

Neither adults nor teenagers are very active in typical Western cultures. Although American teenagers were found to spend a bit more time in moderate and strenuous activity than adults of the same sex, girls spent 95 per cent of their time asleep and in activities classed as very light (2.5 kcal per minute or less) or light (2.5 to 4.9 kcal per minute), and boys spent over 90 percent of their time in light activities.[8] Urban Australian youth spent 78 to 80 percent of their time lying or sitting, 14 to 20 percent in very light activity, and only 1.5 to 4.4 percent in any activity that involved greater energy expenditure than walking.[9]

Work Capacity

The ability to perform work is dependent on energy-yielding processes in muscle cells. To work, muscle cells must have oxygen, which comes from the lungs via the blood and is taken up by the muscle cell. The ability to work can be limited by failure of any one of these processes: inadequate lung capacity, inadequate capability of the heart to pump blood, inadequate oxygen-carrying power of the blood, or failure of the peripheral circulation to supply enough blood to the working muscle. In some disease conditions or in very heavy smokers, lung power may be limiting, but generally it is cardiovascular factors that limit work. During exercise blood is diverted from the organs to the maximum extent feasible to supply the working muscles and the heart. As illustrated in Figure 22–1, the combined effect of diversion of blood circulation and increased heart pumping action augments the blood supply to the muscles by thirtyfold.[10] Anemia is one condition in which oxygen transport is limited. Low blood hemoglobin levels in anemic patients and the sharp drop in hemoglobin occasioned by blood donation in healthy women reduce blood buffering power and capacity to transport oxygen and have a detrimental effect on work performance.[11] In sedentary but normal persons, limitation is usually due to poor cardiovascular fitness, and the heart then has to work very hard to pump blood at levels of work

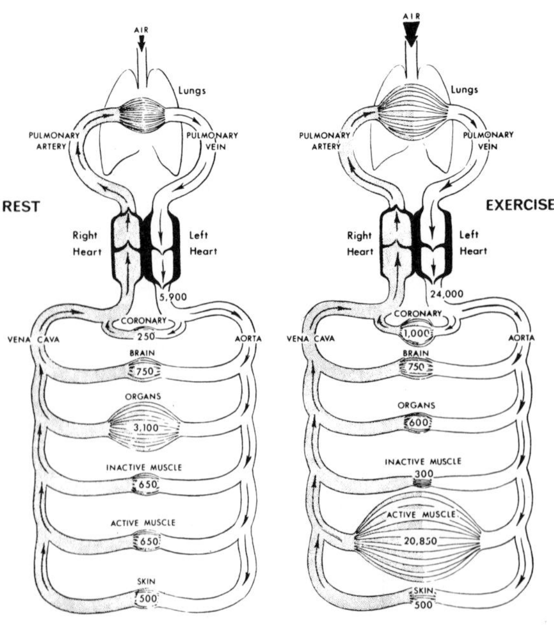

Figure 22–1 Schematic representation of the blood circulation of a sedentary man during standing rest and during exercise at the maximal oxygen uptake. Organs include kidneys, liver, gastrointestinal tract, and others. Blood flow is given in milliliters per minute. (Courtesy of Drs. Mitchell and Blomqvist and the New England Journal of Medicine.[10])

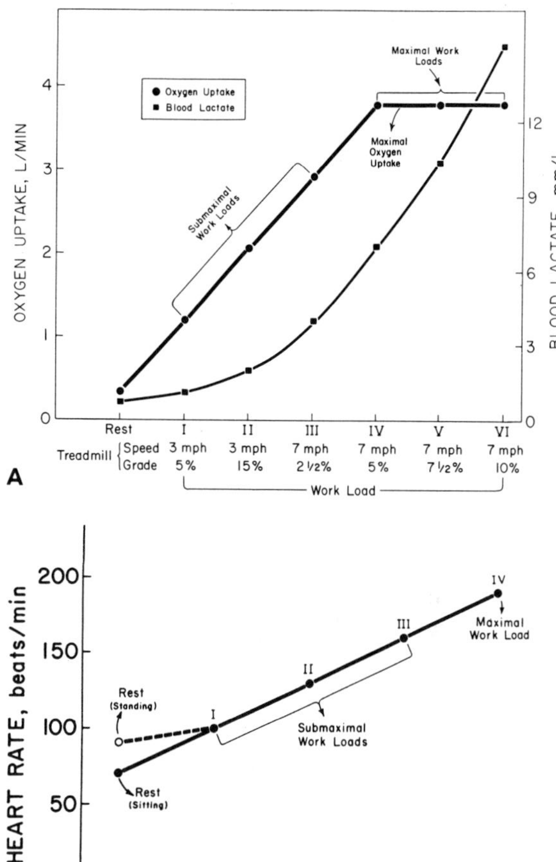

Figure 22–2 **A,** Maximal oxygen uptake determined by means of a motor-driven treadmill. The man does increasingly harder work until the capacity to take in oxygen reaches its limit. After this point, lactic acid rises because there is not enough oxygen to metabolize glycogen completely. **B,** With progressively increasing exercise loads there is a linear relation between heart rate and oxygen uptake.

(Courtesy of Drs. Mitchell and Blomqvist and the New England Journal of Medicine.[10])

that are well tolerated by persons who are more fit.

Since work requires energy expenditure and that involves oxygen, higher work levels are always associated with higher tissue uptake of oxygen and more oxygen removal in respiration. *Maximal oxygen uptake* is the greatest amount of oxygen a person can take in during exercise and so reflects his ability to transport oxygen to his tissues (Fig. 22–2). Thus, maximal oxygen uptake is one index of fitness. For average middle-aged men the maximal oxygen uptake is 35 to 40 ml per kg of body weight per minute, or about 2.5 liters of oxygen per minute. In well-trained young athletes, maximal oxygen uptake is about 70 ml per kg per minute.

When people work at very high rates, oxygen supplied to the tissues is not sufficient to oxidize muscle glycogen completely and an intermediate compound, lactic acid, accumulates. (See section on glycolysis, Chapter 15). After the work is completed, the person continues to breathe heavily and takes up additional oxygen until the lactic acid is completely metabolized and tissue stores are repleted. This is referred to as an *anaerobic work* situation, and the person is said to accumulate an oxygen debt. Man can accumulate a debt equal to 2 to 5 liters of oxygen.

Work at lower intensity that is performed without building up lactic acid in the tissues is called *aerobic work*. For most healthy people, the limit of aerobic work capacity approximates the energy expenditure of a brisk walk and corresponds to use of just over 1 liter of oxygen

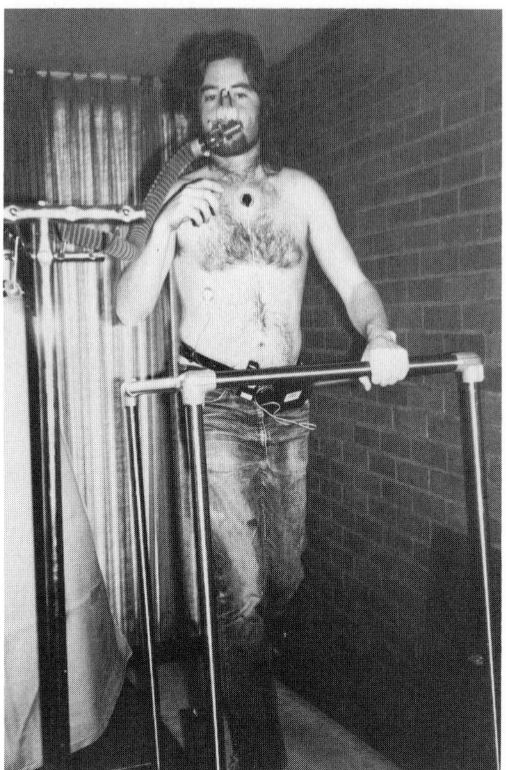

Figure 22–3 Simultaneous measurement of heart rate and oxygen uptake of a subject walking on a motor-driven treadmill. There is a linear relationship between these two parameters and, therefore, between heart rate and energy cost of work at heart rates above 90 beats per minute; at lower heart rates and energy expenditures (sedentary or very light work), the slope is minimal and the error term is large. It is virtually impossible to measure oxygen uptake of people going about their ordinary activities for long periods of time, and investigators have attempted to use heart rate instead to estimate daily energy expenditure. The subject in the photograph is wearing a tape recorder, which is picking up the signal from the electrocardiographic leads on the chest to store information on heart rate; this device could be worn all day with little discomfort or interference with normal activities. (Courtesy of D. Armstrong, University of California, Berkeley.)

or 5 kcal per minute.[2] This is about four to five times the resting metabolic rate (Chapter 2). Work at or below the aerobic capacity is called steady state work because it can be continued steadily for long periods without fatigue.

How long a person can work at a time without a break obviously varies according to the work rate. This is an important consideration in industry, where rest periods must be established, and in endurance sports events, where the work must be paced. If the work task is at or below the aerobic capacity, rest periods are not needed. Durnin and Passmore suggest that rest periods can be calculated simply according to multiples of the aerobic capacity.[12] If the work task requires 7.5 kcal per minute and the aerobic capacity is 5 kcal, then 30 minutes of rest will be needed for every hour worked; if the task is one requiring 10 kcal per minute, then the rest periods will have to be the same length as the work periods. For maximum work output it is best to work and rest for short periods — 10 minutes of work and 5 minutes of rest in climbing a hill, for instance. Otherwise, the work pace must be slowed so that expenditure rate does not exceed the aerobic capacity of the workers. The value of 5 kcal per minute suggests a maximum work output of 2400 kcal per 8 hour work-shift and coincides well with actual observations of sustained hard industrial work, such as coal mining and nonmechanized agriculture.[12] The trained athlete is capable of sustained work at about ten times his resting rate, but he does become fatigued and does accumulate an oxygen debt during this load of work.

In a study of the energy needs of college football players,[13] food eaten at the training table and between meal snacks amounted to 5600 kcal per day during playing season and the men were not gaining weight. The men averaged 80 kg (small, perhaps, but it was the Harvard team), which would indicate an expected energy requirement on the order of 3200 kcal per day if the men had pursued a usual collegiate pattern of moderate activity rather than sports. The difference between ordinary needs and those of the team, 2400 kcal, should be ascribable in some way to football practice and competition. This activity occupied only 2 hours a day, indicating an energy expenditure rate of 1200 kcal per hour, nearly 20 times the basal metabolic rate, which is above a level that is usually sustainable for an extended period. The extra energy need of the team probably reflects in part a continued high rate of metabolism after the exercise was concluded. Benedict's classic research on energy metabolism in the early 1900's included an observation that metabolism during sleep was 25 percent higher when very severe work had been performed 1 hour earlier than when the sleep followed a day of rest; sleeping metabolic rate was still 10 to 15 percent higher as long as 7 hours after severe work. This continued effect of exercise on resting metabolism was mentioned in Chapter 2 and is repeated here as a reminder that calculations of total energy need based on activity categories are only rough approximations. The only satisfactory basis for judging energy need is by maintenance of ideal body weight, because physical work affects the body in ways that have not yet been adequately explained.

Mechanical Work Efficiency

The efficiency with which work is performed can be calculated from the amount of energy metabolized if the amount of mechanical work performed can be measured. In the laboratory this can be accomplished by having the person pedal a stationary bicycle at a stipulated speed against a set resistance, or walk at a given rate and incline on a motor-driven treadmill. *Gross efficiency* is the *ratio of mechanical work performed to the total energy expended. Net efficiency* is the ratio of mechanical work to the increment of the work energy expenditure *above the resting metabolic rate.*

Mechanical work efficiency varies considerably. It is influenced by the type of work performed, previous training or practice, fatigue, the amount of the load, and the speed and conditions under which the work is done. A healthy person performs usual work tasks with about 25 percent net efficiency, which means that he consumes four times as much energy as is represented in the work actually performed. When the person is fit and accustomed to the task (e.g., in trained bicycle riders), efficiencies as high as 33 percent have been obtained. Under unfavorable conditions, such as an unaccustomed task, too heavy a load, too high a rate of speed, inconvenient posture for the task, or fatigue, net mechanical efficiency may fall as low as 10 percent. Low mechanical efficiency means that work is accomplished at a greater cost — that is, more energy and oxygen are needed to produce a given amount of external work, a larger proportion of the energy appearing as heat under these conditions.

Fuel for Muscular Work and Performance Capacity

The source of energy for muscular work is ATP generated from the common metabolic pathways (Chapter 15) or, in short term, from creatine phosphate stored in the muscle. Creatine is a nitrogen-containing compound synthesized in the body from amino acids. It combines with phosphate from ATP in a high-energy linkage, forming creatine phosphate and ADP. When ATP is needed for the initial stages of muscular work, the reverse reaction of creatine phosphate with ADP yields ATP for muscle contraction, and creatine. The latter is again regenerated to creatine phosphate when ATP is abundant.

The nature of the substance undergoing metabolism can be determined by measuring the amount of oxygen used and the amount of carbon dioxide formed during metabolism. If carbohydrate is being metabolized, one molecule of carbon dioxide is formed for every molecule of oxygen used, according to the following equation for glucose:

$$C_6H_{12}O_6 + 6\ O_2 \rightarrow 6\ CO_2 + 6\ H_2O$$

The ratio of carbon dioxide produced to oxygen used is called the *respiratory quotient,* which is abbreviated to RQ. In the glucose example, $6\ CO_2/6\ O_2$ equals an RQ of 1.0. For complete metabolism of fat, the RQ is about 0.7, as illustrated for stearic acid:

$$C_{18}H_{36}O_2 + 26\ O_2 \rightarrow 18\ CO_2 + 18\ H_2O$$

and 18 CO_2/26 O_2 equals 0.7. If the volume and composition of air inhaled and exhaled during work are known, both the energy expended and the composition of the source of energy can be ascertained.

Formerly carbohydrate was thought to be the only energy source for physical work, but present information indicates that carbohydrate plays a dominant role only in heavy exercise when oxygen supply to the muscle becomes limiting. During steady state work, fat provides about half of the energy; with prolonged work (4 hours or more), fatty acid metabolism may reach 60 to 70 percent of the total. The fat utilized comes from lipid pools in the muscle tissue and fatty acids mobilized from adipose tissue and transported to the working muscle by the blood. Protein is not used for work energy to any great extent but certain amino acids have an important role. At rest, the output of the amino acids alanine and glutamine exceeds the input to muscle, and as glucose utilization increases during exercise, there is a parallel rise in muscle alanine output (derived from pyruvate. See Chapter 15). The source of the amino groups used in this synthesis is primarily the branched-chain amino acids (leucine, isoleucine, valine), and their carbon skeletons may contribute importantly to the ATP supply for exercise. The alanine formed is carried to the liver, where it is used for synthesis of glucose (with amino groups disposed of via urea formation and transamination reactions) to help maintain blood sugar during prolonged exercise and to replenish liver glycogen after exercise.[14]

To determine if the metabolic mixture utilized during work does affect work performance, two types of studies have been made. In one, persons were fed a normal diet or one very high in either of the work-energy sources (fat or carbohydrate) for some period of time to foster preferential use of that source during work. Other studies emphasized the composition of meals taken just prior to an event. Carbohydrate has more oxygen in its composition than does fat, and about 10 percent less oxygen is needed per unit of energy when carbohydrate is metabolized, so theoretically preferential utilization of carbohydrate should be beneficial when oxygen limits work.

Diets containing little or no carbohydrate have adverse effects on performance in every study. One experiment compared a diet containing less than 5 percent with one supplying over 90 percent of energy as carbohydrate. Capacity for hard physical work was reduced by one-half with the high-fat diet and increased by one-fourth with the high-carbohydrate regimen, as compared with performance during normal diet periods. Other studies confirm these findings and indicate that one factor involved is the amount of glycogen present in the muscle. Swedish investigators measured performance capacity (work to exhaustion in a standard bicycle test) and obtained samples of muscle by needle biopsy from a group of men fed three diets. Time to exhaustion was 114 minutes for those with a normal diet, 57 minutes when the diet was made up exclusively of high-protein and high-fat foods, and 167 minutes when the diet was high in carbohydrate. After the normal mixed diet, glycogen content was found to be 1.75 gm per 100 gm wet muscle before exercise; after 3 days of carbohydrate-free diet it was 0.63 gm, and after the same period of high-carbohydrate feeding, 3.51 gm.[15]

When men fed a normal mixed diet worked at a rate of about 75 percent of their maximum oxygen uptake, glycogen content of muscle was almost completely depleted in 90 minutes, but blood sugar was satisfactorily maintained. Past this point, evidence indicates that blood sugar falls and constitutes a final limit to performance (Fig. 22–4). Administration of glucose at the point of exhaustion allows work to proceed for an additional period of time.[15]

Diets based on the principle of im-

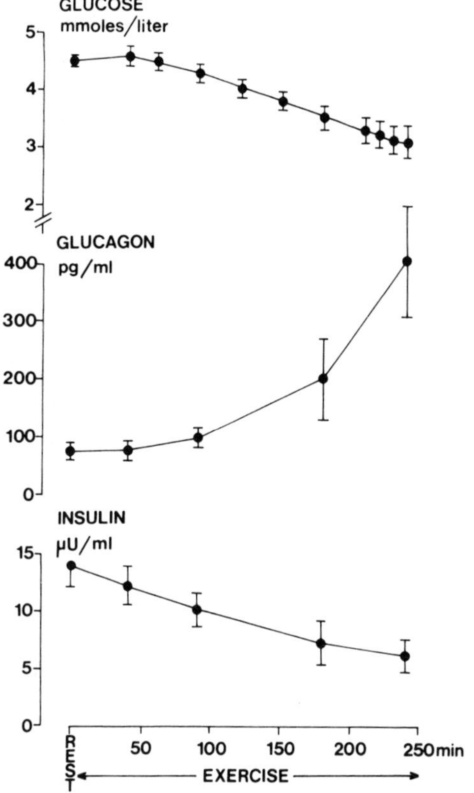

Figure 22–4 Exercise induces a fall in plasma insulin and a rise in plasma glucagon; levels of other hormones that favor maintenance of blood glucose (pituitary growth hormone, epinephrine, norepinephrine, cortisol) also are elevated. In spite of these hormonal responses, in prolonged heavy exercise, hepatic gluconeogenesis and glycolysis fail to keep pace with the accelerated utilization of glucose, and the blood glucose level falls. (Courtesy of P. Felig and J. Wahren and the New England Journal of Medicine.[14])

proving the fuel for muscular work have been developed and enthusiastically adopted in Europe. It is difficult to say if this has a significant effect on the outcome of athletic competition, because there are uncontrollable differences in skills and training between competitors and in environmental factors between events. Also, strength of belief in the efficacy of a treatment may be sufficient to make the treatment effective, a point that is difficult to rule out even in laboratory studies involving subjective acknowledgment of "fatigue." However, this treatment does have a sound basis in theory and a reasonable body of experimental evidence in support of it.

The preparation recommended by Åstrand[15] for competition in endurance events exceeding 30 to 60 minutes' duration is as follows:

1. One week before the competition, exercise to exhaustion the same muscles that will be used in the event. This is done to exhaust the glycogen stores.

2. For the next 3 days eat a diet made up almost exclusively of foods high in protein and fat. (In our opinion it should contain a minimum of 80 gm of carbohydrate). (See Table 22–1). This is to keep the glycogen content low.

3. As the competition nears, add large quantities of carbohydrate to the diet. Åstrand emphasizes that the carbohydrate should be *added* while the intake of protein and fat is maintained.

Åstrand's tests show that muscle glycogen can exceed 4 gm per 100 gm of muscle with this regimen and that total muscle glycogen stores could be as high as 700 gm. This would represent a reserve of about 2800 kcal if completely metabolized or half that if lactic acid were the end-product due to anerobic work metabolism. This is approximately double the usual reserve capacity in trained athletes.

Some notes of warning have been sounded by physicians concerned over possible side effects of carbohydrate loading. They point out that water is deposited along with glycogen, which may cause the muscles to feel heavy and stiff. In an older marathon runner, chest pain and changes in the electrocardiogram occurred when this technique was used; although there is no proof that the diet was the specific causative agent, it was speculated that accumulation of cardiac glycogen might have been a factor.[16] Those who wish to try this method for improving performance would be well advised to do so under supervision and before a competition, so that they and their advisers can determine what the probable effects will be.

Table 22–1 DIETS FOR USE IN THE ÅSTRAND REGIMEN FOR ENHANCED MUSCLE GLYCOGEN STORAGE

Days 4–6 Before an Event	*Days 1–3 Before an Event*
HIGH-ENERGY, LOW-CARBOHYDRATE DIET	VERY HIGH-ENERGY, HIGH-CARBOHYDRATE DIET
Breakfast	
½ grapefruit or ½ c grapefruit juice or berries	1 c orange or pineapple juice
2 eggs	Hot cereal as desired
Generous serving of bacon, ham, or sausage	Eggs and/or hot cakes
Butter or margarine as desired	Generous serving of bacon, ham, or sausage
1 thin slice of whole-wheat bread	Butter or margarine as desired
1 c whole milk or half-and-half	2–4 slices of whole-grain bread
	Chocolate or cocoa as desired
Luncheon and Dinner	
Clear bouillon or ½ c tomato juice	Cream or legume soup or chowder
Large serving of fish, poultry, or liver (> 6 oz)	Large serving of fish, poultry, or liver (> 6 oz)
Mixed green (only) salad or 1 c cooked green vegetable	Added beans or fruits
Salad dressing, butter, or margarine as desired	Salad dressing, butter, or margarine as desired
1 c whole milk or half-and-half	1 c whole milk, half-and-half, or milkshake
Artificially sweetened gelatin with whipped cream (no sugar)	2–4 slices of whole-grain bread or rolls or potato
	Pie, cake, pudding or ice cream
Snacks	
Cheddar cheese	Fruits, especially dates, raisins, apples, bananas
Nuts	More milk or milkshakes
1 slice whole-grain bread	Cookies or candy
Artificially sweetened lemonade	

Studies of the composition of meals taken just before competition do not indicate any special benefit of one mixture of energy sources over another. Glucose has been compared with sucrose, and although there was a small difference in RQ, physical efficiency was the same with the two sugars.[17] Åstrand's practical advice in this connection is that before a competition an athlete should eat according to his own wishes based on the advice of his coach and experience of his own reactions in sports competition. Some additional suggestions are given in the later section on feeding just before work (p. 537).

Nutritional Deficiency and Performance

Among factors known to be detrimental to performance, two are outstanding: *dehydration* and *food deprivation*. Evidence on these points comes from careful laboratory studies and abundant field experience. Of the two, dehydration is the more immediate and serious risk. Normally, voluntary drinking is stimulated when the body water content drops by 1 percent, but during exercise voluntary intake is inhibited and water balance may not be attained until hours or days after a severe bout of work with high rates of water loss as sweat. In a comfortable environment water loss due to sweating during moderate exercise will be about 1 liter per hour; at higher work output or in the heat, loss may be two to four times that rate (Chapter 10). Physical performance begins to deteriorate when the water deficit exceeds 3 percent of body weight.

In spite of this evidence, extremely ill-advised practices are used to meet weight ranges in competitive sports such as wrestling — practices that include withholding water, wearing rubberized apparel and inducing vomiting. The American Medical Association's Committee on Medical Aspects of Sports has this to say about indiscriminate weight control practices: "If weight loss is excessive, the boy's competitive abilities are impaired. If his weight loss is contrived to circumvent a regulation, his ethics have been compromised. If he has an unsuspected metabolic problem or if the weight reduction scheme is extreme, health could be seriously affected."[18]

There is a serious question as to how much weight (other than water) an athlete can safely lose without impairing his performance. Any amount of *excess* fat can be trimmed off to advantage, and reducing weight to the desirable level for height and age is a logical and defensible point. In the famous Minnesota studies of conscientious objectors on a semistarvation regimen, loss of 25 percent of body weight over a 6 month period resulted in diminished work performance, endurance, and strength of the large muscles. Later studies in the same laboratory tested more severely restricted diets of 580 and 1010 kcal per day. The 580 kcal diet was inadequate to maintain blood sugar levels for work and can be dismissed from further consideration. With the higher energy intake, loss of hand strength and lowering of maximal oxygen uptake occurred when the men lost 10 percent or more of body weight. Low work loads can be accomplished for a few days in an emergency, especially if at least 100 gm of carbohydrate, a few grams of salt (such as bouillon cubes), and adequate water are consumed, but this is not compatible with top performance capability.

A sensible plan of weight control, suggested by the AMA Committee, is to undertake ". . . an intensive conditioning program related to the demands of [the sport] for at least four weeks, preferably six, without emphasis on [body] weight. . . . At the end of this period and without altering the daily training routine, [record] weight in a pre-breakfast, post-micturition state. Consider this weight the minimal effective weight for competition as well as certification purposes."[18] A program of this kind that includes sound nutrition education is ideal and is especially important for young people who participate in more than one sport according to the season and for which weight advantages differ, such as football and wrestling. Alternating attempts to gain and lose weight cannot help but be detrimental. Weight can be reduced to a very small extent — at most 200 to 300 gm — by changing to a low-residue diet for 72 hours before an event so that the large bowel is more nearly empty. This means substituting refined cereals for whole grains and reducing the intake of beans and coarse vegetables. Ordinarily, such a diet would not be advised, but a few days of this regimen will not harm a well-nourished person. At this time, it is also reasonable to eliminate from the diet foods that are *highly* salted (chips, ham, pickles) to prevent excess water retention (Chapter 10). However, normal salt intake should be maintained to allow for sweat losses.

Vitamin deficiencies of all kinds are damaging to work performance.[17] How long performance can be maintained when one or more vitamins are omitted from the diet will vary with the amount of tissue reserves of the nutrient the individual has and the role that the specific nutrient plays in work metabolism. On the basis of their participation in the metabolic pathways, lack of the B vitamins would be expected to have the most immediate effects, and this is borne out by investigations of the subject. Lack of thiamin is evident in a few days or weeks, and the symptoms of deficiency appear earlier in men fed a deficient diet who are actively working than in those who are sedentary. This early damage to performance is probably true of most of the B complex vitamins, but effects of lack of vitamin A do not appear for months in previously well-nourished subjects.

Deficiencies of minerals other than sodium (Chapter 10) have not been well-studied, but because of their important role in neuromuscular transmission and as enzyme cofactors, detrimental effects would certainly be expected. The skeleton provides an essential reserve of calcium, which is withdrawn to maintain blood levels of ionized calcium, and the liver holds some stores of the trace minerals, but these are variable according to the quality of the usual diet. When effects of mineral deficiencies other than the electrolytes are examined, one would expect them to appear only after periods of weeks or months, or when there are abnormal losses due to diarrhea or vomiting.

Total deprivation of protein with adequate energy intake for 2 weeks has not been shown to alter performance of fixed work tasks in a laboratory nor to reduce muscular strength. The men do complain of feeling less "fit" subjectively, and the blood volume is reduced somewhat, which would be disadvantageous in high-performance work situations and competitive sports. However, lower levels of protein intake, 50 to 60 gm a day, which are much below intakes of athletes and men engaged in hard physical labor, have not shown to affect adversely the performance of persons who are *already trained.*[17]

Diets During Physical Training

Nutrition is an important feature of any training program. Education of coaches and athletes is needed in regard to both nutritional needs and the role of different foods in the diet. A study of Australian Olympic athletes showed great variability in their diets and in their nutrition knowledge. Intakes of some nutrients were much higher than is required, particularly protein, calcium, and vitamin C, and although these are usually harmless, the diets would not be economical. Some diets were below recommended levels of thiamin if the large energy need of the athletes is taken into account. Records in the competition showed that those whose thiamin intake was adequate placed better, some winning medals, in comparison with the ones whose diets were suboptimal in thiamin content.[19] American athletes generally express a concerned awareness, and many resort to excessive and unnecessary supplementation of the diet with vitamins, minerals, and protein powders.[20]

During training there is an increased need for protein, on the order of 2 gm per kilogram of body weight. Muscle tissue must be built, and there is an increase of plasma protein and of iron-containing muscle and blood proteins. During very strenuous, stressful physical work, the red blood cells become fragile and there is a transient anemia that is corrected after about 2 weeks of training,[21] if the diet is adequate in protein and iron reserves are normal.

The higher energy needs of physical activity must be met, but there is often some loss of body weight and a shift in body composition toward more lean and less fat. This is seen in both military recruits and athletes in training. On the other hand, body weight is apt to increase in persons who are below average weight at the time training begins. Along with increased energy requirements there are increased needs for the B vitamins (see Chapter 8).

The diet must be adequate in all essential nutrients, but there is no evidence that supernormal intakes of nutrients (except as cited previously) will do anything to improve work capacity.[17] There have been hopeful claims for exotic foods such as royal jelly, mysterious benefits have been ascribed to wheat-germ oil and lecithin, and a number of "ergogenic" substances have been tested with a view toward expanding the creatine phosphate pool (glycine, gelatin [which is one-fourth glycine] and creatine *per se*). Salts of the nonessential amino acid, aspartic acid, have also been suggested as improving neuromuscular excitability. None of these has proved to be of benefit in carefully controlled studies. A good diet — one based on meat, milk, fish, poultry and eggs, whole-grain cereals, legumes and nuts, leafy, green vegetables, and other vegetables and fruits — will meet all the nutritional requirements of athletes and persons engaged in hard physical labor. Vitamin pills and special supplements are not needed and should not be relied upon because they may lull the individual into thinking he has met his nutritional needs when in reality he may still be lacking in protein and minerals.

Feeding Just Before and During Work

Industrial experience indicates that frequent feeding is beneficial to work output, which may be due either to meal spacing or to the physical and psychological benefit of rest periods. In any case, more frequent intake of smaller amounts of food may be desirable (Chapter 19). Omission of breakfast does lead to poorer work performance, and blood sugar falls to undesirably low levels with continued deprivation of food.

Eating before athletic competitions has been a subject of lively controversy. Small, balanced meals of 500 to 800 kcal have not been shown to have any adverse effect on a variety of athletic performances conducted in a test situation. The tension and stress of game competition may be another matter, and the experience of seasoned coaches and athletes is a good practical guide. There is general agreement that high protein meals are undesirable just before competition. The usual recommendation is to eat a light, balanced meal high in carbohydrate, which seems to be a sensible approach.

The American Association for Health, Physical Education, and Recreation offers the following suggestions for a meal to be eaten 3 to 4 hours before competition:[22] 1 serving of roasted or broiled meat or poultry; 1 serving of mashed potatoes or a baked potato or ½ cup of macaroni, rice, etc.; 1 serving of vegetables; 1 cup of skim milk; 1 teaspoon of fat spread; 2 teaspoons of jelly or other sweet; 1 serving of fruit or juice; 1 serving of sugar cookies or plain cake. Take 1 or 2 cups of extra beverages and salt the food well.

This group also suggests that a commercial or home-prepared formula may be substituted for a normal meal and is preferred by some athletes. However, these formulas are usually based on milk plus added milk solids, and so are high in lactose content, which is a sugar not well tolerated by many Oriental and African populations and some others (Chapters 3 and 14).

Coffee and tea are best omitted, except by people who are thoroughly habituated to their use. Alcohol is quite deleterious to coordination and judgment.

During competition that involves much sweating, it is essential that water losses be replaced. Sweat is less concentrated in minerals than is plasma, and the fluid used to replace it should be also (Chapter 10). In short-term sports, salt is not a problem, and the fluid given could be water or sweetened lemonade. However, for continued high work output or in severe heat, salt will be needed. Since salt absorption is improved if glucose is present for absorption at the same time, workers and athletes in endurance events should take some carbohydrate as well as salt and water. For this purpose a 0.2 percent salt solution can be drunk or used as the base of a flavored, sweetened beverage, or carbohydrate may be taken in the form of hard candy or fruit jellies along with the salt solution. Workers and climbers may prefer a snack of dried fruits and salted crackers or chips with water or an accustomed beverage. The important consideration is replacement of water and salt, not the form in which these are given.

QUESTIONS AND PROBLEMS

1. What are the advantages of exercise? How does exercise affect body weight? Food intake? Fitness?
2. What factors affect work capacity? What is meant by maximal oxygen uptake? Distinguish between aerobic and an-

aerobic work. How should work and rest cycles be spaced?

3. How much additional energy intake will be required by an athlete? A worker in heavy industry? (Consult the tables in Chapter 2). Do all sports have high energy demands? Make a list of high- and low-energy cost recreations. How much of your time is spent in activities requiring more energy than in walking?

4. What is the fuel for muscular work? How is this determined? Define RQ and tell how it is measured. How much glycogen is present in muscle and what affects this amount? Of what importance is muscle glycogen? Liver glycogen?

5. What effect does nutritional deficiency have on work performance? On fitness and training? Why does dehydration have serious effects on performance? How is dehydration prevented?

6. Make up a menu for a meal to be eaten 3 to 4 hours before a sports event. Devise a liquid formula from inexpensive ingredients that would provide about the same nutrients.

REFERENCES

1. Pollock, M. L., et al.: Effects of walking on body composition and cardiovascular function of middle-aged men. J. Appl. Physiol., *30*:126, 1971.
2. Kuta, I., Parizkova, J., and Dycka, J.: Muscle strength and lean body mass in old men. J. Appl. Physiol., *29*:168, 1970.
3. McDonough, J. R., Kusumi, F., and Bruce, R. A.: Variations in maximal oxygen with physical activity in middle-aged men. Circulation, *41*:743, 1970.
4. Chalmers, J., and Ho, K. C.: Geographical variations in senile osteoporosis. The association with physical activity. J. Bone Joint Surg., *52*:667, 1970.
5. Gendel, E. S.: Pregnancy, fitness and sports. J.A.M.A., *201*:751, 1967.
6. Karvonen, M. J.: Women and men at work. World Health, Jan., 1971, p. 3.
7. Kreitler, H., and Kreitler, S.: Movement and aging: a psychological approach. Med. and Sport, *4*:302, 1970.
8. Huenemann, R. L., et al.: Teen-agers; activities and attitudes towards activity. J. Amer. Dietet. Assoc., *51*:433, 1967.
9. McNaughton, J. W., and Cahn, A. J.: A study of the food intake and activity of a group of urban adolescents. Brit. J. Nutr., *24*:331, 1970.
10. Mitchell, J. H., and Blomqvist, G.: Maximal oxygen uptake. N. Engl. J. Med., *284*:1018, 1971.
11. Anderson, H. T., and Barkue, H.: Iron deficiency and muscular work performance. Scand. J. Lab. Clin. Invest., *25*:supplement 114, 1970; Davies, C.T.M.: Physiological responses to exercise in East African children. 2. The effects of schistosomiasis, anemia and malnutrition. J. Trop. Pediatr., *19*:115, 1973.
12. Durnin, J. V. G. A., and Passmore, R.: *Energy, Work and Leisure.* London, Heinemann Educational Books, Ltd., 1967.
13. Edwards, H. T., Thorndike, A., Jr., and Dill, D. B.: The energy requirement in strenuous muscular exercise. N. Engl. J. Med., *213*:532, 1935.
14. Felig, P., and Wahren, J.: Fuel homeostasis and exercise. N. Engl. J. Med., *293*:1078, 1975.
15. Åstrand, P. O.: Diet and athletic performance. Fed. Proc., *26*:1772, 1967, and Nutr. Today, *3(2)*:9, 1968.
16. Nelson, R. A., and Gastineau, C. F.: Nutrition for athletes. In *The Medical Aspects of Sports: 15.* Ed. by Craig, T. T. Chicago, American Medical Association, 1974; Mirkin, G.: A.M.A. J.A.M.A., *223*:1511, 1973.
17. Mayer, J., and Bullen, B.: Nutrition and athletic performance. Physiol. Rev., *40*:369, 1960.
18. Slocum, D. B., et al.: Wrestling and weight control. J., *201*:541, 1967.
19. Steel, J. E.: A nutritional study of Australian olympic athletes. Med. J. Aust., *2*:119, 1970.
20. Darden, E.: Olympic athletes view vitamins and victories. J. Home Econ., *65(2)*:8, 1973.
21. Yoshimura, H.: Anemia during physical training (sports anemia). Nutr. Rev., *28*:251, 1970.
22. American Alliance for Health, Physical Education, and Recreation: *Nutrition for Athletes: A Handbook for Coaches.* Washington, D.C., 1971.

SUPPLEMENTARY READING

Ahlborg, G., and Felig, P.: Influence of glucose ingestion on fuel-hormone response during prolonged exercise. J. Appl. Physiol., *41*:683, 1976.

Ahrens, R. A., Bishop, C. L., and Berdanier, C. D.: Effect of age and dietary carbohydrate source on the response of rats to forced exercise. J. Nutr., *102*:241, 1972.

Asprey, G. M., Alley, L. E., and Tuttle, W. W.: Effect of eating at various times on subsequent performances in the one-mile free-style swim. Res. Q. Amer. Assoc. Health Phys. Educ. *39*:231, 1968.

Bailey, D. A., et al.: Vitamin C supplementation related to physiological response to exercise in smoking and nonsmoking subjects. Amer. J. Clin. Nutr., *23*:905, 1970.

Balart, L., Moore, M. C., Gremillion, L., and Lopez-S, A.: Serum lipids, dietary intakes, and physical exercise in medical students. J. Amer. Dietet. Assoc., *64*:42, 1974.

Bray, G. A., Whipp, B. J., and Koyal, S. N., The acute effects of food intake on energy expenditure during cycle ergometry. Amer. J. Clin. Nutr., *27*:254, 1974.

Carlson, L. A., Ekelund, L. G., and Olsson, A. G.: Frequency of ischaemic exercise E.C.G. changes in symptom-free men with various forms of primary hyperlipaemia. Lancet, *2*:1, 1975.
Chavez, A., Martinez, C., and Bourges, H.: Nutrition and development of infants from poor rural areas. 2. Nutritional level and physical activity. Nutr. Ret. Internat., *5*:139, 1972.
Cho, M., and Fryer, B. A., What foods do physical education majors and basic nutrition students recommend for athletes? J. Amer. Dietet. Assoc., *65*:541, 1974.
Consolazio, C. F., and Johnson, H. L.: Dietary carbohydrate and work capacity. Amer. J. Clin. Nutr., *25*:85, 1972.
Consolazio, C. F., Johnson, H. J., Nelson, R. A., Dramise, J. G., and Skala, J. H.: Protein metabolism during intensive physical training in the young adult. Amer. J. Clin. Nutr., *28*:29, 1975.
Edgerton, V. R., Bryant, S. L., Gillespie, C. A., and Gardner, G. W.: Iron deficiency anemia and physical performance and activity of rats. J. Nutr., *102*:381, 1972.
Emiola, L., and O'Shea, J. P.: Effects of physical activity and nutrition on bone density measured by radiographic techniques. Nutr. Rpt. Internat., *17*:669, 1978.
Garlaschi, C., et al.: Effect of physical exercise on secretion of growth hormone, glucagon, and cortisol in obese and diabetic children. Diabetes, *24*:758, 1975.
Holloszy, J. O., and Booth, F. W.: Biochemical adaptations to endurance exercise in muscle. Ann. Rev. Physiol., *38*:273, 1976.
Lewis, S., et al.: Effects of physical activity on weight reduction in obese middle-aged women. Amer. J. Clin. Nutr., *29*:151, 1976.
Lincoln, J. E.: Calorie intake, obesity, and physical activity. Amer. J. Clin. Nutr., *25*:390, 1972.
MacDougall, J. D., et al.: Muscle glycogen repletion after high-intensity intermittent exercise. J. Appl. Physiol., *42*:2, 1977.
Martin, B., Robinson, S., and Robertshaw, D.: Influence of diet on leg uptake of glucose during heavy exercise. Amer. J. Clin. Nutr., *31*:62, 1978.
Pařízková, J.: Nutrition, physical fitness and health. *International Series on Sport Sciences*, Vol. 7. Baltimore, University Park Press, 1978.
Shaffer, T. E.: The adolescent athlete. Pediatr. Clin. North Amer., *20*:837, 1973.
Shorey, R. L., Sewell, B., and O'Brien, M.: Efficacy of diet and exercise in the reduction of serum cholesterol and the glyceride in free-living adult males. Amer. J. Clin. Nutr., *29*:512, 1976.
Sidney, K. H., et al.: Endurance training and body composition of the elderly. Amer. J. Clin. Nutr., *30*:326, 1977.
Skubic, V., and Kodgkins, J.: Energy expenditure of women participants in selected individual sports. J. Appl. Physiol., *21*:133, 1966.
Smith, N. J.: Gaining and losing weight in athletics. J.A.M.A., *236*:149, 1976.
Spurr, G. B., Barac-Nieto, M., and Maksud, M. G.: Energy expenditure cutting sugar cane. J. Appl. Physiol., *39*:990, 1975.
Swindells, Y. E.: The influence of activity and size of meals on caloric response in women. Brit. J. Nutr., *27*:65, 1972.
Westerman, R.: Fluid and electrolyte replacement in sweating athletes. J.A.M.A., *212*:1713, 1970.
Yager, J. D., et al.: Effects of various feeding and exercise regimens on rat growth and survival. J. Nutr., *104*:273, 1974.

Articles in Nutrition Reviews

Alcohol metabolism during rest and exercise. *24*:239, 1966.
Exercise and cholesterol catabolism. *28*:211, 1970.
Response of rat heart muscle to exercise. *29*:116, 1971.
Effect of bed rest on bone mineral loss. *30*:11, 1972.
Diet, exercise, and endurance. *30*:86, 1972.
An exercise-induced protein catabolism in man. *30*:108, 1972.
Iron deficiency anemia and physical performance. *30*:236, 1972.
Energy production during exercise. *31*:11, 1973.
Diet, exercise and ketone metabolism. *34*:54, 1976.
Effect of glucose ingestion on substrate utilization during prolonged exercise. *36*:37, 1978.

Chapter 23

Dental Health, Nutrition, and Diet

Dental disease is one of the most widespread and costly diseases in this country. For example, 90 percent of all American children already have dental decay by 4 years of age. The total cost of dental care for this nation is about seven billion dollars a year.

Understanding of the complex causes of the two most important types of dental disease, *dental decay* and *periodontal (gum) disease*, has increased greatly in the past few decades. Awareness of these causes is an important step toward obtaining all the personal benefits of healthy teeth and gums.

There are important interrelationships between oral health and nutrition. First, good nutrition is important for developing and maintaining healthy, sound teeth and gum structures. In turn, healthy dental structures are needed so that an adequate diet may be eaten (see Fig. 23–1).

What exactly is dental disease? Why are "permanent" teeth lost? How can tooth loss and cavities be prevented, and how does diet play a role? In order to answer these questions, this chapter reviews the current concepts regarding the causes of dental decay and periodontal disease, with special emphasis on the role of dietary factors.

NUTRITION ⇄ ORAL HEALTH

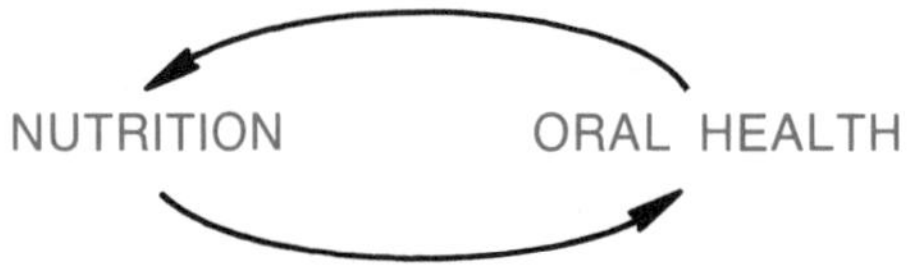

Figure 23–1 Good nutrition is necessary for oral health, and oral health is necessary for good nutrition.

The extent of some of the problems associated with dental decay and periodontal disease — and their secondary result, loss of natural teeth — is demonstrated by the following facts:

1. Over 20 million Americans have *lost all their teeth* (10 percent of the population).

2. At least half of those persons who are 65 or older *have no natural teeth left*.

3. People with *low family income and minimal education* tend to lose teeth earlier and more frequently than people with higher earnings and levels of education.

4. There is an estimated number of one billion unfilled cavities in the American population today — *an average of about five per person*.

5. *Half the children under 15 in the United States have never been to a dentist*, up to 80 percent of this group living in poverty areas.

6. *One-third of the entire population receive no dental care* except, possibly, emergency procedures for relief from pain.

7. *Ninety-six percent of all high*

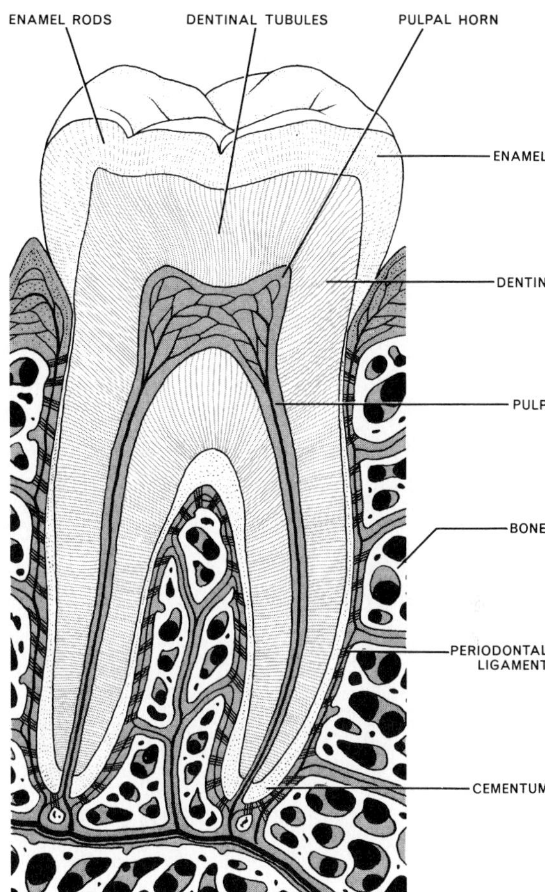

Figure 23–2 The anatomy of the tooth and surrounding structures. (From Morrey, L. W., and Nelsen, R. J.: *Dental Science Handbook.* Washington, D.C., Superintendent of Documents, 1970. Copyright by the American Dental Association. Reprinted by permission.)

school students in the United States have dental decay.

Thus there is an obvious pattern of neglect, including nutritional neglect, surrounding oral health, leading to painful teeth and unhealthy gums. In turn, tooth loss results in the need for artificial replacements of teeth.

DEVELOPMENTAL ANATOMY OF THE TOOTH, AND ROLE OF NUTRITION

The basic structure of the tooth and adjacent gum area is shown in Figure 23–2. The tooth is composed of four separate tissues:

Enamel, the outer layer, is the most durable of all body tissues. It is primarily (95 percent) inorganic in nature, with its major constituents being calcium, phosphorus, magnesium, and carbonate. It can function as a semipermeable membrane.

Dentin, the major part of core of the hard portion of the tooth, is 80 percent inorganic, composed mainly of calcium and phosphorus. It extends almost the entire length of the tooth, and is covered by enamel on the crown and by cementum on the roots. Unlike enamel, it is a very sensitive portion of the tooth.

Cementum is also a calcified tissue that is presumed to be similar in composition to bone and dentin. It acts as a surface for the attachment of the fibers (periodontal ligaments) that hold the tooth to the surrounding tissues.

Pulp, the soft part in the tooth's center, is a vital tissue containing nerves, lymph, blood vessels, and fibrous tissue. It extends for about four-fifths of the

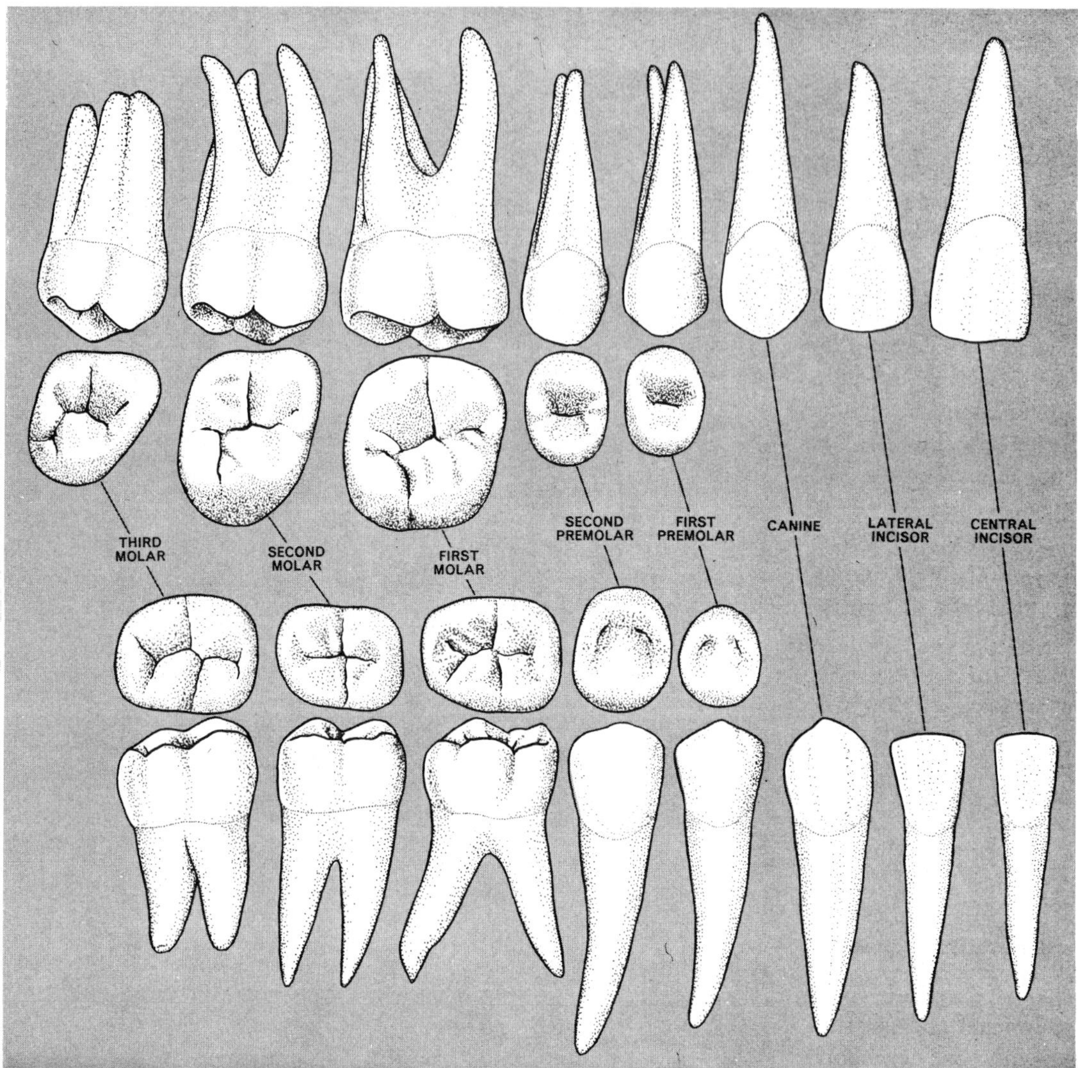

Figure 23–3 The permanent teeth. The incisors are for cutting; the premolars and molars are for grinding food. The canine teeth are used primarily to tear or shred food. (From Morrey, L. W., and Nelsen, R. J.: *Dental Science Handbook.* Washington, D.C., Superintendent of Documents, 1970. Copyright by the American Dental Association. Reprinted by permission.)

length of the tooth, with communication to the general nutritional and nervous systems through the root.

The *periodontal tissues* make up the gums and the tissues that hold the teeth in place. They contain much connective tissue.

Not only *permanent* teeth, but also the *deciduous* or "baby" teeth, the teeth which are lost before the permanent teeth erupt, are important. If these deciduous teeth are lost too early through neglect or any other reason, the spacing of the permanent teeth may be affected, and there may be irregularities in their proper positioning. Also, the deciduous teeth, like the permanent teeth, are important for eating normally, for a healthy appearance, and for proper speech development. A diagram of the permanent teeth is seen in Figure 23–3.

Nutrition plays an important part in future tooth development even prior to birth. The genetic make-up of the individual provides the pattern for the tooth and other oral development, but unless the environment supplies adequate nutrients, the genetic potential is not realized. Thus the pregnant mother must receive generous supplies of calcium, protein, iron, and vitamins, especially A, C, and D (see other sections on these subjects). Examples of how specific nutrients are related to tooth development are the following:

1. Vitamin D aids in absorption and utilization of calcium, promoting the deposition of both calcium and phosphorus in teeth. Excessive vitamin D in pregnant animals leads to badly shaped jaws in the offspring, with resultant faulty bite or malocclusion.

2. Vitamins C and A affect the functional activities of the formative cells. Vitamin C is important for calcification of *dentin* (the inner tooth structure), and vitamin A is necessary for optimal calcification and development of *enamel* (the outer coat of the tooth).

3. In animal studies, specific nutritional deficiencies, or vitamin excesses in some cases, cause defective development of oral structures — for example, cleft palate is seen in offspring when maternal diets are deficient in vitamin E, vitamin A, a number of the B vitamins, and many minerals.

4. Low protein and correspondingly high carbohydrate in the diet of pregnant rats has been shown to be associated with reduction in the size of molars, delay in the eruption of certain teeth, and increased susceptibility to carious lesions.

Thus in experimental animals, there are demonstrated relationships between nutritional factors and microscopic structure, chemical composition, tooth shape and size, eruption time, and susceptibility to caries, as well as to jaw malformations.

Although specific oral and dental malformations resulting from specific nutritional deficiencies have not been experimentally demonstrated in humans, optimal development of the teeth is undoubtedly related to the intake of a balanced and adequate diet. The important role of the nutrient fluoride in tooth development was discussed in Chapter 12 and will also be treated later in this chapter.

DENTAL CARIES

The two major causes of dental ill health and subsequent tooth loss are dental *caries,** or "cavities" as they are generally known, and *periodontal disease*, which refers to disease of the gums and jaw structures that hold the teeth. The first stage of periodontal disease is *gingivitis* or gum inflammation. A severe form of gum disease, involving the bone under the gums, is known as periodontitis.

Tooth loss prior to age 35 years is primarily due to dental caries (see Fig. 23–4). Dental caries does not have a single cause; it is a complex disease involving four major factors: characteristics of the *host* where the teeth are present, actions of specific *bacteria* in the mouth, the presence of certain *substrates* (e.g., sugar) in the diet that are needed for the bacterial

*The word "caries" is derived from the Greek word for "rottenness."

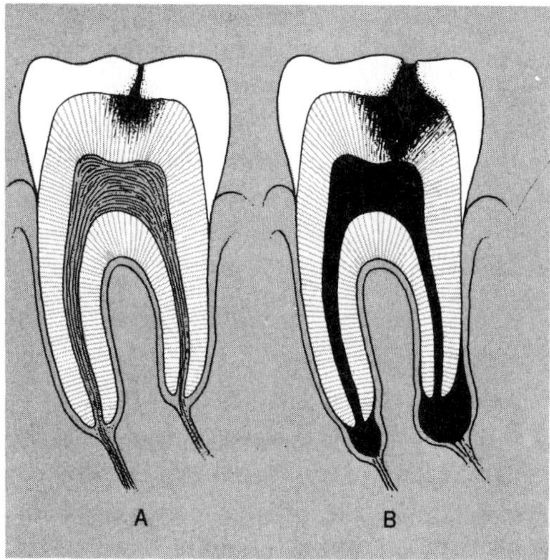

Figure 23–4 The progress of decay; **A,** The bacteria have penetrated the enamel and attacked the softer dentin. **B,** The bacteria have penetrated the dentin and killed the pulp, and infection has spread to the root. At this point the tooth may have to be removed. (From Morrey, L. W., and Nelsen, R. J.: *Dental Science Handbook*. Washington, D.C., Superintendent of Documents, 1970. Copyright by the American Dental Association. Reprinted by permission.)

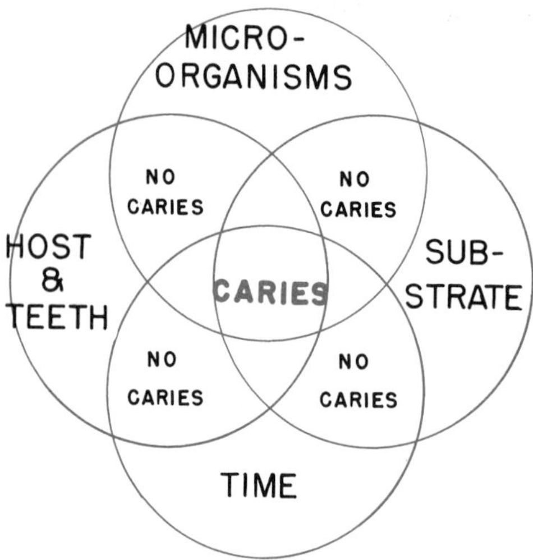

Figure 23–5 The four circles represent the factors involved in the formation of dental caries. All four factors must be acting together (overlapping of the circles) for caries to occur. (From Newbrun, E.: *Etiology of Dental Caries.* San Francisco, University of California, 1971.)

action, and the passage of *time* necessary for the development of caries (see Fig. 23–5). The carious lesion is initiated when enamel is decalcified by acids that are produced by bacteria present in dental plaque and progresses to cavitation when the dentin is invaded and destroyed by bacteria.

Dental caries has been termed one of the oldest diseases of man: Wall paintings depicting dental problems of Cro-Magnon man — 22,000 years ago — have been found. Early theories on the cause of dental decay ranged from invasion by worms to "gangrene" beginning in the inside of the tooth to an imbalance of the four bodily "humours."

In 1600 an English writer[1] noted a relationship between carbohydrate intake and poor teeth, with the following observation: "Overuse" of most confections and sugar plummes . . . rotteth the teeth and maketh them look black." In the early nineteenth century, a chemical theory on the origin of dental caries was postulated. It related carious teeth to "a chemical agent" (acid) produced when food "putrefied" on tooth enamel. Then in the mid-nineteenth century, with the advent of the microscope, bacteria were seen on teeth, and the groundwork was laid for understanding the actual cause of dental caries. It was Miller in 1890 who first demonstrated that the acid-producing action of salivary bacteria on ingested carbohydrates caused decalcification of enamel. An example of an early study that provided proof of the effect of diet on this process is one made in 1938 that showed a significant difference in the number of dental caries between two groups of children — one group that had a balanced diet with no between-meal sweets and no caries; and a second group eating a poor diet, with specifically small quantities of vegetables, fruits, and vitamin D and large amounts of sweets daily, that had an extremely high incidence of caries.[2] This study is one of the many that have documented the role of dietary factors — such as type of food, clearance rate of food, frequency of eating, and "detergent" (leading to reduction in oral debris) effects of foods — in the causation or prevention of caries.

The Effect of Physical Properties of Foods

Physical properties of foods, such as adhesiveness, solubility, and viscosity, may modify the caries-producing potential of foods. Foods that are highly adherent to tooth surfaces and that are slowly soluble contribute to an increase in caries-promoting action.[3] Thus, liquid foods tend to *cause fewer caries* than sticky or retentive foods.

The Effect of Food on the Microbiology of the Oral Cavity

Plaque is an important term to know in discussing dental caries. It is a sticky, nearly colorless layer of gelatinous material that accumulates on a tooth surface, to which it develops a tenacious attachment (Fig. 23–6). It is composed primarily of

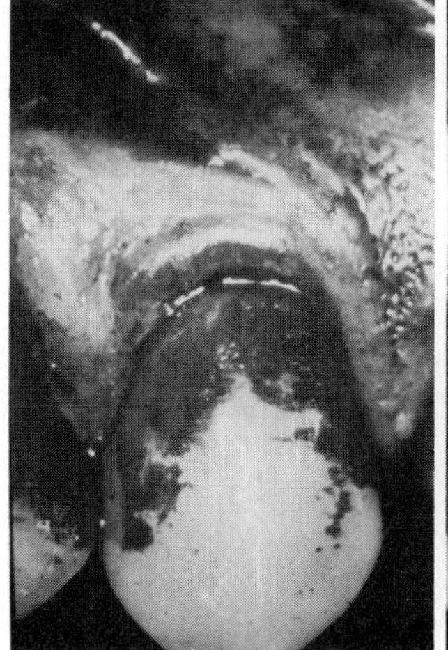
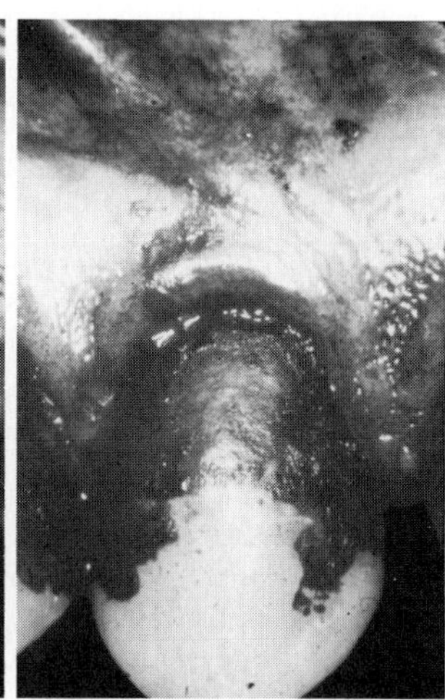

Figure 23–6 Microbial dental plaque stained by a disclosing solution. Dental brushing and flossing is the best method for the removal of plaque. A diet limited in frequency of sucrose intake is important in the prevention of plaque formation.

Bacterial plaque is the cause of most common forms of periodontal disease, as well as being involved in the development of caries. (From Moss, S. (ed.): *Preventive Dentistry,* 1972. Courtesy of Medcom, Inc.)

microcolonies of bacteria and their by-products (see Fig. 23–7). The plaque is colonized by several types of bacteria, both *cariogenic* (those that cause caries and that live mainly on sucrose and other carbohydrates) and noncariogenic. The most important cariogenic bacteria are streptococcal types. These bacteria ferment dietary carbohydrates to form *organic acids,* which, at susceptible sites, initiate the carious lesion by demineralizing the enamel surface.

Caries do not develop in germ-free animals — those reared in the complete absence of bacteria. This is perhaps the most striking evidence that has linked plaque to dental caries. Even when germ-free animals are fed high-carbohydrate, special cariogenic diets, they do not develop caries unless cariogenic bacteria are established in their mouths. Antibiotics, when fed to animals, are effective in reducing the incidence and severity of caries. In addition, children receiving ongoing antibiotic therapy effective against streptococcal bacteria (for example, in certain heart conditions) are known to have fewer caries in their teeth than children not receiving such antibiotics.

Further evidence to implicate the role of bacteria in caries is that specific bacteria have been isolated and cultivated from carious lesions. By inoculating them in germ-free animals, caries have developed. *Streptococcus mutans* and *Streptococcus sanguis* are examples of two common caries-causing bacteria.

Thus dental caries is basically a local disease of the teeth subject to the influence of those dietary components that provide the caries-causing bacteria with their necessary growth material, including a dietary source of essential amino acids, vitamins, and minerals in addition to carbohydrate. Caries is indeed a type of bacterial infection, and a vaccine against this type of dental disease may eventually be an effective preventive measure.

The caries-producing bacterial strains

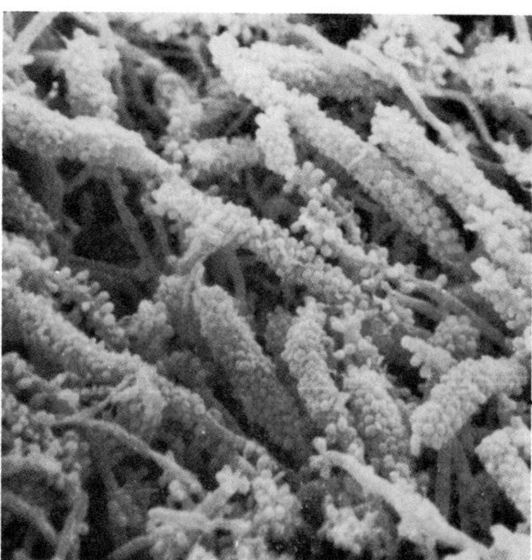

Figure 23–7 Dental plaque, shown here in a scanning electron micrograph, is composed of countless bacteria and contributes to the tooth decay process. (From Jones, S. J.: Dent. Abstr., *17*:8, 1972.)

also have the ability to convert sucrose (or its components glucose or fructose) into the extracellular polysaccharide *dextran* (a complex carbohydrate) and others into an intracellular polysaccharide, *amylopectin.* The dextran so produced is a sticky, insoluble, relatively inert substance that causes plaque to adhere to the teeth and appears to serve as a barrier to buffer systems in the saliva that might otherwise neutralize the acids formed by the bacteria in the plaque. During periods in which the diet is sugar-free, the *intra*cellular polysaccharide of the plaque is available for fermentation and maintenance of acid production. This production of polysaccharides by specific bacteria has been shown to be correlated with the incidence of caries. In fact, organisms that have lost their capacity to make the insoluble extracellular polysaccharides are no longer caries-producing.

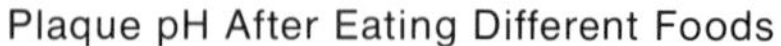

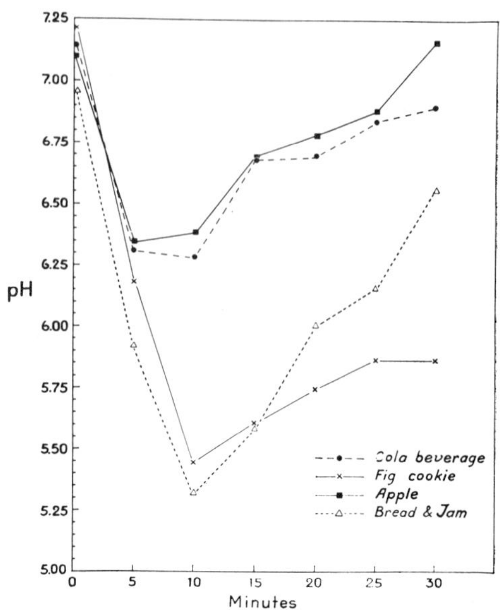

Figure 23–8 Some examples of the changes in plaque pH following eating of different foods. (From Ludwig, T. G., and Bibby, B. G.: J. Dent. Res., *36*:56, 1957.)

The Role of Sucrose and Other Carbohydrates in Dental Caries

The association of food and caries has been known for centuries, ever since it was observed that caries occur almost exclusively on tooth surfaces where self-cleansing mechanisms are least effective. Food is a necessary factor in allowing the cariogenic, dextran-producing plaque bacteria to actually begin causing caries. Dietary carbohydrates, and sucrose in particular, are of primary importance in the processes of bacterial colonization of the tooth surface and production and support of dental decay.

With the aid of carbohydrates to ferment, the plaque bacteria will produce an acid medium, with a pH of about 4.5 to 5.5, by the formation mainly of lactic acid. The drop in plaque pH may remain for up to 2 hours after sucrose ingestion. An example of the pH change observed in plaque after the ingestion of various foods is seen in Figure 23–8.

The important role of sucrose in the etiology of dental decay has been demonstrated by epidemiological and chemical studies as well as by controlled studies on animals and humans. For example:

1. During World War II, sugar consumption in Europe was severely restricted, and caries dropped significantly 2 years therafter. When the sugar intake increased again, caries recurred at previous levels.

2. Rampant caries (especially in the upper front teeth, a rare location) have been observed with frequency in children who fall asleep sucking on a bottle of fruit juice or milk with sugar. This is known as the "nursing bottle syndrome" and is one of the most crippling dental conditions in young children (see Fig. 23–9).

3. A Scandanavian study (the Vipeholm study) is a classic that examined the cariogenicity of various diets in humans.[4] For example, subjects who ate sticky toffee several times a day had 12 times as much caries development as control subjects who did not have this frequent exposure to sugar (Fig. 23–10).

4. In one *in vitro* study, sucrose was

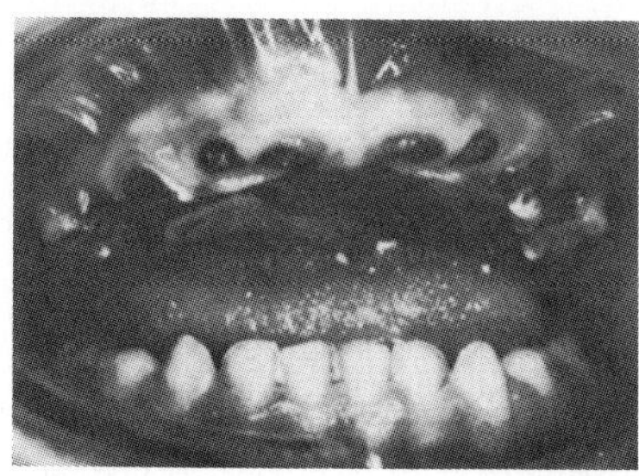

Figure 23–9 Teeth of a 2½ year old child who frequently received apple juice in a baby bottle. Note the nearly complete destruction of upper teeth by caries. (Lower teeth are thought to have been protected because of the position of the tongue and lower lip during sucking.((From Kaplan, H., and Rabbach, V. P.: Apple Juice and Dental Caries. Bambino. Children's Hospital Medical Center, Oakland, California, Winter 1971.)

reported to be the only sugar that would support plaque formation by caries-conducive *streptococci*.

5. People with a genetic defect known as hereditary fructose intolerance will avoid all foods containing sucrose and fructose because eating such foods produces unpleasant symptoms (nausea, vomiting, etc.). Their dental health is excellent, and their teeth often show total absence of dental caries.

6. In one small South Atlantic island, dental decay was virtually nonexistent before the advent of Westernized foods and sweets. Twenty years later, after the inhabitants began consuming an average of 0.5 kg of sugar a week, one-half of permanent molars were carious in those 20 years old and under.

7. England has had a documented increase in sugar consumption of from 20 to 110 pounds per person over the last 100 years, and there has been a nearly parallel rise in caries prevalence.

8. Widely different cavity counts were found in eight countries, and sugar consumption followed the same pattern (with highest caries incidence and sugar intake found in the United States and Central and South America).[5]

9. Sucrose supports the most rapidly progressive caries in the hamster and rat in multiple studies. Fructose, lactose, and, lastly, glucose, also result in caries formation, but with more time than is necessary for sucrose.

10. Maltose, lactose, fructose, and glucose can be used by the plaque bacteria for synthesizing cell wall, capsular, and intracellular polysaccharides, as well as for forming organic acids; but, unlike su-

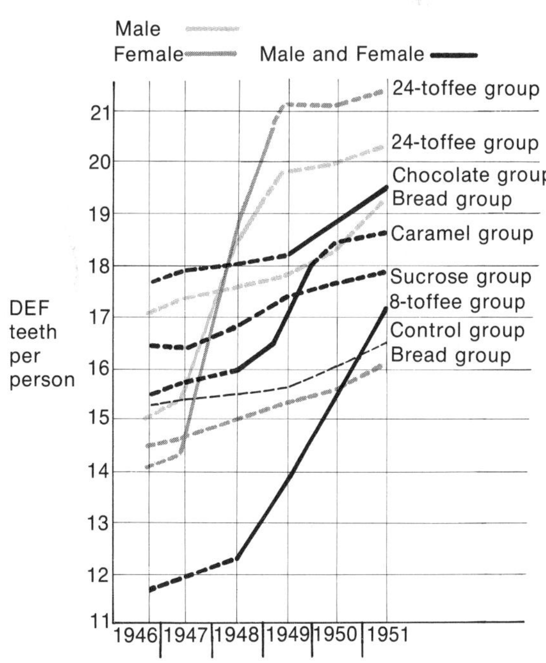

Figure 23–10 Graph of the Vipeholm study, showing the relationship of time of sugar consumption and of type of sugar-containing item to dental caries incidence over a period of 5 years. This study was important in demonstrating that increased frequency of consumption of sugar-containing items that are retained on tooth surfaces is a cause of caries. (From Sweeney, E. A. (ed.): *The Food That Stays: An Update on Nutrition, Diet, Sugar and Caries,* 1977. Courtesy of Medcom, Inc.)

crose, they cannot be utilized in the creation of *extra*cellular polysaccharides. Starches probably cannot diffuse into plaque, as sucrose so easily does, because of the relatively large size of the molecules. Starches are not, however, totally immune from suspicion as caries producers. They may be metabolized by certain (nonstreptococcal) oral bacteria to polysaccharides, which then may become part of the plaque matrix, undergo breakdown by caries-causing bacteria, and thus institute the decay process. See Figure 23–11 for a diagrammatic summary of the metabolism of ingested carbohydrates.

One further observation pertaining to the relationship of nutrition and dental health has been that in extremely poorly nourished populations — for example, overpopulated countries — the incidence of caries has been low. This observation has sometimes been interpreted as evidence for the *lack* of necessary association between a good diet and good teeth. However, these populations had negligible, if any, sucrose in their diet. The lack of this substance permitted their teeth, although probably less than optimally developed and shaped with a lifelong history of malnutrition, to remain free of the effects of the cariogenic plaque bacteria dependent on sucrose, and thus free of caries.

The Role of the Time Factor and the Frequency of Eating

A small area of decalcified enamel, just barely detectable, will generally progress to clinical caries in 1 or 2 years. If, however, careful preventive measures are immediately undertaken (dietary and oral hygiene measures), the development of the caries may be halted, although the eroded spot can never revert to normal.

The age of the tooth plays a part in caries susceptibility. A tooth is most likely to develop caries 2 to 4 years after eruption, when enamel is in the final stages of maturation. When complete enamel maturation has been attained (after 2 to 4 years) the tooth is more resistant to caries formation. This helps to explain why young children and teen-agers (with fairly new deciduous and permanent teeth, respectively) have higher caries rates than individuals of other age groups.

In addition, timing of sugar exposure is related to caries development in that the more often sweets are in contact with the teeth, the longer the exposure to acid decalcification and the higher the caries incidence will be (see Fig. 23–12).

This overriding importance of the *frequency* of exposure to sweets was first documented by the Vipeholm study.[4] Those who ate sweets between meals had more caries than those who ate sweets only at mealtimes, regardless of the total amount of sugar intake per day.

Thus, "snacking" on sugary foods plays a definite role in caries causation.[6] The more frequently sugar is eaten between meals, the greater is the increase in caries. In addition, the longer the sugar substance stays in contact with the teeth, the greater the cariogenicity. (Sticky candy such as taffy and regular chewing gum are examples of prime offenders.)

If sucrose and sticky snacks cannot be avoided in the diet, they should be removed from the teeth as quickly as possible by proper oral hygiene measures.

The Role of Fluoride

Fluoride is at present the only dietary trace element of proven effectiveness in producing decay-resistant teeth in humans. The beneficial effects of fluoride on teeth have been known for over 70 years, and there have been over 10,000 articles on fluoride and dental health printed in the world's scientific journals. At present, fluoridation programs reach over 150 million people throughout the world.

The incidence of dental caries in both the deciduous and the permanent teeth is reduced about 60 percent in children who drink water containing about 1 part per

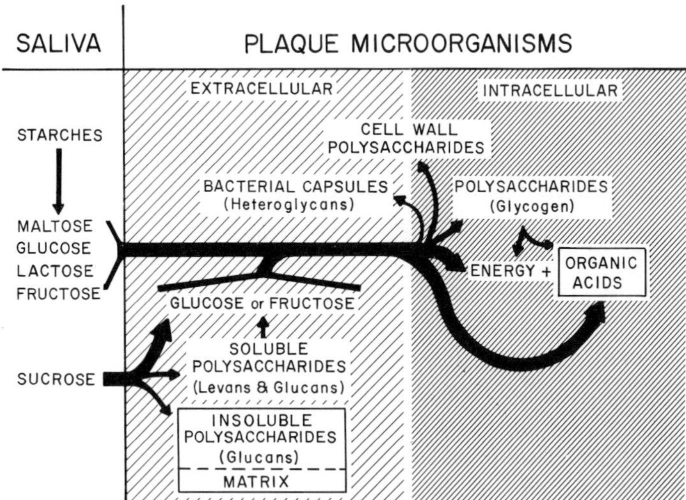

Figure 23–11 Metabolic fate of ingested carbohydrates, showing both extracellular and intracellular end-products. Heavy arrows represent major pathways, and end-products which are particularly harmful to the teeth are shown in the boxes. (From Newbrun, E.: *Etiology of Dental Caries.* San Francisco, University of California, 1971.)

million (1 mg per liter) of fluorine throughout the period of tooth development. See Figure 23–13 for the results of one important study documenting the effects of fluoridation in a community. The caries decrement is smaller when fluoridated water consumption (or dietary fluoride supplementation) is started at a later age. There are also indications that caries inhibition attributable to fluoridated water continues throughout adult life. Most foods contain only trace amounts of fluorides, with the average American diet, exclusive of water, containing 0.2 to 0.5 mg of fluoride. Inclusion of water containing 1 ppm of fluoride thus raises the intake to an estimated 1.5 to 2.0 mg of fluoride per day.

The safety of fluoridation has been

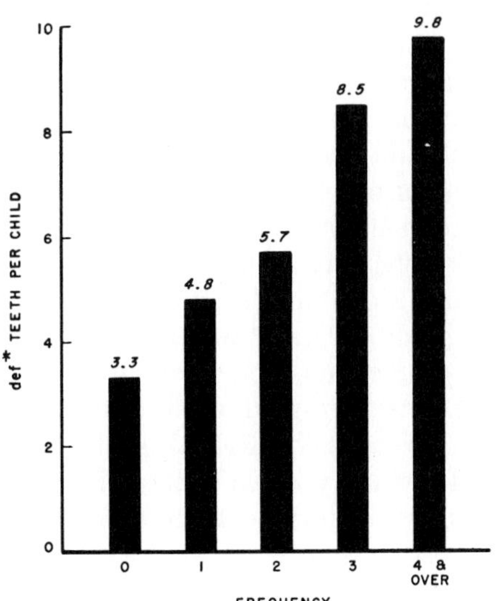

* Includes extracted primary molars.

Figure 23–12 The effect of between-meal eating on caries activity in children. This shows that the more snacks children ate, the higher was the incidence of decay. (From Weiss, R. L., and Trithart, A. H.: Amer. J. Public Health, *50*:1097, 1960.)

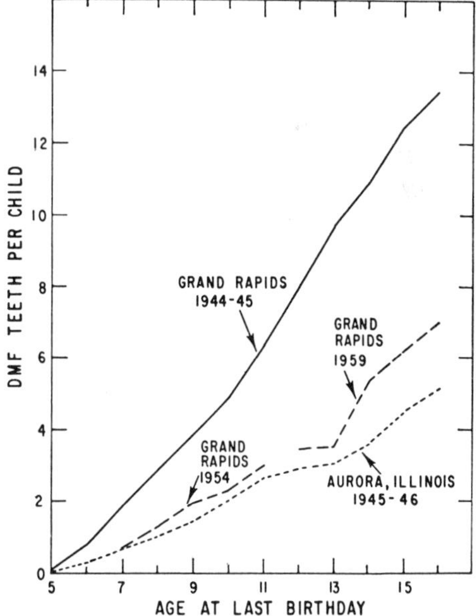

Figure 23–13 This diagram shows the beneficial results of a 15-year period of fluoridation in Grand Rapids, Michigan. It presents the dental caries experience in terms of decayed, missing, and filled teeth ("DMF") per child for Grand Rapids, both before and 15 years after fluoridation, and includes caries data from Aurora, Illinois, a community with natural water fluoridation, for comparison. (From Arnold, F. A., Jr., et al.: J. Amer. Dent. Assoc., *65*:780, 1962.)

well documented by the World Health Organization. Mild, harmless mottling of teeth may occur when water containing as little as 2 ppm or more of fluoride is ingested, but only in the years from 1 to 6. (See also Chapter 12.) Fluoride is cleared very rapidly by the kidneys; thus small amounts do not accumulate in the body in sufficient quantities to produce any health hazard.

The mode of action of fluorides in preventing dental caries is unique and is related to its accumulation in enamel. It renders the structure of the enamel of the tooth more stable and less soluble to acid. There appears to be a lesser protective effect on permanent teeth posteruptively than preeruptively, with the teeth most recently erupted (still not totally "matured") being benefited most. No posteruptive effect on baby teeth has been yet documented. Thus in order to protect the *deciduous* teeth, fluoride must be ingested during the *first year* of life.

The use of fluorine tablets does not appear to be quite as effective as fluoridation of water, perhaps primarily because this method relies on daily cooperation of parent and child. In one study, only 50 percent of families continued giving the pills for the recommended number of years, and this is probably a generous estimate. Fluoride tablets are more costly than community water fluoridation, which costs only 5 to 15 cents per person per year.

The use of fluorides applied topically to the teeth is possible in a practical way by using fluoride-containing toothpastes and mouth rinses. Their use results in a significant preventive value, giving about 20 to 50 percent reduction in incidence of new carious surfaces.

Studies have shown that there are definite reductions in family dental bills after institution of water fluoridation programs at the levels recommended by the United States Public Health Service. For example, the cost of initial dental care of a typical child dropped from 32 dollars to 14 dollars after fluoridation was established in one community. The Head Start Program has found that it must pay from three to ten times as much for dental services for an enrolled child from a nonfluoridated area as it does for such services for a child from a community with fluoridation. It has recently been estimated that fluoridated water would mean a savings of seven million dollars a year in dental bills for the one-half million children in one city in the eastern United States.[7]

With so much evidence regarding the usefulness, safety, and economy of fluoridation, and its unanimous recommendation by scientific bodies,* to what extent is it used in the United States? Unfortunately, not anywhere near 100 percent. The extent to which fluoridation was used in the different states in 1975 is shown in Figure 23–14. The Public Health Service estimates that in 1975 a total of 105 million Americans had access to fluoridated water. This represents about 50 percent of the total United States population, and is an increase by about 6 percent over the 1967 figures.

Further considerations regarding the practicalities of fluoridation of water supplies include the following:

1. In areas where residents do not have access to a community water supply, fluoridation of school water is feasible and should be recommended. Dietary fluoride supplementation during the preschool years is also advised.

2. There is variability in daily water consumption of children. In one study, an average of 300 ml of water was consumed at 1 year of age and about 400 ml at 5 years. The average intake of fluoride from water for these children would be only 0.3 to 0.4 mg a day when water is fluoridated at 1 ppm. Recommendations for fluoride

*The United States Public Health Service was the first to endorse fluoridation, in 1945. Since then it has been endorsed by the American Dental Association, the American Medical Association, the World Health Organization, the American Public Health Association, the American Institute of Nutrition, and the Food and Nutrition Board, among others.

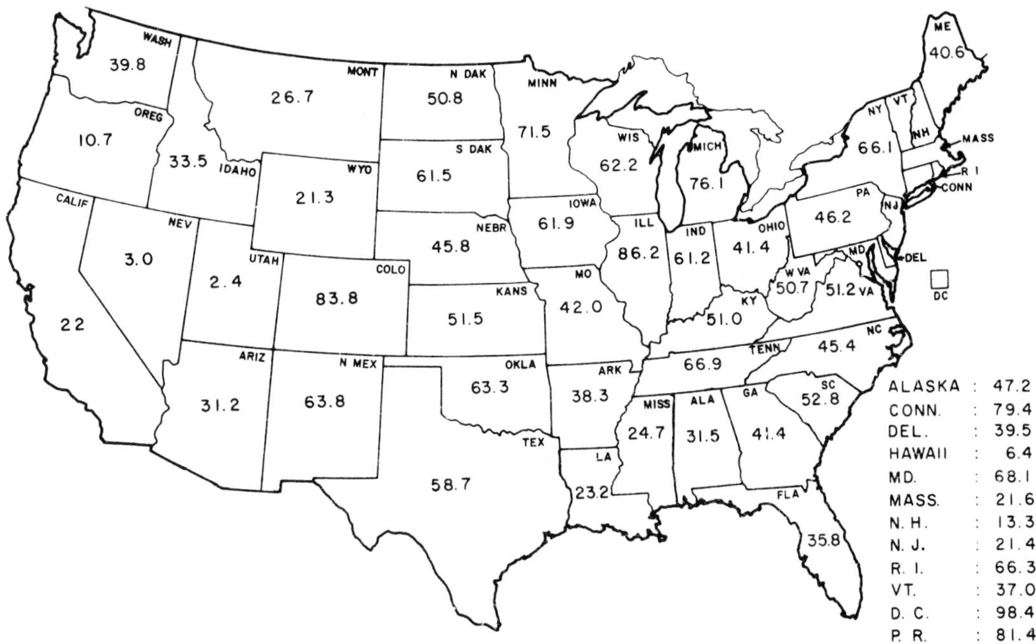

Figure 23–14 Percent of state population using fluoridated water, 1975, as determined by a fluoridation census conducted by the Center for Disease Control. How does your state stand on fluoridation? (From Morbidity and Mortality Weekly Report, *26(27)*:1, 1977.)

supplements depend on fluoride concentration of the water supply as well as the age of the child. These recommendations are summarized in Table 23–1.

3. In hot climates, where there is a high intake of water, fluoridation concentration should be less than in colder climates.

4. The legal validity of fluoridation has been thoroughly tested in the United States in the last decades and has been invariably confirmed. It is thus not considered a "compulsory medication," as opponents charge, but rather as a rightful preventive measure. At least eight states have now passed legislation to require fluoridation in all community water supplies.

Countries in addition to the United States that have fluoridation in a good

Table 23–1 RECOMMENDED FLUORIDE SUPPLEMENTATION*

Fluoride Concentration of Water Supply (ppm)	*Desirable Fluoride Supplementation (mg/day)*				
	AGE 0–6 MO	AGE 6–18 MO	AGE 18–36 MO	AGE 3–6 YR	AGE > 6 YR
<0.2	0	0.25	0.5	0.75	1.0
0.2–0.4	0	0†	0.25	0.5	0.75
0.4–0.6	0	0†	0	0.25	0.5
0.6–0.8	0	0†	0	0	0.25
>0.8	0	0†	0	0	0‡

*From Fomon, S.: *Nutritional Disorders of Children: Prevention, Screening and Follow-Up.* U.S. Dept. of Health, Education, and Welfare, 1976.

†0.25 for breast-fed infants between 6 and 12 months of age.

‡In this age group, the hazard of fluorosis is low, and some additional protection will probably be afforded by fluoride supplementation. However, fluoride supplementation is probably not desirable when drinking water provides more than 1.1 ppm.

number of communities are Australia, Brazil, Canada, Chile, Czechoslovakia, Ireland, the Netherlands, New Zealand, and the U.S.S.R. The further use of added fluoride for drinking water will probably be rapidly increasing throughout the world.

Role of Other Nutritional Factors

It should be added that other nutrients, such as molybdenum and vanadium (as well as vitamin B-6), have been reported to help protect against caries development in the experimental animal. A variety of studies suggest but do not conclusively prove that there are relationships between caries prevalence and a wide variety of trace elements other than fluorine in either humans or experimental animals. More research is needed regarding these possible relationships. The mechanisms for the role of these minerals may have to do with increasing the resistance of enamel or with changing the properties of saliva or plaque.

In animals, phosphate supplementation of food helps to decrease caries susceptibility by lowering the solubility rate of enamel, but this has not been proved in humans. There is no evidence for any direct role of calcium in decreasing caries after the tooth is formed.

Highly acid foods, such as undiluted lemon juice or soft drinks with a high phosphoric acid content, are known to be able to dissolve or etch tooth enamel after long-term contact periods. The usual infrequent short-term exposure, along with the buffering effect of saliva, probably results in little or no damage.

PERIODONTAL DISEASE AND NUTRITION

*Periodontal disease** (disease of the gums and other tissues surrounding the teeth), like caries, is an ancient malady of mankind and one still prevalent throughout the world. Tooth loss after the age of 35 years in this country is usually due to the effects of periodontal disease, because it results in the loss of healthy supporting tissues for viable teeth. Periodontal disease and its effects thus worsen with increasing age, but the potential for advanced disease may start at an early age.

What are the factors that cause poor periodontal health? Local factors in the mouth, such as the state of oral cleanliness and hygiene, and, again, the effect of foods that either encourage or discourage bacterial growth at gingival (gum) margins are all-important. Rates of periodontal disease incidence are highest in populations with the poorest states of oral hygiene (for example, in countries with very few dentists, as well as in segments of the American population with limited access to dental care).

There have been no consistent correlations between specific nutrient intake and periodontal disease. Vitamin A and vitamin E have shown some positive correlations, but firm evidence is lacking. Certain acute periodontal problems — for example, scurvy with its bleeding gums and diseased gums often found in niacin deficiency — do stem from a lack of nutrients in the diet, but these are not examples of classic periodontal disease.

Experimental studies have shown that protein starvation and magnesium deficiency may adversely affect the periodontium in man. An advanced stage of bone and periodontal destruction has been seen with protein deficiency. In addition to contributing to tissue growth and resistance, proteins are also important in the function of the endocrine system, whose hormones play a role in proper maintenance of periodontal tissue. Experimental magnesium lack in animals can cause imperfect development of the alveolar bone, widening of the periodontal membrane, gingival enlargement, and loosening of the teeth. In humans, iron deficiency has been shown to be related to

*From the two Greek words *peri* and *odont*, meaning "around tooth."

unhealthy gingival tissues, especially in females.

In theory, calcium and phosphorus deficiency, if severe enough, could also affect the bone that helps support the tooth.

Bacterial masses, or plaque, are key culprits in periodontal disease. The bacterial accumulations on the tooth surfaces closest to the gingival margins are implicated in this case. In addition, the subsequent accumulation of *calculus* (a mixture of minerals) occurs on the teeth and under loosened gingival margins. These factors lead to inflammation and infection of the periodontal tissues, known as *gingivitis*. This gingivitis, if untreated, is followed by loosening and destruction of the periodontal fibers or ligaments (see Fig. 23–2).

The last stage of periodontal disease is gradual resorption of the alveolar bone that supports the tooth, with consequent tooth loosening and, finally, tooth loss. From this description of the adverse effects of periodontal disease, it is easy to see the detrimental effect that advanced disease will have on the diet. An affected individual will choose foods that are easy to chew but which, unfortunately, are often soft carbohydrates.

Good nutrition, then, is important in the prevention of gingival and periodontal disease because it helps to maintain optimally healthy tissues that are resistant to disease.

Dietary control of sugars and sticky snacks is particularly important because of the key role of bacterial plaque in the process of caries formation. (Review Fig.

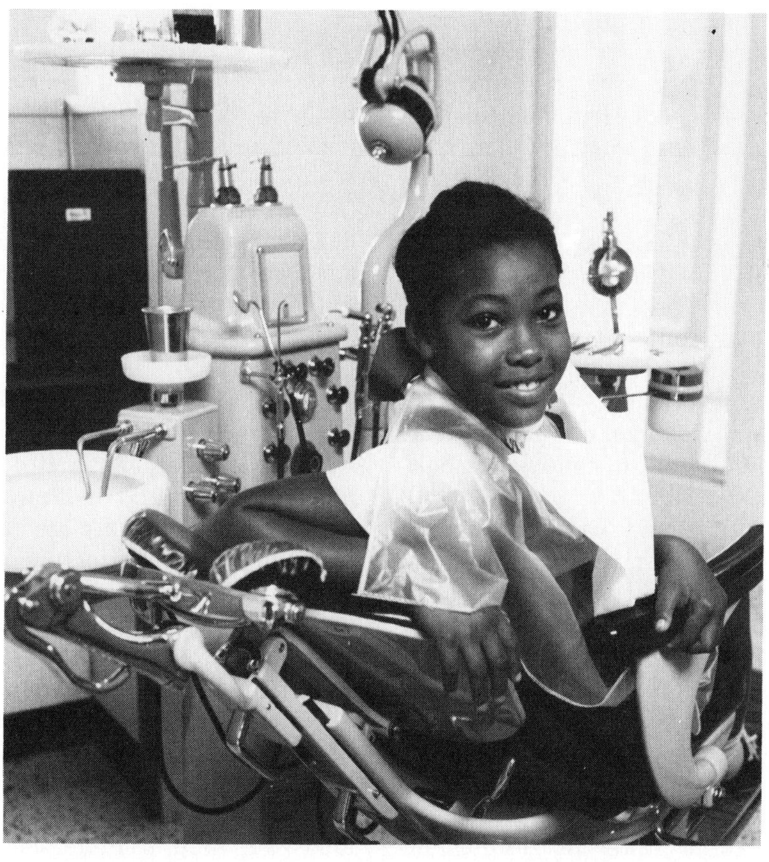

Figure 23–15 Foundations for good oral health are established in childhood. Preventive measures are most effective when instituted early, and these include good eating habits, as well as regular dental care for healthy smiles. (From World Health, Dec. 1973. Courtesy of WHO/P. Almasy.)

23–11.) In addition, certain foods can be of some physical help to those afflicted with periodontal disease. Firm, fibrous foods may help to promote natural cleansing.

PREVENTION OF DENTAL DISEASE

Prevention must be the key to the problem of dental disease (see Fig. 23–15). The four most important factors in prevention are good nutrition, plaque control, fluoridation, and nutrition education.

Preventive oral hygiene measures are important in removing plaque and local irritants, and include proper tooth brushing supplemented by other cleansing aids such as dental floss. If plaque is thus broken up every 24 hours, the activity of the plaque bacteria will be stopped before the underlying enamel begins to decalcify. Tooth brushing is particularly important prior to sleep, for in sleep salivary production decreases, thus reducing the natural salivary buffers that help to partially counteract the effects of the acid-producing bacteria.

The role of diet, and especially of sugars, in dental disease has been discussed in detail. Preventive dietary measures include the following:

1. Avoid foods with the highest caries potentials (Table 23–2).
2. Use cheese, nuts, and raw vegetables and fruits instead of candy and cookies for snacks.
3. Avoid sticky candy, sugared chewing gum, and such candy as "all day suckers," as well as frequent soft drinks.
4. Consume carbohydrates mainly at meals.
5. Use a diet that provides good general nutrition, especially in children, for optimal developmental protection of the teeth.
6. Insure for all an adequate intake of fluoride in either water or supplement form.

Table 23–2 "CARIES-POTENTIALITY" OF REPRESENTATIVE FOODS*

Food	*Total Sugar Content (Percent)*	*"Caries Potentiality"*
Caramel	64.0	27
Honey + bread + butter	19.0	24
Honey	72.8	18
Sweet cookies (biscuits)	9.0	18
Marmalade	65.3	10
Marmalade + bread + butter	16.3	9
Ice cream	2.4	9
Potatoes (boiled)	0.8	7
Potatoes (fried)	3.9	7
White bread + butter	1.5	7
Coarse rye bread + butter	2.3	7
Milk	3.8	6
Apple	7.5	5
Orange	6.5	3
Lemonade	9.3	2
Carrot (boiled)	2.4	1

*Adapted from Dunning, J. M.: *Principles of Dental Public Health.* Cambridge, Mass., Harvard University Press, 1970. Calculated from sugar concentrations in saliva and how long they remained high after eating each specific food. In general, those with the lowest scores should be used instead of those with highest scores if optimal dental health is desired.

Dental disease has been shown to be caused by factors that are accessible, controllable, and correctable, and improvement of individual dental health is within the reach of everyone, with the aid of his dentist. The amount of decay and gingival disease found is really an index of inadequate application of preventive procedures.

QUESTIONS AND PROBLEMS

1. Name the dental structures. What nutrients are found in these structures? Which other nutrients are necessary for formation of these structures?
2. Describe how carbohydrates in the diet play a role in the formation of plaque. Why are the bacteria in plaque an important factor in causing dental caries? What role does sugar play in causing gingivitis?
3. Which foods are associated with a high incidence of dental caries? Which foods are helpful in preventing decay? Why?
4. Plan a lunch that may be carried

from home, that provides one-third of the daily nutrient needs of an 8-year-old child, and that will not foster dental caries.

5. How does fluoride aid in prevention of caries? How may fluoride be administered? Which method is most practical? What is the fluoride level of the water in your community?

REFERENCES

1. Hardwick, J. L.: Brit. Dent. J., *108*:9, 1960.
2. Read, T., and Knowles, E.: Brit. Dent. J., *64*:185, 1938.
3. Caldwell, R. C.: J. Dent. Res., *49*:1293, 1970.
4. Gustafsson, B. E., Quensel, C., Lanke, L. et al.: Acta Odont. Scand., *11*:232, 1954.
5. Dunning, J. M.: *Principles of Dental Public Health.* Cambridge, Mass., Harvard University Press, 1970.
6. Bibby, B. G.: J. Amer. Dental Assoc., *90*:121, 1975.
7. Walsh, D. C.: N. Engl. J. Med., *296*:1118, 1977.

SUPPLEMENTARY READING

General and Reviews

American Dental Association Health Foundation: Symposium: Cariostatic mechanisms of fluorides. Caries Res., *11*: supplement 1, 1977.

Bowen, W. H.: Dental caries. Contemporary Nutrition, *2*:1977. Minneapolis, General Mills Nutrition Department.

Dunning, J. M.: *Principles of Dental Public Health.* Cambridge, Mass., Harvard University Press, 1970.

Dunning, J. M.: *Dental Care for Everyone: Problems and Proposals.* Cambridge, Mass., Harvard University Press, 1976.

Gibbons, R. J., and Van Houte, J.: Dental caries. Ann. Rev. Med., *26*:7136, 1975.

Hartles, R. L., and Leach, S. A.: Effect of diet on dental caries. Brit. Med. Bull., *31*:137, 1975.

McBean, L. D., and Speckmann, E. W.: A review: the importance of nutrition in oral health. J. Amer. Dent. Assoc., *89*:109, 1974.

Molnar, S., and Ward, S. C.: Mineral metabolism and microstructural defects in primate teeth. Amer. J. Phys. Anthropol., *43*:3, 1975.

Morgan, P. M., et al.: Dental health of Louisiana residents based on the Ten-State Nutrition Survey. Pub. Health Rpts., *90*:173, 1975.

Morrey, L. W., and Nelson, R. J. (eds.): *Dental Science Handbook.* Washington, D. C., Superintendent of Documents, 1970.

Newbrun, E. (ed.): Water fluoridation and dietary fluoride. In *Fluorides and Dental Caries.* 2nd Ed. Springfield, Ill., Charles C Thomas, 1975, p. 3.

Newbrun, E.: Diet and dental caries relationships. Adv. Caries Res., *2*: xv, 1974.

Nizel, A. E.: *Preventive Dentistry: Science and Practice.* Philadelphia, W. B. Saunders Co., 1972.

Nizel, A. E.: Nutrition and oral problems. World Rev. Nutr. Dietet., *16*:226, 1973.

Shaw, J. H.: Preeruptive effects of nutrition on teeth. J. Dent. Res., *49*:1238, 1970.

State University of New York: Immunological aspects of dental caries, a symposium. J. Dent. Res., *55*:1976.

Symposium on Nutrition. Dent. Clin. North Amer., *20*:441, 1976.

Ten-State Nutrition Survey 1968–1970, III. Clinical, Anthropometry, Dental. U.S. Dept. of Health, Education, and Welfare Pub. No. (HSM) 72–8131.

World Health Organization: The drive for oral health continues. (nine articles). Geneva, WHO, 1973.

Dental Caries and Sucrose

Bibby, B. G., and Mundorff, S. A.: Enamel demineralization by snack foods. J. Dent. Res., *54*:461, 1975.

Carlsson, J., and Johansson, T.: Sugar and the production of bacteria in the human mouth. Caries Res., *7*:273, 1973.

Fry, A. J., and Grenby, T. H.: The effects of reduced sucrose intake on the formation and composition of dental plaque in a group of men in the Antarctic. Arch. Oral Biol., *17*:873, 1972.

Gawronski, T. H., Staat, R. A., Zaki, H. A., Harris, R. S., and Folke, L. E. A.: Effects of dietary sucrose levels on extracellular polysaccharide metabolism of human dental plaque. J. Dent. Res., *54*:881, 1975.

Koulourides, T., et al.: Cariogenicity of nine sugars tested with an intraoral device in man. Caries Res., *10*:427, 1976.

Retief, D. H., Cleaton-Jones, P. E., and Walker, A. R. P.: Dental caries and sugar intake in South African pupils of 16 to 17 years in four ethnic groups. Brit. Dent. J., *138*:463, 1975.

Staat, R. H., et al.: Effects of dietary sucrose levels on the quantity and microbial composition of human dental plaque. J. Dent. Res., *54*:872, 1975. (also see p. 881).

Tatevossian, A., and Jenkins, G. N.: Sucrose and the role of saccharates in enamel caries. Caries Res., *8*:317, 1974.

Thompson, C. M., et al.: Dental caries: possible sugar substitutes for sucrose. Ecol. Food Nutr., *3*:231, 1974.

van Houte, J., et al.: Role of sucrose in colonization of *streptococcus mutans* in conventional Sprague-Dawley rats. J. Dent. Res., *55*:202, 1976.

Fluoridation

Alternatives to the fluoridation of water. Brit. Med. J., *1*:535, 1975.

American Academy of Pediatrics, Committee on Nutrition: Fluoride as a nutrient. Pediatrics, *49*:456, 1972.

American Dietetic Association: Policy statement on

fluoridation. J. Amer. Dietet. Assoc., *64*:68, 1974.

American Medical Association: Revised statement on fluoridation. J.A.M.A., *231*:1167, 1975.

Austin, K. F., et al.: A statement on the question of allergy to fluoride as used in the fluoridation of community water supplies. J. Allergy, *47*:347, 1971.

Bernhardt, M., and Sprague, B.: Are we depriving our children of healthy teeth? Family Health, 9:31, 1977.

Davies, G. N.: Cost and benefit of fluoride in the prevention of dental caries. WHO Offset Pub. No. 9. Geneva, WHO, 1974.

Domoto, P. K., Faine, R. C., and Rovin, S.: Seattle fluoridation campaign 1973 — prescription for a victory. J. Amer. Dent. Assoc., *91*:583, 1975.

Erickson, J. D.: Mortality in selected cities with fluoridated and nonfluoridated water supplies. N. Engl. J. Med., *298*:1112, 1978.

Erickson, J. D., et al.: Water fluoridation and congenital malformations: no association. J. Amer. Dent. Assoc., *93*:981, 1976.

Ericsson, Y.: Report on the safety of drinking water fluoridation. Caries Res., *8*:16, (supplement), 1974.

Heifetz, S. B., and Horowtiz, H. S.: Effect of school water fluoridation on dental caries: interim results in Seagrove, NC, after four years, J. Amer, Dent. Assoc. *88*:352, 1974.

Hoover, R. N., McKay, F. W., and Fraumeni, J. F. Jr.: Fluoridated drinking water and the occurrence of cancer. J. Natl. Cancer Inst., *57*:757, 1976.

Horowitz, H. S.: Fluoride: research on clinical and public health applications. J. Amer. Dent. Assoc., *87*:1013, 1973.

Horowitz, H. S., and Heifetz, S. B.: The effect of partial defluoridation of a water supply on dental fluorosis — final results in Bartlett, Texas, after 17 years. Amer. J. Pub. Health, *62*:767, 1972.

Horowitz, H. S., Heifetz, S. B., and Law, F. E.: Effect of school water fluoridation on dental caries: final results in Elk Lake, Pa., after 12 years. J. Amer. Dent. Assoc., *84*:832, 1972.

Keene, H. J., Catalanotto, F. A., and Mickel, G. J.: Prevalence of caries free naval recruits from cities with fluoridated and nonfluoridated water supplies. J. Dent. Res., *55*:704, 1976.

National Dairy Council: Nutrition and oral health. Dairy Council Dig., *49*(3):13, 1978.

Newbrun, E.: The safety of water fluoridation. J. Amer. Dent. Assoc., *94*:301, 1977.

Schwab, J. G., and Schwartz, A. D.: Fluoridated water supplies: an inadequate source of fluoride for children. J. Pediatr. *86*:735, 1975.

Shupe, J. L., Leone, N. J., Fletcher, D. C.: *Efficacy and Safety of Fluoridation*. Chicago, American Medical Association, 1975.

Smith, E. H., Jr.: Fluoridation of water supply. J.A.M.A., *230*:1569, 1975.

Wiatrowski, E., et al.: Dietary fluoride intake of infants. Pediatrics, *55*:517, 1975.

Periodontal Disease

Chung, C. S., et al.: Dental plaque and dietary intakes in schoolchildren in Hawaii. J. Dent. Res., *56*:11, 1977.

Freeland, J. H., Cousins, R. J., and Schwartz, R.: Relationship of mineral status and intake to periodontal disease. Amer. J. Clin. Nutr., *29*:745, 1976.

Glickman, I.: Periodontal disease. N. Engl. J. Med., *284*:1071, 1971.

Parfitt, G. J., and Speirs, D. M.: Role of nutrition in the prevention and treatment of periodontal disease. J. Can. Dent. Assoc., *36*:224, 1970.

Slade, E. W., et al.: Vitamin E and periodontal disease. J. Periodont., *47*:352, 1976.

Stahl, S. S.: Nutritional influences on periodontal disease. World Rev. Nutr. Dietet., *13*:277, 1971.

The attack on fluoridation. Consumer's Rpt., *43*:480, 1978.

Vogel, R. I., et al.: The effect of folic acid on gingival health. J. Periodont., *47*:667, 1976.

Other References

Avery, K. T.: The dental health of children of migrant and seasonal agricultural workers. J. Sch. Health, *45*:24, 1975.

Clancy, K. L., et al.: Snack food intake of adolescents and caries development. J. Dent. Res., *45*: 568, 1977.

Delgado, H., Habicht J. P., Yarbrough, C., et al.: Nutritional status and the timing of deciduous tooth eruption. Amer. J. Clin. Nutr., *28*:216, 1975.

Edgar, W. M., et al.: Acid production in plaques after eating snacks: modifying factors in foods. J. Amer. Dent. Assoc., *90*:418, 1975.

Fuller, J. L., and Johnson, W. W.: Citric acid consumption and the human dentition. J. Amer. Dent. Assoc., *95*:80, 1977.

Glass, R. L., and Fleisch, S.: Diet and dental caries: dental caries incidence and the consumption of ready-to-eat cereals. J. Amer. Dent. Assoc., *88*:807, 1974.

Grenby, T. H.: The deposition of dental plaque in young adults on a diet containing chocolate and skim-milk powder. Arch. Oral Biol., *19*:213, 1974.

Kuhnlein, H. V., and Calloway, D. H.: Minerals in human teeth: differences between preindustrial and contemporary Hopi Indians. Amer. J. Clin. Nutr., *30*:883, 1977.

Linn, E. L.: Teenagers' attitudes, knowledge, and behaviors related to oral health. J. Amer. Dent. Assoc., *92*:946, 1976.

Robinson, L. G., et al.: Nutrition counseling and children's dental health. J. Nutr. Ed., *8*:33, 1976.

Rowe, N. H., et al.: Effect of phosphate-enriched ready-to-eat breakfast cereals on dental caries experience in adolescents: a three-year study. J. Amer. Dent. Assoc., *90*:412, 1975.

Rowe, N. H., et al.: The effect of age, sex, race, and economic status on dental caries experience of the permanent dentition. Pediatrics, *57*:457, 1976.

Shank, S. E., and Guthrie, H. A.: Nutritional counseling for prevention of dental caries in adolescents. J. Amer. Dent. Assoc., *92*:378, 1976.

Sharman, I. M.: Fructose and xylitol, the Turku dental studies. Nutr. Food Sci. (U.K.), *43*:20, 1976.

Shelton, P. G., et al.: Nursing bottle caries. Pediatrics, *59*:777, 1977.

Steinberg, A. D., Zimmerman, S. O., and Bramer, M. L.: The Lincoln dental caries study. II. The effect of acidulated carbonated beverages on the incidence of dental caries. J. Amer. Dent. Assoc., *85*:81, 1972.

Tonge, C. H., and McCance, R. A.: Normal development of the jaws and teeth in pigs, and the delay and malocclusion produced by calorie deficiencies. J. Anat., *115*:1, 1973.

Articles in Nutrition Reviews

Protein deficiency and tooth and salivary gland development. *32*:24, 1974.

Malnutrition and oral health of children. *32*:44, 1974.

Dental caries prevalence and trace elements other than fluoride. *32*:120, 1974.

Frequency of eating and dental caries prevalence. *32*:139, 1974.

The role of dietary carbohydrates in plaque formation and oral disease. *33*:353, 1975.

The cause of mottled enamel. *34*:47, 1976.

Domestic water and dental caries. *34*:116, 1976.

Toxic effects of fluoride in enamel formation. *34*:311, 1976.

Evaluation of the caries-producing ability of human foods. *36*:249, 1978.

*Dental Journals for Additional Reading**

Other reliable references to current dental health research and its application are most likely to be found in recent issues of such journals as:

Advances in Caries Research
American Journal of Orthodontics
Archives of Oral Biology
British Dental Journal
Caries Research
Community Dentistry and Oral Epidemiology
Dental Abstracts
Dental Clinics of North America
International Dental Journal
Journal of the American Dental Association
Journal Canadian Dental Association
Journal of Dental Research
Journal of Periodontology
Journal of Periodontal Research
Journal of Public Health Dentistry
Scandinavian Journal of Dental Research

---

*The American Dental Association, 211 E. Chicago Ave., Chicago, Ill. 60611, is a good source of additional applied information.

Chapter 24

Overweight and Underweight

OVERWEIGHT

Obesity is prevalent in all affluent societies. Many people accept as normal the gradual accumulation of weight that so often comes in the later years of life, disregarding the health risks that it brings with it. Some persuade themselves that they are not *much* overweight, just enough to be "pleasingly plump," and that it is more pleasant to indulge in food than to diet. Others are embarrassed by their overweight condition and find it hard to get about, but seem to regard the matter as something determined by fate rather than by themselves. Not all the overweights are middle-aged — some young people, children, and even babies are overweight (Fig. 24–1). The fact that there are obese nutritionists and physicians indicates that neither dietetic information nor knowledge of health risks guarantees adequate control of body weight. Obesity has proved resistant to efforts aimed at either prevention or cure.

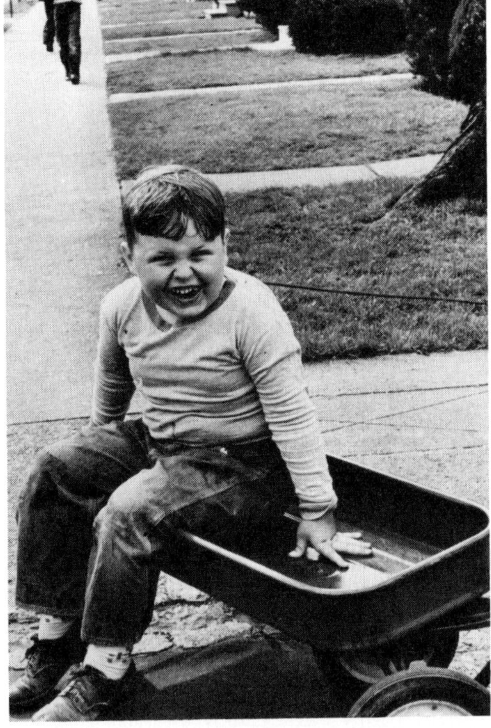

Figure 24–1 Malnutrition of affluence. While poverty is associated with undernutrition and malnutrition — so common in the developing world — the affluent societies are succumbing more and more to the "malnutrition of affluence" caused by overeating. Obesity — a great health hazard — affects almost every third individual in some countries. Dental caries and atherosclerosis are other examples of the adverse effects of affluence. Nutrition education has an important role to play in reversing this dangerous trend. The shadow of obesity hangs over this boy's childhood. In the background may be a mother who, in her mistaken zeal, overfeeds him. (Courtesy of WHO/P. Almasy).

Disadvantages and Dangers of Excess Weight

Obesity carries with it increased risk of illness and death from a number of diseases: heart disease, high blood pressure, stroke, kidney disease, gallstones, cirrho-

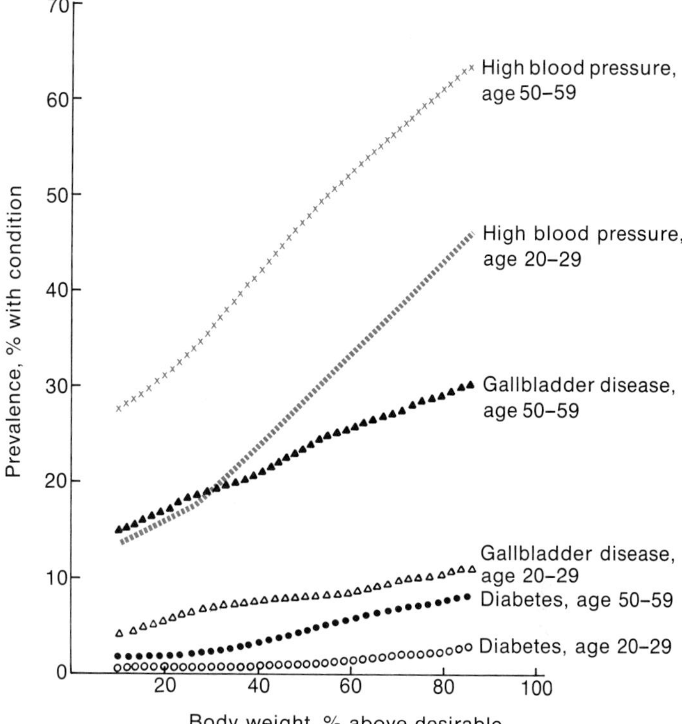

Figure 24–2 Obesity and age-specific occurrence in women with diabetes, gallbladder disease and high blood pressure. Data are for many thousands of weight-conscious women enrolled in a therapeutic TOPS program. (From Rimm, A. A., et al.: Public Health Rpt., *90*:44–51, 1975.)

sis of the liver, and diabetes.[1,2] Overweight people have difficulties with their feet and back because of the added burden of weight on the skeleton, and have, as well, an increased incidence of gout and arthritis.[1] They suffer from shortness of breath, especially on exertion, and have increased surgical risk. Our culture favors a lean look, so the obese are handicapped socially, in employment, and in school admission.

The health hazards that accompany overweight — greater incidence of heart and circulatory diseases and of diabetes — are naturally increased with a larger excess of weight and with advancing years (Fig. 24–2). For instance, in the 40- to 44-year-old age bracket, 20 percent excess over normal weight carries with it a 30 to 40 percent increase in mortality above the expected rate, while a 40 percent excess of weight involves an 80 to 100 percent increase in mortality. Put another way, a 50-year-old man who is 50 pounds overweight has about half the life expectancy of one of the same age who is of normal weight.

Everyone should check his weight occasionally with some tables that show the normal weight for his height. Tables based on the actual *average* weights of the population at various ages are not good for this purpose, because so many otherwise normal people show some degree of overweight after 40 that these figures are too high to represent the *optimum* weight so far as health is concerned. Physicians and life insurance companies now feel that, for the sake of health and longevity, it is best to weigh no more in the years after age 25 or 30 than is normal for height and body build at that age. Table 24–1 gives desirable weights that men and women should maintain at 25 years of age and in later life. An individual who weighs more than 10 percent above the theoretical normal for his height is classed as *overweight*, while one who is 20 percent or more overweight is *obese*.

Obesity in children is common and presents special problems. It handicaps a child socially and in games or sports that involve moving mass in running or jumping. If overweight is not corrected and the

Table 24-1 SUGGESTED WEIGHTS FOR HEIGHTS*

Height		*Median Weight*			
		Men		*Women*	
IN	CM	LB	KG	LB	KG
60	152			109 ± 9	49.5 ± 4
62	158			115 ± 9	52.2 ± 4
64	163	133 ± 11	60.5 ± 5	122 ± 10	55.5 ± 5
66	168	142 ± 11	64.5 ± 5	129 ± 10	58.6 ± 5
68	173	151 ± 14	68.6 ± 6	136 ± 10	61.8 ± 5
70	178	159 ± 14	72.3 ± 6	144 ± 11	65.5 ± 5
72	183	167 ± 15	75.9 ± 7	152 ± 12	69.0 ± 5
74	188	175 ± 15	79.5 ± 7		
76	193	182 ± 16	82.7 ± 7		

*From Food and Nutrition Board: *Recommended Dietary Allowances.* 8th Ed. Washington, D.C., National Academy of Sciences, 1974. Modified from Table 80, Hathaway and Ford, 1960, "Heights and Weights of Adults in the U.S.," *Home Economics Research Report No. 10,* ARS, USDA. Weights were based on those of college men and women. Measurements were made without shoes or other clothing. ± refers to the weight range between the 25th and 75th percentile of each height category.

child trained to practice dietary and physical activity patterns that will keep weight down to normal for his height, he will very likely go on to become an obese adult. A weight-control regimen for a child must be carefully planned to decrease energy to intake while liberally furnishing all nutrients needed for growth — proteins, minerals, and vitamins. Dietary restriction cannot be as drastic or weight readjustment as rapid for children as for adults.

Measurement and Form of Body Fat

Weight tables provide a convenient guide to desirable body weight, but what we are really concerned with is the amount of fat in the body. A football player may be distinctly overweight for height, yet he may be not in the least obese in terms of having excess adipose tissue. Others who are underweight for height may have a larger percentage of adipose tissue than heavier people who are more physically fit. The goal of any reducing program is not to normalize body weight arbitrarily but to reduce to normal the amount of stored fat in the body.

Body fat is stored mainly in the specialized cells of *adipose tissue.* When filled with fat, adipose tissue has about 85 to 90 percent fat, 2 percent protein, and 10 percent water. This fat is formed in the cells from precursors brought in the blood, and fatty acids are released from the cells when there is a demand for energy. Excess fat may be stored in adipose tissue cells that are not yet filled, or new cells will be made if necessary. Insulin is required to store fat, and adrenal and pituitary hormones are involved in mobilizing it in reponse to need. The energy value of adipose tissue is about 8 kcal per gram or 3600 kcal per pound (33.5 MJ per kg.)

A number of ways to measure body fatness have been developed. Many of these are complex, involving use of radioisotopes or elaborate equipment, but others are relatively simple and ingenious. Fat has a lower specific gravity than water; hence, excess tissue fat tends to buoy up the body when immersed in water. This principle has been used to determine the ratio of lean to fatty tissues in the body. The body weight, taken when immersed in water and divided by the weight of the water displaced, is a true index of the relative amount of body fat. Obviously, a low specific gravity of the body indicates a relatively large proportion of body fat, and vice versa.

Estimates of the amount of subcutaneous fat in various parts of the body may also be made from the thickness of folds of skin and fat pinched up in several places (the upper back, abdomen, chest, arms, or legs), as measured accurately by calipers[3] (Fig. 24–3). By mathematical equations, body fat may be estimated from skinfold measurements. Skin measurement can also be used to diagnose obesity (and undernutrition) by using an arbitrary cut-off point for thickness. For example, a 19-year-old male may be classed as obese if a value greater than 100 is obtained when triceps fatfold (mm) is divided by body weight (lbs) and multiplied by 1000.[4] The "educated pinch" has even been suggested for the ordinary layman as a general guide in judging overweight (obesity). If such a skinfold proves to be over an inch (25 mm) in thickness, weight reduction is indicated.

Body fatness may also be calculated from "envelope measurements" of the body (torso, legs, and arms, especially circumference of thigh and buttocks). Young and Blondin[5] found that constants derived from such measurements on individual young women formed a fairly accurate basis for estimating body weight and relative fatness.

Probably the simplest method devised for rating accurately the degree of obesity is the Body Mass Index.[6] This index is easily computed by dividing the body weight by the square of height (W/H^2) (Fig. 24–4).

Causes of Obesity

The chief causes of obesity are overeating and inactivity, usually in combination. People seem not to recognize that they are overeating, yet it is an easy thing to do, especially as one grows older and less inclined to physical exertion. Most Americans exercise little. We tend toward spectator sports, riding in cars, and sitting while we work. Also, we tend to adjust the temperature of our homes and places of work and entertainment and to dress in a way that minimizes the amount of energy used in body temperature regulation. If appetite and former food habits encourage one to take more food than needed, fat accumulates. Only a relatively small excess of food daily may in time add con-

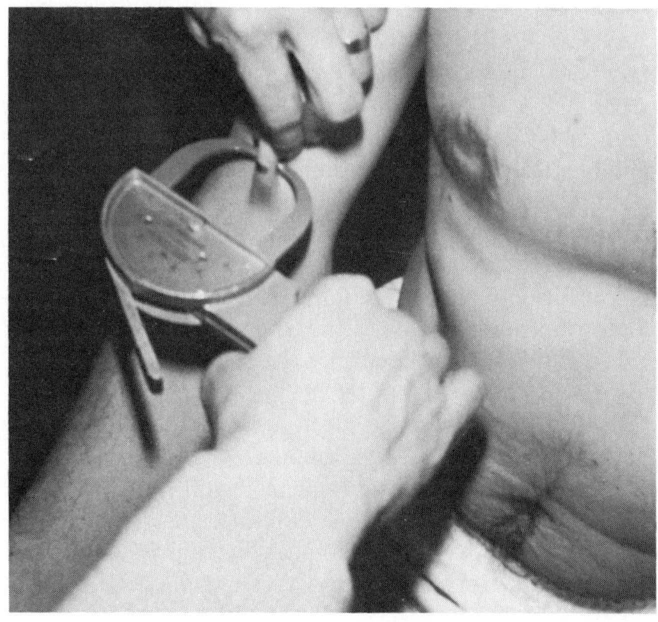

Figure 24–3 Measurement of skinfold thickness. The amount of fat in the body can be estimated reliably from precise measurements of the thickness of the layer of fatty tissue beneath the skin. (Courtesy of Department of Nutritional Sciences, University of California, Berkeley.)

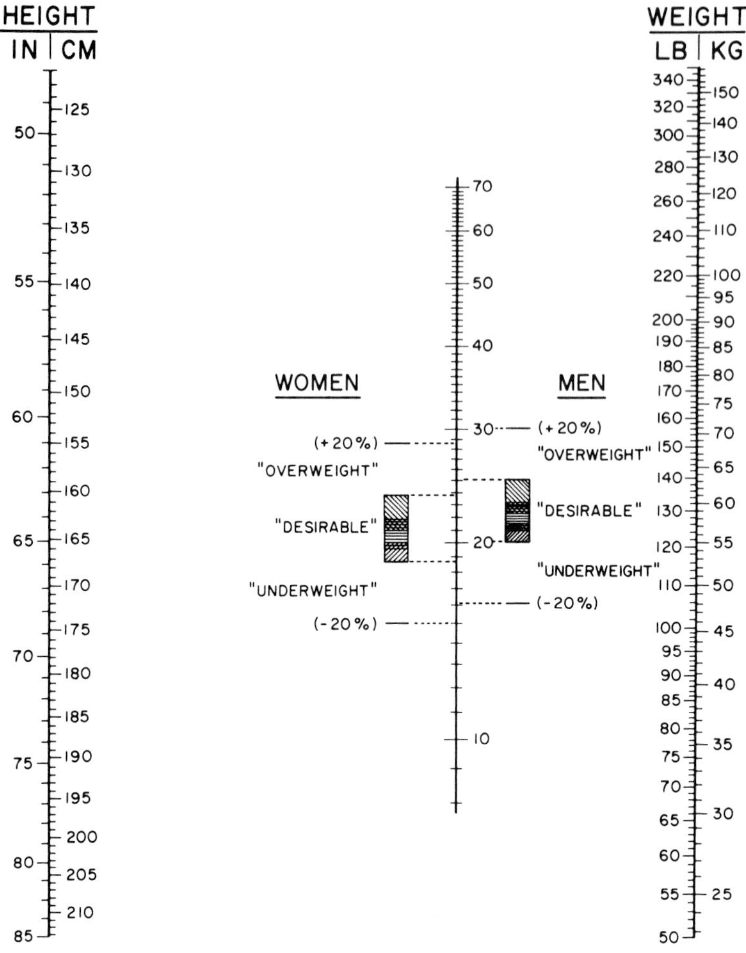

Figure 24–4 Nomograph for body mass index (kg/m²). The ratio weight/height² is read from the central scale. The ranges suggested as "desirable" are from life insurance data. (From Thomas, A. E., McKay, D. A., and Cutlip, M. B.: Amer. J. Clin. Nutr., *29*:302, 304, 1976.)

siderable weight. Excessive portions of food or fat and sugar added to foods may give a *surplus* of energy intake over output that will cause several pounds to be added in a few months, or 20 to 30 pounds extra weight in a few years. For instance, the addition of one martini or 1 ounce of milk chocolate a day adds the energy equivalent of 1 pound of adipose tissue in 3 weeks.

Studies of obese children and adults have revealed that most of them ate about as much as individuals of normal weight but that they were much less active physically. Thus, they were overeating only in terms of their needs. Inactivity is not accompanied by a commensurate decrease in appetite at very low levels of work output in animals or people (Fig. 24–5). Rats become obese if confined to small cages where their movement is restricted, and the standard way for a farmer to finish a steer or fatten a goose for pâté de foie gras is to limit exercise by penning and to provide plenty of food. These same animals — rats, cattle, and fowl — adjust intake to output better when they are free to range and must forage for food. Control of activity alone, e.g., by forcing a rat to run in an activity wheel, allows the animal to remain lean while eating to satisfy its appetite from freely available food. This indicates that of the two factors — food and exercise — exercise is probably the more important. Again, the difference need not be large: just 30 minutes of walking each day can take off 1 pound of adipose tissue in 3 weeks.

People often fail to perceive underactivity and overconsumption as the cause of their weight gain. Instead, they offer such comments as "It is in the family to be stout," or "Something must be the matter with my glands," or "No matter how little I eat, I don't lose weight." In most cases, a family tendency to stoutness has no more mysterious cause than inactivity, combined with a preference for sweets and fatty foods. The dominance of the environmental factors over heredity is demonstrated by Garn's[7] analysis of data from the extensive studies of the population of Tecumseh, Michigan. Garn and his colleagues found essentially the same correlation between skinfold thickness of related and unrelated persons living together (biological and adoptive siblings, husbands and wives, parents and biological and adoptive children). On genetic grounds, the correspondence between dizygotic twins and between twins and siblings should be the same; but the correlation between the twins was much higher (0.7 vs. 0.3), suggesting that the more closely shared environment of the twins altered the expected relationship. Garn concludes that "given fatness similarities between pet-owners and their pets or the far greater fatness similarities between dizygotic twins as compared with siblings, we need not search long for putative control mechanisms of cellular, endocrine, or neurohumoral origin."

On the other hand, it is not unreasonable to acknowledge that some people may have an inherited tendency to put on weight more readily than most people do, just as some strains of animals have slimmer or fatter body conformation (lard hogs versus bacon hogs). Inbreeding has

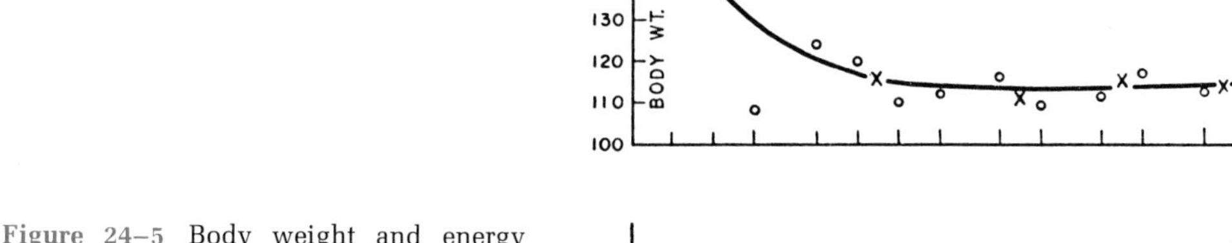

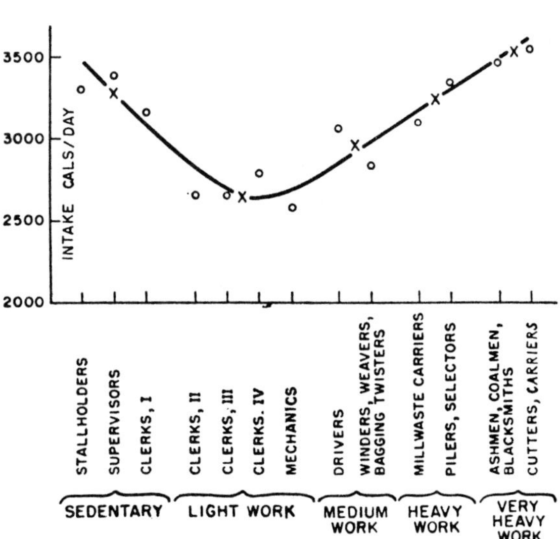

Figure 24–5 Body weight and energy intake as a function of physical activity. (Courtesy of Mayer and Bullen; reprinted from Physiological Reviews.)

produced genetically obese rats and mice, and these have provided many useful clues in research concerning obesity. Before the development of agricultural technology, a tendency to store fat might have had survival value, protecting the individual against starvation during the "hungry" season; and the trait might have persisted. Modern man limits the development of such a genetic characteristic by his taboos on familial marriages.

In some cases, obesity is conditioned by inactivity of some one or more of the endocrine glands (thyroid, pituitary, or sex glands), but these causes are distinctly in the minority. Studies on groups of obese people show that, in most cases, their basal metabolism is about the same per unit of surface area as that of individuals of normal weight.

Psychologists have concluded that some persons overeat to compensate for emotional insecurity or frustration. Such people need to have the cause of their craving for food resolved and to be made aware of the nature and disadvantages of their behavior. People must recognize the advantages to be gained from changing food habits before they are willing to do so, and they must learn to control those aspects of their own behavior that lead to an imbalance between intake and output.

Research on Obesity

The primary causes of obesity in humans are, as we have noted, too much food, too little exercise, or both. These causes really stem from one fundamental cause, an error in regulating the amount of energy eaten in proportion to need. This type of obesity is called *regulatory obesity*. Physiological control of hunger and appetite was considered in Chapter 13. Interesting studies by psychologists have shed new light on this complex problem, and indicate that for some as yet unexplained reason obese people fail to respond to the internal cues that tell a body when food is needed and when it has had enough. What they do respond to is external stimuli, the presence or sight of food. One study showed that overweight college students would eat more of three sandwiches put before them in a test situation than would students who were thin or of normal weight. However, if the subjects had to go to a refrigerator to obtain the sandwiches, the overweight ones ate less than did those of normal weight.[8] This suggests that the overweight students did not recognize biologically how hungry they were or even if they were hungry at all. The obese also approach the process of eating differently; they eat faster and take fewer bites than do persons of normal weight.[9] Palatability is another factor. VanItallie and Hashim made freely available a bland and not distasteful formula diet to adults of normal weight and to overweight ones; the normals soon learned to take enough to maintain their body weight constant, but the overweight ones did not meet their needs and lost weight.[10]

Mayer and his colleagues[2] have described other types of obesity broadly categorized as *metabolic obesity*, in which the rate of fat synthesis is greater than normal or the rate of mobilization of fat from adipose tissue is depressed. One of these is seen in genetically obese-hyperglycemic mice, so called because they are fat and have elevated levels of sugar in the blood. The adipose tissue of these mice differs from normal in having high coenzyme A activity and an increased rate of fat synthesis from acetate precursors (refer to Chapter 15); diminished responsiveness to hormonal triggering of fat release; and an excess amount of a fat-forming enzyme. Mice that have this genetic make-up can be reduced in body weight by food restriction, but they continue to have a higher percentage of body fat than do normal mice of the same body weight.

Yet another theory of obesity may have important implications for the problem that obese people have in staying lean once they have reduced and for the need for a preventive approach to obesity. Studies of adipose tissue of normal, fat, and formerly fat people show that the tissue of the obese has more cells than normal.[11] It is thought that these cells, when lacking in fat, send chemical messages that elicit eating behavior. Thus, if fewer cells were formed — that is, if children were not allowed to become fat by overeating in infancy and the early years of childhood — there would not be a reservoir of demanding adipose cells. (See Chapter 21.)

There is even a possibility that obesity may relate to prenatal food availability.[12] A study of 19-year-old men born during the Dutch famine of World War I shows that obesity rates depend upon the time of exposure to food deprivation. Deprivation during the last trimester of pregnancy and the first few months of life is associated with a low incidence of obesity, indicating that this may be a critical period for development of adipose cells. Obesity rates are higher for those whose deprivation occurred during the first half of pregnancy, the period of hypothalamic differentiation. The degree or duration of deprivation in utero is not known, nor is the later dietary history of these men; nevertheless, the results of this study warrant further study in animals.

Other lines of research raise questions about whether it is possible to express the energy required for weight maintenance with the degree of mathematical accuracy formerly assumed. It may be that the total amount of energy needed depends to some extent on the relative proportions of the three classes of energy nutrients provided in the diet and to some degree on adaptive body mechanisms. Miller and Payne, working with animals, found that the energy intakes required to keep body weight constant varied with individuals over a wide range, which led them to explore the problem in greater depth.[13] Particularly spectacular was an experiment with two pigs, one of which required almost five times the amount of energy for weight maintenance as did the other. This could not be accounted for by differences in digestibility, loss in urine, storage of fat, or physical activity. The pig that required the high energy intake for weight maintenance had a diet containing only half as much protein as did the other. After 40 days, the diets were reversed, and the pig that formerly required high energy adjusted to maintain weight at the lower intake level, and vice versa, showing that the difference was due to the diet rather than to individual differences in the pigs.

Miller and Mumford have reported similar experience in human subjects fed 1400 kcal per day in excess of needs, from diets containing either 2.8 or 15 percent of protein calories.[14] The excess energy consumed was enough to add 5 kg of body weight in theory; the observed mean weight gain of the low-protein group was 1.1 kg and that of the normal diet group was 3.7 kg. The excess caloric intake was disposed of by a sharp increase in heat production associated with work. In effect, energy was wasted as heat. The converse situation exists in genetically obese rats and probably contributes to their obesity. That is, the fat rat has increased efficiency of energy utilization before it becomes obese.[15]

The frequency of eating also affects nutrient utilization in experimental animals,[16] and similar conclusions have been drawn from observations of weight changes in man.[17] Administration of large meals at infrequent intervals is associated with decreased energy need for weight maintenance, increased deposition of body fat, and decreased deposition of body protein, as compared with a "nibbling" pattern of food intake (frequent, small meals). It is known that the body adapts to long-term (days) food deprivation in such a way that a second period of fasting causes less loss of weight and acidosis than does the first fasting experience. It may be that the altered nutrient utilization of animals fed the large meals infrequently represents comparable adaptation to short-term food deprivation (hours).

In conclusion, modern research suggests that obesity may not be a single entity but, rather, one symptom that has many causes. Knowledge of these causes may one day yield effective methods of therapy. Whatever the contributing causes, the final one is always the same: the food intake of that individual is greater than his need. Prevention shows more promise than therapy in dealing with the problem.

Disorders Related to Obesity

Several of the diseases common in adults are associated with obesity, as noted earlier, and these diseases are related to one another. A particular kind of circulatory disorder, atherosclerosis, is common in diabetics; people with atherosclerotic heart disease often have high blood pressure (hypertension); and in both cases they are likely to be obese. However, not all people who have these disorders are obese, and not all people who are obese will inevitably develop these diseases.

Atherosclerosis and Heart Disease. Atherosclerosis is a kind of hardening of the arteries, a degenerative condition in which cholesterol and large lipoproteins are deposited on the interior wall of arteries. When this occurs, the space in the blood vessel is narrowed. A blood clot (thrombus) may form in the narrowed vessel, closing off the supply of blood with its oxygen and nutrients to the organ or tissue served by the blood vessel. If a clot is formed in one of the small arteries that nourish the heart muscle (a coronary vessel), a portion of the muscle will die. If the damage is extensive, the heart may be unable to function and the patient dies. If the damage is small or if the person has a well-developed circulatory system due to regular hard exercise, the heart may be able to continue to pump blood and the muscle will heal. The risk of coronary thrombosis becomes great at about middle age in men and after menopause in women and is increased in persons who have the following characteristics: high levels of blood cholesterol or neutral fat (triglycerides) or both, high blood pressure, family history of heart disease, obesity, sedentary occupation, and cigarette smoking.

Surveys on the fat content of the diet, the blood cholesterol levels, and the incidence of coronary heart disease among peoples in various parts of the world have indicated that levels of blood cholesterol tend to be higher and heart disease more common in the more prosperous nations, where more fats, especially more animal fats, are eaten. (See Chapter 4.) However, because two facts occur coincidentally is not proof that one is the *cause* of the other, and *many factors other than dietary fat and cholesterol* are known to be associated with heart disease. Considerable variation is observed in the blood cholesterol level among normal individuals, irrespective of their diet. There is a familial tendency toward higher levels of cholesterol, and blood cholesterol may also show sudden variations due to emotional or environmental factors. For example, a man may have high blood cholesterol when under tension on his job and 2 weeks later, when relaxed on vacation, have a normal level of this substance in the blood, with no significant change in diet.

Factors such as lack of exercise, overeating, and stress and strain of life decidedly affect the incidence of high blood pressure and heart disease. This was strikingly shown in a joint study by investigators at Harvard University and at Trinity College, Dublin. They collected data on Irish-born men who had emigrated to the Boston area and their brothers who had remained in Ireland, chiefly engaged in agriculture. Although the diet of those in Ireland was higher in total energy, starchy foods, and animal fats (almost twice as much butter), the incidence of heart disease was considerably higher among the urbanized, sedentary American residents than among their paired brothers, who had been living a more active life. Several other studies involving comparisons of occupational groups within a country emphasize the importance of physical activity and energy balance: San Francisco longshoremen have a lower incidence of heart disease than do warehouse workers, London bus conductors than drivers, and British postmen than bank clerks.

Considering the epidemiological evidence and the frequency of the various types of blood lipid disorders, the medical consensus is that people would do well to prevent or correct obesity, take more exercise, and reduce their total fat intake while substituting *moderate* amounts of vegetable fats with high P/S ratios for meat and milk fats.[18] It is equally wise, on nutritional grounds as well as health ones, to reduce the amount of sucrose and increase the amount of starchy and fiber-rich foods in the diet. This does not mean that diets should be so distorted that they constitute a bar to the needed intake of animal foods nor that all gustatory pleasure should be denied — only that moderation should be practiced in the use of animal fats, sweets, and, of course, alcohol.

Hypertension. High blood pressure is thought to have several causes, mainly renal and endocrine in origin. Some hypertensive patients are thin, but the incidence is markedly increased in persons who are obese, for reasons that are obscure. The trait is familial, and environmental factors probably play a role in permitting the potential tendency to become manifest. Epidemiological evidence linking salt and high blood pressure was discussed in Chapter 10, but sodium is only one of a number of possible contributing factors, as has been noted.

Diabetes. When the word "diabetes" is used alone, it refers to a metabolic disease involving inadequate insulin function. The proper name is diabetes mellitus, a combination of the Greek word for "siphon" and the Latin word for "honey," referring to the fact that a dominant symptom of diabetes is excretion of large amounts of urine containing sugar. (See Chapter 15.) The severe disorder, as it occurs in young people, is quite different from the condition that develops at or past middle age, most commonly in obese people.

The reason obesity causes or accompanies maturity-onset diabetes in genetically predisposed individuals is uncertain. It is known that the disorder is less likely to occur in people who remain lean, and the mild form may be controlled simply by reducing weight to normal and increasing the amount of physical exercise. There is no clear evidence that dietary carbohydrate in general or sucrose in particular are causally related to diabetes, although this has been suggested. Normalization of body weight and restriction of sugar in the diet are important aspects of dietary treatment. A possible association of various mineral deficiencies and diabetes exists, because of the role of certain minerals (zinc and chromium) in the formation and utilization of insulin, but there is as yet no evidence that lack of these is a factor in the disease as it commonly occurs.

UNDERWEIGHT

Malnutrition Versus Underweight

The terms *malnutrition* and *underweight* are not synonymous, though the two conditions often occur together. Underweight results from an intake of energy insufficient to meet the body's needs, just as overweight results from a surplus energy intake. Malnutrition is a broader term: It means, literally, *bad* (from *mal*) *nutrition,* whether due to deficiency or excess of one or more nutrients in relation to the tissue needs. The obese person is badly overnourished with respect to energy foods; the emaciated person is underweight owing to supplies of food energy insufficient to meet body needs. Either may also be malnourished relative to other nutrients.

Overweight malnourished persons, either children or adults, usually have enough subcutaneous fat so that they may look well nourished to the superficial observer. This combination of fatness and poor vitamin-mineral status may be found among the poor, whose low income forces them to fill up on the cheaper high-energy foods (white flour, sugar, and lard) and does not allow them to buy enough of the body-building foods (meat, milk, fruits, and vegetables). Such malnourished individuals are also found among the well-to-do who simply prefer to eat the wrong types of food. Their color is usually poor, their flesh flabby, and their bones and teeth of poor quality. They are often anemic and listless, tire quickly, and when seriously ill, are more apt to succumb than persons who have better nourished tissues and greater vitality.

Undernutrition may result from many different causes. Generally, inadequate food intake is the main reason, but there may be a number of contributing factors. Digestion and absorption may be poor. The life-style or environment may cause an individual to have a poor appetite or an aversion to particular foods, or may make him refuse to take food at all. There may be physical injury or organic disease or infection, which affects nutrient utilization loss, or requirements, or any combination of these. In short, anything that interferes with the intake of some essential material, makes the total amount of intake low, or hinders the normal processes by which food it utilized in the body tends to bring about a condition of undernourishment, which will be more or less severe depending on the extent and duration of the conditions.

Underweight and Health Status

Simply being underweight, *without lack of minerals and vitamins,* may or may not be serious, depending on the degree of underweight and the age at which it occurs. The average weights (found in tables) are not necessarily the normal or the best for every individual. There are times when it is advantageous to be somewhat under the average weight for height. This is true of middle-aged or older persons, especially if they have any tendencies to diabetes, high blood pressure, or heart or kidney ailments. Life insurance statistics show that for older adults a slight degree of underweight increases health and life expectancy. This does not mean underweight to the point of emaciation. Some older people, especially those of small means, live on such abstemious diets that serious malnutrition results. However, it is with *children,* and *young adults* that severe underweight is almost sure to be a disadvantage. In general, we may say that to be more than 10 percent below the average weight for one's height and type of body build* usually means lowered vigor.

Normally the body profits from having some stores of fatty tissue, as well as reserves of the other nutrients to draw on in times of extra stress. The fatty tissues serve not only as reserve energy but also as padding about the internal tissues, and organs. The very thin person tends to chill easily, owing to lack of a normal layer of subcutaneous fat and lowered basal metabolism. Such persons are more susceptible to infections, and they are disinclined to any physical exertion, for their bodies are conserving energy. This is what we call living on a lower plane of nutrition.

Chronic Energy Shortage and Starvation

The disadvantages of living on a low level of energy intake were evident in experiments on otherwise healthy people. Benedict studied the effect of sharply re-

*The average weight and height of boys and girls at given ages are found in the Appendix. Adult weights are given on page 560 (and Tables 7 and 8 of the Appendix).

duced energy intake on healthy young men in the early 1900's, and this type of study was repeated during World War II on a group of conscientious objectors at the University of Minnesota by Keys and associates. In both cases, the young men, who had previously taken well over 3000 kcal daily, submitted to a drastic reduction of energy intake until they had lost body weight on an average of 12 percent in the earlier set of experiments and 24 percent in the later ones. Their weight was then kept stable on a somewhat higher but still restricted energy level (1950 kcal in Benedict's group, 1550 kcal in Keys' experiments). At this lower nutritional level, the men reported that they felt well but had less energy and had to drive themselves to do their accustomed tasks, and they tired sooner in various gymnasium tests. Keys' subjects subsisted on the low level of intake for 6 months and developed some more serious symptoms — depression, anemia, edema, slowing of heartbeat, and others. They showed marked lack of endurance, tired easily, and reduced unnecessary movements to a minimum. Both groups reported lowered libido, and the sperm quality was poor in Keys' subjects. When returned to their former level of energy consumption, they recovered their vitality, but it took considerable time to restore them to buoyant health.[19]

Severe undernutrition in previously well-nourished people comes about when there is famine due to crop failure or war, or it may result from serious diseases of the gastrointestinal tract that impair digestion or absorption of food. In some cases it is due to a psychiatric disorder (*anorexia nervosa*). Loss of about 25 percent of body weight is without serious permanent damage in healthy adults of normal weight, but recovery from losses on the order of 50 percent is difficult or impossible. In Europe, during and after the long period of underfeeding in World War II, there was an increase of stillbirths and of babies who died soon after birth (Chapter 20). Wastage of muscle, edema due to lack of plasma protein, and lessened digestive capacity were seen in the severe cases. Tuberculosis and other infectious diseases flared up among both young mothers and children during the postwar years. Even today, among the poor in the teeming populations of Asia, the Middle East, Africa, and South America, there are millions who exist on a very low nutritional level, and we see the results in general misery and disease. (See Chapter 25.)

Undernutrition and Infection

Well-nourished people do not escape infection just because they are well-nourished; good nutrition does not confer any sort of immunity. It is true, though, that nutrition must be satisfactory to maintain the skin and internal membranes that are the first barrier to invading organisms, and that secondary infections do follow deficiency of vitamin A, for example (Chaper 7). In addition, specific nutrients are needed for formation of the antibodies that are the body's internal protection, and suppression of the immune system has been reported in malnourished children and adults, both in those from poor communities where disease is rampant and in hospitalized patients whose disease process has led to malnutrition.*

When the infection is established, nutritional status consistently affects the outcome. Persons who are well nourished are more likely to survive an infection than are those who are weakened because their reserves are too low to support them during a prolonged illness. In the tropics, seemingly healthy individuals often have malaria parasites in the blood or a large population of worms in the intestine. The people are able to cope with these para-

*Exceptions to this generalization occur in the case of some viruses, including the leukemia virus. It has been found that animals deficient in some specific nutrients are more, not less, resistant to invasion. See Chapter 8.

sites, almost to live symbiotically, as long as diets are adequate. But when nutritional status falls, the disease overwhelms them.

Infection also conditions nutritional deficiency. Little children whose diets are barely adequate develop obvious cases of marasmus or kwashiorkor as a result of contracting some ordinary chidhood disease such as measles, whooping cough, or a nonspecific diarrhea. Their reserves are so low that they cannot tolerate the least additional loss from the intestine, the accelerated metabolism of a mild fever, or a few days of nausea or poor intake. The child may die of malnutrition consequent to an infection.

Treatment of Underweight

In order to be effective, treatment must follow two courses:

1. Location and removal of the contributory causes
2. Improvement of the diet.

Under the first heading comes a thorough study of the person's *daily program* to discover whatever faulty food and health habits there may be, and a general *medical examination* to see if there are any physical defects that need to be corrected. These unfavorable factors, which predispose to poor nutrition, must then be remedied. Often, considerable persistence may be needed to determine *all* the causes. *Overfatigue* is one of the most common causes and is easily corrected by longer hours of sleep, rest periods during the day, and reducing the activities that cause fatigue. Poverty is an important contributory factor, especially among the working poor who have hard physical work to perform and often many mouths to feed from a limited supply of food. Mothers of small children are often overtired, and they do not eat if their children are hungry. Persons with more severe undernutrition often require continued observation and study by a physician so that the factors responsible for keeping the person below par physically may be located and treated.

Providing a suitable diet is perhaps the most important single measure for correcting undernutrition — certainly an adequate food supply is indispensable. The corrective diet may be started at once — that is, while one is in the process of locating and clearing up the unfavorable contributory factors. Supplements may be prescribed if specific deficiencies of vitamins and minerals exist.

The body may not be able to take *full* advantage of the diet until all adverse factors are remedied, and the diet given in the meantime should be suited to the physical condition of the individual. Administration of large amounts of food to starved or semistarved persons can have disastrous consequences. The refeeding of concentration camp victims showed that small, frequent feeding of soft, nutritious foods is essential if vomiting, intestinal disturbances, and shock are to be avoided. The weakened organism cannot handle a large metabolic load. The same is true for severely undernourished children.

A body that has been depleted by prolonged underfeeding requires gradually increased feeding and building up in numerous respects. Not only should new deposits of *fat* be laid down, but also the muscles are in need of *protein* for repair and enlargement. Reserve stores of *vitamins* and *minerals* are used up or lost from the body during semistarvation, and an excess of nutrients in the diet is a help in the processes necessary for repair after undernutrition. The diet should be designed to promote gain of any needed lean tissue and a desirable amount of fat according to satisfactory health and aesthetic standards. As soon as the physical condition permits, a controlled exercise program should be instituted to increase anabolism and improve the sense of well-being.

PLANNING THE REDUCING REGIMEN

Total fasting* has been used as a therapeutic measure for grossly obese patients, but it is not to be recommended. Even with large energy reserves available in the body, total lack of food has serious risks. There is loss of potassium and marked loss of sodium with depletion of extracellular fluids and the kidneys do not adequately remove the nitrogenous end-product, uric acid. Some patients have developed gout, and a few have died of heart and liver failure in the course of such treatment.

For the ordinary overweight individual, by far the most satisfactory way to effect weight reduction is simply to cut down sharply on the concentrated energy foods (fats, alcohol, sugars, and starches), while maintaining an otherwise well-balanced and adequate diet. Such a diet does not involve actually going hungry. It can be used over fairly long periods without harm, and it can be continued into the postreducing period (by adding limited amounts of the foods of higher energy value) in order to hold the lower weight one has attained by reducing. It should be, so far as possible, a diet one likes and is willing to use indefinitely, and it should be *inadequate* for body needs *in only one respect* – its *energy* content.

The main things to plan for in any reducing diet are:

1. *Low energy content*
2. At least adequate protein
3. At least fairly low carbohydrate and fat
4. Plenty of minerals and vitamins
5. Good satiety value

Low Energy Intake. Obviously, to accomplish its purpose, a reducing diet must have relatively *low energy content.* The rate at which stored fat is lost will depend on the magnitude of the difference between energy intake and expenditure. For best results it is desirable to increase energy need by increasing physical activity at the same time as intake is lowered. If the diet furnishes 500 to 1000 kcal (2000 to 4000 kJ) less than needed, this should effect a weight loss of about 3 to 6 lb (1.5 to 3 kg) a month. The same rate of weight loss could be brought about by swimming a whole hour every day, without altering food intake. A combination of low-energy diet plus activity accelerates weight reduction, promotes fitness, and prevents tissues from becoming flabby as fat is lost. Contrary to popular belief, increased activity on the part of sedentary persons does not lead to a counterbalancing increase in food intake.[20]

More drastic reduction of energy intake, of course, causes a more rapid loss of weight, but diets below 1000 kcal (4000 kJ) are not recommended because they too severely limit the sources of essential nutrients in the diet. Diets above the 1600 kcal (6400 kJ) level give such slow results in weight loss that they are discouraging to the average adult woman, although men may show good weight loss at that level of intake.

Not only must the choice of foods be right (avoidance of concentrated energy foods), but the size of portions must be limited if intake is to be kept down. For instance, take the case of a woman dieting zealously but fitfully who announced she was having a low-energy breakfast of fruit. She consumed a very large glass of orange juice (10 oz), two large pears, and a bunch of grapes, which meant an intake of at least 500 kcal. One slice of toast with a *small* portion of butter, one egg, and a small glass of juice (4 oz) would have meant only half as much energy. Thus, even foods described as moderately low in energy can raise the intake considerably when taken in large portions. All foods furnish *some* energy, even vinegar,

*Fasting means abstention but usually not total food deprivation. Most often the religious injunction is to abstain from meals before a specified time of day or to omit one component (e.g., meat). During his fasts, Gandhi took fruit juices and sometimes dried fruits, a sensible procedure because some carbohydrate offsets the more serious effects of fasting.

lemon juice, bouillon, tea, and coffee, but in the foods just named the amount is so small as to be ignored in planning the diet.

All between-meal snacks or extras (such as cream, sugar, and salad dressings) taken in or on foods must be counted. This includes cocktails or other alcoholic beverages, because both alcohol and sugar in such drinks furnish energy. A table of approximate caloric content of alcoholic beverages is given in Chapter 3.

Adequate Protein. It is important that the reducing diet provide enough ***protein*** for the maintenance and upkeep of body tissues and that the mixture of proteins taken should provide all essential amino acids. Adults following a slimming diet should have 1 gm of protein per kilogram of body weight, and not less than 50 gm daily for the diet to be adequate. Children need a more liberal protein allowance. Naturally, if one cuts down on the foods that are high in carbohydrates and fats, a greater proportion of the calories tend to be taken as protein. A luxury diet with meat at every meal of the day is unnecessary, but a reducing diet may well include one liberal serving of meat per day, with either a *small* second serving of meat or one of eggs, fish, or poultry. This, together with milk and cheese, provides liberal protein.

Low Carbohydrate and Fat. The exact distribution of calories among protein, carbohydrate, and fat is not critical, except that protein must be adequate and a *certain amount of carbohydrate is desirable.* Diets high in protein or fat, or low in carbohydrate, have been suggested as particularly successful in causing weight reduction, but there is no agreement among experts that any of these has special efficacy in the long run. As a practical matter, fats are usually sharply limited. They are such concentrated sources of energy (2¼ times as much energy per gram as the other two foodstuffs) that only a small quantity can be included without raising the energy intake too high.

On a diet inadequate in energy to meet body needs, the body is constantly burning some of its stored fat. Under these conditions, fats may not be completely oxidized, and the acid intermediate products of their metabolism (keto acids) may accumulate in the body and cause an acidosis, or ketosis. Bloom and Azar found that healthy humans, when fed a diet exclusively of protein and fat, lost 2 pounds daily, but that there were large losses of nitrogen and salt in the urine and the subjects experienced symptoms due to acidosis (ketosis).[21] These symptoms disappeared promptly when carbohydrate was included in the diet.

Others[22] seem to have better success with a high protein-low carbohydrate diet. Weight loss may be more rapid at first on a low carbohydrate diet, but it makes little difference in the end whether reduction of energy intake is brought about by restriction of carbohydrate or fat, in long-term reduction programs.

If small amounts of carbohydrate are included in the reducing diet, acidosis is prevented. An intake of 70 to 100 gm of carbohydrate will suffice. Practically all the energy value of fruits and vegetables and over half that of skim milk comes from the carbohydrates they contain, so that not very much of the more concentrated carbohydrate foods (bread, cereals, and sweets) is needed.

Foods that are high in dietary fiber content are lower in energy yield than the more completely absorbed foods, and they are beneficial in maintaining bowel regularity. Unrefined cereals, legumes, potatoes, and other vegetables provide an excellent variety of nutrients, and the carbohydrate allowance should be derived mainly from these sources.

Minerals and Vitamins. A person on a reducing diet should get his recommended allowance of the various needed *minerals and vitamins* to keep the body in condition while weight loss is going on. This means that any reducing diet should provide liberally for milk, meat, fruits (including citrus or tomatoes), and vegetables. The reduced amounts of bread and

Table 24–2 FOODS FROM WHICH THE REDUCING DIET SHOULD BE BUILT

Foods to Emphasize	*Foods to Avoid*
Clear soups	Alcoholic beverages
Tea and coffee (without sugar or cream)	Soft drinks with added sugar
Milk (especially skim milk or buttermilk)	Fried foods
Fresh fruits and canned or stewed fruits without sugar	Fatty meats
Watery and fibrous vegetables (especially leafy, green, and yellow vegetables)	Rich dressings, sauces, and gravy
Lean meats, fish, and cottage cheese	Rich desserts and pastries
Plain yogurt	Nuts and dried fruits
Small servings of low-energy desserts: e.g., gelatin or fruit	Sugar and sweets
	Cream, fats, and oils

cereals taken should be whole-grain. Skim milk may be substituted for whole milk (it has only about half the energy value). It will furnish the needed calcium and B vitamins but no fat-soluble vitamins. Vitamin A may come from eggs, liver, and the provitamins in green, leafy, and yellow vegetables. These same foods, plus meats, may also serve to meet the need for iron. Many persons who have half starved in order to lose weight rapidly, or who have dieted on very one-sided diets, show the bad effects of this mistake in evidences of lack of vitamins or anemia.

Satiety Value. The satiety value of the diet is very important if hunger is to be avoided. If one took nothing but clear soups, beverages, fruits, and vegetables, he would obtain rapid weight loss but feel very unsatisfied. Meat, poultry, fish, cheese, and eggs have a high satiety value and should be distributed throughout the three meals of the day. Fatty foods, which leave the stomach most slowly and hence have the highest satiety value, must be kept down to small amounts, but a little oil in salad dressing, or a small piece of cheese, may occasionally be included. A small portion of fruit or a simple dessert taken at the end of a meal often does much toward making one feel well fed. Imaginative use of herbs and spices enhances appetite appeal. Some persons are less troubled with hunger if they have a snack between meals or at bedtime (such as an apple or orange, a few crackers, or skim milk), but these must of course be counted in the total day's energy allowance.

Lists of foods around which the reducing diet should be built (foods to use) and those that must be avoided if the energy intake is to be kept low enough to cause appreciable weight loss are given in Table 24–2.

Basic Pattern for Reducing Diet and How to Use It

It is entirely satisfactory for anyone to construct his own reducing diet, using whatever foods he has a preference for in amounts limited to keep the energy content of the diet down to a level at which satisfactory weight loss will be obtained.

In practice, it seems to place too much responsibility on the individual and to be too confusing to leave him entirely without guidance in the selection of a reducing diet. Therefore, we believe it advisable to suggest a ***definite type of meal plan*** for those who desire to reduce, leaving considerable latitude for variety and choice of foods in making up individual menus. Table 24–3 presents a **basic pattern** for the reducing diet, with many of the details on how the pattern may be met left open to choice. The acceptance of a diet built around a smaller number of simple foods is of great help in making one contented on a more or less restricted diet. To be always in quest of new food combinations is likely to keep one's mind on food to such an extent that

Table 24–3 BASIC PATTERN FOR REDUCING DIET APPROXIMATELY 1100 TO 1400 KCAL (4600–5500 KJ)

Total allowance for the day:

2 cups of milk. Each cup of skim milk provides about 85 kcal (350 kJ). Whole milk yields 165 kcal (690 kJ) per cup. 1 oz of Cheddar cheese substitutes for 1 c of milk.

5 oz of lean meat, fish, or poultry, broiled, boiled, or roasted but not fried. All visible fat should be trimmed. Each ounce supplies about 60 to 80 kcal (250–340 kJ); 1 oz of meat equals 1 egg: 3 sardines; 5 shrimp, clams, or oysters; ¼ c tuna fish, salmon, crabmeat, or lobster.

2 or more servings of fruit without added sugar. One serving should be citrus or other fruit high in vitamin C. Each portion listed counts as one serving and provides about 40 to 50 kcal (170–200 kJ).

1	Small apple (2 in diameter)	½	Small mango
½	c applesauce	1	Medium nectarine
2	Fresh apricots or 4 halves dried	1	Small orange or scant ½ c juice
½	Small banana	⅓	Papaya
1	c berries (blackberries, raspberries, strawberries)	1	Medium peach
		1	Small pear
⅔	c blueberries	½	c cubed pineapple or ⅓ c juice
¼	Cantaloupe (6 in diameter)		
10	Large cherries	2	Medium plums or prunes
2	Dates	2	Level tbsp raisins
1	Small dried fig	1	Large tangerine
½	Grapefruit or ½ c juice	1	c dried watermelon or one slice 3 in × 1½ in
12	Grapes or ¼ c juice		
¼	Honeydew melon (7 in diameter)	2	Tomatoes or 1 c juice

2 or more servings of vegetables. At least one serving should be dark green, leafy vegetable. An average (½ c) serving yields 10 to 50 kcal (40–200 kJ). Any vegetable may be used, except peas, corn, and dried beans, which must be substituted for bread. No butter, margarine, salad oil, or regular salad dressing may be added except that included in the total allowance for the day. Lemon juice, vinegar, and low-calorie dressings are acceptable.

3 or 4 servings of whole-grain or enriched bread, or ***substitutes.*** One serving, providing 60 to 80 kcal (250–340 kJ), equals: one slice of bread; one muffin or biscuit (2 in diameter); ½ c cooked cereal, rice, macaroni, spaghetti, or noodles; scant ¾ c dry cereal; 5 saltine crackers; 2 graham crackers; scant ½ c peas or cooked dried beans; ½ ear corn; small potato (2 in diameter) or ½ c mashed; 1½ in cube of sponge or angel food cake without icing.

3 or 4 ***small*** servings of fat. One 50 kcal (200 kJ) serving equals: ½ tbsp butter, margarine, vegetable oil, or other clear fat; 1 slice of drained, crisp bacon; 2 level tbsp light cream (sweet or sour); 1 level tbsp cream cheese or French dressing; 5 olives.

Coffee, tea, lemon juice, herbs, bouillon, and other food items of negligible energy content may be used as desired.

one becomes discontented even with a fairly elaborate diet. The use of a basic food pattern in planning reducing diets may be advantageous in three ways:

1. It permits choice.
2. It guides food selection.
3. It teaches desirable food habits.

All sorts of different menu combinations can be made, if desired, either by altering the foods selected from a given food group or varying the size of servings as needed to raise or lower the level of energy intake. Two sample menus for a day, which conform to the basic food pattern, are given in Table 24–4, and these are planned to meet the needs of young adults who must eat at least some meals away from home.

If the basic food pattern can be adapted to fit the energy level required to produce satisfactory weight loss, it will help to guard the intake of all nutrients other than energy, but it need not be followed slavishly. There will be wide variations among individuals in the restriction needed to produce weight loss, according to the body weight and degree of muscular activity. For a 165 lb man who is moderately active, the 1400 kcal (about 5800 kJ) level would represent a severe reduction below estimated energy needed for weight maintenance, while for an elderly sedentary woman 1400 kcal would be nearly all she needed for maintaining weight and she would probably need to curtail intake even below the 1100 kcal (4600 kJ) level.

Varying the Energy Level of the Reducing Diet

The diet may be adjusted to any required energy level by reducing or using more liberal quantities of the foods of high or moderate energy value. After estimating the proper level of energy that will be required for weight loss in their individual cases (see "General Rules for Reducing Regimen" at the end of the chapter), persons may plan a reducing diet at this energy level by consulting the Table of Nutritive Values of Foods in Average Servings in the Appendix. Foods should be selected from the different food groups as recommended in the basic pattern for a reducing diet given in Table 24–3, limiting the size or number of servings to attain the desired level of energy intake. The menus given in Table 24–4 illustrate diets ranging from 1100 to 1400 kcal (4600 to 5800 kJ). Even with such limited intake, the meals can be made attractive and hunger-satisfying. They will also meet body needs for most essential nutrients (except energy). Although the amounts of fat and carbohydrate are limited, each of the day's menus provides adequate protein (65 to 68 gm) and with the other foods used will probably meet the needs for important vitamins and minerals, except iron for women.

These are only two of a wide variety of possible combinations within the food allowances. Higher levels can easily be arranged either by increasing proportions of the same type of foods or by adding other foods not permissible at lower levels of energy intake.

The actual 24 hour intake of a weight-conscious physician is presented in Table 24–5. This diet provided 1520 kcal and conformed to present recommendations

Table 24–4 SAMPLE MENU PATTERNS FROM THE BASIC REDUCING DIET

Pattern I		*Pattern II*
	BREAKFAST	
Orange juice (1/2 c) Poached egg (1) on Whole-wheat toast (1 slice) Coffee, with skim milk (1/2 c)		Branflakes (3/4 c) with Sliced banana (1/2) and Milk (1/2 c)
	LUNCHEON	
Consommé Shrimp Louis (6 shrimp on large bed of mixed greens with 1 tbsp dressing) Small muffin (1) Canteloupe (1/4) Iced tea with lemon		Tuna fish sandwich (1/4 c tuna fish with 2 tsp salad dressing and lettuce on 2 slices whole-wheat bread) Hard-cooked egg Dill pickle, green pepper, celery strips Radish roses Milk (1 c)
	DINNER	
Broiled lamb chop (3 oz) Small baked potato with sour cream (1 tbsp) and chives Buttered (1/2 tsp) green beans Sliced tomatoes Cheese (1 oz) with saltine crackers (5) Coffee, with skim milk (1/2 c)		Frankfurters (2) with Sauerkraut Buttered (1/2 tsp) carrots Strawberries (1 c) with Sponge cake (1 1/2 inch cube) Coffee with evaporated milk (2 tbsp)

Table 24–5 NUTRIENT CONTENT OF A POORLY SELECTED ENERGY-CONTROLLED DIET

Menu	*Nutrient Yield*	
Breakfast:		
Large glass of orange juice	Energy	1520 kcal
Skim milk	Protein	60 gm
Tea	Fat	50 gm
	Cholesterol	80 mg
	Sucrose	50 gm
Luncheon:		
Split pea soup	Vitamin A	6000 IU
Saltine crackers	Vitamin E	6 mg*
Fruit and cottage cheese salad	Vitamin C	170 mg
Beer (one can)	Thiamin	0.9 mg*
	Riboflavin	1.3 mg*
	Niacin	12 mg*
Dinner:	Vitamin B-6	1.2 mg*
Lean beef steak, small serving	Vitamin B-12	3.5 mcg
Mixed vegetables, seasoned	Folacin, free	0.27 mg
Green salad with dressing (3 tbsp)	Pantothenic acid	3.7 mg
Glass of red wine		
	Sodium	2.5 g
Snack:	Calcium	500 mg*
Small apple	Phosphorus	1000 mg
	Magnesium	200 mg*
	Iron	8 mg*
	Copper	1 mg
	Zinc	10 mg*

*Nutrient is below the RDA for an adult male. Copper and pantothenic acid are also substandard and the Ca/P ratio is 0.5.

regarding fat intake. Note, however, that the diet was below the RDA in a number of nutrients. The reason for this is evident: The diet included 200 kcal in the form of alcohol, 190 kcal from sucrose in the sweetened fruits in the luncheon salad, and about 250 kcal from salad dressing. Over one-third of the total daily energy intake was derived from these three sources, which make little contribution to vitamin and mineral intake. Significant improvement could have been made by simple changes such as substitution of whole-grain cereal for half of the orange juice at breakfast, a bran muffin and glass of skim milk for the saltines and beer at lunch, and a potato for half of the salad dressing at dinner.

Some people may prefer to take a lighter breakfast, or lunch, or both, and use the energy thus saved for a more normal meal with the family at noon or at night. Others may be better able to adhere to the slimming diet if the day's food allowance is divided into five smaller meals (or some reserved for snacks). Care must be taken that the total food taken does not exceed the day's allowance. Some regular system of meals should be adopted and adhered to, for only thus does a reducing diet yield the desired results. Although the level of intake does not have to be *absolutely* the same each day, it is desirable that the meal plan be such that the fluctuations made by choice in foods cause it to vary only within narrow limits, probably not more than 100 to 200 kcal (about 400 to 800 kJ) variations.

When the normal weight is achieved, foods should be added back very gradually, one at a time. Minor increase in weight that is sustained for several days indicates that the additions have been made too rapidly, and the last addition should be deleted. Regular recording of weight is essential as motivation for keeping slim. Experience indicates that very few people who have been truly obese manage to hold to their reduced weight, but rather creep back to the same weight, or more, that they had before they began the reducing regimen. Success is greater if the weight is corrected all the way to the ideal rather than stopping short at some intermediate weight that neither satisfies the ego nor improves the health status in noticeable ways. A vigorous exercise program should be of help, provided the person has found an activity he enjoys. No one knows if the common pattern of weight gain-weight loss-weight regain, etc. (the pattern that Mayer has called the "rhythm method of girth control") is harmful to man. A famine-feast regimen does shorten the life span of genetically obese mice more than if they are allowed to remain obese. In the mice, life span is prolonged by sustained weight reduction.[2]

Adjuncts and Fad Diets

Probably no type of quackery is more profitable at present than the special remedies sold to effect weight reduction and various adjuncts supposed to make weight loss easy and safe. They flourish because the American public has become conscious of the need to do something about overweight but still hopes to do it as painlessly as possible. So the public is credulous about remedies and fad diets that promise "You can eat all you want and still lose weight." Any manufacturer that makes this promise for a product is banking on the fact that his product contains something that reduces appetite. This may be a substance such as cellulose that provides little or no available energy but that helps fill the stomach and satisfy the craving to eat. This type of product is harmless but is expensive and probably ineffective, for laboratory studies indicate that nearly half the diet may be replaced by cellulose without reducing the voluntary energy intake of animals. Other products may contain one of the drugs that depress appetite. There are several that may be prescribed by physicians, but only one or two are allowed to be used without a doctor's prescription. The appetite-depressing drugs that can thus be used in preparations sold on the open market are not potent enough to have any marked effect on appetite, but perhaps taking them has some psychological effect. Truly effective products can be prescribed only by a physician. Administration of "rainbow pills" (usually three — a thyroid hormone, a diuretic agent, and an appetite suppressant) is hazardous to health, and injection of "CG" (chorionic gonadotropin derived from the human placenta) is ineffective in promoting weight loss.[23]

Remedies that promise to reduce weight merely by the patient's lying on a vibrating "couch," or to reduce weight in special places so that unsightly bulges will disappear, are so suspect that Federal agencies are prosecuting promoters for making false claims. The government holds that there is no evidence to show that general weight reduction can be effected by such means alone or that fatty tissue in certain areas can be broken down and gotten rid of by such means as massage. Systematic exercises for certain muscles may firm the muscles and, if accompanied by dietary control, may get rid of extra fat. However, urgent solicitation to enroll at cut rates for exercises or baths at various establishments for weight reduction should be resisted. There can be little or no personal supervision of the exercises, and indiscriminate exercising for an overweight individual who is unused to it and may have back troubles or other ailments can do harm. Baths, including steam baths, can effect little weight reduction except through loss of water from the body, and this can quickly be regained merely by drinking water. The only type of bath that can be a useful adjunct to weight reduction is the cold shower or plunge. This increases the basal metabolism considerably for some time, provided the individual reacts well after a cold shower, but it is rather "heroic" treatment for an overweight person to undergo. Swimming in cold water is an effective way of increasing heat loss and of providing beneficial exercise to improve muscular tone.

Although it is possible to get all the nutrients needed in a well-planned reducing diet, without *extra* care in planning, iron intake will be below the recommended allowance for women. Iron and other supplementary vitamins and minerals may well be a safeguard for persons on drastic or long-continued reducing diets. This is especially true of the fat-soluble vitamins, because fats are sharply curtailed and some persons will not take large amounts of leafy vegetables. In this case, it is better to buy a reputable vitamin preparation, so that the dosage may be known and controlled.

Special diets for reducing are quite in vogue. Popular magazines have all been carrying such planned diets, with menus for a week to a full month. It seems remarkable that people should be so eager to follow menu plans made out by someone who cannot know their food preferences or circumstances or what foods can be obtained readily in local markets. Usually such diets include some foods used less frequently or those prepared in unusual ways. They may be relatively expensive and cause extra work, especially if the rest of the family does not wish to eat the same foods as the reducer. The best of these diets are no more effective than any well-planned reducing diet, though they may suggest variety and avoid monotony in the diet.

For other persons, there is a special appeal in diets that involve a minimum of preparation, such as the "formula diets," which can be bought already mixed in drugstores and food shops. One may lose weight fairly rapidly by subsisting entirely on such a formula (chiefly milk with some sugar added), or the formula diet may be substituted for one or two meals a day, the other meals composed of a variety of foods appropriate to a reducing diet. However, with a bit of planning, one may select a less monotonous and less expensive diet that has the additional advantage of encouraging the improved food habits so necessary for long-term weight control. A breakfast consisting of an ordinary serving of cereal or a slice of toast, a glass of skim milk, and a small glass of fruit juice is easily prepared, is better nutritionally, and yields no more energy than does one can or package of most of the formula preparations.

There are also the peculiar diets based on only a few foods, such as the all-fruit diet, the green vegetable diet, the pineapple and lamb chop diet, the raw tomato and hard-boiled egg diet, etc. These appeal to some people either because they are short cuts in reducing or because they are unusual. Such diets are not only monotonous but also are so one-sided that they are sure to be too low in some of the various nutrients. On any of these diets, the size of portions must be limited (i.e., the total energy intake must be kept down) in order to effect weight reduction.

The "all-protein, modified fast" is the latest entrant in the fad field. Originally, this diet consisted solely of lean meat (supplemented with minerals and vitamins), 400 kcal per day, and was prescribed only under close medical supervision. The theory behind this regimen is that carbohydrate should be avoided so that there is minimal stimulus to insulin secretion and thus less propensity to retain fat and to degrade tissue protein.[24] (See Chapter 15.) Many liquid and powdered protein products flooded the market, and their indiscriminate, unsupervised use has led to serious health problems, including several deaths. The Food and Drug Administration has recommended that these products not be used for weight reduction and has asked for their voluntary withdrawal from the market.

GENERAL RULES FOR REDUCING REGIMEN

1. **Those who should reduce** –

   Normal persons who are 15 percent or more overweight.

   Persons 10 percent overweight, if they have a tendency to heart disease, kidney disease, or diabetes, should reduce to normal weight, or even slightly less.

2. **How to find out the proper level of food intake to use for reducing.**
   Calculate your maintenance level (i.e., the energy intake necessary to maintain weight with normal activity), thus:
   Look up (Table 24–1) the theoretical normal or desirable weight for your height and body build at 25 or 30 years of age.
   Multiple this *ideal* weight (in pounds) by 15 if sedentary and by 20 if active (adults require 15 to 20 kcal per lb per day) (135 to 185 kJ/kg).
   This gives the supposed maintenance level of energy intake.
   Plan the diet to yield 500 to 1000 kcal (about 2000 to 4000 kJ) per day *less* than the maintenance level, depending on how rapidly you want to lose weight.
   EXAMPLE: A woman 5 ft 5 in tall, 25 years old, and of medium frame should weigh about 125 lbs (actually weighs 167 lbs, about 25 percent overweight, and is sedentary).
   125 × 15 = 1875 kcal, minimum maintenance level.
   Reduce energy intake by one-fifth to one-third of maintenance level.
   1875 – 400 = 1475 kcal.
   1875 – 600 = 1275 kcal.
   Reducing diet for this individual should furnish 1300 to 1500 kcal.

3. **How to determine how much to reduce food level in order to get a certain rate of weight loss.**
   One ounce of body fat represents approximately 230 kcal (335 kJ/100 gm) of food.
   If you cut down food intake 500 kcal below maintenance level, you should lose about ¾ lb of fat per week, or 3 lb per month.
   A reduction of 1000 kcal below maintenance level should cause weight to be lost at rate of approximately 6 lb per month.
   You may not lose exactly at the calculated rate each week, especially the first week or two, but in the long run the weight loss will average about that expected, if you stick to your diet.

4. **Weighing and best rate at which to lose.**
   Weigh at least once per week, on the same scales if possible, at about the same time of day, and in clothing of approximately the same weight. Before breakfast is a good time to weigh in. Small fluctuations of weight from day to day have no significance, but steady, gradual loss of weight is what to work for. Keep a written record of your weight, preferably a graph to show your progress (see Fig. 23–3).
   It is not advisable to reduce more rapidly than 1 to 2 lb weight loss per week.
   Too rapid reduction may cause weakness and throws a severe strain on the system for rapid readjustments. It is detrimental to looks, as skin is apt to become wrinkled after the rapid loss of subcutaneous fat, and "crash" dieting leads to loss of hair. Too rapid a weight loss is hard on the disposition, as the very restricted diet necessary will probably cause hunger and irritability or depression.

5. **Exercise**
   It is best to begin exercise gradually, if you have been sedentary. Choose some activity that you enjoy and gradually increase the amount of time spent doing it.
   Try not to ride an elevator less than three floors. Always park your car a short walk from your destination or, better still, ride a bicycle or walk.

6. Necessity of keeping at lower level of food intake after reducing diet.

It should be obvious that, if you go back to the former food and exercise levels on which you gained weight, you will regain the weight that has just been lost unless you increase your physical activity to compensate.

When you have lost the desired amount of weight on a restricted diet, increase the food intake *gradually* until you are eating just enough food to maintain constant weight. Keep the food intake at this new level. If you begin to gain, cut down the diet by a small amount.

DIETS FOR GAINING WEIGHT

A diet suitable for building up a body that has suffered for some time from an insufficient food supply should be planned to provide:

1. A high energy intake — fuel in excess of body needs.
2. Liberal quantities of high-quality protein.
3. An abundant supply of minerals and vitamins.

The first requirement is met by including in the diet liberal amounts of high-energy foods, especially foods rich in *fats* and *starches*, such as butter or margarine, cream, salad dressings, bacon, cereals, bread, cream soups, legumes, nuts, and dried fruits — in short, all foods forbidden to *overweight* individuals. Filling foods that carry little nourishment (e.g., clear soups) should be avoided. Protein of high quality for tissue building and repair is provided by including *milk, eggs,* and *meats* as freely as costs permit. Organ meats, such as liver, which are excellent sources of minerals and vitamins, should be eaten frequently. Even though they may seem to increase the bulk of the diet undesirably, plenty of *fruits* and *vegetables* should be included for their content of mineral elements and vitamins. Milk, eggs, and whole-grain bread and cereals are also valuable sources of minerals and vitamins. Although high energy content is the main objective of the diet, care should be taken that it provides an *abundance of all the other nutritive essentials* as well.

The diet should provide energy in excess of body needs by at least 500 to 1000 kcal (2000 to 4000 kJ). The intake should exceed body needs by one-half to one-third the energy required for maintenance — for example, a person who needs 2100 kcal for maintenance should consume approximately 2800 to 3100 kcal when trying to gain weight. It is often necessary to force one's self to take food in excess of appetite. It is probably easier to accomplish this if the food is divided into more frequent meals, about five to seven a day, taken by clock time rather than by hunger or appetite.

It is easy to increase the energy intake considerably by such devices as an extra square of butter or fortified margarine at each meal (about 220 kcal), liberal use of cream, bacon, and salad dressings (1 tbsp mayonnaise, 2 tbsp thick cream, or 2 heaping tbsp whipped cream each furnishes about 100 kcal), and supplementary nourishment between meals and at bedtime.

The best foods to use for the midmorning or midafternoon lunch are *dairy products and fruit juices.* These can be served in many combinations — for example, plain cold milk enriched with cream, hot malted milk or milk flavored with chocolate or cocoa, egg-nog, or beaten egg in fruit juice, and plain fruit juices with high-energy content (apple, grape, nectars).

An *illustrative menu* is given in Table 24–6. The approximate amount of energy furnished is included to show how rapidly the fuel value of the diet mounts when fats and concentrated starchy foods are included in any considerable quantities. The meals alone, as planned in this diet, furnish over 3100 kcal, or 1000 kcal

Table 24-6 SAMPLE MENU FOR A WOMAN WHO WISHES TO GAIN WEIGHT

	kcal
Breakfast	
Orange juice 6 oz	80
Oatmeal (2/3–3/4 c cooked), with sliced banana (1/2)	115
Cream, (half-and-half) 1/4 c	80
Poached or soft-boiled egg	80
Bacon, 3 slices	155
Whole-wheat toast, 2 slices	120
Butter or margarine, 1 tbsp	100
Jam, 1 tbsp	55
Coffee, with sugar	45
	830
Midmorning	
Apple, 1 (medium)	90
Lunch	
Lettuce wedge, with sliced tomato and avacado (1/4)	95
French dressing, 1 tbsp	60
Creamed chicken (3/4 c), on slice of toast (1)	370
Hard roll, whole-wheat, 1	60
Butter or margarine, 2 tsp	65
Ice cream, 1/2 c	135
Sweetened strawberries	50
Milk, 8 oz	165
	1000
Midafternoon	
Chocolate milk, 1 c	190
Dinner	
Cream of asparagus soup, 3/4 c	130
Crackers, 2	45
Cottage cheese (1/4 c) and fruit cocktail (1/2 c) salad, with 2 tsp mayonnaise	165
Roast lamb, 4 oz	210
Mint jelly, 1 tbsp	55
Baked potato (1 medium)	95
Butter, 1 tbsp	100
Peas, 1/2 c	55
Lemon meringue pie (1/6 of 9 in pie)	360
Coffee, with sugar	45
	1260
Evening	
Milk	165
Sugar cookie	90
	255
Total—approximately	3600

in excess of the energy needs of a 58 kg young woman (2100 kcal) without seeming unduly bulky. Supplementary nourishment between meals (as indicated) may be used to increase the fuel intake by another 500 kcal.

The success of any regimen for increasing weight depends chiefly on getting the individual to use a high-energy diet, while he simultaneously cuts down muscular activity and tenseness by extra rest and relaxation. Those who have little appetite or those who have developed fears that foods cause digestive distress must often force themselves to take food in excess of their natural desires at first. If this is done, the general condition usually improves to such an extent that both the appetite and digestion return to normal. Taking vitamins in tablet form may stimulate appetite and improve well-being if the diet has previously been deficient in those nutrients as well as being inadequate in energy.

Rapid gains in weight should not be the main objective of the program, as such gains are usually due solely to the deposition of *fat* in the body, whereas it is greatly desired that the muscle tissues should also be built up. *Muscle development* is favored by a more gradual gain in weight on a diet containing plenty of the best quality protein (milk, eggs, and meat). Some form of regular *exercise* is the best aid to building up the muscle tissues.

QUESTIONS AND PROBLEMS

1. Give four reasons why persons become overweight. How do you tell how much overweight a person is, and what are the dangers and difficulties of excess weight?

2. Is there any way (or ways) to reduce weight except by restriction of calories in the diet? What foods should be avoided or used only in small amounts in a reducing diet, and why? What foods may be used in quantity, and why? In which nutritive factor (or factors) must the reducing diet be low, and in which should it be adequate or better than adequate? Why? What food groups in the diet assure its adequacy?

3. Following the general meal pattern in Table 24–3, plan a reducing diet that furnishes about 1400 kcal. Revise this diet to drop out 400 kcal.

4. What are the health hazards associated with obesity? With underweight? Are fat people all well nourished? Explain your answer.

5. What are the essential requirements for an effective diet for putting on weight? What kind of a regimen reinforces the good effects of the diet? What benefits may be expected from such a diet and regimen?

6. Plan a fattening and body-building diet that furnishes 3500 kcal for a person with good appetite and digestion. Modify it to give the same energy value for a person whose appetite is poor.

7. Compare your weight with the values given in Table 24–1. What percentage over- or underweight are you? How much will your weight change if you hold all other factors constant but add one 12 oz can of beer each day? Play tennis for 30 minutes?

REFERENCES

1. Rimm, A. A., Werner, L. H., Van Yserloo, B., and Bernstein, R. A.: Relationship of obesity and disease in 73,532 weight-conscious women. Pub. Health Rpts., *90*:44, 1975.
2. Mayer, J.: *Overweight: Causes, Cost and Control.* Englewood Cliffs, N.J., Prentice-Hall, 1968.
3. Seltzer, C. C., and Mayer, J.: A simplified criterion of obesity. Postgrad. Med., *38*:2, 1965.
4. Ruffer, W. A.: Two simple indexes for identifying obesity compared. J. Amer. Dietet. Assoc., *57*:326, 1970.
5. Young, C. M., and Blondin, J.: Estimating body weight and fatness of young women. J. Amer. Dietet. Assoc., *41*:452, 1962.
6. Thomas, A. E., McKay, D. A., and Cutlip, M. B.: A nomograph method for assessing body weight. Amer. J. Clin. Nutr., *29*:302, 1976.
7. Garn, S. M., et al.: Parent-child, sibling and twin comparisons in the study of fatness. Presented at the meeting of the AIN, ASCN, and Nutrition Society of Canada, Michigan State University, Aug. 1976.
8. Nisbett, R. E.: Determinants of food intake in obesity. Science, *159*:1254, 1968.
9. Drabman, R. S., Hammer, D., and Jarvie, G. J.: Eating rates of elementary school children. J. Nutr. Ed., *9*:180, 1977; Stunkard, A., and Kaplan, D.: Eating in public places: a review of reports on the direct observation of eating behavior. Internat. J. Obesity, *1*:89, 1977.
10. Hashim, S. A., and Van Itallie, T. B.: Studies in normal and obese subjects with a monitored food dispensing device. Ann. N.Y. Acad. Sci., *131*:654, 1965.
11. Hirsch, J., Knittle, J. L., and Salans, L. B.: Cell lipid content and cell number in obese and nonobese human adipose tissue. J. Clin. Invest., *45*:1023, 1966.
12. Ravelli, G., Stein, Z. A., and Susser, M. W.: Obesity in young men after famine exposure in utero and early infancy. N. Engl. J. Med., *295*:349, 1976.

13. Miller, D. S., and Payne, P. R.: Weight maintenance and food intake. J. Nutr., *78*:255, 1962.
14. Miller, D. S., and Mumford, P.: Gluttony. 1. An experimental study of overeating low- or high-protein diets. Amer. J. Clin. Nutr., *20*:1212, 1967; Miller, D. S., Mumford, P., and Stock, M. J.: Gluttony. 2. Thermogenesis in overeating man. Amer. J. Clin. Nutr., *20*:1233, 1967.
15. Zucker, L. M.: Efficiency of energy utilization by the Zucker hereditarily obese rat "fatty." Proc. Soc. Exp. Biol. Med., *148*:498, 1975.
16. Mayer, J., et al.: Symposium: Feeding patterns and their biochemical consequences. Fed. Proc., *23*:59, 1964.
17. Fabry, P.: Metabolic consequences of the pattern of food intake. In Code, D.F. (ed.): *Handbook of Physiology*. Section 6, Vol. 1, Chapter 3. Baltimore, The Williams & Wilkins Co. for the American Physiological Society, 1967.
18. Frederickson, D. S., et al.: *Dietary Management of Hyperlipoproteinemia: A Handbook for Physicians*. Bethesda, Md., National Heart and Lung Institute, National Institutes of Health, 1970.
19. Keys, A. B., et al.: *The Biology of Human Starvation*. 2 vols. Minneapolis, University of Minnesota Press, 1950.
20. Janowski, L. W., and Foss, M. L.: The energy intake of sedentary men after moderate exercise. Med. Sci. Sports, *4*:11, 1972.
21. Bloom, W. L., and Azar, G. J.: Similarities of carbohydrate deficiency and fasting. Arch. Intern. Med., *112*:333, 1963.
22. Young, C. M., Scanlan, S. S., Sook Im, H., and Lutwak, L.: Effect on body composition and other parameters in obese young men of carbohydrate level of reduction diet. Amer. J. Clin. Nutr., *24*:290, 1971.
23. Shetty, K. R., and Kalkhoff, R. K.: Human chorionic gonadotropin (HGG) treatment of obesity. Arch. Intern. Med., *137*:151, 1977.
24. Bistrian, B. R., et al.: Effect of a protein-sparing diet and brief fast on nitrogen metabolism in mildly obese subjects. J. Lab. Clin. Med., *89*: 1030, 1972.

SUPPLEMENTARY READING

Alvarez, L. C., Peters, D. J., Murad, H., Wright, E. T., McGhee, G., and Drenick, E. J.: Changes in the epidermis during prolonged fasting. Amer. J. Clin. Nutr., *28*:866, 1975.

AMA Council on Foods and Nutrition: A critique of low-carbohydrate ketogenic weight reduction regimens. J.A.M.A., *224*:1415, 1973.

American Health Foundation: Position statement on diet and coronary heart disease. Prev. Med., *1*:256, 1972.

Bennion, L. J., and Grundy, S. M.: Effects of obesity and caloric intake on biliary lipid metabolism in man. J. Clin. Invest., *58*:996, 1975.

Bray, G. A.: Effect of caloric restriction on energy expenditure in obese patients. Lancet, *2*:397, 1969.

Bray, G. A.: The myth of diet in the management of obesity. Amer. J. Clin. Nutr., *23*:1141, 1970.

Bray, G. A., et al.: Symposium: Experimental models for the study of obesity. Fed. Proc., *36*:137, 1977.

Bray, G. A., et al.: Eating patterns of massively obese individuals. Direct vs. indirect measurements. J. Amer. Dietet. Assoc., *72*:24, 1978.

Bullen, B. A., Reed, R. B., and Mayer, J.: Physical activity of obese and nonobese adolescent girls appraised by motion picture sampling. Amer. J. Clin. Nutr., *14*:211, 1964.

Crisp, A. N., and McGuiness, B.: Jolly fat: relation between obesity and psychoneurosis in general population. Brit. Med. J., *1*:7, 1976.

Drenick, E. J., and Dennin, H. F.: Energy expenditure in fasting obese men. J. Lab. Clin. Med., *81*:421, 1973.

Faloon, W. W., Chairman: Symposium: Jejunoileostomy for obesity. Amer. J. Clin. Nutr., *30*:1, 1977.

Finkelstein, B., and Fryer, B. A.: Meal frequency and weight reduction of young women. Amer. J. Clin. Nutr., *24*:465, 1971.

Garn, S. M., Bailey, S. M., and Higgins, I. T. T.: Fatness similarities in adopted pairs. Amer. J. Clin. Nutr., *29*:1067, 1976.

Genuth, S. M., Castro, J. H., and Vertes, V.: Weight reduction in obesity by outpatient semistarvation. J.A.M.A., *230*:987, 1974.

Goette, D. K., and Odom, R. B.: Alopecia in crash dieters. J.A.M.A., *235*:2622, 1976.

Häger, A., et al.: Adipose tissue cellularity in obese school girls before and after dietary treatment. Amer. J. Clin. Nutr., *31*:68, 1978.

Hannon, B. M., and Lohman, T. G.: The energy cost of overweight in the United States. Amer. J. Physiol., *68*:765, 1978.

Hockaday, T. D. R., et al.: Prospective comparison of modified-fat–high-carbohydrate with standard low-carbohydrate dietary advice in the treatment of diabetes: one year follow-up study. Brit. J. Nutr., *39*:357, 1978.

Jourdan, M., Margen, S., and Bradfield, R. B.: Protein-sparing effect in obese women fed low calorie diets. Amer. J. Clin. Nutr., *27*:3, 1974.

Kaplan, M. L., and Leveille, G. A.: Calorigenic responses in obese and nonobese women. Amer. J. Clin. Nutr., *29*:1108, 1976.

Lewis, S., et al.: Effects of physical activity on weight reduction in obese middle-aged women. Amer. J. Clin. Nutr., *29*:151, 1976.

Lincoln, J. E.: Weight gain after cessation of smoking. J.A.M.A., *210*:1765, 1969.

Mayer, J. (ed.) Obesity. Postgrad. Med., *51*:66–69, 1972.

Metzner, H. L., et al.: The relationship between frequency of eating and adiposity in adult men and women in the Tecumseh Community Health Study. Amer. J. Clin. Nutr., *30*:712, 1977.

Pierson, R. N., Jr., et al.: The assessment of human body composition during reduction: evaluation of a new model for clinical studies. J. Nutr., *106*:1694, 1976.

Schumaker, J. F., and Wagner, M. K.: External-cue responsivity as a function of age at onset of obesity. J. Amer. Dietet. Assoc., *70*:275, 1977.

Sohar, E. and Sneh, E.: Follow-up of obese patients: 14 years after a successful reducing diet. Amer. J. Clin. Nutr., *26*:845, 1973.

Strong, J. P., et al.: Pathology and epidemiology of atherosclerosis, J. Amer. Dietet. Assoc., *62*:262, 1973.

Stunkard, A., et al.: Influence of social class on obesity and thinness in children. JAMA, *221*:579, 1972.

Swenseid, M. E., Mulcare, D. B., and Drenick, E. J.: Nitrogen and weight loss during starvation and realimentation in obesity. J. Amer. Dietet. Assoc., *46*:276, 1965.

Symposium: Control of feeding and the regulation of energy balance. Fed. Proc., *33*:1139, 1974.

Symposium: Obesity in Man. Proc. Nutr. Soc., *32*:169, 1973.

Van Itallie, T. B., and Yang, M.-U.: Diet and weight loss. N. Eng. J. Med., *297*:1158, 1977.

Van Stratum, P., et al.: The effect of dietary carbohydrate:fat ratio on energy intake by adult women. Amer. J. Clin. Nutr., *31*:206, 1978.

Womersley, J., and Durnin, J. V. G. A.: A comparison of the skinfold method with extent of 'overweight' and various weight-height relationships in the assessment of obesity. Brit. J. Nutr., *38*: 271, 1977.

Worthington, B. S., and Taylor, L. E.: Balanced low-calorie vs. high-protein-low-carbohydrate reducing diets. I. Weight loss, nutrient intake, and subjective evaluation. J. Amer. Dietet. Assoc., *64*:47, 1974. II. Biochemical changes. J. Am. Dietet. Assoc., *64*:52, 1974.

Articles in Nutrition Reviews

Comparison of an 800 to 1,000 calorie diet with fasting in weight reduction. *24*:6, 1966.

Sugar and coronary heart disease. *28*:228, 1970.

Dietary obesity in seven strains of rats. *29*:69, 1971.

Cellular growth in the fat adolescent. *29*:158, 1971.

The role of insulin and growth hormone in childhood obesity. *29*:163, 1971.

Adipose cell size and number in experimental human obesity. *30*:60, 1972.

The hematology of anorexia nervosa. *31*:207, 1973.

Anorexigenic substances in rat urine. *32*:123, 1974.

Treatment of massive obesity: rice/reduction diet. *34*:176, 1976.

Intestinal adaptation and hepatic decompensation after jejunoileal bypass for morbid obesity. *35*:43, 1977.

Research on obesity. *35*:249, 1977.

Morbid obesity — long term results of therapeutic fasting. *36*:6, 1978.

Body weight and immunity — a reciprocal relationship? *36*:41, 1978.

The nature of weight loss during short-term fasting. *36*:72, 1978.

Diabetes and obesity: thrifty mutants? *36*:129, 1978.

Anorexia nervosa and hypothalamic endocrine dysfunction. *36*:137, 1978.

Human obesity and adipocyte function. *36*:140, 1978.

Chapter 25

Malnutrition: A Global Perspective

Two types of malnutrition can be found in all countries: the malnutrition of poverty and that of affluence — a convenient classification that calls attention to the characteristic extreme syndromes. At one extreme are the poor, often living in abject misery, for whom undernutrition is only one aspect of general deprivation. At the other extreme are the affluent, whose easy access to food and comfortable lifestyle lead to overnutrition and the diseases associated with it. While both types of malnutrition are found throughout the world, their prevalence and severity differ markedly from country to country. Furthermore, undernutrition is also to be found among people who are in a position to be adequately nourished, and overnutrition occurs among those who are less than truly affluent. Usually, however, discussion of world malnutrition focuses on the two extreme conditions that are readily recognizable and with which we have become familiar through television and other news media. Yet between the extremes of undernutrition and overnutrition — both of which cause death — there is a continuum of deficiency, adequacy, and excess.

Intake and Nutritional State

There is a rather broad range of intakes (depending on the nutrient in question) that can maintain a positive state of health with relatively little of the body's adaptive ability being brought into play. This may be illustrated as follows:

INTAKE	← Deficit			Minimum Requirement	Maximum Allowance	Excess →		
STATE	Death and Disease	Clinical Signs	Biochemical Changes	←HEALTH→ Low Tissue Stores	Tissues Replete	Biochemical Changes	Clinical Signs	Death and Disease

At the upper portion of the allowable range of intakes, all tissue reserves will be filled and daily output in the excreta will be high. If intake exceeds a certain upper limit, adaptive biochemical or physiological processes that can be detected by sophisticated laboratory techniques then develop; at the next stage of excess intake, there will be clinical signs and symptoms of the disordered state, and beyond that, manifest disease and death. The same sequence of events, beginning with depleted reserves, occurs with nutrient intakes at the lower end of the spectrum.

Taking iron as an example, inadequate intake leads first to lowered concentration of iron-transport substances in the blood, then to diminished hemoglobin, and finally to pallor, fatigue, decreased work capacity, and death because of lack of oxygen at the tissue level. With chronically excessive iron intake, transport protein becomes saturated, iron accumulates in the liver, the liver cells are damaged and sometimes so is the heart, and the person may die from failure of the damaged liver or heart. The range of safe intakes is much wider for some nutrients than for others because the body has more ways to dispose of excess and adapt to deficits or because the nutrient does not participate in reactions that are as important to survival. The body state is affected by both present and past intakes, so that diagnosis of malnutrition is more difficult than a single example may indicate. What is important to know is that the body has some capacity to adapt to altered intakes, that there may be hidden evidence of malnourishment before it is clinically noticeable, and that not all body functions may be equally affected by a given degree of deficit or excess at a given time in the life history. Individuals in a borderline state — with adaptive mechanisms operating at near capacity and biochemically detectable but minimal changes in function — may be said to be *at risk* of malnutrition or to be in a subclinical state of malnutrition. The number of persons in this category is many times the number who show clinical signs. Whenever there is a significant number of people with unequivocal clinical malnutrition, a larger segment of the population can be assumed to be at risk. For these people a reduction of intake — or even continued low intake or increase in stress — may lead to open manifestation, or clinical signs, of malnutrition.

WHO ARE THE MALNOURISHED?

Vulnerability to manifest malnutrition is conditioned by various characteristics of a person's situation. Some people are exposed to seasonal fluctuations in the amount and sources of nutrients available and to work stress and disease. Others are exposed to, or are at risk of, natural disaster, or their socioeconomic status makes them subject to loss of income and vulnerable because of poverty. Thus, for these several reasons we may be able to identify sections of a population who in various ways are in danger of manifest malnutrition. Among them some will be undernourished to a lesser degree that will produce no clinical symptoms but that still may affect their reproductive and child-rearing capacity, their resistance to or recovery from disease, their activity and work output, and their attitudes and behavior.

Policies to reduce malnutrition must clearly aim at reducing the numbers who are at risk as well as treating those who are manifestly malnourished. Unless the "at risk" population is reduced, malnutrition will continue to be manifest. Moreover, the consequences of less than severe malnutrition will have a continuing effect on those societies whose demography, disease patterns, work productivity, and social behavior are thus affected (see Figs. 25–1 and 25–2).

Assessment Based on Food Consumption Figures

There are problems in the assessment of nutrition status of populations. Some of

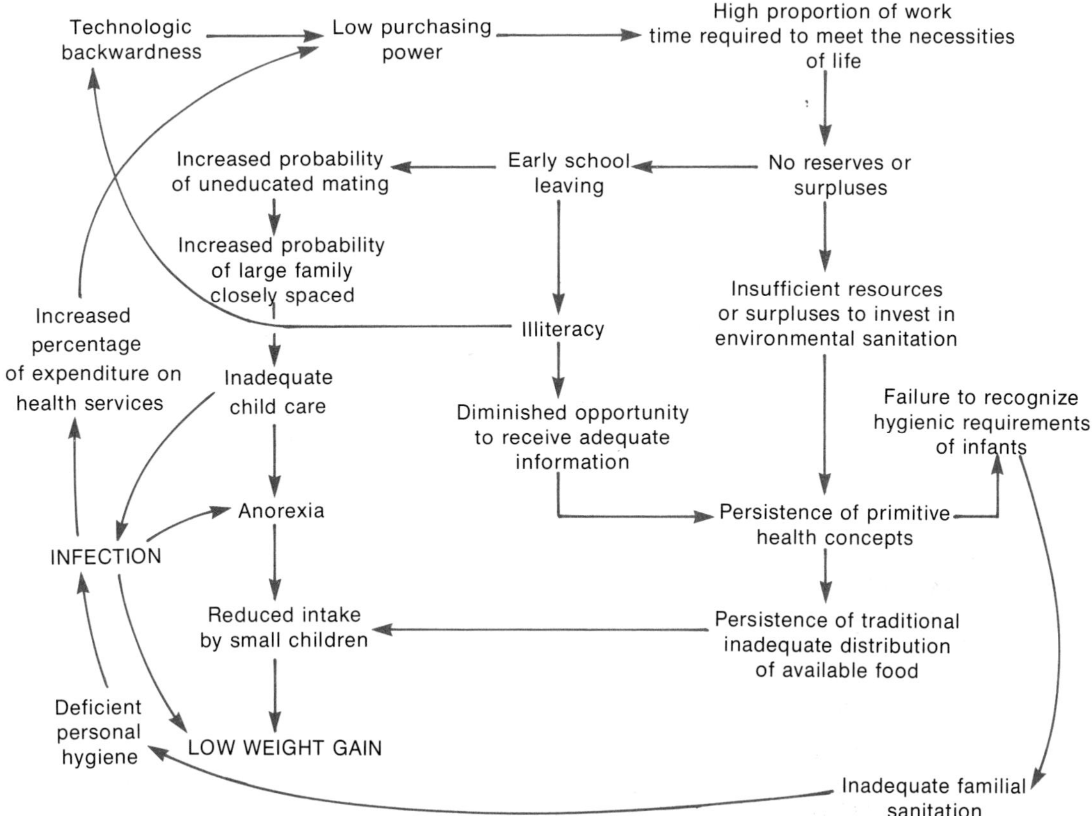

Figure 25–1 This flow chart brings out the interdependence of health, nutrition, and socioeconomic status and the mutually reinforcing and cumulative effects of the contribution of each element to sustaining the poverty condition. The aspects depicted cover only part of the total poverty situation, and there are clearly limits to the effectiveness of attempts to tackle specific aspects of this situation singly. What this diagram does not illustrate is the impact of individual and family poverty, and its characteristic malnutrition, on the community as a whole—the overall impact on demography, disease, work productivity, social activity, attitudes, and social cohesion. While such effects can be inferred as a consequence of malnutrition, the evidence of causal relationships is diffuse and the social effects of malnutrition have, as yet, hardly been researched. (Redrawn from Cravioto, J., and DeLicardie, E. R.: Malnutrition in early childhood. Food Nutr. *No. 4,* 1976.)

the methods that might be used to evaluate the status of individuals, their tissue stores and biochemical indicators especially, are expensive and impractical for application to large populations. Assessment of individual and household food intakes is also expensive. Almost no one eats exactly the same amount and kind of food each day of the week and at all seasons of the year. A single 24 hour record of intake can be quite unrepresentative, but this is the only type of individual intake information it has been deemed feasible to collect in population surveys. Two particularly troublesome deficiencies of such surveys have been identified, in addition to the question of the representativeness of the 24 hour intake. One is the reliability of the information. People may fail to remember or to report accurately; this is particularly true of adults who attempt to recall food intake of their children and of aged or distracted individuals. Generally, there is a tendency to underestimate food intake (Fig. 25–3). A second concern is with the validity of conventional population samples. This is an especially serious problem when con-

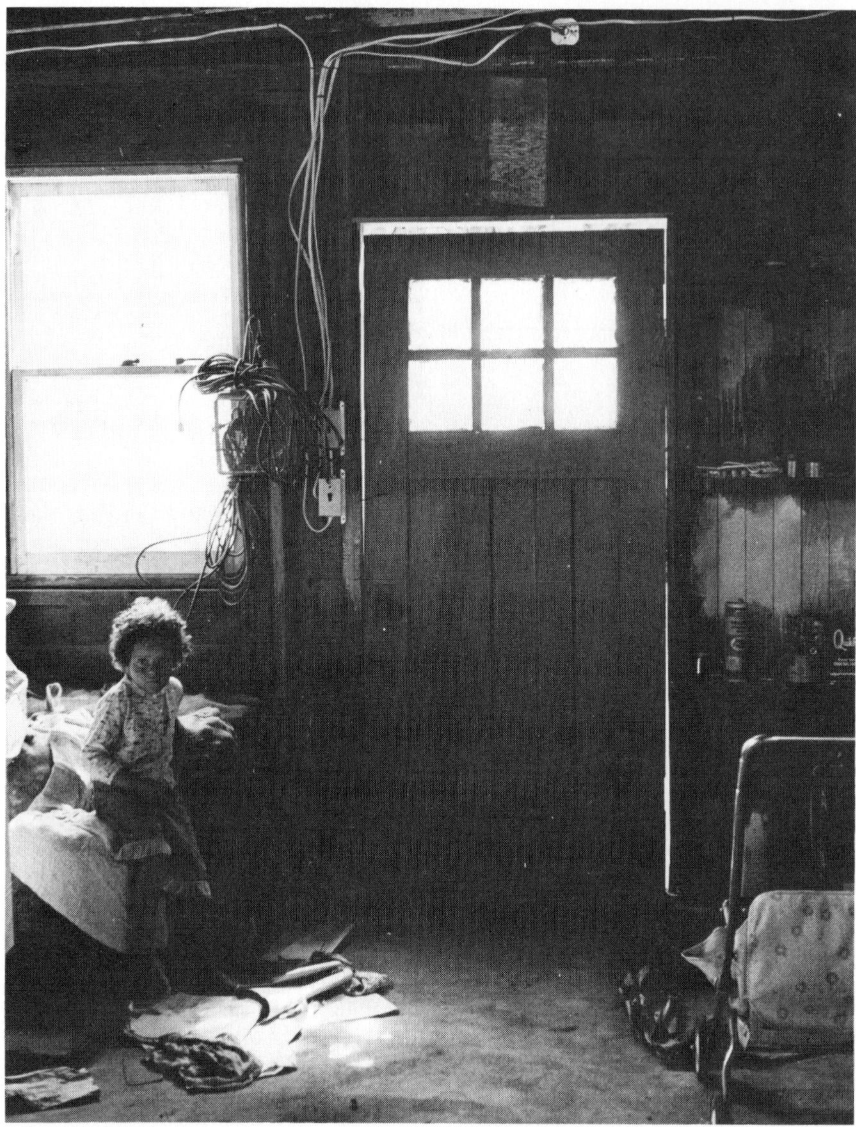

Figure 25–2 Migrant farm worker's housing, Tulare County, California, 1969. The WHO has observed that "Disease and sociopsychological problems are to a great extent determined by the immediate environment of the family — its home. A clean and functional house, not necessarily expensive but adapted to the environment and favoring a healthy way of life for its inhabitants, is an important factor in the prevention of many of the diseases and other problems now afflicting large population groups in rural areas, and even more so in city slums." (Courtesy of Donald Heiny, San Francisco, and University of California, Berkeley.)

clusions are to be drawn about the relationship of nutrient intake to other conditions of life. In a Quebec study[1], for example, out of a sample of 340 households, 104 were absent, 59 refused to participate, and 177 completed the inquiry. However, 63 percent of those from the higher socioeconomic group participated and only 42 percent from the lowest group. The refusal rate of the low economic group was less than that of the more affluent group (14 percent vs. 24 percent), but a much larger number of the low economic group were absent from their homes (44 percent vs. 13 percent). There is no way to determine the extent of bias introduced in the results by low participation rates, but it is likely that the very households one is most concerned about are least well represented in the sample. This problem is, of course, vexing no matter what method of nutritional assessment is used.

Even when intake data are accurate and representative, there are problems in interpretation. In Chapter 19 we discussed briefly the common but erroneous assumption that an individual is nutritionally deficient if his intake falls below some dietary standard. All national and international dietary standards are set at levels judged to cover the needs of almost all healthy persons, i.e., two standard deviations above the average requirement for all nutrients except energy (Fig. 25–4). A comparison between individual intake and a dietary standard can reveal the degree of probability that the individual's needs are not being met. If the habitual intake is far below the standard (about 54 percent of standard for protein, vitamins, and minerals and 70 percent of standard for energy), there is a very low probability that the intake is adequate because only 2.5 percent of the population would have needs that low. When the number of people at any level of nutrient intake less than mean requirement is larger than the predicted number, then there is a corresponding risk that people are undernourished, *if* high intakes are consumed by high requirers and low intakes by low requirers. Even when the individual has free access to food, however, physiological mechanisms do not guarantee that intake, except for energy, meets or exceeds need. Hence, the magnitude of deficiency may actually be larger than the indicated

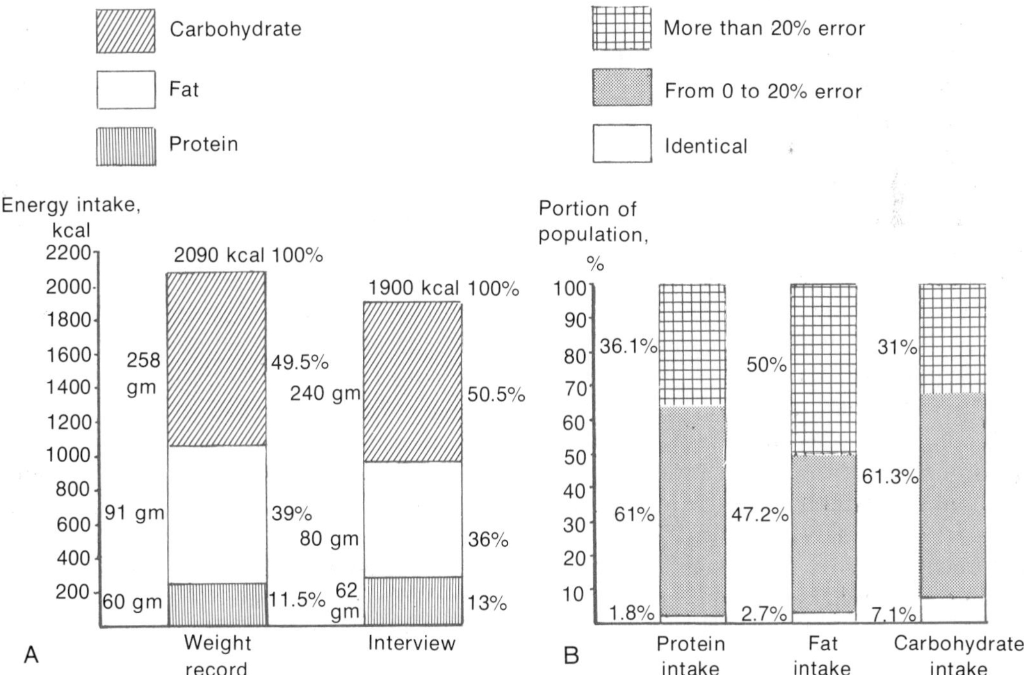

Figure 25–3 Comparison of data on food intake obtained by weighing food and by recall interview. **A,** Mean values for energy, protein, fat, and carbohydrate intake. Note that weighed food intake was 10 percent higher than the interview finding. **B,** Correspondence of the two sets of data for individuals, showing that the estimated intake figure differed from the weighed intake by more than 20 percent in one-third (protein, carbohydrate) to one-half (fat) of the diets examined. (From Debry, G.: Validity of methods of dietary surveys. Ann. Nutr. Alim., *30*:115, 1976.)

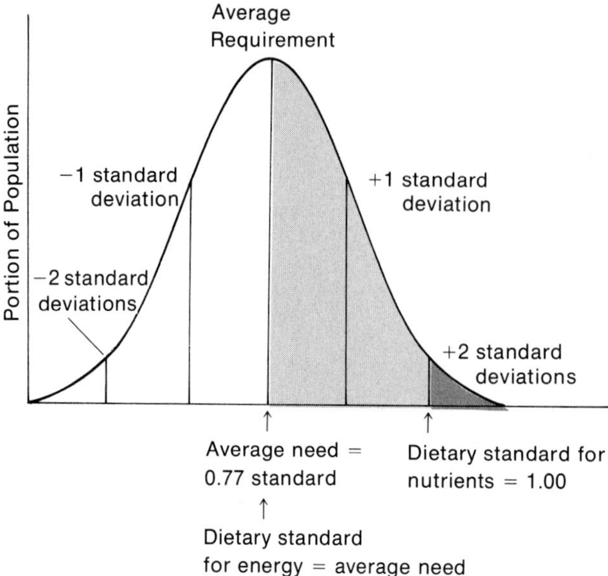

Figure 25–4 Dietary standards for protein, vitamins, and minerals are intended to cover the needs of almost all healthy people in a population; they are set at two standard deviations above the mean requirement where that is known. Thus, only 2½ percent of a normally distributed population of requirers (the darker colored area) will fail to meet their needs if their diets meet the standard. The standard deviation is about 0.15 of the mean requirement in the few instances where valid information exists. Thus the average need is about 77 percent of the standard, and the requirement of half the individuals will be met by intakes at this level. However, the standard for energy is set at the mean requirement, so the needs of half a population are not met (the lighter colored area) by intakes that equal the standard.

statistical risk; it cannot be lower, if the estimate of needs is reliable and if requirement is normally distributed.

Attempts are often made to assess the prevalence of malnutrition in a country by comparing national food consumption data with estimated per capita needs.* Neither of the statistics being compared is fully accurate. For example, consumption statistics may be faulty owing to erroneous data on farm food yields, diversion of food to alcohol production, and so on; per capita needs may include wrong assumptions about physical activity and sizes and ages of the population — even the census figures may be in error. But even if the information were accurate, aggregative data could not provide an accurate diagnosis of malnutrition. These statistics can only indicate whether or not the food consumed would have been sufficient if it had been equitably distributed according to need—an assumption we know to be invalid. Even in affluent societies, foods such as steak and strawberries are not evenly divided among the people, and in the poor countries, the poorest segment does not receive a proportionate share of even the basic staples.

This point is made clear by the data in Table 25–1. As we have noted in the previous chapter, some diseases are characteristically associated with obesity and others with undernutrition. The causes of death in a population reflect these associations. The mortality rate from heart disease and hypertension is high in affluent societies and that from infectious diseases is low; the converse is true of the poorer countries. This contrasting situation is seen also within a country, owing to unequal distribution of food and of health and other welfare services. The Union of South Africa is such an example: the mortality pattern for whites is like that of Canada and the United States, and the pattern for nonwhites is like that seen in the poorer countries of the Americas. Yet the overall per capita nutrient consumption of the Union of South Africa places it in a much better situation than Mexico and Cuba, and on par with Israel.

Prevalence of Malnutrition

The limitations of such aggregative data for estimating the magnitude of the

*Thus the United Nations Food and Agriculture Organization publishes "Food Balance Sheets" for countries and regions of the world.

Table 25-1 MORTALITY PATTERNS AND NATIONAL FOOD COMPUTATION STATISTICS FOR NORTH AND CENTRAL AMERICAN COUNTRIES

Nutrients Consumed per Capita per Day	*FAO 1968 Production Yearbook*	*Canada*	*America* *U.S.*	*Mexico*	*Guatemala*	*Union of South Africa* *Asiatic*	*Colored*	*White*
Energy, kcal	1957–59	3040	3120	2410	2175		2620	
	1963–65	3120	3140	2600	2090		2820	
Protein, gm, total	1957–59	92	92	67	55		74	
	1963–65	95	93	67	55		80	
Animal protein, gm	1957–59	61	65	20	9		24	
	1963–65	62	66	15	9		32	
Legume protein, gm	1957–59	3	4	12	9		3	
	1963–65	3	4	14	6		2	
Cause of Death, Rate per 100,000 Population	***U.N. Demographic Yearbook****							
Tuberculosis	1960	4.8	6.1	26.0	30.6	15.0	101.6	6.3
(respiratory)	1967	3.0	3.6	19.4	25.7	15.3	75.2	5.2
Infectious,	1960	55.4	47.5	423.9	769.1	203.2	453.8	86.4
parasitic diseases	1967	42.4	44.1	246.5	705.9	180.7	361.3	89.3
Infections of the	1960	3.6	2.9	52.7	82.4	16.3	32.5	3.0
newborn	1967	(82.3)†	(97.7)†	(832.6)†	(1584.1)†	(408.9)†	(539.3)†	(92.7)†
Anemia	1960	1.9	2.0	10.0	35.3	3.2	1.9	2.1
	1967	1.8	1.8	9.4	40.0	3.0	2.1	1.6
Gastritis, enteritis,	1960	5.7	4.5	217.2	233.3	62.6	378.7	12.0
colitis	1967	3.6	3.9	92.2	242.8	61.8	341.6	11.4
Arteriosclerotic and	1960	234.9	302.9	13.5	15.5	76.6	74.9	194.4
degenerative heart disease	1967	240.8	320.0	18.8	15.2	78.1	67.6	205.5
Hypertension	1960	27.3	45.8	4.7	5.9	33.6	45.5	24.8
	1967	14.9	33.5	5.0	5.2	33.7	41.8	25.1

*1960 data are for the years 1957–59; 1967 data are for 1962–66.
†Per 100,000 live births.

nutrition problem are now well recognized. Nevertheless, two questions continue to be posed. First, what is the magnitude of the malnutrition problem (nationally and globally)? Second, how great is the deficiency of food supply that must be made good by increases in food production? (See Fig. 25–5.) In attempting to answer these questions, comparisons between estimated intakes and estimated needs continue to be made, though on a more disaggregated basis. Thus, in a World Bank study,[2] Reutlinger and Selowsky attempt to calculate the number of people with different levels of caloric deficiency by using estimates of the relationship between income and calorie consumption and estimates of numbers at different income levels in various countries. Such disaggregation leads to considerable upward revision of previous estimates of the numbers of malnourished based on more aggregative procedures. The estimates quoted here (Table 25–2, Fig. 25–6) have been challenged,* and there is as yet no general agreement about an appropriate definition of nutritional adequacy. Nevertheless, whatever criteria or calculation procedures are used, estimates of the numbers of malnourished in the world are measured in hundreds of millions. Moreover, while

*See Sukhatme, P. V.,[3] and Payne's[4] review of Reutlinger and Selowsky. Sukhatme attempts to establish a new criterion of "inadequacy" with regard to calorie intake. Using this criterion he reduces the estimate for the number of malnourished in one country for which the calculations are presented (Brazil) by half. It should be noted that the FAO, using different reasoning, produced an estimate of 460 million malnourished in the world in 1970 — a figure more in line with Sukhatme's than with Reutlinger and Selowsky's.

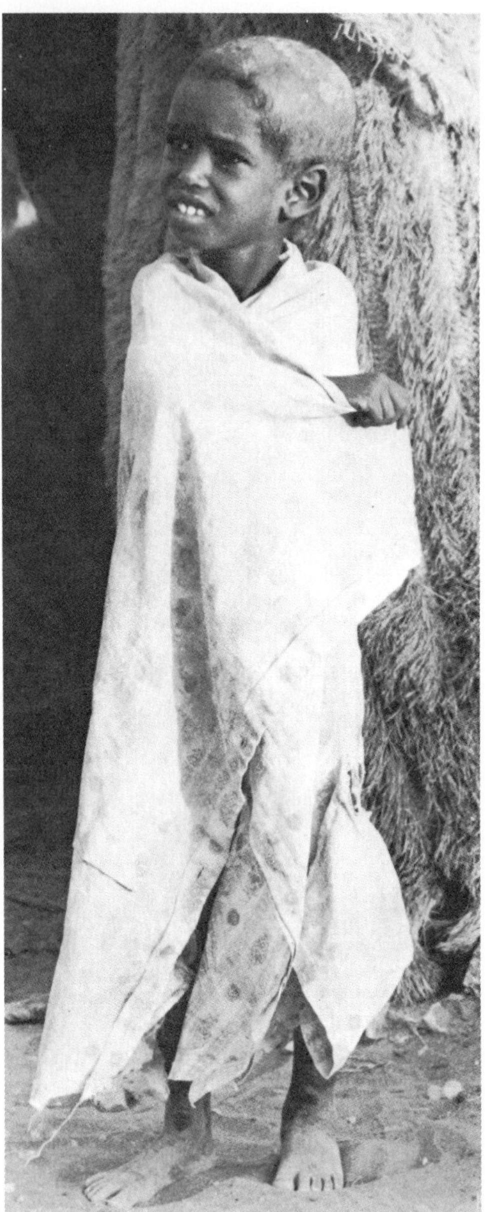

Figure 25–5 In the language of the Iteso people of Eastern Uganda, each month of the year is given a descriptive name. The preharvest month of May, when the granaries are empty, is "the month when the children wait for food." All over the vast savannah areas of Africa, where the main staple foods are cereals and legumes, the lives of millions of people are conditioned to the rhythm of the rains, the harvest, and the preharvest "hungry months" when grain is scarce and when they must look to the perennially available but low-protein cassava for their major source of food.

It is in these hungry months, when the millet crop is growing, that many children, weakened by malnutrition, die of illnesses that well-nourished children would easily survive. (Courtesy of UNICEF/T. S. Satyan.)

the methods used in attempting to predict the number of people who will be malnourished in future years are also crude and questionable, the general expectation is that the numbers, of moderately malnourished at least, will grow.*

While the magnitude of the numbers malnourished poses problems in definition as well as in estimation, it may be necessary to reformulate the question, "How great is the deficiency of food supply that must be made good by an increase in food production?" In posing the question in this way, one makes the assumption that if the caloric value of food supply were increased by at least the sum of individual calorie deficits, then these individual deficits would be corrected. But this is not necessarily so. Increasing food supply may not, in itself, reduce malnutrition. Changing food supply implies changes also in the amounts of labor, fertilizer, and other inputs used in food production, which mean changes in people's incomes (farmers, farm laborers, and employees in fertilizer factories, marketing firms, etc.). This in turn produces changes in the demand for food, in food prices, and in people's consumption. If the increase in food supply is achieved without an accompanying rise in the employment rate, or perhaps even achieved by mechanization or technologies that displace people from employment, then increases in food supply may be associated with little or no reduction in the numbers malnourished. Food prices may fall, and this will ease the position of those whose cash incomes are sustained. But a fall in food prices will adversely affect others: Farmers who normally sell some small percentage of their crop to meet cash needs will be worse off and may have to sell more food and keep less for themselves; farm laborers who find that there is less work being offered by small farmers may be quite badly affected. The most critical fac-

*The FAO estimates that there will be 600 to 800 million malnourished in 1985, which corresponds to their estimate of 460 million in 1970.[5]

Table 25–2 NUMBER OF PEOPLE CONSUMING INSUFFICIENT CALORIES, AND CALORIE DEFICITS IN DEVELOPING COUNTRIES, BY REGIONS, 1965*

Region	*Population with Daily Calorie Deficits*				Total Daily Calorie Deficit
	More Than 250 Calories		*Fewer Than 250 Calories*		
	Millions of People	Average Deficit	Millions of People	Average Deficit	(Thousand Millions)
Low estimate:					
Latin America	55	450	58	131	32
Asia	563	364	173	116	225
Middle East	75	407	16	94	32
Africa	151	380	39	72	61
Total	844		286		350
High estimate:					
Latin America	87	783	26	211	74
Asia	563	503	0	0	283
Middle East	48	906	25	60	45
Africa	151	570	0	0	86
Total	849		51		488

*Adapted from Reutlinger, S., and Selowsky, M.: *Malnutrition and Poverty: Magnitude and Policy Options.* World Bank Occasional Papers, No. 23. Baltimore, Johns Hopkins University Press, 1976.

tor, therefore, is whether the purchasing power of the poorly nourished is increased. When the malnourished are subsistence farmers, their production should be increased or their incomes augmented by greater cash earnings. Thus, while we need to increase food supplies, we need most critically to raise the incomes of the very poor. For this reason, the world food problems cannot be solved simply by increasing the food production of the rich nations. (Or by Americans eating less meat!) Increasing the production of rich or even modestly comfortable farmers in poor countries may also not help much to reduce malnutrition if the increase in production does not create extra incomes for those who are extremely poor. Thus, there may be *no* increase in food supply that alone will eliminate malnutrition. A plan to eradicate malnutrition, however, may include an increased food supply, one that will be available for people to buy when they have enough income to meet their needs.

When people have more than enough to meet their needs, they will spend more on food than is necessary. People with higher incomes buy more expensive foods, including especially animal products whose production has often required considerable amounts of grain. Therefore, as incomes rise, the direct and indirect consumption of food also rises. In addition, as demand for foods increases as a result of rising incomes, so prices increase unless supplies keep pace.

In rich countries, governments are often more concerned about the prospect of falling food prices. As this chapter is being written, measures are being taken to discourage increases in U.S. food grain production, and many major food-producing countries adopt such measures. The fear is that without them prices would be depressed. In the world as a whole we can expect shortages in some places and at some times, and there is even a risk of recurrence of the temporary global shortfall in supply that occurred in 1972–74; but the problem of malnutrition is not a problem of the world's inability to produce food. Even those poor countries where malnutrition is rife mostly have productive potential greatly in excess of their present realized output. But measures to increase output must be related to those designed to raise the economic status of the malnourished. If they are not, there is likely to be only limited

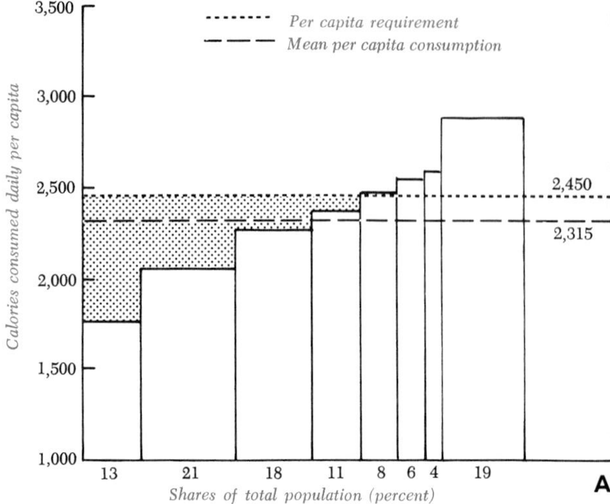

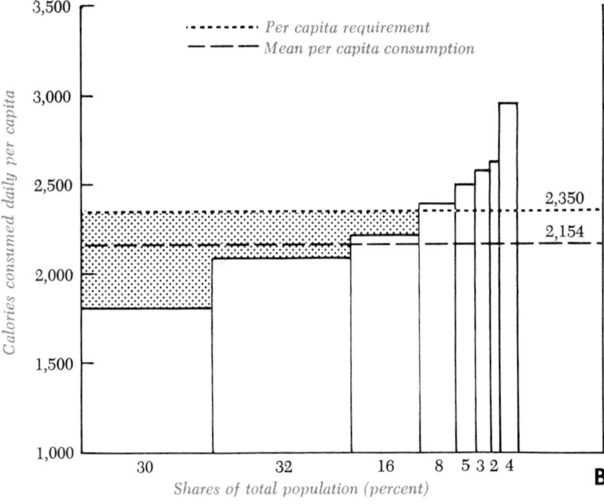

Figure 25–6 Income distribution and calorie consumption, Third World regions, 1965. The relationship between mean per capita consumption and per capita requirement gives only a rough indication of the extent of malnutrition. **A**, Calorie consumption by income groups, Latin America (low estimate). **B**, Calorie consumption by income groups, Asia (low estimate).

success in relieving malnutrition and, in any case, unless production is exported, there will be no market to absorb and sustain the increase in production.

POLICIES AND PROGRAMS FOR REDUCING MALNUTRITION

Policies and programs for reducing malnutrition must address themselves to the correction of manifest malnutrition, to the prevention or amelioration of crises of famine and hunger, which produce episodes of malnutrition; to the improvement of the conditions of those who are "at risk," in order to reduce their numbers; and to the reversal or attenuation of the social and economic trends that are creating "at risk" groups.

Obesity is the present focus of concern with regard to the malnutrition of affluence (see Fig. 25–7), because the disorders associated with it diminish the enjoyment of life, shorten the life span, and impose heavy medical costs on the indi-

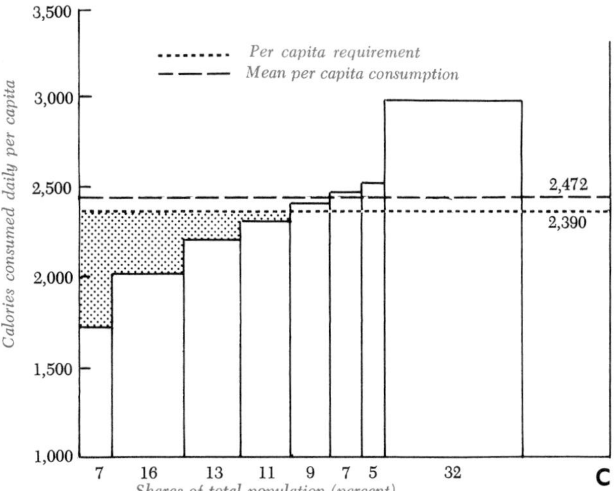

Figure 25–6 *Continued* **C**, Calorie consumption by income groups, Middle East (low estimate). **D**, Calorie consumption by income groups, Africa (low estimate). (From Reutlinger, S., and Selowsky, M.: *Malnutrition and Poverty: Magnitude and Policy Options.* World Bank Occasional Papers, No. 23. Baltimore, Johns Hopkins University Press, 1976.)

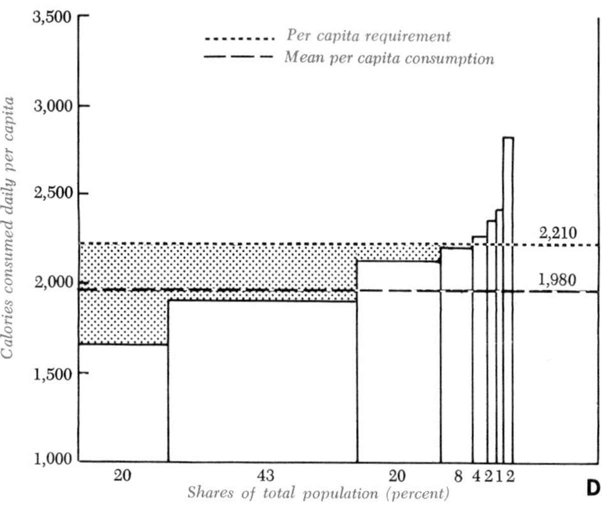

viduals affected and on the society (see Chapter 24). The basic condition of overeating must be remedied. This is clearly a matter of bringing individual energy intake and expenditure into balance. Such a measure requires individuals to change their life styles, and the scope of present programs is limited to efforts to encourage and support individuals in achieving the necessary changes. If it were governmental policy to prevent obesity, then other programs might be devised. Greater emphasis might be placed on encouraging active participant sports and recreations in the school system and in the communities, in lieu of major investment in spectator sports arenas and diversions involving little or no activity. Measures designed to decrease use of personal vehicles might encourage walking. As far as intake is concerned, use of high-energy foods might be reduced by a number of coordinated actions involving taxation, advertising regulation, shelf placement in stores, and improved health education.

The correction of manifest malnutri-

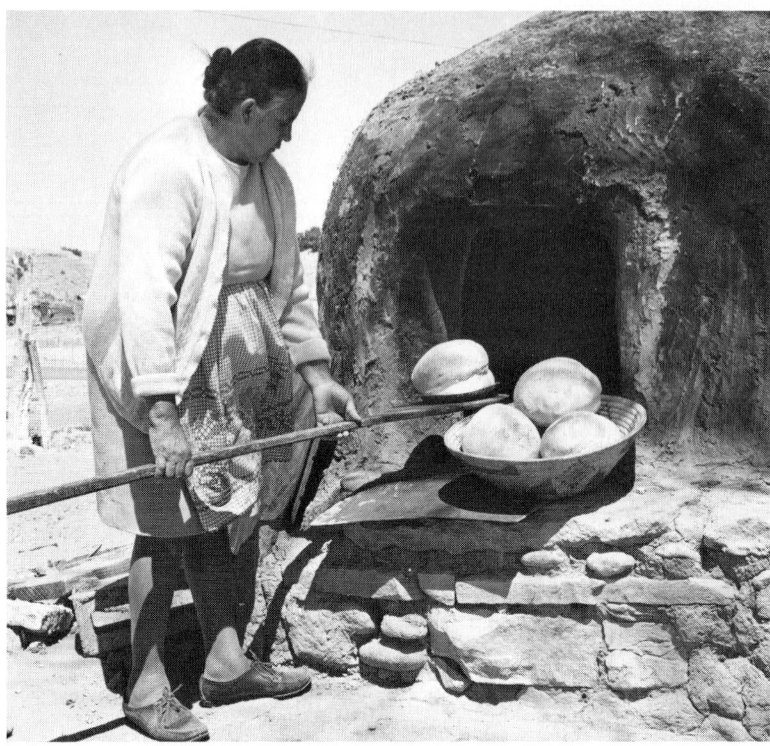

Figure 25–7 Navajo Indian woman baking bread in the traditional way, Navajo Reservation, Arizona. In the United States, obesity is more prevalent among low socioeconomic groups than among the affluent. This is associated with unemployment and lack of recreational facilities and resources; caloric intakes generally are reported to be less than the recommended daily allowances. The food needs of poverty groups are met by a variety of welfare programs that foster, by distribution of commodities or by provision of marginal support to purchase food, reliance on cheap foods. These foods have low nutrient/energy ratios, and the obese poor are often anemic and have low stores of vitamins and minerals. Poor American children are of low height for their age (relative to standards for well-nourished and more economically advantaged children) and are more often of average and above-average weight for height, rather than being thin, but some severely undernourished children are identified as well. (Courtesy of U.S. Department of Agriculture.)

tion, which stems from inadequate intakes, is a very different matter. While it is true that some individuals and families have more success in securing adequate diets than others in similar situations, there are often severe limits to what people can do to help themselves. Nevertheless, the first question to be asked in seeking to develop programs to improve nutrition is, "What can be done by the people themselves to improve their nutrition status?" The answers are likely to vary considerably, depending upon the situation being examined. For example, improvement in infant feeding may require different measures in different situations. While there are common classes of problems (e.g., overdilution of weaning foods), the specific measures designed to meet them will vary and will need to take account of such factors as available foods, mothers' preoccupations, conditions in which food is prepared, possibilities of regular visits to clinics, and so on.

Community health services have, potentially, a major role to play in preventing manifest malnutrition. They might do much by providing prenatal, perinatal, and infant care (including vitamin, mineral, and food supplements, especially during pregnancy; regular weighing and measuring of infants and advice to mothers; and immunization against common childhood diseases, whooping cough and measles especially), as well as by treating the most common ailments (see Fig. 25–8). When accompanied by measures to improve sanitation and drinking water supplies, the net impact of these health services on morbidity and mortality — especially infant mortality — can be considerable. And the cost can be small.* At the same time, it may not be easy to insure that the poorest people, those most susceptible to malnutrition, will be served; a general problem of applied nutrition programs is that it is much easier to make sure that the relatively wealthy are served by these programs than it is to get the program benefits to the poorest.

*Newell[6] reports experiences with community health services, including those of the Indian village of Jamkhed (p. 70), where for 720 people the annual per capita cost of these services was equivalent to 37 cents.

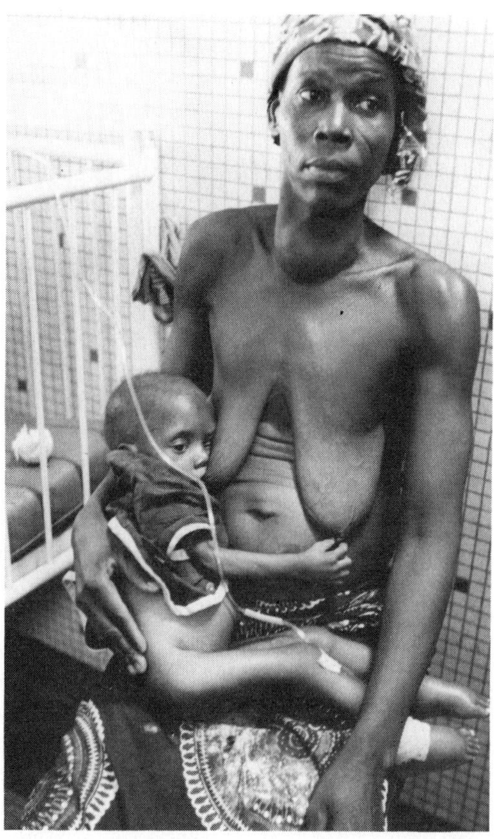

Figure 25–8 Nutrition and infection. These two conditions are a deadly combination. Each aggravates the other, resulting in alarming mortality and morbidity patterns among children in developing countries. Common diseases like diarrhea, respiratory infections, and measles can be fatal for malnourished children. On the other hand, these infections are frequently the main cause of severe malnutrition in children living on a bare subsistence diet, but one that could be adequate for their health if they were not frequently suffering from them. Promotion of nutrition and control of communicable diseases, implemented together, reinforce each other. (From *Guide to Family Health,* Aug.–Sept., 1976. Courtesy of WHO/E. Mandelmann.)

For many households the key question will be how to manage resources in order to secure an adequate food supply through the year or how best to utilize and allocate an inadequate food supply over time and between household members. In some cases, understanding of nutritional requirements is poor and nutrition education is needed. Usually this will be best related to other programs, e.g., community health programs, school and literacy programs, and farmer education. However, not all households, with the resources and the employment opportunities open to them, will be able to provide for themselves adequately and continuously. Thus, the next step concerns the possibilities of social action to provide households with a basis for self-reliance. Clearly, the sorts of actions that might be considered will again vary. Households that have some land may be aided in ways different from those that are landless. But for the most part the problem is one of how to help people so that they are capable of producing their own means of subsistence — that is, how to direct to them the resources and employment opportunities that will enable them to feed themselves.

Whatever the need, it will almost certainly be necessary to examine the specific situations in which malnutrition becomes manifest in order to see what can be done. But there are, nevertheless, measures that can be applied not to specific groups of people but to whole communities or to large sections of the population. Where people eat purchased, centrally processed foods—flour, sugar, salt, tea — it is possible to fortify these with vitamins and minerals if there is a demonstrated need to do so (i.e., if specific deficiency diseases such as anemia, rickets, goiter, and so on are prevalent).

The cost of adding iodine to salt, for example, is very low. Such programs can be very effective. A comprehensive world review of endemic goiter in 1960 produced an estimate of 200 million people suffering from this disease.

Protein-calorie deficiencies are not readily tackled by such means, however. Generally, the diets that people traditionally eat, in the quantities traditionally eaten, provide enough of both protein and energy. When protein-calorie malnutrition (PCM) is a problem among people eating traditional diets, it is usually because people are not eating enough to meet their energy requirement, and they may not, therefore, be eating enough to meet their protein needs either. When energy intakes are too low, there is usually little value in fortifying to increase protein intake. But there have been such fortification schemes, many of which have been based on the fortification of flour with lysine. Experience with such schemes has been disappointing. In particular, they have not been generally successful or appropriate as measures to reduce PCM. In some cases the malnourished were precisely those who did not purchase flour; or, if the malnourished were calorie-deficient, the improvement in protein quality did not significantly affect their status, or, in many cases, overall diets were found to be neither protein-deficient nor, specifically, lysine-deficient. A recent review by Gershoff[7] of experience with cereal grain enrichment programs claims that they have disappointed expectations and concludes "that we lack considerable fundamental information concerning the etiology of malnutrition in developing countries and that this deficiency will have to be corrected before effective public health nutrition programs which will meet their needs can be developed."

The shortcomings of lysine fortification programs apply in part also to attempts to improve the protein quality or content of food grains through breeding new high-protein or high-lysine varieties. Quite apart from the problems (e.g., increased vulnerability to disease during growth or to pests in storage) and costs (e.g., reduced overall caloric yield, increased requirements of fertilizer) experienced with the utilization of these varieties, there is seldom reason for believing that there is any great value to strengthening cereal protein content in this way. Generally, the protein levels of cereal staples are adequate for adults and even for children above 1 year of age. For weanlings, the characteristics that determine whether or not cereal gruels are nutritionally satisfactory are generally the stickiness and texture of the cereals and therefore the degree of dilution found necessary to get babies to eat. Thus, from the point of view of infant feeding, these are characteristics that should receive the attention of plant breeders. But there may be better ways of approaching this problem than through plant breeding. What can and should be done will need to be determined for each situation.

In the past there have been many feeding programs designed to improve the protein intake of the malnourished. Often these have been based on the use of protein-rich foodstuffs provided as supplements — dried skim milk especially has been the basis of reconstituted milk formulas, of biscuits for distribution to children of preschool and school age, or of weaning foods. Concern for the protein content of these foods may have been exaggerated, and such programs have been criticized for being too expensive for poor country governments to sustain independently, and for inducing new habits that are too expensive for poor people to be encouraged to follow. Above all, they have been said to be unnecessary, since, it is claimed, local, traditional diets offered the cheapest and most acceptable sources and were adequate in protein if sufficient food was eaten to meet calorie requirements. (See, for an example, Table 25–3.) Such arguments need to be reviewed in relation to specific situations, but there are

Table 25–3 AN URBAN CASE HISTORY OF CHILDHOOD MALNUTRITION*

"Maria" was 6 years and 11 months of age and lived with her mother and two older brothers and one older sister. The eldest girl in the family was absent from the home and was employed in another town. The father was 78 years of age and lived apart from the family. The mother, 38 years of age, worked as a laundress and was away from the family from about 7 A.M. until about 8 P.M. each day. Meals for the children who stayed at home were prepared by one or other of the older siblings who had also to purchase the foods. Maria either remained at home all day or was taken to a neighboring household or the day nursery of a religious organization.

Maria was born in a hospital, and the mother had remained well during the pregnancy. She had received no prenatal care. The child was born at full term and was of normal size. Maria was breast-fed for 1 year, with the introduction of solid foods, mainly in the form of rice porridge, at the age of 6 months.

The mother and the four children occupied one room of a building situated in a congested area of Manila. Water had to be brought from a public standpipe. There was no toilet, and excreta had to be disposed of in a garbage can.

The mother said that throughout the first year of life Maria had often suffered from fever, for the treatment of which she obtained medicine from a shop or health center. The nature of the fever was not known to the mother. During her second year Maria continued to have fever, and in this year "pertussis" and "bronchitis" were diagnosed. In the following year, when Maria was 3 years of age, she had frequent attacks of diarrhea. The mother said that Maria's ability to walk had been delayed, so that by the age of 3 years she could only crawl.

During her fourth year she was admitted to hospital because of persistent fever and because her feet were swollen. The clinical diagnosis was kwashiorkor and bronchitis. Her weight on admission was recorded as 7.4 kg, which dropped to 6.6 kg when the edema disappeared. She was discharged from hospital after 46 days; her weight then was 8.8 kg. However, Maria continued to have episodes of fever and diarrhea, which continued up to the time of the present study. She had been admitted again to hospital about a year previously because of diarrhea, no mention being made in the hospital of malnutrition.

When seen at the age of almost 7 years, Maria was unable to talk, and she appeared to have photophobia. She was found to be of healthy appearance although small in stature. Her weight was 14 kg and her height was 88 cm; the national standards were 17.3 kg and 105.3 cm for girls age 7 years. (Maria's weight and height are about the 50th centile value for age 2 to 3 years in the United States and about age 5 years in the Philippines.) Examination of one specimen of feces from Maria showed the presence of *Giardia lamblia* (a zooflagellate associated with diarrhea).

Her habitual diet consisted of wheat bread, coffee, sugar, rice, fish, banana inflorescence (sic), coconut oil, green leaves and stalks, soybean paste, and bean sprouts. Average daily intake at the time of the study was 728 kcal, 22 gm protein, 3.7 mg iron, and 627 IU vitamin A.

Analysis:

To meet the U.S. National Research Council's Recommended Dietary Allowance for her chronological age at her observed weight, her intake should have been 1120 kcal, 16.8 gm protein, and 4.6 mg iron. But in order for her growth to catch up, her allowance should be based on her height-age. These are, for ages 5 years and 3 years, per kg body weight: 90 and 100 kcal and 1.5 and 1.8 gm protein, respectively. A corrective intake for Maria would thus be 1260 to 1400 kcal and 21 to 25 gm protein per day. No matter how the daily allowance is computed, the limiting dietary factor appears to be energy, and the solution is more food. Because her reserves are low, owing to chronically low intake and losses from disease, the additional 500 kcal should come from good quality foods. How probable is that?

*Adapted from Bibera, S. B., et al.: Philippine J. Nutr., *24*:105, 1976.

undoubtedly cases in which the criticisms cited have been valid.

Applied nutrition programs of various kinds* will be necessary in the attempt to cure manifest malnutrition, but malnutrition will continue to be manifest unless the "at risk" population can be reduced. Reducing the "at risk" population will call for measures to improve overall nutrition status of those whose status is marginal, measures to increase the resources of those who have insufficient resources to meet the stresses to which they are exposed, and measures to eliminate or alleviate these stresses. Following the World Food Conference in November 1974,† several countries have taken special steps to institute nutrition surveillance measures, one of the purposes of which is to give early warning of impending crises and the emergence of malnutrition. Such measures are clearly required if floods, droughts, and other natural and

*We have in mind here such programs as mother-child care schemes, school feeding programs, fortification programs, and nutrition education programs.

†See Resolution V of The United Nations World Food Conference, Rome, 1974 (Table 25–4).

Table 25-4 RESOLUTION V OF THE UNITED NATIONS WORLD FOOD CONFERENCE (ROME 1974)

THE WORLD FOOD CONFERENCE,

—*considering* that large numbers of people, particularly the less advantaged in many countries, lack adequate and appropriate food resulting in adverse effects on their health, their development and their ability to learn and work for basic livelihood; whereas overconsumption among the affluent not only impairs their health but also contributes to reducing the food availability for less advantaged groups and furthermore large food resources are used to feed animals,

—*recognizing* that malnutrition is closely linked to widespread poverty and inadequate social and institutional structures, and that its effects are aggravated by infectious diseases and the lack of environmental sanitation; and that increased agricultural production and increased incomes may not by themselves lead to improved nutrition; and that to this end a more just and equitable distribution of food and incomes is essential, among nations as well as within countries among their various social categories,

—*recognizing* that information on food consumption patterns and on their consequences for the nutrition and health status of the majority of the population in developing countries is insufficient and inadequate, and that improved knowledge about how to prevent malnutrition through better use of available food resources, including human milk, is essential,

—*considering* the relationship which often exists between children and mothers, malnutrition and too-close pregnancies,

—*recognizing* that food and nutritional aspects are generally not sufficiently taken into account in the formulation of national development plans,

—*considering* the need for improving nutrition in all countries and that the present consumption patterns of the affluent need not be taken as a model,

RECOMMENDS

1. That all governments and the international community as a whole, in pursuance of their determination to eliminate within a decade hunger and malnutrition, formulate and integrate concerted food and nutritional plans and policies aiming at the improvement of consumption patterns in their socioeconomic and agricultural planning, and for that purpose assess the character, extent and degree of malnutrition in all socioeconomic groups as well as the preconditions for improving their nutritional status;

2. That FAO, in cooperation with WHO, UNICEF, WFP, the World Bank, UNDP and Unesco, assisted by PAG, prepare a project proposal for assisting governments to develop intersectoral food and nutrition plans; this proposal to be communicated to the FAO Council at its mid-1975 session through its Food and Nutrition Policy Committee, and to the governing bodies of the other interested agencies;

3. That governments, with their own resources, supplemented with food, financial and technical assistance from multilateral or bilateral external sources, and in close cooperation with agricultural production programmes, initiate new or strengthen existing food and nutrition intervention programmes, on a scale large enough to cover on a continuing basis a substantial part of the vulnerable groups;

4. That governments include nutrition education in the curricula for educational programmes at all levels and that all concerned in the fields of agriculture, health and general education be appropriately trained to enable them to further the nutrition education of the public within their domains;

5. That governments strengthen basic health, family well-being and planning services and improve environmental conditions, including rural water supplies and the elimination of water-borne diseases; and provide treatment and rehabilitation of those suffering from protein-energy malnutrition;

Table continued on opposite page.

social disasters are to be forestalled and their consequences attenuated. Many countries have long-standing regular procedures to this end,* and the attempt to develop these and to provide international support for countries facing such crises is clearly desirable.

But helping people in emergencies is only one of many things that need to be done, for malnutrition is not associated simply with famines and disasters. Somehow the poor and the vulnerable must be made less poor and more self-reliant. To see this as primarily a matter of raising incomes, however, is to oversimplify and to miss the point of what has to be accomplished. If we attempt to forecast future trends in malnutrition, the most significant feature affecting these trends is likely to be the growth in the number of households with insufficient land from which to feed themselves and without employment and earnings adequate to

*India, for example, has a Famine Code dating from the eighteenth century, which defines administrative duties and procedures for forewarning of disaster and for responding to meet it.

Table 25-4 RESOLUTION V OF THE UNITED NATIONS WORLD FOOD CONFERENCE (ROME 1974) *(Continued)*

6. That governments consider the key role of women and take steps to improve their nutrition, their educational levels and their working conditions; and to encourage them and enable them to breast-feed their children:

7. That governments review special feeding programmes within the context of their food and nutrition strategies to determine the desirability and feasibility of undertaking such new programmes, or improving existing ones, particularly among the vulnerable groups (children, pregnant and nursing mothers), but also for shoolchildren, workers and others; such programmes should promote increased local food production and processing thereby stimulating local initiative and employment and should also include an element of nutrition education;

8. That the international agencies, nongovernmental agencies and countries which are in a position to provide funds and foods for this purpose should provide assistance to governments who will request such aid in order to introduce in the period 1975–76 emergency programmes for supplementary feeding of a substantial number of the malnourished children with due attention to basic health and other essential services for the welfare of all children at risk;

9. That governments should explore the desirability and feasibility of meeting nutrient deficiencies, through fortification of staples or other widely consumed foods, with amino acids, protein concentrates, vitamins and minerals, and that, with the assistance of WHO in cooperation with other organizations concerned, should establish a worldwide control programme aimed at substantially reducing deficiencies of Vitamin A, iodine, iron/folate, Vitamin D, riboflavine, and thiamine as quickly as possible;

10. That FAO, in association with other international and nongovernmental organizations concerned, undertake an inventory of vegetable food resources other than cereals, such as roots, tubers, legumes, vegetables and fruits, including also those from unconventional sources, and that it studies the possibility of increasing their production and consumption, particularly in countries where malnutrition prevails;

11. That governments take action to strengthen and modernize consumer education services, food legislation and food control programmes and the relevant aspects of marketing practices, aiming at the protection of the consumer (avoiding false and misleading information from mass media and commercial fraud), and that they increase their support of the Codex Alimentarius Commission;

12. That the joint FAO/WHO food contamination monitoring programme, in cooperation with UNEP, be further developed in order to provide early information to the national authorities for appropiate action;

13. That a global nutrition surveillance system be established by FAO, WHO and UNICEF to monitor the food nutrition conditions of the disadvantaged groups of the population at risk, and to provide a method of rapid and permanent assessment of all factors which influence food consumption patterns and nutritional status;

14. That governments consider establishing facilities and funds for applied nutrition research related to economic, cultural, social and medical aspects of production, processing, preservation, storage, distribution and utilization of food and that FAO, WHO and UNICEF arrange for an internationally coordinated programme in applied nutritional research including establishing priorities, identifying appropriate research centres and generating the necessary fundings;

15. That governments should associate wherever practicable nongovernmental organizations whose programmes include nutrition-related activities with their nutritional efforts, particularly in the areas of food and nutrition programmes, nutrition education and feeding programmes for the most vulnerable groups.

support their families. In part, this is a consequence of growing populations, but the process of economic development itself tends to displace people from land and, in many countries, the rate of growth of jobs is much less than the rate of growth of the labor force. There is nothing new in this. What is new, however, is that whereas in the past the process promoted massive international migrations, such migrations can no longer occur.

Thus, in the long run, the solution of the problem of malnutrition is to be found not in development itself but in the choice of development strategies that aim, as a prime objective, to absorb people productively on the land or in other employment — especially those who would otherwise be very poor. Unless we succeed in this, the numbers at risk will grow and so also will the prevalence of manifest malnutrition. If we succeed in reducing malnutrition in a way that contributes to improved life expectancy, then we may also make a significant contribution to creating the conditions in which birth rates might be reduced and populations brought into equilibrium.

It should be noted that the ideas just presented differ significantly from the current conventional opinions* about the solution to the world's malnutrition problem. Conventionally, the problem is viewed as a failure of food production to keep pace with the growth of population. The solution is therefore seen in terms of measures to promote food supplies and agricultural development. But attempts to solve the problem of malnutrition by focusing on food supply are misguided.

First, it should be noted that in the last 20 years food supplies have grown faster than population. The increase in malnutrition is ascribable to the increase in the number of people neither contributing to nor having a share of this supply. Moreover, while there has been an extraordinary disturbance of world markets resulting from a period of exceptional demands (by Russia especially), which coincided with unusually low yields, and while there has been a major increase in the price of fuel, the world's markets in grains are once again in equilibrium, with prices only modestly higher than they were before 1972 and with experts predicting that prices will stay more or less constant in the future. What this means is that the experts predict that extra supplies will be forthcoming to meet the growth of demand without forcing costs and prices to rise. Predicted increases in demand, however, are largely the increases in demand expected on behalf of the relatively wealthy. The number of poor and malnourished is expected to grow.

The conventional solutions to the problem involve a massive transfer of technology from rich to poor countries in order to increase food production in the poor countries. To this end attempts are made to mobilize political support for rich countries to give, and poor countries to receive, technical assistance and material aid. While such assistance may help to reduce malnutrition, it is of utmost importance that the measures promoted should succeed in absorbing productively those people who cannot now produce, or afford to buy for themselves, the food that they need. If we do not succeed in this, extra food supplies will have little impact on reducing malnutrition. Indeed, if this is not done, the depression in food prices that would result from substantial increases in supply is likely to cause economic depression and the aggravation of malnutrition in many rural areas.

Recognition of these arguments could lead to the identification of new strategies for rural development and for increasing food supplies. Such strategies, when supplemented with community health programs, could have a major effect on reducing malnutrition. Malnutrition is not inevitable. There is food enough and resources enough to eliminate it now. When this is fully comprehended, when the full consequences of poor nutrition are recognized, and when it is more widely understood what needs to be done in order for people to be adequately fed, we can hope that governments, international agencies, and people will insist upon taking the action necessary to eliminate malnutrition.

In opening the Second World Food Congress (The Hague, 1970), A. H. Boerma,[12] then Director-General of the Food and Agriculture Organization, reminded the delegates of the continued existence of two contrasting worlds:

> There is a world of luxury foods, and another where food is the only luxury known.
>
> There is a world of well-appointed homes, and another where people sleep in rat-infested huts or sprawled in their thousands on city streets.
>
> There are those who are free to speculate—and lose —vast fortunes and those who are enslaved to the moneylender for pitifully small sums.
>
> There are those who live for the end of the working week and those who live in hopes of one beginning.

*See, for example, Hopper[8] and Wortman,[9] or Brown[10] or Borgstrom.[11]

This theme was carried through the World Food Conference convened in Rome in 1974, from which a series of resolutions emerged, calling for specific actions to eliminate hunger and malnutrition within a decade (Table 25–4). So far, little progress has been made in reaching the objective, and the time is half gone. Director-General Boerma[12] has urged that

> As a first step, every effort must be made, every device must be used, to make as many people as possible — both the privileged majorities in the richer countries and the privileged minorities in the poorer ones — realize that development is something which is not just morally desirable but in their own best interests — and, even more, in the interests of their children and their children's children. For what future is there for a world of which by far the larger part is in misery and revolt? How can even the privileged enclaves live at ease surrounded by the constant threat — and the enactment — of violence? Where will the richer countries find the new markets they are now starting to scurry for if the others are too poor to buy from them?
>
> What is required is that people everywhere should see the value, not only to others but also to themselves, of thinking in wider terms than those of their own immediate interests. Although for the majority this would amount to nothing less than an internal political revolution within their own minds, recent history has shown that it can be done and that it can produce successful results. Some of the richer countries of the world have now evolved into welfare states, with elaborate systems of social services. And this was as much the result of common sense as of compassion. What is now needed — only more urgently — is that the same kind of thinking that has prevailed in these societies should be applied to produce similar results in what is now a single world society.
>
> In speaking of the changes that are needed in human attitudes toward development, I have so far been talking about individuals. But that is only part of the story. Equally essential are the changes needed in the attitudes of governments. For the structure of world society and the problems confronting it mean that, except for a handful of multinational corporations, it is only governments that are large enough to bring into play sufficient resources sufficiently fast to make a real impact.

In the words of the 35th President of the United States, John F. Kennedy,* "We have the means, we have the capacity to eliminate hunger from the face of the earth in our lifetime. We need only the will." It did not happen in his lifetime; perhaps it will in yours.

REFERENCES

1. Beaudry-Darismé, M. et al.: J. Can. Diet. Assoc., *35*:274, 1974.
2. Reutlinger, S., and Selowsky, M.: *Malnutrition and Poverty: Magnitude and Policy Options.* World Bank Occasional Papers, No. 23. Baltimore, Johns Hopkins University Press, 1976.
3. Sukhatme, P. V.: *Measurement of Poverty Based on Nutritional Needs.* Proceedings, Indian Agricultural Economics Association Conference, 1977.
4. Payne, P. R.: Review of Reutlinger and Selowsky's article. Food Policy, *2*:164, 1977.
5. U.N. World Food Conference, 1974: Extracts of papers. Reprinted in Food and Nutrition, Vol. *1*, No. *1*, 1975. Rome, FAO.
6. Newell, K. W. (ed.): *Health by the People.* Geneva, WHO, 1975.
7. Gershoff, S. N.: *Evaluation of Cereal Grain Enrichment Programs.* Paper, Western Hemisphere Nutrition Congress, Quebec, Canada, August 15, 1977.
8. Hopper, W. D.: The development of agriculture in developing countries. Sci. Amer., *235*:196, 1976.
9. Wortman, S.: Food and agriculture. Sci. Amer., *235*:30, 1976.
10. Brown, L. R., and Eckholm, R. P.: *By Bread Alone.* New York, Praeger Press, 1974.
11. Borgstrom, G.: *The Food and People Dilemma.* North Scituate, Mass., Duxbury Press, Div. of Wadsworth Publishing Co., 1973.
12. Boerma, A. H.: Keynote Address, Second World Food Congress, The Hague, June, 1970. In *FAO Studies in Food and Population.* FAO Economic and Social Development Ser., No. 1, p. 129. Rome, 1976.

SUPPLEMENTARY READINGS

Abelson, P. H. (ed.): *Food: Politics, Economics, Nutrition and Research. A Special Science Compendium.* Washington, D.C., Amer. Assoc. Adv. Sci., 1975.

Beaton, G., and Swiss, L. D.: Evaluation of the nutritional quality of food supplies: prediction of "desirable" or "safe" protein: caloric ratios. Amer. J. Clin, Nutr., *27*:485, 1974.

*Address to the First World Food Congress, Washington, D.C., 1963.

Berg, A.: *The Nutrition Factor: Its Role in National Development.* Washington, D.C., Brookings Institution, 1973.

Berg, A.: The trouble with triage. *New York Times* Magazine, June 15, 1975, p. 26.

Blaxter, K. L., Chairman: Symposium on Famine. Proc. Nutr. Soc., *34*:159, 1975.

Brown, R. E.: *Starving Children: The Tyranny of Hunger.* New York, Springer Publishing Co., 1977.

Burk, M. C., and Pao, E. M.: *Methodology for Large-scale Surveys of Household and Individual Diets.* U.S. Dept. of Agriculture, Home Econ. Res. Rpt. No. 40, 1976.

Chafkin, S. H., and Berg, A. D.: The innocent bystander: some observations on the impact of international financial forces on nutrition. Ecol. Food Nutr., *4*:1, 1975.

Economic Research Service, USDA: *The World Food Situation and Prospects to 1985.* Foreign Agr. Econ. Rpt. No. 98, 1974.

FAO: *Agricultural Commodity Projections 1970–1980.* Rome, 1971.

FAO: *FAO Studies in Food and Population.* FAO Econ. and Soc. Develop. Ser. No. 1, Rome, 1976.

FAO/WHO: *Food and Nutrition Strategies in National Development.* 9th Rpt. Joint FAO/WHO Expert Committee on Nutrition, FAO Nutrition Meetings Rpt. Ser. No. 56, Rome, 1976.

Food and Agriculture. Scientific American Book. San Francisco, W. H. Freeman, 1976.

Forum: Can we afford to eat? Skeptic, No. 10, 1975.

Freeman, H. E., et al.: Relations between nutrition and cognition in rural Guatemala. Amer. J. Pub. Health, *67*:233, 1977.

Gebre-Medhin, M., and Vahlquist, B.: Famine in Ethiopia—the period 1973–75. Nutr. Rev., *35*:194, 1977.

Gomez, F., Galvan, R. R., Cravioto, J., and Frenk, S.: Malnutrition in infancy and childhood with special reference to kwashiorkor. Adv. Pediatr., *7*:131, 1955.

Gongora, J., and Shaw, D. J.: World Food Programme assistance for supplementary feeding programmes. Food Nutr., *3*(2):15, 1977.

Graves, P. L.: Nutrition and infant behavior: a replication study in the Katmandu Valley, Nepal. Amer. J. Clin. Nutr., *31*:541, 1978.

Gustafson, R. A.: Livestock-grain interdependence: implications for policy. Food Policy Review, U.S. Dept. of Agriculture. Pub. ERS/AFPR—1, 1977, p. 119.

Hakim, P., and Solimano, G.: Nutrition and national development, establishing the connection. Food Policy, *1*:249, 1976.

Hakim, P., and Solimano, G.: *Development, Reform and Malnutrition in Chile.* Cambridge, Mass., MIT Press, 1978.

Hanrahan, C. E., and Kennedy, R. M.: International considerations in the development of domestic agricultural and food policy. U.S. Dept. of Agric. Food Policy Review, Pub. ERS/AFPR–1, 1977, p. 130.

Huang, P-C., Lin, H-T, and Tung, T-C: The change of nutrition status of the civilian Chinese population of Taiwan in the recent 16 years. J. Formosan Med. Assoc., *71*:245, 1972.

Ifekwunigwe, A. E.: Emergency assistance. The nature and organization of disaster relief. Food and Nutrition, *2*:6, 1976.

Johnston, B.: Food, health and population in development J. Econ. Lit., *15*:879, 1977.

Jordan, J., et al.: The 1972 Cuban national child growth study as an example of population health monitoring: design and methods. Ann. Hum. Biol., *2*:153, 1975.

Joy, J. L.: Food and nutrition planning. J. Agric. Econ., *24*:165, 1973.

Joy, J. L., and Payne, P. R.: *Food and Nutrition Planning.* FAO Consultants Rpt. Ser. No. 35. Rome, 1975.

Kloth, T. I., et al.: Sahel nutrition survey, 1974. Amer. J. Epidemiol., *103*:383, 1976.

Kutzner, P. L., and Sullivan, T. X.: *Who's Involved with Hunger. An Organization Guide.* Washington, D.C., American Freedom from Hunger Foundation and World Hunger Education Service, 1976.

May, J. M., and McLellan, D. L.: *Studies in Medical Georgraphy.* Vols. 1–14. New York, Hafner Press, 1962–74.

McLaren, D. S.: *Nutrition in the Community.* New York, John Wiley & Sons, 1976.

Mora, J. O., et al.: Nutrition, health and social factors related to intellectual performance. World Rev. Nutr. Diet., *19*:205, 1974.

Olson, R. E. (ed.): *Protein-Calorie Malnutrition.* New York, Academic Press, 1975.

PAG Working Group: Mass communications in nutrition improvement. PAG Bulletin, *6*:1, 1976.

Pariser, E. R., Wallerstein, M. B., Corkery, C. J., and Brown, N. L.: *Fish Protein Concentrate: Panacea for Protein Malnutrition?* Cambridge, Mass., MIT Press, 1978.

Payne, P. R.: Safe protein-calorie ratios in diets. The relative importance of protein and energy intake as causal factors in malnutrition. Amer. J. Clin. Nutr., *28*:281, 1975.

Popkin, B. M., and Solon, F. S.: Income, time, the working mother and child nutriture. Environ. Child Health, *22*:156, 1976.

Puffer, R. R., and Serrano, C. V.: The role of nutritional deficiency in mortality: Findings of the Inter-American investigation of mortality in childhood. PAHO Scientific Publ. No. 262. Washington, D.C., 1973.

Sharples, J. A., and Walker, R. L.: Grain reserves: price instability and the food supply. Agricultural-Food Policy Review, U.S. Dept. of Agriculture Pub. ERS/AFPR–1, 1977, p. 85.

Sukhatme, P. V.: The calorie gap. Ind. J. Nutr. Dietet., *10*:198, 1973.

Symposium: Impact of infection on nutritional status. Amer. J. Clin. Nutr., *30*:1203, 1977.

Teets, R. M., Jr., et al.: *Guide to American Food Programs.* San Francisco, Food Law Center, California Rural Legal Assistance, 1977.

Waterlow, J. C.: Classification and definition of protein-calorie malnutrition. Brit. Med. J., *3*:566, 1972.

WHO: *Nutritional Surveillance.* Report of the Joint FAO/UNICEF/WHO Expert Committee on Methodology of Nutritional Surveillance. WHO Tech. Rpt. Ser. No. 593. Geneva, 1976.

Whyte, R. O.: *Rural Nutrition in China.* London, Oxford University Press, 1972.

Winikoff, B.: Nutrition and National Policy. Cambridge, Mass., MIT Press, 1978.

Appendix

CONTENTS

Table

Table 1A RECOMMENDED DAILY DIETARY ALLOWANCES,* REVISED 1974, FOOD AND NUTRITION BOARD, NATIONAL ACADEMY OF SCIENCES–NATIONAL RESEARCH COUNCIL, DESIGNED FOR THE MAINTENANCE OF GOOD NUTRITION OF PRACTICALLY ALL HEALTHY PEOPLE IN THE U.S.A.

	Age (years)	*Weight*		*Height*				*Fat-Soluble Vitamins*			
								Vitamin A Activity		Vitamin D	Vitamin E Activity¶
	From up to	(kg)	(lbs)	(cm)	(in)	*Energy* (kcal)†	*Protein* (gm)	RE)‡	(IU)	(IU)	(IU)
Infants	0.0–0.5	6	14	60	24	kg × 117	kg × 2.2	420§	1400	400	4
	0.5–1.0	9	20	71	28	kg × 108	kg × 2.0	400	2000	400	5
Children	1–3	13	28	86	34	1300	23	400	2000	400	7
	4–6	20	44	110	44	1800	30	500	2500	400	9
	7–10	30	66	135	54	2400	36	700	3300	400	10
Males	11–14	44	97	158	63	2800	44	1000	5000	400	12
	15–18	61	134	172	69	3000	54	1000	5000	400	15
	19–22	67	147	172	69	3000	54	1000	5000	400	15
	23–50	70	154	172	69	2700	56	1000	5000		15
	51+	70	154	172	69	2400	56	1000	5000		15
Females	11–14	44	97	155	62	2400	44	800	4000	400	12
	15–18	54	119	162	65	2100	48	800	4000	400	12
	19–22	58	128	162	65	2100	46	800	4000	400	12
	23–50	58	128	162	65	2000	46	800	4000		12
	51+	58	128	162	65	1800	46	800	4000		12
Pregnant						+300	+30	1000	5000	400	15
Lactating						+500	+20	1200	6000	400	15

*The allowances are intended to provide for individual variations among most normal persons as they live in the United States under usual environmental stresses. Diets should be based on a variety of common foods in order to provide other nutrients for which human requirements have been less well defined. See text for more detailed discussion of allowances and of nutrients not tabulated.

†Kilojoules (KJ) = 4.2 × kcal.

‡Retinol equivalents.

§Assumed to be all as retinol in milk during the first six months of life. All subsequent intakes are assumed to be one-half as retinol and one-half as β-carotene when calculated from international units. As retinol equivalents, three-fourths are as retinol and one-fourth as β-carotene.

¶Total vitamin E activity, estimated to be 80 percent as α-tocopherol and 20 percent other tocopherols. See text for variation in allowances.

Table 1A RECOMMENDED DAILY DIETARY ALLOWANCES,* REVISED 1974, FOOD AND NUTRITION BOARD, NATIONAL ACADEMY OF SCIENCES–NATIONAL RESEARCH COUNCIL, DESIGNED FOR THE MAINTENANCE OF GOOD NUTRITION OF PRACTICALLY ALL HEALTHY PEOPLE IN THE U.S.A.—(*Continued*)

Water-Soluble Vitamins							*Minerals*					
Ascorbic Acid (mg)	Folacin** (μg)	Niacin†† (mg)	Riboflavin (mg)	Thiamin (mg)	Vitamin B_6 (mg)	Vitamin B_{12} (μg)	Calcium (mg)	Phosphorus (mg)	Iodine (μg)	Iron (mg)	Magnesium (mg)	Zinc (mg)
35	50	5	0.4	0.3	0.3	0.3	360	240	35	10	60	3
35	50	8	0.6	0.5	0.4	0.3	540	400	45	15	70	5
40	100	9	0.8	0.7	0.6	1.0	800	800	60	15	150	10
40	200	12	1.1	0.9	0.9	1.5	800	800	80	10	200	10
40	300	16	1.2	1.2	1.2	2.0	800	800	110	10	250	10
45	400	18	1.5	1.4	1.6	3.0	1200	1200	130	18	350	15
45	400	20	1.8	1.5	2.0	3.0	1200	1200	150	18	400	15
45	400	20	1.8	1.5	2.0	3.0	800	800	140	10	350	15
45	400	18	1.6	1.4	2.0	3.0	800	800	130	10	350	15
45	400	16	1.5	1.2	2.0	3.0	800	800	110	10	350	15
45	400	16	1.3	1.2	1.6	3.0	1200	1200	115	18	300	15
45	400	14	1.4	1.1	2.0	3.0	1200	1200	115	18	300	15
45	400	14	1.4	1.1	2.0	3.0	800	800	100	18	300	15
45	400	13	1.2	1.0	2.0	3.0	800	800	100	18	300	15
45	400	12	1.1	1.0	2.0	3.0	800	800	80	10	300	15
60	800	+2	+0.3	+0.3	2.5	4.0	1200	1200	125	18+‖	450	20
80	600	+4	+0.5	+0.3	2.5	4.0	1200	1200	150	18	450	25

**The folacin allowances refer to dietary sources as determined by *Lactobacillus casei* assay. Pure forms of folacin may be effective in doses less than one-fourth of the RDA.

††Although allowances are expressed as niacin, it is recognized that on the average 1 mg of niacin is derived from each 60 mg of dietary tryptophan.

‖This increased requirement cannot be met by ordinary diets, therefore the use of supplemental iron is recommended.

Table 1B COMPARATIVE DIETARY STANDARDS OF SELECTED COUNTRIES*

Country	*Sex*	*Age (years)*	*Weight (kg)*	*Activity*	*Energy (Kcal)*	*Protein (gm)*	*Calcium (gm)*	*Iron (mg)*	*Vitamin A Activity (IU)*	*Thiamin (mg)*	*Riboflavin (mg)*	*Niacin Equiv. (mg)*	*Vitamin C (mg)*
U.S.A.	M	22	70	*	2800	65	0.8	10	5000	1.4	1.7	18	60
	F	22	58	*	2000	55	0.8	18	5000	1.0	1.5	13	55
Australia	M	25	70	*	2900	70	0.4–0.8	10	2500	1.2	1.5	18	30
	F	25	58	*	2100	58	0.4–0.8	10	2500	0.8	1.1	14	30
Canada (1975)†	M	19–35	70	*	3000	56	0.8	10	5000	1.5	1.8	20	30
	F	19–35	56	*	2100	41	0.7	14	4000	1.1	1.3	14	30
Central America and	M	25	55	Moderate	2700	65	0.45	10	*	1.1	1.6	17.8	60
Panama	F	25	50	activity	2000	60	0.45	10	*	0.8	1.2	13.2	50
Colombia	M	20–29	65	Moderate	2850	68	0.5	10	5000	1.1	1.7	13.8	50
	F	20–29	55	activity	1900	60	0.5	15	5000	0.8	1.1	12.5	50
France	M		65	Moderate	3000	90							
	F		55	activity	2400	75							
India	M	25.4	55	Moderate	2800	55							
	F	21.5	45	activity	2300	45							
Japan‡	M	26–29	56	Moderate	3000	70	0.6	10	2000	1.5	1.5	15	65
	F	26–29	49	activity	2400	60	0.6	10	2000	1.2	1.2	12	60
Netherlands	M	20–29	70	Light	3000	70	1.0	10	5500	1.2	1.8	12	50
	F	20–29	60	activity	2400	60	1.0	12	5500	1.0	1.5	10	50
Norway	M	25	70	None	3400	70	0.8	12	2500	1.7	1.8	17	30
	F	25	60	given	2500	60	0.8	12	2500	1.3	1.5	13	30
Philippines	M	None	53	Moderate	2400	53	0.5	*	5000	1.2	1.2	*	70
	F	Specified	46	activity	1800	46	0.5	*	5000	0.9	0.9	*	70
S. Africa	M	None	73	Moderate	3000	65	0.7	9	4000	1.0	1.6	15	40
	F	Specified	60	activity	2300	55	0.6	12	4000	0.8	1.4	12	40
U.K.	M	20 up	65	Medium	3000	87	0.8	12	5000	1.2	1.8	12	20
	F	20 up	56	activity	2500	73	0.8	12	5000	1.0	1.5	10	20
U.S.S.R.	M			Moderate					5000	2.0	2.5	15	70
	F			activity					5000	2.0	2.5	15	70
E. Germany	M	18–35		Light	2700	85	0.8	10	5000	1.6	1.5	18	70
	F	18–35		work	2300	75	0.8	15	5000	1.4	1.3	15	70
W. Germany	M	25	72	Sedentary	2550	72	0.8	10	5000	1.7	1.8	18	75
	F	25	60	activity	2200	60	0.8	12	5000	1.5	1.8	14	75

*For all footnotes, see original table in Food and Nutrition Board: *Recommended Dietary Allowances.* Publ. 1694. 7th Ed. Washington, D.C., National Academy of Sciences, 1968, pp. 69–71. Also see Trusswell, A. S.: A comparative look at recommended nutrient intakes. Proc. Nutr. Soc. (U.K.), 35:1, 1976 for some more recent values.

†Canadian values corrected to 1975 values (see Table 1D).

‡For revised values (Japan), see Japan. J. Nutr., *34*:51, 1976.

Table 1C FAO/WHO RECOMMENDED INTAKES OF SELECTED NUTRIENTS*

RECOMMENDED DAILY INTAKES OF VITAMIN C, VITAMIN D, VITAMIN B-12, AND FOLACIN

		Vitamin C (mg)	*Vitamin D*[2] *(μg)*[3]	*Vitamin B-12 (μg)*	*Folacin (μg)*
Infants	0– 6 months[1]	20	10	0.3	40
	7–12 months	20	10	0.3	60
Children,	1– 3 years	20	10	0.9	100
	4– 6 years	20	10	1.5	
	7– 9 years	20	2.5	1.5	
	10–12 years	20	2.5	2.0	
Boys, Girls	13–19 years	30	2.5	2.0	200
Adults,	men, women	30	2.5	2.0	200
	pregnancy	50[4]	10[4]	3.0	400
	lactation	50	10	2.5	300

[1]It is accepted that for infants aged 0–6 months breast-feeding by a well-nourished mother is the best way to satisfy the requirements of vitamin C, vitamin B-12 and folacin, but not of vitamin D.

[2]Adequate exposure to sunlight may partially or totally replace dietary vitamin D.

[3]2.5 μg of cholecalciferol are equivalent to 100 IU of vitamin D.

[4]For 2nd and 3rd trimesters.

*From FAO/WHO: *Requirements of Ascorbic Acid, Vitamin D, Vitamin B_{12}, Folate, and Iron.* WHO Technical Report Series No. 452. Geneva, WHO, 1970. Also see *Handbook of Human Nutritional Requirements,* Geneva, WHO, 1974 for a discussion of those values.

Table 1C— *(Continued)* RECOMMENDED DAILY INTAKES OF IRON

		Recommended Intake According to Type of Diet		
		LESS THAN 10% OF CALORIES FROM ANIMAL FOODS (mg)	10–25% OF CALORIES FROM ANIMAL FOODS (mg)	MORE THAN 25% OF CALORIES FROM ANIMAL FOODS (mg)
Infants,	0– 4 months	[1]	[1]	[1]
	5–12 months	10	7	5
Children,	1–12 years	10	7	5
Boys,	13–16 years	18	12	9
Girls,	13–16 years	24	18	12
Adults,	men	9	6	5
	nonmenstruating women	28	19	14
	menstruating women; pregnancy; lactation	See original source, p. 52		

[1] Breast-feeding is assumed to be adequate.

Table 1C– *(Continued)* FAO/WHO RECOMMENDED INTAKES OF SELECTED NUTRIENTS*

RECOMMENDED DAILY INTAKES OF THIAMIN, RIBOFLAVIN, AND NIACIN*

Age	*Thiamin (mg)*	*Riboflavin (mg)*	*Niacin[1] Equivalents (mg)*
0–6 months[2]	–	–	–
7–12 months	0.4	0.6	6.6
1 year	0.5	0.6	7.6
2 years	0.5	0.7	8.6
3 years	0.6	0.8	9.6
4–6 years	0.7	0.9	11.2
7–9 years	0.8	1.2	13.9
10–12 years	1.0	1.4	16.5
13–15 (boys)	1.2	1.7	20.4
(girls)	1.0	1.4	17.2
16–19 (boys)	1.4	2.0	23.8
(girls)	1.0	1.3	15.8
Adults (man)	1.3	1.8	21.1
(woman)	0.9	1.3	15.2

*From FAO/WHO: *Requirements of Vitamin A, Thiamine, Riboflavin, and Niacin.* Geneva, World Health Organization Tech. Rep. Series No. 362, 1967. Recommendations are based on the following intakes per 1000 kcal: thiamin 0.4 mg; riboflavin: 0.55 mg; niacin equivalents: 6.6.

[1]A niacin equivalent is 1 mg niacin or 60 mg L-tryptophan.

[2]For children 0 to 6 months it is accepted that breast-feeding by a well-nourished mother is the best way to satisfy the nutritional requirements for thiamin, riboflavin, and niacin.

Table 1D CANADIAN RECOMMENDED DAILY NUTRIENT INTAKE 1975*

							Water-Soluble Vitamins				
Age	Sex	Weight (kg)	Height (cm)	Energy[a] (kcal)	(M)[b]	Protein (gm)	Thiamin (mg)	Niacin (NE)[f]	Ribo-flavin (mg)	Vitamin B_6[g] (mg)	Folate[h] (μg)
0–6 mo	Both	6	–	kg × 117	kg × 0.49	kg × 2.2(2.0)[e]	0.3	5	0.4	0.3	40
7–11 mo	Both	9	–	kg × 108	kg × 0.45	kg × 1.4	0.5	6	0.6	0.4	60
1–3 yrs	Both	13	90	1400	5.9	22	0.7	9	0.8	0.8	100
4–6 yrs	Both	19	110	1800	7.5	27	0.9	12	1.1	1.3	100
7–9 yrs	M	27	129	2200	9.2	33	1.1	14	1.3	1.6	100
	F	27	128	2000	8.4	33	1.0	13	1.2	1.4	100
10–12 yrs	M	36	144	2500	10.5	41	1.2	17	1.5	1.8	100
	F	38	145	2300	9.6	40	1.1	15	1.4	1.5	100
13–15 yrs	M	51	162	2800	11.7	52	1.4	19	1.7	2.0	200
	F	49	159	2200	9.2	43	1.1	15	1.4	1.5	200
16–18 yrs	M	64	172	3200	13.4	54	1.6	21	2.0	2.0	200
	F	54	161	2100	8.8	43	1.1	14	1.3	1.5	200
19–35 yrs	M	70	176	3000	12.6	56	1.5	20	1.8	2.0	200
	F	56	161	2100	8.8	41	1.1	14	1.3	1.5	200
36–50 yrs	M	70	176	2700	11.3	56	1.4	18	1.7	2.0	200
	F	56	161	1900	7.9	41	1.0	13	1.2	1.5	200
51 + yrs	M	70	176	2300[c]	9.6[c]	56	1.4	18	1.7	2.0	200
	F	56	161	1800[c]	7.5[c]	41	1.0	13	1.2	1.5	200
Pregnancy				+300[d]	1.3[d]	+20	+0.2	+2	+0.3	+0.5	+50
Lactation				+500	2.1	+24	+0.4	+7	+0.6	+0.6	+50

*From Health and Welfare Canada: A look at the dietary standard for Canada. *Dispatch*, No. 39, Feb. 1976.
[a]Recommendations assume characteristic activity pattern for each age group.
[b]Megajoules (10^6 joules). Calculated from the relation 1 kilocalorie = 4.184 kilojoules and rounded to one decimal place.
[c]Recommended energy intake for age 66+ years reduced to 2000 kcal (8.4 MJ) for men and 1500 kcal (6.3 MJ) for women.
[d]Increased energy intake recommended during second and third trimesters. An increase of 100 kcal (418.4 kJ) per day is recommended during the first trimester.
[e]Recommended protein intake of 2.2 gm/kg body wt. for infants age 0–2 mo and 2.0 gm/kg body wt. for those age 3–5 mo. Protein recommendation for infants 0–11 mo assumes consumption of breast milk or protein of equivalent quality.
[f]1 NE (niacin equivalent) is equal to 1 mg of niacin or 60 mg of tryptophan.
[g]Recommendations are based on estimated average daily protein intake of Canadians.
[h]Recommendation given in terms of free folate.

Table 1D CANADIAN RECOMMENDED DAILY NUTRIENT INTAKE 1975*—(*Continued*)

Fat-Soluble Vitamins					*Minerals*					
Vitamin B_{12} (μg)	Vitamin C (mg)	Vitamin A (RE)[j]	Vitamin D (μg cholecalciferol)[k]	Vitamin E (mg d-α-tocopherol)	Calcium (mg)	Phosphorus (mg)	Magnesium (mg)	Iodine (μg)	Iron (mg)	Zinc (mg)
0.3	20[i]	400	10	3	500[m]	250[m]	50[m]	35[m]	7[m]	41[m]
0.3	20	400	10	3	500	400	50	50	7	5
0.9	20	400	10	4	500	500	75	70	8	5
1.5	20	500	5	5	500	500	100	90	9	6
1.5	30	700	2.5[l]	6	700	700	150	110	10	7
1.5	30	700	2.5[l]	6	700	700	150	100	10	7
3.0	30	800	2.5[l]	7	900	900	175	130	11	8
3.0	30	800	2.5[l]	7	1000	1000	200	120	11	9
3.0	30	1000	2.5[l]	9	1200	1200	250	140	13	10
3.0	30	800	2.5[l]	7	800	800	250	110	14	10
3.0	30	1000	2.5[l]	10	1000	1000	300	160	14	12
3.0	30	800	2.5[l]	6	700	700	250	110	14	11
3.0	30	1000	2.5[l]	9	800	800	300	150	10	10
3.0	30	800	2.5[l]	6	700	700	250	110	14	9
3.0	30	1000	2.5[l]	8	800	800	300	140	10	10
3.0	30	800	2.5[l]	6	700	700	250	100	14	9
3.0	30	1000	2.5[l]	8	800	800	300	140	10	10
3.0	30	800	2.5[l]	6	700	700	250	100	9	9
+1.0	+20	+100	+2.5[l]	+1	+500	+500	+25	+15	+1[n]	+3
+0.5	+30	+400	+2.5[l]	+2	+500	+500	+75	+25	+1[n]	+7

[i]Considerably higher levels may be prudent for infants during the first week of life to guard against neonatal tyrosinemia.

[j]1 RE (retinol equivalent) corresponds to a biological activity in humans equal to 1 μg retinol (3.33 IU) or 6 μg β-carotene (10 IU).

[k]One μg cholecalciferol is equivalent to 1 μg ergocalciferol (40 IU vitamin D activity).

[l]Most older children and adults receive vitamin D from irradiation, but 2.5 μg daily is recommended. This intake should be increased to 5.0 μg daily during pregnancy and lactation and for those confined indoors or otherwise deprived of sunlight for extended periods.

[m]The intake of breast-fed infants may be less than the recommendation but is considered to be adequate.

[n]A recommended total intake of 15 mg daily during pregnancy and lactation assumes the presence of adequate stores of iron. If stores are suspected of being inadequate, additional iron as a supplement is recommended.

INTRODUCTORY NOTES FOR TABLE 2

Values for foods and nutrients are taken mainly from Adams, C.F.: *Nutritive Value of American Foods in Common Units.* U.S.D.A. Agriculture Handbook No. 456, 1975, updated, as available, from revised U.S.D.A. Handbook No. 8 (Vols. I and II, 1976). The following are primary sources used for values not included in those Handbooks:

Magnesium: Watt, B.K., and Merrill, A.L.: *Composition of Foods–Raw, Processed, Prepared.* U.S.D.A. Agriculture Handbook No. 8, 1963.

Zinc: Murphy, E.W., Willis, B.W., and Watt, B.K.: Provisional tables on the zinc content of foods. J. Amer. Dietet. Assoc., *66*:345, 1975; Freeland, J.H., and Cousins, R.J.: Zinc content of selected foods. J. Amer. Dietet. Assoc., *68*:526, 1976.

Copper: Pennington, J.T. and Calloway, D.H.: Copper content of foods. J. Amer. Dietet. Assoc., *63*:143, 1973.

Vitamin B-6, pantothenic acid, and vitamin B-12: Orr, M.L.: *Pantothenic Acid, Vitamin B-6 and Vitamin B-12 in Foods.* U.S.D.A. Home Econ. Res. Rpt. No. 36, 1969.

Folacin: Perloff, B.P., and Butrum, R.R.: Folacin in selected foods. J. Amer. Dietet. Assoc., *70*:161, 1977; Hoppner, K., Lampi, B., and Perrin, D.E.: The free and total folate activity in foods available in the Canadian market. Can. Instit. Food Sci. Tech. J., *5*:60, 1972; Hurdle, A.D.F., Barton, D., and Searles, I.H.: A method for measuring folate in foods and its application to a hospital diet. Am. J. Clin. Nutr., *21*:1202, 1968; Toepfer, E.W., Zook, E.G., Orr, M.L., and Richardson, L.R.: *Folic Acid Content of Foods.* U.S.D.A. Agriculture Handbook No. 29, 1951.

A few values were abstracted from Pennington, J.A.: *Dietary Nutrient Guide.* Westport, Conn., Avi Publishing Co., 1976, and from Church, C.F., and Church, H.N.: *Bowes and Church's Food Values of Portions Commonly Used.* 12th Ed., Philadelphia, J.B. Lippincott Co., 1975.

Values for some commercial foods were taken from information published by manufacturers for professional use. This information did not generally include data on the lesser studied nutrients, and in many cases we have assigned values to these from counterpart items.

We have provided information on some food combinations that are widely used (sandwiches, salads). Data represent our summation of ingredients or values given by fast-food purveyors.

Most values have been rounded because these figures are, at best, merely representative of foods typically consumed. The exact nutrient yield is affected by serving size, variety and breed, animal diets and plant fertilizers, environmental factors, and conditions of processing, storage, and the like. The data provided here should be used with this in mind.

Notes and a supplementary reading list are found at the end of Table 2.

NOTES FOR TABLE 2

[1] Symbols used are: tr=trace; u=unknown but thought to be present; 0=absent or below detection limit.
[2] In bleached asparagus, vitamin A activity is 80 IU.
[3] All canned foods listed, except fruits, have salt added according to commercial practice, unless otherwise noted.
[4] Guiness stout; value for American beer is unknown.
[5] Made with yellow maize-corn meal.
[6] Sara Lee, information mainly from manufacturer.
[7] Based on green variety.
[8] If added, approximately 1400 IU vitamin A and approximately 10 mg vitamin C per 1 oz portion.
[9] Yellow variety; white products have essentially no vitamin A activity.
[10] Campbell's, information mainly from manufacturer.
[11] No salt added.
[12] Vitamin A–fortified fluid milk has 500 IU per cup.
[13] Buttermilk has 320 mg sodium per cup.
[14] McDonald's, information mainly from manufacturer.
[15] Red Barn, information mainly from manufacturer.
[16] Total folacin.
[17] Franco American, information mainly from manufacturer.
[18] Aunt Jemima, information mainly from manufacturer.
[19] Unless recipe includes milk or eggs.

SUPPLEMENTARY READING FOR TABLE 2

FAO: *Amino Acid Content of Foods and Biological Data on Proteins.* FAO Nutritional Study No. 24. Rome, 1970.

Paul, A.A., and Southgate, D.A.T.: *McCance and Widdowson's The Composition of Foods.* 4th rev. ed. London, HMSO, 1978.

Posati, L.P., Kinsella, J.E., and Watt, B.K.: Comprehensive evaluation of fatty acids in foods. I. Dairy products. J. Amer. Dietet. Assoc., *66*:482, 1975.

Watt, B.K., Gebhardt, S.E., Murphy, E.W., and Butrum, R.R.: Food composition tables for the 70's. J. Amer. Dietet. Assoc., *64*:257, 1974.

Yuk, A.W., Chan Chim, Wheeler, E.F., and Leppington, I.M.: Variation in the apparent nutrient content of foods: a study of sampling error. Brit. J. Nutr., *34*:391, 1975.

Food	Weight	Approximate Measure	Energy	Protein	Fat	Total Carbo-hydrate	Minerals								Vitamins								
	gm		Kcal	gm	gm	gm	Calcium mg	Phos-phorus mg	Mag-nesium mg	Sodium mg	Potas-sium mg	Zinc mg	Copper mg	Iron mg	Total Vitamin A Activity IU	Thia-min mg	Ribo-flavin mg	Niacin mg	Vitamin B-6 mg	Panto-thenic Acid mg	Folacin (free) mcg	Vitamin B-12 mcg	Vitamin C mg
Almonds, chopped	15	12–15 nuts, 2 tbsp	90	3.0	8.0	3	35	75	40	1	115	0.2	0.1	0.7	0	0.04	0.1	0.5	0.02	0.07	5	0	tr
Apples, raw with skin	150	1 medium 3/lb	80	0.3	0.8	20	10	15	10	1	150	0.08	0.1	0.4	100	0.04	0.03	0.1	0.04	0.2	5	0	6
Apple juice, canned, no sugar added	125	1/2 c	60	0.1	tr	15	10	10	5	1	125	0.04	.01	0.6	u	0.01	0.02	0.1	0.04	0.1	1	0	1
Applesauce, sweetened	125	1/2 c	120	0.3	0.1	30	5	5	5	3	100	0.1	.01	0.6	50	0.03	0.01	tr	0.04	0.1	1	0	1
Apricots																							
Fresh	100	2–3 medium	50	1.0	0.2	13	15	25	10	1	280	0.04	0.1	0.5	2700	0.03	0.04	0.6	0.07	0.2	u	0	10
Canned, heavy syrup	120	4 halves, 2 tbsp juice	100	0.7	0.1	25	15	20	10	1	235	0.04	0.1	0.4	2000	0.02	0.02	0.5	0.06	0.1	u	0	5
water pack	100	4 halves, 2 tbsp juice	40	0.7	0.1	10	10	15	10	1	245	0.03	0.1	0.3	1800	0.02	0.02	0.4	0.06	0.1	u	0	4
Dried, sulfured, raw	30	4–6 medium halves	80	1.5	0.2	20	20	30	20	1	295	0.04	0.1	1.7	3300	tr	0.05	1.0	0.05	0.2	3	0	4
Apricot nectar, canned	125	1/2 c	70	0.4	0.1	18	10	15	5	tr	190	u	u	0.3	1200	0.01	0.01	0.3	0.04	0.10	u	0	4
Artichokes, French, boiled	120	1 large (300 g as purchased)	30	3.0	0.2	12	60	85	u	35	360	0.4	0.4	1.3	200	0.08	0.05	0.8	0.30	0.60	u	0	10
Asparagus,[2]																							
Fresh, green, cooked	100	1/2 c cut, 6–7 spears	20	2.0	0.2	4	20	50	15	1	185	0.3	0.1	0.6	900[2]	0.2	0.2	1.5	0.2	0.6	60	0	25
Canned, salt added[3]	100	1/2 c cut, 6–7 spears	20	2.0	0.4	3	20	50	15	235	165	0.8	0.1	1.9	800[2]	0.06	0.1	0.8	0.06	0.2	25	0	15
Avocados	125	1/2 fruit, 4 in long	190	2.0	18.0	7	10	45	55	5	680	0.5	0.5	0.7	350	0.1	0.2	2.0	0.4	1.1	40	0	15
Baby foods																							
Dinners	130	Contents 4½ oz jar																					
beef-noodle			60	3.5	1.5	9	15	35	u	150	205	u	0.1	0.6	790	0.03	0.06	0.6	0.04	0.2	u	0.3	3
beef-vegetable			110	9.5	4.5	8	15	110	u	115	145	u	0.1	1.5	1410	0.09	0.2	2.0	0.10	0.3	4	0.3	3
vegetable-beef-cereal			70	3.5	2.0	10	20	50	u	150	185	u	0.1	1.0	3580	0.04	0.05	1.0	0.05	0.2	u	0.2	1
Fruits and desserts	135	Contents 4¾ oz jar																					
banana-pineapple			110	0.5	0.1	30	30	15	u	10	100	u	0.1	0.3	40	0.01	0.01	0.1	0.06	0.2	1	0.05	3
custard pudding			130	3.0	2.5	25	80	80	u	80	120	u	0.06	0.4	130	0.03	0.2	0.1	0.02	0.3	u	0.2	1
fruit pudding			130	1.5	1.0	30	35	45	u	15	100	u	0.1	0.4	140	0.04	0.07	0.1	0.02	0.2	u	0.08	4
Bacon, broiled, drained	25	2 strips, thick	140	6.5	12.5	1	3	55	5	245	60	1.2	0.1	0.8	0	0.1	0.08	1.0	0.03	0.08	0.1	0.2	0
Bagels	60	4 in diameter	180	6.5	2.0	30	10	50	u	u	u	0.6	0.2	1.3	30	0.15	0.11	1.3	u	u	u	0	0
Bamboo shoots	100	3/4 c	25	2.5	0.3	5	13	60	u	u	530	u	u	0.5	20	0.15	0.07	0.6	u	u	u	0	4

Bananas	120	1 medium	100	1.5	0.2	25	10	30	55	1	440	0.3	0.2	0.8	250	0.06	0.07	0.8	0.6	0.3	25	0	10
Beans																							
Canned, with pork and tomato sauce	130	1/2 c	160	8.0	3.5	25	70	115	35	590	270	1.0	0.2	2.3	150	0.10	0.04	0.8	0.4	0.1	10	0	3
Canned, with pork and sweet sauce	130	1/2 c	190	8.0	6.0	25	80	145	35	485	u	1.0	0.3	3.0	u	0.08	0.05	0.7	0.1	0.1	10	0	3
Lima, fresh or frozen, boiled	85	1/2 c	95	6.5	0.4	17	40	105	55	2	360	0.9	0.4	2.2	250	0.20	0.08	1.0	0.1	0.2	8	0	15
Red, canned	125	1/2 c	120	7.0	0.5	20	35	140	35	4	335	1.0	0.2	2.3	tr	0.06	0.05	0.8	0.4	0.1	10	0	0
Refried	120	1/2 c	230	8.5	12.5	25	50	165	35	340	360	1.0	0.2	2.3	tr	0.30	0.07	0.8	0.2	0.2	20	0	0
Snap, green, fresh or frozen, boiled	65	1/2 c	15	1.0	0.2	3	55	25	15	2	95	0.2	0.08	0.4	350	0.05	0.06	0.3	0.04	0.1	5	0	8
canned	65	1/2 c	15	1.0	0.2	3	55	25	15	150	60	0.2	0.08	1.0	300	0.02	0.04	0.2	0.03	tr	5	0	2
Soybeans, mature, dry, cooked	90	1/2 c (1 oz, dry wt.)	120	10.0	5.0	10	65	160	80	2	490	0.6	0.3	2.5	20	0.20	0.08	0.6	u	u	20	0	0
Bean sprouts. See *Sprouts*.																							
Beef																							
Corned, canned	80	2 slices each, 3 in x 2 in x ¼ in	170	20.0	9.5	0	15	85	20	u	u	2.5	u	3.4	tr	0.02	0.20	3.0	0.08	0.5	2	1.5	0
hash, with potatoes	110	1/2 c	200	10.0	12.5	12	15	75	20	595	220	1.4	u	2.2	tr	0.01	0.10	2.5	0.08	0.6	u	0.8	0
Dried, creamed	120	1/2 c	190	10.0	12.5	9	130	170	40	880	190	1.8	u	1.0	450	0.08	0.20	0.8	0.60	0.7	u	u	1
Hamburger, broiled, lean, 21% fat	85	4/lb, raw wt.	240	20.0	16.5	0	10	160	20	50	220	3.7	0.07	2.6	30	0.07	0.20	4.5	0.4	0.3	3	1.5	0
very lean, 10% fat	85	4/lb, raw wt.	190	23.0	9.5	0	10	195	20	60	260	4.9	0.09	3.0	20	0.08	0.20	5.0	0.4	0.3	3	1.5	0
Roast, chuck, braised	85	3 oz	240	23.0	16.5	0	10	115	20	40	185	3.7	0.07	2.9	30	0.04	0.20	3.5	u	u	3	1.5	0
rib, U.S. choice	85	3 oz	380	17.0	33.5	0	10	160	20	40	190	3.1	0.07	2.2	70	0.05	0.10	3.0	0.3	0.3	3	1.5	0
Steak, broiled																							
round with fat	85	3 oz	220	24.5	13.0	0	10	215	25	60	270	5.0	0.09	3.0	20	0.07	0.20	5.0	0.3	0.4	3	2.2	0
sirloin with fat	85	3 oz	330	20.0	27.0	0	10	160	20	50	220	3.7	0.07	2.5	50	0.05	0.20	4.0	u	u	3	1.5	0
Beef stew, with vegetables	245	1 c	220	15.5	10.5	15	30	185	50	90	615	2.4	0.05	2.9	2400	0.15	0.15	4.7	0.3	0.2	7	1.6	15
Beer	360	12 oz bottle	150	1.0	0	14	20	110	35	25	90	0.1	0.2	tr	0	0.01	0.10	2.0	0.2	0.3	25[4]	0	0
Beet greens, boiled	75	1/2 c	15	1.0	0.2	2	70	20	80	55	240	0.5	0.1	1.4	3700	0.05	0.10	0.2	0.08	0.2	u	0	10
Beets, sliced, canned	85	1/2 c	30	1.0	0.1	8	15	15	15	200	135	0.3	0.1	0.6	20	0.01	0.03	0.1	0.04	0.1	30	0	2
Beverages. See *Carbonated beverages*, individual entries, and Table 3–5, Chapter 3.																							
Biscuits, from mix, enriched	30	1 of 2 in diameter	90	2.0	3.0	15	20	65	5	270	30	0.3	0.09	0.6	tr	0.08	0.07	0.6	0.01	0.1	2	0	0
Blackberries, boysenberries, etc., raw	70	1/2 c	40	0.8	0.6	9	25	15	20	1	120	0.05	0.1	0.6	150	0.02	0.03	0.3	0.04	0.2	2	0	15
Blueberries, raw	70	1/2 c	45	0.5	0.4	11	10	10	4	1	60	0.05	0.08	0.8	80	0.02	0.04	0.4	0.05	0.1	2	0	10
Bokchay. See *Pakchoy*.																							
Brazil nuts, raw	30	6 large nuts	180	4.0	19.0	3	55	195	65	tr	205	1.4	0.4	1.0	tr	0.30	0.03	0.5	0.05	0.1	tr	0	0
Bread																							
Boston brown, canned	45	1 slice, ½ in thick	95	2.5	0.6	20	40	70	u	115	130	u	u	0.9	30	0.05	0.03	0.5	u	u	u	0	0
Corn, from mix	55	2½ in square	180	4.0	6.0	30	135	210	u	265	60	u	u	0.8	150[5]	0.10	0.10	0.8	u	u	u	u	0

Food	Weight	Approximate Measure	Energy	Protein	Fat	Total Carbo-hydrate	Minerals: Calcium	Phos-phorus	Mag-nesium	Sodium	Potas-sium	Zinc	Copper	Iron	Vitamins: Total Vitamin A Activity	Thia-min	Ribo-flavin	Niacin	Vitamin B-6	Panto-thenic Acid	Folacin (free)	Vitamin B-12	Vitamin C
	gm		Kcal	gm	gm	gm	mg	mg	mg	mg	mg	mg	mg	mg	IU	mg	mg	mg	mg	mg	mcg	mcg	mg
Bread, continued																							
Cracked wheat	25	1 slice	65	2.2	0.6	13	20	30	10	130	35	0.3	0.05	0.3	tr	0.03	0.02	0.3	0.02	0.2	3	0[19]	0
French, Vienna, Italian, enriched	25	1 slice	70	2.3	0.8	14	10	20	5	145	20	0.5	0.09	0.6	0	0.07	0.06	0.6	0.02	0.1	3	0	0
Fry bread, Indian, enriched	60	1 piece, medium	200	4.0	7.5	28	80	50	u	305	35	u	u	1.0	0	0.10	0.09	1.3	0.02	0.2	10	0	0
Raisin, not enriched	25	1 slice	65	1.5	0.7	13	20	20	5	90	60	0.3	0.05	0.3	tr	0.01	0.02	0.2	0.01	0.1	3	0[19]	0
Rye, American	25	1 slice	65	2.5	0.3	13	15	40	10	140	35	0.4	0.05	0.4	0	0.05	0.02	0.4	0.02	0.1	2	0	0
White, not enriched	25	1 slice	70	2.2	0.8	13	20	25	5	130	25	0.2	0.05	0.2	tr	0.02	0.02	0.3	0.01	0.1	3	0[19]	0
enriched	25	1 slice	70	2.2	0.8	13	20	25	5	130	25	0.2	0.05	0.6	tr	0.06	0.05	0.6	0.01	0.1	3	0[19]	0
Whole-wheat	25	1 slice	65	2.5	0.8	12	25	60	10	130	70	0.4	0.05	0.8	tr	0.06	0.03	0.7	0.04	0.2	9	0[19]	0
Broccoli, fresh or frozen, boiled	85	1/2 c	20	2.5	0.2	4	70	50	15	8	205	0.2	0.07	0.6	1900	0.07	0.20	0.6	0.1	0.4	20	0	70
Brussels sprouts, fresh or frozen, boiled	85	4 large sprouts	30	3.5	0.3	5	25	60	15	8	230	0.3	0.08	0.9	440	0.07	0.12	0.7	0.4	1.1	15	0	70
Butter, salted	5	1 tsp or pat (90/lb)	35	tr	4.0	tr	1	1	tr	40	1	tr	0	tr	150	tr	tr	tr	0	0	0	tr	0
	15	1 tbsp	100	0.1	11.5	0.1	3	3	tr	120	3	tr	0	tr	450	tr	tr	tr	0	0	0	tr	0
Cabbage, green, headed																							
Raw, shredded	70	1 c	17	0.9	0.1	4	35	20	10	15	165	0.3	0.08	0.3	90	0.04	0.04	0.2	0.1	0.1	20	0	35
Cooked, chopped	70	1/2 c	15	0.8	0.2	3	30	15	10	10	120	0.3	0.02	0.2	100	0.03	0.03	0.2	0.09	0.1	2	0	25
Cakes																							
Angel food	40	2 in sector of 10 in cake	105	2.5	0.1	25	40	50	10	60	25	0.1	0.02	0.1	0	tr	0.04	tr	tr	0.08	1	tr	0
Cheese cake, frozen[6]	85	1/10 of cake	225	6.5	12.5	24	80	80	30	170	90	u	0.04	0.5	200	0.05	0.1	0.3	u	u	u	u	tr
Chocolate, with chocolate icing	90	2 in sector of 8 in cake	310	4.0	11.5	55	55	95	20	240	120	1.1	0.3	0.7	150	0.03	0.07	0.3	0.07	0.4	3	0.1	0
Gingerbread	65	2¾ in square	170	2.0	4.5	30	55	65	u	190	175	u	u	1.0	tr	0.02	0.06	0.5	u	u	u	u	0
Cupcake, iced	50	1 medium	190	2.0	6.0	30	60	95	u	160	55	u	u	0.4	80	0.02	0.05	0.1	u	u	u	u	0
Pound cake	30	3½ in x 3 in x ½ in	140	1.5	9.0	14	6	25	5	35	20	0.2	0.02	0.2	80	0.01	0.03	0.1	0.01	0.09	2	u	0
Yellow with chocolate icing	70	2 in sector of 8 in cake	230	3.0	8.0	40	65	125	15	160	75	0.3	0.07	0.4	100	0.01	0.06	0.1	0.03	0.2	2	u	0
Candy																							
Caramels	30	1 oz	120	1.0	3.0	20	40	35	u	65	55	u	0.01	0.4	tr	0.01	0.05	0.1	tr	0	u	u	0
Chocolate bar																							
plain milk chocolate	30	1 oz	140	2.0	9.0	16	65	65	20	25	110	0.1	0.3	0.3	80	0.02	0.10	0.1	tr	0.03	1	u	0
with almonds	30	1 oz	150	2.5	10.0	14	65	75	u	25	125	0.1	u	0.5	70	0.02	0.10	0.2	tr	u	1	u	0
Fudge with nuts	30	1 oz	120	1.0	5.0	20	20	30	u	50	50	u	u	0.3	tr	0.01	0.03	0.1	u	u	u	tr	0
Hard	30	1 oz	110	0	0.3	30	6	2	u	10	1	u	0.03	0.5	0	0	0	0	0	0	0	0	0
Marshmallow	30	1 oz, 4 large	90	0.6	tr	25	5	2	u	10	2	0.01	0.06	0.5	0	0	tr	tr	u	u	0	0	0
Peanut brittle	30	1 oz.	120	1.5	3.0	25	10	25	u	10	45	u	u	0.7	0	0.05	0.01	1.0	u	u	u	0	0
Cantaloupe. See *Melons*.																							
Carbonated beverages sweet	170	6 oz	65	0	0	17	0	0	0	0	0	0	0	0	0	0	0	0	0	0	0	0	0

Carrots																							
Raw	80	1 carrot, 7 1/2 in x 1 1/8 in	30	0.8	0.1	7	25	25	15	35	245	0.3	0.07	0.5	7900	0.04	0.04	0.4	0.1	0.2	10	0	6
Boiled	70	1/2 c diced	20	0.5	0.3	10	25	20	4	25	160	0.2	0.07	0.4	7600	0.04	0.04	0.4	0.02	0.2	2	0	4
Cashews, roasted	30	1 oz	160	5.0	13.0	8	10	105	80	60	130	1.3	0.2	1.1	30	0.1	0.07	0.5	0.1	0.4	2	0	0
Cauliflower																							
Raw	50	1/2 c whole flower buds	15	1.5	0.1	3	10	30	12	5	150	u	0.1	0.6	60	0.1	0.1	0.7	0.1	0.5	15	0	75
Boiled	60	1/2 c	15	1.5	0.2	3	15	25	8	10	130	u	0.1	0.4	40	0.06	0.05	0.4	0.1	0.5	2	0	35
Celery																							
Raw	80	2 large stalks	15	0.8	0.1	3	30	20	17	100	270	u	0.09	0.2	200[7]	0.02	0.02	0.2	0.05	0.3	5	0	8
Boiled	75	1/2 c diced	10	0.6	0.1	2	25	15	u	65	180	u	0.08	0.2	200[7]	0.02	0.02	0.2	0.05	0.3	u	0	4
Cereals, breakfast																							
Ready-to-eat																							
bran flakes, 40% enr.	35	1 c	100	3.5	0.6	30	20	125	u	205	135	1.3	0.4	12.4	0[8]	0.4	0.5	4.0	0.1	0.3	6	0	0[8]
corn flakes, enriched	25	1 c	95	2.0	0.1	20	4	10	4	250	30	0.07	0.03	0.6	0[8]	0.3	0.4	3.0	0.02	0.05	3	0	0[8]
granola	50	1/2 c	215	5.7	9.6	29	30	170	60	3	180	1.0	0.4	1.6	0	0.16	0.08	1.1	0.06	0.45	20	tr	0
rice, puffed, enriched	15	1 c	60	0.9	0.1	13	3	15	u	tr	15	0.2	0.03	0.3	0	0.07	0.01	0.7	0.01	0.06	1	0	0
wheat flakes, enriched	30	1 c	100	3.0	0.5	25	10	85	30	310	80	0.7	0.3	1.1	0[8]	0.4	0.4	3.5	0.09	0.1	3	0	0[8]
wheat, shredded	50	1 c of spn-sized	180	5.0	1.0	40	20	195	65	2	175	1.4	0.4	1.8	0	0.1	0.06	2.0	0.1	0.4	5	0	0
Cooked, 1 oz. dry wt., salt added																							
cornmeal and grits,																							
unenriched	120	1/2 c	60	1.5	0.2	13	1	15	10	130	20	0.1	0.06	0.2	70[9]	0.02	0.01	0.1	0.04	0.2	2	0	0
enriched	120	1/2 c	60	1.5	0.2	13	1	15	10	130	20	0.1	0.06	0.5	70[9]	0.07	0.05	0.6	0.04	0.2	2	0	0
oatmeal	120	1/2 c	65	2.5	1.0	12	10	70	30	260	75	0.6	0.04	0.7	0	0.10	0.02	0.1	0.04	0.4	5	0	0
wheat, farina																							
light, enriched (e.g., Cream of Wheat)	120	1/2 c	50	1.5	0.1	10	5	15	4	175	10	0.07	0.04	0.4	0	0.05	0.04	0.5	0.02	0.1	5	0	0
whole-meal (e.g,. Ralston)	120	1/2 c	55	2.0	0.4	12	10	65	35	260	60	0.6	0.3	0.6	0	0.08	0.02	0.8	0.1	0.2	10	0	0
Chard, Swiss, boiled	70	1/2 c	15	1.5	0.2	2	55	20	45	60	230	u	u	1.3	3900	0.03	0.08	0.3	u	0.1	u	0	0
Cheese																							
Natural																							
blue, Roquefort	30	1 oz	100	6.0	8.0	0.7	150	110	7	395	75	0.8	0.04	0.1	200	0.01	0.1	0.3	0.05	0.5	0.3	0.3	0
cheddar	30	1 oz	115	7.0	9.5	0.4	205	145	8	175	30	0.9	0.04	0.2	300	0.01	0.1	tr	0.02	0.1	0.3	0.2	0
cottage, creamed	110	1/2 c	120	14.0	5.0	3.0	70	150	6	455	95	0.4	0.02	0.2	180	0.02	0.2	0.1	0.2	0.15	15[16]	0.7	0
cream	30	2 tbsp	100	2.0	10.0	0.8	25	30	2	85	35	0.2	0.01	0.3	400	tr	0.06	tr	0.01	0.1	0.2	0.1	0
Parmesan	30	1 oz	130	12.0	8.5	1.0	390	230	15	455	30	0.8	0.1	0.3	200	0.01	0.1	0.1	0.03	0.1	0.3	u	0
Swiss	30	1 oz	110	8.0	8.0	1.0	270	170	10	75	30	1.1	0.04	0.1	250	tr	0.1	tr	0.02	0.1	0.3	0.5	0
Pasturized, processed																							
American	30	1 oz	110	6.0	9.0	0.5	175	210	6	405	45	0.8	0.05	0.1	350	0.01	0.1	tr	0.02	0.1	0.9	0.2	0
cheese spread	30	1 oz	80	4.5	6.0	2	160	200	8	380	70	0.7	u	0.1	200	0.01	0.1	tr	0.03	0.2	u	0.1	0
Cheese fondue	100	2/3 c	260	15.0	18.5	10	320	295	u	540	165	u	0.04	1.2	900	0.06	0.3	0.2	u	u	u	u	0
Cherries																							
Raw, sweet	75	10 cherries	45	0.9	0.2	12	15	15	10	1	130	0.1	0.1	0.3	70	0.03	0.04	0.3	0.02	0.2	4	0	7
Red, canned																							
heavy syrup	130	1/2 c with syrup	100	1.0	0.2	25	20	15	10	2	160	u	0.06	0.4	80	0.02	0.02	0.2	0.06	0.1	tr	0	4
water pack	120	1/2 c with juice	50	1.0	0.2	13	20	15	10	2	160	u	0.06	0.4	80	0.04	0.02	0.2	u	u	tr	0	4

Food	Weight gm	Approximate Measure	Energy Kcal	Protein gm	Fat gm	Total Carbohydrate gm	Minerals								Vitamins								
							Calcium mg	Phosphorus mg	Magnesium mg	Sodium mg	Potassium mg	Zinc mg	Copper mg	Iron mg	Total Vitamin A Activity IU	Thiamin mg	Riboflavin mg	Niacin mg	Vitamin B-6 mg	Pantothenic Acid mg	Folacin (free) mcg	Vitamin B-12 mcg	Vitamin C mg
Chicken																							
Canned, flesh only	100	1/2 c	200	22.5	12.0	0	20	255	20	u	140	2	0.2	1.6	250	0.04	0.1	4.5	0.3	0.8	2	0.8	0
Creamed	120	1/2 c	210	17.5	12.0	7	85	140	u	u	u	u	u	1.1	300	0.04	0.2	4.0	u	u	u	u	tr
Fried																							
breast	95	1/2 breast	160	25.5	5.0	1	9	220	10	u	u	0.8	0.1	1.3	70	0.04	0.2	11.5	0.6	0.8	2	0.4	0
leg	55	1 medium	90	12.0	4.0	0.4	6	90	10	u	u	1.4	0.1	0.9	50	0.03	0.2	2.5	0.3	0.2	3	0.2	0
thigh	65	1 medium	120	15.0	6.0	1	7	120	10	u	u	1.6	0.1	1.2	100	0.03	0.2	3.5	0.4	0.5	3	0.3	0
Roasted, light meat, without skin	100	3½ oz	170	31.5	3.0	0	12	265	u	65	410	0.9	0.1	1.4	60	0.04	0.1	11.5	0.7	0.8	3	0.4	0
Chickpeas or *garbanzos*, cooked without salt	125	1/2 c (30 gm, dry wt.)	110	6.0	1.0	18	45	106	u	10	240	2.7	u	2.1	15	0.1	0.03	0.6	0.2	0.4	7	0	0
Chili con carne, with beans, canned	255	1 c	340	19.0	15.5	30	80	320	65	1355	595	4.2	0.8	4.3	150	0.08	0.20	3.3	0.3	0.4	10	u	tr
Chili powder, chilis. See *Peppers.*																							
Chili relleno (stuffed pepper)	110	1 pepper	190	10.5	14.0	6	225	195	u	465	270	u	u	1.3	1600	0.08	0.2	0.8	0.1	0.7	15	1.0	55
Chocolate, bitter or baking	30	1 oz	140	3.0	15.0	8	20	110	u	1	235	0.7	0.8	1.9	20	0.01	0.07	0.4	0.01	0.06	4	0	0
Sweet, milk. See *Candy.*																							
Chow mein, canned, chicken without noodles	250	1 c	95	6.5	0.3	18	45	85	45	725	420	1.2	0.3	1.3	150	0.05	0.10	1.0	0.4	1.2	10	1.6	15
Clams, canned, with liquid	100	3½ oz, 1/2 c	50	8.0	0.7	3	55	135	115	u	140	1.2	0	4.0	u	0.01	0.1	1.0	0.08	0.3	3	20	u
Cocoa, dry	5	1 tbsp	15	0.9	1.0	3	5	35	20	tr	80	0.3	0.2	0.6	tr	0.01	0.02	0.1	tr	tr	1	0	0
Coconut, dry, unsweetened	30	1 oz	180	2.0	17.5	6	5	50	u	u	160	u	0.2	0.9	0	0.02	0.01	0.2	0.01	0.06	u	0	0
Coffee, instant, regular dry powder	2.5	1 tbsp	3	tr	tr	1	4	10	10	2	80	0.01	0.02	0.1	0	0	0.01	0.8	0.02	u	u	0	0
Collards, boiled	70	1/2 c	20	2.0	0.4	4	110	30	30	35	170	0.5	0.2	0.4	3900	0.1	0.2	0.8	0.1	0.3	25	0	35
Cookies																							
Commercial assortment	35	4 cookies	170	1.5	7.0	25	10	55	5	125	25	0.2	0.05	0.2	30	0.01	0.02	0.1	0.02	0.1	1	0	0
Fig bar	55	4 cookies	200	2.0	3.0	40	45	35	15	140	110	0.6	0.1	0.6	60	0.02	0.04	0.2	0.05	0.2	2	0	tr
Oatmeal with raisins	50	4 cookies	235	3.0	8.0	40	10	55	u	85	190	0.6	0.06	1.5	30	0.06	0.04	0.3	u	u	2	u	tr
Corn, sweet, yellow																							
Fresh or frozen, boiled	80	1/2 c	70	2.5	0.8	15	2	75	25	tr	135	0.3	0.08	0.5	350	0.09	0.08	1.0	0.2	0.3	2	0	6
Canned, whole kernel	80	1/2 c	70	2.0	0.6	16	4	40	15	195	80	0.3	0.05	0.4	300	0.02	0.04	0.8	0.2	0.2	2	0	4
Cream style	130	1/2 c	110	2.5	0.8	25	4	70	25	300	125	0.6	0.08	0.8	400	0.04	0.06	1.5	0.3	0.4	2	0	6

Corn fritter	35	1 fritter 2 in x 1½ in	130	2.5	8.0	14	20	55	u	165	45	u	u	0.6	150	0.06	0.07	0.6	u	u	u	u	tr
Corn syrup	20	1 tbsp	60	0	0	15	10	3	u	15	1	u	0.07	u	0	0	0	0	0	0	0	0	0
Cowpeas or *blackeye peas*																							
Immature	80	1/2 c	90	7.0	0.6	15	20	120	15	1	310	0.6	0.2	1.7	300	0.2	0.09	1.0	0.04	0.2	20	0	15
Mature, dry, cooked	125	1/2c,(1ozdry wt.)	95	6.5	0.4	17	20	120	u	10	285	2.0	0.2	1.6	10	0.2	0.05	0.5	0.07	0.3	20	0	u
Crabmeat	100	1/2 c, packed	100	18.0	2.0	0.6	45	185	u	u	90	4.5	1.0	0.8	2300	0.2	0.08	3.0	0.3	0.6	2	10	2
Crackers																							
Butter (e.g., Ritz)	15	5 round	75	1.1	3.0	11	25	40	u	180	20	u	0.03	0.1	30	tr	tr	0.1	u	u	u	0	0
Graham	15	1 cracker 5 in x 2½ in	55	1.0	1.0	10	5	20	5	95	55	0.2	0.03	0.2	0	0.01	0.03	0.2	0.01	0.08	4	0	0
Rye wafer (e.g., Rykrisp)	15	2 wafers	40	1.5	0.2	10	5	50	u	110	u	u	0.04	0.5	0	0.04	0.03	0.2	u	u	u	0	0
Saltines	10	4 each, 2 in square	50	1.0	1.5	8	2	10	3	125	15	0.05	0.02	0.1	0	tr	tr	0.1	0.01	0.05	2	0	0
Cranberry jelly, or *sauce*, canned	35	1/8 c	50	tr	tr	13	2	1	u	tr	10	tr	u	tr	10	tr	tr	tr	0.01	u	u	0	tr
Cream																							
Half-and-half	60	1/4 c or 4 tbsp	80	2.0	7.0	3	65	55	8	25	80	0.3	0.07	tr	300	0.02	0.08	0.02	0.02	0.2	1	0.2	tr
Heavy, whipping	60	1/4 c; 1/2 c whipped vol	210	1.0	22.0	2	45	35	4	20	45	0.1	0.06	tr	850	0.01	0.08	0.02	0.01	0.2	0.6	0.1	tr
Light, for coffee	60	1/4 c, 4 tbsp	120	2.0	12.0	2	60	50	5	25	75	0.2	0.06	tr	450	0.02	0.08	tr	0.02	0.2	0.6	0.1	tr
Sour	60	1/4 c, 4 tbsp	130	1.5	11.0	2	60	50	5	25	80	0.2	0.06	tr	450	0.02	0.09	0.05	0.01	0.2	7	0.1	tr
Cream substitutes																							
Coffee whitener	3	1 tsp or packet	15	0.1	0.8	2	1	12	tr	5	20	0.02	u	tr	5	0	0	0	0	0	0	0	0
Whipped topping, frozen	10	2 tbsp	30	0.1	2.5	2	1	1	tr	2	2	tr	u	tr	80	0	0	0	0	0	0	0	0
Cucumber, raw, peeled	80	1/2 small	10	0.4	0.1	2	15	15	5	4	125	0.08	0.04	0.2	tr	0.02	0.03	0.2	0.03	0.2	10	0	8
Custard, baked	130	1/2 c	150	7.0	7.5	15	150	155	u	105	195	u	0.1	0.6	450	0.06	0.2	0.2	u	u	4	u	0
Dandelion greens, boiled	50	1/2 c	20	1.0	0.3	3	75	20	20	25	120	u	u	1.0	6100	0.07	0.08	u	u	u	u	0	10
Dasheen (Japanese taro), raw	100	1 1/3 corms	100	2.0	0.2	25	30	60	u	5	515	u	u	1.0	20	0.1	0.04	1.1	u	u	u	0	4
Dates, dried	80	10, pitted	220	2.0	0.4	60	45	50	45	1	520	u	0.2	2.4	40	0.07	0.08	2.0	0.1	0.6	10	0	0
Doughnuts																							
Cake type	40	1 average	160	2.0	8.0	20	15	80	5	210	40	0.2	0.04	0.6	30	0.07	0.07	0.5	0.02	0.2	3	0	0
Yeast, raised	40	1 average	180	2.5	11.0	16	15	30	5	100	35	0.3	0.04	0.6	30	0.07	0.07	0.6	0.02	0.2	4	0	0
Eggnog	250	1 c	340	9.5	19.0	34	330	275	45	140	420	1.1	u	0.5	900	0.08	0.5	0.3	0.1	1.1	2	1.1	3
Eggs, chicken																							
Whole, raw or hard cooked	50	1 large	80	6.0	5.5	0.6	30	90	6	60	65	0.7	0.05	1.0	300	0.04	0.15	tr	0.06	0.9	25	0.6	0
white	33	1 white	15	3.5	tr	0.4	4	4	3	50	45	tr	0.01	tr	0	tr	0.09	tr	tr	0.07	1	0.02	0
yolk	17	1 yolk	65	3.0	5.0	tr	25	85	3	10	15	0.6	0.05	0.9	300	0.04	0.07	tr	0.05	0.9	25	0.6	0
Scrambled	140	2 eggs	190	12.0	14.0	30	95	195	15	310	170	1.4	0.07	1.9	600	0.07	0.30	0.1	0.1	1.8	50	1.3	tr
Eggplant, boiled	100	1/2 c diced	20	1.0	0.2	4	10	20	15	1	150	u	0.1	0.6	10	0.05	0.04	0.5	0.08	0.2	2	0	3

Food	Weight	Approximate Measure	Energy	Protein	Fat	Total Carbo-hydrate	Minerals								Vitamins								
	gm		Kcal	gm	gm	gm	Calcium mg	Phos-phorus mg	Mag-nesium mg	Sodium mg	Potas-sium mg	Zinc mg	Copper mg	Iron mg	Total Vitamin A Activity IU	Thia-min mg	Ribo-flavin mg	Niacin mg	Vitamin B-6 mg	Panto-thenic Acid mg	Folacin (free) mcg	Vitamin B-12 mcg	Vitamin C mg
Enchiladas, beef																							
Frozen, commercial[10]	200	7 oz portion	240	15.0	8.5	25	20	190	u	725	155	u	u	2.5	600	0.1	0.2	3.0	u	u	u	u	u
Home recipe	190	2 enchiladas	365	32.0	16.7	22	450	480	u	510	585	u	u	5	6000	0.1	0.4	6.0	0.8	0.7	10	2	10
Fats, shortening, solid	100	1/2 c	880	0	100.0	0	0	0	0	0	0	0	0	0	0	0	0	0	0	0	0	0	0
or oil	12	1 tbsp	110	0	12.0	0	0	0	0	0	0	0	0	0	0	0	0	0	0	0	0	0	0
Figs, fresh	100	2 medium	80	1.0	0.4	20	35	20	20	2	195	u	0.07	0.6	80	0.06	0.06	0.4	0.1	0.3	u	0	2
Dried	30	2 small	80	1.5	0.4	20	40	25	20	u	190	u	0.08	0.6	20	0.03	0.03	0.2	0.05	0.1	1	0	0
Fish																							
Cod, steak, sautéed	110	4 oz	180	30.0	6.0	0	30	285	30	115[11]	420	0.9	0.2	1.0	200	0.08	0.1	3.0	0.3	0.3	10	0.9	0
Fish sticks, breaded	110	4 sticks	200	19.0	10.0	7	10	190	20	u	u	0.3	0.2	0.4	0	0.04	0.08	2.0	0.06	0.3	10	1.1	0
Haddock, fried	110	4 oz	180	22.0	7.0	6	45	270	30	195[11]	385	1.1	0.2	1.3	u	0.04	0.08	3.5	0.2	0.1	5	1.4	2
Mackerel, sautéed	105	3 average	250	23.0	17.0	0	5	295	30	u	u	1.0	0.2	1.3	550	0.2	0.3	8.0	0.7	0.9	5	9.4	0
Salmon,																							
steak, broiled	145	1 average 6 in x 2 in	230	35.0	9.0	0	u	530	60	150[11]	565	2.4	1.2	1.5	200	0.2	0.08	12.5	1.0	1.9	6	5.8	0
canned, pink	110	1/2 c	160	23.0	6.0	0	215	315	30	425	395	1.0	0.3	0.9	80	0.04	0.2	9.0	0.3	0.6	10	7.6	0
red	110	1/2 c	190	22.0	10.0	0	285	380	30	575	380	1.0	0.3	1.3	250	0.04	0.2	8.0	0.3	0.6	10	7.6	0
Sardines																							
canned in oil	85	3 oz drained	170	20.5	9.0	0	370	425	35	700	500	2.4	0.03	2.4	200	0.03	0.2	4.5	0.2	0.7	10	8.5	0
Sole or flounder, fillet, baked	100	3 oz	200	30.0	8.0	0	25	345	30	235[11]	585	1.0	0.07	1.4	u	0.07	0.08	2.5	0.2	0.8	10	1.2	2
Swordfish, broiled	100	3 oz	170	26.5	6.0	0	25	260	u	u	u	u	u	1.3	2000	0.04	0.05	10.5	u	0.2	u	1.0	0
Tuna, raw	100	1/2 c	135	27.5	3.0	0	5	175	30	35[11]	180	0.5	0.5	1.3	50	0.02	0.05	6.6	0.9	0.5	3	3.0	7
canned in oil	100	1/2 c	200	28.0	8.0	0	10	230	25	u	u	1.0	0.1	1.9	80	0.05	0.1	12.0	0.4	0.3	8	2.2	0
in water	100	1/2 c	130	28.0	0.8	0	15	190	25	865	275	u	u	1.6	80	0.05	0.1	13.0	0.4	0.3	8	2.2	0
Flour, wheat																							
White, all purpose																							
unenriched	115	1 c	420	12.0	1.0	90	20	100	30	2	110	0.8	0.2	0.9	0	0.07	0.06	1.0	0.07	0.5	20	0	0
enriched	115	1 c	420	12.0	1.0	90	20	100	30	2	110	0.8	0.2	3.3	0	0.5	0.3	4.0	0.07	0.5	20	0	0
Whole-grain	120	1 c	400	16.0	2.5	85	50	445	135	4	445	2.9	0.6	4.0	0	0.7	0.1	5.0	0.4	1.3	35	0	0
French toast, frozen[10]	65	1 slice	130	5.0	4.3	18	50	85	u	305	80	u	u	1.3	250	0.1	0.1	0.7	u	u	u	u	0
Frozen dinners																							
Chicken, fried, with potatoes, mixed vegetables	310	11 oz dinner	570	28.0	29.0	48	70	350	60	1075	350	3.0	0.4	3.2	1800	0.2	0.6	16.0	0.9	1.6	20	0.7	10
Meat loaf with tomato sauce, potatoes, peas	310	11 oz dinner	410	25.0	21.0	30	60	365	60	1225	360	3.5	0.5	4.0	1300	0.3	0.4	5.5	0.7	0.9	20	1.1	10
Turkey with gravy, potatoes, peas	310	11 oz dinner	340	25.0	9.0	40	80	260	65	1200	530	3.0	0.4	3.3	400	0.2	0.3	7.0	0.8	1.8	30	0.6	10
Fruit cocktail	130	1/2 c	95	0.5	0.2	25	10	15	40	5	205	u	0.04	0.5	200	0.02	0.02	0.5	0.04	u	u	0	2
Gelatin, dry	8	1 tbsp or packet	30	7.0	0	0	u	u	2	1	u	u	0.1	u	0	0	0	0	0	0	0	0	0
Gelatin dessert, plain	120	1/2 c	70	2.0	0	17	u	u	2	u	u	0.02	0.03	u	0	0	0	0	0	0	0	0	0

Grapefruit, raw	100	1/2 medium	40	0.5	0.1	10	15	15	12	1	130	0.1	0.04	0.4	80	0.04	0.02	0.2	0.03	0.3	8	0	35
Grapefruit juice, canned																							
Unsweetened	180	3/4 c	75	0.9	0.2	18	15	25	22	2	300	u	0.02	0.7	20	0.06	0.04	0.4	0.02	0.2	15	0	65
Sweetened	180	3/4 c	100	0.9	0.2	25	15	25	20	2	300	u	0.02	0.7	20	0.06	0.04	0.4	u	u	15	0	60
Grapes, raw																							
Slip-skin	100	20 grapes	45	0.8	0.8	10	10	10	10	2	105	0.17	0.1	0.2	80	0.02	0.02	0.2	0.08	0.08	4	0	2
Adherent skin	100	20 grapes	70	0.6	0.4	17	10	20	6	4	175	0.3	0.1	0.4	100	0.06	0.04	0.4	0.08	0.08	4	0	4
Grape juice	190	3/4 c	120	0.4	tr	30	20	20	25	4	220	u	0.03	0.6	u	0.08	0.04	0.4	0.04	0.08	4	0	tr
Guacamole	120	1/2 c	140	2.1	12.8	7	15	40	u	165	565	u	0.3	0.7	550	0.10	0.2	1.6	0.4	0.9	30	0	35
Ham, baked	85	3 oz	250	18.0	19.0	0	10	145	15	635	200	3.4	0.3	2.2	0	0.4	0.2	3.0	0.3	0.3	1	0.4	0
Hominy grits. See *Cereal*, cooked.																							
Honey, strained	20	1 tbsp	65	0.1	0	17	1	1	1	1	10	0.02	0.03	0.1	0	tr	0.01	0.1	tr	0.04	0	0	tr
Ice cream, vanilla																							
Plain, 10% fat	65	1/2 c	135	2.5	7.0	15	90	70	10	60	130	0.7	0.02	0.05	300	0.02	0.2	0.05	0.03	0.3	1	0.3	0
Rich, 16% fat	75	1/2 c	175	2.0	12.0	16	75	60	8	50	110	0.6	0.02	0.05	450	0.02	0.15	0.05	0.03	0.3	1	0.3	0
Ice milk, vanilla	65	1/2 c	90	2.5	3.0	15	90	65	10	50	130	0.3	u	0.09	100	0.04	0.2	0.05	0.04	0.3	1	0.4	0
Ices, water, lime	95	1/2 c	120	0.4	tr	30	tr	tr	u	tr	3	u	u	tr	0	tr	tr	tr	0	0	0	0	0
Jams and *jellies*	20	1 tbsp	55	0.1	tr	14	4	2	1	2	20	0.1	0.02	0.2	tr	tr	0.01	tr	0.01	0.02	1	0	tr
Kale, boiled without stems	55	1/2 c	20	2.5	0.4	3	105	30	18	25	120	u	u	0.9	4600	0.06	0.1	0.9	0.2	0.6	25	0	50
Kidney, braised	100	3 1/2 oz	250	33.0	12.0	0.8	20	240	20	250	320	2.4	0.1	13.0	1100	0.5	4.8	10.5	0.4	3.8	60	30	u
Kohlrabi, boiled	80	1/2 c, diced	20	1.5	0.1	4	25	35	30	5	215	u	u	0.2	15	0.05	0.02	0.2	0.1	0.5	u	0	35
Kumquat, raw	20	1 medium	10	0.2	tr	3	10	4	u	1	45	u	u	0.1	100	0.01	0.02	u	u	u	u	0	7
Lamb, choice grade																							
Chop, loin, broiled																							
lean and fat	95	1 average	340	21.0	28.0	0	10	165	15	50	235	u	0.1	1.2	u	0.1	0.2	5.0	0.3	0.5	1	2.0	0
lean only	65	1 average	120	18.0	5.0	0	10	140	15	45	205	3.0	0.1	1.3	u	0.1	0.2	4.0	0.2	0.4	1	1.4	0
Leg, roasted																							
lean only	85	3 oz	160	24.0	6.0	0	10	200	15	60	275	3.6	0.05	1.9	u	0.1	0.3	5.5	0.2	0.5	1	1.8	0
Shoulder, roasted																							
lean and fat	85	3 oz	280	18.5	23.0	0	10	145	15	45	205	u	0.1	1.0	u	0.1	0.2	4.0	0.2	0.5	1	1.8	0
Lard. See *Fats.*																							
Lasagna, frozen[6]	225	8 oz serving	380	27.0	12.4	43	310	470	55	1100	740	1.4	u	5.6	1300	0.4	0.4	4.5	u	u	u	u	15
Lemon juice, fresh	15	1 tbsp	5	0.1	tr	1	1	2	1	tr	20	tr	0.01	tr	tr	tr	tr	tr	0.01	0.02	u	0	7
Lemonade, from frozen concentrate	250	1 c	110	0.1	tr	30	2	3	2	1	40	0.02	0.02	0.1	10	0.01	0.02	0.2	0.01	0.03	5	0	15
Lentils, dried, cooked	100	1/2 c	110	8.0	tr	19	25	120	20	u	250	1.0	0.3	2.1	20	0.07	0.06	0.6	u	u	6	0	0

Food	Weight gm	Approximate Measure	Energy Kcal	Protein gm	Fat gm	Total Carbo-hydrate gm	Minerals: Calcium mg	Phos-phorus mg	Mag-nesium mg	Sodium mg	Potas-sium mg	Zinc mg	Copper mg	Iron mg	Vitamins: Total Vitamin A Activity IU	Thia-min mg	Ribo-flavin mg	Niacin mg	Vitamin B-6 mg	Panto-thenic Acid mg	Folacin (free) mcg	Vitamin B-12 mcg	Vitamin C mg
Lettuce, raw																							
Head, solid (iceberg type)	90	1/6 head	10	0.8	0.1	3	20	20	10	10	160	0.4	0.08	0.5	300	0.05	0.05	0.3	0.05	0.2	30	0	5
Loose leaf, romaine, cos	55	1 c, chopped	10	0.7	0.2	2	35	15	10	5	145	0.2	0.05	0.8	1000	0.03	0.04	0.2	0.03	0.1	30	0	10
Liver																							
Beef, fried	85	3 oz	200	22.5	9.0	4	10	405	15	155	325	4.3	2.5	7.5	45,400	0.2	3.6	14.0	0.7	6.5	70	68.0	25
Calf, fried	85	3 oz	220	25.0	11.2	3	10	455	20	100	385	5.2	6.5	12.1	27,800	0.2	3.5	14.0	0.6	6.5	70	51.0	30
Chicken, simmered	70	1/2 c, chopped	120	18.5	3.0	2	10	110	u	40	105	2.4	0.2	6.0	8600	0.1	1.9	8.0	0.5	4.2	u	17.5	10
Lobster, northern, cooked	95	2/3 c meat	90	18.0	1.5	0.3	65	185	20	205	175	2.1	1.6	0.8	u	0.1	0.07	u	u	1.4	8	0.5	u
Lychee nuts, raw	150	10 nuts	60	0.8	0.3	15	5	40	u	3	155	u	u	0.4	0	u	0.05	u	u	u	u	0	40
Macaroni and other pastas, cooked																							
Unenriched	130	1 c	190	6.5	0.7	40	15	85	25	1[11]	105	0.6	0.03	0.7	0	0.03	0.03	0.5	0.03	0.2	5	0	0
Enriched	130	1 c	190	6.5	0.7	40	15	85	25	1[11]	105	0.6	0.03	1.4	0	0.2	0.1	2.0	0.03	0.2	5	0	0
Macaroni with cheese, casserole, baked	200	1 c	430	17.0	22.0	40	360	320	50	1085	240	1.3	0.08	1.8	850	0.2	0.4	2.0	0.09	0.4	10	0.8	0
Mangos, raw	165	1c, diced	110	1.0	0.7	30	15	20	30	10	310	0.8	0.2	0.7	7900	0.08	0.08	2.0	u	0.3	u	0	60
Margarine	5	1 tsp, 1 pat (90/lb)	35	tr	4	tr	1	1	tr	50	1	0.01	tr	0	160	0	0	0	0	0	0	0	0
Melons																							
Cantaloupe	160	1/2 melon or 1 c, cubed	50	1.0	0.2	12	20	25	20	20	400	0.1	0.06	0.6	5400	0.06	0.05	1.0	0.1	0.4	50	0	55
Honeydew	170	1/8 melon or 1 c, cubed	55	1.4	0.5	13	25	25	u	20	425	0.1	0.06	0.7	70	0.07	0.05	1.0	u	u	u	0	40
Watermelon	425	1/16 melon (2lb with rind)	110	2.0	0.9	25	30	45	35	5	425	u	0.3	2.1	2500	0.1	0.1	0.9	0.3	1.2	8	0	30
Milk, cow																							
Whole, fluid	245	1 c	155	8.0	8.5	11	290	225	30	120	370	1.0	0.08	0.1	350	0.09	0.4	0.2	0.1	0.8	10[16]	0.9	2
2%, low-fat	245	1 c	140	10.0	5.0	14	350	275	40	145	450	1.1	0.08	0.1	200[12]	0.1	0.5	0.2	0.1	0.9	15[16]	1.0	2
Skim, nonfat, or buttermilk	245	1 c	90	8.5	0.4	12	300	245	3	125[13]	400	1.0	0.08	0.1	10[12]	0.09	0.4	0.2	0.1	0.8	15[16]	1.0	2
Chocolate, low-fat	250	1 c	180	8.0	5.0	26	285	255	30	150	420	1.0	u	0.6	200[12]	0.1	0.4	0.3	0.1	0.7	10[16]	0.8	2
Dried, instant																							
whole	30	1/4 c	160	8.5	8.5	12	290	250	25	120	425	1.0	0.06	0.1	300	0.09	0.4	0.2	0.09	0.7	10[16]	1.0	2
nonfat	35	1/4 c	125	12.0	0.2	13	445	345	40	190	600	1.5	0.1	0.1	10	0.09	0.5	0.3	0.1	1.1	15[16]	1.4	2
Evaporated	250	1 c	340	17.5	20.0	25	660	510	60	265	765	1.9	0.2	0.4	600	0.1	0.8	0.5	0.1	1.6	20[16]	0.4	3
Condensed, sweetened	40	1 fl oz	120	3.0	3.5	20	105	95	10	50	140	0.4	0.08	0.1	100	0.03	0.2	0.1	0.02	0.3	4[16]	0.2	tr
Milk, human, U.S.	30	1 fl oz	21	0.3	1.3	2.1	10	4	1	5	16	0.05	0.01	0.01	70	0.004	0.01	0.1	0.003	0.07	2[16]	0.02	2
Milkshakes, commercial	270	10 fl oz	320	11.0	7.0	50	365	340	30	300	600	0.5	0.04	0.3	300	0.08	0.5	0.4	0.1	1.0	15[16]	0.6	tr

Molasses																							
Light	20	1 tbsp	50	0	0	13	35	10	9	3	185	u	u	0.9	0	0.01	0.01	tr	u	u	u	0	0
Medium	20	1 tbsp	50	0	0	12	60	15	16	5	215	0.9	0.3	1.2	0	u	0.02	0.2	0.04	0.07	2	0	0
Blackstrap	20	1 tbsp	45	tr	0	11	135	15	52	20	585	u	u	3.2	0	0.02	0.04	0.4	u	u	u	0	0
Muffins																							
Bran	40	1 muffin	100	3.0	4.0	15	55	160	u	180	170	u	u	1.5	100	0.06	0.1	1.5	u	u	u	u	0
Cornmeal	40	1 muffin	130	3.0	4.0	19	40	70	20	190	55	u	u	0.7	100[5]	0.08	0.09	0.6	u	u	u	u	0
Plain or blueberry	40	1 muffin	120	3.0	4.0	17	40	60	10	175	50	0.5	0.09	0.6	50	0.07	0.09	0.6	0.02	0.2	3	0.1	0
Mushrooms, raw	35	1/2 c, sliced	10	1.0	0.1	2	2	40	5	5	145	0.1	0.04	0.3	tr	0.04	0.2	1.5	0.04	0.8	7	0	1
Mustard greens, boiled	70	1/2 c	15	1.5	0.3	3	95	20	10	10	155	0.2	0.06	1.2	4100	0.06	0.1	0.4	0.09	0.1	u	0	35
Mustard, prepared, yellow	5	1 tsp	4	0.2	0.2	0.3	4	4	2	65	5	0.03	0.02	0.1	0	u	u	u	u	u	u	0	0
Noodles, egg, cooked,																							
Unenriched	105	2/3 c	130	4.5	1.5	25	10	65	25	2	45	0.6	0.02	0.6	70	0.03	0.02	0.4	0.02	0.2	2	tr	0
Enriched	105	2/3 c	130	4.5	1.5	25	10	65	25	2	45	0.6	0.02	0.9	70	0.10	0.09	1.3	0.02	0.2	2	tr	0
Oils. See *Fats*.																							
Okra, boiled	105	10 pods	30	2.0	0.3	6	100	45	40	2	185	u	0.1	0.5	500	0.1	0.2	1.0	0.08	0.2	10	0	20
Olives																							
Green	25	5 large	20	0.2	2.5	0.2	10	4	5	465	10	0.02	0.09	0.3	60	u	u	u	0.01	0	3	0	0
Ripe	25	5 large	35	0.2	4.0	0.6	20	4	u	150	5	0.07	0.09	0.4	20	tr	tr	u	tr	tr	u	0	0
Onions																							
Green, raw, bulb and top	25	1/4 c, chopped or 3 onions	10	0.4	tr	2	15	10	3	1	60	0.07	0.01	0.3	500	0.01	0.01	0.1	u	0.4	10	0	8
Mature, dry	85	1/2 c, chopped	30	1.5	0.1	7	25	30	10	10	135	0.3	0.1	0.4	35[9]	0.02	0.04	0.2	0.1	0.1	8	0	8
raw	10	1 tbsp, 1/8 onion	4	0.2	tr	0.9	3	4	1	1	15	0.03	0.01	0.1	tr	tr	tr	tr	0.01	0.01	1	0	1
boiled	105	1/2 c, sliced	30	1.0	0.1	7	25	30	10	10	115	0.6	0.08	0.4	40[9]	0.03	0.03	0.2	0.1	0.1	10	0	8
Oranges, raw	140	1 medium	80	1.8	0.1	18	60	30	30	1	270	0.3	0.09	0.6	280	0.14	0.06	0.6	0.08	0.4	45	0	85
Orange juice, fresh or frozen	185	3/4 c	85	1.5	0.4	19	20	30	20	2	370	0.04	0.09	0.4	400	0.2	0.05	0.8	0.07	0.4	65	0	95
Oysters, raw																							
Eastern	120	6 oysters	80	10.0	2.0	4	115	170	40	90	145	90.0	4.0	6.6	350	0.2	0.2	3.0	0.6	0.3	u	21.6	u
Pacific	120	6 oysters	110	12.5	2.5	8	100	185	30	u	u	10.8	4.0	8.6	u	0.1	u	1.6	u	u	u	u	35
Pakchoy, raw	100	2/3 c	15	1.0	0.1	3	165	45	u	25	305	u	u	0.8	3000	0.05	0.1	0.8	u	u	u	0	25
Pancakes, plain	110	4, ea. 4 in diam.	245	7.5	10.0	35	230	280	15	610	170	0.9	0.06	1.2	300	0.2	0.2	0.8	0.4	0.8	10	u	0
Papaya, raw	225	1/2 fruit or 1 c, cubed	60	0.9	0.2	15	30	25	u	4	355	u	0.02	0.4	2700	0.06	0.06	0.4	u	0.5	u	0	85
Parsley, raw	5	1 tbsp, chopped	2	0.1	tr	0.3	5	2	2	2	25	u	0.02	0.2	300	tr	0.01	tr	0.01	0.02	2	0	6
Peaches, without skin																							
Raw, yellow	115	1 medium	40	0.6	0.1	10	10	20	12	1	200	0.2	0.06	0.5	1300	0.02	0.05	1.0	0.03	0.2	2	0	7
Canned, heavy syrup	150	2 halves and 3 tbsp juice	120	0.6	0.2	30	5	20	9	4	200	0.1	0.1	0.4	650	0.02	0.04	1.0	0.03	0.08	u	0	4
water pack	155	2 halves and 3 tbsp juice	50	0.6	0.2	12	5	20	9	4	210	u	0.08	0.4	700	0.02	0.04	1.0	u	u	u	0	4
Dried, sulfured, uncooked	65	5 halves	170	2.0	0.4	45	30	75	30	10	620	u	u	3.9	2500	tr	0.1	3.5	0.06	u	u	0	10

Food	Weight	Approximate Measure	Energy	Protein	Fat	Total Carbo-hydrate	Minerals								Vitamins								
	gm		Kcal	gm	gm	gm	Calcium mg	Phos-phorus mg	Mag-nesium mg	Sodium mg	Potas-sium mg	Zinc mg	Copper mg	Iron mg	Total Vitamin A Activity IU	Thia-min mg	Ribo-flavin mg	Niacin mg	Vitamin B-6 mg	Panto-thenic Acid mg	Folacin (free) mcg	Vitamin B-12 mcg	Vitamin C mg
Peanuts, roasted, salted	30	1oz, 30 nuts	65	7.5	14.0	5	20	115	50	120	190	0.9	0.1	0.6	0	0.09	0.04	4.9	0.1	0.6	8	0	0
Peanut butter	15	1 tbsp	95	4.0	8.0	3	10	60	25	95	100	0.4	0.09	0.3	0	0.02	0.02	2.4	0.05	0.3	3	0	0
Pears																							
Raw, with skin	180	1, 3½ in x 2½ in	100	1.0	0.7	25	15	20	15	3	215	u	0.3	0.5	30	0.03	0.07	0.2	0.03	0.1	9	0	7
Canned, syrup	150	2 halves and 3 tbsp juice	115	0.4	0.4	30	10	10	7	2	130	u	0.06	0.4	tr	0.02	0.04	0.2	0.02	0.3	9	0	2
water pack	155	2 halves and 3 tbsp juice	50	0.4	0.4	13	10	10	7	2	135	u	0.08	0.4	tr	0.02	0.04	0.2	u	u	u	0	2
Peas																							
Green, frozen, boiled	80	1/2 c	55	4.0	0.2	9	15	70	15	90	110	0.6	0.2	1.5	500	0.2	0.1	2.2	0.1	0.3	14	0	15
Canned, drained	85	1/2 c	75	4.0	0.4	14	20	65	10	200	80	0.7	0.1	1.6	500	0.08	0.05	0.7	0.04	0.1	5	0	7
Split, dry, cooked	100	1/2 c (1 oz, dry wt.)	115	8.0	0.3	20	10	90	8	15[11]	295	1.1	0.07	1.7	40	0.2	0.09	0.9	0.04	0.6	20	0	0
Peas and carrots, frozen, boiled	80	1/2 c	40	2.5	0.2	8	20	45	15	65	125	u	u	0.9	7400	0.2	0.05	1.0	0.08	0.2	u	0	6
Pecans	30	1 oz, 20 halves	200	2.5	20.0	4	20	80	40	tr	170	u	0.3	0.7	40	0.2	0.04	0.3	0.05	0.5	4	0	1
Peppers, hot (chili)																							
Green, canned sauce	15	1 tbsp	3	0.1	tr	1	1	2	u	u	u	u	u	0.1	100	tr	tr	0.1	u	u	u	0	10
Red, dry, chili powder	3	1 tsp	8	0.3	0.4	1	7	8	4	25	50	0.07	u	0.4	900	0.01	0.02	0.2	u	u	u	0	2
Peppers, sweet																							
Green, raw	75	1/2 c, chopped	15	0.9	0.1	4	5	15	15	10	155	0.2	0.07	0.5	300	0.06	0.06	0.4	0.2	0.2	5	0	95
Red, raw	90	1 medium	25	1.0	0.2	5	10	20	u	u	u	u	u	0.4	3300	0.06	0.06	0.4	u	0.2	20	0	150
Pickles, cucumber																							
Dill	135	1 large	15	0.9	0.3	3	35	30	1	1930	270	0.4	0.03	1.4	150	tr	0.03	tr	0.01	0.3	4	0	8
Sweet	35	1 medium	50	0.2	0.1	13	4	5	tr	u	u	0.05	0.07	0.4	30	tr	0.01	tr	tr	0.07	1	0	2
Relish, sweet	15	1 tbsp	20	0.1	0.1	5	3	2	u	105	u	0.01	0.05	0.1	u	0	0	0	u	u	0	0	tr
Pies																							
Apple, berry, rhubarb	160	1/6 of 9 in pie	400	3.5	17.5	60	15	35	5	475	125	0.1	0.1	0.5	50	0.03	0.03	0.6	0.06	0.2	3	0	2
Cherry, peach	160	1/6 of 9 in pie	410	4.0	18.0	60	20	40	u	480	165	0.06	0.1	0.5	700	0.03	0.03	0.8	u	u	u	0	tr
Cream, pudding type with meringue	150	1/6 of 9 in pie	380	7.5	18.0	50	105	150	u	390	210	u	u	1.1	300	0.05	0.20	0.3	u	1.4	u	u	tr
Custard	150	1/6 of 9 in pie	330	9.5	17.0	35	145	170	u	u	u	u	u	0.9	350	0.08	0.30	0.5	u	u	u	u	0
Lemon meringue	140	1/6 of 9 in pie	360	5.0	14.5	55	20	70	u	395	70	u	u	0.7	250	0.04	0.10	0.3	u	u	3	u	4
Mince	160	1/6 of 9 in pie	430	4.0	18.0	65	45	60	u	710	280	u	0.1	1.6	tr	0.10	0.06	0.6	u	u	u	u	2
Pecan	140	1/6 of 9 in pie	580	7.0	31.5	70	65	140	u	305	170	u	u	3.9	200	0.20	0.10	0.4	u	u	u	u	tr
Pumpkin	150	1/6 of 9 in pie	320	6.0	17.0	35	80	105	10	325	245	0.6	0.08	0.8	3800	0.05	0.20	0.8	0.06	0.8	5	u	tr
Sweet potato	150	1/6 of 9 in pie	325	7.0	17.0	36	105	130	u	330	250	u	u	0.8	3600	0.08	0.20	0.5	u	u	u	u	6
Pineapple, diced or crushed																							
Raw	155	1 c	80	0.6	0.3	20	25	10	20	2	225	0.3	0.1	0.8	100	0.1	0.05	0.3	0.1	0.2	15	0	25
Canned, in heavy syrup	130	1/2 c solids and liquid	95	0.4	0.2	25	15	6	10	2	120	0.3	0.2	0.4	60	0.1	0.02	0.2	0.1	0.1	3	0	9

Pineapple, continued																							
in juice	125	1/2 c solids and liquid	70	0.4	0.2	17	15	8	15	1	180	0.3	0.1	0.6	80	0.1	0.04	0.2	0.1	0.2	u	0	15
water pack	125	1/2 c solids and liquid	50	0.4	0.1	13	15	5	u	1	120	u	u	0.4	60	0.1	0.02	0.2	u	u	u	0	8
Pineapple juice	190	3/4 c	105	0.8	0.6	25	30	15	20	2	280	u	0.1	0.6	100	0.1	0.04	0.4	0.2	0.2	u	0	15
Pinenuts, piñon	30	1 oz, 4 tbsp	180	3.5	17.0	6	3	170	u	u	u	u	u	1.5	10	0.4	0.07	1.3	u	u	u	u	tr
Pizza, cheese	65	1/8 of 14 in pizza	150	8.0	5.5	18	145	125	20	455	85	0.8	0.2	0.7	400	0.04	0.1	0.7	u	u	u	u	5
Sausage	65	1/8 of 14 in pizza	160	5.0	6.0	20	10	60	u	490	115	0.8	u	0.8	400	0.06	0.08	1.0	u	u	u	u	6
Plantain	265	1 banana 11 in x 2 in	310	3.0	1.0	82	20	80	u	15	1010	u	u	1.8	u	0.2	0.1	1.6	u	0.7	u	0	35
Plums, raw	70	1 medium	30	0.3	0.1	8	10	10	6	1	110	u	0.07	0.3	150	0.02	0.02	0.3	0.04	0.1	1	0	4
Canned, purple in heavy syrup	140	3 and 3 tbsp syrup	110	0.5	0.1	30	10	15	7	1	190	u	u	1.2	500	0.03	0.03	0.5	0.04	0.1	u	0	3
Popcorn with oil and salt	10	1 c	40	0.9	2.0	5	1	20	10	175	u	0.2	0.03	0.2	u	u	0.01	0.2	0.02	0.04	0	0	0
Pork																							
Chop, broiled																							
lean and fat	80	1 medium	300	19.5	24.5	0	10	210	15	45	215	u	u	2.7	0	0.8	0.2	4.5	0.3	0.5	3	0.4	0
lean only	50	1 medium	110	13.0	6.5	0	5	135	10	30	145	1.5	0.04	1.6	0	0.5	0.1	2.9	0.1	0.2	2	0.2	0
Loin, roasted																							
lean and fat	85	2½ in x 2½ in x ¾ in	310	21.0	24.0	0	10	220	20	50	235	u	0.05	2.7	0	0.8	0.2	4.8	0.3	0.5	1	0.5	0
Spareribs, braised	90	yield from ½ lb, raw wt.	400	18.5	35.0	0	15	220	u	65	300	u	u	4.7	0	0.8	0.4	6.1	u	u	u	0.6	0
Potatoes																							
Baked	200	1 large	140	4.0	0.2	35	15	100	45	5[11]	780	0.4	0.3	1.1	tr	0.2	0.07	2.7	0.5	0.8	20	0	30
Boiled, pared before cooking	135	1 medium	90	2.5	0.1	20	10	55	u	3[11]	385	0.4	0.1	0.7	tr	0.1	0.05	1.6	0.5	0.8	15	0	20
French-fried																							
commercial[14]	70	1 "order"	220	3.0	10.2	28	9	70	20	120	u	u	u	0.4	tr	0.1	0.04	2.4	0.2	u	5	0	9
frozen, reheated	100	20 strips	220	3.5	8.4	35	10	90	30	4[11]	660	0.3	0.3	0.8	tr	0.1	0.02	2.6	0.2	0.5	10	0	20
Mashed with milk	100	1/2 c	100	2.0	4.5	13	25	50	15	350	260	0.1	0.1	0.4	200	0.08	0.05	1.0	0.1	0.2	10	0	10
Potato chips	20	10 chips, 2 in diameter each	115	1.0	8.0	10	10	30	10	200	225	0.2	0.04	0.4	tr	0.04	0.01	1.0	0.04	0.1	2	0	3
Potato salad. See *Salads.*																							
Pretzels	30	10, 3-ring pretzels	120	3.0	1.5	25	5	40	u	500	80	0.3	0.04	0.5	0	0.01	0.02	0.4	0.01	0.2	u	tr	0
Prunes, dried, raw	50	5	130	1.0	0.3	35	25	40	u	4	355	u	0.1	2.0	800	0.04	0.08	0.8	0.1	0.2	tr	0	2
Cooked without sugar	125	1/2 c	120	1.0	0.3	35	25	40	u	4	350	u	0.2	1.9	800	0.04	0.08	0.8	u	u	u	0	1
Prune juice, canned	190	3/4 c	150	0.8	0.2	35	25	40	u	4	450	tr	0.04	2.0	800	0.02	0.02	0.8	u	u	u	u	4
Puddings																							
Almendrado	65	1/3 c and 2 tbsp sauce	100	2.7	4.3	14	35	50	u	35	50	u	u	0.3	250	0.02	0.08	0.03	0.02	0.3	8	0.4	tr
Apple Brown Betty	110	1/2 c	160	1.5	4.0	30	20	25	5	165	110	u	u	0.6	100	0.06	0.04	0.4	u	u	u	u	1
Capirotada	155	1/2 c	385	10.8	14.0	58	230	200	u	335	355	u	u	2.5	250	0.10	0.20	3.0	0.10	0.4	6	0.3	0
Chocolate, instant, packaged	130	1/2 c	160	5.0	3.0	30	185	120	u	160	170	u	u	0.4	150	0.04	0.20	0.2	u	u	u	u	0

Food	Weight gm	Approximate Measure	Energy Kcal	Protein gm	Fat gm	Total Carbo-hydrate gm	Minerals								Vitamins								
							Calcium mg	Phos-phorus mg	Mag-nesium mg	Sodium mg	Potas-sium mg	Zinc mg	Copper mg	Iron mg	Total Vitamin A Activity IU	Thia-min mg	Ribo-flavin mg	Niacin mg	Vitamin B-6 mg	Panto-thenic Acid mg	Folacin (free) mcg	Vitamin B-12 mcg	Vitamin C mg
Puddings, continued																							
Custard	130	1/2 c	150	7.0	7.5	15	150	155	u	105	195	u	u	0.6	450	0.06	0.2	0.2	u	u	4	u	tr
Rice with raisins	130	1/2 c	200	5.0	4.0	35	130	125	u	95	235	0.4	0.04	0.6	150	0.04	0.2	0.2	u	u	5	u	tr
Tapioca	80	1/2 c	110	4.0	4.0	14	85	90	u	130	110	u	0.04	0.4	250	0.04	0.2	0.1	u	u	2	u	0
Vanilla, home recipe	130	1/2 c	140	4.5	5.0	20	150	115	u	85	175	u	0.05	tr	200	0.04	0.2	0.2	u	u	u	u	0
Pumpkin, canned	245	1 c	80	2.5	0.7	19	60	65	30	5[11]	560	u	0.3	1.0	15,700	0.07	0.1	1.5	0.1	1.0	4	0	10
Radishes, raw	45	5 large	7	0.4	tr	1	10	10	7	10	130	0.1	0.04	0.4	5	0.01	0.01	0.1	0.03	0.08	10	0	10
Raisins	35	1/4 c	100	0.9	0.1	30	20	35	10	10	275	0.06	0.08	1.3	10	0.04	0.03	0.2	0.08	0.2	1	0	tr
Rhubarb, cooked with sugar	135	1/2 c	190	0.7	0.2	50	105	20	20	2	275	0.1	0.1	0.8	100	0.02	0.07	0.4	0.03	0.09	10	0	8
Rice cooked, salt added																							
Brown	130	2/3 c	160	3.5	0.8	35	15	95	40	370	90	0.8	0.1	0.7	0	0.1	0.03	1.8	0.2	0.5	10	0	0
White, enriched	135	2/3 c	150	3.0	0.1	35	15	85	10	515	40	0.5	0.07	1.2	0	0.2	0.01	1.4	0.05	0.3	1	0	0
Precooked, instant	110	2/3 c	120	2.5	tr	25	3	20	u	300	u	0.2	u	0.9	0	0.1	u	1.1	u	u	u	0	0
Rolls and *buns*																							
Danish pastry	65	1, of 4 in diameter	270	5.0	15.5	30	35	70	15	240	75	u	u	0.6	200	0.04	0.1	0.5	u	u	5	u	tr
Hamburger or frank-furter bun, enriched	40	1 average	120	3.5	2.0	20	30	35	10	200	40	0.2	0.08	0.8	tr	0.1	0.07	0.9	u	u	5	u	0
Hard rolls, enriched	50	1 large	160	5.0	1.5	30	25	45	15	315	50	0.6	u	1.2	tr	0.1	0.1	1.4	u	u	6	0	0
Plain pan rolls, white, enriched	30	1 small	85	2.5	1.5	15	20	25	10	140	25	0.4	u	0.5	tr	0.08	0.05	0.6	0.01	0.09	4	u	0
Rutabagas, boiled	85	1/2 c, cubed	30	0.8	0.1	7	50	25	12	4	140	u	u	0.2	500	0.05	0.05	0.7	0.08	0.1	u	0	20
Salads																							
Chef's (lettuce w/ham, cheese, dressing)[15]	u	1 serving	285	13.0	24.0	3	150	185	u	u	u	u	u	2.2	1250	0.2	0.2	1.2	u	u	u	u	13
Potato, home recipe	125	1/2 c	120	3.5	3.5	20	40	80	u	650	400	0.3	u	0.8	150	0.1	0.09	1.4	u	u	u	u	14
Tuna fish	100	1/2 c	170	15.0	10.0	4	20	145	u	u	u	u	u	1.3	250	0.04	0.1	5.1	u	u	u	u	1
Salad dressings																							
Blue cheese	15	1 tbsp	75	0.7	8.0	1	10	10	u	165	5	0.04	u	tr	30	tr	0.02	tr	u	u	u	tr	tr
French, regular	15	1 tbsp	65	0.1	6.0	3	2	2	2	220	15	0.01	u	0.1	u	u	u	u	u	u	u	0	u
low-calorie	15	1 tbsp	15	0.1	0.7	3	2	2	u	125	15	u	u	0.1	u	u	u	u	u	u	u	0	u
Italian, regular	15	1 tbsp	85	tr	9.0	1.0	2	1	1	315	2	0.02	0.1	tr	tr	tr	tr	tr	0	0	0	0	0
low-calorie	15	1 tbsp	10	tr	0.7	0.4	tr	1	u	120	2	u	u	tr	tr	tr	tr	tr	0	0	0	0	0
Mayonnaise	15	1 tbsp	100	0.2	11.0	0.3	3	4	tr	85	5	0.02	0.04	0.1	40	tr	0.01	tr	u	0.02	0	0	0
Salad dressing	15	1 tbsp	65	0.2	6.5	2.0	2	4	tr	90	1	0.08	u	tr	30	tr	tr	tr	0	0.02	0	0	0
Thousand Island, or Louie-type	15	1 tbsp	80	0.1	8.0	2.5	2	3	u	110	20	0.02	u	0.1	50	tr	tr	tr	u	u	u	u	tr
Salmon. See *Fish*.																							

Sandwiches																							
Bacon, lettuce, tomato on white bread	150	1 average	280	7.0	15.5	30	55	90	u	u	u	u	u	1.5	850	0.2	0.1	1.5	u	u	u	u	15
Egg salad on white bread	140	1 average	280	10.5	12.5	30	70	155	u	u	u	u	u	2.4	600	0.2	0.02	1.0	u	u	u	u	2
Fish fillet, fried on bun[14]	135	1 average	410	15.0	21.5	37	95	235	20	760	u	u	u	1.6	80	0.2	0.4	2.9	0.1	u	20[16]	0.8	2
Ham and cheese on white bread[15]	u	1 average	350	20.0	19.0	30	215	240	u	u	u	u	u	3.1	300	0.4	0.3	2.5	u	u	u	u	0
Hamburger on bun[14]	95	1 regular	250	13.0	9.6	28	50	120	15	540	u	u	u	2.6	160	0.2	0.4	3.7	0.1	u	20[16]	0.8	4
"Big Mac"[14]	185	1 large	560	26.0	32.0	40	160	290	30	1060	u	u	u	3.8	200	0.8	0.6	6.5	0.2	u	30[16]	1.5	5
Tuna salad on white bread	105	1 average	280	11.0	14.0	25	50	135	u	u	u	u	u	1.2	250	0.1	0.1	4.0	u	u	u	u	1
Sashimi. See *Fish,* tuna, raw.																							
Sardines. See *Fish.*																							
Sauces																							
Butterscotch	45	2 tbsp	200	0.5	7.0	35	40	25	u	u	u	u	u	1.4	300	tr	tr	tr	u	u	u	0	0
Cheese	40	2 tbsp	65	3.0	5.0	2	90	65	u	u	u	u	u	0.1	200	0.01	0.08	0.1	u	u	u	u	tr
Chocolate																							
thin syrup	40	2 tbsp	100	0.9	0.8	25	7	35	u	u	u	u	0.2	0.6	tr	0.01	0.03	0.2	u	u	u	0	0
fudge type	40	2 tbsp	125	2.0	5.0	20	50	60	u	35	105	u	u	0.5	60	0.02	0.08	0.2	u	u	u	tr	0
Custard	70	1/4 c	85	3.5	4.0	10	80	80	u	u	u	u	u	0.4	250	0.04	0.2	0.1	u	u	u	u	tr
Hard sauce	20	2 tbsp	95	0.1	5.5	12	2	1	u	u	u	u	u	tr	250	tr	tr	tr	0	0	0	0	0
Hollandaise	50	1/4 c scant	180	2.0	18.5	0.4	25	80	u	u	u	u	u	0.9	1000	0.03	0.04	tr	u	u	u	u	tr
Soy	35	2 tbsp	25	2.0	0.5	4	30	40	u	2665	135	u	u	1.7	0	0.01	0.09	0.1	u	u	u	0	0
Tartar	15	1 tbsp	75	0.2	8.0	0.6	3	4	u	100	10	u	u	0.1	30	tr	tr	tr	u	u	u	u	tr
Tomato catsup	15	1 tbsp	15	0.3	0.1	4	3	10	3	155	55	0.04	0.09	0.1	200	0.01	0.01	0.2	0.02	u	tr	0	2
White, medium	125	1/2 c	200	5.0	15.5	11	145	115	20	475	175	0.5	0.05	0.2	600	0.05	0.2	0.2	0.06	0.8	1	0.2	1
Sauerkraut, canned	120	1/2 c	20	1.0	0.2	5	40	20	u	880	165	1.0	0.1	0.6	60	0.04	0.04	0.2	0.2	0.1	u	0	16
Sausages																							
Bologna	30	1 slice, 4¼ in x 1/8 in	85	3.5	8.0	0.3	2	35	u	370	65	0.5	tr	0.5	0	0.05	0.06	0.7	0.03	u	1	u	0
Frankfurter (all-meat)	45	1 average	135	5.5	12.0	0.7	2	45	u	u	u	0.7	0.04	0.7	0	0.07	0.09	1.1	0.06	0.2	1	0.6	0
Liverwurst	30	1 oz	85	4.5	7.0	0.5	3	70	5	u	u	2.2	0.9	1.5	1800	0.06	0.4	1.6	0.06	0.8	6	4.2	tr
Luncheon meat, pork, cured	30	1 oz	85	4.5	7.0	0.4	3	30	u	350	65	u	0.02	0.6	0	0.09	0.06	0.9	u	0.2	1	u	0
Pork sausage, links	40	3 links	185	7.0	17.0	tr	3	60	5	375	105	0.2	0.06	0.9	0	0.3	0.1	1.5	0.07	0.3	1	0.2	0
Salami, dry	30	3 small slices	130	6.5	11.0	0.3	4	80	u	u	u	u	u	1.0	0	0.1	0.07	1.5	0.04	u	1	u	0
Vienna, canned	50	3 sausages	115	6.5	9.5	0.1	3	75	u	u	u	u	u	0.9	0	0.03	0.06	1.2	0.04	u	1	u	0
Scallops																							
Breaded, fried	95	3½ oz	180	17.0	8.0	10	u	u	u	u	u	u	0.1	u	0	u	u	u	u	0.1	15	u	0
Steamed	95	3½ oz	105	22.0	1.5	3	110	320	u	250	455	u	0.1	2.8	0	u	0.06	1.3	u	u	18	1.1	u
Sesame seeds, hulled	40	1/4 c	220	7.0	20.0	7	40	220	7	u	u	u	0.6	0.9	0	0.07	0.05	2.0	u	u	25	0	0
Sherbet, orange	95	1/2 c	135	1.0	2.0	30	50	75	8	45	100	0.6	0.02	0.1	90	0.01	0.04	tr	0.01	tr	7[16]	0.1	2
Shrimp, canned	85	3 oz	100	20.5	0.9	0.6	100	225	45	u	105	1.8	0.1	2.7	60	0.01	0.03	1.5	0.05	0.2	6	u	0
French-fried	85	3 oz	190	17.5	9.5	8	60	160	40	160	195	0.8	0.3	1.8	u	0.03	0.06	2.5	0.05	0.3	5	0.6	0
Soups																							
Albondiga (meatballs in tomato broth)	240	1 c with 4 meatballs	340	18.5	21.4	17	25	175	u	180	460	u	u	3.6	500	0.2	0.2	5.0	0.6	0.7	10	1.2	8

Food	Weight gm	Approximate Measure	Energy Kcal	Protein gm	Fat gm	Total Carbo-hydrate gm	Minerals: Calcium mg	Phos-phorus mg	Mag-nesium mg	Sodium mg	Potas-sium mg	Zinc mg	Copper mg	Iron mg	Vitamins: Total Vitamin A Activity IU	Thia-min mg	Ribo-flavin mg	Niacin mg	Vitamin B-6 mg	Panto-thenic Acid mg	Folacin (free) mcg	Vitamin B-12 mcg	Vitamin C mg
Soups, continued																							
Bean, with pork	250	1 c	170	8.0	6.0	22	65	130	u	1010	395	u	u	2.3	650	0.1	0.08	1.0	u	u	u	u	3
Bouillon, broth, consomme	240	1 c	30	5.0	0	3	tr	30	u	780	130	u	0.02	0.5	tr	tr	0.02	1.0	u	u	u	u	0
Cream soups, canned,																							
diluted with water	240	1 c	65	2.5	1.5	10	25	40	u	985	120	u	u	0.7	300	0.05	0.1	0.7	u	u	u	u	u
diluted with milk	245	1 c	150	7.0	6.0	17	175	160	u	1070	300	u	u	0.7	500	0.07	0.3	0.7	u	u	10	u	tr
Chicken noodle, from dry mix	240	1 c	55	2.0	1.5	8	7	20	u	580	20	0.1	0.1	0.2	50	0.07	0.05	0.5	u	u	u	u	0
Clam chowder, Manhattan	245	1 c	80	2.0	2.5	12	35	45	u	940	185	1.4	u	1.0	900	0.02	0.02	1.0	u	u	8	u	u
Onion	240	1 c	35	1.5	1.0	6	10	10	u	690	60	0.07	u	0.2	tr	tr	tr	tr	u	u	u	u	2
Split pea	245	1 c	140	8.5	3.0	20	30	150	15	940	270	1.0	0.2	1.5	450	0.2	0.2	1.5	0.1	0.2	2	0.4	tr
Tomato	245	1 c	90	2.0	2.5	16	15	35	15	970	230	0.2	0.2	0.7	1000	0.05	0.05	1.0	0.05	0.2	5	0	10
Vegetable beef	245	1 c	80	5.0	2.0	10	10	50	25	1050	160	0.4	0.1	0.7	2700	0.05	0.05	1.0	0.07	0.2	5	u	u
Spaghetti																							
Canned, with tomato sauce and meatballs[17]	210	1 can, 7½ oz	250	10.4	12.8	23	20	120	u	1035	375	u	0.3	2.2	1030	0.15	0.2	3.4	u	u	u	u	u
Home recipe, with tomato sauce																							
with cheese	250	1 c	260	9.0	9.0	35	80	135	30	955	410	0.2	0.3	2.3	1100	0.2	0.2	2.5	0.1	0.8	2	0.6	15
with meatballs	250	1 c	330	18.5	11.5	40	125	235	40	1010	665	3.5	0.4	3.7	1600	0.2	0.3	4.0	0.4	0.5	15	0.6	20
Spinach, fresh or frozen, boiled	90	1/2 c	20	2.5	0.2	3	90	40	60	50	300	0.5	0.1	2.0	7300	0.06	0.1	0.4	0.2	0.2	60	0	20
Sprouts, raw																							
Alfalfa	100	1 c, packed	40	5.0	0.6	5	30	u	u	u	u	1.0	u	1.4	u	0.1	0.2	1.5	u	u	u	0	15
Mung bean	100	1 c	35	4.0	0.2	7	20	65	u	5	235	0.9	u	1.4	20	0.1	0.1	0.8	u	u	u	0	20
Soybean	100	1 c	50	6.5	1.5	6	50	70	u	u	u	1.6	u	1.1	80	0.2	0.2	0.8	u	u	u	0	15
Squash																							
Summer, boiled	90	1/2 c	10	0.8	0.1	3	20	20	15	1	125	0.2	0.07	0.4	350	0.04	0.07	0.7	0.2	0.1	2	0	9
Winter																							
baked	100	1/2 c	65	2.0	0.4	15	30	50	17	1	470	u	u	0.8	430	0.05	0.1	0.7	0.09	0.3	u	0	15
boiled	120	1/2 c	45	1.5	0.4	10	25	40	17	1	315	u	u	0.6	4300	0.05	0.1	0.5	0.1	0.3	u	0	10
Strawberries																							
Fresh	100	2/3 c whole	35	0.7	0.5	8	20	20	12	1	165	0.08	u	1.0	60	0.03	0.07	0.6	0.06	0.3	15	0	60
Frozen, sweetened	170	2/3 c	160	0.7	0.3	40	20	25	14	2	180	u	u	1.0	50	0.03	0.1	0.9	0.07	0.2	15	0	95
Sugar																							
Brown	220	1 c, packed	820	0	0	210	185	40	u	65	755	u	0.7	7.5	0	0.02	0.07	0.4	u	u	u	0	0
White																							
granulated	200	1 c	770	0	0	200	0	0	0	2	5	0.1	0.04	0.2	0	0	0	0	0	0	0	0	0
	4	1 tsp	15	0	0	4	0	0	0	tr	tr	tr	tr	tr	0	0	0	0	0	0	0	0	0
powdered	8	1 tbsp	30	0	0	8	0	0	0	tr	tr	tr	tr	tr	0	0	0	0	0	0	0	0	0
Sunflower seeds, hulled	35	1/4 c	200	8.5	17.0	7	45	305	13	10	335	u	0.6	2.6	20	0.7	0.08	2.0	0.4	0.5	u	0	0

Sweet potatoes																							
Baked in skin	145	1 potato, 5 in x 2 in	160	2.5	0.6	35	45	65	45	15	340	1.0	0.2	1.0	9200	0.1	0.08	0.8	0.05	1.0	10	0	25
Boiled in skin	130	1/2 c mashed	150	2.0	0.5	35	40	60	u	15	620	u	0.2	0.9	9200	0.1	0.08	0.8	0.3	1.0	9	0	20
Candied	105	1/2 medium	180	1.5	3.5	35	40	45	u	45	200	u	0.06	0.9	6600	0.06	0.04	0.4	u	u	7	0	10
Syrup, maple-flavored, artificial	20	1 tbsp	50	0	0	13	20	2	u	2	35	tr	0.08	0.2	0	0	0	0	0	0	0	0	0
Tacos, beef	80	1 taco	160	11.0	8.5	9	135	160	u	200	210	u	u	2.0	530	0.07	0.1	2.3	0.3	0.3	25	0.7	3
Tamales, canned	100	3½ oz	140	4.5	7.0	14	20	40	10	665	u	0.9	0.05	1.2	u	u	u	u	u	u	u	u	u
Home recipe, chicken	130	2 tamales	275	8.3	23.7	8	100	60	u	60	90	u	u	0.9	2800	0.05	0.1	2.7	0.2	0.3	1	0.1	7
Tea, instant	1	1/2 tsp	3	0	0	1	tr	u	4	u	45	u	u	tr	0	0	tr	tr	u	u	u	0	0
Tofu, soybean curd	120	1 piece, 2½ in x 2¾ in x 1 in	85	9.5	5.0	3	155	150	130	10	50	u	u	2.3	0	0.07	0.04	0.1	u	u	u	0	0
Tomatoes, raw	135	1 medium	25	1.5	0.2	6	15	35	20	4	300	0.3	0.1	0.6	1100	0.07	0.05	0.9	0.1	0.4	25	0	30
Canned	120	1/2 c	25	1.0	0.2	5	5	25	15	155	260	0.2	0.2	0.6	1100	0.06	0.04	0.8	0.1	0.3	10	0	20
Tomato juice, canned	180	3/4 c	35	1.5	0.2	8	15	35	20	365	415	u	0.1	1.6	1500	0.09	0.05	1.5	0.3	0.4	18	0	30
Tomato paste	130	1/2 c	110	4.5	0.5	25	35	90	25	50[11]	1120	u	0.9	4.6	4300	0.3	0.2	4.0	0.5	0.6	25	0	65
Tongue, beef, braised	100	3½ oz	250	21.5	17.0	0.4	5	120	16	60	165	u	0.07	2.2	0	0.05	0.3	3.5	0.1	2.0	u	u	0
Tortillas																							
Corn, lime-treated	30	1, of 6 in diameter	65	1.5	0.6	14	60	40	30	u	u	0.03	0.06	0.9	tr	0.04	0.02	0.3	0.02	0.03	tr	0	0
White flour	30	1, of 6 in diameter	110	3.0	1.0	20	4	50	15	250	30	u	u	1.0	0	0.08	0.04	0.5	0.02	0.03	5	0	0
Tostada with beans and small portion of cheese	210	1 tostada	335	11.6	17.6	35	195	245	u	350	425	u	u	3.2	1650	0.3	0.2	1.3	0.2	0.4	10	0.2	10
Tuna. See *Fish*.																							
Turkey, roasted																							
Light meat	85	2 slices, each 4 in x 2 in x ¼ in	150	28.0	3.5	0	7	200	20	70	350	1.8	0.2	1.0	u	0.04	0.1	9.5	0.3	0.5	3	0.4	0
Dark meat	85	4 slices, each 2½ in x 1½ in x ¼ in	170	25.5	7.0	0	7	200	20	85	340	3.7	0.2	2.0	u	0.03	0.2	3.5	0.3	1.0	7	0.4	0
Turnips, boiled	80	1/2 c, cubed	20	0.6	0.2	4	25	20	10	25	145	0.07	0.03	0.3	tr	0.03	0.04	0.2	0.06	0.08	u	0	15
Turnip greens, boiled	70	1/2 c	15	1.5	0.2	3	135	25	20	u	u	u	u	0.8	4600	0.1	0.2	0.4	0.7	0.1	u	0	50
Veal cutlet, broiled	85	3 oz	180	23.0	9.5	0	10	195	20	55	260	4.1	0.04	2.7	0	0.06	0.2	4.5	0.3	0.8	15	1.6	0
Vinegar, cider	15	1 tbsp	2	tr	0	1	1	1	u	tr	15	0.02	0.01	0.1	0	0	0	0	0	0	0	0	0
Waffles																							
Made from mix	75	1, of 7 in diameter	210	6.5	8.0	25	180	260	20	515	145	u	u	1.0	200	0.1	0.2	0.7	u	0.5	u	u	0
Frozen[18]	45	2 sections	120	3.0	4.0	16	130	195	u	340	u	u	u	0.5	u	0.04	0.05	0.5	u	u	u	u	0
Walnuts, English	100	1 c halves	650	15.0	64.0	16	100	380	135	2	450	2.8	0.9	3.1	30	0.3	0.1	0.9	0.7	0.9	45[16]	0	2
	15	2 tbsp, chopped	100	2.5	10.0	3	15	60	20	tr	70	0.4	0.1	0.4	10	0.06	0.02	0.2	0.1	0.1	5[16]	0	tr

Food	Weight gm	Approximate Measure	Energy Kcal	Protein gm	Fat gm	Total Carbohydrate gm	Minerals: Calcium mg	Phosphorus mg	Magnesium mg	Sodium mg	Potassium mg	Zinc mg	Copper mg	Iron mg	Vitamins: Total Vitamin A Activity IU	Thiamin mg	Riboflavin mg	Niacin mg	Vitamin B-6 mg	Pantothenic Acid mg	Folacin (free) mcg	Vitamin B-12 mcg	Vitamin C mg
Watercress, raw	35	10 sprigs	5	0.8	0.1	1	55	20	5	20	100	u	0.03	0.6	1700	0.03	0.06	0.3	0.04	0.1	70[16]	0	30
Wheat bran, crude	30	1 oz	60	4.5	1.0	17	35	355	135	3	315	2.7	0.4	4.2	0	0.2	0.1	6.0	0.2	0.1	u	0	0
Wheat germ, raw	30	1 oz	100	7.5	3.0	13	20	315	90	tr	230	1.7	0.7	2.6	u	0.6	0.2	1.0	0.3	0.9	80	0	0
Toasted	30	1 oz	120	9.0	3.5	15	15	350	90	tr	285	1.7	0.7	2.5	50	0.5	0.2	1.5	0.3	0.4	u	0	0
Wine, dessert (18.8%)	105	3½ fl oz	140	0.1	0	8	10	u	5	4	75	0.1	0.08	0.4	u	0.01	0.02	0.2	0.04	0	0	0	0
Table (12.2%)	100	3½ fl oz	85	0.1	0	4	10	10	10	5	95	0.1	0.01	0.4	u	tr	0.01	0.1	0.04	0	0	0	0
Yeast																							
Dry, active	5	1 tbsp	20	2.5	0.1	3	3	90	3	4	140	u	0.2	1.1	tr	0.2	0.4	2.5	0.1	0.6	7	0	0
Brewer's, debittered	5	1 tbsp	25	3.0	0.1	3	15	140	10	10	150	u	u	1.4	tr	1.2	0.3	3.0	0.1	0.6	9	0	0
Yogurt																							
Low-fat																							
plain	230	8 fl oz carton	145	12.0	3.5	16	415	325	40	160	530	2.0	u	0.2	150	0.1	0.5	0.3	0.1	1.3	25[16]	1.3	2
fruit, sweetened	230	8 fl oz carton	225	9.0	2.6	42	315	245	30	120	400	1.5	u	0.1	110	0.08	0.4	0.2	0.1	1.0	20[16]	1.0	1
Regular																							
plain	230	8 fl oz carton	140	8.0	7.5	11	275	215	25	105	350	1.3	u	0.1	280	0.07	0.3	0.2	0.1	0.9	20[16]	0.8	2

Table 3 CIVILIAN PER CAPITA AVAILABILITY OF MAJOR FOOD COMMODITIES (RETAIL WEIGHT) AND CIVILIAN POPULATION, SELECTED YEARS*

Commodity†	*1960*	*1970*	*1975*	*1977***
Meats:	134.1	151.4	145.4	154.8
Beef	64.3	84.1	88.9	93.2
Veal	5.2	2.4	3.5	3.2
Lamb and mutton	4.3	2.9	1.8	1.5
Pork (excluding lard)	60.3	62.0	51.2	56.9
Fish (edible weight)	10.3	11.8	12.2	12.8
Poultry products:				
Eggs	42.4	39.5	35.4	34.5
Chicken (ready-to-cook)	27.8	40.5	40.3	44.3
Turkey (ready-to-cook)	6.2	8.0	8.6	9.2
Dairy products:				
Cheese	8.3	11.5	14.5	16.3
Condensed and evaporated milk	13.7	7.1	5.0	4.4
Fluid milk and cream (product weight)	321.0	296.0	291.1	289.4
Ice cream (product weight)	18.3	17.7	18.7	17.7
Fats and oils – total, fat content	45.3	53.0	53.3	54.4
Butter (actual weight)	7.5	5.3	4.8	4.4
Margarine (actual weight)	9.4	11.0	11.2	11.6
Lard	7.6	4.7	4.0	3.5
Shortening	12.6	17.3	17.3	17.5
Other edible fats and oils	11.5	18.2	20.3	21.6
Fruits:				
Fresh	90.0	79.1	81.3	82.4
Citrus	32.5	27.9	28.7	25.2
Noncitrus	57.5	51.2	52.6	57.2
Processed:				
Canned fruit	22.6	23.3	19.3	19.5
Canned juice	13.0	14.6	15.3	13.7
Frozen (including juices)	9.1	9.8	12.6	12.4
Chilled citrus juices	2.1	4.7	5.7	5.8
Dried	3.1	2.7	3.0	2.6
Vegetables:				
Fresh‡	96.0	91.0	93.9	93.1
Canned, excluding potatoes and sweet potatoes	43.4	51.2	52.1	52.8
Frozen, excluding potatoes	7.0	9.6	9.7	9.7
Potatoes, (including fresh equivalent of processed)	105.0	115.3	120.3	120.7
Sweet potatoes, (including fresh equivalent of processed)	6.5	5.2	5.3	5.0

Table continued on following page.

*From National Food Review. Washington, D.C., U.S. Dept. of Agriculture, April, 1978, p. 53.

†Quantity in pounds, retail weight unless otherwise shown. Wastage not deducted. Data on calendar year basis except for dried fruits, fresh citrus fruits, peanuts, and rice, which are on a crop-year basis.

‡Commercial production for sale as fresh produce.

Table 3 CIVILIAN PER CAPITAL AVAILABILITY OF MAJOR FOOD COMMODITIES (RETAIL WEIGHT) AND CIVILIAN POPULATION, SELECTED YEARS*—(*Continued*)

Grains:				
Wheat flour§	118	110	107	107
Rice	6.1	6.7	7.7	7.6
Other:				
Coffee	11.6	10.5	9.0	6.9
Tea	0.6	0.7	0.8	.9
Cocoa	2.9	3.1	2.6	2.7
Peanuts (shelled)	4.9	5.9	6.5	6.5
Dry edible beans	7.3	5.9	6.5	6.0
Melons	23.2	21.2	17.5	19.0
Sugar (refined)	97.4	101.8	90.2	95.7
Civilian population¶	178.1	201.7	211.4	214.7

§White, whole-wheat, and semolina flour, including use in bakery products.
¶July 1 civilian population used to derive per capita figures except for sugar, dried fruits, peanuts, and rice.
**Preliminary.

Table 4 CONVERSION FACTORS FOR WEIGHTS AND MEASURES*

To Change	*To*	*Multiply By*
Inches	Centimeters	2.54
Feet	Meters	.305
Miles	Kilometers	1.609
Meters	Inches	39.37
Kilometers	Miles	.621
Fluid ounces	Cubic centimeters	29.57
Quarts	Liters	.946
Cubic centimeters	Fluid ounces	.034
Liters	Quarts	1.057
Grains	Milligrams	64.799
Ounces (av.)	Grams	28.35
Pounds (av.)	Kilograms	.454
Ounces (troy)	Grams	31.103
Pounds (troy)	Kilograms	.373
Grams	Grains	15.432
Kilograms	Pounds	2.205
Kilocalories	KiloJoules	4.184
Kilocalories	MegaJoules	.004

*Also see Chapter 1, Table 1–2.

Table 5 PERCENTILES* FOR HEIGHT AND WEIGHT FOR BOYS 0–18 YEARS†

Age	*Body Weight, kg* 3*	50*	97*	*Height, cm* 3*	50*	97*
0–3 months	3.72	4.56	6.01	51.55	55.50	59.15
3–6 months	5.58	6.65	8.44	59.90	63.40	67.05
6–9 months	6.94	8.32	10.25	65.35	68.80	73.15
9–12 months	7.96	9.57	11.72	69.50	73.20	78.10
1–2 years	9.57	11.43	14.29	77.50	81.80	88.20
2–3 years	11.43	13.61	16.78	86.90	92.10	99.50
3–4 years	12.93	15.56	18.82	94.30	99.80	106.50
4–5 years	14.33	17.42	21.50	100.60	106.70	114.30
5–6 years	16.56	20.68	25.92	105.30	114.40	122.85
6–7 years	18.48	23.22	29.71	111.25	120.80	129.80
7–8 years	20.64	25.90	33.86	116.80	127.10	136.80
8–9 years	22.79	28.62	38.38	121.90	132.80	142.75
9–10 years	24.78	31.30	43.04	126.45	137.90	147.80
10–11 years	26.90	33.93	48.02	131.05	142.30	152.35
11–12 years	29.26	36.74	53.50	135.75	146.90	158.15
12–13 years	31.57	40.23	59.47	140.15	152.30	165.70
13–14 years	34.43	45.50	65.46	144.30	158.90	173.30
14–15 years	38.80	51.66	70.80	149.05	165.30	180.95
15–16 years	44.16	56.65	75.32	154.10	169.70	183.70
16–17 years	48.51	60.33	78.50	157.75	172.70	186.10
17–18 years	50.69	62.41	80.42	159.30	174.10	187.10

*The percentile refers to the percent of subjects below the given weight or height.
†From Nelson, W. E., et al. (eds.): *Textbook of Pediatrics.* 9th Ed. Philadelphia, W. B. Saunders Co., 1969.

Table 6 PERCENTILES* FOR HEIGHT AND WEIGHT FOR GIRLS 0–18 YEARS†

Age	*Body Weight, kg* 3*	50*	97*	*Height, cm* 3*	50*	97*
0–3 months	3.54	4.49	5.51	51.45	54.85	58.35
3–6 months	5.10	6.44	7.92	58.45	62.35	65.95
6–9 months	6.30	7.98	10.02	63.25	67.65	71.45
9–12 months	7.24	9.23	11.64	67.15	72.15	76.45
1–2 years	8.80	11.11	14.02	74.90	80.90	86.70
2–3 years	10.70	13.43	17.33	84.50	91.40	98.70
3–4 years	12.47	15.38	20.55	92.00	99.50	108.00
4–5 years	13.98	17.46	23.09	98.10	106.80	116.20
5–6 years	16.08	19.96	25.06	105.30	112.80	121.70
6–7 years	17.30	22.41	28.58	111.00	119.10	128.55
7–8 years	19.64	25.04	33.16	116.55	125.20	134.55
8–9 years	21.41	27.67	38.28	121.35	130.50	140.40
9–10 years	23.20	30.44	43.50	125.65	135.80	146.35
10–11 years	25.20	33.79	48.72	130.00	141.70	153.35
11–12 years	27.56	37.74	54.56	135.05	148.10	161.00
12–13 years	30.80	42.37	61.24	140.75	154.30	166.50
13–14 years	35.22	47.04	66.48	145.95	158.40	169.55
14–15 years	39.03	50.35	69.40	149.20	160.40	171.15
15–16 years	41.00	52.30	70.96	150.50	161.70	171.80
16–17 years	42.12	53.57	71.94	150.90	162.40	172.10
17–18 years	42.73	54.20	72.62	151.00	162.50	172.00

*The percentile refers to the percent of subjects below the given weight or height.
†From Nelson, W. E., et al. (eds.): *Textbook of Pediatrics.* 9th Ed. Philadelphia, W. B. Saunders Co., 1969.

Table 7 AVERAGE WEIGHTS OF MEN*

Graduated Weights (in Indoor Clothing) in Pounds

Age Groups

Height	15–16	17–19	20–24	25–29	30–39	40–49	50–59	60–69
5′ 0″	98	113	122	128	131	134	136	133
1″	102	116	125	131	134	137	139	136
2″	107	119	128	134	137	140	142	139
3″	112	123	132	138	141	144	145	142
4″	117	127	136	141	145	148	149	146
5″	122	131	139	144	149	152	153	150
6″	127	135	142	148	153	156	157	154
7″	132	139	145	151	157	161	162	159
8″	137	143	149	155	161	165	166	163
9″	142	147	153	159	165	169	170	168
10″	146	151	157	163	170	174	175	173
11″	150	155	161	167	174	178	180	178
6′ 0″	154	160	166	172	179	183	185	183
1″	159	164	170	177	183	187	189	188
2″	164	168	174	182	188	192	194	193
3″	169	172	178	186	193	197	199	198
4″	†	176	181	190	199	203	205	204

*Excerpted from *Build and Blood Pressure Study,* Society of Actuaries, October 1959. (*Note:* Average weights and *desirable* weights are not the same. For information on desirable weights, see Chapter 24 of this book, the most recent Recommended Dietary Allowances booklet (1979), and Bray, G. A. (ed.): *Obesity in Perspective,* DHEW Publ. No. (NIH)75-708.)

†Average weights omitted in classes having too few cases.

Table 8 AVERAGE WEIGHTS OF WOMEN*

Graduated Weights (in Indoor Clothing) in Pounds

Age Groups

Height	15–16	17–19	20–24	25–29	30–39	40–49	50–59	60–69
4′10″	97	99	102	107	115	122	125	127
11″	100	102	105	110	117	124	127	129
5′ 0″	103	105	108	113	120	127	130	131
1″	107	109	112	116	123	130	133	134
2″	111	113	115	119	126	133	136	137
3″	114	116	118	122	129	136	140	141
4″	117	120	121	125	132	140	144	145
5″	121	124	125	129	135	143	148	149
6″	125	127	129	133	139	147	152	153
7″	128	130	132	136	142	151	156	157
8″	132	134	136	140	146	155	160	161
9″	136	138	140	144	150	159	164	165
10″	†	142	144	148	154	164	169	†
11″	†	147	149	153	159	169	174	†
6′ 0″	†	152	154	158	164	174	180	†

*Excerpted from *Build and Blood Pressure Study,* Society of Actuaries, October 1959. (Also see footnote in Table 7.)

†Average weights omitted in classes having too few cases.

Table 9 INTRODUCTION TO SOME BASIC ORGANIC GROUPS AND COMPOUNDS

Classification and Distinguishing Chemical Group	***Examples***

Hydrocarbon

Composed of only hydrogen (H) and carbon (C)

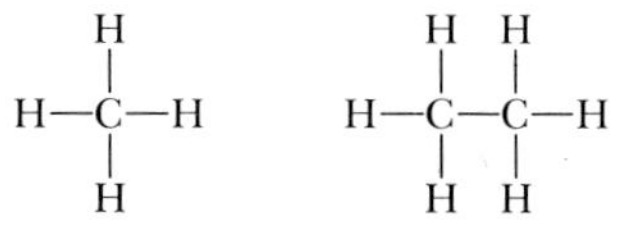

```
     H              H   H
     |              |   |
  H—C—H          H—C—C—H
     |              |   |
     H              H   H

  Methane          Ethane
```

Alcohol

Hydroxyl group, (oxygen = "O") R—OH

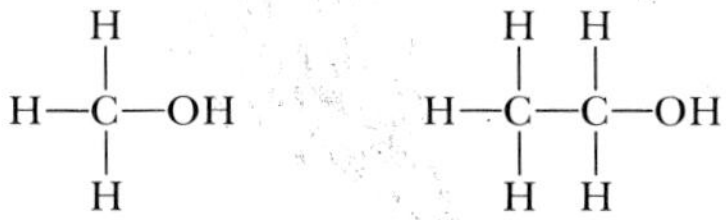

```
     H              H   H
     |              |   |
  H—C—OH         H—C—C—OH
     |              |   |
     H              H   H
  Methanol       Ethanol (in alcoholic beverages)
```

Carboxylic acid

Carboxyl group,

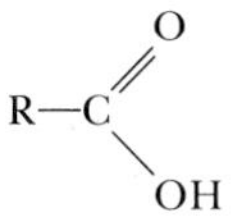

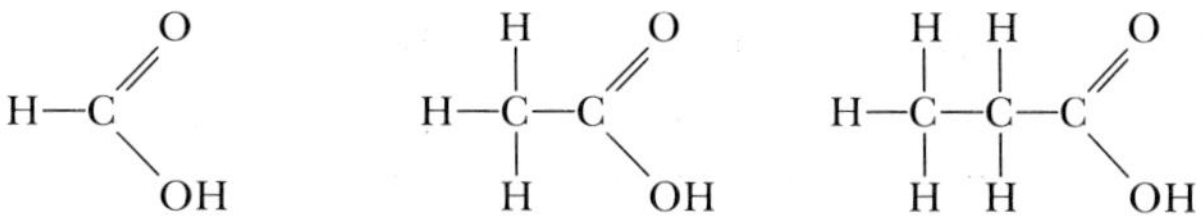

```
       O            O           H     O          H  H     O
      //           //           |    //          |  |    //
  R—C          H—C          H—C—C          H—C—C—C
      \            \            |    \           |  |    \
       OH           OH          H     OH         H  H     OH
               Formic acid    Acetic acid       Propionic acid
```

Aldehyde

Carbonyl group with hydrogen attached,

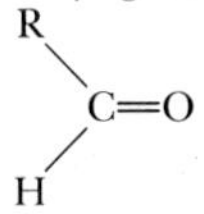

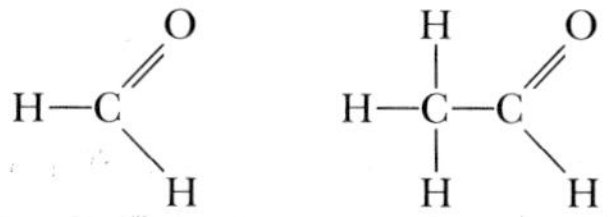

```
  R                          O            H    O
   \                        //            |   //
    C=O                 H—C          H—C—C
   /                        \             |   \
  H                          H            H    H
                      Formaldehyde     Acetaldehyde
```

Ketone

Carbonyl group,

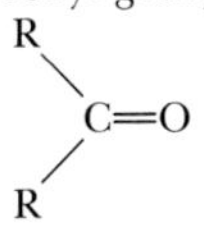

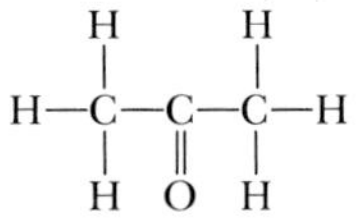

```
  R                      H       H
   \                     |       |
    C=O               H—C—C—C—H
   /                     |  ||  |
  R                      H  O   H
                          Acetone
```

Examples of other common biological compounds containing more than one of the above groups:

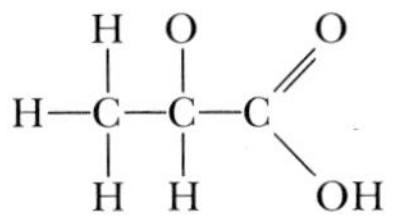

```
                               H    O
                               |   //
                            H—C—C
                               |   \
                               |    OH
  H  O    O                    |    O               O       O
  |  |   //                    |   //                \\    //
H—C—C—C                  HO—C—C                     C—C
  |  |   \                     |   \                /    \
  H  H    OH                   |    OH            HO      OH
                               |    O
                               |   //
                            H—C—C
                               |   \
                               H    OH
  Lactic acid              Citric acid             Oxalic acid
```

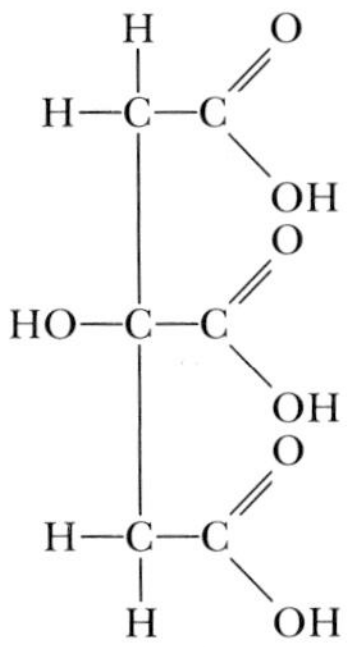

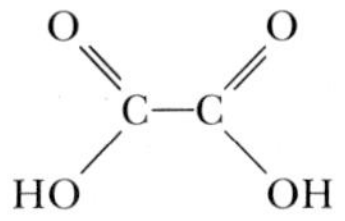

"R" represents the remainder of the molecule.

Table 10 STRUCTURE AND MELTING POINTS OF SOME COMMON FATTY ACIDS

Number of Carbon Atoms	*Fatty Acids*		*Melting Point in °C*
Saturated			
4	Butyric	C_3H_7COOH	−7.9
6	Caproic	$C_5H_{11}COOH$	−3.4
10	Capric	$C_9H_{19}COOH$	31.6
16	Palmitic	$C_{15}H_{31}COOH$	62.9
18	Stearic	$C_{17}H_{35}COOH$	69.6
Unsaturated			
18	Oleic	$CH_3(CH_2)_7CH{=}CH(CH_2)_7COOH$	16.3
18	Linoleic	$CH_3(CH_2)_4CH{=}CHCH_2CH{=}CH(CH_2)_7COOH$	−5.0
18	Linolenic	$CH_3CH_2CH{=}CHCH_2CH{=}CHCH_2CH{=}CH(CH_2)_7COOH$	−11.0
20	Arachidonic	$CH_3(CH_2)_4(CH{=}CHCH_2)_4(CH_2)_2COOH$	−49.5

Table 11 STRUCTURAL FORMULAS OF THE MOST COMMON AMINO ACIDS*

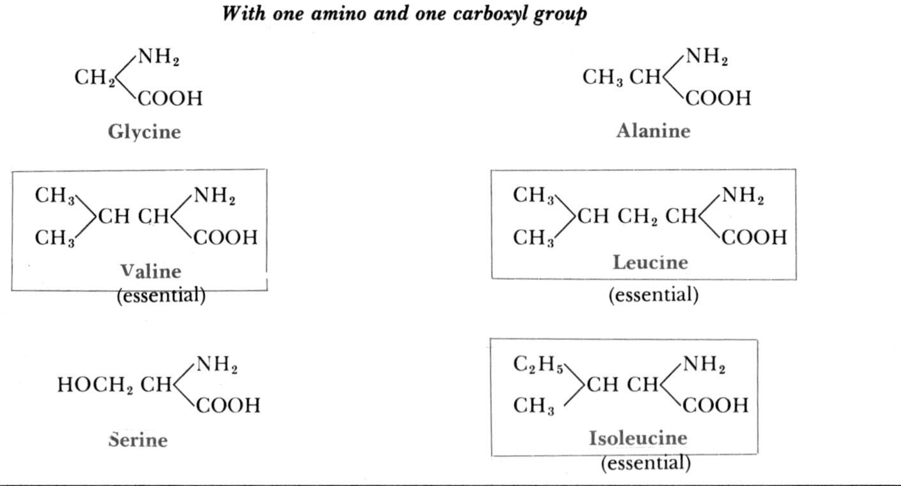

*Each of the essential amino acids is marked so. Histidine and perhaps arginine are needed only by growing children, not by adults (see Chapter 5).

Table 11 STRUCTURAL FORMULAS OF THE MOST COMMON AMINO ACIDS (*Continued*)

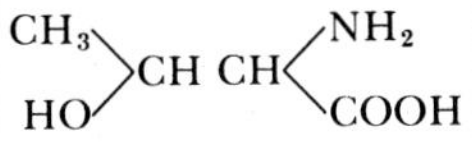

$CH_3(HO)>CH\ CH<(NH_2)(COOH)$

Threonine

(essential)

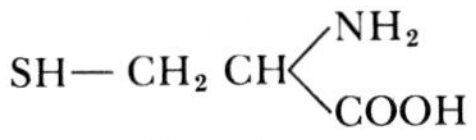

$SH—CH_2\ CH<(NH_2)(COOH)$

Cysteine

$CH_3SCH_2\ CH_2\ CH<(NH_2)(COOH)$

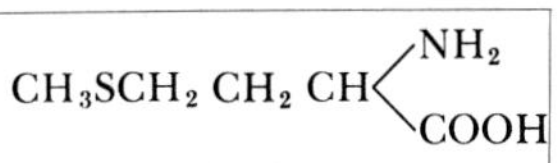

Methionine

(essential)

With two amino and two Carboxyl groups

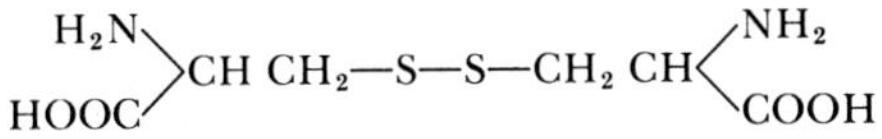

$H_2N(HOOC)>CH\ CH_2—S—S—CH_2\ CH<(NH_2)(COOH)$

Cystine

With heterocyclic group

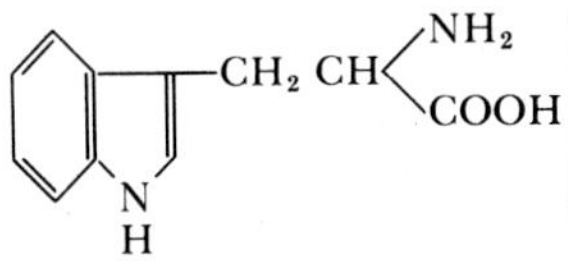

Indole ring (N, H) $—CH_2\ CH<(NH_2)(COOH)$

Tryptophan

(essential)

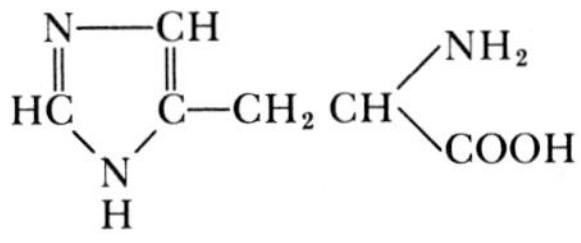

N—CH, HC, C—CH_2 CH<(NH_2)(COOH), N, H

Histidine

(essential)

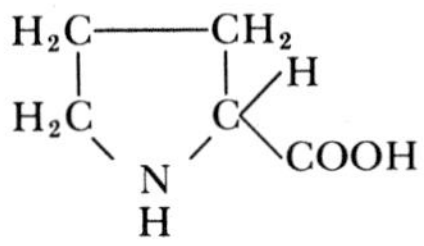

H_2C—CH_2, H_2C, C<(H)(COOH), N, H

Proline

H, HOC—CH_2, H_2C, C<(H)(COOH), N, H

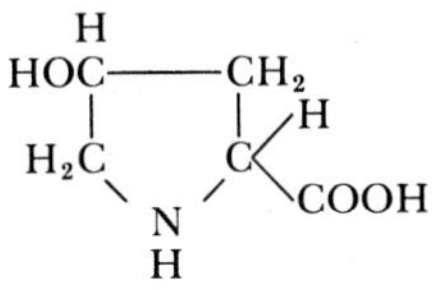

Hydroxyproline

Table 11 STRUCTURAL FORMULAS OF THE MOST COMMON AMINO ACIDS (*Continued*)

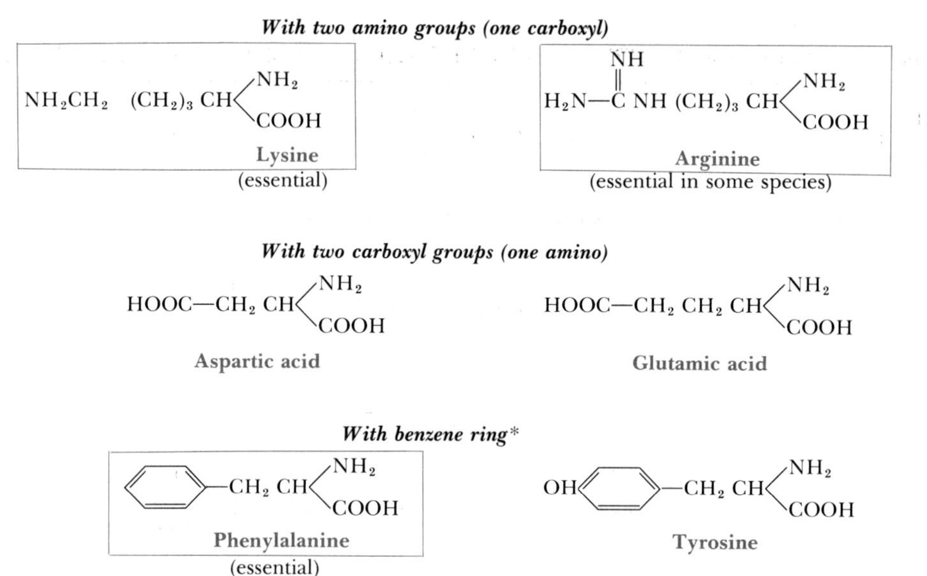

*For simplification, the benzene ring is often represented by a hexagon. It should be understood that there is a carbon atom (C) at each of the six points of the hexagon with hydrogen atoms attached, except where the valence bond is attached to the remainder of the molecule. The benzyl radical may also be represented as:

C_6H_5— or HC(H)=C(H)—C—, with the ring closed by HC=C(H)—C(H) (H's above and below each C)

In the heterocyclic groups, simplified representations of which are used in formulas on the following page, there are also carbon atoms at each point unless otherwise indicated (e.g., N), with hydrogen atoms attached as needed to satisfy valences.

Table 12 STRUCTURES OF WATER-SOLUBLE VITAMINS

Ascorbic Acid: Vitamin C

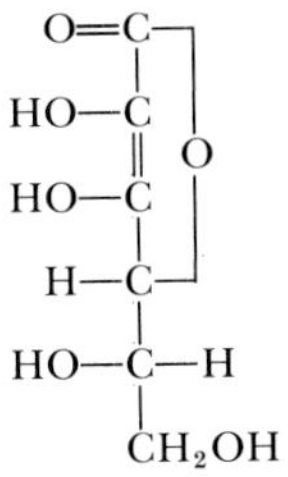

O=C—, HO—C, HO—C, H—C (lactone ring through O), HO—C—H, CH_2OH

Riboflavin

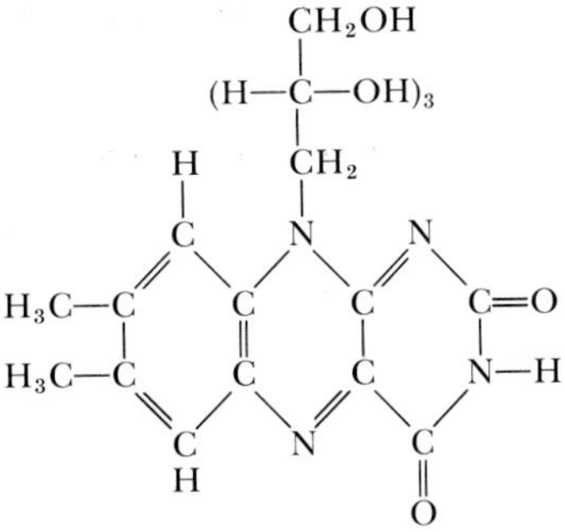

CH_2OH, $(H—C—OH)_3$, CH_2, H_3C—C, H_3C—C, N—H, C=O

Thiamin: Vitamin B-1

NH_2, CH_3, C=C—CH_2CH_2OH, H_3C—C, CH H, C—S, H, Cl^-

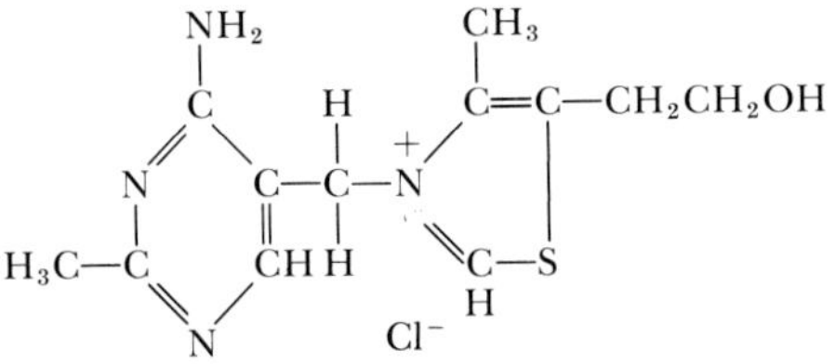

Niacin

Nicotinic Acid

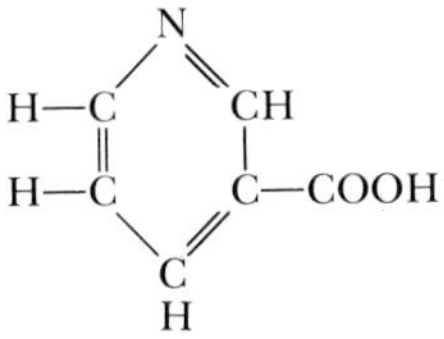

N, H—C, CH, H—C, C—COOH, C, H

Nicotinamide

N, H—C, CH, H—C, C—$CONH_2$, C, H

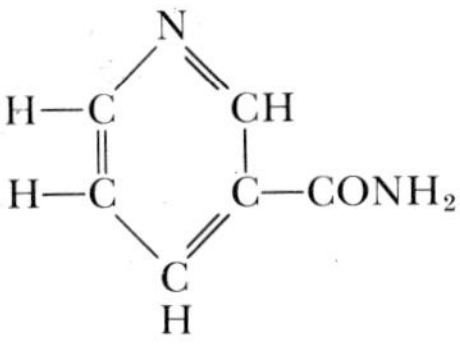

Vitamin B-6 Group

Pyridoxine

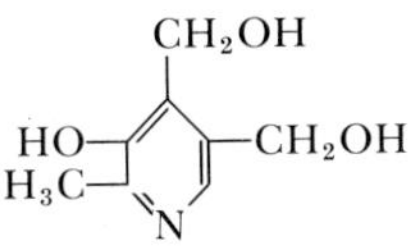

CH_2OH, HO—, —CH_2OH, H_3C—, N

Pyridoxal

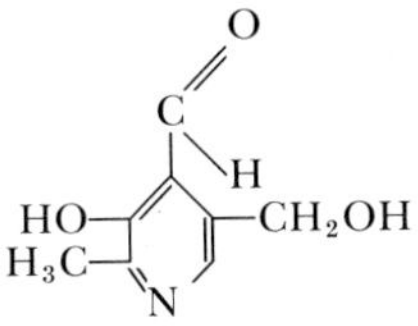

O, C, H, HO—, —CH_2OH, H_3C—, N

Pyridoxamine

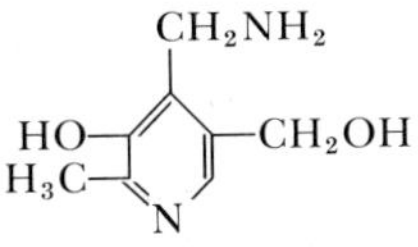

CH_2NH_2, HO—, —CH_2OH, H_3C—, N

Pantothenic Acid

HO—CH₂—C(CH₃)₂—CH(OH)—C(=O)—NH—CH₂—CH₂—COOH

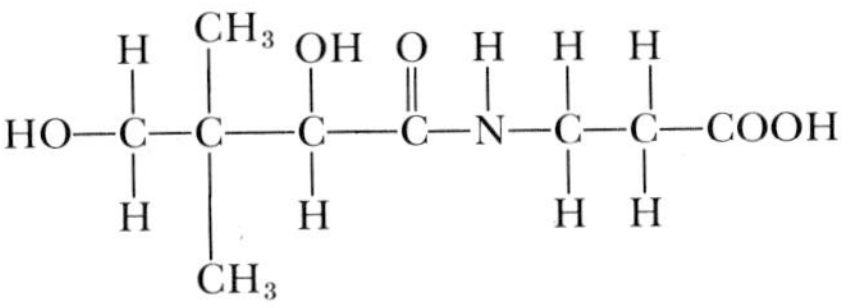

Table continued on following page.

Table 12 STRUCTURES OF WATER-SOLUBLE VITAMINS *(Continued)*

Folacin

(represented by monopteroylglutamic acid)

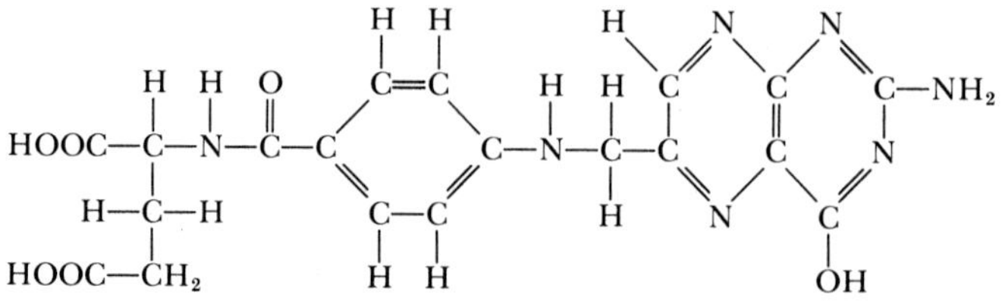

H H H N N
H H O C=C H H C C C—NH_2
HOOC—C—N—C—C C—N—C—C C N
H—C—H C—C H N C
HOOC—CH_2 H H OH

Biotin

O
C
HN NH
H—C——C—H
CH_2—CH_2—CH_2CH_2COOH
H_2—C C
S H

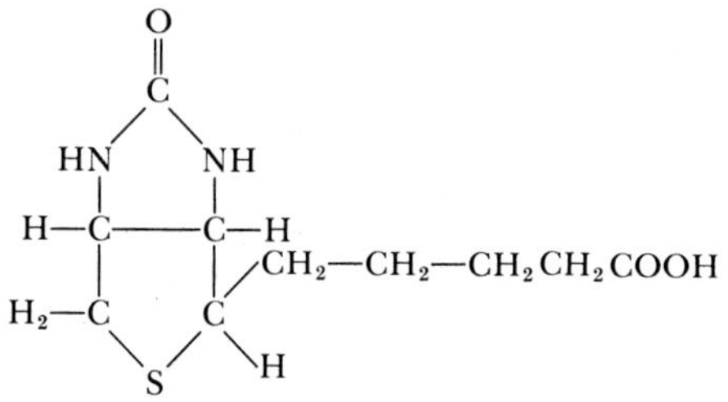

Vitamin B-12

(represented by cyanocobalamin)

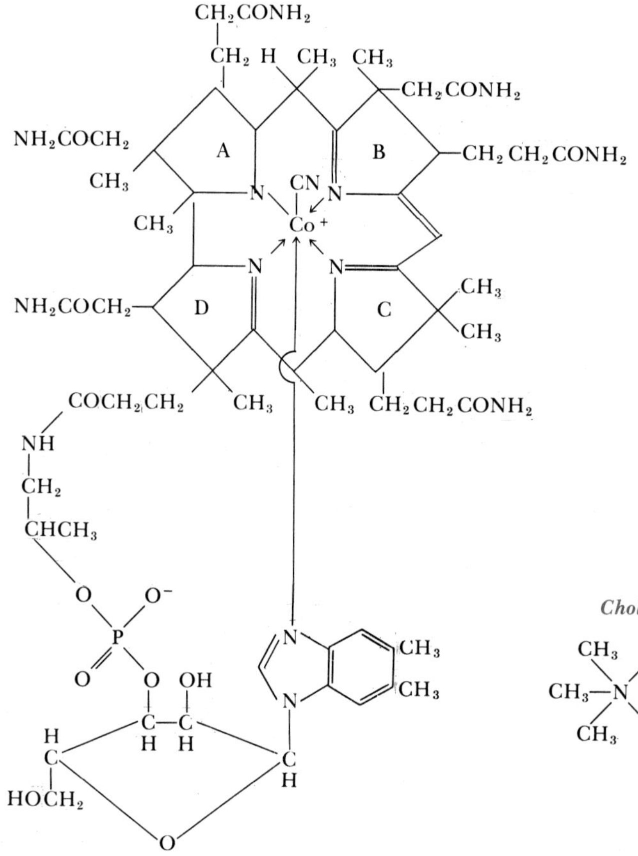

CH_2CONH_2
CH_2 H CH_3 CH_3
—CH_2CONH_2
NH_2COCH_2 A B —$CH_2CH_2CONH_2$
CH_3 N CN N
CH_3 Co^+
N N CH_3
NH_2COCH_2— D C CH_3
$COCH_2CH_2$ CH_3 CH_3 $CH_2CH_2CONH_2$
NH
CH_2
$CHCH_3$
O O^-
P N CH_3
O O OH CH_3
N
H C—C
C H H C
H
$HOCH_2$
O

Choline

CH_3 CH_2CH_2OH
CH_3—N
CH_3 OH

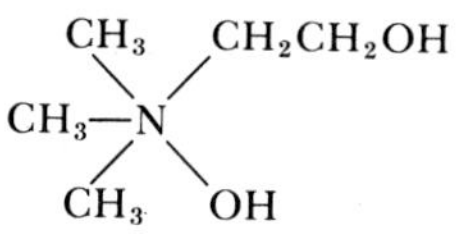

Table 13 STRUCTURES OF FAT-SOLUBLE VITAMINS

Vitamin A
(represented by retinol)

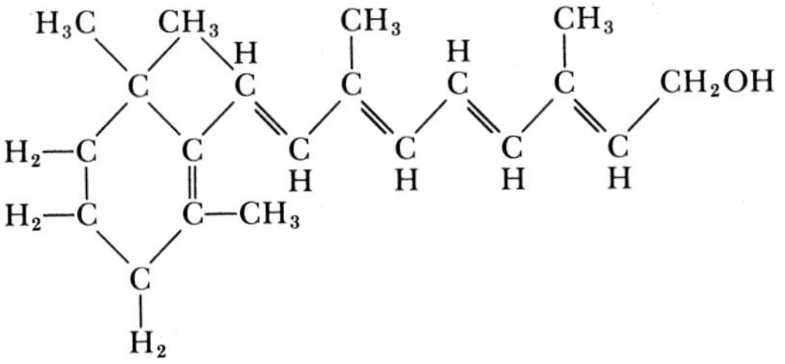

Beta-carotene
(provitamin A)

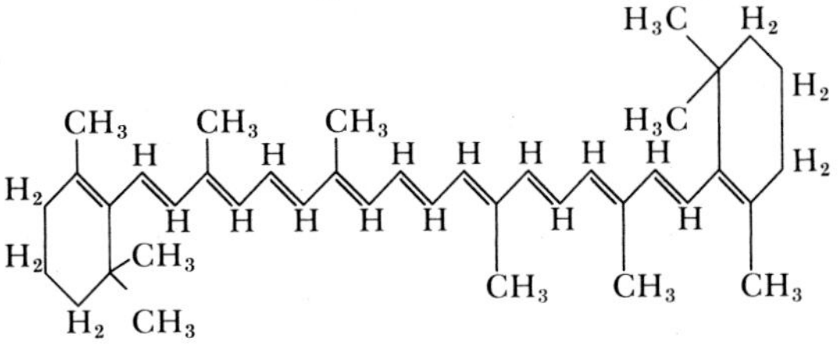

Vitamin D
(represented by cholecalciferol, vitamin D_3)*

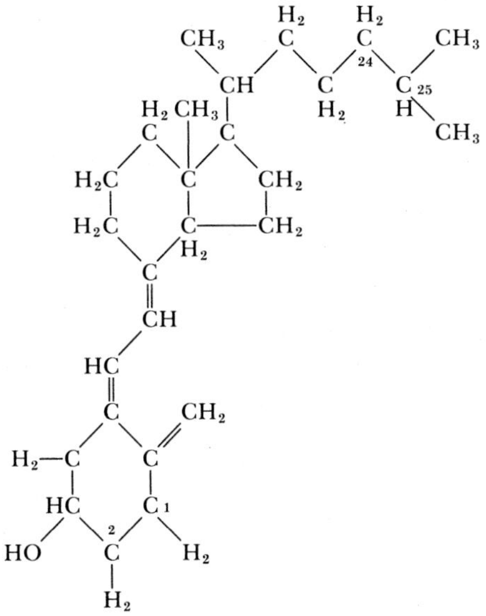

*The numbers of the carbon atoms involved in the biosynthesis of vitamin D hormone are shown.

Vitamin E
(represented by alpha-tocopherol)

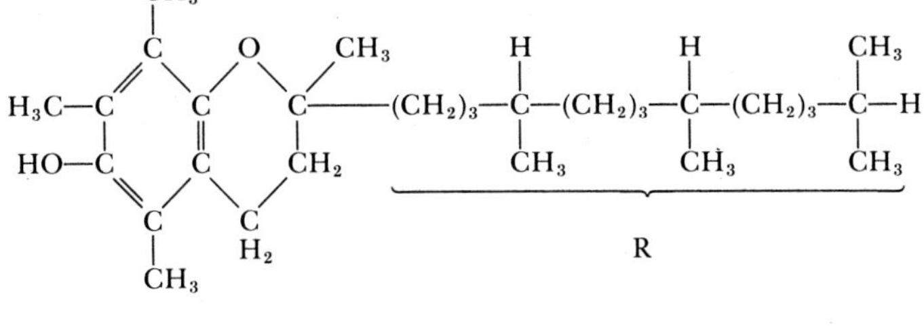

R

Vitamin K
(represented by phytylmenaquinone, vitamin K_1)

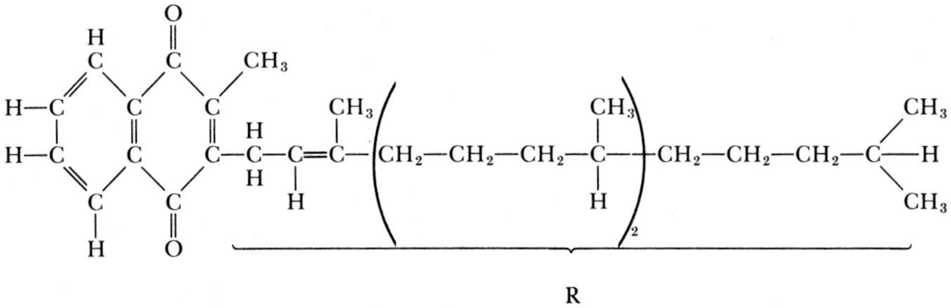

R

Table 14 TABLE OF CURRENT GUIDELINES FOR CRITERIA OF NUTRITIONAL STATUS FOR LABORATORY EVALUATION

Nutrient and Units	Age of Subject (years)	Criteria of Status		
		Deficient	Marginal	Acceptance
*Hemoglobin (gm/100 ml)	6–23 mos.	Up to 9.0	9.0– 9.9	10.0+
	2–5	Up to 10.0	10.0–10.9	11.0+
	6–12	Up to 10.0	10.0–11.4	11.5+
	13–16M	Up to 12.0	12.0–12.9	13.0+
	13–16F	Up to 10.0	10.0–11.4	11.5+
	16+M	Up to 12.0	12.0–13.9	14.0+
	16+F	Up to 10.0	10.0–11.9	12.0+
	Pregnant (after 6+ mos.)	Up to 9.5	9.5–10.9	11.0+
*Hematocrit (Packed cell volume in percent)	Up to 2	Up to 28	28–30	31+
	2–5	Up to 30	30–33	34+
	6–12	Up to 30	30–35	36+
	13–16M	Up to 37	37–39	40+
	13–16F	Up to 31	31–35	36+
	16+M	Up to 37	37–43	44+
	16+F	Up to 31	31–37	37+
	Pregnant	Up to 30	30–32	33+
*Serum Albumin (gm/100 ml)	Up to 1	–	Up to 2.5	2.5+
	1–5	–	Up to 3.0	3.0+
	6–16	–	Up to 3.5	3.5+
	16+	Up to 2.8	2.8–3.4	3.5+
	Pregnant	Up to 3.0	3.0–3.4	3.5+
*Serum Protein (gm/100 ml)	Up to 1	–	Up to 5.0	5.0+
	1–5	–	Up to 5.5	5.5+
	6–16	–	Up to 6.0	6.0+
	16+	Up to 6.0	6.0–6.4	6.5+
	Pregnant	Up to 5.5	5.5–5.9	6.0+
*Serum Ascorbic Acid (mg/100 ml)	All ages	Up to 0.1	0.1–0.19	0.2+
*Plasma vitamin A (mcg/100 ml)	All ages	Up to 10	10–19	20+
*Plasma Carotene (mcg/100 ml)	All ages	Up to 20	20–39	40+
	Pregnant	–	40–79	80+
*Serum Iron (mcg/100 ml)	Up to 2	Up to 30	–	30+
	2–5	Up to 40	–	40+
	6–12	Up to 50	–	50+
	12+M	Up to 60	–	60+
	12+F	Up to 40	–	40+
*Transferrin Saturation (percent)	Up to 2	Up to 15.0	–	15.0+
	2–12	Up to 20.0	–	20.0+
	12+M	Up to 20.0	–	20.0+
	12+F	Up to 15.0	–	15.0+
**Serum Folacin (ng/ml)	All ages	Up to 2.0	2.1–5.9	6.0+
**Serum vitamin B_{12} (pg/ml)	All ages	Up to 100	–	100+

Table continued on following page.

Table 14 TABLE OF CURRENT GUIDELINES FOR CRITERIA OF NUTRITIONAL STATUS FOR LABORATORY EVALUATION—(*Continued*)

Nutrient and Units	*Age of Subject (years)*	*Criteria of Status*		
		DEFICIENT	MARGINAL	ACCEPTANCE
*Thiamine in Urine (mcg/g creatinine)	1–3	Up to 120	120–175	175+
	4–5	Up to 85	85–120	120+
	6–9	Up to 70	70–180	180+
	10–15	Up to 55	55–150	150+
	16+	Up to 27	27–65	65+
	Pregnant	Up to 21	21–49	50+
*Riboflavin in Urine (mcg/g creatinine)	1–3	Up to 150	150–499	500+
	4–5	Up to 100	100–299	300+
	6–9	Up to 85	85–269	270+
	10–16	Up to 70	70–199	200+
	16+	Up to 27	27–79	80+
	Pregnant	Up to 30	30–89	90+
**RBC Transketolase-TPP-effect (ratio)	All ages	25+	15–25	Up to 15
**RBC Glutathione Reductase-FAD-effect (ratio)	All ages	1.2+	–	Up to 1.2
**Tryptophan Load (mg Xanthurenic acid excreted)	Adults (Dose: 100 mg/kg body weight)	25+(6 hrs.) 75+(24 hrs.)	– –	Up to 25 Up to 75
**Urinary Pyridoxine (mcg/g creatinine)	1–3	Up to 90	–	90+
	4–6	Up to 80	–	80+
	7–9	Up to 60	–	60+
	10–12	Up to 40	–	40+
	13–15	Up to 30	–	30+
	16+	Up to 20	–	20+
*Urinary N'methyl nicotinamide (mg/g creatinine)	All ages	Up to 0.2	0.2–5.59	0.6+
	Pregnant	Up to 0.8	0.8–2.49	2.5+
**Urinary Pantothenic Acid (mcg)	All ages	Up to 200	–	200+
**Plasma vitamin E (mg/100 ml)	All ages	Up to 0.2	0.2–0.6	0.6+
**Transaminase Index (ratio)				
†EGOT	Adult	2.0+	–	Up to 2.0
‡EGPT	Adult	1.25+	–	Up to 1.25

From Christakis, G. (ed.): Nutritional assessment in health programs. Amer. J. Pub. Health, 63 (Suppl.): 34–35, 1973.

*Adapted from the Ten State Nutrition Survey.
**Criteria may vary with different methodology.
†Erythrocyte Glutamic Oxalacetic Transaminase.
‡Erythrocyte Glutamic Pyruvic Transaminase.

Table 15 STANDARDS FOR DIETARY INTAKE* AND BLOOD† DATA

Age, sex, and physiological state		*Calories (per kg)*	*Protein (gm per kg)*	*Calcium (mg)*	*Iron (mg)*	*Vitamin A‡ (IU)*	*Vitamin C (mg)*	*B Vitamins (All Ages)*	*Acceptable Hemoglobin (gm/100 ml)†*	*Acceptable Hematocrit (%)†*
AGE AND SEX										
1–5 years:										
12–23 months,								Thiamin,		
male and female		90	1.9	450	15	2000	40	0.4 mg	≥10.0	≥31
24–47 months,								per 1000		
male and female		86	1.7	450	15	2000	40	calories	≥11.0	≥34
48–71 months,										
male and female		82	1.5	450	10	2000	40		≥11.0	≥34
6–7 years, male and female		82	1.3	450	10	2500	40		≥11.5	≥36
8–9 years, male and female		82	1.3	450	10	2500	40	Riboflavin,	≥11.5	≥36
10–12 years	Male	68	1.2	650	10	2500	40	0.55 mg	≥11.5	≥36
	Female	64	1.2	650	18	2500	40	per 1000	≥11.5	≥36
13–16 years	Male	60	1.2	650	18	3500	50	calories	≥13.0	≥40
	Female	48	1.2	650	18	3500	50		≥11.5	≥36
17–19 years	Male	44	1.1	550	18	3500	55	Niacin,	≥14.0	≥44
	Female	35	1.1	550	18	3500	50	6.6 mg	≥12.0	≥38
20–29 years	Male	40	1.0	400	10	3500	60	per 1000	14.0	≥44
	Female	35	1.0	600	18	3500	55	calories	≥12.0	≥38
30–39 years	Male	38	1.0	400	10	3500	60		≥14.0	≥44
	Female	33	1.0	600	18	3500	55		≥12.0	≥38
40–49 years	Male	37	1.0	400	10	3500	60		≥14.0	≥44
	Female	31	1.0	600	18	3500	55		≥12.0	≥38
50–54 years	Male	36	1.0	400	10	3500	60		≥14.0	≥44
	Female	30	1.0	600	18	3500	55		≥12.0	≥38
55–59 years	Male	36	1.0	400	10	3500	60		≥14.0	≥44
	Female	30	1.0	600	10	3500	55		≥12.0	≥38
60–69 years	Male	34	1.0	400	10	3500	60		≥14.0	≥44
	Female	29	1.0	600	10	3500	55		≥12.0	≥38
70 years and over	Male	34	1.0	400	10	3500	60		≥14.0	≥44
	Female	29	1.0	600	10	3500	55		≥12.0	≥38
PHYSIOLOGICAL STATE										
Pregnancy (5th month and beyond), add to basic standard		200	20	200		1000	5§			
Lactating, add to basic standard		1000	25	500		1000	5			

*Standards for evaluation of dietary intake used in the Health and Nutrition Examination.
Survey, by age, sex, and physiological state: United States, 1971–1974. DHEW. Pub. No. (HRA) 77-1647, July, 1977, p. 74.

†Guidelines for classification and interpretation of group blood data collected as part of the Ten State Nutrition Survey: 1968–1970.

‡Assumed 70 percent carotene, 30 percent retinol.

§For all pregnancies.

Table 16 NUTRIENTS AVAILABLE FOR CONSUMPTION, PER CAPITA PER DAY, SELECTED PERIODS*

Nutrient	*Unit*	*Average 1957–59*	*1967*	*1975*	*1976*	*1977*†
Food energy	Cal	3,140	3,210	3,250	3,380	3,380
Protein	Gm	95	99	99	103	103
Fat	Gm	143	150	152	159	159
Carbohydrate	Gm	375	374	377	390	391
Calcium	Gm	.98	.95	.92	.95	.94
Phosphorus	Gm	1.53	1.54	1.53	1.57	1.57
Iron	Mg	16.3	17.3	18.2	18.7	18.6
Magnesium	Mg	347	343	341	349	347
Vitamin A value	IU	8,100	7,900	8,100	8,200	8,200
Thiamin	Mg	1.84	1.91	2.03	2.08	2.09
Riboflavin	Mg	2.30	2.36	2.44	2.52	2.50
Niacin	Mg	21.1	22.9	24.8	25.5	25.6
Vitamin B_6	Mg	1.99	2.13	2.21	2.28	2.29
Vitamin B_{12}	Mcg	8.9	9.6	9.6	9.7	9.7
Ascorbic acid	Mg	140	104	118	118	116

*From National Food Review (USDA), Jan. 1978, p. 13. Quantities of nutrients computed by Agricultural Research Service, Consumer and Food Economics Institute, on the basis of estimates of per capita food consumption (retail weight), including estimates of produce of home gardens, prepared by the Economic Research Service. No deduction made in nutrient estimates for loss or waste of food in the home, use for pet food, or for destruction or loss of nutrients during the preparation of food. Civilian consumption. Data include iron, thiamin, riboflavin, and niacin added to flour and cereal products; other nutrients added primarily as follows: Vitamin A value to margarine, milk of all types, milk extenders; vitamin B_6 to cereals, meal replacements, infant formulas; vitamin B_{12} to cereals; ascorbic acid to fruit juices and drinks, flavored beverages and dessert powders, milk extenders, and cereals. Quantities of added nutrients for 1960–66 were estimated in part by Consumer and Food Economics Institute. Nutrient data reflect revision of potato series 1956 to present.

†Preliminary.

Table 17 PERIODIC CHART OF THE ELEMENTS

From Ternay, A. L.: *Contemporary Organic Chemistry.* Philadelphia, W. B. Saunders Company, 1976.

PERIODIC CHART OF THE ELEMENTS

1A	2A	3B	4B	5B	6B	7B	8B	8B	8B	1B	2B	3A	4A	5A	6A	7A	8A
																1 **H** 1.00797 ±0.00001	2 **He** 4.0026 ±0.00005
3 **Li** 6.939 ±0.0005	4 **Be** 9.0122 ±0.00005											5 **B** 10.811 ±0.003	6 **C** 12.01115 ±0.00005	7 **N** 14.0067 ±0.00005	8 **O** 15.9994 ±0.0001	9 **F** 18.9984 ±0.00005	10 **Ne** 20.183 ±0.0005
11 **Na** 22.9898 ±0.00005	12 **Mg** 24.312 ±0.0005											13 **Al** 26.9815 ±0.00005	14 **Si** 28.086 ±0.001	15 **P** 30.9738 ±0.00005	16 **S** 32.064 ±0.003	17 **Cl** 35.453 ±0.001	18 **Ar** 39.948 ±0.0005
19 **K** 39.102 ±0.0005	20 **Ca** 40.08 ±0.005	21 **Sc** 44.956 ±0.0005	22 **Ti** 47.90 ±0.005	23 **V** 50.942 ±0.0005	24 **Cr** 51.996 ±0.001	25 **Mn** 54.9380 ±0.00005	26 **Fe** 55.847 ±0.003	27 **Co** 58.9332 ±0.00005	28 **Ni** 58.71 ±0.005	29 **Cu** 63.54 ±0.005	30 **Zn** 65.37 ±0.005	31 **Ga** 69.72 ±0.005	32 **Ge** 72.59 ±0.005	33 **As** 74.9216 ±0.00005	34 **Se** 78.96 ±0.005	35 **Br** 79.909 ±0.002	36 **Kr** 83.80 ±0.005
37 **Rb** 85.47 ±0.005	38 **Sr** 87.62 ±0.005	39 **Y** 88.905 ±0.0005	40 **Zr** 91.22 ±0.005	41 **Nb** 92.906 ±0.0005	42 **Mo** 95.94 ±0.005	43 **Tc** (99)	44 **Ru** 101.07 ±0.005	45 **Rh** 102.905 ±0.0005	46 **Pd** 106.4 ±0.05	47 **Ag** 107.870 ±0.003	48 **Cd** 112.40 ±0.005	49 **In** 114.82 ±0.005	50 **Sn** 118.69 ±0.005	51 **Sb** 121.75 ±0.005	52 **Te** 127.60 ±0.005	53 **I** 126.9044 ±0.00005	54 **Xe** 131.30 ±0.005
55 **Cs** 132.905 ±0.0005	56 **Ba** 137.34 ±0.005	57 ***La** 138.91 ±0.005	72 **Hf** 178.49 ±0.005	73 **Ta** 180.948 ±0.0005	74 **W** 183.85 ±0.005	75 **Re** 186.2 ±0.05	76 **Os** 190.2 ±0.05	77 **Ir** 192.2 ±0.05	78 **Pt** 195.09 ±0.005	79 **Au** 196.967 ±0.0005	80 **Hg** 200.59 ±0.005	81 **Tl** 204.37 ±0.005	82 **Pb** 207.19 ±0.005	83 **Bi** 208.980 ±0.0005	84 **Po** (210)	85 **At** (210)	86 **Rn** (222)
87 **Fr** (223)	88 **Ra** 226.05	89 **†Ac** (227)	104 (257)	105													

*Lanthanum Series

58 **Ce** 140.12 ±0.005	59 **Pr** 140.907 ±0.0005	60 **Nd** 144.24 ±0.005	61 **Pm** (147)	62 **Sm** 150.35 ±0.005	63 **Eu** 151.96 ±0.005	64 **Gd** 157.25 ±0.005	65 **Tb** 158.924 ±0.0005	66 **Dy** 162.50 ±0.005	67 **Ho** 164.930 ±0.0005	68 **Er** 167.26 ±0.005	69 **Tm** 168.934 ±0.0005	70 **Yb** 173.04 ±0.005	71 **Lu** 174.97 ±0.005

†Actinium Series

90 **Th** 232.038 ±0.0005	91 **Pa** (231)	92 **U** 238.03 ±0.005	93 **Np** (237)	94 **Pu** (242)	95 **Am** (243)	96 **Cm** (247)	97 **Bk** (249)	98 **Cf** (249)	99 **Es** (254)	100 **Fm** (253)	101 **Md** (256)	102 **No** (253)	103 **Lr** (257)

Printed in U S A

Atomic Weights are based on C^{12}—12.0000 and Conform to the 1961 Values

Table 18

From Brescia, F., et al.: *Chemistry: A Modern Introduction.* 2nd Ed. Philadelphia, W. B. Saunders Company, 1978.

INTERNATIONAL TABLE OF ATOMIC WEIGHTS (1973)

Based on relative atomic mass of $^{12}C = 12$. Includes 1975 corrected values.

The following values apply to elements as they exist in materials of terrestrial origin and to certain artificial elements. When used with the due regard to footnotes, they are reliable to ±1 in the last digit, or ±3 when followed by an asterisk (*). Value in parentheses is the mass number of the isotope of longest half-life.

	Symbol	*Atomic number*	*Atomic weight*
Actinium	Ac	89	(227)
Aluminum	Al	13	26.98154[a]
Americium	Am	95	(243)
Antimony	Sb	51	121.75*
Argon	Ar	18	39.948[b,c,d,g]
Arsenic	As	33	74.9216[a]
Astatine	At	85	(210)
Barium	Ba	56	137.33
Berkelium	Bk	97	(247)
Beryllium	Be	4	9.01218[a]
Bismuth	Bi	83	208.9804[a]
Boron	B	5	10.81[c,d,e]
Bromine	Br	35	79.904[c]
Cadmium	Cd	48	112.41
Calcium	Ca	20	40.08[g]
Californium	Cf	98	(251)
Carbon	C	6	12.011[b,d]
Cerium	Ce	58	140.12
Cesium	Cs	55	132.9054[a]
Chlorine	Cl	17	35.453[c]
Chromium	Cr	24	51.996[c]
Cobalt	Co	27	58.9332[a]
Copper	Cu	29	63.546*[c,d]
Curium	Cm	96	(247)
Dysprosium	Dy	66	162.50*
Einsteinium	Es	99	(254)
Erbium	Er	68	167.26*
Europium	Eu	63	151.96
Fermium	Fm	100	(257)
Fluorine	F	9	18.998403[a]
Francium	Fr	87	(223)
Gadolinium	Gd	64	157.25*
Gallium	Ga	31	69.72
Germanium	Ge	32	72.58*
Gold	Au	79	196.9665[a]
Hafnium	Hf	72	178.49*
Helium	He	2	4.00260[b,c]
Holmium	Ho	67	164.9304[a]
Hydrogen	H	1	1.0079[b,d]
Indium	In	49	114.82
Iodine	I	53	126.9045[a]
Iridium	Ir	77	192.22*
Iron	Fe	26	55.847*
Krypton	Kr	36	83.80[e]
Lanthanum	La	57	138.9055*[b]
Lawrencium	Lr	103	(260)
Lead	Pb	82	207.2[d,g]
Lithium	Li	3	6.941*[c,d,e,g]
Lutetium	Lu	71	174.967 *
Magnesium	Mg	12	24.305[c,g]
Manganese	Mn	25	54.9380[a]
Mendelevium	Md	101	(258)
Mercury	Hg	80	200.59*
Molybdenum	Mo	42	95.94
Neodymium	Nd	60	144.24*
Neon	Ne	10	20.179*[c,e]
Neptunium	Np	93	237.0482[f]
Nickel	Ni	28	58.70
Niobium	Nb	41	92.9064[a]
Nitrogen	N	7	14.0067[b,c]
Nobelium	No	102	(255)
Osmium	Os	76	190.2[g]
Oxygen	O	8	15.9994[b,c,d]
Palladium	Pd	46	106.4
Phosphorus	P	15	30.97376[a]
Platinum	Pt	78	195.09*
Plutonium	Pu	94	(244)
Polonium	Po	84	(209)
Potassium	K	19	39.0983*
Praseodymium	Pr	59	140.9077[a]
Promethium	Pm	61	(145)
Protactinium	Pa	91	231.0359[a,f]
Radium	Ra	88	226.0254[f,g]
Radon	Rn	86	(222)
Rhenium	Re	75	186.207[c]
Rhodium	Rh	45	102.9055[a]
Rubidium	Rb	37	85.4678*[c]
Ruthenium	Ru	44	101.07*
Samarium	Sm	62	150.4
Scandium	Sc	21	44.9559[a]
Selenium	Se	34	78.96*
Silicon	Si	14	28.0855*[d]
Silver	Ag	47	107.868[c]
Sodium	Na	11	22.9877[a]
Strontium	Sr	38	87.62[g]
Sulfur	S	16	32.06[d]
Tantalum	Ta	73	180.9479*[b]
Technetium	Tc	43	(97)
Tellurium	Te	52	127.60*
Terbium	Tb	65	158.9254[a]
Thallium	Tl	81	204.37*
Thorium	Th	90	232.0381[f,g]
Thulium	Tm	69	168.9342[a]
Tin	Sn	50	118.69*
Titanium	Ti	22	47.90*
Tungsten	W	74	183.85*
Uranium	U	92	238.029[b,c,e,g]
Vanadium	V	23	50.9415[b,c]
Wolfram	W	74	183.85*
Xenon	Xe	54	131.30[e]
Ytterbium	Yb	70	173.04*
Yttrium	Y	39	88.9059[a]
Zinc	Zn	30	65.38
Zirconium	Zr	40	91.22

[a] Elements with only one stable nuclide.

[b] Element with one predominant isotope (about 99 to 100% abundance).

[c] Element for which the atomic weight is based on calibrated measurements.

[d] Element for which known variation in isotopic abundance in terrestrial samples limits the precision of the atomic weight given.

[e] Element for which users are cautioned against the possibility of large variations in atomic weight due to inadvertent or undisclosed artificial isotopic separation in commercially available materials.

[f] Most commonly available long-lived isotope.

[g] In some geological specimens this element has a highly anomalous isotopic composition, corresponding to an atomic weight significantly different from that given.

Index

Page numbers in *italics* refer to illustrations;
(t) indicates tables.